Disorders of Voluntary Muscle

The seventh edition of *Disorders of Voluntary Muscle* has been rewritten and redesigned with the needs of the clinician and clinical scientist in mind. It contains up-to-date information on the aetiology and pathogenesis of diseases of skeletal muscles, including the mitochondrial myopathies, ion-channel disorder, muscular dystrophies and dysimmune myopathies. It covers the many recently identified diseases of muscle and emphasizes the progress that has been made in diagnosis and treatment.

As background to the clinical coverage, the new edition also has chapters summarizing advances in molecular and developmental biology, immunopathology, mitochondrial biology, ion-channel dynamics, cell membrane and signal transduction science, and imaging technology.

Combining essential new knowledge with the fundamentals of history taking and clinical examination, this extensively illustrated book will continue to be the mainstay for practising physicians and biomedical scientists concerned with muscle disease.

George Karpati is Isaac Walton Killam Professor in the Department of Neurology and Neurosurgery, and Professor of Pediatrics at McGill University, Montreal.

David Hilton-Jones is Consultant Neurologist in the Department of Clinical Neurology, University of Oxford, and Clinical Director of the Muscle and Nerve Centre at the Radcliffe Infirmary, Oxford.

Robert C. Griggs is Edward A. and Alma Vollertsen Rykenboer Professor of Neurophysiology, Professor of Neurology, Medicine, Pathology and Pediatrics, and Chairman of Neurology at the University of Rochester Medical Center, Rochester, NY. He is editor of *Neurology*.

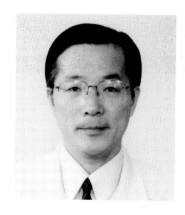

Dedication
Kiichi Arahata (1946–2000)

Kiichi Arahata, one of the world's leading investigators of muscle diseases, died December 20, 2000 shortly before the publication of this text. Kiichi contributed an authoritative chapter on Emery–Dreifuss muscular dystrophy to this edition, a masterful summary of all facets of the disease – much of the recent literature by Kiichi himself.

Kiichi was Director of the Department of Neuromuscular Research at the National Institute of Neuroscience, NCNP, Tokyo, Japan. During a highly productive but all-too-short research career, Kiichi made many major discoveries on muscle diseases: analysis of mechanisms of muscle injury by cytotoxic lymphocytes; precise immunolocalization in normal and dystrophic muscles of dystrophin, emerin and dysferlin; and the identification of pathogenic mutations in 7-integrin in a congenital muscular dystrophy. He made contributions to our understanding of Duchenne, facioscapulohumeral, myotonic and different forms of limb girdle dystrophy. Throughout his career, Kiichi earned the respect, admiration and affection of all who worked with him.

Kiichi's research repertoire expanded as the field of muscle diseases grew. Beginning his career with Andrew Engel working on immunopathology, he ultimately developed extraordinary expertise in the molecular pathobiology of muscular dystrophies – a range of capabilities beautifully illustrated by his chapter.

All three editors know from their long and rewarding interactions with Kiichi that he combined an intense, productive research career with a warm personality. He was a man of great kindness and charm. We dedicate this volume to our friend.

George Karpati, MD
David Hilton-Jones, MD
Robert C. Griggs, MD

Disorders of Voluntary Muscle

Seventh Edition

Edited by

George Karpati

McGill University, Montréal, Québec, Canada

David Hilton-Jones

University of Oxford and Radcliffe Infirmary, Oxford, UK

Robert C. Griggs

University of Rochester, Rochester, NY, USA

Foreword by

Lord Walton of Detchant

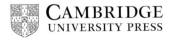

PUBLISHED BY THE PRESS SYNDICATE OF THE UNIVERSITY OF CAMBRIDGE
The Pitt Building, Trumpington Street, Cambridge, United Kingdom

CAMBRIDGE UNIVERSITY PRESS
The Edinburgh Building, Cambridge CB2 2RU, UK
40 West 20th Street, New York, NY 10011-4211, USA
10 Stamford Road, Oakleigh, VIC 3166, Australia
Ruiz de Alarcón 13, 28014 Madrid, Spain
Dock House, The Waterfront, Cape Town 8001, South Africa

http://www.cambridge.org

First published 1964, J & A Churchill Ltd
Second edition 1969
Third edition 1974
Fourth edition 1981, Longman Group Ltd
Fifth edition 1988
Sixth edition 1994, Longman Group Ltd
Seventh edition 2001

Printed in the United Kingdom at the University Press, Cambridge

Typeface Utopia 8.5/12 pt   *System* QuarkXPress™ [SE]

A catalogue record for this book is available from the British Library

Library of Congress Cataloguing in Publication data
Disorders of voluntary muscle / edited by George Karpati, David Hilton-Jones, and
Robert C. Griggs; Foreword by Lord Walton of Detchant – 7th ed.
    p.   cm
Includes bibliographical references and index.
ISBN 0 521 65062 3 (HB : alk.paper)

1. Muscles – Diseases.   I. Karpati, George. II. Hilton-Jones, David. III. Griggs, Robert
C., 1939–   .
[DNLM: 1. Muscular Diseases. 2. Muscle, Skeletal – Physiopathology.
3. Neuromuscular Diseases. WE 550 D612 2001]
RC925.D535 2001
616.7'4 – dc21   00-046748 CIP

ISBN 0 521 65062 3 hardback

Contents

Contributors

Ali Al-Mudallal

Departments of Neurology and Neurosciences, Case Western Reserve University School of Medicine and the Department of Veterans Affairs Medical Center in Cleveland, University Hospitals of Cleveland, 11100 Euclid Avenue, Cleveland, OH 44106, USA

Louise V. B. Anderson

Department of Experimental Neurology, School of Neurosciences and Psychiatry, University Medical School, Newcastle-upon-Tyne NE2 4HH, UK

the late Kiichi Arahata

formerly of the Department of Neuromuscular Research, National Institute of Neuroscience, NCNP, 4-1-1 Ogawa-higashi, Kodaira, Tokyo 187-8502, Japan

Zohar Argov

Department of Neurology, The Hebrew University, Hadassah Medical School, Jerusalem, Israel 91120

Richard L. Barbano

Department of Neurology, University of Rochester School of Medicine, 601 Elmwood Ave, Rochester, NY 14642, USA

Robert L. Barchi

Department of Neurological Sciences and Neurology, University of Pennsylvania School of Medicine, Philadelphia, PA 19104, USA

Richard J. Barohn

Department of Neurology, University of Texas Southwestern Medical Center at Dallas, 5323 Harry Hines Blvd, Dallas, TX 75235-8897, USA

Kimby N. Barton
Banting and Best Department of Medical Research, University of Toronto, Charles H. Best Institute, 112 College St, Toronto, Ontario, Canada M5G1L6

Jacques S. Beckmann
Genethon, BP 60, 1 rue de l'Internationale, 91002 Ivry, Cedex, France

David Beeson
Neurosciences Group, Institute of Molecular Medicine, John Radcliffe Hospital, Oxford OX3 9DS, UK

Saïd Bendahhou
Howard Hughes Medical Institute, Departments of Neurology and Human Genetics, 4420 Eccles Institute of Human Genetics, University of Utah, 15 North 2030 East, Salt Lake City, UT 84112-5531, USA

Bernard Brais
Centre de Recherche du Centre Hospitalier de l'Université de Montréal (CHUM), Campus Notre-Dame, 1560 rue Sherbrooke est, Montréal, Québec, H2L 4M1, Canada

Michael H. Brooke
University of Alberta-MacKenzie HSC, Division of Neurology, 8th Ave and 112 St, Edmonton, Alberta T6G 2B7 Canada

Susan C. Brown
Neuromuscular Unit, Department of Pediatrics, Imperial College of Science, Technology and Medicine, Hammersmith Hospital, Du Cane Road, London, W12 0NN, UK

Robert, E. Burke
Laboratory of Neural Control, National Institute of Neurological Disorders and Stroke, National Institutes of Health, Bethesda, MD 302892-4455, USA

Kate Bushby
Departments of Biochemistry and Genetics, 19/20 Claremont Place, Newcastle-upon-Tyne NE2 4AA, UK

Salvatore Carbonetto
Centre for Research in Neuroscience, McGill University, Montréal, Québec, Canada

Stirling Carpenter
Rua Diogo Afonso 19, I.F., 4100 Porto, Portugal

Patrick Chinnery
The Medical School, University of Newcastle-upon-Tyne, Newcastle-upon-Tyne NE2 4HH, UK

Barry J. Cooper
Department of Biomedical Sciences, College of Veterinary Medicine, Cornell University, Ithaca, NY, USA

Marinos C. Dalakas
National Institutes of Health, 9000 Rockville Pike, Bethesda, MD 20892, USA

George Dickson
School of Biological Sciences, Royal Holloway College – University of London, Egham, TW20 0EX, UK

Victor Dubowitz
Dubowitz Neuromuscular Centre, Imperial School of Medicine, Hammersmith Hospital, Du Cane Road, London W12 0NN, UK

Michel Fardeau
Institute de Myologie, Groupe Hospitalier Pitie Salpetriere, 47–83 boulevard de l'Hôpital, F-75013 Paris, France

James L. Fleckenstein
Department of Radiology, University of Texas Southwestern Medical Center at Dallas, 5323 Harry Hines Blvd, Dallas, Texas 75235-8897, USA Dallas, TX, USA

Hans H. Goebel
Department of Neuropathology, Johannes Gutenberg University, Langenbeckstrausse 1, D-55131 Mainz, Germany

Robert C. Griggs
Neuromuscular Disease Center, Department of Neurology, University of Rochester School of Medicine and Dentistry, 601 Elmwood Ave, Rochester, NY 14642, USA

Peter S. Harper
Institute of Medical Genetics, University of Wales College of Medicine, Heath Park, Cardiff CF14 4XN, UK

David Hilton-Jones
Department of Clinical Neurology, University of Oxford and Muscle and Nerve Centre, Radcliffe Infirmary, Oxford OX2 6HE UK

Eric P. Hoffman
Research Center for Genetic Medicine, Children's
National Medical Center, Washington DC 20010, USA

Paul C. Holland
Montreal Neurological Institute and Centre for Research
in Neuroscience, McGill University, Montréal, Québec,
Canada

Henry J. Kaminski
Department of Neurology, Case Western Reserve
University School of Medicine and the Department of
Veterans Affairs Medical Center in Cleveland, University
Hospitals of Cleveland, 11100 Euclid Ave, Cleveland, OH
44106, USA

Jean-Claude Kaplan
Service de Biochimie et Genetique Moleculaire, Hopital
Cochin-Maternites, 123 boulevard de Port-Royal, Paris,
France

George Karpati
Departments of Neurology and Neurosurgery, McGill
University and Montreal Neurological Institute, 3801
University St, Montréal, Québec, H3A 2BA, Canada

John T. Kissel
Department of Neurology, Division of Neuromuscular
Disease, Ohio State University, Columbus, OH 43210, USA

John M. Land
Departments of Clinical Biochemistry and
Neurochemistry, National Hospital for Neurology and
Neurosurgery, Institute of Neurology, Queen Square,
London WC1N 3BG, UK

Russell Lane
West London Neurosciences Centre, Charing Cross
Hospital and the Division of Clinical Neurosciences and
Psychological Medicine, Imperial College of Science,
Technology and Medicine, University of London, London,
UK

Raffaele Lodi
Dipartimento di Medicina Clinica e Biotecnologia
Applicata, University of Bologna, Bologna, Italy

Eric L. Logigian
University of Rochester School of Medicine, Department
of Neurology, 601 Elmwood Ave, Rochester, NY 14642,
USA

David H. MacLennan
Banting and Best Department of Medical Research,
University of Toronto, Charles H. Best Institute, 112
College St, Toronto, Ontario, Canada M5G1L6

Giovanni Meola
Ospedale Clinic San Donato, Division of Neurology,
Via Morandi 30 – San Donato Milanese, Milan,
20097 Italy

Jeffrey B. Miller
Myogenesis Research Laboratory, Massachusetts General
Hospital and Program in Neuroscience, Harvard Medical
School, Massachusetts General Hospital, 149 13th St,
Charlestown, MA 02129, USA

Richard T. Moxley III
University of Rochester School of Medicine, Department
of Neurology, 601 Elmwood Ave, Rochester, NY 14642,
USA

John Newsom-Davis
Department of Clinical Neurology, University of Oxford
and Radcliffe Infirmary, Oxford, OX2 6HE, UK

Louis J. Ptáček
Howard Hughes Medical Institute, Departments of
Neurology and Human Genetics, 4420 Eccles Institute of
Human Genetics, University of Utah, 15 North 2030 East,
Salt Lake City, UT 84112-5531, USA

Robert L. Ruff
Departments of Neurology and Neurosciences, Case
Western Reserve University School of Medicine and the
Department of Veterans Affairs Medical Center in
Cleveland, University Hospitals of Cleveland, 11100
Euclid Ave, Cleveland, OH 44106, USA

Caroline A. Sewry
Dubowitz Neuromuscular Centre, Imperial College
School of Medicine, Hammersmith Hospital, Du Cane
Road, London W12 0NN and the Robert Jones and Agnes
Hunt Orthopaedic and District Hospital NHS Trust,
Oswestry, SY10 7AG, UK

John M. Shoffner
MetaMetrix Clinical Laboratory, 4855 Peachtree Industrial
Estate, Norcross, GA 30092 and Children's Healthcare of
Atlanta, Molecular Medicine Laboratory, 5455 Meridian
Mark Road NE, Suite 530, Atlanta, GA 30342, USA

Eric A. Shoubridge
Montreal Neurological Institute and Department of
Human Genetics, McGill University, Montréal, Québec,
Canada

Rabi Tawil
Neuromuscular Disease Center, Department of
Neurology, University of Rochester School of Medicine
and Dentistry, 601 Elmwood Ave, Rochester, NY 14642,
USA

Doris J. Taylor
MRC Biochemical and Clinical Magnetic Resonance Unit,
John Radcliffe Hospital and the Department of
Biochemistry, University of Oxford, Oxford OX3 9DU, UK

Douglas Turnbull
The Medical School, University of Newcastle-upon-Tyne,
Newcastle-upon-Tyne NE2 4HH, UK

Angela Vincent
Neurosciences Group, Institute of Molecular Medicine,
John Radcliffe Hospital, Oxford OX3 9DS, UK

Thomas Voit
Department of Pediatrics and Pediatric Neurology,
University of Essen, Germany

Lord Walton of Detchant
13 Norham Gardens, Oxford
OX2 6PS, UK

Frank S. Walsh
SmithKline Beecham Pharmaceuticals, New Frontiers
Science Park, Third Ave, Harlow CM19 5AW, UK

Preface to the Seventh Edition

This is the Seventh Edition of *Disorders of Voluntary Muscle*. It is practically a total re-write of the Sixth Edition, published in 1994, since the intervening time has brought an avalanche of exciting new developments in the myopathies. The new edition has the latest information on the aetiology and pathogenesis of diseases of skeletal muscles, including the mitochondrial myopathies, ion channel disorders, the muscular dystrophies caused by deficiencies of surface membrane-related cytoskeletal molecules and the dysimmune myopathies. It adds the many new muscle diseases that have recently been identified, such as those causing congenital neuromuscular transmission defects and limb girdle syndrome. It emphasizes the major progress that has taken place in diagnostics and treatment of muscle disease.

The new edition also adds chapters and sections that provide the clinician–scientist with pertinent summaries of the scientific advances in molecular biology, developmental biology, immunopathology, mitochondrial biology, ion channel dynamics, cell membrane and signal transduction science and imaging technology. These chapters provide background for the important clinical developments of the past decade.

The Editors have retained essential information on history taking and physical examination and informative illustrations. By making this information succinct, we have been able to add important new knowledge while keeping the book manageable in size.

The Editors have worked to present the material in a clinician-friendly format aimed at practising physicians in neurology, orthopaedics, paediatrics, rheumatology, physiatry (physiotherapy) and other disciplines. The main aim of this book is to enable the practising physician to maintain a state-of-the-art ability to diagnose and treat diseases of skeletal muscles with a sufficient understanding of their scientific basis. The book will also be a concise but comprehensive text for medical and graduate science students, residents as well as scientists, who wish to familiarize themselves with muscle disease.

We have reorganized the chapters and omitted material no longer pertinent to allow us to add new ones. Chapters on neurophysiology have been substantially condensed but they still contain essential clinical information and add exciting new data on ion channel function.

We thank our authors for their superb scientific and clinical presentations. Their skilful and dedicated work and the publisher's efficient management will keep *Disorders of Voluntary Muscle* at the forefront of works on muscle diseases well into the 21st century and continue the excellent tradition that it enjoyed under the stewardship of Lord Walton during the past 36 years.

The editors

Foreword

Fifty years ago, the late Professor F. J. Nattrass of Newcastle upon Tyne invited me, as a young trainee neurologist, to join him in a programme of research into muscular dystrophy and related neuromuscular disorders. The next few years were among the most exciting and fruitful of my career as I strove to identify and examine personally all the patients with muscular dystrophy and other forms of neuromuscular disease in the northeast of England. This work led to the publication of several papers, including our joint publication entitled The Classification, Natural History and Treatment of the Myopathies, published in *Brain* in 1954. My interest in this field was further enriched by an eventful year of work with Professor Raymond D. Adams at the Massachusetts General Hospital in Boston, followed by a period of research under Dr E. A. Carmichael in the neurological research unit at the National Hospital, Queen Square. I was especially moved during this period by the effects of muscular dystrophy upon patients and their families, and particularly upon those suffering from what had previously been called pseudohypertrophic muscular dystrophy, but which we renamed the Duchenne type. I, therefore, became determined that research into neuromuscular disease would become a personal lifetime priority, and I was fortunate in being able to obtain research grants first from the Muscular Dystrophy Associations of America, subsequently from the Muscular Dystrophy Association of Canada, and later still from the embryo Muscular Dystrophy Group of Great Britain, which Professor Nattrass and I founded in the 1950s. Later grants from the Medical Research Council, the Wellcome Trust and a number of other organizations enabled me and my colleagues to establish a major unit for the clinical management and investigation of neuromuscular disease in Newcastle upon Tyne.

In 1962, I was approached by Mr J. Rivers of J. and A. Churchill Ltd, who asked me whether I would consider editing a book on neuromuscular disease in order to bring to the attention of a wider audience of neurologists, paediatricians and others some of the information that had been derived from our research programme and from the burgeoning research in this rapidly developing field carried out in many other parts of the world. It was thus that *Disorders of Voluntary Muscle* was born and the first edition was published in 1964. At that time, I thought that the volume was a very substantial one, but little did I realise the extent to which exciting developments in basic medical science and in clinical care and molecular genetics would enhance the field. Inevitably, therefore, each successive edition became larger than the one before, and each required substantial restructuring in the light of new developments.

I was happy to edit the first five editions personally, but the vast expansion of relevant knowledge convinced me that it was important to recruit co-editors and I was delighted that in the preparation of the sixth edition, Professor George Karpati and Dr David Hilton-Jones joined me. Subsequently, the time came to consider the future of the book and I recognized that, as I was no longer in clinical practice nor personally involved in research, the time had come for me to relinquish the editorship of the book. It was a matter of very great pleasure when I learned that George Karpati and David Hilton-Jones were willing to continue to edit the book and that they had recruited Robert C. Griggs as a co-editor.

I believe that they have done a wonderful job in restructuring the volume in the light of current understanding of neuromuscular function in health and disease, and I could not possibly be more thrilled in recognizing, as I am sure they have, that the long-term future of this work is now assured. The contributions made by many workers across the world to our increased understanding of disease and improved patient care shine forth from the pages of this volume, derived from advances in physiology, biochemistry, molecular genetics and so many more fields that it would be difficult to enumerate them all. I am delighted to see that so many international experts not previously involved in writing for the book have been recruited, and I am satisfied that this volume, prepared in a clear and attractive format, beautifully illustrated and attractively written, will prove to be a great success. At a time when prospects of gene therapy for many inherited disorders of the neuromuscular system are becoming increasingly bright, when developments arising out of stem cell research engender substantial hope for future developments in therapy, and when research and care in the field of neuromuscular disease has developed an increasingly high profile among doctors and scientists across the world, the publication of this seventh edition is, I believe, to be warmly welcomed.

Lord Walton of Detchant

Oxford
March 2001

Part I

The scientific basis of muscle disease

The structure and function of motor units

Robert E. Burke

Introduction

Movements, whether voluntary or reflex, are produced by muscles acting on the skeleton or soft tissues. The founder of modern neurophysiology, Sir Charles Sherrington, recognized that the control of muscle by motoneurons within the central nervous system (CNS) required an anatomical substrate. Accordingly, he proposed that each motoneuron innervates a group of individual muscle fibres, such that each muscle fibre receives innervation from one, and only one, motoneuron. This assumption has been shown to be true in normal muscles (Brown and Matthews, 1960). Sherrington introduced the term 'motor unit' for the combination of motoneuron and the muscle fibres innervated by it (Liddell and Sherrington, 1925). Later it became convenient to introduce the term 'muscle unit' to denote the group of muscle fibres innervated by a given motoneuron (Burke, 1967).

The motoneuron and its muscle unit are inseparable in function because each action potential in the neuron normally activates all muscle unit fibres. Thus motor units are the indivisible quantal elements in all movements. They are also remarkable biological amplifiers; a single action potential in a motoneuron axon triggers an enormous release of chemical and mechanical energy within its muscle unit, which is physically much larger than the motoneuron and its axon (Fig. 1.1). In addition, motoneurons exert powerful 'trophic' control over the properties of their muscle unit fibres, which represents a different kind of amplification and which is exerted over a long time span. A full understanding of disorders of voluntary muscle, therefore, requires some attention to the fact that muscles are really collections of muscle units arranged for common mechanical action.

Anatomy of motor units

Motoneurons

Motoneurons are the only CNS neurons with axons that leave the CNS to innervate non-neuronal tissue. There are three kinds of motoneuron in mammals. Alpha, or skeletomotor, neurons are large cells (Burke et al., 1982) that exclusively innervate the large, extrafusal striated muscle fibres that make up the bulk of muscle tissue. Gamma, or fusimotor, neurons are considerably smaller (Moschovakis et al., 1991) and exclusively innervate one or more of the three types of small, highly specialized intrafusal muscle fibre within the muscle spindle stretch receptor organs that are present in virtually all somatic muscles (Matthews, 1972). They will not be considered further in this chapter. A third class of motoneuron, called beta, or skeletofusimotor, neurons innervate both intra- and extrafusal muscle fibres (Bessou et al., 1965). Beta motoneurons have been found in higher primates (Murthy et al., 1982) and it is quite likely that they occur also in humans. Because beta motoneurons are difficult to identify in physiological experiments, there is little direct evidence about their properties. What little is available indicates that the properties of these cells and their extrafusal muscle units are essentially the same as those of alpha motoneurons (Burke and Tsairis, 1977). The two categories will, therefore, not be distinguished in what follows.

Although alpha motoneurons have extensive dendritic trees that receive synaptic input over their entire extent (Brännström, 1993), their membrane properties are such that synaptic information is effectively delivered to the initial segment of the motor axon where action potentials are initiated (Eccles, 1957). Motoneuron axons have large diameters and correspondingly fast conducting velocities (50 to 120 m/s in cat), which ensures that centrally generated

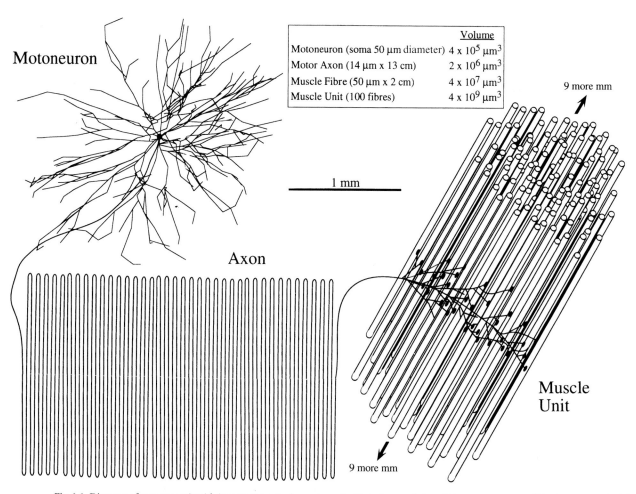

Motoneuron

	Volume
Motoneuron (soma 50 μm diameter)	4×10^5 μm^3
Motor Axon (14 μm x 13 cm)	2×10^6 μm^3
Muscle Fibre (50 μm x 2 cm)	4×10^7 μm^3
Muscle Unit (100 fibres)	4×10^9 μm^3

9 more mm

1 mm

Axon

9 more mm

Muscle
Unit

Fig. 1.1. Diagram of a motor unit with its components drawn to scale. Note the small size of the motoneuron cell body compared with its extensive dendritic tree and very long motor axon. The volume of a single muscle fibre is more than tenfold greater than the total volume of cytoplasm in the motoneuron plus its axon.

spike trains are rapidly and accurately transmitted over the relatively long distances that the axons travel to the periphery. The length and diameter of these motor axons is such that the volume of axoplasm may exceed the volume in the cell body and dendrites by tenfold or more (Fig. 1.1). The large size of motoneuron cell bodies presumably results, in part, from the metabolic demands required to support such a very large peripheral apparatus.

The motoneurons that innervate a given muscle are located in contiguous cell columns, called motor nuclei (Burke et al., 1977), that occupy predictable positions within the ventrolateral grey matter of the spinal cord in animals (Rexed, 1952; Fetcho, 1987) and humans (Sharrard, 1955). There is some tendency for the motoneurons that innervate muscle units in a given location within the target muscle to cluster in particular regions along the

length of the motor cell column (Swett et al., 1970; Weeks and English, 1987).

Neuromuscular junctions

As the myelinated motor axons near their target muscle, they begin to divide into tens or hundreds of terminal branches (Eccles and Sherrington, 1930), which lose their myelin sheaths as they near the neuromuscular junctions (NMJs). In normal adult somatic muscles there is only one NMJ per muscle fibre; as a result, the innervation pattern within a motor unit is private to one motoneuron (Brown and Matthews, 1960). The NMJ on a given fibre is located approximately equidistant from the ends of the muscle fibre, ensuring that activation of that fibre spreads equally to both ends. The NMJs are large and highly specialized

(a) Pinnate Muscle

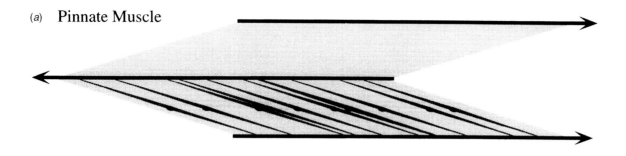

(b) Interdigitated Muscle

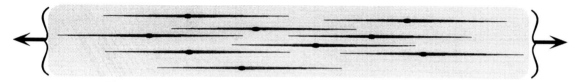

Fig. 1.2. The two basic designs of muscle architecture. (*a*) Pinnate arrangement of muscle fibres in parallel arrays that run at an angle (the angle of pinnation) between aponeuroses of origin and aponeurosis of insertion. The fibres of an individual muscle unit are depicted in the lower half, with central neuromuscular junctions aligned along the axis of muscle belly. All of the muscle unit fibres contribute to the effective cross-sectional area of the muscle unit in force generation. (*b*) An interdigitated muscle, showing tapered muscle unit fibres and their neuromuscular junctions scattered along the muscle belly in irregular arrays. Forces produced by the individual fibres are transmitted to the tendons of origin and insertion by an internal connective tissue stroma. Note that the effective cross-sectional area of the muscle unit is less than its total cross-sectional area.

synapses that normally liberate far more acetylcholine transmitter than is required for fibre activation, ensuring a high safety factor so that all muscle unit fibres are activated by every action potential in the motor axon (Paton and Waud, 1967). Finally, NMJs exhibit different structural specializations, which are related to the type of muscle fibre on which they terminate (Padykula and Gauthier, 1970; Prakash et al., 1996).

Muscles and muscle units

Muscles are essentially collections of muscle units bound together by connective tissue. This tissue delivers active forces to the points of anatomical origin and insertion. One of the constraints that affect the internal architecture of different muscles is the fact that most individual muscle fibres are only 3–6 cm in length, even in large muscles. This length limitation is thought to reflect the need for sarcomeres along the entire fibre to be simultaneously active despite the relatively slow conduction of action potentials along the muscle fibre (2–10 m/s, depending on fibre diameter; Loeb et al., 1987). Accordingly, many limb and trunk muscle have fibres that are considerably shorter than the muscle length described by gross anatomy.

There are two general ways of packing short muscle fibres to make a longer muscle belly (Gans, 1982). Pinnate muscles have fibres in parallel bundles, often arranged at an angle in a feather-like pattern (hence the name) along tendinous aponeuroses of origin and insertion (Fig. 1.2*a*). Some pinnate muscles have multiple aponeuroses, which divide the muscle belly into compartments, sometimes with different force vectors (English and Ledbetter, 1982). Pinnate muscles have a relatively limited range of excursion and a correspondingly narrow length–tension relationship, which is constrained by the number of sarcomeres in series. However, they can deliver large output forces because they pack a large number of muscle fibres and, therefore, sarcomeres in parallel. At the other extreme, the fibres in interdigitated muscles are organized in connective tissue fascicles in serial arrays staggered along the longitudinal axis, beginning and ending at different locations on a web-like intramuscular stroma (Fig. 1.2*b*; Loeb et al., 1987; Trotter, 1993). Muscles with serially interdigitated fibres are more extensible and generate active forces over wider ranges of physiological length than pinnate muscles, because they have more sarcomeres in series. The price of this extended range of action is that maximum force output is limited because only a fraction of

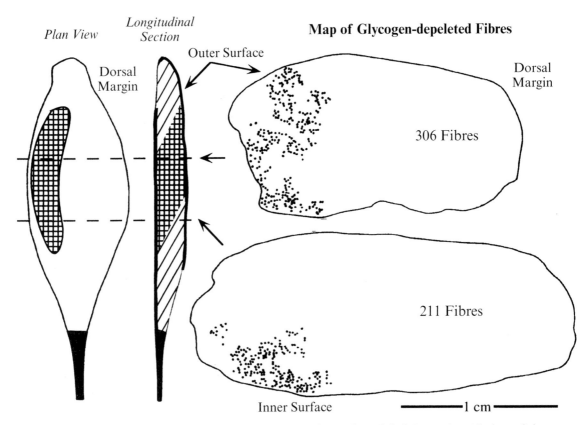

Fig. 1.3. The distribution of glycogen-depleted fibres in a type FR muscle unit (fast twitch, fatigue resistant) in the medial gastrocnemius muscle of a cat. The cross-hatched areas in the whole muscle diagrams on the left indicate the extent of the muscle unit territory, which occupied only a fraction of the muscle volume. The diagonal hatching on the longitudinal section denotes the angulation of fibres in this unipinnate muscle. Maps of the spatial distribution of depleted fibres at two levels along the muscle belly are shown on the right. Note the irregular boundaries of the unit territory but relatively even distribution of fibres within it. (Adapted from Fig. 2 in Burke and Tsairis, 1973.)

the total sarcomeres actually exert force in parallel. As might be expected, some muscles exhibit mixtures of these designs (e.g. tibialis anterior in the cat; Roy et al., 1995). A few long, strap-like muscles, such as semitendinosus and biceps femoris, have two or more bellies arranged in series separated by tendinous inscriptions (Bodine et al., 1982; Chanaud et al., 1991a). Such complex internal organizations undoubtedly have important functional consequences (e.g. English, 1984; Chanaud et al., 1991b; Schieber et al., 1997).

It is obvious that the arrangement of fibres within a muscle unit must accommodate to the internal architecture of the parent muscle. The spatial distribution of fibres within an individual muscle unit can be studied directly by depleting them of endogenous glycogen by prolonged stimulation (Edström and Kugelberg, 1968; Burke et al., 1971). In pinnate muscles, muscle unit fibres are scattered more or less evenly through territories that are relatively

large, although smaller than the total cross-section of the muscle (Fig. 1.3). Although relatively few unit fibres occur immediately adjacent to one another (Kugelberg et al., 1970; Burke and Tsairis, 1973), statistical studies suggest that the fibre distributions in single units are basically random (Bodine-Fowler et al., 1990). Individual muscle units in some multicompartment muscles are distributed only within one compartment (English and Weeks, 1984), while in others, particularly in the forelimb, fibres belonging to some muscle units are found in different compartments (Schieber et al., 1997). Evidence from electromyographic (EMG) studies of single fibres in humans suggest that motor units in human muscles display similar patterns of spatial organization (Garnett et al., 1979; Stålberg and Antoni, 1980).

Although there is less information about the dispersion of muscle unit fibres in interdigitated muscles, the available data indicate that fibres within a given muscle unit occur in many of the fascicles scattered along the length of the muscle (Fig. 1.2*b*) (Lev-Tov et al., 1988; Smits et al., 1994). In the cat sartorius muscle, however, muscle units are distributed asymmetrically along the length of the muscle belly, undoubtedly complicating transmission of force between origin and insertion (Thomson et al., 1991).

Innervation ratio

The 'size' of a motor unit is usually envisioned in terms of the number of fibres in its muscle unit (the innervation ratio). As might be expected, innervation ratios vary with muscle size. Mean innervation ratios can be calculated by dividing estimates of the number of total muscle fibres by the number of large efferent motor axons (Eccles and Sherrington, 1930). Such average innervation ratios in humans vary with the size of the muscle, from less than 12 in intrinsic extraocular muscles to over a thousand in large limb and trunk muscles (Buchthal, 1961; Enoka, 1995; McComas, 1998). Direct estimates of innervation ratios in individual motor units using glycogen depletion in animal muscles have shown considerable variation from unit to unit within a given muscle (Burke and Tsairis, 1973), which is a major factor that accounts for variation in output force (Bodine et al., 1987; Rafuse et al., 1997).

Functional types of motor unit

For more than a century, it has been known that somatic muscles in most mammals fall into two general groups, called 'red' and 'white', which have slow and fast, respectively contraction times (Ranvier, 1874). About the same time, Grützner (1884) described histological differences between muscle fibres that suggested the presence of fast and slow twitch fibres within the same muscle. However, physiological evidence that nominally fast muscles contain some muscle units with relatively slow contraction times is more recent (Gordon and Phillips, 1953; Bessou et al., 1963; Wuerker et al., 1965). It is now clear that most muscles, in fact, are made up of individual muscle units with wide ranges of contraction speeds and force outputs; pure fast or slow muscles are exceptional (for reviews see Burke, 1981; McDonagh et al., 1980a; Hoyle, 1983; Enoka, 1995).

Consequently it is necessary to take account of the identity of the active motor units to understand how the CNS controls movement. Motor unit 'identity' is best determined by patterns of physiological and structural proper-

ties of the muscle unit portion, which are often codified as motor unit 'type' (Burke, 1967, Burke et al., 1973).

Definition of motor unit types

The speed of muscle unit contraction has been a major criterion in classifying motor units, although muscle units also differ in many other mechanical properties (e.g. twitch and tetanic force outputs, resistance to fatigue during repetitive activation, and the ratio of twitch to tetanic force; see Burke, 1981). These features exhibit continuous distributions that initially made it problematic to define distinct groups (e.g. Wuerker et al., 1965). However, two criteria have been found that permit relatively clear separation of motor units in large limb muscles of cats into fast and slow groups: a 'fatigue index' based on the decline in output force during a defined sequence of intermittent tetanization and a 'sag property' based on the shape of unfused isometric tetanic contractions (Figs. 1.4 and 1.5) (Burke et al., 1971, 1973; Dum and Kennedy, 1980; McDonagh et al., 1980a,b). The same criteria have been used with somewhat more variable success in classifying motor units in rat muscles (e.g. Kanda and Hashizume, 1992; Tötösy de Zepetnek et al., 1992). Using these criteria (Fig. 1.4), three main motor units types can be defined: type FF (fast twitch, fatigable), type FR (fast twitch, fatigue resistant) and type S (slow twitch, fatigue resistant). Some fast twitch units exhibit fatigue resistance intermediate between those of FF and FR units and are, therefore, referred to as F(int) or FI (Burke and Tsairis, 1973; McDonagh et al., 1980a; Botterman et al., 1985).

Clearly distinguishable FF, FR and S motor unit groups are not apparent in all motor unit populations. For example, early work on small lumbrical muscles of the cat showed that the distribution of properties of their motor units do not suggest distinct categories (Bessou et al., 1963). By comparison, recent work on rat lumbrical motor units indicates that they can be divided into type FR and S using criteria similar to those in the cat, with no fatigue-sensitive FF units evident (Gates et al., 1991). All classification schemes have advantages and disadvantages. The main advantage of the FF–FR–S categories is that they have proven to be useful in organizing a rather large body of information (Fig. 1.4 and Table 1.1; Burke, 1981). The disadvantage of such schemes is that they can lead to overly rigid thinking. Virtually all of the properties of motor units exhibit continuous distributions that vary with muscle, species and experimental methods. It is, therefore, advisable to view the notion of motor unit types as simply a convenient way to encapsulate correlated information.

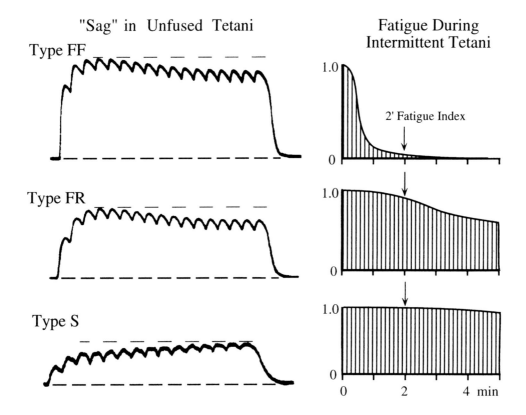

Fig. 1.4. Mechanical responses from three muscle units to illustrate the properties used to identify motor unit type: FF, fast twitch, fatigable; FR, fast twitch, fatigue resistant; and S, slow twitch, fatigue resistant. The records in the left column are unfused tetani produced by repetitive stimulation at intervals near 1.25 times the respective twitch contraction times. The FF and FR unit responses show an early maximum force and subsequent 'sag'. The graphs on the left show the peak force produced by a sequence of short unfused tetani produced by 13 stimulus pulses at 40 Hz, delivered every second for 5 min (duty cycle 0.33). The fatigue index is calculated as the ratio of the peak tetanic force after 2 min of repetitive stimulation (arrows) divided by the force produced by the first tetanus. The fatigue index of the type FF units was less than 0.25 while those of the FR and S units were greater than 0.75. The two properties taken together serve to distinguish four groups, the fourth, called F(int), having fatigue indices between 0.25 and 0.75 and 'sag' in unfused tetani (see Fig. 1.5).

The association of motor unit types with muscle fibre types

The development of reliable histochemical methods for studying muscle in the 1960s showed that many nominally 'white' muscles in fact contain not two but three different kinds of muscle fibre, based on the density and arrangement of mitochondria (Stein and Padykula, 1962). Later, differences based on pH effects on myosin ATPase activity were used to identify three types of muscle fibre (Guth and Samaha, 1969), which are now widely referred to as types I, IIA and IIB (Brooke and Kaiser, 1970). These fibre types also exhibit associated patterns of oxidative and glycolytic metabolic enzyme activities, as well as ultrastructural differences (Table 1.1; see Chapter 13). The development of molecular markers has complicated this simple scheme because a wide variety of myosin isoforms is expressed in both types I and II fibres, with a corresponding proliferation of fibre types (Pette and Staron, 1990).

The glycogen depletion method was first used successfully to identify the fibres of individual rat motor units by Edström and Kugelberg (1968), enabling them to describe the association between the mechanical and histochemical characteristics of two types of fast-twitch muscle unit. Burke and coworkers (1971, 1973) later used the same

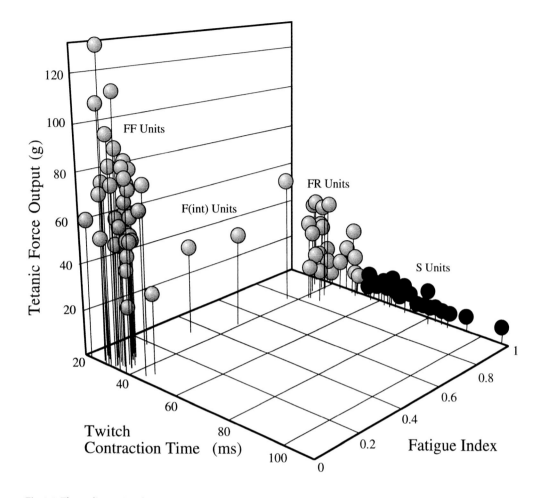

Fig. 1.5. Three-dimensional scatter diagram showing four attributes of a sample of cat gastrocnemius muscle units. Presence of 'sag' in unfused tetani (see Fig. 1.4) is denoted by lightly stippled spheres and absence by dark spheres. The data cluster into three main groups in the four-dimensional space, with two units showing fatigue indices intermediate between the FF and FR clusters. Note that the distributions of tetanic force show overlaps between the FF and FR clusters, and between the FR and S clusters, while twitch contraction times of FF and FR clusters also show large overlap. The type clusters emerge clearly only when all four properties are considered together. See Fig. 1.4 for abbreviations. (Adapted from Burke et al., 1973.)

approach to examine the histochemistry of fibres within the full range of physiologically identified FF, FR and S units in the cat gastrocnemius muscle, finding a perfect match with histochemical types IIB, IIA and I, respectively (Fig. 1.5 and Table 1.1; see also Dum and Kennedy, 1980; McDonagh et al., 1980b; Hamm et al., 1988). They also found some evidence that fibres in the minority F(int) unit type are histochemically distinct from the three main types (Burke et al., 1973; McDonagh et al., 1980b). Recent work with antibodies to myosin heavy chain (MHC) isoforms

has identified a third type II fibre, called type IIX (Schiaffino et al., 1989). Glycogen-depletion studies in rat muscles are divided as to which physiological type of muscle unit is associated with MHC-IIX fibres; some associate it with type FR units (Gates et al., 1991; de Ruiter et al., 1996; see also Sieck et al., 1995) while others find type IIX fibres in muscle units with type F(int) properties (Larsson et al., 1991; Zardini and Parry, 1998). In contrast, a recent study of glycogen-depleted muscle units in the cat diaphragm and tibialis posterior found that MHC-IIX is

Table 1.1. Summary of correlations between motor unit and muscle fibre characteristics in cat muscle

Properties	Motor Unit Types			Reference
	FF	FR	S	
Motor unit properties				
Twitch contraction time	Fast	Fast	Slow	Burke et al., 1973
Maximum tetanic force	High	Moderate	Small	
Fatigue resistance	Low	Moderate/high	Very high	
'Sag'	Yes	Yes	No	
Fibre types	IIB	IIA	I	Burke et al., 1973
Myosin-ATPase (pH 9.4)	High	High	Low	
Myosin-ATPase (pH 4.6)	Medium	Low	High	
Oxidative capacity	Low	Medium/high	High	
Glycolytic capacity	High	High	Low	
Glycogen	High	High	Low	
Motoneurons				
Axon conduction velocity	Fast	Fast	Slower	Emonet-Denand et al., 1988
Afterhyperpolarization duration	Short	Short	Longer	Zengel et al., 1985
Rheobase	High	Medium	Low	Fleshman et al., 1981a; Zengel et al., 1985
Input resistance	Low	Higher	Highest	Fleshman et al., 1981a; Zengel et al., 1985
Membrane area	Large	Smaller	Smallest	Burke et al., 1982
Synaptic organization				
Monosynaptic group Ia EPSPs	Small	Larger	Largest	Burke et al., 1976a,b; Fleshman et al., 1981b
Disynaptic group Ia IPSPs	Small	Larger	Largest	Burke et al., 1976a,b
Recurrent (Renshaw) IPSPs	Small	Larger	Largest	Friedman et al., 1981
Distal cutaneous afferents	Mainly EPSP	Mainly EPSP	Mainly IPSP	Burke et al., 1970a
Rubrospinal effects	Mainly EPSP	Mainly EPSP	Mainly IPSP	Burke et al., 1970a; Powers et al., 1993

Notes:

FF, fast twitch, fatigable; FR, fast twitch, fatigue resistant; S, slow twitch, fatigue resistant; EPSP, excitatory postsynaptic potential; IPSP, inhibitory postsynaptic potential.

characteristic of fibres in type FF and some F(int) muscle units; fibres of type FF units showed little or no expression of MHC-IIB (Sieck et al., 1996). To complicate matters further, some individual muscle fibres in normal muscles express multiple myosin isoforms (Pette and Staron, 1990; Gates et al., 1991; Larsson et al., 1991; Sieck et al., 1996; Rivero et al., 1998). It is possible that some of the variation in properties such as contraction time within a given motor unit type (e.g. Fig. 1.4) are associated with different combinations of myosin isoforms, but this remains to be investigated systematically.

Fibres that belong to the same muscle unit have the same fibre type by myosin ATPase activity (Edström and Kugelberg, 1968; Burke et al., 1973; McDonagh et al., 1980b; Sieck et al., 1996) and MHC isoforms (Larsson et al., 1991; Unguez et al., 1995; Sieck et al., 1996). The individual muscle fibres within a muscle unit also appear to have

similar metabolic enzyme capacities (Nemeth et al., 1986, 1991; Nemeth, 1990). Some studies using quantitative histochemistry of fibres belonging to single muscle units suggest more variance than expected in metabolic enzyme content (Martin et al., 1988; Larsson, 1992); but more recent work by Sieck and colleagues (1996) provides strong evidence favouring metabolic uniformity. It is, therefore, assumed that muscle unit fibres also have essentially identical mechanical properties (Nemeth et al., 1991).

Functional correlates of fibre and motor unit types

The fact that fast-twitch muscle unit fibres exhibit greater ATPase activity at alkaline pH than slow-twitch fibres suggest that this association is causal (Barany, 1967; Bottinelli et al., 1996). However, it is now clear that myosin isoform is only one of many factors that control intrinsic shortening speed: differences in the contractile regulatory proteins (e.g. troponin and tropomyosin; Pette and Staron, 1990), the proteins involved in intrafibre Ca^{2+} regulation (Fiehn and Peter, 1971; Heilmann and Pette, 1979; Hochachka, 1994) and the structure of the sarcoplasmic reticulum (Eisenberg, 1983) also play important roles. It seems likely that the 'sag' property, which differs sharply in fast and slow units, is produced by interactions among these factors (Burke et al., 1976a; Burke, 1990).

Resistance to fatigue is directly related to the oxidative capacity of the different fibre types (Table 1.1; Burke et al., 1973; Kugelberg and Lindegren, 1979), as well as to their mitochondrial content (Eisenberg, 1983) and local capillary supply (Romanul, 1965). These correlations are certainly causally related. Muscle fibres of all types adapt to endurance exercise with increasing aerobic enzyme content and capillarization, accompanied by increased fatigue resistance and often some reduction in fibre diameter (for reviews see Saltin and Gollnick (1983) and Booth and Baldwin (1996)). All of these changes revert quickly and completely to baseline during de-training (Brown et al., 1989). Myosin isoforms are much more resistant to change with functional usage, and for this reason myosin characteristics are preferred for fibre typing (Brooke and Kaiser, 1970). Despite the wide variety of structural and metabolic protein isoforms (e.g. Pette and Staron, 1990), the number of combinations found in the basic fibre types is relatively constrained, presumably because of the complex interactions between the different systems that make up a functioning muscle fibre (Hochachka, 1994).

The forces produced by individual muscle units during high-frequency tetanization can vary over two orders of magnitude in large limb muscles in animals, and this variation is correlated with motor unit type (Fig. 1.4 and Table 1.1). Force output is a function of the 'effective' cross-sectional area of the muscle unit fibres that are active in parallel multiplied by the specific force output of that fibre type per unit area. The effective cross-section is, in turn, given by the average area of the individual fibres in the muscle unit multiplied by the effective innervation ratio, which can approximate the actual innervation ratio in pinnate muscles (Burke and Tsairis, 1973) but is less in interdigitated muscles, which have unit fibres in serial arrays (Fig. 1.2b). In many animals, type I and IIA fibres have considerably smaller fibre areas than type IIB, making fibre area an important component of the equation. There is some controversy about whether specific force output, which cannot be measured directly, differs between units with types I and II muscle fibres. Some indirect estimates suggest that specific force output in type S unit fibres may be less than half that of type FF or FR units (Burke and

Tsairis, 1973; McDonagh et al., 1980a; Burke, 1981) while other work indicates a smaller disparity, apprroximately 20–30% less (e.g. Bodine et al., 1987; Bottinelli et al., 1996). In any case, the effective innervation ratio probably accounts for much of the variation in force output within a given motor unit type, with the other factors perhaps having more contribution to the intertype differences (Burke, 1981, 1990).

Motor units in human muscles

There is a wealth of information available from EMG studies in humans about the behaviour of motor units in normal and diseased muscle, and it has been known for some time that fast- and slow-twitch muscle fibres coexist in human muscle (Eberstein and Goodgold, 1968). However, for obvious technical reasons, it is difficult to examine the mechanical responses of individual muscle units under the controlled conditions possible in animal experiments. Denny-Brown and Pennybacker (1939) were the first to record individual twitches from human motor units in patients with motor neuron disease, using an indirect pneumatic transducer. Buchthal and Schmalbruch (1970) used a mechanical transducer attached to a needle inserted into tendons, plus intramuscular stimulation of 'small nerve branches', to demonstrate that small groups of human motor units in normal muscles generate a wide range of twitch speeds, which varied in relation to the predominant local fibre type (see also Sica and McComas, 1971).

The introduction of 'spike-triggered' computer averaging into clinical neurophysiology made it possible to record the responses of individual motor units with greater assurance (Milner-Brown et al., 1973a). In this technique, isolated unit EMG discharges during steady voluntary contractions are used to trigger an averaging computer, with the appendage (e.g. a finger) attached to a force transducer. Unfortunately the recorded 'twitch' responses are not isolated twitches but rather components of unfused tetani, leading to errors in estimating twitch forces and contraction times (Milner-Brown et al., 1973a; Calancie and Bawa, 1986). Refinements to intramuscular stimulation of single motor axons have been used in order to overcome this limitation (Taylor and Stephens, 1976; Thomas et al., 1990). However, the compliant mechanical linkage between active muscle fibres and force transducer in most human studies, as well mechanical interference from circulatory and respiratory rhythms (Buchthal and Schmalbruch, 1970; Westling et al., 1990), remains a problem that can significantly degrade the mechanical responses observed (see Thomas et al., 1990).

Despite these technical problems, the interrelations found in some studies between contraction speed, force output and (when examined) resistance to fatigue are generally similar to those from animal muscle (Stephens and Usherwood, 1977; Garnett et al., 1979; Romaiguère et al., 1989), although this is not a universal finding (Elek et al., 1992; Macefield et al., 1996). The histochemical characteristics of muscle fibres in humans, and the admixture of fibre types in most muscles, are basically the same as found in other mammals (Brooke and Kaiser, 1970; Essen et al., 1975). Although it remains to be seen whether human motor units can be typed in the same way as those in animal muscle, the available evidence strongly suggests that the basic characteristics of human motor units are similar to those in the cat and rat.

Motoneurons and synaptic specializations

In view of the differences between muscle units in physiological and histochemical properties (Fig. 1.5 and Table 1.1), it is not surprising that the motoneurons that innervate them exhibit corresponding specializations (Table 1.1; reviewed by Burke (1981) and Binder et al. (1996)). Motoneurons that innervate type S muscle units have, in general, slower axonal conduction velocities, longer durations of postspike hyperpolarized after-potentials (AHPs), and higher whole cell input resistance values than the cells that innervate either FR or FF muscle units. The AHP duration is particularly important because it is a key factor that controls the maximum rate of motoneuron firing; motoneurons of type S units generally fire more slowly than those of FR or FF units.

When examined with intracellular labelling methods, the motoneurons of type S units tend to be smaller in membrane area than type FF cells; type FR motoneurons are intermediate in size (Burke et al., 1982). There is, however, no systematic difference between axonal conduction velocities of FF and FR unit groups (Emonet-Denand et al., 1988). Although the distributions of motoneuron properties are continuous and exhibit large overlaps when sorted according to muscle unit type, the relative excitability of the motoneurons to depolarizing currents injected directly, measured as the rheobase (the amount of current required to produce action potentials reliably), is more closely related to unit type than other measures (Fleshman et al., 1981a). In fact, using rheobase and input resistance together, Zengel and coworkers (1985) were able to predict muscle unit type in about 95% of their sample of cat gastrocnemius motor units. The rheobase data imply that intrinsic motoneuron excitability varies as S>FR>FF, which has important

implications for the recruitment order of motor units (see below).

The strength of several synaptic inputs to motoneurons show type-related differences that are undoubtedly related to the way in which the various types are used during activity. For example, the average amplitudes of monosynaptic excitatory postsynaptic potentials (EPSPs) produced in motoneurons by group Ia muscle spindle afferents, which are largely responsible for the stretch reflex, are ordered as S>FR>FF (Table 1.1, see also Fig. 1.7 below) (Burke et al., 1976b). The same ordering is evident with the disynaptic inhibition produced by stimulation of group Ia afferents from antagonist muscles (Burke et al., 1976b) and with disynaptic recurrent inhibition produced by Renshaw interneurons activated fom motor axon collaterals (Friedman et al., 1981). Estimates of effective synaptic current from these sources in provisionally type-identified motoneurons have led to similar conclusions (Binder et al., 1996). Assessment of relative synaptic efficacy of polysynaptic input systems is more problematic and will be discussed later. However, as implied in Fig. 1.6, the organization of synaptic efficacy is a key factor that controls the function of motor unit populations.

Motor units and the control of muscle force

Recruitment

The primary mechanism that controls whole muscle force output by the CNS is the recruitment and derecruitment of active motor units (Liddell and Sherrington, 1925). Much of our information about this process comes from observations in human muscles (e.g. Milner-Brown et al., 1973b; Desmedt and Godaux, 1977; 1981). Under many conditions, small force units are the first to be recruited (Denny-Brown and Pennybacker, 1939), followed by larger and larger units as force demand increases (Burke, 1981; Kernell, 1992). The term 'size principle' has come into wide use to encapsulate this orderly recruitment sequence (Henneman and Mendell, 1981). When directly tested by studying recruitment order in pairs of motor units, the smaller force unit exhibits the lower functional threshold in a high proportion of trials (Zajac and Faden, 1985; Zajac, 1990). In fact several of the interrelated properties of motor units (Table 1.1) can predict relative excitability equally well (Cope and Clark, 1991), so size-ordered recruitment is more-or-less equivalent to type-ordered recruitment. For example, if recruitment were to occur strictly in order of increasing force output, most of the early recruited units would be fatigue-resistant type S, followed

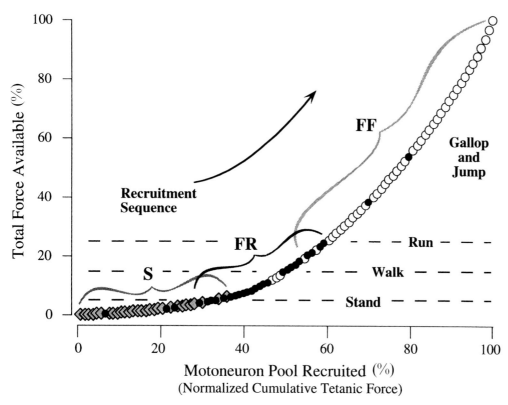

Fig. 1.6. The nonlinear increase in force output (ordinate) from the cat medial gastrocnemius (MG) muscle if its motor unit population were recruited (abscissa) strictly in order of the force produced by each motor unit. The initial stage of recruitment is dominated by type S units (grey diamonds) up to approximately 30% of the pool, which produces in aggregate about 5% of the total force available. As indicated by the lowest horizontal dashed line, the MG muscle produces this force range in the Achilles tendon during quiet standing in normal adult cats. The next region, between 30 and 60% of the pool, is dominated by type FR units (filled circles). Recruitment of types FR and S units together produce about 25% of the total force available, which is the range found during walking and running on a treadmill. The final region (above 60% recruitment) is dominated by type FF units, with force rising more steeply because of the larger individual forces of FF units. Forces in this range are seen in the MG muscle only during galloping and jumping. Despite being pooled from different animals, the motor unit types exhibit relatively little overlap when arranged in this way. See Fig. 1.4 for abbreviations. (The motor unit data are from Burke et al. (1976b) and the MG tendon force data are from Walmsley et al. (1978).)

by type FR, and finally by type FF (Fig. 1.6). The diagram would change little if recruitment were ordered by motor unit type alone. The same basic sequence, although with greater overlaps, would occur if units were recruited strictly in order of decreasing amplitude of monosynaptic group Ia EPSPs (Fig. 1.7). Clearly, gradations of intrinsic motoneuron excitability (i.e. rheobase; Table 1.1) would give the same general pattern. There is abundant evidence that organization of synaptic input and intrinsic motoneuron properties are both critical to recruitment control. In the case of group Ia excitation (and presumably other inputs as well), both factors cooperate to produce size-ordered recruitment (Burke, 1981; Binder et al., 1996).

There are mechanical as well as metabolic advantages to size-ordered recruitment (Table 1.2). In type S motor units, slow contraction, small unit force and fatigue resistance are all advantageous properties for motor units active during sustained, precisely graded actions at modest total force, such as are needed for postural maintenance. There is also evidence that type I muscle fibres are metabolically more efficient during isometric force production than when shortening (Barclay et al., 1993). At the other extreme, the large force, fatigable type FF motor units are clearly best suited for rapid, large force contractions that are intermittent and occur relatively infrequently, to be paid for metabolically by subsequent reformation of stored

Table 1.2. Functional specializations of motor unit types

	Motor unit types		
Functions	FF	FR	S
Usual recruitment threshold	High	Intermediate	Low
Duty cycle	Short/intermittent	Intermediate	Long/continuous
Fatigue resistance	Low	Medium/high	High
Metabolic cost at rest	Low	Medium/high	High
Metabolic optimum action	Shortening	Shortening	Isometric
Force gradation with recruitment	Coarse	Intermediate	Fine

Notes:
FF, fast twitch, fatigable; FR, fast twitch, fatigue resistant; S, slow twitch, fatigue resistant.

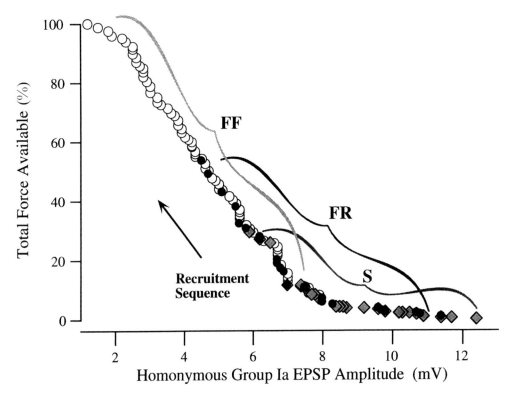

Fig. 1.7. This graph is based on the same data set as in Fig. 1.6 but arranged assuming that medial gastrocnemius motor unit recruitment occurs strictly in order of *decreasing* amplitude of group Ia excitatory postsynaptic potentials (EPSPs, abscissa; data from Burke et al. (1976b)). A nonlinear relation similar to that in Fig. 1.6 is evident, although with considerably more overlap between the motor unit types in different regions of the recruitment sequence. Given the fact that intrinsic motoneuron excitability varies as $S > FR > FF$ (see text), some of these overlaps might be smaller in reality. See Fig. 1.4 for abbreviations.

glycogen. The type FR units occupy a middle ground, combining relatively rapid contraction and moderate force increments with considerable resistance to fatigue and the ability to use either aerobic or anaerobic metabolic pathways.

The composition of the motor unit population in the cat medial gastrocnemius can be matched against the forces actually produced by that muscle during unrestrained activity (Fig. 1.6) (Walmsley et al., 1978). Given size-ordered recruitment, this comparison suggests that the type S population is sufficient to generate the relatively small forces needed to maintain quiet standing, while walking and running require additional participation of the type FR population. Activation of the type FF population is required only during infrequent actions such as gallop and jumping. The motor unit pools of other hindlimb muscles in the cat exhibit differences in composition that fit the mechanical demands as well as the life style of these sedentary predators that must gallop and jump only occasionally (McDonagh et al., 1980a; Dum et al., 1982; Emonet-Denand et al., 1988). The matter of lifestyle is well illustrated by considering the gastrocnemius motor unit pool in the striped skunk (van de Graaff et al., 1977). This muscle contains only types S and FR motor units, as befits a scavanging animal that has no serious predators and neither runs nor jumps but rather must range over long distances to find food.

In many cat muscles, type IIB fibres make up 50–70% of muscle bulk but probably have a very low duty cycle (i.e. are seldom used). It seems likely that the size and proportion of type FF motor units that are represented by this bulk represent an evolutionary compromise between occasional demand for large output forces and the need to minimize the metabolic cost of muscle maintenance. Muscle fibres of high oxidative activity have a higher resting blood flow (Ong et al., 1988) and, by inference, higher rates of oxygen and substrate extraction than fibres with low oxidative capacity. Therefore, the metabolic cost of type S and FR muscle units is probably considerably higher than that of type FF units even at rest, making the latter relatively cheap to maintain.

Selective recruitment of high-threshold motor units

The fact that synaptic input is a critical element in the control of motor unit recruitment is evident in the considerable degree of stochastic variability in the relative firing thresholds of motoneurons observed even in simple monosynaptic stretch reflexes, which can be explained only by corresponding fluctuations in synaptic drive (Rall and Hunt, 1956; Gossard et al., 1994). However, the idea

that large, fast-twitch motor units might be selectively recruited before, or even without, recruitment of normally lower-threshold smaller units is controversial (Calancie and Bawa, 1990; Burke, 1991; Cope and Pinter, 1995). Selective activation of fast muscle with suppression of slow muscle activity has been observed during electrical stimulation of the brainstem (Denny-Brown, 1929) and occurs during rapidly alternating movements such as paw shaking in the cat (Smith et al., 1980) and rapid elbow movements in humans (Kuo and Clamann, 1981). It has also been found during slow voluntary lengthening at a controlled rate against a constant load (Nardone and Schieppati, 1988).

Selective recruitment of relatively high-threshold motor units within a single muscle has been more difficult to demonstrate (Burke, 1991). For example, selective activation of high-threshold motor units has been found in some examples of ballistic contractions in humans (Grimby and Hannerz, 1977) but not in others (Desmedt and Godaux, 1977). Garnett et al. (1979) found marked reversals of force thresholds in ordinarily high- versus low-threshold motor units in the human first dorsal interosseus muscle during non-noxious electrical stimulation of the index finger (see also Kanda and Desmedt, 1983). A similar behaviour has been seen in individual motor units in cat ankle extensors during stimulation of certain skin regions (Kanda et al., 1977; Gossard et al., 1994; but cf. Clark et al., 1993), which was attributed to the tendency for some distal skin regions to excite fast-twitch and inhibit slow-twitch units in this animal (Burke et al., 1970a). In a more straightforward functional situation, Nardone and coworkers (1989) observed selective recruitment of high-threshold units in human gastrocnemius muscle during voluntary lengthening at a controlled rate against a constant load.

There is evidence that certain supraspinal systems, notably the rubrospinal tract, tend to excite relatively high-threshhold motoneurons while inhibiting low-threshold cells (Burke et al., 1970a; Powers et al., 1993; Binder et al., 1996). As shown in Fig. 1.8a, this pattern is opposite to that found in group Ia excitation (Fig. 1.7) and many other spinal reflex systems (Burke, 1981). There are two potential advantages to such competing control systems. First, low-threshold, slow-twitch motor units are also slow to relax. Bypassing them in rapid alternating actions and in controlled active lengthening thus may be functionally important (Smith et al., 1980; Nardone et al., 1989). Second, large fractions of the motor unit pool are recruited virtually simultaneously during very rapid, 'ballistic' contractions (Desmedt and Godaux, 1977). Such synchronous activation would be facilitated by conjoint action of the two systems shown in Fig. 1.8a by narrowing the threshold

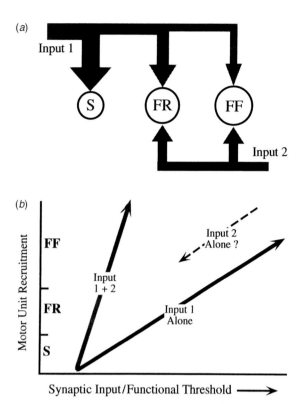

Fig. 1.8. Two possible patterns of organization of synaptic input to a mixed motor unit pool. (*a*) A number of synaptic systems are organized so as to produce excitation of motoneurons in the sequence: FF < FR < S (input 1), while a few produce predominant excitation mainly in FF and FR motoneurons (input 2). (*b*) Increasing synaptic drive from input systems with the strength distribution shown by input 1 would produce the size-ordered recruitment that is observed in many movements. In contrast, if drive were from systems arranged like input 2 alone, there could be selective recruitment of the fast-twitch units such as found in some exceptional situations (dashed arrow). If the motor unit pool were driven by both input systems, the threshold difference between low- and high-threshold units would be narrowed, facilitating the simultaneous activation of the entire motor unit pool that has been found in very rapid, forceful movements.

differences between high- and low-threshold units in the pool (Fig. 1.8*b*).

Control of muscle unit force by motoneuron firing rates and patterns

When excited by gradually rising synaptic depolarization, motoneurons fire with quite regular frequencies that increase from minimum rates of approximately 5–10 Hz to maximum frequencies of 25–40 Hz, depending on the

muscle involved (Burke, 1981). As noted above, motoneuron firing frequencies are constrained by the AHPs that follow each action potential (Kernell, 1992), which fits their functional role in activating muscle units that are inherently slow and highly nonlinear devices. One aspect of this nonlinear behaviour is illustrated in Fig. 1.9. The maximum tension, P_t, that can be produced by an individual muscle unit at different motoneuron firing frequencies varies in a sigmoidal fashion, starting at the force produced by isolated twitches (long interspike intervals) to a maximum that is five to ten times higher when activated at high frequencies (short intervals). This tetanic force reaches 75 to 80% of the maximum possible when motoneuron firing intervals equal the time at which the twitch responses reach their maximum force (twitch contraction time).

It is also instructive to estimate motor unit output as the force–time integral under a sequence of responses during isometric tetani at different stimulation frequencies (Fig. 1.9, inset), which is roughly equivalent to the work that the unit would generate if the muscle were free to contract (Burke et al., 1976a). When plotted against the interval between the stimulation pulses (Fig. 1.9, A_{10} from ten successive responses), the force–time curve reaches a fairly sharp peak at interstimulus intervals near the twitch contraction time in both fast- and slow-twitch units (Burke et al., 1976a). Therefore, if a muscle unit twitch contraction time is 33 ms (fairly typical of type FF or FR units; Fig. 1.4), its optimum frequency for work output would be about 30 Hz, while for a type S unit with a twitch contraction time of 80 ms, the optimum would be 12.5 Hz. These frequencies are well within the range actually observed for animal and human motor units.

The highly nonlinear behaviour of individual muscle units during constant frequency activation (Fig. 1.9) illustrates the dependence of muscle unit force output on its short-term activation history. Enhancement as well as reduction (i.e. fatigue) of force output reflect longer-term activation history. For example, repeated bursts of stimulation at relatively high frequency induce increases in force output and changes in the shape of mechanical responses, called post-tetanic potentiation (PTP), that can last for many seconds to minutes (Fig. 1.10*a,b*). Twitch responses are very sensitive to PTP, as can be seen in comparing the first components (dotted falling phases) in unfused tetani in Fig. 1.10*a,b*.

Muscle units are remarkably sensitive to the pattern of stimulus intervals as well as to their rate. For example, a single short interval, or doublet, inserted into an otherwise low-frequency stimulus train can produce sustained enhancement of isometric force production, referred to as

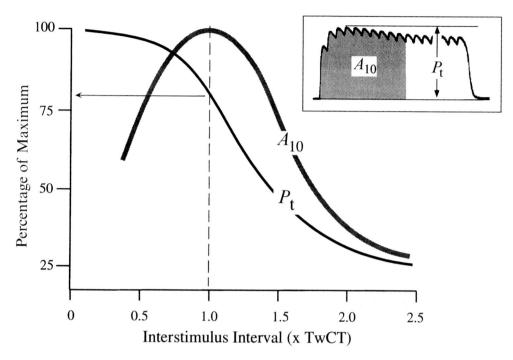

Fig. 1.9. The relation between motoneuron firing intervals (abscissa; the reciprocal of firing frequency) and two measures of muscle unit output. The peak amplitude in tetanic contractions (P_t; thinner curve) rises monotonically as firing intervals decrease, to reach about 80% of maximum for both fast- and slow-twitch muscle units with stimulus intervals around the twitch contraction time (TwCT). Alternatively, integrating the isometric force responses to a given number of stimuli (A_n, where $n = 10$ in the example shown in the inset) produces a curve (A_{10}) that has a fairly sharp peak when stimulus intervals are near the twitch contraction time. The force–time integral is a useful estimator for the work that a muscle would do if free to contract. Similar curves are produced by fast- and slow-twitch muscle units when plotted against stimulus interval normalized by twitch contraction time. (Adapted from Figs. 2 and 3 in Burke et al., 1976a.)

a 'catch property', in both fast- and slow-twitch muscle units (Fig. 1.10; Burke et al., 1970b, 1976a). The effect of an initial doublet in type FF or FR muscle units enhances force output for a few hundred milliseconds but the force profile returns to the baseline level because the 'sag' property curtails the duration of catch in these units (Fig. 1.10a). Fig. 1.10b shows, in the same unit, that catch enhancement is markedly reduced when the unit responses are enhanced through PTP, an effect also observed in type S units. Catch enhancement can be quite prolonged in type S units because they have little or no 'sag' to curtail it. In Fig. 1.10c, different levels of sustained force were produced by changing only one or two intervals within otherwise constant (low) frequency tetani, showing that catch enhancement does not require closely spaced doublet firing. Doublet firing is found in normal human motor units (Denslow, 1948), particularly at the onset of rapid, forceful contractions and presumably result in similar nonlinear force

enhancements (Desmedt and Godaux, 1977; cf. Macefield et al., 1996); consequently, it is possible that similar pattern-related modulation of unit force may occur in humans. Clearly, pattern as well as average rate of motoneuron firing provide significant modulation of force output from individual motor units.

Plasticity of muscle fibre and motor unit types

Muscle displays a remarkable ability to adapt to altered conditions. For example, adaptation to exercise has been studied intensively in humans and animals because of the wide interest in optimizing fitness and athletic performance (for reviews see Saltin and Gollnick (1983) and Booth and Baldwin (1996)). Endurance exercise training produces marked increases in oxidative enzyme capacity and capillary perfusion in muscle fibres of all fibre types,

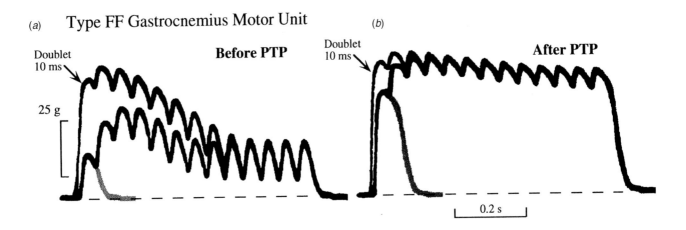

(a) **Type FF Gastrocnemius Motor Unit**

Doublet
10 ms

Before PTP

25 g

(b)

Doublet
10 ms

After PTP

0.2 s

(c) **Type S Gastrocnemius Motor Unit**

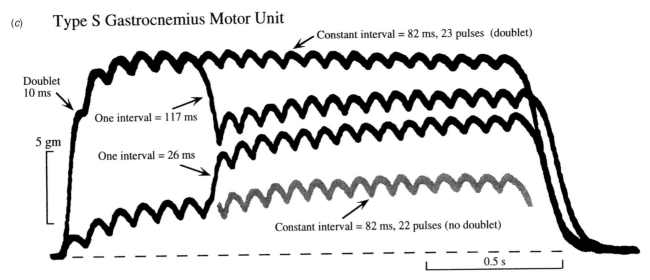

Constant interval = 82 ms, 23 pulses (doublet)

Doublet
10 ms

One interval = 117 ms

5 gm

One interval = 26 ms

Constant interval = 82 ms, 22 pulses (no doublet)

0.5 s

Fig. 1.10. Force enhancement, or 'catch', produced by changing one or two stimulus intervals in unfused tetanic responses produced by fast- and slow-twitch muscle units when stimulated by otherwise constant low-frequency stimulus trains. (a) Photographically superimposed isometric unfused tetanic responses produced by a fast-twitch muscle unit in a cat gastrocnemius muscle unit by a low-frequency stimulus train, with (larger response) and without a single extra pulse (doublet) at the onset. The enhanced force produced by the doublet decayed to the baseline force with the same time course as the 'sag' evident in the basic response. (b) Responses with and without an initial doublet after repeated tetanization of the muscle unit to produce post-tetanic potentiation (PTP). The responses with and without the initial doublet are larger than before PTP and the force enhancement produced by the doublet is correspondingly much reduced. Note also the marked difference produced by PTP in the first 'twitch' responses in each tetanic sequence (grey traces show twitch falling phases). (c) Photographically superimposed responses from a type S muscle unit in cat gastrocnemius showing persistent 'catch' enhancement produced by an initial doublet in otherwise constant low-frequency trains (interval 82 ms = 11.5 Hz; compare with grey trace that denotes to output in the absence of the doublet). The traces with intermediate forces were produced by altering one interval in the first third of responses with and without an initial doublet, showing that sustained force was modulated over a threefold range by small changes in stimulus pattern. ((a,b) Adapted from Burke et al. (1976) and (c) from Burke et al. (1970).)

although there is little or no interconversion between histochemically defined type I and II fibre types (Saltin and Gollnick, 1983). There is, however, evidence that MHC isoforms can respond to different forms of exercise training (Booth and Baldwin, 1996). In animal studies, the interrelations between muscle unit properties that are used to recognize motor unit 'types' are robust in the face of altered conditions that produce muscle atrophy, such as chronic immobilization (Mayer et al., 1981), spinal cord transsection (Mayer et al., 1984; Pierotti et al., 1991) or compensatory hypertrophy (Walsh et al., 1978). The available evidence indicates that there are no major shifts or interconversions between motor unit types with altered conditions of usage within the physiological range (i.e. when innervation remains intact and muscles are not artificially stimulated).

Altered conditions outside the physiological range

The situation is quite different when conditions outside of the normal physiological range are imposed, such as re-innervation of a denervated muscle. The classic example is cross-reinnervation of a predominately fast muscle (e.g. the flexor digitorum longus (FDL) of the cat) by the motor axons that originally innervated a predominately slow muscle (soleus). This slow-to-fast reinnervation causes the FDL to become markedly slower (Buller et al., 1960) and its motor unit population switches quite completely to type S (Dum et al., 1985a). However, the effect is not symmetrical. Although fast-to-slow cross-reinnervation of the soleus by FDL motor axons produces some speeding of the soleus contraction (Buller et al., 1960), the cross-reinnervated soleus muscle fibres remain histochemically type I, even though they co-express a form of fast-twitch myosin as well as slow myosin (Gauthier et al., 1983). Cross-reinnervated soleus motor units, like the whole muscle, exhibit shorter than normal twitch contraction times but otherwise retain type S characteristics (Dum et al., 1985b). The muscle fibres in the histochemically mixed FDL and homogeneous soleus clearly display different degrees of plasticity when reinnervated by foreign motoneurons. The interpretation of such cross-reinnervation experiments is complicated because the foreign motoneurons do not change their activity patterns, which forces the cross-reinnervated muscle units to function under very different conditions of loading than their normal patterns (O'Donovan et al., 1985).

Self-reinnervation of a denervated muscle is a simpler situation. To a large but variable extent (depending on the conditions used), the normal muscle fibre and motor unit types reform in self-reinnervated muscles (Dum et al.,

1985a; Rafuse and Gordon, 1998), although wider ranges of tetanic force output and innervation ratios are evident. However, the normal spatial distribution of fibres is disorganized, with more clustering of unit fibres than in normal units (Kugelberg et al., 1970; Dum et al., 1985a; Rafuse and Gordon, 1996). Some studies have found histochemical uniformity within a given muscle unit after reinnervation (Kugelberg et al., 1970; Dum et al., 1985a,b; see also Gauthier et al., 1983), but more recent studies report some degree of nonuniformity of myosin isoforms in some fibres of the same glycogen-depleted muscle units after self-reinnervation (Unguez et al., 1993; Rafuse and Gordon, 1998). Such observations, like those after cross-reinnervation, suggest that some muscle fibres are more resistant than others to re-specification when innervated by a foreign motoneuron, for reasons that remain unclear.

Prolonged repetitive electrical stimulation of normally innervated as well as denervated muscles produces slowed contraction times and increased resistance to fatigue, which is associated with increases in oxidative capacity and capillarity, and loss of total force output (for review see Pette and Vrbova (1992)). These adaptations begin shortly after the onset of chronic stimulation and before evident transformations in myosin isoforms (Pette et al., 1975), although the latter eventually occur (Pette and Vrbova, 1992). The transformation of fast fibres into slow is the general result of imposed electrical stimulation, irrespective of the frequency of chronic stimulation (Eerbeek et al., 1984; Kernell et al., 1987), and the effect is completely reversible on cessation of imposed stimulation (Brown et al., 1989). The reverse transformation (i.e. slow to fast) occurs only under a more limited set of conditions (very short bursts of high-frequency stimulation in denervated muscle; Lømo et al., 1980; Pette and Vrbova, 1992).

The effect of chronic electrical stimulation, both indirectly through the nerve and directly in the muscle, on individual motor units has been studied in cat medial gastrocnemius muscle (Gordon et al., 1997). This work showed essentially complete conversion of all tested motor units to physiological type S and of muscle fibres to type I, although the histochemical characteristics were not identical to those of type I fibres in the control muscles. The type S units in stimulated muscles contracted more slowly than the original population of type S units. Chronic stimulation also produced changes in the innervating motoneurons in the direction expected of cells that innervate type S muscle units (Munson et al., 1997).

The dramatic muscle fibre conversions produced by self- and cross-reinnervation are good evidence that the innervating motoneuron exerts powerful, albeit less than total, control over the expression of the features that make up muscle fibre 'type'. It is clear that usage, or duty cycle, is an important component in this control, but the classic notion of 'trophic substances' (Buller et al., 1960), perhaps acting in bidirectional streams between motoneuron and muscle unit, remains as a viable adjunct mechanism. There is growing evidence that muscle fibre types are specified early in development, well before they are innervated (Sanes, 1987), which may account for some of the evident resistance of some muscle fibres to complete transformation.

References

Barany, M. (1967). ATPase activity of myosin correlated with speed of muscle shortening. *J. Gen. Physiol.* **50**, 197–216.

Barclay, C. J., Constable, J. K. and Gibbs, C. L. (1993). Energetics of fast- and slow-twitch muscles of the mouse. *J. Physiol. (Lond.)* **472**, 61–80.

Bessou, P., Emonet-Denand, F. and Laporte, Y. (1963). Relation entre la vitesse de conduction des fibres nerveuses motrices at la tempe de contraction de leurs unites motrices. *C. R. Acad. Sci., Ser. D (Paris)* **256**, 5625–5627.

Bessou, P., Emonet-Denand, F. and Laporte, Y. (1965). Motor fibres innervating extrafusal and intrafusal muscle fibres in the cat. *J. Physiol. (Lond.)* **180**, 649–672.

Binder, M. D., Heckman, C. J. and Powers, R. K. (1996). The physiological control of motoneuron activity. In: *Handbook of Physiology*, Sect. 12: *Exercise: Regulation and Integration of Multiple Systems*, eds. L. B. Rowell and J. T. Shepherd, pp. 3–53. New York: Oxford University Press.

Bodine, S. C., Roy, R. R., Meadows, D. A. et al. (1982). Architectural, histochemical, and contractile characteristics of a unique biarticular muscle: the cat semitendinosus. *J. Neurophysiol.* **48**, 192–201.

Bodine, S. C., Roy, R., Eldred, E. and Edgerton, V. (1987). Maximal force as a function of anatomical features of motor units in the cat tibialis anterior. *J. Neurophysiol.* **57**, 1730–1745.

Bodine-Fowler, S., Garfinkel, A., Roy, R. and Edgerton, V. (1990). Spatial distribution of muscle fibers within the territory of a motor unit. *Muscle and Nerve* **13**, 1133–1145.

Booth, F. W. and Baldwin, K. M. (1996). Muscle plasticity: energy demand and supply processes. In: *Handbook of Physiology*, Sect. 12: *Exercise: Regulation and Integration of Multiple Systems*, eds. L. B. Rowell and J. T. Shepherd, pp. 1075–1123. New York: Oxford University Press.

Botterman, B. R., Iwamoto, G. A. and Gonyea, J. (1985). Classification of motor units in flexor carpi radialis muscle of the cat. *J. Neurophysiol.* **54**, 656–690.

Bottinelli, R., Canepari, M., Pelligrino, M. A. and Reggiani, C. (1996). Force–velocity properties of human skeletal muscle fibres: myosin heavy chain isoform and temperature dependence. *J. Physiol. (Lond.)* **495**, 573–586.

Brännström, T. (1993). Quantitative synaptology of functionally different types of cat medial gastrocnemius alpha-motoneurons. *J. Comp. Neurol.* **330**, 439–454.

Brooke, M. H. and Kaiser, K. K. (1970). Muscle fibre types: how many and what kind? *Arch. Neurol. (Chicago)* **23**, 369–379.

Brown, J. M. C., Henriksson, J. and Salmons, S. (1989). Restoration of fast muscle characteristics following cessation of chronic stimulation: physiological, histochemical and metabolic changes during slow-to-fast transformation. *Proc. R. Soc. Lond. B Biol. Sci.* **235**, 321–346.

Brown, M. C. and Matthews, P. B. C. (1960). An investigation into the possible existence of polyneuronal innervation of individual skeletal muscle fibres in certain hind-limb muscles of the cat. *J. Physiol. (Lond.)* **151**, 436–457.

Buchthal, F. (1961). The general concept of the motor unit. *Res. Publ. Assoc. Res. Nervous Mental Dis.* **38**, 3–30.

Buchthal, F. and Schmalbruch, H. (1970). Contraction times and fibre types in intact human muscles. *Acta Physiol. Scand.* **79**, 435–452.

Buller, A. J., Eccles, J. C. and Eccles, R. M. (1960). Interactions between motoneurones and muscles in respect of the characteristic speeds of their responses. *J. Physiol. (Lond.)* **150**, 417–439.

Burke, R. E. (1967). Motor unit types of cat triceps surae muscle. *J. Physiol. (Lond.)* **193**, 141–160.

Burke, R. E. (1981). Motor units: anatomy, physiology and functional organization. In: *Handbook of Physiology*, Sect. 1: *The Nervous System*, Vol. II. *Motor Control*, Part 1, ed. V. B. Brooks, pp. 345–422. Washington, DC: American Physiological Society.

Burke, R. E. (1990). Motor unit types: some history and unsettled issues. In: *The Segmental Motor System*, eds. M. Binder and L. Mendell, pp. 207–221. New York: Oxford University Press.

Burke, R. E. (1991). Selective recruitment of motor units. In: *Motor Control: Concepts and Issues*, eds. D. R. Humphrey and H.-J. Freund, pp. 5–21. Chichester: John Wiley.

Burke, R. E. and Tsairis, P. (1973). Anatomy and innervation ratios in motor units of cat gastrocnemius. *J. Physiol. (Lond)* **234**, 749–765.

Burke, R. E. and Tsairis, P. (1977). Histochemical and physiological profile of a skeletofusimotor (beta) unit in cat soleus muscle. *Brain Res.* **129**, 341–345.

Burke, R. E., Jankowska, E. and ten Bruggencate, G. (1970a). A comparison of peripheral and rubrospinal synaptic input to slow and fast twitch motor units of triceps surae. *J. Physiol. (Lond.)* **207**, 709–732.

Burke, R. E., Rudomin, P. and Zajac, F. E. (1970b). Catch property in single mammalian motor units. *Science* **168**, 122–124.

Burke, R. E., Levine, D. N., Zajac, F. E., Tsairis, P. and Engel, W. K. (1971). Mammalian motor units: physiological-histochemical correlation in three types in cat gastrocnemius. *Science* **174**, 709–712.

Burke, R. E., Levine, D. N., Tsairis, P. and Zajac, F. E. (1973). Physiological types and histochemical profiles in motor units of the cat gastrocnemius. *J. Physiol. (Lond.)* **234**, 723–748.

Burke, R. E., Rudomin, P. and Zajac, F. E. (1976a). The effect of activation history on tension production by individual muscle units. *Brain Res.* **109**, 515–529.

Burke, R. E., Rymer, W. Z. and Walsh, J. V. (1976b). Relative strength of synaptic input from short latency pathways to motor units of defined type in cat medial gastrocnemius. *J. Neurophysiol.* **39**, 447–458.

Burke, R. E., Strick, P. L., Kanda, K., Kim, C. C. and Walmsley, B. (1977). Anatomy of medial gastrocnemius and soleus motor nuclei in cat spinal cord. *J. Neurophysiol.* **40**, 667–680.

Burke, R. E., Dum, R. P., Fleshman, J. W. et al. (1982). An HRP study of the relation between cell size and motor unit type in cat ankle extensor motoneurons. *J. Comp. Neurol.* **209**, 17–28.

Calancie, B. and Bawa, P. (1986). Limitations of the spike triggered averaging technique. *Muscle and Nerve* **9**, 78–83.

Calancie, B. and Bawa, P. (1990). Motor unit recruitment in humans. In: *The Segmental Motor System*, eds. M. D. Binder and L. M. Mendell, pp. 75–95. New York: Oxford University Press.

Chanaud, C. M., Pratt, C. A. and Loeb, G. E. (1991a). Functionally complex muscles of the cat hindlimb. 2. Mechanical and architectural heterogenity within the biceps-femoris. *Exp. Brain Res.* **85**, 257–270.

Chanaud, C. M., Pratt, C. A. and Loeb, G. E. (1991b). Functionally complex muscles of the cat hindlimb. 5. The roles of histochemical fiber-type regionalization and mechanical heterogeneity in differential muscle activation. *Exp. Brain Res.* **85**, 300–313.

Clark, B. D., Dacko, S. M. and Cope, T. C. (1993). Cutaneous stimulation fails to alter motor unit recuitment in the decerebrate cat. *J. Neurophysiol.* **70**, 1433–1439.

Cope, T. C. and Clark, B. D. (1991). Motor-unit recruitment in the decerebrate cat: several unit properties are equally good predictors of order. *J. Neurophysiol.* **66**, 1127–1138.

Cope, T. C. and Pinter, M. J. (1995). The size principle: still working after all these years. *News Physiol. Sci.* **10**, 280–286.

Denny-Brown, D. (1929). On the nature of postural reflexes. *Proc. R. Soc., Ser. B Biol. Sci.* **104**, 252–301.

Denny-Brown, D. and Pennybacker, J. B. (1939). Fibrillation and fasciculation in voluntary muscle. *Brain* **61**, 311–334.

Denslow, J. S. (1948). Double disharges in human motor units. *J. Neurophysiol.* **11**, 209–215.

de Ruiter, C. J., De Haan, A. and Sargeant, A. J. (1996). Fast-twitch muscle unit properties in different rat medial gastrocnemius muscle compartments. *J. Neurophysiol.* **75**, 2243–2234.

Desmedt, J. E. and Godaux, E. (1977). Ballistic contractions in man: Characteristic recruitment pattern of single motor units of the tibialis anterior muscle. *J. Physiol. (Lond.)* **264**, 673–694.

Desmedt, J. E. and Godaux, E. (1981). Spinal motoneuron recruitment in man: Rank deordering with direction but not with speed of voluntary movement. *Science* **214**, 933–936.

Dum, R. P. and Kennedy, T. T. (1980). Physiological and histochemical characteristics of motor units in cat tibialis anterior and extensor digitorum longus muscles. *J. Neurophysiol.* **43**, 1615–1630.

Dum, R. P., Burke, R. E., O'Donovan, M. J., Toop, J. and Hodgson, J. A. (1982). Motor unit organization in the flexor digitorum longus muscle of the cat. *J. Neurophysiol.* **47**, 1108–1125.

Dum, R. P., O'Donovan, M. J., Toop, J. and Burke, R. E. (1985a). Cross-reinnervated motor units in cat muscle: 1. Flexor digitorum longus muscle units reinnervated by soleus motoneurons. *J. Neurophysiol.* **54**, 818–836.

Dum, R. P., O'Donovan, M. J., Toop, J., Tsairis, P., Pinter, M. J. and Burke, R. E. (1985b). Cross-reinnervated motor units in cat muscle: 2. Soleus muscle units reinnervated by flexor digitorum longus motoneurons. *J. Neurophysiol.* **54**, 837–851.

Eberstein, A. and Goodgold, J. (1968). Slow and fast twitch fibers in human skeletal muscle. *Am. J. Physiol.* **215**, 535–541.

Eccles, J. C. (1957). *The Physiology of Nerve Cells*. Baltimore: The Johns Hopkins Press.

Eccles, J. C. and Sherrington, C. S. (1930). Numbers and contraction values of individual motor units examined in some muscles of the limbs. *Proc. R. Soc. Lond. B Biol. Sci.* **106**, 326–357.

Edström, L. and Kugelberg, E. (1968). Histochemical composition, distribution of fibres and fatiguability of single motor units. Anterior tibial muscle of the rat. *J. Neurol. Neurosurg. Psychiatry* **31**, 424–433.

Eerbeek, O., Kernell, D. and Verhey, B. A. (1984). Effects of fast and slow patterns of tonic long-term stimulation on contractile properties of fast muscle in the cat. *J. Physiol. (Lond.)* **352**, 73–90.

Eisenberg, B. R. (1983). Quantitative ultrastructure of mammalian skeletal muscle. In: *Handbook of Physiology*, Sect. 10, *Skeletal Muscle*, eds. L. D. Peachey and R. Adrian, pp. 73–112. Bethesda, MD: American Physiological Society.

Elek, J. M., Kossev, A., Dengler, R., Schubert, M., Wohlfahrt, K. and Wolf, W. (1992). Parameters of human motor unit twitches obtained by intramuscular microstimulation. *Neuromusc. Disord.* **2**, 261–267.

Emonet-Denand, F., Hunt, C., Petit, J. and Pollin, B. (1988). Proportion of fatigue-resistant motor units in hindlimb muscles of cat and their relation to axonal conduction velocity. *J. Physiol. (Lond.)* **400**, 135–158.

English, A. W. (1984). An electromyographic analysis of compartments in cat lateral gastrocnemius muscle during unrestrained locomotion. *J. Neurophysiol.* **52**, 114–125.

English, A. W. and Ledbetter, W. D. (1982). Anatomy and innervation patterns of cat lateral gastrocnemius and plantaris muscles. *Am. J. Anat.* **164**, 67–77.

English, A. W. and Weeks, O. I. (1984). Compartmentalization of single muscle units in cat lateral gastrocnemius. *Exp. Brain Res.* **56**, 361–368.

Enoka, R. M. (1995). Morphological features and activation patterns of motor units. *J. Clin. Neurophysiol.* **12**, 538–559.

Essen, B., Jansson, E., Henriksson, J., Taylor, A. W. and Saltin, B. (1975). Metabolic characteristics of fibre types in human skeletal muscle. *Acta Physiol. Scand.* **95**, 153–165.

Fetcho, J. R. (1987). A review of the organization and evolution of motoneurons innervating the axial musculature of vertebrates. *Brain Res. Rev.* **12**, 243–280.

Fiehn, W. and Peter, J. B. (1971). Properties of the fragmented sarcoplasmic reticulum from fast-twitch and show-twitch muscles. *J. Clin. Invest.* **50**, 570–573.

Fleshman, J. W., Munson, J. B., Sypert, G. W. and Friedman, W. A. (1981a). Rheobase, input resistance, and motor-unit type in medial gastrocnemius motoneurons in the cat. *J. Neurophysiol.* **46**, 1326–1338.

Fleshman, J. W., Munson, J. B. and Sypert, G. W. (1981b). Homonymous projection of individual group Ia-fibers to physiologically characterized medial gastrocnemius motoneuron in the cat. *J. Neurophysiol.* **46**, 1339–1348.

Friedman, W. A., Sypert, G. W., Munson, J. B. and Fleshman, J. W. (1981). Recurrent inhibition in type-identified motoneurons. *J. Neurophysiol.* **46**, 1349–1359.

Gans, C. (1982). Fiber architecture and muscle function. In: *Exercise and Sport Sciences Reviews*, ed. R. J. Terjung, pp. 160–207. Philadelphia, PA: The Franklin Institute.

Garnett, R., O'Donovan, M., Stephens, J. and Taylor, A. (1979). Motor unit organization of human medial gastrocnemius. *J. Physiol. (Lond.)* **287**, 33–43.

Gates, H. J., Ridge, R. M. A. P. and Rowlerson, A. (1991) motor units of the fourth deep lumbrical muscle of the adult rat – isometric contractions and fibre type compositions. *J. Physiol. (Lond.)* **443**, 193–215.

Gauthier, G. F., Burke, R. E., Lowey, S. and Hobbs, A. W. (1983). Myosin isozymes in normal and cross-reinnervated cat skeletal muscle fibers. *J. Cell Biol.* **97**, 756–771.

Gordon, G. and Phillips, C. G. (1953). Slow and rapid components in a flexor muscle. *Q. J. Exp. Physiol.* **38**, 35–45.

Gordon, T., Tyreman, N., Rafuse, V. F. and Munson, J. B. (1997). Fast-to-slow conversion following chronic low-frequency activation of medial gastrocnemius muscle in cats. I. Muscle and motor unit properties. *J. Neurophysiol.* **77**, 2585–2604.

Gossard, J.-P., Floeter, M. K., Kawai, Y., Burke, R. E., Chang, T. and Schiff, S. J. (1994). Fluctuations of excitability in the monosynaptic reflex pathway to lumbar motoneurons in the cat. *J. Neurophysiol.* **72**, 1227–1239.

Grimby, L. and Hannerz, J. (1977). Firing rate and recruitment order of toe extensor motor units in different modes of voluntary contraction. *J. Physiol. (Lond.)* **264**, 865–879.

Grützner, P. (1884). Zur anatomie und physiologie der quergestreiften muskeln. *Recl. Zool. Suisse* **1**, 665–684.

Guth, L. and Samaha, F. J. (1969). Qualitative differences between actomyosin ATPase of slow and fast memmalian muscle. *Exp. Neurol.* **25**, 138–152.

Hamm, T. M., Nemeth, P. M., Solanki, L., Gordon, D. A., Reinking, R. M. and Stuart, D. G. (1988). Association between biochemical and physiological properties in single motor units. *Muscle and Nerve* **11**, 245–254.

Heilmann, C. and Pette, D. (1979). Molecular transformations in sarcoplasmic reticulum of fast-twitch muscle by electro-stimulation. *Eur. J. Biochem.* **93**, 437–446.

Henneman, E. and Mendell, L. M. (1981). Functional organization of motoneuron pool and its inputs. In: *Handbook of Physiology*, Sect. I. *The Nervous System*. Vol. II, *Motor Control*, Part 1, ed. V. B. Brooks, pp. 423–507. Bethesda, MD: American Physiological Society.

Hochachka, P. W. (1994). *Muscles as Molecular and Metabolic Machines*. Boca Raton, FL: CRC Press.

Hoyle, G. (1983). *Muscles and Their Neural Control*. New York: Wiley.

Kanda, K. and Desmedt, J. E. (1983). Cutaneous facilitation of large motor units and motor control of human fingers in precision grip. In: *Advances in Neurology: Motor Control Mechanisms in Health and Disease*, ed. J. E. Desmedt, pp. 253–261. New York: Raven Press.

Kanda, K. and Hashizume, K. (1992). Factors causing difference in force output among motor units in the rat medial gastrocnemius muscle. *J. Physiol. (Lond.)* **448**, 677–695.

Kanda, K., Burke, R. E. and Walmsley, B. (1977). Differential control of fast and slow twitch motor units in the decerebrate cat. *Exp. Brain Res.* **29**, 57–74.

Kernell, D. (1992). Organized variability in the neuromuscular system – a survey of task-related adaptations. *Arch. Ital. Biol.* **130**, 19–66.

Kernell, D., Eerbeek, O., Verhey, B. A. and Donselaar, Y. (1987). Effects of physiological amounts of high- and low-rate chronic stimulation on fast-twitch muscle of the cat hindlimb. I. Speed- and force-related properties. *J. Neurophysiol.* **58**, 598–613.

Kugelberg, E. and Lindegren, B. (1979). Transmission and contraction fatigue of rat motor units in relation to succinate dehydrogenase activity of motor unit fibres. *J. Physiol. (Lond.)* **288**, 285–300.

Kugelberg, E., Edström, L. and Abbruzzese, M. (1970). Mapping of motor units in experimentally reinnervated rat muscle. *J. Neurol. Neurosurg. Psychiatry* **33**, 319–329.

Kuo, K. H. M. and Clamann, H. P. (1981). Coactivation of synergistic muscles of different fiber types in fast and slow contractions. *Am. J. Phys. Med.* **60**, 219–238.

Larsson, L. (1992). Is the motor unit uniform? *Acta Physiol. Scand.* **144**, 143–154.

Larsson, L., Ansved, T., Edström, L., Gorza, L. and Schiaffino, S. (1991). Effects of age on physiological, immunohistochemical and biochemical properties of fast-twitch single motor units in the rat. *J. Physiol. (Lond.)* **443**, 257–275.

Lev-Tov, A., Pratt, C. A. and Burke, R. E. (1988). The motor unit population of the cat tenuissimus muscle. *J. Neurophysiol.* **59**, 1129–1142.

Liddell, E. G. T. and Sherrington, C. S. (1925). Recruitment and some other factors of reflex inhibition. *Proc. R. Soc., Ser. B Biol. Sci.* **97**, 488–518.

Loeb, G. E., Pratt, C. A., Chanaud, C. M. and Richmond, F. J. R. (1987). Distribution and innervation of short, interdigitated muscle fibers in parallel-fibered muscles of the cat hindlimb. *J. Morphol.* **191**, 1–15.

Lømo, T., Westgaard, R. H. and Engebretsen, L. (1980). Different stimulation patterns affect contractile properties of denervated rat soleus muscles. In: *Plasticity of Muscle*, ed. D. Pette, pp. 297–309. Berlin: Walter de Gruyter.

Macefield, V. G., Fuglevand, A. J. and Bigland-Ritchie, B. (1996). Contractile properties of single motor units in human toe extensors assessed by intraneural motor axon stimulation. *J. Neurophysiol.* **75**, 2509–2519.

Martin, T. P., Bodine-Fowler, S., Roy, R. R., Eldred, E. and Edgerton, V. R. (1988). Metabolic and fiber size properties of cat tibialis anterior motor units. *Am. J. Physiol.* **255**, C43–C50.

Matthews, P. B. C. (1972). *Mammalian Muscle Receptors and their Central Actions.* London: Arnold.

Mayer, R. F., Burke, R. E., Toop, J., Kanda, K. and Walmsley, B. (1981). The effect of long-term immobilization on the motor unit population of the cat medial gastrocnemius muscle. *Neuroscience* **6**, 725–739.

Mayer, R. F., Burke, R. E., Toop, J., Walmsley, B. and Hodgson, J. A. (1984). The effect of spinal cord transection on motor units in cat medial gastrocnemius muscles. *Muscle Nerve* **7**, 23–31.

McComas, A. J. (1998). Motor units: how many, how large, what kind? *J. Electromyogr. Kinesiol.* **8**, 391–402.

McDonagh, J. C., Binder, M. D., Reinking, R. M. and Stuart, D. G. (1980a). A commentary on muscle unit properties in cat hindlimb muscles. *J. Morphol.* **166**, 217–230.

McDonagh, J. C., Binder, M. D., Reinking, R. M. and Stuart, D. G. (1980b). Tetrapartite classification of motor units of cat tibialis anterior. *J. Neurophysiol.* **44**, 696–712.

Milner-Brown, H. S., Stein, R. B. and Yemm, R. (1973a). The contractile properties of human motor units during voluntary isometric contractions. *J. Physiol. (Lond.)* **228**, 285–306.

Milner-Brown, H. S., Stein, R. B. and Yemm, R. (1973b). The orderly recruitment of human motor units during voluntary isometric contractions. *J. Physiol. (Lond.)* **230**, 359–370.

Moschovakis, A. K., Burke, R. E. and Fyffe, R. E. W. (1991). The size and dendritic structure of HRP-labelled gamma motoneurons in the cat spinal cord. *J. Comp. Neurol.* **311**, 531–545.

Munson, J. B., Foehring, R. C., Mendell, L. M. and Gordon, T. (1997). Fast-to-slow conversion following chronic low-frequency actiovation of medial gastrocnemius muscle in cats. II. Motoneuron properties. *J. Neurophysiol.* **77**, 2605–2615.

Murthy, K. S. K., Ledbetter, W. D., Eidelberg, E., Cameron, W. E. and Petit, J. (1982). Histochemical evidence for the existence of skeletofusimotor (β) innervation in the primate. *Exp. Brain Res.* **46**, 186–190.

Nardone, A. and Schieppati, M. (1988). Shift of activity from slow to fast muscle during voluntary lengthening contractions of the triceps surae muscles in humans. *J. Physiol. (Lond.)* **395**, 363–381.

Nardone, A., Romano, C. and Schieppati, M. (1989). Selective recruitment of high-threshold human motor units during voluntary isotonic lengthening of active muscles. *J. Physiol. (Lond.)* **409**, 451–471.

Nemeth, P. M. (1990). Metabolic fiber types and influences on their transformation. In: *The Segmental Motor System*, eds. M. D. Binder and L. M. Mendell, pp. 258–277. New York: Oxford University Press.

Nemeth, P. M., Solanski, L., Gordon, D. A., Hamm, T. M., Reinking, R. M. and Stuart, D. G. (1986). Uniformity of metabolic enzymes within individual motor units. *J. Neurosci.* **6**, 892–898.

Nemeth, P. M., Rosser, B. W. C. and Wilkinson, R. S. (1991). Metabolic and contractile uniformity of isolated motor unit fibres of snake muscle. *J. Physiol. (Lond.)* **434**, 41–55.

O'Donovan, M. J., Pinter, M. J., Dum, R. P. and Burke, R. E. (1985). Kinesiological studies of self- and cross-reinnervated FDL and soleus muscles in freely-moving cats. *J. Neurophysiol.* **54**, 852–866.

Ong, T., Hayes, D. and Armstrong, R. (1988). Distribution of microspheres in plantaris muscles of resting and exercising rats as a function of fiber type. *Am. J. Anat.* **182**, 318–324.

Padykula, H. A. and Gauthier, G. F. (1970). The ultrastructure of the neuromuscular junctions of mammalian red, white, and intermediate skeletal muscle fibers. *J. Cell. Biol.* **46**, 27–41.

Paton, W. D. M. and Waud, D. R. (1967). The margin of safety of neuromuscular transmission. *J. Physiol. (Lond.)* **191**, 59–90.

Pette, D. and Staron, R. S. (1990). Cellular and molecular diversities of mammalian skeletal muscle fibers. *Rev. Physiol. Biochem. Pharmacol.* **116**, 2–76.

Pette, D. and Vrbova, G. (1992). Adaptation of mammalian skeletal muscle fibers to chronic electrical stimulation. *Rev. Physiol. Biochem. Pharmacol.* **120**, 115–202.

Pette, D., Ramirez, B. U., Müller, W., Simon, R., Exner, G. U. and Hildebrand, R. (1975). Influence of intermittent long-term stimulation of contractile, histochemical and metabolic properties of fibre populations in fast and slow rabbit muscles. *Pflü gers Arch.* **361**, 1–7.

Pierotti, D. J., Roy, R. R., Bodine-Fowler, S. C., Hodgson, J. A. and Edgerton, V. R. (1991). Mechanical and morphological properties of chronically inactive cat tibialis anterior motor units. *J. Physiol. (Lond.)* **444**, 175–192.

Powers, R. K., Robinson, F. R., Konodi, M. A. and Binder, M. D. (1993). Distribution of rubrospinal synaptic input to cat triceps surae motoneurons. *J. Neurophysiol.* **70**, 1460–1468.

Prakash, Y. S., Miller, S. M., Huang, M. and Sieck, G. C. (1996). Morphology of diaphragm neuromuscular junctions on different fibre types. *J. Neurocytol.* **25**, 88–100.

Rafuse, V. F. and Gordon, T. (1996). Self-reinnervated cat medial gastrocnemius muscles. II. Analysis of the mechanisms and significance of fiber type grouping in reinnervated muscles. *J. Neurophysiol.* **75**, 282–297.

Rafuse, V. F. and Gordon, T. (1998). Incomplete rematching of nerve and muscle properties in motor units after extensive nerve injuries in cat hindlimb muscle. *J. Physiol. (Lond.)* **509**, 909–926.

Rafuse, V. F., Pattullo, M. C. and Gordon, T. (1997). Innervation ratio and motor unit force in large muscles: a study of chronically stimulated cat medial gastrocnemius. *J. Physiol. (Lond.)* **499**, 809–823.

Rall, W. and Hunt, C. C. (1956). Analysis of reflex variability in terms of partially correlated excitability fluctuations in a population of motoneurons. *J. Gen. Physiol.* **39**, 397–422.

Ranvier, L. (1874). De quelques faits relatifs à l'histologie et à la physiologie des muscles striés. *Arch. Physiol. Norm. Pathol.* **1**, 5–18.

Rexed, B. (1952). The cytoarchitectonic organization of the spinal cord in the cat. *J. Comp. Neurol.* **96**, 415–496.

Rivero, J.-L. L., Talmadge, R. J. and Edgerton, V. R. (1998). Fibre size and metabolic properties of myosin heavy chain-based fibre types in rat skeletal muscle. *J. Muscle Res. Cell Motil.* **19**, 733–742.

Romaiguère, P., Vedel, J.-P., Pagni, S. and Zenatti, A. (1989). Physiological properties of the motor units of the wrist extensor muscles in man. *Exp. Brain Res.* **78**, 51–61.

Romanul, F. C. A. (1965). Capillary supply and metabolism of muscle fibers. *Arch. Neurol.* **12**, 497–509.

Roy, R. R., Garfinkel, A., Ounjian, M., Jayne, J., Hirahara, A., Hsu, E. and Edgerton, V. R. (1995). Three-dimensional structure of cat tibialis anterior motor units. *Muscle Nerve* **18**, 1187–1195.

Saltin, B. and Gollnick, P. D. (1983). Skeletal muscle adaptability: significance for metabolism and performance. In: *Handbook of Physiology*, Sect. 10, *Skeletal Muscle.*, eds. L. Peachey and R. H. Adrian, pp. 555–631. Bethesda, MD: American Physiological Society.

Sanes, J. R. (1987). Cell lineages and the origin of muscle fiber types. *Trends Neurosci.* **10**, 219–223.

Schiaffino, S., Gorze, L., Sartore, S. et al. (1989). Three mysoin heavy chain isoforms in type 2 skeletal muscle fibers. *J. Muscle Res. Cell Motil.* **10**, 197–205.

Schieber, M. H., Chua, M., Petit, J. and Hunt, C. C. (1997). Tension distribution of single motor units in multitendoned muscles: comparison of a homologous digit muscle in cats and monkeys. *J. Neurosci.* **17**, 1734–1747.

Sharrard, W. J. W. (1955). The distribution of the permanent paralysis in the lower limb in poliomyelitis. *J. Bone Joint Surg.* **37**, 540–558.

Sica, R. E. P. and McComas, A. J. (1971). Fast and slow twitch units in a human muscle. *J. Neurol. Neurosurg. Psychiatry* **34**, 113–120.

Sieck, G. C., Zhan, W. Z., Prakash, Y. S., Daood, M. J. and Watchko, J. F. (1995). SDH and actomyosin ATPase activities of different fiber types in rat diaphragm muscle. *J. Appl. Physiol.* **79**, 1629–1639.

Sieck, G. C., Fournier, M., Prakash, Y. S. and Blanco, C. E. (1996). Myosin phenotype and SDH enzyme variability among motor unit fibers. *J. Appl. Physiol.* **80**, 2179–2189.

Smith, J. L., Betts, B., Edgerton, V. R. and Zernicke, R. F. (1980). Rapid ankle extension during paw shakes: selective recruitment of fast ankle extensors. *J. Neurophysiol.* **43**, 612–620.

Smits, E., Rose, P. K., Gordon, T. and Richmond, F. J. R. (1994). Organization of single motor units in feline sartorius. *J. Neurophysiol.* **72**, 1885–1896.

Stålberg, E. and Antoni, L. (1980). Electrophysiological cross section of the motor unit. *J. Neurol. Neurosurg. Psychiatry* **43**, 496–474.

Stein, J. M. and Padykula, H. A. (1962). Histochemical classification of individual skeletal muscle fibers of the rat. *Am. J. Anat.* **110**, 103–124.

Stephens, J. A. and Usherwood, T. P. (1977). The mechanical properties of human motor units with special reference to their fatiguability and recruitment threshold. *Brain Res.* **125**, 91–97.

Swett, J., Eldred, E. and Buchwald, J. S. (1970). Somatotopic cord-to-muscle relations in efferent innervation of cat gastrocnemius. *Am. J. Physiol.* **219**, 762–766.

Taylor, A. and Stephens, J. A. (1976). Study of human motor unit contractions by controlled intramuscular microstimulation. *Brain Res.* **117**, 331–335.

Thomas, C., Bigland-Ritchie, B., Westling, G. and Johansson, R. (1990). A comparison of human thenar motor-unit properties studied by intraneural motor-axon stimulation and spike triggered averaging. *J. Neurophysiol.* **64**, 1347–1351.

Thomson, D. B., Scott, S. H. and Richmond, F. J. R. (1991). Neuromuscular organization of feling anterior sartorius: I. Asymmetrical distribution of motor units. *J. Morphol.* **210**, 147–162.

Tötösy de Zepetnek, J. E., Zung, H. V., Erdebil, S. and Gordon, T. (1992). Motor-unit categorization based on contractile and histochemical properties: a glycogen depletion analysis of normal and reinnervated rat tibialis anterior muscle. *J. Neurophysiol.* **67**, 1404–1415.

Trotter, J. A. (1993). Functional morphology of force transmission in skeletal muscle – a brief review. *Acta Anat.* **146**, 205–222.

Unguez, G. A., Bodine-Fowler, S., Roy, R. R., Pierotti, D. J. and Edgerton, V. R. (1993). Evidence of incomplete neural control of motor unit properties in cat tibialis anterior after self-reinnervation. *J. Physiol. (Lond.)* **472**, 103–125.

Unguez, G. A., Roy, R. R., Pierotti, D. A., Bodine-Fowler, S. and Edgerton, V. R. (1995). Further evidence of incomplete neural control of muscle properties in cat tibialis anterior motor units. *Am. J. Physiol.* **268**, C527–C534.

van de Graaff, K. M., Frederick, E. C., Williamson, R. G. and Goslow, G. E., Jr (1977). Motor units and fiber types of primary ankle extensors of the skunk *Mephitis mephitis*. *J. Neurophysiol.* **40**, 1424–1431.

Walmsley, B., Hodgson, J. A. and Burke, R. E. (1978). Forces produced by medial gastrocnemius and soleus muscles during locomotion in freely moving cats. *J. Neurophysiol.* **41**, 1203–1216.

Walsh, J. V., Burke, R. E., Rymer, W. Z. and Tsairis, P. (1978). The effect of compensatory hypertrophy studied in individual motor units in the medial gastrocnemius muscle of the cat. *J. Neurophysiol.* **41**, 496–508.

Weeks, O. I. and English, A. W. (1987). Cat triceps surae motor nuclei are organized topologically. *Exp. Neurol.* **96**, 163–177.

Westling, G., Johansson, R. S., Thomas, C. K. and Bigland-Ritchie, B. (1990). Measurement of contractile and electrical properties of single human thenar motor units in response to intraneural motor-axon stimulation. *J. Neurophysiol.* **64**, 1331–1338.

Wuerker, R. B., McPhedran, A. M. and Henneman, E. (1965). Properties of motor units in a heterogeneous pale muscle (m. gastrocnemius) of the cat. *J. Neurophysiol.* **28**, 85–99.

Zajac, F. E. (1990). Coupling of recruitment order to the force produced by motor units: The 'size principle hypothesis' revisited. In: *The Segmental Motor System*, ed. M. Binder and L. Mendell, pp. 96–111. New York: Oxford University Press.

Zajac, F. E. and Faden, J. S. (1985). Relationship among recruitment order, axonal conduction velocity, and muscle-unit properties of type-identified motor units in cat plantaris muscle. *J. Neurophysiol.* **53**, 1303–1322.

Zardini, D. M. and Parry, D. J. (1998). Physiological characteristics of identified motor units in the mouse extensor digitorum longus muscle: an in vitro approach. *Can. J. Physiol. Pharmacol.* **76**, 68–71.

Zengel, J. E., Reid, S. A., Sypert, G. W. and Munson, J. B. (1985). Membrane electrical properties and prediction of motor-unit type of cat medial gastrocnemius motoneurons in the cat. *J. Neurophysiol.* **53**, 1323–1344.

2

Developmental biology of skeletal muscle

Jeffrey B. Miller

Introduction

Many of the molecular and cellular events that choreograph skeletal muscle development have been identified in the past few years. The combined results from studies of muscle gene regulation, somite formation, cell signalling, the cell cycle and neuromuscular interactions have produced clear insights into the mechanisms that control muscle formation and lifelong function. In addition, there have been truly remarkable advances in the molecular genetics of neuromuscular diseases. Indeed, the gene defects that produce a large proportion of neuromuscular diseases have now been identified (Brown, 1998). Optimism reigns as methods to improve the function of diseased, injured and aged muscle now appear possible, if not yet proven in humans. This chapter reviews the cellular and molecular biology of myogenesis.

The cell biology of skeletal muscle is unique. The terminally differentiated cells of skeletal muscles are very large, multinucleate muscle fibres (myofibres). Myofibres form when mononucleate myoblasts cease replicating and fuse with each other to form multinucleate cells that express muscle-specific proteins such as myosin and the other members of the contractile apparatus. Muscle fibres form in distinct stages (Fig. 2.1) (reviewed in Kelly, 1983; Stockdale, 1997; Miller et al., 1999).

Cells with myogenic potential are first found in the somites, at about embryonic day 8.5 (E8.5) in the mouse and at about 6–8 weeks in utero for the human. The first myosin-expressing cells appear in somites, though these somitic myocytes are atypically mononucleate. In the head, limbs and trunk, multinucleate myofibres form in several distinct waves. The first or primary myofibres form from the nearly simultaneous fusion of many myoblasts (Harris et al., 1989). Almost simultaneously with their formation, the primary myofibres are contacted by motor neurons and functional neuromuscular junctions are established (Dennis et al., 1981; Duxson et al., 1989).

As myogenesis proceeds, secondary muscle fibres begin to form parallel to each primary fibre; as a result a rosette of several small, newly formed secondary fibres surrounds each large primary fibre. Secondary fibres begin to form near the sites where primary myotubes are contacted by motor neurons (Duxson et al., 1989). Primary and secondary fibres are initially contained within a single basal lamina and are electrically coupled (Kelly, 1983). At later stages of postnatal growth and development, primary and secondary fibres grow by additional myoblast fusion, become morphologically indistinguishable as they become the same size and develop individual basal laminae (Harris et al., 1989). In large organisms, including humans, primary and secondary myogenesis is followed by a tertiary wave of myofibre formation that can continue well past the time of birth (Draeger et al., 1987; Wilson et al., 1992).

An important feature of myogenesis is the formation of specialized types of fast and slow muscle fibres which are arrayed in distinctive patterns in different muscles. Most mammalian muscles, including those of humans, contain a mixture of fibre types, including those that contract relatively slowly (slow type I), and those that contract more rapidly (fast type IIA, IIB, and IIX) (Fig. 2.2). The masticatory muscles (e.g. the masseter) and extraocular muscles have particularly complex fibre type compositions (Stal et al., 1994). Primary myotubes survive into adulthood and most appear to become slow type I fibres, though some may also become fast type IIB fibres (Zhang and McLennan, 1998). The maximum contraction rate of a skeletal muscle fibre is determined both by the ATPase activity of the myosin heavy chain (MHC) isoform(s) expressed in the fibre and by the myosin light chain (MLC) isoforms that form the complete myosin hexamer (Schiaffino and Reggiani, 1994). In addition to differences in contractile

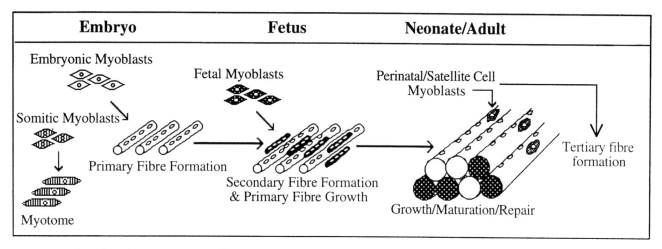

| Embryo | Fetus | Neonate/Adult |

Fig. 2.1. An outline of vertebrate myogenesis. Different types of myoblast appear in the initial stages of muscle fibre formation and diversification; general features of myogenesis include the generation of multiple types of myoblast and the nerve-independent formation of different types of primary and secondary myotube. Based on their time of appearance and properties in vitro, the diverse types of myoblast are proposed to have distinct roles in the initial formation of primary and secondary myotubes. Though not illustrated, nerves are required for maturation and maintenance of muscle fibres, as described in the text. Some details of myoblast diversity vary between birds and mammals (Miller, 1992; Stockdale, 1997). In large mammals, there is an additional, tertiary period of myofibre formation, which follows secondary fibre formation (Draeger et al., 1987; Wilson et al., 1992).

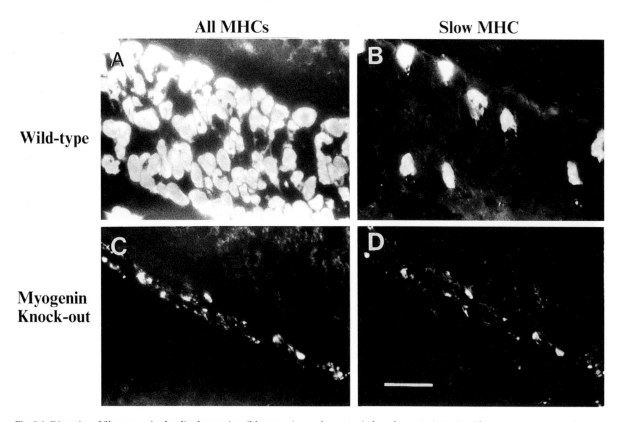

Fig. 2.2. Diversity of fibre types in the diaphragm in wild-type mice and myogenin knock-out ($-/-$) mice. Fluorescent staining is for either the slow isoform of myosin heavy chain (slow MHC) or all isoforms of myosin heavy chain (all MHCs). The samples are transverse sections from embryonic day 19 mice. Note that about 10% of the myofibres in the wild type contains the slow MHC isoform, whereas the remaining myofibres do not. There is a dramatic decrease in myofibre formation in myogenin knock-out mice. Note that only a few, very small MHC-positive cells are found in the myogenin-null diaphragm (see Zhu and Miller, 1997). Scale bar = 45 μm.

Table 2.1. Myogenesis and the four muscle regulatory factors

Genotype	Skeletal muscle phenotype	References
MyoD (−/−)	Delayed limb myogenesis, impaired regeneration	Megeney et al., 1996; Kablar et al., 1997
Myf5 (−/−)	Delayed back muscle development; rib defects	Braun et al., 1992; Kablar et al., 1997
MyoD (−/−) and Myf5 (−/−)	No muscle cells form	Rudnicki et al., 1993
Myogenin (−/−)	Drastic reduction of myofibre numbers	Hasty et al., 1993; Nabeshima et al., 1993
MRF4 (−/−)	Variable, depending on Myf5 level[a]	Olson et al., 1996
MyoD (−/−) and MRF4 (−/−)	Similar to myogenin (−/−)	Rawls et al., 1998

Notes:

[a] The muscle defects seen in three different MRF4 (−/−) strains range from mild to severe, apparently because each MRF4 knock-out
 also causes, by *cis*-acting mechanisms, a decrease in expression from nearby *myf5* (Yoon et al., 1997).

protein isoforms, myofibres can differ in metabolism (e.g. oxidative versus glycolytic), fatigue resistance and relaxation rates. As described below, the functional differences among myofibres are produced during embryonic, fetal and postnatal development by a complex array of cellular mechanisms.

Myogenesis and the somites

The somites are the source of myogenic cells that will form the skeletal muscles of the trunk and limbs (Chevallier et al., 1977; Christ et al., 1977; Ordahl and LeDouarin, 1992; Lee and Sze, 1993). (Many head muscles, in contrast, form from nonsomitic, paraxial mesoderm that lies rostral to the somites (Couly et al., 1992, 1993).) Somites form as epithelial balls but soon subdivide into sclerotomal, dermatomal and myotomal compartments (Gossler and Hrabe de Angelis, 1998). Myogenic cells in the somites form in a spatially and temporally organized sequence, with cells expressing muscle regulatory factors (MRFs) first appearing along the dorsomedial lip of the dermomyotome, followed by an ordered appearance of myocytes in the spatially distinct myotome (Smith, T.H. et al., 1994; Denetclaw et al., 1997; Kahane et al, 1998). Despite this apparent link between somite structure and myogenesis, complete morphogenesis of the somites is not required for the formation of myogenic cells.

One demonstration of how myogenesis can be unlinked from somitogenesis comes from studies of the gene *paraxis*. The Paraxis protein is a bHLH (basic helix-loop-helix) transcription factor that is expressed throughout the epithelial ball stage of somites but later becomes restricted to the dermomyotome (Burgess et al., 1995, 1996; Sosic et al., 1997). In the absence of Paraxis, epithelial balls fail to form and there are defects in patterning of the axial skeleton and muscles. Myogenic cells, however, are sti ll produced and form

segmented structures reminiscent of myotomes (Burgess et al., 1996). This work also confirms that the forming somites are responding to an underlying segmentation that precedes the initial epithelial ball stage of somite formation (cf. Packard and Meier, 1983; Palmeirim et al., 1997).

Another mesodermally expressed bHLH protein is Mesp2 (Saga et al., 1997). In Mesp2-null mouse embryos, somitogenesis is disrupted and the initial epithelial ball stage somites fail to form (Saga et al., 1997). Nonetheless, myogenic cells form and make segmented myotomes in Mesp2-null embryos, much as in Paraxis-null embryos. Remarkably, despite the absence of the epithelial ball stage of somitogenesis, Mesp2-null embryos do make apparently normal-looking dermomyotomes. This uncoupling of dermomyotome and epithelial ball formation is unexpected and suggests a separate origin for the cells in the epithelium of the dermomyotome. A similar lack of the epithelial ball stage with normal dermomyotomes is seen in dII1-null embryos, which lack one member of the Delta homologue family of ligands that interact with the Notch family of receptors (Hrabe de Angelis et al., 1997). Notch is itself a regulator of myogenesis, as constitutively active Notch receptors inhibit myogenesis (Kopan et al., 1994).

Signalling and early myogenesis

Studies of myogenesis in knock-out mice and in co-cultures of embryonic tissues have identified transcription factor networks and possible intercellular signalling pathways that control myogenic cell origins (reviewed in Molkentin and Olson, 1996; Borycki and Emerson, 1997; Tajbakhsh and Cossu, 1997).

Myogenesis is controlled to a large extent by four muscle-specific transcription factors, Myf5, MyoD, MRF4 and myogenin, that form a family of regulatory factors, the MRFs (Table 2.1). Mice that lack either MyoD or Myf5 are capable of at least some myofibre formation in vivo (Braun et al., 1992; Rudnicki et al., 1992), whereas mice that lack both MyoD and Myf5 make no myogenic cells (Rudnicki et al., 1993). Inactivation of Myf5 also leads to rib defects (Braun et al, 1992). Surprisingly, portions of the ribs are formed by cells from the dermomyotome, rather than the sclerotome (Kato and Aoyama, 1998), so the lack of Myf5 may directly inhibit formation of rib precursor cells. A lack of myogenin leads to a drastic reduction in numbers of myofibres, though myoblasts appear to form normally (Hasty et al., 1993; Nabeshima et al., 1993). Though individual knock-outs of MyoD and MRF4 produce relatively mild muscle phenotypes (Olson et al., 1996; Kablar et al., 1997), double knock-out of MyoD and MRF4 leads to a drastic reduction of myofibre numbers similar to that seen in myogenin knock-outs (Rawls et al., 1998).

Another transcription factor involved in somitic myogenesis is the *paired*-related protein Pax3. In the somites, Pax3 is initially expressed throughout the epithelium but then becomes restricted to the migratory myogenic cells in the ventrolateral region of the dermomyotome (Bober et al., 1994; Goulding et al., 1994; Williams and Ordahl, 1994). Pax3 plays a critical role in successful myogenesis, as confirmed by the failure of *splotch* mutant embryos of mice, which lack Pax3, to make muscles that require migratory precursors. The limb muscles, in particular, are completely absent in Pax3-deficient mice as a result of lack of migration from the somite, even though Pax3-deficient cells are capable of myogenesis (Daston et al., 1996). Myogenic cell migration requires hepatocyte growth factor/scatter factor (HGF/SF) and its receptor, c-Met (Bladt et al., 1995). Expression of c-Met in myogenic cells of the somites requires Pax3, providing an explanation for the lack of migration by Pax3-deficient cells (Daston et al., 1996; Epstein et al., 1996). Mice that lack either c-Met or HGF/SF have muscle-deficient phenotypes that are similar to the Pax3-deficient mutants (Bladt et al., 1995; Schmidt et al., 1995; Uehara et al., 1995).

MyoD, Myf5 and Pax3 appear to participate in a cross-regulatory network. MyoD expression is significantly delayed in Myf5(−/−) mice (Kablar et al., 1997), suggesting that Myf5 is involved in early activation of MyoD. Furthermore, no MyoD is expressed in the bodies of mice that lack both Pax3 and Myf5. These results imply that, whereas Myf5 is required for early activation of MyoD, Pax3 is needed for later activation or maintenance of MyoD expression (Tajbakhsh et al., 1997). In addition, Myf5 expression appears to be independent of Pax3 expression, except in the ventrolateral domain of interlimb somites (Tajbakhsh et al., 1997). Therefore, Myf5 and Pax3 may define distinct molecular pathways in the activation of MyoD.

A Pax3-independent pathway regulates formation of the anterior head muscles. Unlike the epaxial and hypaxial muscles, the head muscles are not derived from the somites but rather are formed from unsegmented paraxial mesoderm that lies rostral to the somites (Couly et al., 1993). Head muscle development does, however, require either MyoD or Myf5, as shown by the lack of head muscles in double mutants that lack both MyoD and Myf5 (Rudnicki et al., 1993). In Pax3(−/−) mice, head muscles appear normal, except for those tongue muscles and the hypoglossal muscle that originate in the somites (Franz et al., 1993). In the absence of both Pax3 and Myf5, the body muscles fail to form, but the anterior head muscles appear normal (Tajbakhsh et al., 1997).

Several proteins may mediate positional signals that direct formation of epaxial and hypaxial myogenic cells. In particular, a combination of Sonic hedgehog (Shh) and Wnt family members can substitute for neural tube/notochord tissue to induce myogenesis in somitic mesoderm explants (Münsterberg et al., 1995). Studies of Shh(−/−) mice suggest, however, that it is only the epaxial lineage of myogenic cells in the dorsomedial region of the somite that require Shh (Chiang et al., 1996; Reshef et al., 1998). Thus, Shh-dependent signals appear to induce the Myf5-dependent myogenic cells in the dorsomedial somite, but do not induce the MyoD-dependent myogenic cells in the ventrolateral somite.

Signalling in the bone morphogenetic protein (BMP) pathway also appears to regulate somitic myogenesis, possibly by restricting Pax3 action (Fig. 2.3). Wnt1, which in combination with Shh induces dorsomedial myogenesis (Münsterberg et al., 1995; Reshef et al., 1998), is expressed in the neural tube adjacent to the dorsomedial lip of the somite, where it induces expression of Noggin in the neighbouring somites (Hirsinger et al., 1997; Reshef et al., 1998). Noggin is a protein that binds to and inactivates BMPs, and it also induces myogenesis in somite/ectoderm co-cultures. In contrast, BMP4 alone inhibits myogenesis in these co-cultures (Reshef et al., 1998). Consistent with a role for BMP4 as an inhibitor of myogenesis, ectopic expression of Noggin leads to an expanded region of MyoD expression in somites, presumably by relieving BMP4 inhibition of myogenesis (Reshef et al., 1998). Noggin may well act in combination with follistatin, another BMP antagonist, which is also expressed in developing somites and is required for normal muscle development (Matzuk et al., 1995; Amthor et al., 1996). Further complexity is added by the finding that members of the basic fibroblast growth factor (bFGF) and transforming growth factor (TGFβ) families can be potent inducers of myogenesis in explants of chicken embryo paraxial mesoderm (Stern et al., 1997).

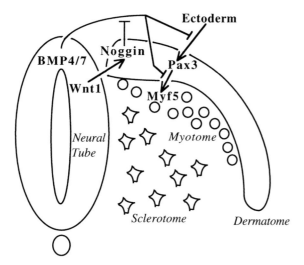

Fig. 2.3. Possible regulatory pathways that may regulate formation of the somitic myotome. Signals from ectoderm and axial tissues (neural tube) appear to activate Pax3 expression, and Pax3 subsequently induces Myf5. Myf5 is the first of the muscle regulatory factors (MRF) to be expressed in the somite of the mouse, and Myf5 expression begins in the dorsomedial lip of the dermamyotome (Smith et al., 1994). Signals from bone morphogenetic proteins (BMP) may block induction of Pax3, but BMP action is blocked by Noggin. Wnt signals from the dorsal neural tube induce Noggin expression at the dorsomedial lip of the dermamyotome; Noggin probably acts with other BMP antagonists (e.g., follistatin) to lift BMP-mediated inhibition of Myf5 expression, thus initiating the formation of myosin-containing somitic myocytes. (Adapted from Reshef et al., 1998.)

The intracellular pathways affected by intercellular signals appear to be mediated through the calcium-dependent kinase (CDK) inhibitors p21^{CIP1} and p57^{KIP2} and the retinoblastoma (Rb) protein (Zhang et al., 1999). The p21^{CIP1} and p57^{KIP2} proteins function to inhibit cyclin/CDK complexes, which cooperate to control cell cycling through phosphorylation and inactivation of the Rb protein. Double knock-out of p21^{CIP1} and p57^{KIP2} leads to a nearly complete lack of myofibres (Zhang et al., 1999), which is a phenotype closely similar to that of myogenin knock-outs (Hasty et al., 1993; Nabeshima et al., 1993). Mice lacking the Rb protein also show defects in myogenesis (Novitch et al., 1996). Therefore, these proteins regulate myoblast cell cycle exit, and this cessation of myoblast proliferation is required for terminal differentiation and the formation of myofibres in which the nuclei are not normally mitotic.

Myoblasts and myogenic cell lineages

Myoblasts, which fuse with each other to form terminally differentiated myofibres, are the penultimate cell in the myogenic cell lineage. Myoblasts are mononucleate cells that do not express skeletal muscle myosin but usually do express desmin and one or more of the four MRFs (George-Weinstein et al., 1993; Smith et al., 1993). Proper spatial and temporal expression of the MRFs is critical for successful myogenesis (Weintraub, 1993; Arnold and Braun, 1996; Molkentin and Olson, 1996; Yun and Wold, 1996; Firulli and Olson, 1997; Abmayr and Keller, 1998). The MRFs share structural homologies and are to a large extent functionally interchangeable in vivo (Wang et al., 1996; Wang and Jaenisch, 1997; Zhu and Miller, 1997). The MRFs interact with each other and with other proteins, most notably members of the MEF2 family (reviewed in Molkentin and Olson, 1996).

The four MRFs are expressed in a defined sequence in myogenic cells. In mouse cells, Myf5 and MyoD are typically the earliest MRFs expressed, followed by myogenin and, lastly, MRF4 (Smith et al., 1993; Smith T. H. et al., 1994; Cornelison and Wold, 1997). This expression sequence identifies early (Myf5/MyoD) and late (MRF4/myogenin) stages in the life of a myoblast. Myoblasts appear to be capable of proliferation at early stages but become nonmitotic at later stages when the cells express both myogenin and the *cdk* inhibitor p21 (Walsh and Perlman, 1997). Consequently, the term 'myoblast' covers a heterogeneous group of cells that can have distinct patterns of gene expression and are at different points in the progression of genetic events that culminate in terminal differentiation.

Several types of experiment have shown that, just as there are multiple types of myofibre, there are also multiple types of myoblast, and these are most abundant at different stages of development (Fig. 2.1). Experimentally distinct types of avian and mammalian myoblasts have been identified (Hauschka et al., 1979; Cossu and Molinaro, 1987, Smith and Miller, 1992; Edom-Vovard et al., 1998). The four major types of mouse myoblast are termed somitic, embryonic, fetal and perinatal/satellite cell myoblasts to indicate site of origin and time of appearance (Cossu and Molinaro, 1987; Miller, 1992) (Fig. 2.1). Different myoblast types can be distinguished based on their differing responses to growth factors (e.g. to TGFβ) and metabolic inhibitors (e.g. phorbol esters), and on the differing morphologies and gene expression patterns of the myotubes they form (Smith and Miller, 1992; Cusella-de Angelis et al., 1994; Zappelli et al., 1996; Edom-Vovard et al., 1998). In mammals, there are distinct subtypes of satellite cell myoblasts that coexist in perinatal and adult animals (Rosenblatt et al., 1996; Barjot et al., 1998; Yang et al., 1998). Satellite cell myoblasts that lie next to slow muscle fibres generally form myofibres that express slow myosin; in contrast, satellite cells adjacent to fast fibres form myofibres that do not express slow myosin (Rosenblatt et al., 1996). The fast and slow subtypes of satellite cells remain stably committed to form distinct types of myotube and do not change fates, even when the muscles in which they reside have been converted to the opposite phenotype by electrical stimulation or cross-reinnervation (Barjot et al., 1998).

These results suggest that at least early stages of the formation of fast and slow muscle fibres may depend on distinct types of myoblast, thus providing a possible explanation for the finding that the initial stages of muscle fibre diversification do not require innervation (Butler et al., 1982; Crow and Stockdale, 1986; Condon et al., 1990).

In addition to the temporally distinct populations of myoblasts, there also appear to be spatially distinct populations of myoblasts during development. Analyses of quail–chicken chimaerae have shown that trunk and limb muscles have different developmental origins than the anterior head muscles (Fig. 2.4). In both avian and mammalian embryos, the skeletal muscles of the trunk and limbs form from myoblasts that arise in the embryonic somites and then migrate to muscle-forming regions (Chevallier et al., 1977; Christ et al., 1977; Ordahl and LeDouarin, 1992; Lee and Sze, 1993). Myoblasts derived from somites also form the extrinsic and intrinsic muscles of the tongue, as well as the jaw-opening muscles that attach to the hyoid (Couly et al., 1993). In contrast to the somite-derived muscles, the muscles of the anterior head, including jaw-closing masticatory muscles such as the masseter, pterygoid and temporalis, appear to arise from myogenic cells that form in the prechordal mesoderm, which is the nonsomitic, paraxial mesoderm that lies adjacent to the cephalic neural tube in the developing head but is rostral to the somites (Couly et al., 1992, 1993; Faerman et al., 1995).

There is a further complexity in the origins of muscle derived from somites. Dorsal muscles of the back (epaxial muscles) are formed from a different lineage of myogenic cells than are muscles of the limbs and ventral ribs (hypaxial muscles), as shown by the quail–chicken transplantation experiments of Ordahl and Le Douarin (1992). Myogenic cells that form the back muscles arise in the dorsomedial portion of somites nearest to the neural tube, whereas those that form the limb and ribs arise in the ventrolateral portion of the somites (Ordahl and Le Douarin, 1992). Cells from the ventrolateral portion of the limb-level somites migrate from the somites into the limbs to form

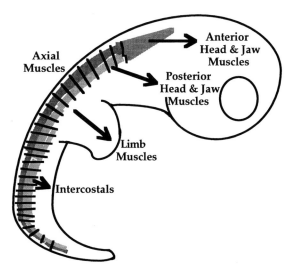

Fig. 2.4. Muscle in different parts of the animal originate in spatially distinct domains. Limb and intercostal (hypaxial) muscles are formed by myogenic cells that originate in the ventrolateral domains of the somites and then migrate to areas of muscle development (Ordahl and LeDouarin, 1992). See text for further details.

the limb muscles (Milaire, 1976; Ordahl and Le Douarin, 1992; Lee and Sze, 1993).

The dorsal (epaxial) and ventral (hypaxial) muscle cell lineages are clearly distinguishable by their distinct patterns of MRF expression. Myf5 is initially expressed in only the dorsomedial portion of the dermomyotome of mouse somites, which is the source of epaxial muscle precursors, whereas MyoD is initially expressed in only the ventrolateral portion, which is the source of hypaxial muscle precursors (Ordahl and Le Douarin, 1992; Smith T. H. et al., 1994). Both Myf5 and MyoD are initially expressed in columnar epithelial cells of the limb-level somites (dorsomedial lip for Myf5, ventromedial lip for MyoD), with later expression of both in somitic myoblasts and myocytes located in the myotome. Unlike many cell types, epithelial cells of the somite do not appear to respond to MRF expression by induction of terminal differentiation. MHC, a marker of terminal differentiation, has not been found to be expressed in somitic epithelial cells, even when these cells express Myf5 or MyoD in normal embryos (Smith T. H. et al., 1994) or myogenin or MRF4 in transgenic mice (Block et al., 1996). This finding raises the possibility that somitic epithelial cells have an active mechanism for post-translational inhibition of MRF family function, perhaps through the Noggin/BMP pathway discussed above.

As shown by analyses of knock-out mice, the spatially and temporally distinct expression patterns of Myf5, MyoD and MRF4 are functionally important. In Myf5-deficient mouse embryos, for example, dorsal (epaxial) muscle development is delayed for 2–3 days, whereas limb (hypaxial) muscle development occurs on a normal schedule (Braun et al., 1994; Kablar et al., 1997). In MyoD-deficient mouse embryos, the opposite pattern is found: limb muscle development and expression of Myf5 are delayed, but dorsal muscle development occurs at the normal time (Kablar et al., 1997). The central region of the somite, between the Myf5- and MyoD-dependent domains, also appears to be distinct. Myogenic cells in this central portion of the somite initially express MRF4, but not Myf5 or MyoD (Smith T. H. et al., 1994), and, in the absence of MRF4, terminally differentiated myocytes fail to form at these central sites (Patapoutian et al., 1995a).

Muscle stem cells

Several lines of evidence suggest that MRF-expressing myoblasts are the progeny of a distinct class of MRF-negative muscle stem cells (Dominov et al., 1998; Beauchamp et al., 1999; Miller et al., 1999; Gussoni et al., 1999). A muscle stem cell does not express muscle markers (e.g. the MRFs) but is able to produce both new muscle stem cells (i.e. is capable of self-renewal) and progeny destined to become myoblasts and myofibres (definition adapted from Slack (1991) and Wolpert et al. (1997)).

One piece of evidence for muscle stem cells has been provided by serial subcloning assays. When cells in an individual clonal muscle colony are dissociated, the resulting cells, which are all the progeny of a single cell, can be re-cultured individually (Rutz and Hauschka, 1982; Miller and Stockdale, 1986a,b; Baroffio et al., 1996). Some of these subcloned cells remain mononucleate and can form new muscle colonies, though the number of new muscle colonies is always much less than the number of mononucleate, potential founder cells in the original colony (Rutz and Hauschka, 1982; Baroffio et al., 1996). This result suggests that only a small number of the clonally related cells have the properties of stem cells and are capable of muscle colony formation.

Muscle stem cells have also been identified by lineage tracing in the somites of mouse embryos (Nicolas et al., 1996). From these experiments, Nicolas et al. (1996) concluded that the muscle cells of the myotome are produced from a unique, spatially organized pool of self-renewing stem cells. They also concluded that stem cells produce progeny by asymmetric divisions, in which one daughter retains stem cell properties and the other becomes a myotomal cell. The stem cell daughter that becomes a myoto-

mal cell appears to have a limited proliferative capacity; individual myotomes typically contained fewer than 16 labelled cells (compared with ~1000 total muscle cells/myotome) (Nicolas et al., 1996).

Gene expression patterns identify a stage in the myogenic cell lineage that occurs prior to MRF expression and may represent the muscle stem cell. For example, myogenic cells in the perinatal/satellite cell lineage do not express any of the MRFs unless activated in response to injury or culturing (Smith et al., 1993; Maley et al., 1994; Smith C. K. et al., 1994; Yablonka-Reuveni and Rivera, 1994; Koishi et al., 1995; Cornelison and Wold, 1997). One protein that is expressed by MRF-negative satellite cells, however, is myocyte nuclear factor-alpha (MNFα) (Garry et al., 1997; Yang et al., 1997). MNFα is a member of the winged-helix family of transcription factors, and it binds to promoter regions of several muscle-specific genes. In uninjured muscle, the MNFα protein is found only in the nuclei of satellite cells.

A second gene expressed by quiescent satellite cells is c-*met* (Cornelison and Wold, 1997), which gives rise to the HGF/SF receptor (see above). HGF/SF is a mitogen for satellite cells (Tatsumi et al., 1998), and signalling through c-*met* is required for successful myogenic cell migration (Bladt et al., 1995). Cornelison and Wold (1997) found that all tested satellite cells express the mRNA and protein from c-*met*, even at the quiescent stage when none of the MRFs are expressed. In contrast to c-Met, M-cadherin is expressed by less than 20% of the quiescent satellite cells. As the satellite cells generate myotubes in culture, all cells continue to express c-Met, and expression of M-cadherin and one or more of the MRFs expands to a large fraction of the cells. By 96h of culture, a small fraction of the satellite cells remain negative for MRF. The activated satellite cells begin MRF expression rather asynchronously over a 72h period, suggesting either that the progenitors of MRF-expressing cells are heterogeneous or that MRF-negative cells continue to produce new cohorts of MRF-negative progeny that will progress to MRF expression.

Another protein associated with the pre-MRF stage of myogenesis is Bcl-2 (Dominov et al., 1998). Bcl-2, which is an inhibitor of apoptosis (Reed, 1997), is expressed by <10% of the mononucleate cells in muscle cell cultures. Bcl-2 expression is limited to a subset of mononucleate cells and is not co-expressed with late markers of myogenesis including myogenin, MRF4 and myosin. These results suggest that Bcl-2 identifies an early, predominantly pre-MRF, stage of myogenesis in cultured satellite cells and muscle cell lines. Perhaps, as in other cell types (Reed, 1997), Bcl-2 acts to inhibit apoptosis of these possible

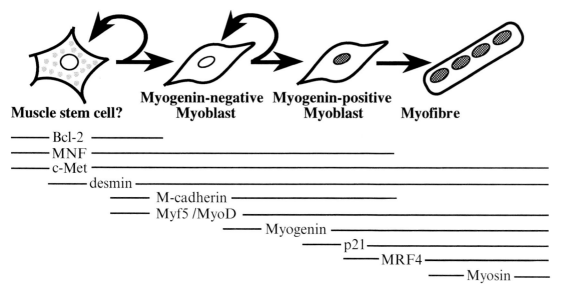

Fig. 2.5. Proposed stages in the perinatal/adult satellite cell lineage (modified from Dominov et al. (1998) and Miller et al. (1999)). Horizontal lines indicate the steps of myogenesis during which particular marker genes are expressed. Bcl-2 expression may coincide with a proposed muscle stem cell stage and turn off in the early myoblast stage. Though c-Met and MNF (myocyte nuclear factor) are also expressed in the proposed muscle stem cell, expression of these and each of the additional markers continues into the myofibre stage of differentiation, whereas Bcl-2 expression stops prior to myogenin expression. Though myogenesis is shown as proceeding only in one direction, it is possible that some myogenin-expressing myoblasts are able, prior to p21 expression (Walsh and Perlman, 1997), to return to a myogenin-negative stage, indicating that these cells are capable of self-renewal.

muscle stem cells. Bcl-2 might also act as a regulator of muscle stem cell cycle progression by inducing cells to enter a quiescent G_0/G_1 state, as found in lymphocytes and fibroblasts (Vairo et al. 1996; Huang et al., 1997; O'Reilly et al. 1997; Reed, 1997).

Taken together, the gene expression patterns and functional assays suggest that the cells in the perinatal/satellite cell lineage proceed through distinct steps of myogenesis beginning with a muscle stem cell (Fig. 2.5). This model appears to be consistent with experiments showing that satellite cells in vivo are in at least two distinct lineage 'compartments' (Schultz, 1996). About 80% of the satellite cells in growing rat leg muscles had dividing times of approximately 32 h and were responsible chiefly for providing nuclei to growing myofibres, whereas the remaining 20% of the cells divided more slowly and appeared to generate new satellite cells (Schultz, 1996). The larger group of rapidly dividing, myofibre-forming cells identified by Schultz (1996) might correspond to mitotic myoblasts (Fig. 2.5). In contrast, the smaller group of more slowly dividing cells that give rise to new satellite cells might correspond to muscle stem cells.

Finally, two recent sets of experiments firmly identify muscle stem cells. First, Beauchamp et al. (1999) showed that all of the muscle fibres that are formed by transplanted myoblasts are actually formed by the progeny of only a tiny fraction (<5%) of the transplanted cells. This minority population of cells divides slowly in tissue culture but is rapidly proliferative after grafting, suggesting a subpopulation with stem cell-like characteristics.

In addition, Gussoni et al. (1999) have used a powerful fluorescence-activated cell sorting technique to identify a novel population of muscle-derived stem cells. These cells, which represent <5% of muscle-derived mononucleate cells, show low Hoechst dye staining. When injected into irradiated *mdx* mice, these rare cells can reconstitute the haematopoietic compartment of the transplanted recipients and can also incorporate into muscle fibres leading to the partial restoration of dystrophin expression in the affected muscle. These studies suggest multipotent muscle stem cells reside in skeletal muscle tissue throughout life.

Myogenesis and motor innervation

Though early stages of myofibre diversification are largely independent of innervation, interaction with motor neurons is required to complete postnatal fibre formation and for the final diversification of fibre types (reviewed in

Miller, 1991; Grinnell, 1995; Sohal, 1995; Stockdale, 1997; Burden, 1998; Kernell, 1998). The matching of muscle fibres and appropriate motor neurons depends on local interactions between the two types of cell, whereas the earlier phases of myogenesis and motor neuron formation are largely autonomous (Sohal, 1995; Landmesser, 1996). Different muscle fibre types form in the absence of innervation, so motor neurons innervate an intrinsically heterogeneous population of muscle fibres.

Several studies suggest that individual motor neurons may preferentially innervate specific types of muscle fibre. For example, Fladby and Jansen (1990) found that motor neurons in the mouse, even shortly after birth, innervated predominately, though not exclusively, only one type of muscle fibre. The initial small complement of aberrant synapses was eliminated by 5–15 days after birth. Cell surface differences between fast and slow muscle fibres might account for specificity of innervation. Motor neurons show different branching patterns, selective fasciculations and different angles of projection across fast and slow muscle fibres (Dahm and Landmesser, 1988; Milner et al., 1998). Fast (mostly derived from secondary fibres) and slow (mostly derived from primary fibres) muscle fibres also differ in surface components including laminin, vascular cell adhesion molecule 1 and neural cell adhesion molecule (Schafer and Stockdale, 1987; Dahm and Landmesser, 1988; Bleisch et al., 1989; Rosen et al., 1992). The results of Fladby and Jansen (1990), as well as other studies (Soileau et al., 1987; Desypris and Parry, 1990; Rafuse et al., 1996), suggest that individual motor neurons preferentially innervate a particular fibre type (or prospective fibre type in the case of fibres that have not reached their final MHC expression pattern), though the specificity is not absolute and some aberrant synapses may be made and later eliminated. This model requires that different types of motor neuron must form in early embryonic development; indeed, motor neurons that project to axial, dorsal and ventral muscles have distinct expression patterns of the LIM class of transcription factors (reviewed in Lumsden, 1995; Tanabe and Jessell, 1996).

Specificity in rostrocaudal patterning in neuromuscular development is suggested by studies showing that motor neurons from different levels of the spinal cord preferentially reinnervate or maintain synapses with particular groups of muscle fibres. As examples, rat intercostal muscles are selectively reinnervated by motor neurons from the appropriate spinal cord level (Wigston and Sanes, 1985), and thoracic motor neurons can be made to innervate wing muscles in the chicken embryo, but these inappropriate connections are lost after an initial period of seemingly normal innervation (Butler et al., 1986; O'Brien et al., 1990). In addition, a rostrocaudal gradient in muscle-specific expression of a MLC promoter fragment demonstrates that muscles have rostrocaudal identity (Grieshammer et al., 1995; Rao et al., 1996). This conclusion is also supported by the finding that the MLC 3F promoter is activated through different promoter elements in different muscles (Rao et al., 1996). Finally, targeted inactivation of *hoxc-8* leads to mice with altered segment identities and patterned neuromuscular deficits that are consistent with a requirement for rostrocaudal matching of motor neurons and muscles during normal development (Tiret et al., 1998).

Myogenesis is therefore a process in which temporally and spatially distinct types of myoblasts arise and participate, with motor neurons, in the formation of diverse types of myofibre.

Ageing and regeneration

Myofibre regeneration and repair is important in diseased and injured muscles and appears to occur also in ageing muscles (reviewed by Anderson, 1998; Cannon, 1998; Grounds, 1998). Regeneration is carried out by the satellite cells, a group of mononucleate, myogenic cells that reside next to and within the same basal lamina as their neighbouring myofibres (Mauro, 1961; Bischoff and Heintz, 1994). In uninjured muscle, satellite cells divide rarely or not at all, and they do not express any of the MRFs, though, as discussed above, they do express c-Met and MNFα. Muscle injury, however, leads to activation of the satellite cells and they begin to divide rapidly, express MRFs (Koishi et al., 1995) and either form new myofibres or fuse with, and thus repair, injured myofibres.

Muscles in aged animals have fewer myofibres and correspondingly less strength than the muscles of young animals. Aged muscles often have only two-thirds as many fibres as young muscles and show particularly large losses of fast type IIB fibres and an increase in proportion of slow type I fibres (Tzankoff and Norris, 1977; Grimby et al., 1982; Larrson and Edström, 1986; Brooks and Faulkner, 1988; Musaro et al., 1995). Ageing or multiple rounds of regeneration in dystrophic muscle also produces satellite cells that have a decreased capacity for proliferation compared with satellite cells from younger or healthy muscle (Webster and Blau, 1990). In addition, the satellite cells from some muscles, such as the masseter, appear to have less regeneration capacity than satellite cells from limb muscles (Pavlath et al., 1998). The decrease in proliferative capacity upon ageing is correlated with decreases in telomere length. Satellite cells from aged muscle, though not the nonmitotic nuclei within myofibres, have shorter telomeres than satellite cells from young muscles (Decary et al., 1997).

Recent experiments have shown that it is possible to alter muscle ageing and regeneration in response to injury by application of exogenous growth factors. In particular, expression of insulin growth factor 1 (IGF1) from an adeno-associated virus vector injected into skeletal muscle leads to an increase of muscle mass and strength and prevents ageing-related muscle changes in old adult mice (Barton-Davis et al., 1998). In older treated mice, muscle mass and fibre type distributions were similar to those in young adults. Barton-Davis et al. (1998) suggest that exogenous IGF1 produced from the gene vector may stimulate muscle regeneration by promoting the proliferation of satellite cells, though other mechanisms of IGF1 action, including actions on nonmuscle cells, may be important as well. Also, the regeneration of mouse muscle after experimental contusions can be improved by application of IGF1, bFGF and nerve growth factor (Kasemkijwattana et al., 1998). These results show that muscle function during ageing and injury repair can be improved by exogenous application of selected growth factors, thus opening fertile ground for additional work in therapeutic approaches to amelioration of myofibre loss during ageing, disease and injury in humans.

Malleable cell fates and myogenesis

At first glance, myogenesis appears linear: stem cells make myoblasts, and myoblasts make myofibres. Unexpectedly, however, myogenesis can be much more complex, because cells that ordinarily are nonmyogenic can become muscle cells under some conditions (reviewed, Cossu, 1997); conversely, cells that ordinarily are destined to become muscle can adopt different fates under some conditions.

The dermal fibroblast is one example of a cell type with unexpected myogenic potential. Dermal fibroblasts sometimes fuse with myogenic cells to form mosaic myotubes in culture and can form myofibres when injected into mouse muscles (Chaudhari et al., 1989; Gibson et al., 1995; Salvatori et al., 1995). Three additional examples of unexpectedly myogenic cells include bone marrow cells, neural tube epithelial cells, and pregastrulation chicken epiblast cells. Bone marrow contains a population of cells that can be converted to myogenesis by 5-azacytidine treatment in vitro (Wakitani et al., 1995), and bone marrow cells can also contribute nuclei to regenerated myofibres in vivo without such treatment (Ferrari et al., 1998). Bone marrow

is known to contain a rare population of mesenchymal stem cells that can give rise to bone, cartilage and lung parenchymal cells (Pereira et al., 1995); whether it is these mesenchymal stem cells that also give rise to the myogenic cells remains to be determined. In other experiments, Tajbakhsh et al. (1994) found that a small percentage of cells derived from the neural epithelium of the embryonic mouse neural tube are myogenic in culture. Finally, cells from normally nonmyogenic regions of the chicken epiblast become myogenic at high frequency when cultured at low density in serum-free medium (George-Weinstein et al., 1996). Myogenesis by epiblast cells can be repressed by signals from neighbouring tissues (George-Weinstein et al., 1996).

Just as nonmuscle cells can sometimes become myogenic, cells that normally are myogenic sometimes display an unexpected ability to adopt new fates. As one example, cells of the C2C12 mouse muscle cell line, as well as primary mouse muscle cells, can become osteogenic upon treatment with BMP2 (Katagari et al., 1994). Such osteogenic conversion has not been seen in the absence of treatment. C2C12 and primary muscle cells can also become adipogenic when treated with long-chain fatty acids or thiazolidinediones, which also are potent activators of differentiation of preadipose cells (Grimaldi et al., 1997). In the developing mouse oesophagus, fetal skeletal muscle cells appear to transform into smooth muscle cells (Patapoutian et al., 1995b). Primary cells from embryonic chicken pectoral muscles normally form only muscle cells in culture; however, a subpopulation of these cells can produce chondrocytes when grown at high, though not low, density (Stringa et al., 1997). In addition, cells in the mouse somite that are normally destined to express Myf5 and form muscle cells will convert to dermis or cartilage cells when Myf5 protein expression is prevented (Tajbakhsh et al., 1996).

The stages of myogenesis at which muscle cells retain malleable fates remain to be determined. Perhaps late-stage myoblasts (i.e. positive for myogenin and p21) will prove to be less likely to change fates than MRF-negative stem cells or early myoblasts. Because cells that normally are only myogenic are able to adopt different fates when given the proper signals, it is possible that cells in the early steps of the myogenic cell lineage are, in fact, multipotent stem cells, rather than strictly unipotent muscle stem cells. Several permanent cell lines, including the P19 mouse cell line, are multipotent and able to differentiate into limited combinations of nerve, fat, cartilage, smooth muscle, cardiac and skeletal muscle cells depending on intercellular interactions and extracellular signals (e.g. Angello et al., 1997; Grepin et al., 1997).

Summary

Myogenic cells originate in the paraxial mesoderm under control of signals from neighbouring tissues. The newly formed myogenic cells, however, are not all alike; distinct mechanisms underlie the formation of myogenic cells in different regions of the embryo (e.g. head, epaxial, hypaxial). Within each of these spatially distinct centres of myogenesis, a sequence of temporally distinct myogenic cell lineages appears. That is, at different stages of embryonic, fetal and perinatal/adult life, distinct types of experimentally distinguishable myoblast are most abundant (Fig. 2.1). Further work is needed to identify the mechanisms that lead to the distinctions among these temporally separated lineages of myogenic cells and to examine their possible roles in the formation and repair of different myofibre types.

The lineage relationships among the temporally distinct myoblasts have not been fully determined. It seems likely, however, that distinct populations of stem cells may give rise to different myogenic cell lineages. In birds, for example, the early embryonic myoblasts never give rise to the later fetal type of myoblast (Rutz and Hauschka, 1982). Within the quail fetal lineage, however, a single progenitor cell can give rise to two distinct types of fetal myoblast (Schafer et al., 1987). Whether particular intercellular signals in the somites generate all, or only a subset, of the different myogenic cell lineages and their subtypes remains to be determined.

Myogenic cells proceed through a sequence of events, beginning with a muscle stem cell stage, continuing through early (myogenin-negative) and late (myogenin-positive) myoblast stages, and finishing with formation of terminally differentiated, multinucleate myofibres (Fig. 2.5). Under the model of the satellite cell lineage in Fig. 2.5, Bcl-2-expressing cells should have stem cell capability, but myogenin-expressing cells should not. It is clearly necessary to test this model in detail and also to identify new genes or patterns of gene expression that identify cells at different stages of the lineage.

Factors have not yet been identified that specifically affect muscle stem cells, perhaps by altering division rates or the ratio of asymmetric to symmetric divisions. One possibility is Shh, as recent work (Duprez et al., 1998) has shown that Shh administration increases the domain occupied by Pax3-expressing cells and their MyoD-expressing descendents in developing limbs. These results are consistent with the idea that Shh is a mitogen for Pax3-expressing cells that are destined to become muscle cells but have not yet progressed to the myoblast stage of MRF expression. HGF/SF is also a mitogen for satellite cells in the adult and is found in injured muscle (Tatsumi et al., 1998), suggesting that HGF/SF acts through the c-met receptors found on satellite cells (Cornelison and Wold, 1997) to increase myoblast formation and myofibre regeneration in injured muscles. Identification of the cellular target(s) for IGF1 and how IGF1 actions are modified by other growth factors may guide the design of treatments to improve muscle function after injury and during ageing.

With increased understanding of cellular, genetic and molecular mechanisms of skeletal muscle development and disease, molecular therapies for muscle disorders have become much more likely. Much current work, therefore, is directed to improving gene transfer and expression in skeletal muscle, both to replace mutated versions of endogenous genes and to modify skeletal muscle function and repair by local application of modulatory factors (Blau and Springer, 1995). Molecular targets might include defective disease gene products, the apoptosis signalling and execution pathways, the cell cycle/differentiation decision and growth factor pathways. For different disorders, it may be useful to target processes that modulate myoblast, myofibre, motor neuron, vascular, immune system or connective tissue function. As our understanding of myogenesis continues to improve, we will also improve our chances to ameliorate the muscle damage occurring during injury, ageing and disease.

Acknowledgements

The author's work is supported by grants from the Muscular Dystrophy Association of the USA, the National Institute of Arthritis and Musculoskeletal and Skin Diseases, and the National Institute for Dental Research.

References

Abmayr, S. M. and Keller, C. A. (1998). Drosophila myogenesis and insights into the role of nautilus. *Curr. Top. Dev. Biol.* **38**, 35–80.

Amthor, H., Connolly, D., Patel, K. et al. (1996). The expression and regulation of follistatin and a follistatin-like gene during avian somite compartmentalization and myogenesis. *Dev. Biol.* **178**, 343–362.

Anderson, J. E. (1998). Murray L. Barr Award Lecture. Studies of the dynamics of skeletal muscle regeneration: the mouse came back! *Biochem. Cell Biol.* **76**, 13–26.

Angello, J. C., Stern, H. M. and Hauschka, S. D. (1997). P19 embryonal carcinoma cells: a model system for studying neural tube induction of skeletal myogenesis. *Dev. Biol.* **192**, 93–98.

Arnold, H.-H. and Braun, T. (1996). Targeted inactivation of myogenic factor genes reveals their role during mouse myogenesis: a review. *Int. J. Dev. Biol.* **40**, 345–353.

Barjot, C., Roaunet, P., Vigneron, P., Janmot, C., d'Albis, A. and Bacou, F. (1998). Transformation of slow- or fast-twitch rabbit muscles after cross-reinnervation of low frequency stimulation does not alter the in vitro properties of their satellite cell. *J. Musc. Res. Cell Motil.* **19**, 25–32.

Baroffio, A., Hamann, M., Bernheim, L., Bochatonpiallat, M. L., Gabbiani, G. and Bader, C. R. (1996). Identification of self-renewing myoblasts in the progeny of single human muscle satellite cells. *Differentiation* **60**, 47–57.

Barton-Davis, E. R., Shoturma, D. I., Musaro, A., Rosenthal, N. and Sweeney, H. L. (1998). Viral mediated expression of insulin-like growth factor I blocks the ageing-related loss of skeletal muscle function. *Proc. Natl. Acad. Sci. USA* **95**, 15603–15607.

Beauchamp, J. R., Morgan, J. E., Pagel, C. N. and Partridge, T. A. (1999). Dynamics of myoblast transplantation reveal a discrete minority of precursors with stem cell-like properties as the myogenic source. *J. Cell Biol.* **144**, 1113–1122

Bischoff, R. and Heintz, C. (1994). Enhancement of skeletal muscle regeneration. *Dev. Dynam.* **201**, 41–54.

Bladt, F., Riethmacher, D., Isenmann, S., Aguzzi, A. and Birchmeier, C. (1995). Essential role for the c-Met receptor in the migration of myogenic precursor cells into the limb bud. *Nature* **376**, 768–771.

Blau, H. M. and Springer, M. L. (1995). Muscle-mediated gene therapy. *N. Engl. J. Med.* **333**, 1554–1556.

Bleisch, W., Scharff, C. and Nottebohm, F. (1989). Neural cell adhesion molecule (N-CAM) is elevated in adult avian slow muscle fibers with multiple terminals. *Proc. Nat. Acad. Sci. USA* **86**, 6403–6407.

Block, N. E., Zhu, Z., Kachinsky, A. M., Dominov, J. A. and Miller, J. B. (1996). Acceleration of somitic myogenesis and cell lineage-specific activation of muscle gene expression in embryos of myogenin promoter-MRF4 transgenic mice. *Dev. Dynam.* **207**, 382–394.

Bober, E., Franz, T., Arnold, H.-H., Gruss, P. and Tremblay, P. (1994). Pax-3 is required for the development of limb muscles: a possible role for the migration of dermomyotomal muscle progenitor cells. *Development* **120**, 603–612.

Borycki, A. G. and Emerson, C. P. (1997). Muscle determination: another key player in myogenesis? *Curr. Biol.* **7**, R620–R623.

Bruan, T., Rudnicki, M. A., Arnold, H.-H. and Jaenisch, R. (1992). Targeted inactivation of the muscle regulatory gene *myf-5* results in abnormal rib development and perinatal death. *Cell* **71**, 369–382.

Braun, T. and Arnold, H.-H. (1994). ES-cells carrying two inactivated myf-5 alleles form skeletal muscle cells: activation of an alternative myf-5-independent differentiation pathway. *Dev. Biol.* **164**, 24–36.

Braun, T., Bober, E., Rudnicki, M. A., Jaenisch, R. and Arnold, H.-H. (1994). MyoD expression marks the onset of skeletal myogenesis in Myf-5 mutant mice. *Development* **120**, 3083–3092.

Brooks, S. V. and Faulkner, J. A. (1988). Contractile properties of skeletal muscles from young, adult and aged mice. *J. Physiol. (Lond.)* **404**, 71–82.

Brown, R. H. Jr (1998). Dystrophin-associated proteins and the muscular dystrophies. *Annu. Rev. Med.* **48**, 457–466.

Burden, S. J. (1998). The formation of neuromuscular synapses. *Genes Dev.* **12**, 133–148.

Burgess, R., Cserjesi, P., Ligon, K. L. and Olson, E. N. (1995). Paraxis: a basic helix-loop-helix protein expressed in paraxial mesoderm and developing somites. *Dev. Biol.* **168**, 296–306.

Burgess, R., Rawls, A., Brown, D., Bradley, A. and Olson E. N. (1996). Requirement of the paraxis gene for somite formation and musculoskeletal patterning. *Nature* **384**, 570–573.

Butler, J., Cosmos, E. and Brierly, J. (1982). Differentiation of muscle fiber types in aneurogenic brachial muscles of the chick embryo. *J. Exp. Zool.* **224**, 65–80.

Butler, J., Cauwenbergs, P. and Cosmos, E. (1986). Fate of brachial muscles of the chick embryo innervated by inappropriate nerves: structural, functional and histochemical analyses. *J. Embryol. Exp. Morphol.* **95**, 147–168.

Cannon, J. G. 1998. Intrinsic and extrinsic factors in muscle ageing. *Ann. N. Y. Acad. Sci.* **854**, 72–77

Chaudhari, N., Delay, R. and Beam, K. G. (1989). Restoration of normal function in genetically defective myotubes by spontaneous fusion with fibroblasts. *Nature* **341**, 445–447.

Chevallier, A., Kieny, M. and Mauger, A. (1977). Limb-somite relationship: origin of the limb musculature. *J. Embryol. Exp. Morphol.* **41**, 245–258.

Chiang, C., Y. Litingtung, E., Lee, K. E. et al. (1996). Cyclopia and defective axial patterning in mice lacking Sonic hedgehog gene function. *Nature* **383**, 407–413.

Christ, B., Jacob, H. J. and Jacob, M. (1977). Experimental analysis of the origin of the wing musculature in avian embryos. *Anat. Embryol.* **150**, 171–186.

Condon, K., Silberstein, L., Blau, H. and Thompson, W. J. (1990). Differentiation of fiber types in aneural musculature of the prenatal rat hindlimb. *Dev. Biol.* **138**, 275–295.

Cornelison, D. D. and Wold, B. J. (1997). Single-cell analysis of regulatory gene expression in quiescent and activated mouse skeletal muscle satellite cells. *Dev. Biol.* **191**, 270–283.

Cossu, G. (1997). Unorthodox myogenesis: possible developmental significance and implications for tissue histogenesis and regeneration. *Histol. Histopath.* **12**, 755–760.

Cossu, G. and Molinaro, M. (1987). Cell heterogeneity in the myogenic lineage. *Curr. Top. Dev. Biol.* **23**, 185–208.

Couly, G. F., Coltey, P. M and LeDouarin, L. M (1992). The developmental fate of the cephalic mesoderm in quail-chick chimeras. *Development* **114**, 1–15.

Couly, G. F., Coltey, P. M. and LeDouarin, L. M. (1993). The triple origin of the skull in higher vertebrates: a study in quail-chick chimeras. *Development* **117**, 409–429.

Crow, M. T. and Stockdale, F. E. (1986). Myosin expression and specialization of the earliest muscle fibers of the developing avian limb. *Dev. Biol.* **113**, 238–254.

Cusella-de Angelis, M. G., Molinari, S., Le Donne, A. et al. (1994). Differential response of embryonic and fetal myoblasts to TGF beta: a possible regulatory mechanism of skeletal muscle histogenesis. *Development* **120**, 925–933.

Dahm, L. M. and Landmesser, L. T. (1988). The regulation of intramuscular nerve branching during normal development and following activity blockade. *Dev. Biol.* **130**, 621–644.

Daston, G., Lamar, E., Olivier, M. and Goulding, M. (1996). Pax-3 is necessary for migration but not differentiation of limb muscle precursors in the mouse. *Development* **122**, 1017–1027.

Decary, S., Mouly, V., Hamida, C. B., Sautet, A., Barbet, J. P. and Butler-Browne, G. S. (1997). Replicative potential and telomere length in human skeletal muscle: implications for satellite cell-mediated gene therapy. *Hum. Gene Ther.* **8**, 1429–1438.

Denetclaw, W. F. Jr., Christ, B. and Ordahl, C. P. (1997). Location and growth of epaxial myotome precursor cells. *Development* **124**, 1601–1610.

Dennis, M. J., Ziskind-Conhaim, L. and Harris, A. J. (1981). Development of neuromuscular junctions in rat embryos. *Dev. Biol.* **81**, 266–279

Desypris, G. and Parry, D. J. (1990). Relative efficacy of slow and fast alpha-motoneurons to reinnervate mouse soleus muscle. *Am. J. Physiol.* **258**, C62–C70.

Dominov, J. A., Dunn, J. J. and Miller, J. B. (1998). Bcl-2 expression identifies an early stage of myogenesis and promotes clonal expansion of muscle cell. *J. Cell Biol.* **142**, 537–544.

Draeger, A., Weeds, A. G. and Fitzsimons, R. B. (1987). Primary, secondary and tertiary myotubes in developing skeletal muscle: a new approach to the analysis of human myogenesis. *J. Neurol. Sci.* **81**, 19–43.

Duprez, D., Fournier-Thibault, C. and Le Douarin, M. (1998). Sonic hedgehog induces proliferation of committed skeletal muscle cells in the chick limb. *Development* **125**, 495–505.

Duxson, M. J., Usson, Y. and Harris, A. J. (1989). The origin of secondary myotubes in mammalian skeletal muscles: ultrastructural studies. *Development* **107**, 743–750.

Edom-Vovard, F., Mouly, V., Barbet, J. P. and Butler-Browne, G. S. (1998). The four populations of myoblasts involved in human limb muscle formation are present from the onset of primary myotube formation. *J. Cell Sci.* **112**, 191–199.

Epstein, J. A., Shapiro, D. N., Cheng, J., Lam, P. Y. and Maas, R. L. (1996). Pax3 modulates expression of the c-Met receptor during limb muscle development. *Proc. Natl. Acad. Sci. USA* **93**, 4213–4218.

Faerman, A., Goldhamer, D., Puzis, R., Emerson, C. P. Jr. and Shani, M. (1995). The distal human myoD enhancer sequences direct unique muscle-specific patterns of lacZ expression during mouse development. *Dev. Biol.* **171**, 27–38.

Ferrari, G., Cusella-de Angelis, G., Coletta, M. et al. (1998). Muscle regeneration by bone marrow-derived myogenic progenitors. *Science* **279**, 1528–1530.

Firulli, A. B. and Olson, E. N. (1997). Modular regulation of muscle gene transcription: a mechanism for muscle cell diversity. *Trends Genet.* **13**, 364–369.

Fladby, T. and Jansen, J. K. (1990). Development of homogeneous fast and slow motor units in the neonatal mouse soleus muscle. *Development* **109**, 723–732.

Franz, T., Kothary, R., Surani, M. A., Halata, Z. and Grim, M. (1993). The *splotch* mutation interferes with muscle development in the limbs. *Anat. Embryol.* **187**, 153–160.

Garry, D. J. Yang, Q., Bassel-Duby, R. and Williams, R. S. (1997). Persistent expression of MNF identifies myogenic stem cells in postnatal muscles. *Dev. Biol.* **188**, 280–294.

George-Weinstein, M., Foster, R. F., Gerhart, J. V. and Kaufman, S. J. (1993). In vitro and in vivo expression of alpha 7 integrin and desmin define the primary and secondary myogenic lineages. *Dev. Biol.* **156**, 209–229.

George-Weinstein, M., Gerhart, J., Reed, R. et al. (1996). Skeletal myogenesis: the preferred pathway of chick embryo cells in vitro. *Dev. Biol.* **173**, 279–291.

Gibson, A. J., Karasinski, J., Relvas, J. et al. (1995). Dermal fibroblasts convert to a myogenic lineage in *mdx* mouse muscle. *J. Cell Sci.* **108**, 207–214.

Gossler, A. and Hrabe de Angelis, M. (1998). Somitogenesis. *Curr. Top. Dev. Biol.* **38**, 225–287.

Goulding, M., Lumsden, A. and Paquette, A. J. (1994). Regulation of Pax-3 expression in the dermomyotome and its role in muscle development. *Development* **120**, 957–971.

Grepin, C., Nemer, G. and Nemer, M. (1997). Enhanced cardiogenesis in embryonic stem cells overexpressing the GATA-4 transcription factor. *Development* **124**, 2387–2395.

Grieshammer, U., McGrew, M. J. and Rosenthal, N. (1995). Role of methylation in maintenance of positionally restricted transgene expression in developing muscle. *Development* **121**, 2245–2253.

Grimaldi, P. A., Teboul, L., Inadera, H., Gaillard, D. and Amri, E. Z. (1997). Trans-differentiation of myoblasts to adipoblasts: triggering effects of fatty acids and thiazolidinediones. *Prostaglandins Leukot. Essent. Fatty Acids* **57**, 71–75.

Grimby, G., Danneskiold-Samsoe, B., Hvid, K. and Saltin, B. (1982) Morphology and enzymatic capacity in arm and leg muscles in 78–81 year old men and women. *Acta Physiol. Scand.* **115**, 125–134.

Grinnell, A. D. (1995). Dynamics of nerve-muscle interaction in developing and mature neuromuscular junctions. *Physiol. Rev.* **75**, 789–834.

Grounds, M. D. (1998). Age-associated changes in the response of skeletal muscle cells to exercise and regeneration. *Ann. N. Y. Acad. Sci.* **854**, 78–91.

Gussoni, E., Soneoka, Y., Strickland, C. D. et al. (1999). Dystrophin expression in the mdx mouse restored by stem cell transplantation. *Nature* **401**, 390–394

Harris, A. J., Duxson, M. J., Fitzsimons, R. B. and Rieger, F. (1989). Myonuclear birthdates distinguish the origins of primary and secondary myotubes in embryonic mammalian skeletal muscles. *Development* **107**, 771–784

Hasty, P., Bradley, A., Morris, J. H. et al. (1993). Muscle deficiency and neonatal death in mice with a targeted mutation in the myogenin gene. *Nature* **364**, 501–506.

Hauschka, S. D., Linkhart, T. A., Clegg, C. and Merrill, G. (1979). Clonal studies of human and mouse muscle. In: *Muscle Regeneration*, ed. A. Mauro, pp. 311–322. New York: Raven.

Hirsinger, E., Duprez, D., Jouve, C., Malapert, P., Cooke, J. and Pourquie, O. (1997). Noggin acts downstream of Wnt and Sonic Hedgehog to antagonize BMP4 in avian somite patterning. *Development* **124**, 4605–4614.

Hrabe de Angelis, M., McIntyre, J. II and Gossler, A. (1997). Maintenance of somite borders in mice requires the delta homologue DII1. *Nature* **386**, 717–721.

Huang, D. C. S., O'Reilly, L. A., Strasser, A. and Cory, S. (1997). The anti-apoptosis function of Bcl-2 can be genetically separated from its inhibitory effect on cell cycle entry. *EMBO J.* **16**, 4628–4638.

Kablar, B., Krastel, K., Ying, C., Asakura, A., Tapscott, S. J. and Rudnicki, M. A. (1997). MyoD and Myf-5 differentially regulate the development of limb versus trunk skeletal muscle. *Development* **124**, 4729–4738.

Kahane, N., Cinnamon, Y. and Kalcheim, C. (1998). The cellular mechanism by which the dermomyotome contributes to the second wave of myotome development. *Development* **125**, 4259–4271.

Kasemkijwattana, C., Menetrey, J., Somogyl, G. et al. (1998). Development of approaches to improve the healing following muscle contusion. *Cell Transplant* **7**, 585–598.

Katagiri, T., Yamaguchi, A., Komaki, M. et al. (1994). Bone morphogenetic protein-2 converts the differentiation pathway of C2C12 myoblasts into the osteoblast lineage. *J. Cell Biol.* **127**, 1755–1766.

Kato, N. and Aoyama, H. (1998). Dermomyotomal origin of the ribs as revealed by extirpation and transplantation experiments in chick and quail embryos. *Development* **125**, 3437–3443.

Kelly, A. M. (1983). Emergence of specialization in skeletal muscle. In: *Handbook of Physiology*, ed. L. D. Peachey, Sect. 10, pp. 507–537. Baltimore, MD: Williams & Wilkins.

Kernell, D. (1998). Muscle regionalization. *Can. J. Appl. Physiol.* **23**, 1–22.

Koishi, K., Zhang, M., McLennan, I. S. and Harris, A. J. (1995). MyoD protein accumulates in satellite cells and is neurally regulated in regenerating myotubes and skeletal muscle fibers. *Dev. Dynam.* **202**, 244–254.

Kopan, R., Nye, J. S. and Weintraub, H. (1994).The intracellular domain of mouse Notch: a constitutively activated repressor of myogenesis directed at the basic helix-loop-helix region of MyoD. *Development* **120**, 2385–2396.

Landmesser, L. (1996). Cell adhesion/recognition molecule-mediated steps during the guidance of commissural and motor axons. *Prog. Brain Res.* **108**, 109–116.

Larrson, L. and Edström, L. (1986) Effects of age on enzyme-histochemical fibre spectra and contractile properties of fast- and slow-twitch skeletal muscles in the rat. *J. Neurol. Sci.* **76**, 69–89.

Lee, K. and Sze, L. (1993). Role of the brachial somites in the development of the appendicular musculature in rat embryos. *Dev. Dynam.* **198**, 86–96.

Lumsden, A. (1995). Neural development. A 'LIM' code for motor neurons. *Curr. Biol.* **5**, 491–495.

Maley, M. A., Fan, Y., Beilharz, M. W. and Grounds, M. D. (1994). Intrinsic differences in MyoD and myogenin expression between primary cultures of SJL/J and BALB/C skeletal muscle. *Exp. Cell Res.* **211**, 99–107.

Maroto, M., Reshef, R., Münsterberg, A. E., Koester, S., Goulding, M. and Lassar, A. B. (1997). Ectopic Pax-3 activates MyoD and myf-5 expression in embryonic mesoderm and neural tissue. *Cell* **89**, 139–148.

Matzuk, M. M., Lu, N., Vogel, H., Sellheyer, K., Roop, D. R. and Bradley, A. (1995). Multiple defects and perinatal death in mice deficient in follistatin. *Nature* **374**, 360–363.

Mauro, A. (1961). Satellite cells of skeletal muscle fibers. *J. Biophys. Biochem. Cytol.* **9**, 493–495.

Megeney, L. A., Kablar, B., Garrett, K., Anderson, J. E. and Rudnicki, M. A. (1996). MyoD is required for myogenic stem cell function in adult skeletal muscle. *Genes Dev.* **10**, 1173–1183.

Milaire, J. (1976). Contribution cellulaire des somites a la genèse des bourgeons de membres postérieurs chez la souris. *Arch. Biol. (Brux.)* **87**, 315–343.

Miller, J. B. (1991). Myoblasts, myosins, MyoDs, and the diversification of muscle fibers. *Neuromusc. Disord.* **1**, 7–17.

Miller , J. B. (1992). Myoblast diversity in skeletal myogenesis: How much and to what end? *Cell* **69**, 1–3.

Miller, J. B. and Stockdale, F. E. (1986a). Developmental origins of skeletal muscle fibers: clonal analysis of myogenic cell lineages based on fast and slow myosin heavy chain expression. *Proc. Nat. Acad. Sci.* **83**, 3860–3864.

Miller, J. B. and Stockdale, F. E. (1986b). Developmental regulation of the multiple myogenic cell lineages of the avian embryo. *J. Cell Biol.* **103**, 2197–2208.

Miller, J. B., Schaefer, L. and Dominov, J. A. (1999). Seeking muscle stem cells. *Curr. Top. Dev. Biol.* **43**, 191–219.

Milner, L. D., Rafuse, V. F. and Landmesser, L. T. (1998). Selective fasciculation and divergent pathfinding decisions of embryonic chick motor axons projecting to fast and slow muscle regions. *J. Neurosci.* **18**, 3297–3313.

Molkentin, J. D. and Olson, E. N. (1996). Defining the regulatory networks for muscle development. *Curr. Opin. Genet. Dev.* **6**, 445–453.

Münsterberg, A. E., Kitajewski, J., Bumcrot, D. A., McMahon, A. P. and Lassar, A. B. (1995). Combinatorial signalling by Sonic hedgehog and Wnt family members induces myogenic bHLH gene expression in the somite. *Genes Dev.* **9**, 2911–2922.

Musaro, A., Cusella De Angelis, M. G., Germani, A., Ciccarelli, C., Molinaro, M. and Zani, B. M. (1995). Enhanced expression of myogenic regulatory genes in aging skeletal muscle. *Exp. Cell Res.* **221**, 241–248.

Nabeshima, Y., Hanaoka, K., Hayasaka, M. et al. (1993). Myogenin gene disruption results in perinatal lethality because of severe muscle defect. *Nature* **364**, 532–535.

Nicolas, J. F., Mathis, L. and Bonnerot, C. (1996). Evidence in the mouse for self-renewing stem cells in the formation of a segmented longitudinal structure, the myotome. *Development* **122**, 2933–2946.

Novitch, B. G., Mulligan, G. J., Jacks, T. and Lassar, A. B. (1996). Skeletal muscle cells lacking the retinoblastoma protein display defects in muscle gene expression and accumulate in S and G2 phases of the cell cycle. *J. Cell Biol.* **135**, 441–456.

O'Brien, M. K., Landmesser, L. and Oppenheim, R. W. (1990). Development and survival of thoracic motoneurons and hind-limb musculature following transplantation of the thoracic neural tube to the lumbar region in the chick embryo: functional aspects. *J. Neurobiol.* **21**, 341–355.

Olson, E. N., Arnold, H. H., Rigby, P. W. and Wold, B. J. (1996). Know your neighbors: three phenotypes in null mutants of the myogenic bHLH gene MRF4. *Cell* **85**, 1–4.

Ordahl, C. P. and LeDouarin, N. (1992). Two myogenic lineages within the developing somite. *Development* **114**, 339–353.

O'Reilly, L. A., Harris, A. W., Tarlinton, D. M., Corcoran, L. M. and Strasser, A. (1997). Expression of a *bcl-2* transgene reduces proliferation and slows turnover of developing B lymphocytes in vivo. *J. Immunol.* **159**, 2301–2311.

Packard, D. S. Jr. and Meier, S. (1983). An experimental study of the somitomeric organization of the avian segmental plate. *Dev. Biol.* **97**, 91–202.

Palmeirim, I., Henrique, D., Ish-Horowicz, D. and Pourquie, O. (1997). Avian hairy gene expression identifies a molecular clock linked to vertebrate segmentation and somitogenesis. *Cell* **91**, 639–648.

Patapoutian, A., Yoon, J. K., Miner, J. H., Wang, S., Stark, K. and Wold, B. (1995a). Disruption of the mouse MRF4 gene identifies multiple waves of myogenesis in the myotome. *Development* **121**, 3347–3358.

Patapoutian, A., Wold, B. J. and Wagner, R. A. (1995b). Evidence for developmentally programmed transdifferentiation in mouse esophageal muscle. *Science* **270**, 1818–1821.

Pavlath, G. K., Thaloor, D., Rando, T. A., Cheong, M., English, A. W. and Zheng, B. (1998). Heterogeneity among muscle precursor cells in adult skeletal muscles with differing regenerative capacities. *Dev. Dynam.* **212**, 495–508.

Pereira, R. F., Halford, K. W., O'Hara, M. D. et al. (1995). Cultured adherent cells from marrow can serve as long-lasting precursor cells for bone, cartilage, and lung in irradiated mice. *Proc. Natl. Acad. Sci. USA* **92**, 4857–4861.

Rafuse, V. F., Milner, L. D. and Landmesser, L. T. (1996). Selective innervation of fast and slow muscle regions during early chick neuromuscular development. *J. Neurosci.* **16**, 6864–6877.

Rao, M. V., Donoghue, M. J., Merlie, J. P. and Sanes, J. R. (1996). Distinct regulatory elements control muscle-specific, fiber-type-selective, and axially graded expression of a myosin light-chain gene in transgenic mice. *Mol. Cell. Biol.* **16**, 3909–3922.

Rawls, A., Valdez, M. R., Zhang, W., Richardson, J., Klein, W. H. and Olson, E. N. (1998). Overlapping functions of the myogenic bHLH genes MRF4 and MyoD revealed in double mutant mice. *Development* **125**, 2349–2358.

Reed, J. C. (1997). Double identity for proteins of the Bcl-2 family. *Nature* **387**, 773–776.

Reshef, R., Maroto, M. and Lassar, A. B. (1998). Regulation of dorsal somitic cell fates: BMPs and Noggin control the timing and pattern of myogenic regulator expression. *Genes Dev.* **12**, 290–303.

Rosen, G. D., Sanes, J. R., LaChance, R., Cunningham, J. M., Roman, J. and Dean, D. C. (1992). Roles for the integrin VLA-4 and its counter receptor VCAM-1 in myogenesis. *Cell* **69**, 1107–1119.

Rosenblatt, J. D., Parry, D. J. and Partridge, T. A. (1996). Phenotype of adult mouse muscle myoblasts reflects their fiber type of origin. *Differentiation* **60**, 39–45.

Rudnicki, M. A., Braun, T., Hinuma, S. and Jaenisch, R. (1992). Inactivation of MyoD in mice leads to upregulation of the myogenic HLH gene myf-5 and results in apparently normal muscle development. *Cell* **71**, 383–390.

Rudnicki, M. A., Schnegelsberg, P., Stead, R. H., Braun, T., Arnold, H.-H. and Jaenisch, R. (1993). MyoD or myf-5 is required for the formation of skeletal muscle. *Cell* **75**, 1351–1360.

Rutz, R. and Hauschka, S. D. (1982). Clonal analysis of vertebrate myogenesis. VII. Heritability of muscle colony type through sequential subclonal passages in vitro. *Dev. Biol.* **91**, 399–411.

Saga, Y., Hata, N., Koseki, H. and Taketo, M. M. (1997). *mesp2*: a novel mouse gene expressed in the presegmented mesoderm and essential for segmentation initiation. *Genes Dev.* **11**, 1827–1839.

Salvatori, G., Lattanzi, L., Coletta, M., Aguanno, S. et al. (1995). Myogenic conversion of mammalian fibroblasts induced by differentiating muscle cells. *J. Cell Sci.* **108**, 2733–2739.

Schafer, D. A. and Stockdale, F. E. (1987). Identification of sarcolemma-associated antigens with differential distributions on fast and slow skeletal muscle fibers. *J. Cell Biol.* **104**, 967–979.

Schafer, D. A., Miller, J. B. and Stockdale, F. E. (1987). Cell diversification within the myogenic lineage: in vitro generation of two types of myoblasts from a single myogenic progenitor cell. *Cell* **48**, 659–670.

Schiaffino, S. and Reggiani, C. (1994). Myosin isoforms in mammalian skeletal muscle. *Am. J. Physiol.* **161**, 493–501.

Schmidt, C., Bladt, F., Goedecke, S. et al. (1995). Scatter factor/hepatocyte growth factor is essential for liver development. *Nature* **373**, 699–702.

Schultz, E. (1996). Satellite cell proliferative compartments in growing skeletal muscles. *Dev. Biol.* **175**, 84–94.

Slack, J. M. W. (1991). *From Egg to Embryo*, 2nd edn. Cambridge: Cambridge University Press.

Smith, C. K. 2nd, Janney, M. J. and Allen, R. E. (1994). Temporal expression of myogenic regulatory genes during activation, proliferation, and differentiation of rat skeletal muscle satellite cells. *J. Cell. Physiol.* **159**, 379–385.

Smith, T. H. and Miller, J. B. (1992). Distinct myogenic programs of embryonic and fetal mouse muscle cells: Expression of the perinatal myosin heavy chain isoform. *Dev. Biol.* **149**, 16–26.

Smith, T. H., Block, N. E., Rhodes, S. J., Konieczny, S. F. and Miller, J. B. (1993). A unique pattern of expression of the four muscle regulatory factors distinguishes somitic from embryonic, fetal, and newborn mouse myogenic cells. *Development* **117**, 1125–1133.

Smith, T. H., Kachinsky, A. M. and Miller, J. B. (1994). Somite subdomains, muscle cell origins, and the four muscle regulatory factor proteins. *J. Cell Biol.* **127**, 95–105.

Sohal, G. S. (1995). Embryonic development of nerve and muscle. *Muscle Nerve* **18**, 2–14.

Soileau, L. C., Silberstein, L., Blau, H. M. and Thompson, W. J. (1987). Reinnervation of muscle fiber types in the newborn rat soleus. *J. Neurosci.* **7**, 4176–9414.

Sosic, D., Brand-Saberi, B., Schmidt, C., Christ, B. and Olson, E. N. (1997). Regulation of paraxis expression and somite formation by ectoderm- and neural tube-derived signals. *Dev. Biol.* **185**, 229–243.

Stal, P., Eriksson, P. O., Schiaffino, S., Butler-Browne, G. S. and Thornell, L. E. (1994). Differences in myosin composition between human oro-facial, masticatory and limb muscles: enzyme-, immunohisto- and biochemical studies. *J. Muscle Res. Cell Motil.* **15**, 517–534.

Stern, H. M., Lin-Jones, J. and Hauschka, S. D. (1997). Synergistic interactions between bFGF and a TGF-beta family member may mediate myogenic signals from the neural tube. *Development* **124**, 3511–3523.

Stockdale, F. E. (1997). Mechanisms of formation of muscle fiber types. *Cell Struct. Func.* **22**, 37–43.

Stringa, E., Love, J. M., McBride, S. C., Suyama, E. and Tuan, R. S. (1997). In vitro characterization of chondrogenic cells isolated from chick embryonic muscle using peanut agglutinin affinity chromatography. *Exp. Cell Res.* **232**, 287–294.

Tajbakhsh, S. and Cossu, G. (1997). Establishing myogenic identity during somitogenesis. *Curr. Opin. Genet. Dev.* **7**, 634–641.

Tajbakhsh, S., Vivarelli, E., Cusella-de Angelis, G., Rocancourt, D., Buckingham, M. and Cossu, G. (1994). A population of myogenic cells derived from the mouse neural tube. *Neuron.* **13**, 813–821.

Tajbakhsh, S., Rocancourt, D. and Buckingham, M. (1996). Myogenic progenitor cells failing to respond to positional cues adopt non-myogenic fates in *myf-5* null mice. *Nature* **384**, 266–270.

Tajbakhsh, S., Rocancourt, D., Cossu, G. and Buckingham, M. (1997). Redefining the genetic hierarchies controlling skeletal myogenesis: Pax-3 and Myf-5 act upstream of MyoD. *Cell* **89**, 127–138.

Tanabe, Y. and Jessell, T. M. (1996). Diversity and pattern in the developing spinal cord. *Science* **274**, 1115–1123.

Tatsumi, R., Anderson, J. E., Nevoret, C. J., Halevy, O. and Allen, R. E. (1998). HGF/SF is present in normal adult skeletal muscle and is capable of activating satellite cells. *Dev. Biol.* **194**, 114–128.

Tiret, L., Le Mouellic, H., Maury, M. and Brulet, P. (1998). Increased apoptosis of motoneurons and altered somatotopic maps in the brachial spinal cord of Hoxc-8-deficient mice. *Development* **125**, 279–291.

Tzankoff, S. P. and Norris, A. H. (1977). Effect of muscle mass decrease on age-related BMR changes. *J. Appl. Physiol.* **43**, 1001–1006.

Uehara, Y., Minowa, O., Mori, C. et al. (1995). Placental defect and embryonic lethality in mice lacking hepatocyte growth factor/scatter factor. *Nature* **373**, 702–705.

Vairo, G., Inner, K. M. and Adams, J. M. (1996). Bcl-2 has a cell cycle inhibitory function separable from its enhancement of cell survival. *Oncogene* **13**, 1511–1519.

Wakitani, S., Saito, T. and Caplan, A. I. (1995). Myogenic cells derived from rat bone marrow mesenchymal stem cells exposed to 5-azacytidine. *Muscle Nerve* **18**, 1417–1426.

Walsh, K. and Perlman, H. (1997). Cell cycle exit upon myogenic differentiation. *Curr. Opin. Genet. Dev.* **7**, 597–602.

Wang, Y. and Jaenisch, R. (1997). Myogenin can substitute for myf5 in promoting myogenesis but less efficiently. *Development* **124**, 2507–2513.

Wang, Y., Schnegelsberg, P. N., Dausman, J. and Jaenisch R. (1996). Functional redundancy of the muscle-specific transcription factors myf5 and myogenin. *Nature* **379**, 823–825.

Webster, C. and Blau, H. M. (1990). Accelerated age-related decline in replicative life-span of Duchenne muscular dystrophy myoblasts: implications for cell and gene therapy. *Somat. Cell Mol. Genet.* **16**, 557–565.

Weintraub, H. (1993). The MyoD family and myogenesis: Redundancy, networks, and thresholds. *Cell* **75**, 1241–1244.

Wigston, D. J. and Sanes, J. R. (1985). Selective reinnervation of intercostal muscles transplanted from different segmental levels to a common site. *J. Neurosci.* **5**, 1208–1221.

Williams, B. A. and Ordahl, C. P. (1994). Pax-3 expression in segmental mesoderm marks early stages in myogenic cell specification. *Development* **120**, 785–796.

Wilson, S. J., McEwan, J. C., Sheard, P. W. and Harris, A. J. (1992). Early stages of myogenesis in a large mammal: formation of successive generations of myotubes in sheep tibialis cranialis muscle. *J. Muscle Res. Cell Motil.* **13**, 534–550.

Wolpert, L., Beddington, R., Brockes, J., Jessell, T., Lawrence, P. and Meyerowitz, E. (1997). *Principles of Development.* Oxford: Oxford University Press and Current Biology.

Yablonka-Reuveni, Z. and Rivera, A. J. (1994). Temporal expression of regulatory and structural muscle proteins during myogenesis of satellite cells on isolated adult rat fibers. *Dev. Biol.* **164**, 588–603.

Yang, J., Kelly, R., Daood, M., Ontell, M., Watchko, J. and Ontell, M. (1998). Alteration in myosatellite cell commitment with muscle maturation. *Dev. Dynam.* **211**, 141–152.

Yang, Q., Bassel-Duby, R. and Williams, R. S. (1997). Transient expression of a winged-helix protein, MNF-beta, during myogenesis. *Mol. Cell. Biol.* **17**, 5236–5243.

Yoon, J. K., Olson, E. N., Arnold, H. H. and Wold, B. J. (1997). Different MRF4 knockout alleles differentially disrupt myf-5 expression: *cis*-regulatory interactions at the *mrf4/myf-5* locus. *Dev. Biol.* **188**, 349–362.

Yun, K. and Wold, B. (1996). Skeletal muscle determination and differentiation: story of a core regulatory network and its context. *Curr. Opin. Cell Biol.* **8**, 877–889.

Zappelli, F., Willems, D., Osada, S. et al. (1996). The inhibition of differentiation caused by TGFbeta in fetal myoblasts is dependent upon selective expression of PKCtheta: a possible molecular basis for myoblast diversification during limb histogenesis. *Dev. Biol.* **180**, 156–164.

Zhang, M. and McLennan, I. S. (1998). Primary myotubes preferentially mature into either the fastest or slowest muscle fibers. *Dev. Dynam.* **213**, 147–157.

Zhang, P., Wong, C., Liu, D., Finegold, M., Harper, J. W. and Elledge, S. J. (1999). p21CIP1 and p57KIP2 control muscle differentiation at the myogenin step. *Genes Dev.* **13**, 213–224.

Zhu Z. and Miller, J. B. (1997). MRF4 can substitute for myogenin during early stages of myogenesis. *Dev. Dynam.* **209**, 233–241.

3

The molecular and cellular biology of muscle

Susan C. Brown, Frank S. Walsh and George Dickson

Introduction

One of the most important breakthroughs in recent years has been the discovery of dystrophin as the protein missing in Duchenne muscular dystrophy (DMD). This work provided increased impetus to discover other gene defects associated with various forms of neuromuscular disease and focused attention on the muscle fibre cytoskeleton and the importance of the linkages it maintains with the extracellular matrix. A variety of adhesion receptors allow cells to interact with the surrounding extracellular matrix. The integrin family of receptors are well known in this regard and have been shown to mediate a wide range of responses, including cell growth, gene expression and differentiation in a variety of cell types (Hynes, 1992). In recent years, the search for the underlying cause of muscular dystrophy has identified a group of proteins and glycoproteins that appear to fulfil a similar role (Ervasti and Campbell, 1991). Dystrophin was the first protein of this group to be identified (Hoffman et al., 1987) and the transmembrane complex with which it associates is now referred to as the dystrophin-associated protein complex (DAPC; Campbell et al., 1991). Mutations in several components of this complex are now known to be involved in the pathogenesis of several forms of muscular dystrophy (Campbell, 1995). More recently, attention has focused on the role of nuclear envelope components in the pathogenesis of neuromuscular disorders. Alterations in the genes for emerin and lamin A/C have now been shown to be the underlying cause of X-linked and autosomal dominant Emery–Dreifuss muscular dystrophy (EDMD), respectively (Nagano et al., 1996; Bonne et al., 1999). In terms of our understanding of the underlying causes of many of the muscular dystrophies, these discoveries represent landmarks. The development of strategies to alleviate the consequences of this group of diseases is one of the major challenges for the future. This chapter gives a broad outline of the cell biology of skeletal muscle and then goes on to discuss how characteristics of this highly specialized tissue may be used to develop gene-based therapies for neuromuscular disease.

Muscle development

Embryologically skeletal muscle develops from the somatic mesoderm, the trunk and body-wall muscles originating from the metamerically segmented paraxial myotomes and the limb muscles from the unsegmented splanchnopleure (Landon, 1992). Differentiation follows a proximo-distal and cephalo-caudal progression. Somites are observed in the mouse embryo from about day 8 (total gestational period around 21 days). In the human embryo, condensations of mesenchyme are apparent at the sites of the future muscle masses by 6 weeks of gestation. By 8 weeks, the primordia of most individual muscles are clearly defined. Multipotential stem cells in the mesoderm give rise to the so-called myoblasts, which eventually fuse to form multinucleated myotubes and ultimately muscle fibres. Myoblast differentiation is controlled by a family of muscle-specific basic helix-loop-helix (bHLH) transcription factors that activate muscle genes by binding E-box elements (CANNTG) as heterodimers with ubiquitous bHLH proteins called E proteins (Lassar and Munsterberg, 1994). As myoblasts pass through the myogenic pathway, they express distinct sets of muscle-specific proteins. For example, desmin, Myf5 and MyoD are expressed at a relatively early stage, whereas myogenin, myogenin regulatory factor 4 (MRF4) and myosin are expressed during the later stages. MyoD and Myf5 play overlapping roles in the specification of myoblasts; consequently, in the absence of one of the two factors, myogenesis is unaffected, whereas in the absence of both no myoblasts are formed (Arnold and Winter, 1988). By contrast, myogenin is essential for muscle differentiation and in its absence the ability of myoblasts to differentiate is impaired. MRF4 and MyoD also have overlapping functions in the differentiation pathway (Rawls et al., 1999).

While bHLH proteins are expressed in proliferating, undifferentiated myoblasts, they fail to activate muscle differentiation until myoblasts exit the cell cycle and become postmitotic. The reasons for this seem to be the existence of a diverse number of powerful mechanisms that act to restrict transcriptional activity until the appropriate stage of development. Peptide growth factors such as transforming growth factor β (TGFβ), the bone morphogenetic proteins (BMPs) and the fibroblast growth factors (FGFs) are known to inhibit myogenesis by blocking the expression and transcriptional activity of myogenic factors. Nuclear factors such as the inhibitory HLH protein Id and the immediate early gene products Fos and Jun have also been attributed with a role, as have changes in phosphorylation of the myogenic factors (Arnold and Winter, 1998). In addition, more recent work has identified MyoR, another bHLH protein able to form heterodimers with E proteins. This factor acts as a transcriptional repressor and inhibitor of myogenesis (Lu et al., 1999) and is expressed predominantly during primary myotube formation (see below). There is also evidence to suggest that the Cdk inhibitors p21 (CIP1) and p57 (KIP2) are co-ordinately regulated to trigger both cell-cycle exit and a muscle-specific programme of gene expression (Zhang et al., 1999).

The fusion of successive populations of postmitotic myoblasts gives rise to successive generations of myotubes (Kelly and Zacks, 1969a). The first to form are the primary myotubes arising from the near synchronous fusion of myoblasts (Ontell and Kozeka, 1984). These myotubes are characterized by their centrally located nuclei, containing prominent nucleoli, and syncytial cytoplasm rich in ribosomes, sarcotubular membranes, glycogen granules, lipid droplets and scattered groups of myofilaments (Landon, 1992). Primaries form at around embryonic days 13–14 (E13–14) in the mouse and E3–8 in the chick. During the early stages of muscle formation, these myotubes form small groups enclosed within a common basal lamina (Fig. 3.1), although as differentiation proceeds mononucleated cells intervene and a basal lamina is deposited around each individual myotube. The synthesis of the basal lamina is thought to be the result of cooperation between the myotube and surrounding mononucleated cells. Once formed, primary myotubes increase rapidly in length, girth and nuclear content. Unlike later myotube generations, they stretch the entire length of the newly formed muscle (i.e.

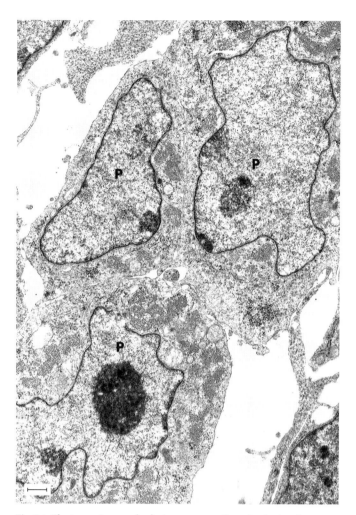

Fig. 3.1. Electron micrograph of a transverse section of a cluster of primary myotubes in the m. biceps of a mouse embryo at 15 days of gestation. The large centrally located nuclei and scattered groups of myofibrils are evident in each primary myotube, which all appear to be at a similar stage of differentiation. Scale bar = 5 μm. P, primary myotube.

from tendon to tendon) (Ontell and Kozeka, 1984). Acetylcholinesterase and acetylcholine receptor (AChR) aggregations appear in multiple bands across the muscle shortly after primary myotube formation. The number of the bands and their pattern of distribution across the muscles is preserved in the adult muscle (Wilson et al., 1992).

There is short time period between primary myotube formation and the waves of fusion associated with secondary myotube formation. The reasons for this are at present unclear but may relate to some alteration in the adhesive properties of the primary myotube since it must now support the alignment and fusion of successive generations of postmitotic myoblasts. Secondary myotube

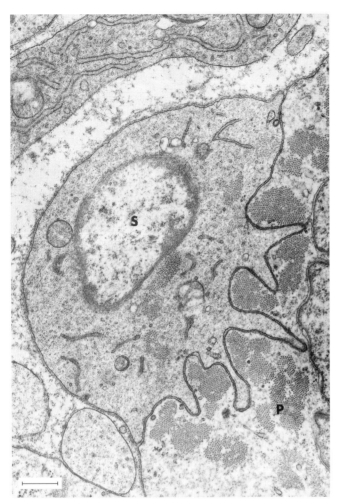

Fig. 3.2. Electron micrograph of a transverse section through a primary and secondary myotube showing the finger-like processes that the secondary myotube characteristically inserts into the primary during the early stages of its development. Scale bar = 5 μm. P, primary myotube; S, secondary myotube.

formation is initiated at around E16–17 in the mouse and E8–14 in the chicken. Fusion takes place preferentially around the sites of innervation. One striking feature of the initial stages of secondary myotube development is the finger-like extensions that the secondary myotube inserts into the primary myotube (Fig. 3.2) (Landon, 1992). These may facilitate the attachment of the relatively immature secondary myotube to the primary myotube at a time when the latter is innervated and contractile. Secondaries are initially enclosed within the basal lamina of the primary myotube, although as development proceeds each myotube attains its own basal lamina and separates from the parent primary myotube seemingly aided by the intervention of mononucleated cells.

Primary and secondary myotubes may be distinguished both by their size (during the early stages) and their myosin heavy chain (MHC) profiles (later stages). Maturation of the primaries to muscle fibres (i.e. peripheral migration of the nuclei, synthesis of contractile proteins, maturation of the T-tubule system, sarcoplasmic reticulum (SR) and the establishment of motor innervation) occurs concurrently with the formation of secondary myotubes. Primary myotube development is independent of innervation, but subsequent secondary myotube generations are considerably depleted in the absence of innervation (Harris, 1981). A single primary myotube may support the development of a variable number of secondaries; the rate of myotube formation is, therefore, the highest during secondary myogenesis. This pattern of development is similar in all mammals, although there is evidence that in larger animals the process of muscle fibre generation is more complex. For example, secondary myotubes may themselves act as a scaffold for subsequent myotube generations, since calculations for sheep tibialis cranialis show that the ratio of adult muscle fibre to primary myotube number is approximately 70:1 (Wilson et al., 1992). It is also apparent that, while adult fibre number is largely determined by the time of birth in small mammals, fibre formation continues until the fourth postnatal month in the human (Montgomery, 1962). Interactions between the extracellular matrix and the developing myotube are thought to play a major role in muscle fibre formation. The importance of the integrin family of receptors was initially demonstrated by studies on the myospheroid mutant in *Drosophila*. This mutant fails to produce an integrin β-subunit and consequently displays grossly abnormal muscle morphology owing to weaknesses at the tendon attachments and abnormal myofibrillar organization (Volk et al., 1990). The α_{7A}-, α_{7B}-, α_v- and β_{1D}-integrins are the major integrin receptors involved in striated muscle (see Berthier and Blaineau (1997) for review). The $\alpha_7\beta_1$-integrin is a laminin receptor on the surface of both myoblasts and muscle fibres. Alternative forms of both the α_7- and β_1-chains are expressed in a developmentally regulated fashion during myogenesis (Burkin and Kaufman, 1999). These isoforms localize at specific sites and appear to play a role in the migration and proliferation of myoblasts, the formation of the neuromuscular junction (NMJ) and the myotendinous, junction (MTJ) (Bao et al., 1993) and the adhesion between muscle fibres that is essential to the generation of contractile force. Perhaps not surprisingly, the $\alpha_7\beta_1$-integrin appears to be both directly and indirectly related to several muscle diseases (Burkin and Kaufman, 1999).

The DAPC is another means by which muscle fibres bind to laminin. Utrophin, the autosomal homologue of dystrophin (Love et al., 1989; Khurana et al., 1990),

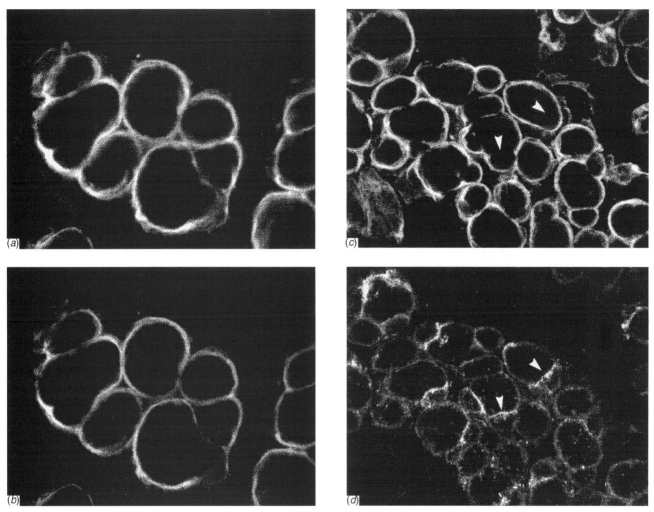

Fig. 3.3. Confocal image (single optical section) showing the distribution of dystrophin and laminin in human muscle at 16 weeks of gestation. Clusters of myotubes consisting of a primary and a variable number of adherent secondary myotubes are evident. (*a*) Laminin delineates the forming basal laminae and can be seen to surround each myotube cluster. (*b*) Immunostaining with antibodies to dystrophin on the same section show that at this stage of development dystrophin localization at the membrane reflects that of laminin deposition on the myotube surface. (*c,d*) Double staining of muscle with antibodies against laminin (*c*) and neural cell adhesion molecule (NCAM) (*d*) highlight the areas of membrane between adjacent primary and secondary myotubes that display high levels of NCAM but no laminin deposition. Overall these images show that dystrophin expression at the membrane is accompanied by the deposition of laminin on the myotube surface.

associates with a similar or identical complex to dystrophin and so is also able to mediate the link between the muscle fibre cytoskeleton and laminin in the basement membrane. Utrophin is often thought of as a developmental isoform of dystrophin in that it is expressed at the myotube membrane by 9 weeks of gestation in the human, although there is some variability both between and within individual myotubes (Clerk et al., 1993). Immunolabelling of utrophin becomes more uniform at around 17–18 weeks of gestation when expression is maximal, after which there is a marked decline such that by 26 weeks sarcolemmal staining is negligible (Clerk et al., 1993). Dystrophin tran-

scripts accumulate with those of myosin, and the protein is evident from 9 weeks of gestation in the human (Clerk et al., 1992). While dystrophin is membrane associated in both primary and secondary myotube generations, it appears to be absent from those areas not in direct contact with the extracellular matrix (Brown and Dickson, 1996). For example, while both laminin and dystrophin co-localize during early secondary myotube development (Fig. 3.3*a*), staining with antibodies to laminin and neural cell adhesion molecule (NCAM) reveal areas of membrane apposition between the primary and secondary myotube that contain no dystrophin (Fig. 3.3*b*).

NCAM is a member of the immunoglobulin (Ig) super-family of recognition molecules and operates via a homophilic (self) binding mechanism. In addition to the above, it is also involved in muscle–neuron interactions and, as a consequence, its expression is regulated by the state of innervation. The switch from myoblast to myotube is associated with an upregulation of expression of the gene for NCAM such that there is approximately four to five times more NCAM on myotubes than myoblasts. NCAM is present on both primary and secondary myotubes, although as development proceeds there is a progressive loss of the protein such that in adult muscle the main site of expression is at the NMJ (Moore and Walsh, 1986). In this location, NCAM may perform an adhesive and/or signalling function since an upregulation of NCAM is observed transiently in myofibres during the early phases of regeneration and when the myofibres are dennervated.

Myofibrils appear early after the fusion of myoblasts to form myotubes. Intermyofibrillar organization in adult muscle is thought to be maintained by intermediate filaments composed principally of desmin. During myotube differentiation, desmin filaments shift from being predominantly longitudinal to a perpendicular orientation (Tokuyasu et al., 1985), a process that is paralleled by alignment of the Z discs and the peripheral location of the muscle nuclei. Precursors of the Z discs, referred to as the I–Z–I bodies, invariably contain the proteins titin, nebulin α-actin and α-actinin. Titin is the third most abundant protein in adult muscle and is thought to act as a molecular ruler for sarcomere assembly and turnover by providing spatially defined binding sites for other sarcomeric proteins over the distance of an entire half-sarcomere. Protein interactions in the N-terminal regions of titin are thought to be crucial for Z-disc formation (Mayans et al., 1998). In attempts to analyse this further, recent work has identified a protein called telethonin, which has been found to interact in a conformation-dependent way with the N-terminal region of titin (Mues et al., 1998). In adult muscle, the structure and location of titin is such that it is thought to act as a molecular spring maintaining the structural integrity of the contracting myofibrils (Gregorio et al., 1999).

The first evidence of innervation of the proximal limb muscles in the human fetus occurs around the 10th week of gestation, although patches of acetylcholinesterase are present from the eighth week. Recent work suggests that these patches accumulate at sites of nerve–muscle contact via their interaction with a dystroglycan–perlecan complex (Peng et al., 1999). The nerve fibres enter the developing muscle and ramify among the myotubes, making contact within the central region of the target myotube. These early contacts are structurally very simply and the extensive

folding of the muscle fibre postsynaptic membrane evident in the adult is noticeably absent (Kelly and Zacks, 1969b). Formation of the NMJ involves a number of steps that are dependent on communication between the nerve and muscle fibre. A crucial step in the differentiation of the postsynaptic membrane is the accumulation of AChR into high-density aggregates. There is now much evidence to suggest that agrin orchestrates this (Ruegg & Bixby, 1998). Agrin is a protein with a predicted molecular mass of 225 kDa, consisting of an array of modules homologous to domains found in other basal lamina proteins. Its localization in the basal lamina is mediated by high-affinity binding to the laminins, especially laminin-2 and laminin-4, the two forms present in the synaptic lamina. Agrin acts via a receptor complex that includes MuSK a muscle-specific receptor tyrosine kinase and MASC, a myotube-specific accessory component. In the absence of either agrin or MuSK, synapse formation is blocked. Another important component in this system is the intracellular peripheral membrane protein rapsyn, which couples agrin-mediated MuSK activation to AChR phosphorylation (Glass and Yancopoulos, 1997). Mice deficient in agrin, MuSK or rapsyn fail to form NMJs (Gautam et al., 1995; for review see Sanes et al., 1998).

Electrical stimulation of skeletal muscle results in a release of Ca^{2+} from the SR and a transient increase in the level of intracellular Ca^{2+}, which then activates the contractile machinery. This process is referred to as excitation–contraction coupling (E–C coupling) and involves two closely interrelated sets of internal membrane systems, namely the transverse tubules (T-tubules) and the SR. The dihydropyridine receptor (DHP) in the T-tubule membrane acts as a voltage sensor and is coupled to the calcium release channel of the SR, otherwise known as the ryanodine receptor. In adult muscle, the SR ensheathes the myofibrillar apparatus and plays a central role in the storage, release and subsequent uptake of Ca^{2+} via the SR endoplasmic ATPases (SERCAs). The distribution of SERCA and ryanodine receptors may be visualized immunocytochemically in cultured mouse myotubes, where they can be seen to display a striated pattern once the myotubes become spontaneously contractile (Fig. 3.4). During myogenesis, a transition from the Ca^{2+} regulation system of presumptive myoblasts with general housekeeping functions to the highly specialized E–C coupling system of the adult muscle fibre occurs and is characterized by a shift from an inositol 1,4,5-trisphosphate-mediated to a ryanodine-sensitive system of Ca^{2+} release. Functional differentiation of E–C coupling is reached when myotubes respond to electrical stimulation with a visible twitch.

The DHP receptor in the T-tubule membrane and the ryanodine receptor of the SR are both identifiable from the earliest stages of myotube differentiation. The SR arises from the rough endoplasmic reticulum and the T-tubules from caveolin-containing precursor elements, which themselves may arise from invaginations of the sarcolemma although this is not yet proven (Parton et al., 1997). However, while the components are present from the earliest stages of myofibrillogenesis, their organization and location shows marked changes during the transition from myotube to muscle fibre (Takekura et al., 1994). For example, the Ca^{2+} release units are initially assembled at the surface membrane of the myotube. With maturation, these disappear and junctions appear between the developing transverse tubule network and the SR giving rise to the so called triadic junctions (triads take their name from the fact that they are composed of one T-tubule and two terminal cisternae of the SR). This stage occurs simultaneously in primary and secondary myotubes despite their differences in the maturation. There then follows a prolonged period during which the density of the SR increases, the triads locate to the A–I junction and fibre type differences become apparent. Slow- and fast-twitch fibre types display marked differences in the extent and arrangement of the SR. This pattern of development ensures that the complexity of the system and its ability to deliver Ca^{2+} throughout the entire fibre develops in parallel with the formation of myofibrils (Takekura et al., 1994). The SR ultimately ensheathes the myofibrillar apparatus and plays a central role in the storage, release and subsequent uptake of cytosolic Ca^{2+} via the SERCAs.

Fibre type differentiation

Adult muscle fibres are diverse biochemically and can be divided into a number of fibre types characterized by unique patterns of enzymes or contractile protein isoforms. There has been considerable debate over whether this reflects an intrinsic diversity in the myoblast populations during development. This has been largely addressed using single-cell myoblast cloning methods in conjunction with antibody detection of MHC isoforms. Recent work on cells isolated from human limbs at different stages of develoment shows that from as early as seven weeks of gestation (i.e. at the time at which primary myotubes are beginning to form in vivo), four distinct myoblast types are evident. As development proceeds, the characteristics of each remain the same but their relative numbers change (Edom-Vovard et al., 1999). These findings are consistent with the hypothesis that initial diversity may result from

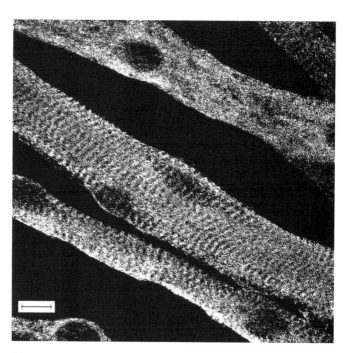

(a)

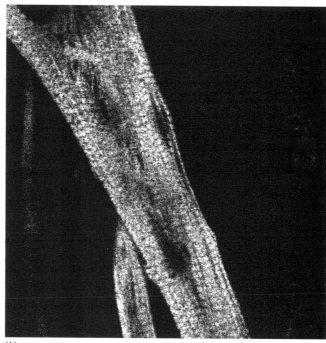

(b)

Fig. 3.4. Confocal image (single optical slice) of contractile cultured mouse myotubes immunostained for two components of the machinery for Ca^{2+} uptake and release: (a) the sarcoplasmic endoplasmic reticulum ATPase (SERCA) and (b) the ryanodine receptor. Note the regular striated arrangement of each in the myotube at this stage of differentiation. Scale bar for a and $b = 10\,\mu m$.

the existence of different populations of myoblasts with distinct MHC phenotypes.

Fast muscle fibres (type II) express a type of myosin that hydrolyses ATP rapidly and generates high levels of force. This, coupled with the bursts of high-frequency stimulation that these fibres receive from the innervating motor neurons, induces rapid but brief movements. These fibres fatigue rapidly because they use glycolytic metabolism to generate ATP quickly. Slow fibres (type I) are involved in more prolonged movements and are stimulated at continuous low frequencies. They express the slow isoform of myosin, which hydrolyses ATP more slowly, and use oxidative metabolism to generate ATP. The firing patterns determine the expression of genes specific to fibre types, as cross-innervation experiments showed many years ago. Most mature fibres express either the slow or the fast isoforms, although in disease muscle co-expression of one or more isoforms in the same fibre is common. As to how this is determined at the cellular level still remains to be resolved, although recent work implicates signalling pathways involving the NFAT (nuclear factor of activated T cells) transcription factors (Chin et al., 1998).

The contractile apparatus and associated proteins

The contractile sarcomeric cytoskeleton consists of the thin (principal component actin) and thick (principal component myosin) myofilaments (Fig. 3.5). The Z discs not only mark the limits of each sarcomere but may also contribute to the mechanical characteristics of the fibre. In accordance with this, the width of the Z disc varies with species, muscle (skeletal or cardiac) and fibre type (reviewed in Stromer, 1995). Alpha-actinin is a major structural component of the Z disc and is thought to permit interactions with an array of other integral and peripheral Z-disc proteins. Both vinculin and filamin are also present at the level of the Z disc but their role in this region remains unclear (Stromer, 1995). Desmin intermediate filaments are located at the periphery of myofibrils and are most numerous at the level of the Z disc, where they form lateral links between individual myofibrils and also between peripheral myofibrils and the sarcolemma. Given this location, desmin has been attributed with a role in transmitting tension and preventing a breakdown of force transmission between adjacent sarcomeres. This is supported by observations of desmin null mice, which show necrosis and focal regeneration by two weeks of age, particularly in muscles that are continually used such as the diaphragm and soleus (Li et al., 1997).

An electron dense M line at the centre of the A band includes three to five major sets of primary M bridges, which connect thick myosin filaments at their centres (for review see Stromer, 1995). These M bridges are thought to add stability to the A band and their pattern varies between fibre type, age, species and muscle. Additional M-line components include myomesin (185 kDa), M protein (165 kDa) and skelemin (215 kDa) although their precise role in forming any of the M-line structure is at present unclear. Other proteins associated with the myofibrillar sarcomere are titin, nebulin and tropomyosin. A single molecule of titin extends from the Z disc to the M-line region. The labelling patterns obtained with monoclonal antibodies specific for defined regions of the molecule indicate that the N-terminal 80 kDa of titin spans the entire Z-disc region such that titin filaments from opposite sarcomeres overlap. Between 800 and 1500 kDa of titin is located within the I band depending on the isoform. The C-terminal 2000 kDa of titin is located in the A band, this region being rendered inextensible by its association with the myosin thick filament. Approximately 200 kDa of the final C-terminal region of the protein locates to the M line, with the kinase domain at the periphery. As in the Z discs, titin filaments from opposite half-sarcomeres fully overlap within the M-line region, where they are interconnected via other sarcomeric components.

A fourth structural filament system is formed by nebulin, a protein specific to skeletal muscle. Inextensible filaments of nebulin are anchored at the Z disc and span the length of the thin filaments. The molecular mass of nebulin varies between 600 and 900 kDa depending on the tissue, species and developmental stage. This size correlates with the length of thin filaments in different skeletal muscles, which together with the presence of highly periodical features in the primary structure has led to the suggestion that nebulin regulates thin filament length. The C-terminal region of nebulin is thought to anchor the nebulin filament within the Z disc, although unlike actin and titin, which span the entire Z disc, nebulin inserts only within the periphery. Polymers of tropomyosin, which coil around and stabilize the actin filaments, and also thought to be absent from the central Z-disc region, possibly because α actinin inhibits tropomyosin binding to actin. This arrangement suggests that the C-terminal region of nebulin may determine where tropomyosin binding of the actin filament terminates. Titin and nebulin at the Z disc both contain differentially expressed repeat families referred to as Z repeats. In vitro studies indicate that the Z repeats bind the extreme C-terminal 10 kDa of α-actinin. The differential expression of the Z repeats might, therefore, be expected to result, in a variable number of

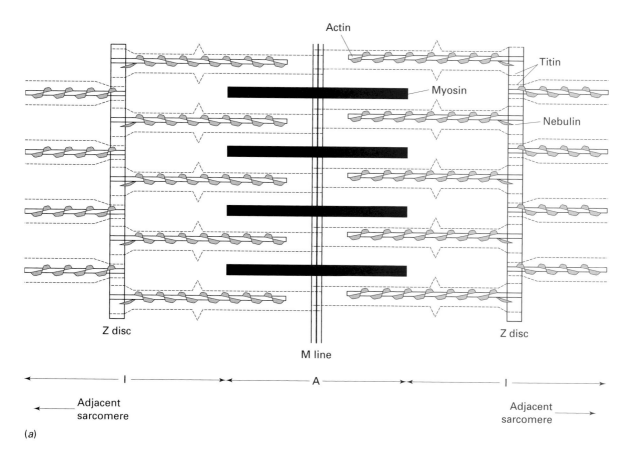

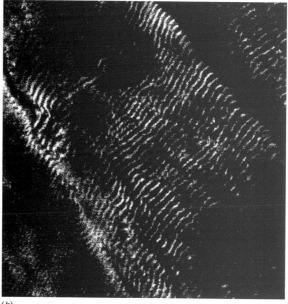

Fig. 3.5. Sarcomere structure. (*a*) Diagrammatic representation of a single sarcomere showing the A bands that contain the myosin thick filaments (thick black lines) and the I bands that contain the actin thin filaments. Overlapping thin filaments from adjacent sarcomeres are anchored in the Z disc, while the thick filaments are anchored in the M line. The N-terminal regions of titin (indicated by dotted lines) from adjacent sarcomeres overlap in the Z disc and also in the M line. The C-terminal ends of nebulin (indicated in grey) insert into the Z disc while their N-terminal ends are located at or near to the ends of the thin actin filaments (*b*) Confocal image (single optical slice) of a longitudinal section of human muscle immunostained for titin.

cross-links with α-actinin within the Z disc. This may influence the mechanical properties of the Z disc and be the molecular basis for the variation in this structure noted between different fibre types (Gregorio et al., 1999).

Mutations in the genes encoding nebulin and α-tropomyosin (*TPM3*) have been shown to cause nemaline myopathy. The congenital nemaline myopathies are rare hereditary muscle disorders characterized by the presence in the muscle fibres of nemaline bodies, consisting of proteins derived from the Z disc and the thin filaments.

Hypertrophied Z discs characterize this disease and are formed by extended overlap zones of thin filaments from adjacent sacrcomeres (see Stromer (1995) for review). Recent immunofluorescence studies with antibodies specific to the C-terminal region of nebulin indicate that some mutations may cause protein truncation and a loss of fibre-type diversity, factors that may be relevant to the disease pathogenesis (Pelin et al., 1999).

Calpain (Ca^{2+}-dependent cysteine protease) is a major intracellular protease thought to regulate cellular function by hydrolysing substrates. The u- and m-calpains exist as heterodimers consisting of a unique large catalytic subunit and a common small regulatory subunit. The calpains can be classified into two groups, ubiquitous and tissue-specific species. The p94 isoform (calpain 3 or nCL-1, which stands for novel calpain large subunit) is a specific member of the calpain family expressed predominantly in skeletal muscle, where its mRNA is at least 10 times more abundant than those for the u and m-calpain large subunits. Defects in the gene for p94 are now known to be the cause of limb-girdle muscular dystrophy type 2A (LGMD2A), suggesting that a p94-specific function is indispensable for normal muscle activity (Richard et al., 1999). While p94 is expressed abundantly at the mRNA level in skeletal muscle, little is detectable as protein because of its very rapid autolysis, which distinguishes it from other cysteine proteases including other calpains. It does associate with titin, implying a regulatory role in myofibril turnover. The loss of p94 protease activity rather than its autolytic activity underlie the pathogenesis of LGMD2A (Ono et al., 1998). Interestingly, recent work has shown the presence of myonuclear apoptosis in LGMD2A. Apoptosis, or programmed cell death, is an active process fundamental to the development and homeostasis of multicellular organisms. A wide variety of stimuli, such as ultraviolet radiation, ionizing radiation, heat shock and oxidative stress, has been shown to be active in stimulating this process in a number of different cell types. In LGMD2A, myofibre apoptosis was linked to an altered subcellular distribution of the transcription factors IκBα and NF-κB, resulting in sarcoplasmic sequestration of NF-κB (Baghdiguian et al., 1999). It does, nonetheless, remain to be shown whether this incidence of apoptosis contributes significantly to the disease pathogenesis.

The muscle fibre nucleus and associated proteins

The intermediate filaments are major structural proteins encoded by a large multigene family (McLean and Lane, 1995). Five classes are recognized on the basis of similarities in their rod domains. Their expression is tissue specific, strongly suggesting that intermediate filament type is related to function in individual tissues. Nuclear lamins are members of the intermediate filament family and are the most abundant components of the 10–50 nm thick fibrous layer underlying the inner nuclear membrane. Lamins interact with chromatin and integral proteins of the inner nuclear membrane such as the lamin B receptor, lamin-associated proteins (LAPs) and emerin. Nuclear lamins are inherently polymorphic and their genetic variation is further increased by post-translational modification specific to particular cells and stages of the cell cycle, a diversity that is mirrored by the range of lamin-associated proteins. As to whether this heterogeneity provides flexibility to the laminae of different cell types remains to be determined, but it is of particular relevance given that alterations in either emerin or lamin A seem to be specifically deleterious to muscle tissue (Nagano, 1996; Bonne et al., 1999).

Mutations in the gene for lamin A/C are associated with autosomal dominant EDMD (Bonne et al., 1999). This disease is characterized by slowly progressive muscle wasting and weakness, and a cardiomyopathy. Together with mutations in the gene for emerin (see below), these observations underscore the potential importance of the nuclear envelope components in the pathogenesis of neuromuscular disorders. Moreover, the newly found relationship between nuclear function and genetic disease in muscle promises to lead to increased insight into normal nuclear processes. Interactions between the nuclear membrane and lamins are highly modulated during mitosis. The A-type lamins are completely disassembled and dissociated from the nuclear envelope whereas the B-type lamins remain associated with membranous structures. The precise role of these proteins in the postmitotic nucleus of the muscle fibre remains however, to be elucidated.

Emerin is a 34 kDa inner nuclear membrane protein encoded in humans by the gene *EMD* located on Xq28. Genetic defects in this protein have been shown to be the underlying cause of X-linked EDMD (Bione et al., 1994; Manilal et al., 1999). The majority of mutations identified predict no emerin expression, although a small number of in-frame deletions and missense mutations have now been identified. Human emerin mRNA shows ubiquitous tissue distribution, with the highest expression in skeletal and cardiac muscle (Bione et al., 1994). Emerin possesses at least two nonoverlapping targeting sequences, which are involved in targeting it to the nuclear envelope. The first of these is in the N-terminal domain and the second is in the C-terminal 36 residues, which includes the transmembrane region. Mutant forms from patients with EDMD have been shown to exhibit aberrant cell cycle-dependent phosphorylated forms of emerin (Ellis et al., 1998). Interactions between nuclear membrane components, nuclear lamina and chromatin are important for maintaining the structure of the nuclear membrane–chromatin organization during interphase and for assembly and reformation of the nuclear membrane during mitosis. However, as to why mutations in this gene are particularly deleterious to striated muscle remains to be elucidated. One hypothesis is that the nuclear membrane of skeletal and cardiac muscle also lacks lamin B_1, and so the additional absence of emerin may be particularly damaging (Manilal et al., 1999).

Adult skeletal muscle exhibits a remarkable capacity for regeneration following damage, an ability that results from a population of precursor or satellite cells. Satellite cells reside between the basement membrane and sarcolemma of individual muscle fibres (Mauro, 1961; Brown and Stickland, 1993). In adult muscle, these cells are normally quiescent; however, after muscle fibre damage, they become activated to migrate, proliferate and differentiate, thereby effecting repair and regeneration in the appropriate areas (Bischoff, 1997). In many aspects, regeneration in the adult recapitulates muscle development. However, the precise origins and lineage of satellite cells are ill-defined. Recent data suggest that cultures of myoblasts contain distinct subpopulations defined by their behaviour in vitro and divergent responses when these cells are grafted into muscle. By examining the fate of myoblasts transplanted into muscles of dystrophic mice, Beauchamp et al., (1999) have recently demonstrated the existence of a lineage that divides only slowly in vitro but which is rapidly proliferative after grafting, implying the existence of a subpopulation of cells with stem cell-like characteristics. In terms of attempts to develop myoblast transplantation for genetic modification of adult muscle, these findings represent an important step forward (Bauchamp et al., 1999). More recently, controversial evidence of the existence of a circulating reserve of myogenic stem cells derived from the bone marrow has been reported, which may have important therapeutic consequences (Ferrari et al., 1998; see also below).

The neuromuscular and myotendinous junctions

The NMJ and the MTJ together with the costameres all define cytoskeletal domains that effectively anchor submembranous actin filaments by means of multimolecular complexes. At least some of these complexes also act as receptors for extracellular matrix proteins, thus providing important linkages between the cytoskeleton of the muscle fibre and its surrounding extracellular matrix. The MTJ is a highly specialized structure that serves to transmit force from the contractile apparatus to the tendon. The cytoplasmic side of the sarcolemma in this region also contains talin, vinculin and dystrophin. Desmin is present but is located at least 30 nm from the sarcolemma and, therefore, is farther from the membrane than talin, vinculin and dystrophin. On the basis of this, it has been suggested that desmin filaments may serve as a separate force-transmitting system (reviewed in Stromer, 1995). The MTJ appears to be not only a preferential site for lesion during acute mechanical stress but also the site of muscle fibre growth during development. The presence of nicotinic AChRs at the MTJ is as yet unexplained, although it has been suggested that they may play a role in promoting the fusion of myogenic cells during muscle fibre repair (Bernheim et al., 1996).

At the adult vertebrate NMJ, nicotinic AChRs are clustered at high density on the crests of the postsynaptic folds in precise register with presynaptic sites of acetylcholine release. In the depths of the postjunctional folds, immediately adjacent to these receptor clusters, voltage-gated sodium channels are present at a density ten times that of nonsynaptic areas (Sealock et al., 1991; Bewick et al., 1992). These distributions are essential in ensuring rapid, efficient synaptic transmission and the initiation of the action potential in the postsynaptic muscle fibre (Martin, 1994). Dystrophin and utrophin both complex with dystroglycan at the NMJ. However, utrophin is confined to the crests of the postsynaptic folds in close association with the AChR clusters, whereas dystrophin is found in the depths of the folds, a region that is sparse in AChRs but enriched in sodium channels.

The high concentration of AChRs at the synapse arises in part from the selective transcription of the genes for the AChR subunits. This has been attributed to the nerve-derived molecule ARIA (AChR-inducing activity), which acts via the activation of the ErbB receptor tyrosine kinases (Ruegg and Bixby 1998). The signalling processes that determine the clustering of the sodium channels at the NMJ are less well defined. However, recent work attributes the syntrophins with linking the channels to the actin cytoskeleton and the extracellular matrix via their association with the DAPC (see below). The synaptic cleft contains a specific basal lamina that accumulates a number of NMJ-restricted proteins, including acetylcholinesterase, s-laminins, agrin and ARIA. Recent work indicates that the behaviour of Schwann cells and motor neurons can be regulated directly by the local laminin composition (Cho et al., 1998; Patton et al., 1998). The precise geometric relationship of these cells at the NMJ may, therefore, reflect the unique composition of the basal lamina.

Interactions between the muscle fibre and its surrounding extracellular matrix

Adult skeletal muscle fibres must withstand repeated cycles of contraction and relaxation throughout their entire lifetime, for which they have developed a highly specialized system of linking the cortical cytoskeleton with components of the extracellular matrix. The underlying cause of a number of different muscular dystrophies is now known to be a defect in either the linkages that the fibre maintains between the cytoskeleton and matrix or in specific matrix components (Campbell, 1995). While the following discussion considers some of the essential components of this system separately, it should be remembered that it is the complete assembly that provides the fibre with dynamic structural integrity not only to withstand the stresses of activity but also to adapt to them.

A complex matrix comprising laminins, fibronectin, collagens, entactin and perlecan, in addition to growth factors and agrin, surrounds each fibre. The laminins are heterotrimeric cross-shaped molecules made up of various combinations of three chains, α, β, and γ, with the major laminin variant present in adult skeletal muscle fibres, referred to as merosin, being composed of $\alpha_2\beta_1\gamma_1$ chains. Merosin is associated with muscle fibres by a least two mechanisms. One of these is the DAPC, which has been extensively studied in recent years as a consequence of its disruption being the underlying cause of several forms of muscular dystrophy. The other is an integrin-mediated system. Integrins are a large family of transmembrane glycoproteins that consist of noncovalently linked heterodimers each composed of an α- and a β-chain (Hynes, 1992). Different α- and β-subunits are expressed on skeletal muscle cells at different times and subcellular locations. The $\alpha_7\beta_1$-integrin is a transmembrane receptor for laminin and links the extracellular matrix with the cytoskeleton, as does the DAPC. Enhanced expression of $\alpha_7\beta_1$-mediated linkage of the extracellular matrix is seen in DMD and may compensate for the absence of the dystrophin-mediated linkage (Hodges et al., 1997). By contrast, downregulation of expression may contribute to the development of pathology in congenital laminin deficiencies (Burkin and Kaufman, 1999).

The cysteine-rich and C-terminal domains of dystro-phin associate with a large complex of sarcolemmal proteins collectively known as the DAPC (Ervasti and Campbell, 1991). The DAPC consists of dystroglycan, sarcoglycan and syntrophin subcomplexes (Tinsley et al., 1994) plus sarcospan, a recently identified 25 kDa component (Crosbie et al., 1997).

The extracellular proteoglycan α-dystroglycan is able to bind to the G domain of laminin, and to merosin and agrin in the extracellular matrix. Beta-dystroglycan is a transmembrane protein, the extreme C-terminus of which forms a unique binding site for the cysteine-rich region of dystrophin. Thus the subsarcolemmal cytoskeleton of the muscle fibre is linked in a complex manner with the extracellular matrix, which is essential for normal physiological function (Henry and Campbell, 1996). This link appears also to be essential in other nonmuscle cell systems, as gene-targeted disruption of the gene for dystroglycan in the mouse results in embryos that fail to progress beyond the early egg cylinder stage (Williamson et al., 1997; Durbeej et al., 1998). Detailed analyses of the reasons for this strongly suggest that dystroglycan plays an essential role in basement membrane formation by nucleating diverse laminin isoforms on cell surfaces. This is supported by recent tissue culture studies in which it was shown that dystroglycan plays a primary role in nucleating laminin at the cell surface during the early stages of basement membrane formation (Henry and Campbell, 1998). A number of mutations affecting the sarcoglycan complex are now known to be the underlying cause of various forms of muscular dystrophy. The syntrophins are a biochemically heterogeneous group of 58 kDa intracellular membrane-associated dystrophin-binding proteins but they have not yet been shown to be the cause of any form of neuromuscular disease. They directly associate as a complex with the C-terminal domain of dystrophin, probably at multiple interaction sites. At present, one acidic syntrophin (α_1) and two basic syntrophins (β_1 and β_2) have been identified in muscle. The α_1-form is most abundant in heart and skeletal muscle and is located to the sarcolemma; the β_1- and β_2-syntrophins are more widely expressed.

This arrangement of the DAPC has been widely hypothesized to play a role in maintaining the structural integrity of the sarcolemma during repeated cycles of contraction and relaxation (Petrof et al., 1993). Observations of apparently increased fragility of dystrophin-deficient membranes and increased sarcolemmal permeability have lent support to this idea (Menke and Jockusch, 1991; Menke et al., 1993; Pasternak et al., 1995). However, it has become increasingly clear that this complex may also act as a mediator of at least one signal transduction pathway (Brown et al., 1999). Evidence in support of this comes from the observation that nNOS (neuronal nitric oxide synthase) binds directly to α_1-syntrophin via a PDZ motif. In the absence of dystrophin, both activity and expression of nNOS are greatly reduced. The physiological consequences of this remained unclear until it was shown that nitric oxide production from nNOS opposes adrenergic vasoconstriction. This was found to be compromised in both the dystrophin-deficient *mdx* mouse and the nNOS null mutant (Thomas et al., 1998). Therefore, the absence of this enzyme renders these animals less able to match muscle blood flow to increases in metabolic activity.

Costameres were first described by Pardo et al. (1983) and are thought to allow for the transmission of force laterally along the fibre to the extracellular matrix, to adjacent fibres and, ultimately, to the tendon (Pardo et al, 1983; Minetti et al., 1992; Porter et al., 1992). These vinculin-rich areas appear like stripes flanking the level of the Z lines and overlying the I band. Their name comes from the rib-like pattern apparent after immunostaining for vinculin (Latin: *costa*, rib; Greek: *meros*, part). Interestingly, many proteins display an apparent costameric pattern when detected immunocytochemically. These include dystrophin, b-dystroglycan, α-, β- and γ-sarcoglycan, β_1-integrin, vinculin, paxillin, nNOS, caveolin 3, talin, spectrin and γ-actin. Given the number of proteins involved, it seems likely that the role of the costameric lattice will turn out to be more complex than originally thought.

Myoblast and gene transfer approaches to therapy

As discussed in the previous sections, combined advances in understanding the molecular genetics of disease and the molecular cell biology of skeletal muscle has led to elucidation of the molecular basis of an increasing number of inherited neuromuscular disorders. These insights have, in turn, given rise to new hypotheses on potential therapeutic approaches. In particular, the related concepts of muscle gene therapy (Marshall and Leiden, 1998; Dunckley and Dickson, 2001; Karpati et al., 1999; Murphy and Dickson, 1999) and myoblast transfer therapy (Blau and Springer, 1995; Partridge and Davies, 1995; Braun et al., 1999) have received considerable attention. The basic premise linking these two approaches is the genetic modification of patient skeletal muscle tissues either by virtue of the natural genetic composition of donor implanted myoblasts or via direct in vivo or indirect ex vivo genetic modification of autologous cells.

The concept of myoblast transplantation therapy for primary inherited myopathies exploits the ability of exogenous myoblasts to incorporate into postnatal skeletal muscle during regeneration (Partridge et al., 1989; Gussoni et al., 1997; Law et al., 1997a,b; Qu et al., 1998; Vilquin et al., 1999). In the early 1990s, several clinical trials of myoblast transfer therapy were conducted in patients with DMD. With the exception of one centre (Law et al., 1997b), these proved ineffective in restoring dystrophin expression in DMD muscle (Thomson, 1992). Despite the fact that recent re-evaluation of muscle biopsies taken at the time of the initial trials have shown evidence for low-level survival of implanted myoblasts (using in situ polymerase chain reaction for donor-specific chromosomal sequence elements; Gussoni et al., 1997), the field of donor myoblast transfer and the true identity of the skeletal muscle stem cell remains highly controversial (Partridge, 1997; Beauchamp et al., 1999). In terms of the biology of muscle stem cells, significant interest has been generated from the recent observation that bone marrow transplantation in experimental animals can result in the apparent migration of a haematopoietic cell population to skeletal muscle sites and their incorporation into myofibres (Ferrari et al., 1998). Indeed, fluorescence-activated cell sorting studies indicate the existence of a reciprocal population of muscle-derived mononuclear cells that can repopulate lethally irradiated animals (E. Gussoni et al. (1999), personal communication). It remains to be defined whether these unexpected observations are indicative of a fundamental physiological mechanism to recruit muscle stem cells from a circulating haematopoietic population, and indeed potentially vice versa. In any event, retrospective analyses of rare patients with inherited myopathies who have undergone an unrelated therapeutic episode of bone marrow transplantation will be important to determine whether this phenomenon may provide a therapeutic avenue to treat inherited muscle diseases.

In muscle-directed recombinant gene therapy, a range of options have been proposed for various inherited myopathies, including the muscular dystrophies and metabolic myopathies (Dunckley and Dickson, 2001; Karpati et al., 1999; Murphy and Dickson, 1999). The general concept has been to provide gain-of-function gene augmentation therapies to affected myofibres by delivery of a recombinant gene via viral or non-viral delivery vectors (Jooss et al., 1998; Hu et al., 1999). However, in the case of the metabolic myopathy Pompe's disease (α-glucosidase deficiency), an intriguing approach utilizing liver expression of secreted gene product, which can be taken up via high levels of mannose receptors in skeletal and cardiac muscle, has shown good efficiency in animal models (Amalfitano et al., 1998 and A. Amalfitano et al. (1999) personal communication). In the muscular dystrophies, approaches to gene therapy are moving toward phase I clinical experiments. In transgenic mouse studies, it has been clearly demonstrated that recombinant dystrophin or its homologue utrophin, expressed in *mdx* mouse, results in effective elimination of muscle pathology (Cox et al., 1993; Wells et al., 1995; Tinsley et al., 1996, 1998). A range of somatic gene-transfer systems is under development to deliver genes to muscle including helper-dependent and helper-independent adenovirus (HD- and HI-AV; Acsadi et al., 1996; Floyd et al., 1998; Guibinga et al., 1998; Holt et al., 1998; Yuasa et al., 1998; Chen et al., 1999), integrating retroviral vectors (RVs; Fassati et al., 1997a,b, 1998), adeno-associated virus (AAV; Xiao et al., 1996; Fisher et al., 1997; Monahan et al., 1998; Greelish et al., 1999; Herzog et al., 1999) and simple 'naked' bacterial plasmid vectors (Decrouy et al., 1997, 1998). Phase I clinical trials with dystrophin plasmid, dystrophin HD-AV vectors and sarcoglycan AAV vectors have been proposed by groups in France and the USA (Hughes et al., Chamberlain et al., S. Braun et al., personal communications at the MDG Workshop on Gene Therapy, Cambridge, 1999). However, in the area of muscle-directed gene therapy for recessive neuromuscular disorders, a number of interlinked considerations remain to be optimized: the nature of the recombinant gene, the gene delivery vector, the route of administration and the host response in terms of longevity of transgene expression and adverse immunological reactions.

Various recombinant cDNAs have been utilized for dystrophin gene augmentation for DMD. The full-length cDNA (~13.9 kb: Ascadi et al., 1991; Dickson et al., 1991) can only be delivered by high-capacity vectors such as HD-AVs (Clemens et al., 1996; Hauser et al., 1997). A minidystrophin gene of ~6.3 kb modelled on a mild Becker muscular dystrophy phenotype (England et al., 1990) and encoding a highly function dystrophin of some 220 kDa has been widely examined in preclinical experimental animal studies using RV (Fassati et al., 1997a,b, 1998) and HI-AV vectors (Vincent et al., 1993; Acsadi et al., 1996). Finally microdystrophin cDNAs of some 4 kb in size incorporating significant deletion of putative nonfunctional regions of dystrophin and compatible with AAV vector technology have been engineered but remain to be fully characterized functionally (Yuasa et al., 1998; Dickson et al., unpublished data).

The use of replication-defective RV and HI-AV vectors to deliver the 6.3 kb minidystrophin cDNA into skeletal muscle of the *mdx* mouse (Vincent et al., 1993; Acsadi et al., 1996; Dickson 1996a,b) or GRMD dog (McHowell et al., 1998) has yielded 20–80% transduction of fibres within a 2–3 mm radius of the injection site (Fig. 3.6). Strong sarco-

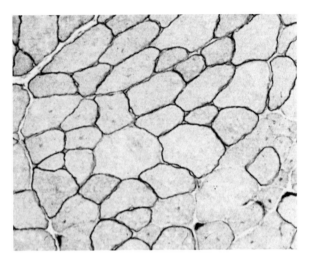

Fig. 3.6. Adenovirus-mediated transduction and expression of a human dystrophin minigene in *nude-mdx* skeletal muscle by direct in vivo injection of helper-independent vector particles. Cryosection of transduced muscle is stained for recombinant dystrophin.

lemmal dystrophin expression, re-establishment of the DAPC complex and reversal of pathophysiology was obtained for small muscles of the *mdx* mouse (Deconinck et al., 1997b; Karpati et al., 1999). Intramuscular delivery of full-length dystrophin HI-AV vectors has produced similar results, with apparent reduction in adverse host immune reactions (Clemens et al., 1996; Chen et al., 1999). However, it is apparent that mature myofibres are relatively refractory to AV infection, and it remains likely that transduction here is occurring via immature regenerating fibres or indeed activated satellite cells (Feero et al., 1997; Nalbantoglu et al., 1999). The AAV vector system is based on a nonpathogenic parvovirus that exhibits attractive properties as a muscle gene-transfer system (Xiao et al., 1996; Fisher et al., 1997; Monahan et al., 1998; Greelish et al., 1999; Herzog et al., 1999): notably, the ability to transduce mature fibres and an apparent paucity of deleterious immune responses to transgene neoantigens. The limited capacity of AAV vectors for foreign DNA represents a major drawback for dystrophin gene transfer unless microdystrophin constructs prove effective. However, AAV may prove ideal for gene therapy of recessive sarcoglycanopathies since the sarcoglycan cDNAs are relatively small. Preclinical studies in the cardiomyopathic hamster, a model of sarcoglycan deficiency, have shown the feasibility of the gene therapy approach with AV vectors (Holt et al., 1998). The recent studies of Greelish et al. (1999) with a sarcoglycan–AAV vector clearly indicate a possible approach for broad loco-regional gene therapy using intra-arterial delivery of AAV in combination with administration of capillary dilating and permeabilizing agents. This group of researchers, in collaboration with clinical investigators at Ohio State University, has submitted phase I treatment protocols to the US regulatory authorities for permission to proceed to gene therapy trials in patients with LGMD using sarcoglycan–AAV vectors (H. Stedman, personal communication). The issue of systemic gene therapy vector delivery remains, however, a crucial issue. Based upon successful studies in the *mdx* mouse using intramuscular implants of cells that are releasing dystrophin–RV vectors, Parrish et al. (1999) have proposed an interesting approach to employ ex vivo engineered monocyte/macrophage cells as a systemic cellular vehicle, which will home to sites of pathology in widespread dystrophic muscles. The aim here is ex vivo engineering of autologous monocyte cells to act as transient producers of dystrophin–RV vectors. It is proposed that, following subsequent systemic infusion, a proportion of the engineered cells will traffic to widespread sites of muscle necrosis and regeneration and mediate permanent transduction of local muscle satellite cell populations by dystrophin–RV vectors.

Finally, the work of Davies et al. (Deconinck et al., 1997a; Tinsley, 1998; Tinsley et al., 1996, 1998) has clearly shown that overexpression of utrophin in *mdx* skeletal muscle can rescue dystrophin-deficient fibres. Utrophin is an autosomal homologue of dystrophin expressed in a range of tissues including embryonic skeletal muscle. It has been proposed that therapeutic overexpression of the endogenous gene for utrophin could be induced pharmacologically by transcriptional activation; random screening of chemical libraries for appropriate lead compounds from which to derive small molecule transcriptional activators is in progress but has not yet been fruitful (Tinsley, 1998). Alternatively, gene therapy with utrophin–AV vectors in *mdx* muscle has proved effective, with apparent reduced immunological complications compared with corresponding dystrophin gene delivery systems because, potentially, utrophin does not represent a neo-antigen in a dystrophin-deficient host (Gilbert et al., 1998; Ohtsuka et al., 1998). In summary, induced overexpression of utrophin in dystrophin-deficient muscle represents an attractive potential therapeutic strategy for DMD.

During the period that this edition goes to press, early phase I clinical experiments for the sarcoglycanopathies using AAV vectors and for DMD using HI-AV and plasmid vectors are likely to be approved and instigated. These studies will provide baseline data on safety profiles of these vectors and immune responses following delivery by an intramuscular route in human patients. However, development of generalized systemic administration modalities and the logistics and feasibility of pharmaceutical scale-up vector production remain major technological and experimental challenges. While enormous progress has been made in addressing the complex requirements for successful gene therapy of the muscular dystrophies and other recessive inherited myopathies, we are still a significant distance from a clinically useful genetic medicine.

References

Acsadi, G., Dickson, G., Love, D. R. et al. (1991). Human dystrophin expression in *mdx* mice after intramuscular injection of DNA constructs. *Nature* **352**, 815–818.

Acsadi, G., Lochmuller, H., Jani, A. et al. (1996). Dystrophin expression in muscles of *mdx* mice after adenovirus-mediated in vivo gene transfer. *Hum. Gene Ther.* **7**, 129–140.

Amalfitano, A., Hauser, M. A., Hu, H. M., Serra, D., Begy, C. R. and Chamberlain, J. S. (1998). Production and characterization of improved adenovirus vectors with the E1, E2b, and E3 genes deleted. *J. Virol.* **72**, 926–933.

Arnold, H. H. and Winter, B. (1998). Muscle differentiation: more complexity to the network of myogenic regulators. *Curr. Opin. Genet. Dev.* **8**, 539–544.

Baghdiguian, S., Richard, M. M., Pons, F. et al. (1999). Calpain 3 deficiency is associated with myonuclear apoptosis and profound perturbation of the IκB α/NF-κB pathway in limb-girdle muscular dystrophy type 2A. *Nat. Med.* **5**, 503.

Bao, Z. Z., Lakonishok, M., Kaufman, S. and Horwitz, A. F. (1993). α7β1 integrin is a component of the myotendinous junction on skeletal muscle. *J. Cell Sci.* **106**, 579–589.

Beauchamp, J. R., Morgan, J. E., Pagel, C. N. and Partridge, T. A. (1999). Dynamics of myoblast transplantation reveal a discrete minority of precursors with stem cell-like properties as the myogenic source. *J. Cell Biol.* **144**, 1113–1121.

Bernheim, L., Hamann, M., Liu, J. H., Fischer-Lougheed, J. and Bader, C. R. (1996). Role of nicotinic acetylcholine receptors at the vertebrate myotendinous junction: a hypothesis. *Neuromus. Dis.* **6**, 211–214.

Berthier, C. and Blaineau, S. (1997). Supramolecular organization of the subsarcolemmal cytoskeleton of adult skeletal muscle fibres: a review. *Biol. Cell* **89**, 413–434.

Bewick, G. S, Nicolson, L. B., Young, C, Odonnell, E. and Slater, C. R. (1992). Different distributions of dystrophin and related proteins at nerve muscle junctions. *Neuroreport.* **3**, 857–868.

Bione, S., Maestrini, E., Rivella, S. et al. (1994). Identification of a novel X-linked gene responsible for Emery–Dreifuss muscular-dystrophy. *Nat. Genet.* **8**, 323–327.

Bischoff, R. (1997). Chemotaxis of skeletal muscle satellite cells. *Dev. Dynam.* **208**, 505–515.

Blau, H. M. and Springer, M. L. (1995). Muscle-mediated gene-therapy. *N. Engl. J. Med.* **333**, 1554–1556.

Bonne, G., Di Barletta, M. R., Varnous, S. et al. (1999). Mutations in the gene encoding lamin A/C cause autosomal dominant Emery-Dreifuss muscular dystrophy. *Nat. Genet.* **21**, 285–288.

Braun, S., Thioudellet, C., Perraud, E. et al. (1999). Gene transfer into canine myoblasts. *Cytotechnology* **30**, 181–189.

Brown, S. C. and Dickson, G. (1996). Dystroglycan complexes and their role in muscle development. *Basic Appl. Myol.* **6**, 449–456.

Brown, S. C. and Stickland, N. C. (1993). Satellite cell content in muscle of large and small mice. *J. Anat.* **183**, 91–96.

Brown, S. C., Fassati, A., Popplewell, L. et al. (1999). Dystrophic phenotype induced in vitro by antibody blockade of muscle α-dystroglycan–laminin interaction. *J. Cell Sci.* **112**, 209–216.

Burkin, D. J. and Kaufman, S. J. (1999). The $\alpha_7\beta_1$ integrin in muscle development and disease. *Cell Tissue Res.* **296**, 183–190.

Campbell, K. P. (1995). Three muscular dystrophies: loss of cyto-skeleton–extracellular matrix linkage. *Cell* **80**, 675–679.

Campbell, K. P., Ervasti, J. M., Ohlendieck, K., Beskrovnaya-Ibraghimov, O. and Matsumura, K. (1991). Molecular characterization of the dystrophin-associated glycoproteins. *Am. J. Hum. Genet.* **49**, 4.

Chen, H. H., Mack, L. M., Choi, S. Y., Ontell, M., Kochanek, S. and Clemens, P. R. (1999). DNA from both high-capacity and first-generation adenoviral vectors remains intact in skeletal muscle. *Hum. Gene Ther.* **10**, 365–373.

Chin, E. R., Olson, E. N., Richardson, J. A. et al. (1998). A calcineurin-dependent transcriptional pathway controls skele-tal muscle fibre type. *Genes Dev.* **12**, 2499–2509.

Cho, S. I., Ko, J., Patton, B. L., Sanes, J. R. and Chiu, A. Y. (1998). Motor neurons and Schwann cells distinguish between synaptic and extrasynaptic isoforms of laminin. *J. Neurobiol.* **37**, 339–358.

Clemens, P. R., Kochanek, S., Sunada, Y. et al. (1996). In vivo muscle gene transfer of full-length dystrophin with an adenoviral vector that lacks all viral genes. *Gene Ther.* **3**, 965–972.

Clerk, A,. Strong, P. and Sewry C. (1992). Characterisation of dystro-phin during development of human skeletal muscle. *Development* **114**, 395–402.

Clerk, A., Morris, G. E., Dubowitz, V., Davies, K. E. and Sewry, C. A. (1993). Dystrophin-related protein, utrophin, in normal and dystrophic human fetal skeletal muscle. *Histochem. J.* **25**, 554–561.

Cox, G. A., Cole, N. M., Matsumura, K et al. (1993). Overexpression of dystrophin in transgenic *mdx* mice eliminates dystrophic symptoms without toxicity. *Nature* **364**, 725–729.

Crosbie, R. H., Heighway, J., Venzke, D. P., Lee, J. C. and Campbell, K. P. (1997). Sarcospan, the 25–kDa transmembrane component of the dystrophin–glycoprotein complex. *J. Biol. Chem.* **272**, 31221–31224.

Deconinck, A. E., Rafael, J. A., Skinner, J. A. et al. (1997a). Utrophin-dystrophin-deficient mice as a model for Duchenne muscular dystrophy. *Cell* **90**, 717–727.

Deconinck, N., Tinsley, J., DeBacker, F. et al. (1997b). Expression of truncated utrophin leads to major functional improvements in dystrophin-deficient muscles of mice. *Nat. Med.* **3**, 1216–1221.

Decrouy, A., Renaud, J. M., Davis, H. L., Lunde, J. A., Dickson, G. and Jasmin, B. J. (1997). Mini-dystrophin gene transfer in *mdx*4(cv) diaphragm muscle fibers increases sarcolemmal stability. *Gene Ther.* **4**, 401–408.

Decrouy, A., Renaud, J. M., Lunde, J. A., Dickson, G. and Jasmin, B. J. (1998). Mini- and full-length dystrophin gene transfer induces the recovery of nitric oxide synthase at the sarcolemma of *mdx*4(cv) skeletal muscle fibers. *Gene Ther.* **5**, 59–64.

Dickson, G. (1996a). Gene therapy of Duchenne muscular dystro-phy. *Chem. Indust.* **8**, 294–297.

Dickson, G. (1996b). Gene transfer to muscle. *Biochem. Soc. Trans.* **24**, 514–519.

Dickson, G., Love, D. R., Davies, K. E., Wells, K. E., Piper, T. A. and Walsh, F. S. (1991). Human dystrophin gene-transfer: production and expression of a functional recombinant DNA-based gene. *Hum. Genet.* **88**, 53–58.

Dunckley, M. G. and Dickson, G. (2001). Options for the develop-ment of gene-based therapy of Duchenne muscular dystrophy. In: *Muscular Dystrophy: Methods and Protocols*, eds. K. Bushby, and L. Anderson. New Jersey: Humana Press, in press.

Durbeej, M., Henry, M. D. and Campbell, K. P. (1998). Dystroglycan in development and disease. *Curr. Opin. Cell Biol.* **10**, 594–601.

Edom-Vovard, F., Mouly, V., Barbet, J. P. and Butler-Browne, G. S. (1999). The four populations of myoblasts involved in human limb muscle formation are present from the onset of primary myotube formation. *J. Cell Sci.* **112**, 191–199.

Ellis, J. A., Craxton, M., Yates, J. R. W. and Kendrick-Jones, J. (1998). Aberrant intracellular targeting and cell cycle-dependent phos-phorylation of emerin contribute to the Emery–Dreifuss muscu-lar dystrophy phenotype. *J. Cell Sci.* **111**, 781–792.

England, S. B., Nicholson, L. V. B., Johnson, M. A. et al. (1990). Very mild muscular dystrophy associated with the deletion of 46–percent of dystrophin. *Nature* **343**, 180–182.

Ervasti, J. M. and Campbell, K. P. (1991). Membrane organization of the dystrophin–glycoprotein complex. *Cell* **66**, 1121–1131.

Fassati, A., Wells, D. J., Serpente, P. S. et al. (1997a). Genetic correc-tion of dystrophin deficiency and skeletal muscle remodeling in adult mdx mouse via transplantation of retroviral producer cells. *J. Clin. Invest.* **100**, 620–628.

Fassati, A., Murphy, S. and Dickson, G. (1997b). Gene therapy of Duchenne muscular dystrophy. *Adv. Genet.* **35**, 117–153.

Fassati, A., Bardoni, A., Sironi, M. et al. (1998). Insertion of two independent enhancers in the long terminal repeat of a self-inactivating vector results in high-titer retroviral vectors with tissue-specific expression. *Hum. Gene Ther.* **9**, 2459–2468.

Feero, W. G., Rosenblatt, J. D., Huard, J. et al. (1997). Viral gene delivery to skeletal muscle: insights on maturation-dependent loss of fiber infectivity for adenovirus and herpes simplex type 1 viral vectors. *Hum. Gene Ther.* **8**, 371–380.

Ferrari, G., Cusella-DeAngelis, G., Coletta, M. et al. (1998). Muscle regeneration by bone marrow derived myogenic progenitors. *Science* **279**, 1528–1530.

Fisher, K. J., Jooss, K., Alston, J. et al. (1997). Recombinant adeno-associated virus for muscle directed gene therapy. *Nat. Med.* **3**, 306–312.

Floyd, S. S., Clemens, P. R., Ontell, M. R. et al. (1998). Ex vivo gene transfer using adenovirus-mediated full-length dystrophin delivery to dystrophic muscles. *Gene Ther.* 5, 19–30.

Gautam, M., Noakes, P. G., Mudd, J. et al. (1995). Failure of postsynaptic specialization to develop at neuromuscular junctions of rapsyn-deficient mice. *Nature* 377, 232–236.

Gilbert, R., Nalbanoglu, J., Tinsley, J. M., Massie, B., Davies, K. E. and Karpati, G. (1998) Efficient utrophin expression following adenovirus gene transfer in dystrophic muscle. *Biochem. Biophys. Res. Commun.* 242, 244–247.

Glass, D. J. and Yancopoulos, G. D. (1997). Sequential roles of agrin, MuSK and rapsyn during neuromuscular junction formation. *Curr. Opin. Neurol.* 7, 379–384.

Greelish, J. P., Su, L. T., Lankford, E. B. et al. (1999). Stable restoration of the sarcoglycan complex in dystrophic muscle perfused with histamine and a recombinant adeno-associated viral vector. *Nat. Med.* 5, 439–443.

Gregorio, C. C., Granzier, H., Sorimachi, H. and Labeit, S. (1999). Muscle assembly: a titanic achievement? *Curr. Opin. Cell Biol.* 11, 18–25.

Guibinga, G. H., Lochmuller, H., Massie, B., Nalbantoglu, J., Karpati, G. and Petrof, B. J. (1998). Combinatorial blockade of calcineurin and CD28 signalling facilitates primary and secondary therapeutic gene transfer by adenovirus vectors in dystrophic (*mdx*) mouse muscles. *J. Virol.* 72, 4601–4609.

Gussoni, E., Blau, H. M. and Kunkel, L. M. (1997). The fate of individual myoblasts after transplantation into muscles of DMD patients. *Nat. Med.* 3, 970–977.

Harris, A. J. (1981). Embryonic growth and innervation of rat skeletal muscles. 1. Neural regulation of muscle fibre numbers. *Philos. Trans. R. Soc. Lond. Ser B* 293, 257–277.

Hauser, M. A., Amalfitano, A., KumarSingh, R., Hauschka, S. D. and Chamberlain, J. S. (1997). Improved adenoviral vectors for gene therapy of Duchenne muscular dystrophy. *Neuromusc. Disord.* 7, 277–283.

Henry, M. D. and Campbell, K. P. (1996). Dystroglycan – an extracellular-matrix receptor-linked to the cytoskeleton. *Curr. Opin. Cell Biol.* 8, 625–631.

Henry, M. D. and Campbell, K. P. (1998). A role for dystroglycan in basement membrane assembly. *Cell* 95, 859–970.

Herzog, R. W., Yang, E. Y., Couto, L. B. et al. (1999). Long-term correction of canine hemophilia B by gene transfer of blood coagulation factor IX mediated by adeno-associated viral vector. *Nat. Med.* 5, 56–63.

Hodges, B. L., Hayashi, Y. K., Nonaka, I., Wang, W., Arahata, K. and Kaufman, S. J. (1997). Altered expression of the alpha 7 beta 1 integrin in human and murine muscular dystrophies. *J. Cell Sci.* 110, 2873–2881.

Hoffman, E. P., Brown, R. H. and Kunkel, L. M. (1987). Dystrophin – the protein product of the Duchenne muscular dystrophy locus. *Cell* 51, 919–928.

Holt, K. H., Lim, L. E., Straub, V. et al. (1998). Functional rescue of the sarcoglycan complex in the BIO 14. 6 hamster using delta-sarcoglycan gene transfer. *Mol. Cell* 1, 841–848.

Hu, H. M., Serra, D. and Amalfitano, A. (1999). Persistence of an [E1(−), polymerase(−)] adenovirus vector despite transduction of a neoantigen into immune-competent mice. *Hum. Gene Ther.* 10, 355–364.

Hynes, R. O. (1992). Integrins: versatility, modulation and signaling in cell adhesion. *Cell* 69, 11–25.

Jooss, K., Yang, Y. P., Fisher, K. J. and Wilson, J. M. (1998). Transduction of dendritic cells by DNA viral vectors directs the immune response to transgene products in muscle fibers. *J. Virol.* 72, 4212–4223.

Karpati, G., Pari, G. and Molnar, M. J. (1999). Molecular therapy for genetic muscle diseases – status 1999. *Clin. Genet.* 55, 1–8.

Kelly, A. M. and Zacks, S. I. (1969a). The histogenesis of rat intercostal muscle. *J. Cell Biol.* 42, 135–153.

Kelly, A. M. and Zacks, S. I. (1969b). The fine structure of motor endplate morphogenesis. *J. Cell Biol.* 42, 154–169.

Khurana, T. S., Hoffman, E. P. and Kunkel, L. M. (1990). Identification of a chromosome-6–encoded dystrophin-related protein. *J. Biol. Chem.* 265, 16717–16720.

Landon, D. N. (1992). Skeletal muscle – normal morphology, development and innervation. In: *Skeletal Muscle Pathology*, eds. F. L. Mastaglia and Lord Walton of Detchant, pp. 1–94. Edinburgh: Churchill Livingstone.

Lassar, A. and Munsterberg, A. (1994). Wiring diagrams – regulatory circuits and the control of skeletal myogenesis. *Curr. Opin. Cell Biol.* 6, 432–442.

Law, P. K., Goodwin, T. G., Fang, Q. et al. (1997a). Human gene therapy with myoblast transfer. *Transplant. Proc.* 29, 2234–2237.

Law, P. K., Goodwin, T. G., Fang, Q. W. et al. (1997b). First human myoblast transfer therapy continues to show dystrophin after 6 years. *Cell Transplant.* 6, 95–100.

Li, Z., Mericskay, M., Agbulut, O. et al. (1997). Desmin is essential for the tensile strength and integrity of myofibrils but not for myogenic commitment, differentiation, and fusion of skeletal muscle. *J. Cell Biol.* 139, 129–144.

Love, D. R., Hill, D. F., Dickson, G. et al. (1989). An autosomal transcript in skeletal-muscle with homology to dystrophin. *Nature* 339, 55–58.

Lu, J. R., Webb, R., Richardson, J. A. and Olson, E. N. (1999). MyoR: a muscle-restricted basic helix-loop-helix transcription factor that antagonizes the actions of MyoD. *Proc. Natl. Acad. Sci. USA* 96, 552–557.

Manilal, S., Sewry, C. A., Pereboev, A. et al. (1999). Distribution of emerin and lamins in the heart and implications for Emery–Dreifuss muscular dystrophy. *Hum. Mol. Genet.* 8, 353–359.

Marshall, D. J. and Leiden, J. M. (1998). Recent advances in skeletal-muscle-based gene therapy. *Curr. Opin. Genet. Dev.* 8, 360–365.

Martin, A. R. (1994). Amplification of neuromuscular transmission by postjunctional folds. *Proc. R. Soc. Ser. B* 258, 321–326.

Mauro, A. L. (1961). Satellite cell of skeletal muscle fibres. *J. Biophys. Biochem. Cytol.* 9, 493–495.

Mayans, O., van der Ven, P. F. M., Wilm, M. et al. (1998). Structural basis for activation of the titin kinase domain during myofibrillogenesis. *Nature* 395, 863–869.

McClean, W. H. and Lane, E. B. (1995). Intermediate filaments in disease. *Curr. Opin. Cell Biol.* **7**, 118–125.

McHowell, J. M., Fletcher, S., Ohara, A., Johnsen, R. D., Lloyd, F. and Kakulas, B. A. (1998). Direct dystrophin and reporter gene transfer into dog muscle in vivo. *Muscle Nerve* **21**, 159–165.

Menke, A. and Jockusch, H. (1991). Decreased osmotic stability of dystrophin-less muscle-cells from the *mdx* mouse. *Nature* **349**, 69–71.

Menke, A., Brinkmeier, H., Naumann, T., Rudel, R. and Jockusch, H. (1993). Duchenne myotubes are more susceptible to hypoosmotic shock than dystrophin expressing human controls. *J. Musc. Res. Cell Motil.* **14**, 258–259.

Minetti, C., Tanji, K. and Bonilla, E. (1992). Immunological study of vinculin in Duchenne muscular-dystrophy. *Neurology* **42**, 1751–1754.

Monahan, P. E., Samulski, R. J., Tazelaar, J. et al. (1998). Direct intramuscular injection with recombinant AAV vectors results in sustained expression in a dog model of haemophilia. *Gene Ther.* **5**, 40–49.

Montgomery, R. D. (1962). Growth of human striated muscle. *Nature* **195**, 194–196.

Moore, S. E., and Walsh, F. S. (1986). Nerve dependent regulation of neural cell-adhesion molecule expression in skeletal-muscle. *Neuroscience* **18**, 499–505.

Mues, A., van der Ven, P. F. M., Young, P., Furst, D. O. and Gautel, M. (1998). Two immunoglobulin-like domains of the Z-disc portion of titin interact in a conformation-dependent way with telethonin. *FEBS Lett.* **428**, 111–114.

Murphy, S. and Dickson, G. (1999). Gene therapy approaches to Duchenne muscular dystrophy. In: *Gene Therapy Technologies and Regulations: From Laboratory to Clinic*, ed. A. Meager. Chichester, UK: Wiley.

Nagano, A., Koga, R., Ogawa, M. et al. (1996). Emerin deficiency at the nuclear membrane in patients with Emery–Dreifuss muscular dystrophy. *Nat. Genet.* **12**, 254–259.

Nalbantoglu, J., Pari, G., Karpati, G. and Holland, P. C. (1999). Expression of the primary coxsackie and adenovirus receptor is downregulated during skeletal muscle maturation and limits the efficacy of adenovirus-mediated gene delivery to muscle cells. *Hum. Gene Ther.* **10**, 1009–1019.

Ohtsuka, Y., Udaka, K., Yamashiro, Y., Yagita, H. and Okumura, K. (1998). Dystrophin acts as a transplantation rejection antigen in dystrophin-deficient mice: implication for gene therapy. *J. Immunol.* **160**, 4635–4640.

Ono, Y., Shimada, H., Sorimachi, H. et al. (1998). Functional defects of a muscle-specific calpain, p94, caused by mutations associated with limb-girdle muscular dystrophy type 2A. *J. Biol. Chem.* **273**, 17073–17078.

Ontell, M. and Kozeka, K. (1984). The organogenesis of murine striated muscle: a cytoarchitectural study. *Am. J. Anat.* **171**, 133–148.

Pardo, J., Siliciano, D. and Craig, S. (1983). A vinculin-containing cortical lattice in skeletal muscle. Transverse lattice elements ('costameres') mark sites of attachment between myofibrils and the sarcolemma. *Proc. Natl. Acad. Sci. USA* **80**, 1008–1012.

Parrish, E., Peltekian, E., Dickson, G., Epstein, A. L. and Garcia, L. (1999). Cell engineering for muscle gene therapy: extemporaneous production of retroviral vector packaging macrophages using defective herpes simplex virus type 1 vectors harbouring *gag, pol, env* genes. *Cytotechnology* **30**, 173–180.

Parton, R. G., Way, M., Zorzi, N. and Stang, E. (1997). Caveolin-3 associates with developing T-tubules during muscle differentiation. *J. Cell Biol.* **136**, 137–154.

Partridge, T. A. (1997). Untitled – Response. *Cell Transplant.* **6**, 198.

Partridge, T. A. and Davies, K. E. (1995). Myoblast-based gene therapies. *Br. Med. Bull.* **51**, 123–137.

Partridge, T. A., Morgan, J. E, Coulton, G. R., Hoffman, E. P. and Kunkel, L. M. (1989). Conversion of mdx myofibres from dystrophin negative to positive by injection of normal myoblasts. *Nature* **337**, 176–179.

Pasternak, C., Wong, S. and Elson, E. L. (1995). Mechanical function of dystrophin in muscle-cells. *J. Cell Biol.* **128**, 355–361.

Patton, B. L., Chiu, A. Y. and Sanes, J. R. (1998). Synaptic laminin prevents glial entry into the synaptic cleft. *Nature* **393**, 698–701.

Pelin, K., Hilpela, P., Donner, K. et al. (1999). Mutations in the nebulin gene associated with autosomal recessive nemaline myopathy. *Proc. Natl. Acad. Sci. USA* **96**, 2305–2310.

Peng, H. B., Xie, H., Rossi, S. and Rotundo, R. (1999). Acetylcholinesterase clustering at the neuromuscular junction involves perlecan and dystroglycan. *J. Cell Biol.* **145**, 911–921.

Petrof, B. J., Shrager, J. B., Stedman, H. H., Kelly, A. M. and Sweeney, H. L. (1993). Dystrophin protects the sarcolemma from stresses developed during muscle-contraction. *Proc. Natl. Acad. Sci. USA* **90**, 3710–3715.

Porter, G. A., Dmytrenko, G. M., Winkelmann, J. C. and Bloch, R. J. (1992). Dystrophin colocalizes with beta-spectrin in distinct subsarcolemmal domains in mammalian skeletal-muscle. *J. Cell Biol.* **117**, 997–1005.

Qu, Z. Q., Balkir, L., van Deutekom, J. T., Robbins, P. D., Pruchnic, R. and Huard, J. (1998). Development of approaches to improve cell survival in myoblast transfer therapy. *J. Cell Biol.* **142**, 1257–1267.

Rawls, A., Valdez, M., Zhang, W., Richardson, J., Klein, W. and Olson, E. (1999). Overlapping functions of the myogenic bHLH genes for MRF4 and MyoD revealed in double mutant mice. *Development* **125**, 2349–2358.

Richard, I., Roudaut, C., Saenz, A. et al. (1999). Calpainopathy – a survey of mutations and polymorphisms. *Am. J. Hum. Genet.* **64**, 1524–1540.

Ruegg, M. A. and Bixby, J. L. (1998). Agrin orchestrates synaptic differentiation at the vertebrate neuromuscular junction. *TINS* **21**, 22–27.

Sanes, J. R., Apel, E. D., Burgess, R. W. et al. (1998). Development of the neuromuscular junction: genetic analysis in mice. *J. Physiol. (Paris)* **92**, 167–172.

Sealock, R., Butler, M. H., Kramarcy, N. R. et al. (1991). Localization of dystrophin relative to acetylcholine-receptor domains in electric tissue and adult and cultured skeletal muscle. *J. Cell Biol.* **113**, 1133–1144.

Stromer, M. H. (1995). Immunocytochemistry of the muscle cell cytoskeleton. *Microsc. Res. Tech.* **31**, 95–105.

Takekura, H., Sun, X. and Franzini-Armstrong, C. (1994). Development of the excitation–contraction coupling apparatus in skeletal muscle: peripheral and internal calcium release units are formed sequentially. *J. Musc. Res. Cell Motil.* **15**, 102–118.

Thomas, G. D., Sander, M., Lau, K. S., Huang, P. L., Stull, J. T. and Victor, R. G. (1998). Impaired metabolic modulation of alpha-adrenergic vasoconstriction in dystrophin-deficient skeletal muscle. *Proc. Natl. Acad. Sci. USA* **95**, 15090–15095.

Thomson, L. (1992). Cell transplant results under fire. *Science* **257**, 472.

Tinsley, J. (1998). Utrophin or dystrophin: which is the better potential gene therapeutics agent for Duchenne muscular dystrophy? *Curr. Res. Mol. Therapeut.* **1**, 695–701.

Tinsley, J. M., Blake, D. J., Zuellig, R. and Davies, K. E. (1994). Increasing complexity of the dystrophin-associated protein complex. *Proc. Natl. Acad. Sci. USA* **91**, 8307–8313.

Tinsley, J. M., Potter, A., Phelps, S. R., Fisher, R., Trickett, J. I. and Davies, K. E. (1996). Amelioration of the dystrophic phenotype of *mdx* mice using a truncated utrophin transgene. *Nature* **384**, 349–353.

Tinsley, J., Deconinck, N., Fisher, R. et al. (1998). Expression of full-length utrophin prevents muscular dystrophy in *mdx* mice. *Nat. Med.* **4**, 1441–1444.

Tokuyasu, K. T., Maher, P. A. and Singer, S. J. (1985). Distributions of vimentin and desmin in developing chick myotubes in vivo. II Immuno-electron microscopic study. *J. Cell Biol.* **100**, 1157–1166.

Vilquin, J. T., Guerette, B., Puymirat, J. et al. (1999). Myoblast transplantation leads to the expression of the laminin alpha 2 chain in normal and dystrophic (*dy/dy*) mouse muscles. *Gene Ther.* **6**, 792–800.

Vincent, N., Ragot, T., Gilgenkrantz, H. et al. (1993). Long term correction of mouse dystrophic degeneration by adenovirus-mediated transfer of a mini-dystrophin gene. *Nat. Genet.* **5**, 130–134.

Volk, T., Fessler, L. I. and Fessler, J. H. (1990). A role for integrin in the formation of sarcomeric cytoarchitecture. *Cell* **63**, 525–536.

Wells, D. J., Wells, K. E., Asante, E. A. et al. (1995). Expression of human full-length and minidystrophin in transgenic mdx mice – implications for gene-therapy of duchenne muscular-dystrophy. *Hum. Mol. Genet.* **4**, 1245–1250.

Williamson, R. A., Henry, M. D., Daniels, K. J. et al. (1997). Dystroglycan is essential for early embryonic development: disruption of Reichert's membrane in Dag1-null mice. *Hum. Mol. Genet.* **6**, 831–841.

Wilson, S. J., Mcewan, J. C., Sheard, P. W. and Harris, A. (1992). Early stages of myogenesis in a large mammal: formation of successive generations of myotubes in sheep tibialis cranialis muscle. *J. Musc. Res. Cell Motil.* **13**, 534–550.

Xiao, X. A., Li, J. A., Samulski, R. J. (1996). Efficient long-term gene transfer into muscle tissue of immunocompetent mice by adeno-associated virus vector. *J. Virol.* **72**, 8098–8108.

Yuasa, K., Miyagoe, Y., Yamamoto, K., Nabeshima, Y., Dickson, G. and Takeda, S. (1998). Effective restoration of dystrophin-associated proteins in vivo by adenovirus-mediated transfer of truncated dystrophin cDNAs. *FEBS Lett.* **425**, 329–336.

Zhang, P. M., Wong, C., Liu, D., Finegold, M., Harper, J. W. and Elledge, S. J. (1999). p21(CIP1) and p57(KIP2) control muscle differentiation at the myogenin step. *Genes Dev.* **13**, 213–224.

4

The molecular basis of muscle disease

Louise V. B. Anderson

Introduction

When myoblasts fuse to become myotubes and, eventually, mature muscle fibres, the organization and control of gene and protein expression changes. While myoblasts are single cells with individual nuclei that are capable of division, mature muscle fibres are multinucleate syncytia, which have turned from division to differentiation. The degree of coordination that is required for effective gene expression becomes very obvious when one considers that a 1 cm segment from a single muscle fibre may contain over 1000 myonuclei. Terminally differentiated fibres have particular problems: they are very large (a single fibre from a human sartorius muscle may be over 30 cm long with a volume of cytoplasm that totals several microlitres), very long lived (repairing rather than reproducing) and very complex, with a well-defined organization of overlapping thick and thin filaments to form the contractile apparatus. The fibres interact with nerves at neuromuscular junctions, and these regions require localized concentrations of particular proteins. Superimposed upon this is the need to respond to changing requirements and altered patterns of activity – after birth for example, or during intensive training for a sporting activity. The aim of this chapter is to describe how skeletal muscle generates diverse forms of protein to cope with these changing requirements, to review the categories of factors that may control or influence the choice of protein expressed and to highlight how abnormal gene and protein expression is implicated in muscle disease.

Unlike the prokaryotic genes of bacteria, the eukaryotic genes of higher animals have exons or expressed sequences that are interspersed with noncoding introns. Skeletal muscle contains the largest gene identified to date (dystrophin, ~2 500 000 base pairs (bp)), the longest intron (~180 000 bp) and the largest number of exons (~79). The gene with the largest number of exon permutations identified so far – 32 different combinations for exons 4–8 – occurs in one of the troponin T genes. Vertebrate striated muscle also has the longest known single-chain protein (titin, with a molecular mass of ~3000 kDa). Single titin molecules are long enough to stretch from the Z disc to the M line, a length of over 1 μm in resting muscle; they may form the template for the assembly of other proteins into the thick filament.

Individual nuclei may exert control over the proteins expressed in their immediate vicinity, and the restricted distribution of some proteins, particularly at neuromuscular junctions, led to the concept of 'nuclear domains' where protein synthesis was compartmentalized and controlled by individual nuclei within the syncytium (Pavlath et al., 1989). However, it now appears that a protein and its respective mRNA are not always found in exactly the same place, suggesting less-restricted control than once thought. Furthermore, recent evidence suggests that all the nuclei within a fibre do not express 'housekeeping' muscle genes (e.g. α-skeletal actin, troponin I slow) all the time. The number of transcriptionally active nuclei appears to vary with requirement (during development, following injury). Therefore, in a mature fibre, despite the uniform protein composition of the contractile apparatus along the length of the fibre, transcription is only occurring in a proportion of nuclei at any one time (Newlands et al., 1998).

The flow diagram in Fig. 4.1 indicates the hierarchical stages in the production of a protein, with the opportunities that can arise to generate diversity or alter expression. Genes that are encoded by mitochondrial DNA are not considered in this chapter. Each of the factors or mechanisms that can alter the diversity of protein expression is considered in turn in the following sections.

Chromosomes and DNA conformation

The DNA in metaphase chromosomes, such as those seen in a karyotype, is highly condensed relative to the extended linear length. Such highly coiled and condensed DNA, whether present in chromosomes or in the heterochromatin of interphase nuclei, is almost never transcriptionally active. Whereas the DNA in chromosomes and heterochromatin has a packing ratio in the range 1000–10 000, the DNA from which mRNAs are transcribed in interphase nuclei has a packing ratio of only 1–10. In more recent years, the term 'nuclear domains' has also been used to describe specific domains within nuclei whereby DNA is orientated so that related gene loci are close to each other. In this way the DNA containing groups of genes that are required in, for example, skeletal muscle will be spatially related within skeletal muscle nuclei. It is suggested that this encourages efficient synthesis and processing of related gene transcripts (Schul et al., 1998; Stein et al., 1998).

A classic example of the regulatory power of chromatin configuration is in X-chromosome inactivation, in which one of the two chromosomes in cells that are genetically female is rendered constitutively heterochromatic (appearing in the nucleus as 'Barr bodies') so that almost none of the genes on inactivated X chromosomes are transcribed. One practical aspect of X inactivation involves women who are carriers of X-linked diseases. In any cell, the active X chromosome may be either the normal or abnormal one. If, by chance, there is a non-random distribution and a high proportion of active abnormal X, the carriers themselves may show some features of the disease. Thus women who carry mutations of the dystrophin gene may manifest the clinical signs of muscular dystrophy (Hoffman et al., 1992). This may be particularly striking in female identical twin carriers, where one may manifest severe clinical symptoms while the other does not. The severely affected twin appears to have skewed or non-random X-inactivation patterns and a high proportion of their muscle fibres have the mutant X active (Lupski et al., 1991). The possible effects of X inactivation on dystrophin expression in female carriers are demonstrated in Fig. 4.2, which shows the normal uniform dystrophin labelling at the periphery of muscle fibres, the absence of dystrophin in the muscle of a patient with Duchenne muscular dystrophy (DMD), and a mixture of the two types of labelling in a manifesting carrier who has the normal X active in the dystrophin-positive fibres and the mutated X active in the dystrophin-negative fibres.

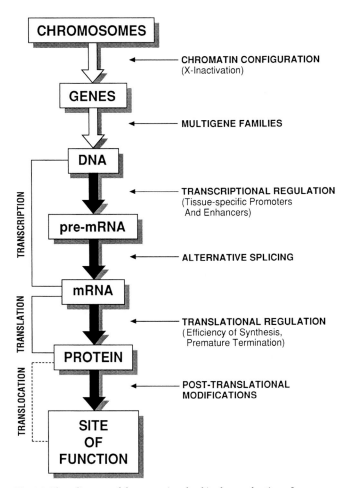

Fig. 4.1. Flow diagram of the stages involved in the production of a protein and the opportunities that arise to generate diversity or alter expression. Filled arrows indicate the formal stages of protein synthesis. Transcription and translation always occur; translocation may be required to transport a newly synthesized protein to its site of function.

Multigene families

In evolutionary terms, current multigene families arose from gene duplications that were found to be advantageous (or at least not disadvantageous) and were, therefore, selected in subsequent generations. In some instances, the genes remained clustered, but if the duplication event was followed by crossing over and recombination between nonhomologous chromosomes, the genes were translocated to a different chromosome. Pseudogenes are evolutionary 'blind alleys', which may be derived from a duplication event that then mutated into a gene

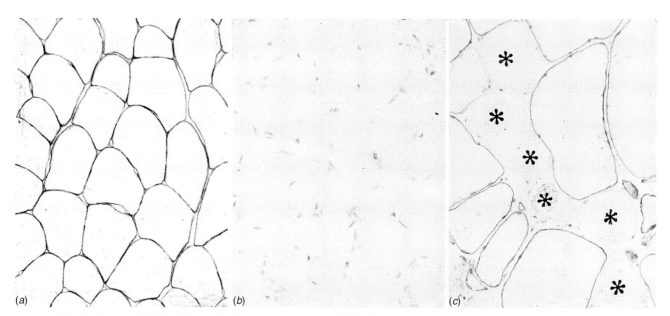

Fig. 4.2. Immunolabelling of dystrophin in transverse sections of skeletal muscle. (*a*) Control shows uniform labelling at the periphery of all fibres. (*b*) Labelling in a patient with Duchenne muscular dystrophy (DMD) who has a mutation of the Xp21 locus and dystrophin-negative muscle fibres. (*c*) A manifesting carrier of DMD has a mixture of dystrophin-positive and dystrophin-negative fibres. Fibres that do not express dystrophin (indicated with asterisks) have the normal X chromosome inactive; as a result, protein expression is controlled by the defective X chromosome bearing the DMD mutation. (Indirect peroxidase labelling, magnification ×165; photographs by courtesy of Dr Margaret Johnson and Mr Martin Barron.)

which was missing some or all of the signals required for successful transcription, splicing or translation (see p. 183 in Strachan and Read, 1996).

Skeletal muscle shares some common features with other excitable tissues (cardiac and smooth muscle, tissues of the nervous system) and many of the proteins in adult skeletal muscle have homologous counterparts (chains, subunits, isoforms) in these other tissues. One obvious way to generate protein diversity is to have different genes encoding related products, and skeletal muscle has many examples of multigene families.

Genes on different chromosomes

Members of the myosin superfamily are found in a multitude of organisms from humans to *Dictyostelium*, plants and yeast. Current nomenclature includes 12 classes, with class II containing the most common human skeletal, cardiac and smooth muscle isoforms (Sellers et al., 1996). Class VII contains an unconventional form of myosin (VIIA) that is implicated in human nonsyndromic recessive deafness and Usher 1B syndrome (Liu et al., 1997; Weil et al., 1997). Conventional myosin is a hexameric ATPase composed of two heavy chains (MHC), two nonphosphor-

ylated alkali light chains and two phosphorylatable regulatory light chains (MLC). Each of the three myosin subunits is encoded by multigene families that are specifically expressed according to tissue, developmental stage or physiological requirement. In humans, genes for skeletal muscle MHCs have been assigned to chromosomes 17 and 7, those for cardiac MHCs to chromosome 14, a smooth muscle isoform on chromosome 16, and nonmuscle isoforms to chromosomes 22 and 17. Among the MLCs, fast skeletal MLC1/3 is assigned to chromosome 2, cardiac MLCs have been mapped to chromosomes 3, 12 and 17, with a cardiac-like isoform assigned to chromosome 8 (see OMIM http://www.ncbi.nlm.nih.gov/omim).

Other examples of human multigene families with protein isoforms in muscle include actin, α-actinin, tropomyosin, the troponins, the acetylcholine receptor (AChR) subunits, various ion channels, the caveolins, extracellular matrix proteins (including the laminins, the tenascins and collagen) and several cell adhesion molecules (including the cadherins and the integrins). Among the different chromosomes, chromosome 17 has the largest concentration of genes that are expressed in muscle, but analysis within cytogenetic bands reveals that locations 6p21, 10q22, 12q24, 14q31 and 19p13 have a significant excess of such genes. However, only about 3% of the currently known genes are expressed exclusively in muscle (Bortoluzzi et al., 1998).

Gene clusters

Some members of gene families are organized together on the same chromosome, rather than being on different chromosomes. In humans, the genes for several adult, perinatal and embryonic isoforms of skeletal muscle MHC (*MYH1, MYH2, MYH3, MYH4* and *MYH8*) are clustered on the short arm of chromosome 17 while those for both the α- and β-isoforms of cardiac MHC (*MYH6* and *MYH7*) are assigned to the long arm of chromosome 14. Although the skeletal MHC genes are physically linked to each other and are sequentially expressed during development, they do not appear to be activated in a coordinate manner, and transcription of each gene is independently regulated, as in the corresponding rodent gene cluster. The genes coding for the α-, γ- and δ-subunits of the skeletal muscle AChR have all been localized to a region of 2q and the genes for a group of myogenic determination factors (*myf*) are also clustered, on chromosome 12 (see OMIM http://www.ncbi.nlm.nih.gov/omim).

Genes within genes

Where does an isoform end and a new protein begin? Isoforms are derived from a common gene and generally represent subtle variations on a theme with an overall structure/function that is not vastly different from the basic molecule. Alternatively, proteins that are products of different genes but which share a family resemblance in terms of structure or function are said to be homologues. Therefore α-actinin, α- and β-spectrin, dystrophin and utrophin are homologous members of the family of rod-like actin-binding proteins. Several examples now exist, however, of proteins that are encoded by parts of the same gene but which have such vastly different size, structure (and therefore presumably function) and tissue distribution that it is tempting to regard them as different proteins. Many of these 'genes within genes' result from rather extreme forms of alternative splicing and are initiated by their own promoters.

Calcitonin and calcitonin gene-related peptide (CGRP) are two products from the same gene, primarily derived by alternative splicing (Fig. 4.3). Calcitonin is produced in the thyroid, and acts as a circulating regulator of calcium homeostasis, whereas CGRP is produced by neurons and is locally active as a neuromodulator and neurohormone. The sequence for the mature calcitonin polypeptide is entirely contained within exon 4 of the gene, whereas the

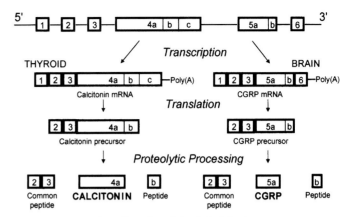

Fig. 4.3. Representation of how the calcitonin/calcitonin gene-related protein (CGRP) gene produces two different protein products via a combination of alternative splicing, different 3′ polyadenylation sites and proteolytic processing.

protein sequence for CGRP is entirely within exon 5 (Rosenfeld et al., 1983). An intronic element after exon 4 may regulate polyadenylation of an embedded alternative 3′ terminal exon to produce calcitonin in a tissue-specific manner (Lou and Gagel, 1998).

Dystrophin, the protein product of the gene that is defective in Duchenne/Becker muscular dystrophy (Hoffman et al., 1987) has a 'standard' molecule of about 427 kDa, which is primarily expressed in skeletal and cardiac muscle and, to a lesser extent, in smooth muscle and brain. However, by utilizing a set of eight different promoters, alternative polyadenylation sites and alternative exon splicing, a whole range of protein molecules of various sizes are produced in different tissues. Other examples of alternative gene products include calspermin and telokin. Calspermin is a small acidic protein identified in rat testis that represents the independent expression of the C-terminus of a calcium/calmodulin-dependent protein kinase found in cerebellar granule cells (Ohmstede et al., 1991). Similarly, the C-terminal domain of smooth muscle MLC kinase (MLCK) is expressed as one or more separate proteins named telokin (Ito et al., 1989) or kinase-related protein (Collinge et al., 1992).

Recently, a preliminary study identified a small independent transcript (designated ORF2) within intron 11 of the gene for dystrophin. Interestingly, the transcript is also expressed in cardiac and skeletal muscle like dystrophin (Ferlini and Muntoni, 1998). Similarly, the gene encoding the vesicular acetylcholine transporter is embedded within the first intron of the gene encoding choline acetyltransferase (Mallet et al., 1998). Both of these examples involve transcription in the same orientation. In contrast, three

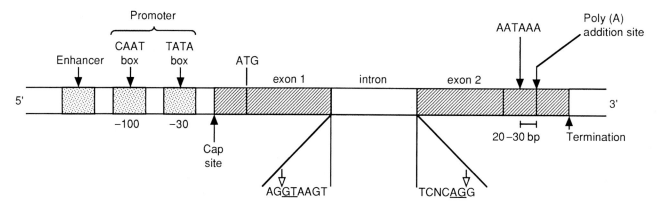

Fig. 4.4. Organization of a class II gene. A typical gene is characterized by a promoter region at the 5′ end and the presence of introns. In some cases, the CAAT and TATA consensus sequences are absent. Transcription factor-binding sites are found at the 5′ end of the gene as are many enhancer elements. The exon-intron splice sites are indicated with open arrows. The left junction (splice donor) and right junction (splice acceptor) consensus sequences are shown with the most invariant dinucleotides underlined. See text for other details. (This diagram is modified from an illustration in *Gene Structure and Transcription – In Focus*, 2nd edn, ed. Beebee, T. and Burke, J. (1992), with permission of IRL/Oxford University Press.)

small genes, each with two exons, have been located within intron 27 of the neurofibromatosis type 1 gene (*NF1*). In this case, however, the genes are transcribed from the opposite DNA strand to that used for *NF1* (i.e. the *NF1* anti-sense strand) (see p. 160 of Strachan and Read, 1996).

Control of transcription

Eukaryotic genes are of three types, each transcribed by a different RNA polymerase. Class I genes are tandemly linked ribosomal RNA genes, which are clustered in the nucleolus. Classical class II genes produce mRNA and are characterized by a promoter region at the 5′ end and the presence of introns. Enhancers are commonly found at the 5′ end, although they may be internal or downstream of the gene (Fig. 4.4). Transcription factor-binding sites are also found at the 5′ end of the gene. Class III genes, which includes those producing transfer RNA (tRNA), are physically small and characterized by internal promoters (reviewed by Beebee and Burke, 1992; Lewin, 1997).

Transcription of class II genes starts with the core promoter, which is located just upstream of the transcript start site or 'cap site', so named because the 5′ ends of eukaryotic mRNAs are modified or capped by the addition of a methylated G residue (see Fig. 4.4). Elements in the promoter are recognized, and bound in turn, by the initiation proteins TFIID, TFIIA, TFIIB (the class-specific RNA polymerase pol II), TFIIE and TFIIF. Once assembled, this very large complex (with a total molecular mass of over 900 kDa) is poised to unwind the DNA template locally and initiate transcription. Initiation requires the hydrolysis of an ATP molecule and the formation of a 'rapid start complex'. Elongation of the primary transcript commences with the phosphorylation of pol II and is accompanied by the binding of another protein, TFIIS. The rate of transcription depends upon the binding of yet more regulatory factors. A sequence that codes for the polyadenylation signal (AATAAA) is found just before the end of the transcript. The end of the pre-mRNA is clipped and a stabilizing poly(A) tail is added to the mature mRNA about 20–30 bp after this signal (see Fig. 4.4).

Cis-acting elements

Although the same genes are present in all cells, utilization of specific *cis*-acting DNA sequences and *trans*-acting factors allows gene transcription to be regulated in a tissue- or developmental stage-specific manner. *Cis*-acting modulators exert an effect on their own gene (e.g. promoters and enhancers), whereas *trans*-acting factors or proteins are not an integral part of the gene themselves. Among the best characterized of the general *cis* elements are the TATA box (frequently required for the correct initiation at the transcription start site) and the CAAT and/or GC boxes (which play a role in controlling the frequency of initiation) (Beebee and Burke, 1992; Strachan and Read, 1996). Recent studies have suggested that elements around the TATA box may confer some tissue-specific regulation in muscle, thereby converting a generic promoter to a more specific one (Diagana et al., 1997). Specific patterns of DNA methylation around promoter regions may also play a role in controlling tissue- or developmental-specific promotion of gene expression (Edwards, 1990).

A number of muscle-associated regulatory elements have been described. The best characterized of these is the CArG box, originally identified in the promoters of cardiac and skeletal muscle α-actin but found subsequently, by deletion and mutational analysis, to be required for the muscle-specific activation of genes for MLC, troponin T, troponin C, creatine kinase and dystrophin (Wasserman and Fickett, 1998). Multiple CArG boxes may be present, which interact with each other and with the initiating TATA sequence. In addition to the conventional position upstream of the cap site, cis-acting enhancers may also be found after the first exon (Klamut et al., 1996), where they may direct expression in skeletal versus cardiac muscle (Fabre-Suver and Hauschka, 1996; Klamut et al., 1997) and at the 3' end of the gene (Donoghue et al., 1988). Another potentially 'muscle-specific' promoter element is the MCAT (muscle-CAT) consensus CATTCCT. Disruption of only one or two of these sequence elements can abolish the ability to direct muscle-specific transcription (Mar and Ordahl, 1988).

The promoters or enhancers of many muscle genes also contain a consensus sequence referred to as an E-box (CANNTG), which forms the binding site for many of the basic helix-loop-helix (bHLH) regulatory factors described in the next section. Multiple E-boxes or their homologues are found in the 5' regions of genes for MHC, troponin I, muscle creatine kinase and the AChR subunits. The gene for the immature AChR γ-subunit contains two adjacent CANNTG sequence motifs that appear to be essential for muscle-specific transcriptional activity. The gene for the mature ε-subunit carries only a single CANNTG motif, which is not required for the positive expression in muscle cells but is necessary for repressing transcription in non-muscle cells (Numberger et al., 1991). Promoter elements may also play a role in restricting transcription to synaptic nuclei (Klarsfeld et al., 1999). Within the gene for utrophin, the promoter contains the core sequences of both an N-box and an E-box, elements of which appear to direct the synapse-specific expression of AChR subunits by enhancing the expression at the neuromuscular junction while acting as a 'silencer' in the extrajunctional regions (Dennis et al., 1996).

Many tissue-specific promoters are associated with alternative 5' exons. Figure 4.5 illustrates the eight promoters that have been identified to date for dystrophin isoforms (the isoforms are named by size and, for full-size forms, location, e.g. Dp427m is the dystrophin protein of 427 kDa found in muscle). The most 5' promoter (initiating isoform Dp427l) was identified in lymphoblastoid cells,

although dystrophin protein is not detected there (Nishio et al., 1994). The next promoter is active in brain, and transcripts for this isoform, Dp427c, have been localized to cortical and hippocampal neurons (Nudel et al., 1989); however the loss of this promoter does not seem to be associated with intellectual impairment (Den Dunnen et al., 1991). The brain promoter appears to be quite restricted in its activity compared with the next promoter (initiating the major Dp427m isoform), which is active in skeletal, cardiac and smooth muscle and, to a lesser extent, in some neurons and cultured glial cells. This promoter is 'leaky', and low-level transcription, considered to be illegitimate or ectopic, may occur in fibroblasts and lymphocytes (Chelly et al., 1990). Mutations involving the dystrophin muscle promoter have been implicated in X-linked dilated cardiomyopathy, a disease without the extensive skeletal muscle involvement of a muscular dystrophy (Muntoni et al., 1995a). The Dp427m muscle promoter contains a TATA box, a GC-rich motif and several conserved motifs that have been found in muscle-specific genes (Klamut et al., 1990; Gilgenkrantz et al., 1992). In contrast, the brain promoter does not contain any of these elements and may use a less-defined 'initiator' element instead (Makover et al., 1991). The fourth 5' promoter (initiating Dp427p) is located in the first intron of the Dp427m gene and controls expression in the cerebellum, particularly in Purkinje cells (Górecki et al., 1992). Transcripts from the Dp427p promoter have been found to be subject to alternative splicing that is developmentally regulated in the brain (cortex as well as cerebellum), and low levels were found differentially expressed in skeletal versus cardiac muscle tissues. This indicates that Dp427p may have a broader scope of expression, regulation and complexity than previously appreciated (Holder et al., 1996). In total, dystrophin expression levels in brain are 1–2% of those in muscle. Among the smaller isoforms, Dp260 is initiated with a promoter located in intron 29 of the major muscle isoform. It was identified in the retina after observing reduced b-wave amplitude in the dark-adapted state in boys with DMD. Dp260 expression is found in the outer plexiform layer of the retina and has also been reported in brain and cardiac muscle (D'Souza et al., 1995). The Dp140 transcript is expressed from a promoter located within intron 44 of Dp427m, yet the first translated exon is number 51; therefore, unlike all the other isoforms it has no unique N-terminus. Dp140 is found throughout the central nervous system and in kidney, but not in skeletal or cardiac muscle (Lidov et al., 1995; Lidov and Kunkel, 1998). Dp116 is expressed from a promoter in intron 55 of Dp427m and appears exclusively in adult peripheral nerve, along the Schwann cell membrane (Byers et al., 1993). The Dp71

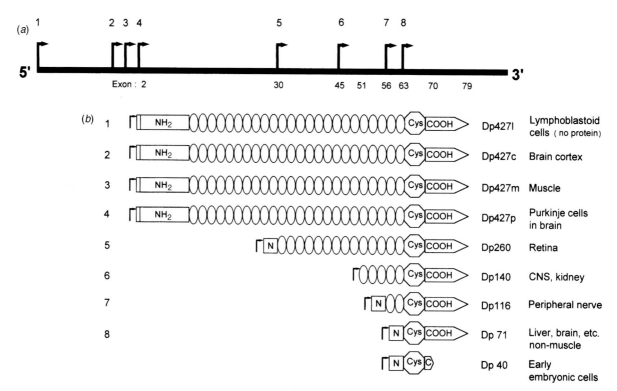

Fig. 4.5. Diagrammatic representation of the eight alternative promoters and major products of the dystrophin gene. (*a*) The relative positions of the promoters are shown along the gene. (*b*) A schematic of the molecules produced. The isoforms are named after their size and, for the full-size forms, location (i.e. Dp427m is the dystrophin protein of 427 kDa found in muscle). The unique first exons (coding for up to 31 amino acid residues) are indicated by boxes after the promoter arrows. The largest isoforms then share a common N-domain (NH$_2$) coded by exons 2–10. Ovals represent up to 24 triple-helical repeats (exons 10–64), and this is followed by a region (exons 65–67) that is relatively rich in cystein residues (Cys), terminating in a C-domain (COOH) coded by exons 68–79. The numerous variations produced by cassette-type alternative splicing are not shown. See text for further detail.

isoform promoter is located in intron 62 of Dp427m and is subject to alternative splicing at the C-terminus (Rapaport et al., 1992; Austin et al., 1995). Dp71 is not found in adult skeletal muscle but may be more abundant than Dp427m in brain, tissues containing smooth muscle (stomach, lung, skin and testis) and many fetal tissues. It is also found in tissues where the full-length protein is not generally synthesized: liver, kidney and spleen, plus hepatoma, lymphoblastoid and Schwannoma cell lines (Bar et al., 1990; Blake et al., 1992; Rapaport et al., 1992). Dp71 may also have a special role in retinal function, since it has recently been specifically localized to the inner limiting membrane of the retina, in addition to Dp260 in the outer plexiform layer (Howard et al., 1998). Involvement of Dp71 with the actin cytoskeleton during myogenesis also suggests a role for Dp71 during development that is distinct from Dp427m (Howard et al., 1999). Furthermore, it has been suggested that altered expression of smaller isoforms that occur in the brain (Dp71, Dp140) may be related to the cognitive

impairment associated with DMD (Moizard et al., 1998). Dp40 uses the Dp71 promoter in intron 62 plus an alternative polyadenylation site located after exon 70 of Dp427m. This isoform is expressed in the same tissues as Dp71, but the specific Dp40 transcript has also been uniquely identified in early embryonic stem cells (Tinsley et al., 1993). Dp40 is also known as apo-dystrophin-3, apo-dystrophin-1 being Dp71 and apo-dystrophin-2 being Dp116. An excellent summary of the generation and expression of all the dystrophin isoforms identified to date is available on the Leiden Muscular Dystrophy pages© (http://www.dmd.nl/).

Trans-acting factors

Of the *trans*-factors that may bind to promoter or enhancer elements in muscle, the best studied is the family of myogenic regulatory factors (MRFs) that includes MyoD, myogenin, Myf5 and MRF4. The genes for these four proteins have a common three-exon structure and are expressed exclusively in skeletal muscle cell lineages. They are part of the bHLH superfamily of regulatory transcription factors, which all have a DNA-binding basic sequence adjacent to a helix-loop-helix domain that is required for the formation of dimers. These proteins function in pairs to activate transcription by binding to their target sites. In muscle, the MRFs form heterodimers with other bHLH proteins, the ubiquitous E-proteins, and activate transcription by binding to the E-boxes (reviewed in Megeney and Rudnicki, 1995; Buonanno and Rosenthal, 1996). In addition, synergistic interactions with the myocyte enhancing factor-2 (MEF2) group of transcription factors may further refine the target site specificity of myogenic factors (Molkentin et al., 1995). Conversely, when another bHLH protein, Id (inhibitor of differentiation), binds to the E-protein E12, dimerization with MyoD family members is prevented and transcription is inhibited (Benezra et al., 1990). Proliferin, a protein with homology to prolactin and growth hormone, has also been identified as a selective inhibitor of bHLH *trans*-activators in the actin multigene family (Muscat et al., 1991).

Analysis of the MRFs during embryogenesis has revealed that MyoD and Myf5 are primary factors, as they are required for determination of myoblasts, while myogenin and MRF4 are secondary factors, since they appear to function during terminal differentiation (Megeney and Rudnicki, 1995). The effects of targeted disruption of the genes encoding these myogenic factors further emphasize their complex interactions. Mice with null mutations of the *myf5* locus have delayed myotome differentiation, but otherwise muscle development proceeds normally. Surprisingly, rib formation is also disrupted in these mice. Mice carrying a null mutation of the *myoD* locus have only defects of satellite cell regeneration. However, double knock-out mice, lacking both factors, have no skeletal muscle at all and are completely devoid of myoblasts. Disruption of the *myogenin* gene locus produces a more predictable phenotype in which the muscle beds contain myoblasts but terminal differentiation is largely blocked and muscles fail to form (reviewed in Buonanno and Rosenthal, 1996). Skeletal, cardiac and smooth muscle may each require different subprogrammes of gene regulation, involving complex patterns of activation or inhibition initiated by the binding of these transcription factors to specific promoters and enhancers (Firulli and Olson, 1997). Regeneration of skeletal muscle involves complicated interactions between the transcription factors and a variety of growth factors that stimulate or inhibit at the different stages of proliferation and differentiation (Chambers and McDermott, 1996).

RNA splicing

Constitutive splicing

Precise excision of intron sequences from the primary pre-mRNA transcript and concomitant ligation of the exons is accomplished in the nucleus through a sequence of splicing processes. In a simple gene, each exon present is incorporated into one mature mRNA transcript through the invariant joining of consecutive pairs of donor and acceptor splice sites, thereby producing a single gene product from each transcriptional unit (reviewed in Adams et al., 1996; Cooper and Mattox, 1997; Lewin, 1997). Clearly, any alteration in the amino acid sequences that mark the intron/exon boundaries could cause aberrant splicing in the mature transcript.

Alternative splicing

In many genes expressed in muscle, constitutive RNA splicing is enriched by varieties of alternative splicing that generate multiple forms of protein from a single gene (see reviews by Breitbart et al., 1987; Nadal-Ginard et al., 1991; Chabot, 1996). Figure 4.6 illustrates the various mechanisms that result in the production of alternative transcripts. Splicing enhancers have been identified that assist the splicing of introns containing weak splice sites. These appear to aid the inclusion of appropriate exons, possibly acting in a tissue-specific manner. Originally these elements were described as purine-rich exon sequences, but enhancers can also reside within introns, and nonpurine-rich enhancer elements have also been identified (Dye et al., 1998).

Combinatorial cassette exons

While exons that are included in all transcripts are constitutive, individual whole exons that may, or may not, be included are said to be combinatorial cassettes (Breitbart et al., 1987). Troponin T, which is a component of the Ca^{2+}-sensitive complex that regulates the interactions of tropomyosin with the actin filaments in striated muscle, contains several such exons. The rat fast skeletal troponin T gene contains a group of five exons that may be assembled together in 32 different combinations (Breitbart et al., 1987). The default splicing pattern is the exclusion of exons 4–8, and their inclusion is controlled by the state of differentiation and physiological demand. This extreme heterogeneity may be important in modulating interactions of troponin T within the troponin–tropomyosin complex, although several different transcripts may be detected at the same time in the same fibre (Breitbart and Nadal-Ginard, 1989).

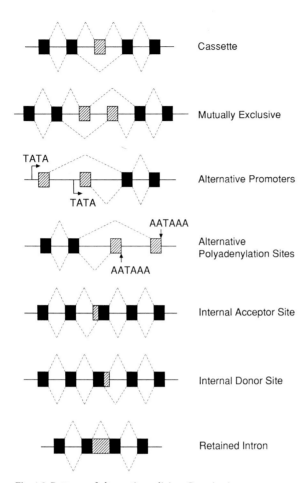

Fig. 4.6. Patterns of alternative splicing. Constitutive exons (black), alternative sequences (striped) and introns (solid lines) are spliced according to different pathways (dotted lines). Alternative promoters (TATA) and polyadenylation signals (AATAAA) are indicated. (This diagram has been redrawn and reproduced, with permission, from the *Annual Review of Biochemistry* Vol. 56, 1987, by Annual Reviews Inc.)

The neural cell adhesion molecule (NCAM) is expressed in mature neurons, glia and skeletal muscle, after transient expression in a number of early embryonic structures. In skeletal muscle, NCAM is implicated in several aspects of myogenesis including innervation and synaptogenesis. The human gene for NCAM is extensively spliced and processed in a tissue-specific manner, and a block of four exons (the smallest exon coding for a single amino acid) are spliced between exons 12 and 13 of the brain transcript to form a 'muscle-specific domain' in the extracellular domain of the molecule (Dickson et al., 1987). Vinculin is another protein associated with cell–cell interactions, and a larger form of the protein, meta-vinculin, is found only in

smooth and skeletal muscle. Like NCAM, this 'muscle specificity' is generated by the splicing of an additional exon into the basic transcript (Koteliansky et al., 1992). Similarly, a striated muscle-specific form of β_1-integrin, β_{1D}, is generated by the inclusion of an additional exon between 6 and 7 of the normal transcript (Zhidkova et al., 1995).

Agrin is an extracellular matrix protein that plays a central role in nerve–muscle synapse formation. It is highly concentrated in the synaptic basal lamina, where it is involved in AChR clustering. This activity is regulated by alternative splicing and the use of cassette exons in a region near the C-terminus. Four isoforms are generated: two are active in cluster formation by themselves but the other two require some form of interaction with proteoglycans in the basal lamina (e.g. α-dystroglycan, laminin, MuSK (a muscle-specific receptor tyrosine kinase), heparin) before they are active. The inclusion of an insert of eight amino acid residues at the 'z' splice site can enhance agrin's clustering activity over 1000-fold. The z insert is always accompanied by the presence of a four amino acid residue insert at the 'y' splice site (Ferns et al., 1992; Deyst et al., 1998). Agrin splice variants also play their role in collateral synaptogenic events such as the formation of presynaptic membrane folds and the localized transcription of AChR subunit mRNAs (Deyst et al., 1998; Meier et al., 1998a).

A number of alternatively spliced transcripts have been identified in the gene for dystrophin. In addition to promoters with initial exons, a number of splice variants have been detected in the C-terminal domain. These involve the removal of exons 68, 71, 78, 71–78, 71–72–78, 71–72–73–74 or 71–72–73–74–78, and the variation seems to be most extensive in nonmuscle tissues, particularly in the brain, kidney, retina and other synaptic sites, including Purkinje conduction fibres in the heart. Patterns of alternative splicing in the proximal half of the gene have also been identified (summarized on the Leiden Muscular Dystrophy pages© http://www.dmd.nl/).

Dystrophin is a very good example of a protein with many variants on a theme. However, the multiplicity of gene products is nothing compared with that of the neurexins. The neurexins are recently identified neuronal cell-surface proteins that are estimated to have more than 1000 isoforms, generated by alternative splicing of transcripts from six promoters in three genes. The different isoforms are expressed in various subsets of neurones within the brain (Missler et al., 1998). They share nearly identical, short, cytoplasmic C-terminal and transmembrane domains, exposing highly variable extracellular sequences on the cell surface. Neurexins are thought to be receptors for a number of cell-signalling proteins (e.g. neurexophi-lin), to act as cell-adhesion molecules or to interact with the extracellular matrix. They also bind to another group of cell-surface receptors, the neuroligins. The extensive alternative splicing in the neurexins might regulate their binding to ligands and increase the number of potential interactions (Missler and Sudhof, 1998).

Mutually exclusive exons

Exons that are never spliced together in the same transcript are mutually exclusive. Skeletal muscle tropomyosin contains α- and β-subunits which are assembled into homo- and heterodimers in variable proportions depending on the fibre type. The gene for human α-tropomyosin has two mutually exclusive versions of exon 5, one of which is expressed specifically in skeletal muscle (Graham et al., 1992). Other genes expressed in muscle that have mutually exclusive exons include MLC1–3, pyruvate kinase and phosphorylase kinase.

A number of different mechanisms have been proposed to account for alternative splice site selection in these genes. These include the relative strengths of 5′ and 3′ splice sites; intron size; the pyrimidine content of the 3′ splice site; the location, number and sequence of branch-points; intron sequences between a 3′ splice site and upstream branchpoint, exon sequences and sequence-specific RNA-binding proteins (Nadal-Ginard et al., 1991).

Alternative promoters and/or polyadenylation sites

Alternative 5′ and 3′ end sequences arise through the differential utilization of promoters or cleavage sites, each associated with their own exons. This can generate variability in the amino acid sequences of the N- and C-terminal domains, which, in turn, may regulate interactions with other proteins, in a tissue-specific manner (Sonenberg, 1996; Edwalds-Gilbert et al., 1997). In dystrophin, for example, a total of eight tissue-related promoters have been identified (see Fig. 4.5), with alternative 3′ exons generating other tissue and developmentally regulated isoforms. Similarly, calcitonin and CGRP utilize alternative polyadelylation sites (see Fig. 4.3).

Human erythrocyte and skeletal muscle β-spectrin are transcribed from the same gene, but in skeletal muscle the C-terminal exon of the erythrocyte form (which is involved in phosphorylation-dependent interactions of the α- and β-subunit) is spliced out and replaced with four longer exons (Winkelmann et al., 1990). The presence of such a different C-terminal domain in skeletal muscle β-spectrin may indicate an association with a different membrane protein complex to that found in erythrocytes. The use of alternative polyadenylation sites also confers distinct syn-aptic properties to α-dystrobrevin: the 84 kDa α-dystro-brevin-1 preferentially binds to utrophin at the neuromuscular junction, whereas the 65 kDa α-dystrobrevin-2 preferentially binds to dystrophin at the extrajunctional membrane as well as in the depths of the postjunctional folds (Blake et al., 1996; Peters et al., 1998).

Alternative acceptor and donor splice sites

Many of the examples already cited include the utilization of alternative splice sites. The alternative production of calcitonin in thyroid C cells and CGRP in neurons of the central and peripheral nervous system is primarily regulated by cis-active elements near the calcitonin-specific 3′-splice junction (Emeson et al., 1989). Similarly, the transcripts for erythroid and nonerythroid β-spectrin differ in C-terminal splice site selection (Winkelmann et al., 1990), some of the sodium channel isoforms in brain, cardiac and skeletal muscle utilize alternative donor splice sites (Schaller et al., 1992), as do isoforms of the AChR β-subunit (Goldman and Tamai, 1989).

Retained introns

Retained introns are not a very common occurrence in mammals, but examples may be found in the genes for fibronectin (Kornblihtt et al., 1996), for acetylcholineste-rase in haematopoietic cells (Li et al., 1991) and for several tumour-associated proteins (Goodison et al., 1998; Lupetti et al., 1998). In the nervous system, examples include the glial platelet-derived growth factor (Tong et al., 1987), tau microtubule-associated proteins (Sadot et al., 1994), a tyrosine phosphatase receptor that is involved in neural development (Zhang and Longo, 1995) and periaxin, a protein that appears to play a role in the initiation of myelin deposition in peripheral nerves (Dytrych et al., 1998).

Translation

Proteins are synthesized from the N- to the C-terminus on ribosomes that move along the mRNA. In eukaryotes, mRNA translation starts with Met-tRNA binding to the 40S subunit of a ribosome together with initiation factors and guanosine 5′-diphosphate (GDP). This initiation complex then binds the mRNA at the cap structure and scans along until the initiation codon AUG is reached (see Fig. 4.4). The 60S ribosomal subunit then binds and elongation of the polypeptide chain ensues. To become a substrate for protein synthesis, free amino acids are activated by coupling with the adenylic moiety of ATP and covalent linkage to tRNA via aminoacyl-tRNA synthetase. The resulting aminoacyl-tRNA is used by the ribosome as a substrate and the energy of the chemical bond between the amino acid residue and tRNA is used for forming a peptide bond (Spirin, 1986).

The efficiency of translation may depend on several factors, including sequences in the 5′ untranslated region immediately preceding the initiation codon transcript secondary structures formed in the vicinity of the initiation codon, and motifs in the 3′ untranslated region. Translational efficiency is a useful regulatory process. For example, although there are two genes for adult haemoglobin α-chain and only one for the β-chain, reduced efficiency of transcription and, particularly, of translation ensures that there is not a significant overproduction of α-chains for assembly with β-chains in the final $\alpha_2\beta_2$ complex (Arnstein and Cox, 1992). Similarly, increased iron levels stimulate the synthesis of ferritin, without any corresponding increase in ferritin mRNA, while decreased iron levels stimulate the production of transferrin receptor without effect on its mRNA (Strachan and Read, 1996).

Open reading frame

The instruction to synthesize each amino acid (or to terminate synthesis) is defined by a triplet of RNA nucleotides, or codon. The open reading frame is the name given to the alignment, usually starting with the AUG initiation codon, that will divide the mRNA nucleotide sequence into triplets which are potentially translatable (reviewed in Lewin, 1997).

In some genes, a truncated isoform of the full-length protein is produced by the introduction of a premature stop codon. Thus a novel secreted form of NCAM is produced in skeletal muscle and brain by the inclusion of a discrete exon which induces a premature in-frame stop codon. The truncated polypeptide lacks either of the C-terminal hydrophobic domains necessary for interaction with the plasma membrane (Gower et al., 1988). Similarly, vascular smooth muscle expresses a truncated isoform of the Na^+/K^+/ATPase α_1-subunit, which may play a role in active ion transport (Medford et al., 1991). Premature termination of translation is one of the most common forms of pathogenic mutation.

Co- and post-translational processing

During or following synthesis, polypeptide chains may be modified in various ways to produce mature forms of protein. Such processing may involve proteolytic cleavage; covalent alterations to the carbon chains of certain amino acids like proline, lysine or glutamic acid; or chemical sub-stitution of amino acid residues by sugars or acyl, carboxyl, alkyl, methyl, phosphate or sulphate groups (reviewed in Arnstein and Cox, 1992; Strachan and Read, 1996). In some cases, more than one class of processing takes place.

Proteolytic cleavage

Cleavage by proteolytic enzymes is a common processing event among the precursors of many hormones and enzymes (e.g. insulin, adrenocorticotrophin/β-lipotrophin) or neuroendocrine peptides (e.g. substance P, enkephalin) (see Hall, 1992). Most secreted proteins have a signal sequence that is cleaved following translocation across the outer cell membrane (Lewin, 1997). Proteins of the nuclear membrane may also have signal sequences that aid location. The gene for lamin A/C (defective in autosomal dominant Emery–Dreifuss muscular dystrophy) produces two protein products by alternative splicing: prelamin A and lamin C. Prelamin A is isoprenylated at a consensus cysteine residue at the C-terminus and this appears to be required before cleavage of the C-terminal tail and insertion of the mature lamin A protein into the nuclear membrane (Lin and Worman, 1993).

In skeletal muscle, dystroglycan is processed into two of the dystrophin-associated glycoproteins (DAGs) that form part of the complex at the muscle membrane (Straub and Campbell, 1997; Durbeej et al., 1998). A 97 kDa precursor polypeptide is synthesized, which is then split into two polypeptides of about 56 and 41 kDa (Fig. 4.7). The 56 kDa polypeptide undergoes extensive O-glycosylation, forming a mature 156 kDa protein that is an extracellular laminin-binding component of the DAG complex. A putative N-terminal signal peptide, which may be used to ensure translocation, may also be cleaved. The 41 kDa polypeptide undergoes some N-glycosylation to form a mature 43 kDa protein with a single transmembrane domain and a cytoplasmic tail (Ibraghimov-Beskrovnaya et al., 1992).

Modification of side chains

Various covalent modifications to amino acid residues occur in muscle proteins. Disulphide bonds, between or within chains, are important for the tertiary and quaternary structure of some proteins. The anchorage of acetylcholinesterase to the extracellular matrix is achieved via disulphide bridges (Silman and Futerman, 1987). The hydroxylation of certain proline and lysine residues occurs in the biosynthesis of collagen for the extracellular matrix of muscle (Pihlajaniemi et al., 1991). Similarly, some proteins involved in Ca^{2+}-dependent interactions have been found to contain glutamate residues (Glu) that have been modified by post-translational carboxylation to

γ-carboxyglutamate (Gla), which is able to chelate Ca^{2+} (Arnstein and Cox, 1992).

Chemical substitution of residues

Mono- or oligosaccharide chains may be attached via the amino group of asparagine (N-glycosylation), or through the hydroxyl group of serine, threonine or hydroxylysine residues (O-glycosylation). As mentioned above, most of the proteins in the dystrophin-associated complex are glycosylated, α-dystroglycan so extensively that its apparent molecular mass increases nearly threefold. The extent of glycosylation may vary between muscle and nonmuscle tissues (Ibraghimov-Beskrovnaya et al., 1992). The muscle-specific domain of the NCAM has O-linked oligosaccharides (Walsh et al., 1989), which may have functional significance in terms of an extended structure that would lift the NCAM molecule above the glycocalyx of muscle cells to a position where it could more effectively mediate specific interactions (Walsh and Doherty, 1991).

Many skeletal muscle proteins contain phosphate groups linked to the hydroxyl groups of tyrosine, serine or threonine residues. Kinase-mediated protein phosphorylation is the most common post-translational modification, and reversible phosphorylation modifies the action of many enzymes, mediators and regulatory factors involved in movement, cell growth and metabolic regulation (Arnstein and Cox, 1992). In skeletal muscle, there are many phosphorylatable proteins such as the regulatory MLCs, desmin, vimentin, dystrophin and dystrobrevin. It is thought that cell cycle-dependent phosphorylation of emerin may contribute to the Emery–Dreifuss muscular dystrophy phenotype (Ellis et al., 1998). Agrin-induced AChR clustering at the neuromuscular junction requires tyrosine phosphorylation (Ferns et al., 1996; Meier et al., 1998b) and rapsyn may modify clustering by regulating phosphorylation (Qu et al., 1996). The pattern of phosphoprotein expression is different in fast- and slow-twitch muscles, and this appears to be controlled by neuronal activity rather than by trophic factors (Nicholson et al., 1990). In myotonic dystrophy, the causal mutation is in a gene for protein kinase, and defective protein phosphorylation may play a role in the disease (Dunne et al., 1994). In contrast to phosphorylation, methylation is not a frequent modification. Nevertheless, both skeletal muscle myosin and actin in muscle undergo this process (Huszar, 1975).

Acylation of a variety of specific proteins by fatty acids is a common post-translational modification. The binding of lipid to vinculin is implicated in the reversible association of the protein with plasma membranes (Burn and Berger, 1987), and the cotranslational myristoylation of the AChR-associated 43 kDa protein rapsyn affects the affinity with

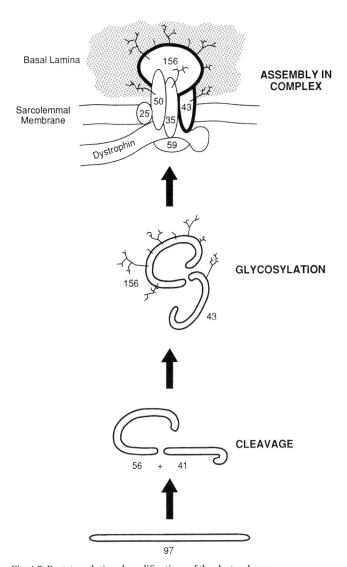

Fig. 4.7. Post-translational modifications of the dystroglycan polypeptide (97 kDa) to produce two mature proteins of 156 and 43 kDa.

which the protein is anchored in the plasma membrane (Musil et al., 1988). Prenylation is used to attach proteins to the plasma membrane or to internal membranes. Of the two products of the gene for lamin A/C, only prelamin A can be modified by isoprenylation (Lin and Worman, 1993). A number of membrane-associated proteins are attached to the cell surface via glycosyl-phosphatidylinositol (GPI) anchors (Low 1989). Addition of the GPI anchor involves cleavage of the original polypeptide chain near the C-terminus and the generation of a new C-terminus linked to the anchor. In this way, the hydrophobic anchorage of acetylcholinesterase in the lipid bilayer of muscle

Table 4.1. How abnormal gene expression can arise

Gene change	Example
Whole gene/adjacent genes deleted	Spinal muscular atrophy
Whole gene/adjacent genes duplicated	Charcot–Marie–Tooth disease
Contraction of tandem repeats	Facioscapulohumeral muscular dystrophy
Expansion of repeated triplet motifs	Myotonic dystrophy, Friedreich ataxia, Huntington's disease
Single/multiple exons deleted	Duchenne/Becker muscular dystrophy
Single/multiple exons duplicated	Duchenne/Becker muscular dystrophy
Single/few base pairs removed	Common
Single/few base pairs inserted	Common
Point mutations (missense, nonsense and splice-site mutations)	Very common

plasma membranes is achieved by the covalent attachment of single phosphatidylinositol residues (Silman and Futerman, 1987). Similarly, most of the NCAM in skeletal muscle is a GPI-anchored isoform, while the larger isoforms of NCAM in neurons have transmembrane domains (Walsh and Doherty, 1991).

Targeting and translocation

There are two main routes for proteins to arrive at their site of function, involving the synthesis of polypeptides either by ribosomes bound to the endoplasmic reticulum or by free cytosolic ribosomes. In the first pathway, protein synthesis is accompanied by insertion of the nascent protein into the membrane of the endoplasmic reticulum followed by translocation into the lumen. After any processing that is required, the protein is transported through the Golgi network to various destinations depending on the particular protein. The second major route involves synthesis on ribosomes that are not bound to membranes. Many water-soluble globular proteins destined for housekeeping use in the cytoplasm use this pathway (Austin and Westwood, 1991).

In the environment that a protein encounters inside the cell, there are many possibilities for incorrect interactions with other macromolecules, and 'chaperones' keep the nascent polypeptide, literally, on the straight and narrow. Chaperones are additional proteins that help assembly and folding but which are not part of the final structure. They form stable complexes with precursor proteins, preventing them from folding prematurely and maintaining an open conformation for translocation across membranes (Csermely et al., 1998).

The transcription and translation of proteins that are composed of several subunits encoded by different genes is coordinated. The five subunits of mature AChR, $\alpha_2\beta\delta\varepsilon$,

($\alpha_2\beta\gamma\delta$ in immature form) are translocated to the inside of the endoplasmic reticulum. Here they are assembled into $\alpha\varepsilon$ (or $\alpha\gamma$) and $\alpha\delta$ heterodimers, which associate with the β-subunit and with each other to gain the correct stoichiometry. The fully assembled functional unit then enters the Golgi apparatus and is transported to the muscle membrane (Blount et al., 1990).

When things go wrong: types of gene mutation

Having considered the pattern of normal protein synthesis in skeletal muscle, it is pertinent to consider what can go wrong in the system. There is a wide range of possibilities and Table 4.1 outlines the various ways abnormal gene expression can arise. Mutations in one gene may exert an effect on those around it, possibly by altering DNA conformation or DNA–protein interactions. The trinucleotide expansion of myotonic dystrophy protein kinase may be like this (Moreira et al., 1998), and so might deletions in the tandem repeat region of chromosome 4 that are associated with facioscapulohumeral muscular dystrophy (Tawil et al., 1998). In the spinal muscular atrophies, the critical region in 5q13 contains an inverted repeat harbouring several genes, including the survival motor neuron (*SMN*) gene and those for the neuronal apoptosis inhibitory protein (NAIP) and p44, a transcription factor subunit. Mutations in this region are complicated and may involve interconversion between the main gene involved, *SMN*, and the centromeric copy of this gene (Campbell et al., 1997). Expression of more than one gene may be involved in generating the clinical phenotype, and there is evidence that the product(s) of *SMN* may be involved in both apoptosis and pre-mRNA splicing (Lefebvre et al., 1998). A duplication of a 1.5 Mb genomic region encompassing the gene for the peripheral myelin protein 22 is found on

Table 4.2. Effect of mutations on protein synthesis

Mutation type	Description
Premature termination	
Nonsense	Point mutation where one base is exchanged for another and a stop codon replaces a codon for an amino acid
Splice site mutation	Point mutation occurs which alters splicing of introns and exons: exon not included; the reading frame is disrupted, giving rise to incorrect amino acids and/or stop codon
Frame-shifting deletion/ insertion/duplication	Codons altered: incorrect amino acids incorporated then a newly generated stop codon
Normal termination	
Missense	Point mutation causes an incorrect amino acid to be substituted; resultant changes in charge or shape may alter functional sites
Splice site mutation	Point mutation occurs that alters splicing of introns and exons: exons not included; the reading frame is maintained but functional sites may be altered
In frame deletion/ duplication	Codons maintained as whole amino acids are removed/repeated

chromosome 17p11.2–12 in Charcot–Marie–Tooth disease type 1A (CMT1A), whereas the reciprocal deletion is associated with hereditary neuropathy with liability to pressure palsies (HNPP). Since most patients with CMT1A harbour three copies of the gene *PMP22*, and most patients with HNPP carry only a single copy, a gene dosage effect has been proposed as a mechanism for both diseases (Hanemann and Muller, 1998).

Most intragenic mutations commonly fall into two basic categories: those where the translational open reading frame is disrupted, and those where it is maintained (Table 4.2). With premature termination, the mRNA frequently shows reduced stability and little or no protein is detected. Alternatively, a truncated protein may be synthesized (i.e. up to the newly generated stop codon) but this smaller-sized protein is often unstable and rapidly degraded (as in DMD; Koenig et al., 1989; Bulman et al., 1991).

Missense mutations may cause erroneous mRNA splicing. A variant of osteogenesis imperfecta is caused by a point mutation that alters a constitutive splice site in one of the pro-α-chains of type I collagen. This results in the skipping of exon 28 and, although the open reading frame is maintained, the loss of this exon prohibits subunit assembly and results in a lethal phenotype (Tromp and Prockop, 1988). In dystrophin Kobe, the deletion of 52 bp near the 5′ splice donor site within exon 19 of the dystrophin gene leads to the skipping of exon 19 during mRNA splicing, to disruption of the open reading frame and to premature termination of translation. Although this deletion does not affect the splice site directly, it abolishes the formation of an intra-exonic hairpin structure that the wild-type dystrophin mRNA precursor is able to produce in its secondary structure. The hairpin structures were also found in a further 22 separate exons, indicating that they may be essential components for constitutive splicing of dystrophin mRNA (Matsuo et al., 1992). Defective RNA splicing and exon skipping is also the basis of dystrophin-deficiency in Golden Retriever dogs (Sharp et al., 1992).

Low levels of mRNA and protein can also result from mutations that affect the promoter or enhancer elements of a gene (as in X-linked dilated cardiomyopathy; Muntoni et al., 1995a,b). With normal termination, the generation of missense mutations or small in-frame deletions and insertions may affect the folding of a polypeptide chain such that it is unable to interact with chaperone molecules and be transported to its correct site of function: such molecules are usually removed in the 'quality control' system of the endoplasmic reticulum (Edwards and Swallow, 1997). Alternatively, abnormal folding in one protein could destroy subunit or complex formation with other proteins, resulting in a general instability and removal of all the molecules involved (as in the sarcoglycanopathies (Barresi et al., 1997) or hypertrophic cardiomyopathy (Becker et al., 1997)). A misfolded protein could also be synthesized as normal and arrive safely at its site of action but then be unable to function correctly owing to altered reactive sites or motifs. Protein levels might appear normal in this case or even show an increase through the excessive accumulation of protein (as in Alzheimer's or Huntington's diseases; Askansas and Engel, 1998; Walling et al., 1998). Small, or missense, mutations can alter sites used for post-translational modifications. This could result in a nonfunctional mature protein because of abnormal proteolysis, phosphorylation or glycosylation (as in factor VIII; Kaufman and Pipe, 1997). All of these problems are regarded as loss-of-function, but occasionally, the altered structure of a mutated protein is reflected in a gain-of-function. In these cases, substrate preferences might be altered so that an enzyme has a less-restricted activity (as in motor neuron disease; Gurney et al., 1998). Finally, mutations that might be innocuous in themselves can become pathogenic on certain genetic backgrounds, or in combination with other missense changes or polymorphisms (reviewed in Edwards and Swallow, 1997).

Conclusion

In this chapter, examples have been given of the ways gene and protein expression can be modified intrinsically to generate diversity. In addition, it is clear that a number of external factors can influence gene and protein expression in skeletal muscle. These include stages of development, regeneration (in which developmental patterns of gene expression may be re-expressed), innervation, load bearing (activity and exercise) and a variety of hormones including thyroid hormones, insulin, insulin-like growth factors and growth hormone. In the past, research has tended to polarize to the study of genes *or* proteins, but recent advances in the techniques of molecular biology have made it possible to integrate these approaches. For example, it is now common to use techniques that permit the simultaneous demonstration of mRNA and protein expression by a combination of in situ hybridization and immunocytochemistry (Chiu et al., 1996; Muller-Ladner et al., 1996; Andersen and Schiaffino, 1997).

The last few years has also witnessed a huge increase in the generation of transgenic and knock-out mice, whereby gene expression in mouse embryonic stem cells is manipulated so that a target gene is modified or silenced. By disabling a specific gene it is feasible to generate a murine model of a genetic disease, and by studying the effects of the absence of a protein, the function of the native protein might be deduced. A few recent examples include the genes for myotonic dystrophy, motor neuron disease, desmin, utrophin/dystrophin, β_1-integrin and the various molecules associated with AChR clustering (Aguzzi et al., 1996; Reddy et al., 1996; Capetanaki et al., 1997; Deconinck 1997; Baudoin et al., 1998; Sanes et al., 1998). Alternatively, if an animal model with a defective gene already exists, it may be possible to correct the defect by introducing a functional gene via an assortment of routes. Gene therapy experiments of this type have been undertaken in animal models of cystic fibrosis (Cohen et al., 1998), Parkinson's disease (Raymon et al., 1997; Prasad et al., 1998), Alzheimer's disease (Winkler et al., 1998), haemophilia (Herzog and High, 1998) and DMD (Fassati et al., 1997; Howell et al., 1998; Yang et al., 1998; Yuasa et al., 1998).

One advantage of gene families is that the depletion of one member protein might be compensated for by the upregulation of another. This is the basis of the proposed therapeutic upregulation of utrophin to replace dystrophin in DMD (Tinsley and Davies, 1993; Deconinck et al., 1997). Low levels of dystrophin are often detected in boys with DMD and frame-shifting mutations, and it appears that the underlying exonic deletion is extended so that the reading frame is restored and a Becker-like protein produced in some muscle fibres (Nicholson, 1993). Consequently, another possible therapeutic approach is via antisense oligoribonucleotides, to increase exon skipping and thereby improve the phenotype of affected patients (Dunckley et al., 1998).

In summary, skeletal muscle has much to offer those interested in gene and protein expression, and there are many exciting areas of research currently under development that are likely to provide us with a much greater understanding of the complex nature of muscle gene and protein expression.

References

Adams, M. D., Rudner, D. Z. and Rio, D. C. (1996). Biochemistry and regulation of pre-mRNA splicing. *Curr. Opin. Cell Biol.* **8**, 331–339.

Aguzzi, A., Brandner, S., Marino, S. and Steinbach, J. P. (1996). Transgenic and knockout mice in the study of neurodegenerative diseases. *J. Mol. Med.* **74**, 111–126.

Andersen, J. L. and Schiaffino, S. (1997). Mismatch between myosin heavy chain mRNA and protein distribution in human skeletal muscle fibers. *Am. J. Physiology.: Cell Physiol.* **272**, C1881–C1889.

Arnstein, H. R. V. and Cox, R. A. (1992). *Protein Biosynthesis – In Focus.* Oxford: IRL/Oxford University Press.

Askanas, V. and Engel, W. K. (1998). Does overexpression of βAPP in ageing muscle have a pathogenic role and a relevance to Alzheimer's disease? Clues from inclusion body myositis, cultured human muscle, and transgenic mice. *Am. J. Pathol.* **153**, 1673–1677.

Austin, B. M. and Westwood, O. M. R. (1991). *Protein Targeting and Secretion – In Focus.* Oxford: IRL/Oxford University Press.

Austin, R. C., Howard, P. L., D'Souza, V. N., Klamut, H. J. and Ray, P. N. (1995). Cloning and characterization of alternatively spliced isoforms of Dp71. *Hum. Mol. Genet.* **4**, 1475–1483.

Bar, S., Barnea, E., Levy, Z., Neuman, S., Yaffe, D. and Nudel, U. (1990). A novel product of the Duchenne muscular dystrophy gene which greatly differs from the known isoforms in its structure and tissue distribution. *Biochem. J.* **272**, 557–560.

Barresi, R., Confalonieri, V., Lanfossi, M. et al. (1997). Concomitant deficiency of β- and γ-sarcoglycans in 20 α-sarcoglycan (adhalin)-deficient patients: immunohistochemical analysis and clinical aspects. *Acta Neuropath.* **94**, 28–35.

Baudoin, C., Goumans, M. J., Mummery, C. and Sonnenberg, A. (1998). Knockout and knockin of the β1 exon D define distinct roles for integrin splice variants in heart function and embryonic development. *Genes Devel.* **12**, 1202–1216.

Becker, K. D., Gottshall, K. R., Hickey, R., Perriard, J. C. and Chien, K. R. (1997). Point mutations in human β cardiac myosin heavy chain have differential effects on sarcomeric structure and assembly: an ATP binding site change disrupts both thick and thin filaments, whereas hypertrophic cardiomyopathy mutations display normal assembly. *J. Cell Biol.* **137**, 131–140.

Beebee, T. and Burke, J. (1992). *Gene Structure and Transcription – In Focus*, 2nd edn. Oxford: IRL/Oxford University Press.

Benezra, R., Davis, R. L., Lockshon, D., Turner, D. L. and Weintraub, H. (1990). The protein Id: a negative regulator of helix-loop-helix DNA binding proteins. *Cell* **61**, 49–59.

Blake, D. J., Love, D. R., Tinsley, J. et al. (1992). Characterisation of a 4.8 kb transcript from the Duchenne muscular dsytrophy locus expressed in Schwannoma cells. *Hum. Mol. Genet.* **1**, 103–109.

Blake, D. J., Nawrotzki, R., Peters, M. F., Froehner, S. C. and Davies, K. E. (1996). Isoform diversity of dystrobrevin, the murine 87-kDa postsynaptic protein. *J. Biol. Chem.* **271**, 7802–7810.

Blount, P., Smith, M. M. and Merlie, J. P. (1990). Assembly intermediates of the mouse muscle nicotinic acetylcholine receptor in stably transfected fibroblasts. *J. Cell Biol.* **111**, 2601–2611.

Bortoluzzi, S., Rampoldi, L., Simionati, B. et al. (1998). A comprehensive, high-resolution genomic transcript map of human skeletal muscle. *Genome Res.* **8**, 817–825.

Breitbart, R. E. and Nadal-Ginard, B. (1989). Tissue specific alternative splicing in the troponin T multigene family. In: *Tissue Specific Gene Expression*, ed. R. Renkawitz, pp. 199–215. Weinheim: VCH Verlagsgesellschaft.

Breitbart, R. E., Andreadis, A. and Nadal-Ginard, B. (1987). Alternative splicing, a ubiquitous mechanism for the generation of multiple protein isoforms from single genes. *Ann. Rev. Biochem.* **56**, 467–495.

Bulman, D. E., Gangopadhyay, S. B., Bebchuck, K. G., Worton, R. G. and Ray, P. N. (1991). Point mutation in the human dystrophin gene: identification through Western blot analysis. *Genomics* **10**, 457–460.

Buonanno, A. and Rosenthal, N. (1996). Molecular control of muscle diversity and plasticity. *Devel. Genet.* **19**, 95–107.

Burn, P. and Berger, M. M. (1987). The cytoskeletal protein vinculin contains transformation-sensitive, covalently bound lipid. *Science* **235**, 476–479.

Byers, T. J., Lidov, H. G. W. and Kunkel, L. M. (1993). An alternative dystrophin transcript specific to peripheral nerve. *Nat. Genet.* **4**, 77–81.

Campbell, L., Potter, A., Ignatius, J., Dubowitz, V. and Davies K. (1997). Genomic variation and gene conversion in spinal muscular atrophy: implications for disease process and clinical phenotype. *Am. J. Hum. Genet.* **61**, 40–50.

Capetanaki, Y., Milner, D. J. and Weitzer, G. (1997). Desmin in muscle formation and maintenance: knockouts and consequences. *Cell Struct. Func.* **22**, 103–116.

Chabot, B. (1996). Directing alternative splicing: cast and scenarios. *Trends Genet.* **12**, 472–478.

Chambers, R. L. and McDermott, J. C. (1996). Molecular basis of skeletal muscle regeneration. *Can. J. App. Physiology* **21**, 155–184.

Chelly, J., Hamard, G., Koulakoff, A., Kaplan, J.-C., Kahn, A. and Berwald-Netter, Y. (1990). Dystrophin gene transcribed from different promoters in neuronal and glial cells. *Nature* **344**, 64–65.

Chiu, K. P., Duca, K. A., Berman, S. A., Sullivan, T. and Bursztajn, S. (1996). A novel in situ double-labelling method for simultaneous detection of mRNA and expressed protein or two different mRNAs. *J. Neurosci. Meth.* **66**, 69–79.

Cohen, J. C., Morrow, S. L., Cork, R. J., Delcarpio, J. B. and Larson, J. E. (1998). Molecular pathophysiology of cystic fibrosis based on the rescued knockout mouse model. *Mol. Genet. Metab.* **64**, 108–118.

Collinge, M., Matrisian, P. E., Zimmer, W. E. et al. (1992). Structure and expression of a calcium binding protein gene contained within a calmodulin regulated protein kinase gene. *Mol. Cell. Biol.* **12**, 2359–2371.

Cooper, T. A. and Mattox, W. (1997). The regulation of splice-site selection, and its role in human disease. *Am. J. Hum. Genet.* **61**, 259–266.

Csermely, P., Schnaider, T., Soti, C., Prohászka, Z. and Nardai, G. (1998). The 90-kDa molecular chaperone family: structure, function, and clinical applications. A comprehensive review. *Pharmacol. Therapeut.* **79**, 129–168.

D'Souza, V. N., Nguyen thi Man, Morris, G. E., Karges, W., Pillers, D.-A. M. and Ray, P. N. (1995). A novel dystrophin isoform is required for normal retinal electrophysiology. *Hum. Mol. Genet.* **4**, 837–842.

Deconinck, A. E. (1997). Utrophin/dystrophin-deficient mice as a model for Duchenne muscular dystrophy. *Cell* **90**, 717–727.

Deconinck, N., Tinsley, J., de Backer, F. et al. (1997). Expression of truncated utrophin leads to major functional improvements in dystrophin-deficient muscles of mice. *Nat. Med.* **3**, 1216–1221.

Den Dunnen, J. T., Casula, L., Kakover, A. et al. (1991). Mapping of dystrophin brain promoter: a deletion of this region is compatible with normal intellect. *Neuromusc. Disord.* **1**, 327–331.

Dennis, C. L., Tinsley, J. M., Deconinck, A. E. and Davies, K. E. (1996). Molecular and functional analysis of the utrophin promoter. *Nucleic Acids Res.* **24**, 1646–1652.

Deyst, K. A., McKechnie, B. A. and Fallon, J. R. (1998). The role of alternative splicing in regulating agrin binding to muscle cells. *Dev. Brain Res.* **110**, 185–191.

Diagana, T. T., North, D. L., Jabet, C., Fiszman, M. Y., Takeda, S. and Whalen, R. G. (1997). The transcriptional activity of a muscle-specific promoter depends critically on the structure of the TATA element and its binding protein. *J. Mol. Biol.* **265**, 480–493.

Dickson, G., Gower, H. J., Barton, C. H. et al. (1987). Human muscle neural cell adhesion molecule (NCAM): identification of a muscle-specific sequence in the extracellular domain. *Cell* **50**, 1119–1130.

Donoghue, M., Ernst, H., Wetworth, B., Nadal-Ginard, B. and Rosenthal, N. (1988). A muscle-specific enhancer is located at the 3′ end of the myosin light-chain 1/3 gene locus. *Genes Devel.* **2**, 1779–1790.

Dunckley, M. G., Manoharan, M., Villiet, P., Eperon, I. C. and Dickson, G. (1998). Modification of splicing in the dystrophin gene in cultured *mdx* muscle cells by antisense oligoribonucleotides. *Hum. Mol. Genet.* **7**, 1083–1090.

Dunne, P. W., Walch, E. T. and Epstein, H. F. (1994). Phosphorylation reactions of recombinant human myotonic dystrophy protein kinase and their inhibition. *Biochemistry* **33**, 10809–10814.

Durbeej, M., Henry, M. D. and Campbell, K. P. (1998). Dystroglycan in development and disease. *Curr. Opin. Cell Biol.* **10**, 594–601.

Dye, D. E., Buvoli, M., Mayer, S. A. and Lin, C.-H. (1998). Enhancer elements activate the weak 3′ splice site of α-tropomyosin exon 2. *RNA* **4**, 1523–1536.

Dytrych, L., Sherman, D. L., Gillespie, C. S. and Brophy, P. J. (1998). Two PDZ domain proteins encoded by the murine periaxin gene are the result of alternative intron retention and are differentially targeted in Schwann cells. *J. Biol. Chem.* **273**, 5794–5800.

Edwalds-Gilbert, G., Veraldi, K. L. and Milcarek, C. (1997). Alternative poly(A) site selection in complex transcription units: means to an end? *Nucl. Acids Res.* **25**, 2547–2561.

Edwards, Y. H. (1990). CpG islands in genes showing tissue-specific expression. *Phil. Trans. R. Soc.Lond. B Biol. Sci.* **326**, 207–215.

Edwards, Y. H. and Swallow, D. M. (1997). Mutation and protein dysfunction. In: *Protein Dysfunction and Human Genetic Disease*, eds. D. M. Swallow and Y. H. Edwards, pp. 1–14. Oxford: BIOS.

Ellis, J. A., Craxton, M., Yates, J. R. and Kendrick-Jones, J. (1998). Aberrant intracellular targeting and cell cycle-dependent phosphorylation of emerin contribute to the Emery–Dreifuss muscular dystrophy phenotype. *J. Cell Sci.* **111**, 781–792.

Emeson, R. B., Hedjran, F., Yeakley, J. M., Guise, J. W. and Rosenfeld, M. G. (1989). Alternative production of calcitonin and CGRP mRNA is regulated at the calcitonin-specific splice acceptor. *Nature* **341**, 76–80.

Fabre-Suver, C. and Hauschka, S. D. (1996). A novel site in the muscle creatine kinase enhancer is required for expression in skeletal but not cardiac muscle. *J. Biol. Chem.* **271**, 4646–4652.

Fassati, A., Wells, D. J., Serpente, P. A. S. et al. (1997). Genetic correction of dystrophin deficiency and skeletal muscle remodeling in adult *mdx* mouse via transplantation of retroviral producer cells. *J. Clin. Invest.* **100**, 620–628.

Ferlini, A. and Muntoni, F. (1998). The 5′ region of intron 11 of the dystrophin gene contains target sequences for mobile elements and three overlapping ORFs. *Biochem. Biophys. Res. Commun.* **242**, 401–406.

Ferns, M., Deiner, M. and Hall, Z. (1996). Agrin-induced acetylcholine receptor clustering in mammalian muscle requires tyrosine phosphorylation. *J. Cell Biol.* **132**, 937–944.

Ferns, M., Hoch, W., Campanelli, J. T., Rupp, F., Hall, Z. W. and Scheller, R. H. (1992). RNA splicing regulates agrin-mediated acetylcholine receptor clustering activity on cultured myotubes. *Neuron* **8**, 1079–1086.

Firulli, A. B. and Olson, E. N. (1997). Modular regulation of muscle gene transcription: a mechanism for muscle cell diversity. *Trends Genet.* **13**, 364–369.

Gilgenkrantz, H., Hugnot, J.-P., Lambert, M., Chafey, P., Kaplan, J.-C. and Kahn, A. (1992). Postitive and negative regulatory DNA elements including a CCArGG box are involved in the cell type-specific expression of the human muscle dystrophin gene. *J. Biol. Chem.* **267**, 10823–10830.

Goldman, D. and Tamai, K. (1989). Coordinate regulation of RNAs encoding two isoforms of the rat muscle nicotinic acetylcholine receptor β-subunit. *Nucl. Acids Res.* **17**, 3049–3056.

Goodison, S., Yoshida, K., Churchman, M. and Tarin, D. (1998). Multiple intron retention occurs in tumor cell CD44 mRNA processing. *Am. J. Pathol.* **153**, 1221–1228.

Górecki, D. C., Monaco, A. P., Derry, J. M., Walker, A. P., Barnard, E. A. and Barnard, P. J. (1992). Expression of four alternative dystrophin transcripts in brain regions regulated by different promoters. *Hum. Mol. Genet.* **1**, 505–510.

Gower, H. J., Barton, C. H., Elsom, V. L., Thompson, J., Moore, S. E. and Walsh, F. S. (1988).Alternative splicing generates a secreted form of NCAM in muscle and brain. *Cell* **55**, 955–964.

Graham, I. R., Hamshere, M. and Eperon, I. C. (1992). Alternative splicing of a human α-tropomyosin muscle-specific exon: identification of determining sequences. *Mol. Cell. Biol.* **12**, 3872–3882.

Gurney, M. E., Liu, R., Althaus, J. S., Hall, E. D. and Becker, D. A. (1998). Mutant CuZn superoxide dismutase in motor neuron disease. *J. Inher. Metab. Dis.* **21**, 587–597.

Hall, Z. W. (1992). *An Introduction to Molecular Neurobiology.* Sunderland, MA: Sinauer Associates.

Haneman, C. O. and Muller, H. W. (1998). Pathogenesis of Charcot–Marie–Tooth 1A (CMT1A) neuropathy. *Trends Neurosci.* **21**, 282–286.

Herzog, R. W. and High, K. A. (1998). Problems and prospects in gene therapy for hemophilia. *Curr. Opin. Hematol.* **5**, 321–326.

Hoffman, E. P., Brown, R. H. and Kunkel, L. M. (1987). Dystrophin: the protein product of the Duchenne muscular dystrophy locus. *Cell* **51**, 919–928.

Hoffman, E. P., Arahata, K., Minetti, C., Bonilla, E. and Rowland, L. P. (1992). Dystrophinopathy in isolated cases of myopathy in females. *Neurology* **42**, 967–975.

Holder, E., Maeda, M. and Bies, R. D. (1996). Expression and regulation of the dystrophin Purkinje promoter in human skeletal muscle, heart, and brain. *Hum. Genet.* **97**, 232–239.

Howard, P. L., Dally, G. Y., Wong, M. H. et al. (1998). Localization of dystrophin isoform Dp71 to the inner limiting membrane of the retina suggests a unique functional contribution of Dp71 in the retina. *Hum. Mol. Genet.* **7**, 1385–1391.

Howard, P. L., Dally, G. Y., Ditta, S. D. et al. (1999). Dystrophin isoforms Dp71 and Dp427 have distinct roles in myogenic cells. *Muscle Nerve* **22**, 16–27.

Howell, J. M., Lochmüller, H., O'Hara, A. et al. (1998). High-level dystrophin expression after adenovirus-mediated dystrophin minigene transfer to skeletal muscle of dystrophic dogs: prolongation of expression with immunosuppression. *Hum. Gene Ther.* **9**, 629–634.

Huszar, G. (1975). Tissue-specific biosynthesis of ε-N-monomethyllysine and ε-N-trimethyllysine in skeletal and cardiac muscle myosin: a model for the cell-free study of post-translational amino acid modifications in proteins. *J. Mol. Biol.* **94**, 311–326.

Ibraghimov-Beskrovnaya, O., Ervasti, J. M., Leveille, C. J., Slaughter, C. A., Sernett, S. W. and Campbell, K. P. (1992). Primary structure of dystrophin-associated glycoproteins linking dystrophin to the extracellular matrix. *Nature* **355**, 696–702.

Ito, M., Dabrowska, R., Guerriero, V. and Hartshorne, D. J. (1989). Identification in turkey gizzard of an acidic protein related to the C-terminal portion of smooth muscle myosin light chain kinase. *J. Biol. Chem.* **264**, 13971–13974.

Kaufman, R. J. and Pipe, S. W. (1997). Factor VIII and haemophilia A. In: *Protein Dysfunction and Human Genetic Disease*, ed. D. M. Swallow and Y. H. Edwards, pp. 77–98. Oxford: BIOS Scientific.

Klamut, H. J., Gangopadhyay, S. B., Worton, R. G. and Ray, P. N. (1990). Molecular and functional analysis of the muscle-specific promoter region of the Duchenne muscular dystrophy gene. *Mol. Cell. Biol.* **10**, 193–205.

Klamut, H. J., Bosnoyan-Collins, L. O., Worton, R. G., Ray, P. N. and Davis, H. L. (1996). Identification of a transcriptional enhancer within muscle intron 1 of the human dystrophin gene. *Hum. Mol. Genet.* **5**, 1599–1606.

Klamut, H. J., Bosnoyan-Collins, L. O., Worton, R. G. and Ray, P. N. (1997). A muscle-specific enhancer within intron 1 of the human dystrophin gene is functionally dependent on single MEF-1/E box and MEF-2/AT-rich sequence motifs. *Nucl. Acids Res.* **25**, 1618–1625.

Klarsfeld, A., Bessereau, J. L., Salmon, A. M., Triller, A., Babinet, C. and Changeux, J. P. (1999). An acetylcholine receptor α-subunit promoter conferring preferential synaptic expression in muscle of transgenic mice. *EMBO* **10**, 625–632.

Koenig, M., Beggs, A. H., Moyer, M. et al. (1989). The molecular basis for Duchenne versus Becker muscular dystrophy: correlation of severity with type of deletion. *Am. J. Hum. Genet.* **45**, 498–506.

Kornblihtt, A. R., Pesce, C. G., Alonso, C. R. et al. (1996). The fibronectin gene as a model for splicing and transcription studies. *FASEB J.* **10**, 248–257.

Koteliansky, V. E., Ogryzko, E. P., Zhidkova, N. I. et al. (1992). An additional exon in the human vinculin gene specifically encodes meta-vinculin-specific difference peptide: crossspecies comparison reveals variable and conserved motifs in the meta-vinculin insert. *Eur. J. Biochem.* **204**, 767–772.

Lefebre, S., Bürglen, L., Frézal, J. et al. (1998). The role of the SMN gene in proximal spinal muscular atrophy. *Hum. Mol. Genet.* **7**, 1531–1536.

Lewin, B. (1997). *Genes VI*. Oxford: Oxford University Press.

Li, Y., Camp, S., Rachinsky, T. L., Getman, D. and Taylor, P. (1991). Gene structure of mammalian acetylcholinesterase: alternative exons dictate tissue-specific expression. *J. Biol. Chem.* **266**, 23083–23090.

Lidov, H. G. W. and Kunkel, L. M. (1998). Dystrophin and Dp140 in the adult rodent kidney. *Lab. Invest.* **78**, 1543–1551.

Lidov, H. G. W., Selig, S. and Kunkel, L. M. (1995). Dp140: a novel 140 kDa CNS transcript from the dystrophin locus. *Hum. Mol. Genet.* **4**, 329–335.

Lin, F. and Worman, H. J. (1993). Structural organization of the human gene encoding nuclear lamin A and nuclear lamin C. *J. Biol. Chem.* **268**, 16321–16326.

Liu, X. Z., Walsh, J., Mburu, P. et al. (1997). Mutations in the myosin VIIA gene cause non-syndromic recessive deafness. *Nat. Genet.* **16**, 188–190.

Lou, H. and Gagel, R. F. (1998). Alternative RNA processing – its role in regulating expression of calcitonin/calcitonin gene-related peptide. *J. Endocrinol.* **156**, 401–405.

Low, M. G. (1989). Glycosyl-phosphatidylinositol: a versatile anchor for cell surface proteins. *FASEB J.* **3**, 1600–1608.

Lupetti, R., Pisarra, P., Verrecchia, A. et al. (1998). Translation of a retained intron in tyrosinase-related protein (TRP) 2 mRNA generates a new cytotoxic T lymphocyte (CTL)-defined and shared human melanoma antigen not expressed in normal cells of the melanocytic lineage. *J. Exp. Med.* **188**, 1005–1016.

Lupski, J. R., Garcia, C. A., Zoghbi, H. Y., Hoffman, E. P. and Fenwick, R. G. (1991). Discordance of muscular dystrophy in monozygotic female twins: evidence supporting asymmetric splitting of the inner cell mass in a manifesting carrier of Duchenne dystrophy. *Am. J. Med.Genet.* **40**, 354–364.

Makover, A., Zuk, D., Breakstone, J., Yaffe, D. and Nudel, U. (1991). Brain-type and muscle-type promotors of the dystrophin gene differ greatly in structure. *Neuromusc. Disord.* **1**, 39–45.

Mallet, J., Houhou, L., Pajak, F. et al. (1998). The cholinergic locus: ChAT and VAChT genes. *J. Physiol. (Paris)* **92**, 145–147.

Mar, J. H. and Ordahl, C. P. (1988). A conserved CATTCCT motif is required for skeletal muscle-specific activity of the cardiac troponin T gene promoter. *Proc. Nat. Acad. Sci. USA* **85**, 6404–6408.

Matsuo, M., Nishio, H., Kitoh, Y., Francke, U. and Nakamura, H. (1992). Partial deletion of a dystrophin gene leads to exon skipping and to loss of an intra-exon hairpin structure from the predicted mRNA precursor. *Biochem. Biophys. Res. Commun.* **182**, 495–500.

Medford, R. M., Hyman, R., Ahmad, M. et al. (1991). Vascular smooth muscle expresses a truncated Na^+,K^+-ATPase α-1 subunit isoform. *J. Biol. Chem.* **266**, 18308–18312.

Megeney, L. A. and Rudnicki, M. A. (1995). Determination versus differentiation and the MyoD family of transcription factors. *Biochem. Cell Biol.* **73**, 723–732.

Meier, T., Masciulli, F., Moore, C. et al. (1998a). Agrin can mediate acetylcholine receptor gene expression in muscle by aggregation of muscle-derived neuregulins. *J. Cell Biol.* **141**, 715–726.

Meier, T., Ruegg, M. A., Wallace, B. G. (1998b). Muscle-specific agrin isoforms reduce phosphorylation of AChR γ and δ subunits in cultured muscle cells. *Mol. Cell. Neurosci.* **11**, 206–216.

Missler, M. and Sudhof, T. C. (1998). Neurexins: three genes and 1001 products. *Trends Genet.* **14**, 20–26.

Missler, M., Fernandez-Chacon, R. and Sudhof, T. C. (1998). The making of neurexins. *J. Neurochem.* **71**, 1339–1347.

Moizard, M. P., Billard, C., Toutain, A., Berret, F., Marmin, N. and Moraine, C. (1998). Are Dp71 and Dp140 brain dystrophin isoforms related to cognitive impairment in Duchenne muscular dystrophy? *Am. J. Med. Genet.* **80**, 32–41.

Molkentin, J. D., Black, B. L., Martin, J. F. and Olson, E. N. (1995). Cooperative activation of muscle gene expression by MEF2 and myogenic bHLH proteins. *Cell* **83**, 1125–1136.

Moreira, E. S., Vainzof, M., Marie, S. K., Nigro, V., Zatz, M. and Passos-Bueno, M. R. (1998). A first missense mutation in the δ sarcoglycan gene associated with a severe phenotype and frequency of limb-girdle muscular dystrophy type 2F (LGMD2F) in Brazilian sarcoglycanopathies. *J. Med. Genet.* **35**, 951–953.

Muller-Ladner, U., Kriegsmann, J., Gay, R. E. and Gay, S. (1996). A one-day double-labelling technique for tissue specimens: immunogold-silver staining for in situ hybridization combined with alkaline phosphatase-anti-alkaline phosphatase (APAAP) immunohistochemistry for antigens. *Histochem. J.* **28**, 133–134.

Muntoni, F., Melis, M. A., Ganau, A. and Dubowitz, V. (1995a). Transcription of the dystrophin gene in normal tissues and in skeletal muscle of a family with X-linked dilated cardiomyopathy. *Am. J. Hum. Genet.* **56**, 151–157.

Muntoni, F., Wilson, L., Marrosu, G. et al. (1995b). A mutation in the dystrophin gene selectively affecting dystrophin expression in the heart. *J. Clin. Invest.* **96**, 693–699.

Muscat, G. E. O., Gobius, K. and Emery, J. (1991). Proliferin, a pro-lactin/growth hormone-like peptide represses myogenic-specific transcription by the suppression of an essential serum-response factor-like DNA-binding activity. *Mol. Endocrinol.* **5**, 802–814.

Musil, L. S., Carr, C., Cohen, J. B. and Merlie, J. P. (1988). Acetylcholine receptor-associated 43K protein contains covalently bound myristate. *J. Cell Biol.* **107**, 1113–1121.

Nadal-Ginard, B., Smith, C. W., Patton, J. G. and Breitbart, R. E. (1991). Alternative splicing is an efficient mechanism for the generation of protein diversity: contractile protein genes as a model system. *Adv. Enzyme Regul.* **31**, 261–286.

Newlands, S., Levitt, L. K., Robinson, C. S. et al. (1998). Transcription occurs in pulses in muscle fibres. *Genes Devel.* **12**, 2748–2758.

Nicholson, G. A., Hawkins, S. and McLeod, J. G. (1990). Effect of neural activity on skeletal muscle phosphoproteins. *Muscle Nerve* **13**, 675–680.

Nicholson, L. V. B. (1993). The 'rescue' of dystrophin synthesis in boys with Duchenne muscular dystrophy. *Neuromusc. Disorders* **3**, 525–532.

Nishio, H., Takeshima, Y., Narita, N. et al. (1994). Identification of a novel first exon in the human dystrophin gene and of a new promoter located more than 500 kb upstream of the nearest known promoter. *J. Clin. Invest.* **94**, 1037–1042.

Nudel, U., Zuk, D., Einat, P. et al. (1989). Duchenne muscular dystrophy gene product is not identical in muscle and brain. *Nature* **337**, 76–78.

Numberger, M., Durr, I., Kues, W., Koenen, M. and Witzemann, V. (1991). Different mechanisms regulate muscle-specific AChR γ- and ε-subunit gene expression. *EMBO J.* **10**, 2957–2964.

Ohmstede, C.-A., Bland, M. M., Merrill, B. M. and Sahyoun, N. (1991). Relationship of genes encoding Ca^{2+}/calmodulindependent protein kinase Gr and calspermin: a gene within a gene. *Proc. Natl. Acad. Sci. USA* **88**, 5784–5788.

Pavlath, G. K., Rich, K., Webster, S. G. and Blau, H. M. (1989). Localization of muscle gene products in nuclear domains. *Nature* **337**, 570–573.

Peters, M. F., Sadoulet-Puccio, H. M., Grady, M. R. et al. (1998). Differential membrane localization and intermolecular associations of α-dystrobrevin isoforms in skeletal muscle. *J. Cell Biol.* **142**, 1269–1278.

Pihlajaniemi, T., Myllyla, R. and Kivirikko, K. I. (1991). Prolyl 4-hydroxylase and its role in collagen synthesis. *J. Hepatol.* **13**(suppl. 3), S2–S7.

Prasad, K. N., Clarkson, E. D., La Rosa, F. G., Edwards-Prasad, J. and Freed, C. R. (1998). Efficacy of grafted immortalized dopamine neurons in an animal model of Parkinsonism: a review. *Mol. Genet. Metab.* **65**, 1–9.

Qu, Z. C., Apel, E. D,. Doherty, C. A., Hoffman, P. W., Merlie, J. P. and Huganir, R. L. (1996). The synapse-associated protein rapsyn regulates tyrosine phosphorylation of proteins colocalized at nicotinic acetylcholine receptor clusters. *Mol. Cell. Neurosci.* **8**, 171–184.

Rapaport, D., Lederfein, D., Den Dunnen, J. T. et al. (1992). Characterization and cell type distribution of a novel, major transcript of the Duchenne muscular dystrophy gene. *Differentiation* **49**, 187–193.

Raymon, H. K., Thode, S. and Gage, F. H. (1997). Application of ex vivo gene therapy in the treatment of Parkinson's disease. *Exp. Neurol.* **144**, 82–91.

Reddy, S., Smith, D. B. J., Rich, M. M. et al. (1996). Mice lacking the myotonic dystrophy protein kinase develop a late onset progressive myopathy. *Nat. Genet.* **13**, 325–335.

Rosenfeld, M. G., Mermod, J. J., Amara, S. G. et al. (1983). Production of a novel neuropeptide encoded by the calcitonin gene via tissue-specific RNA processing. *Nature* **304**, 129–135.

Sadot, E., Marx, R., Barg, J., Behar, L. and Ginzburg, I. (1994). Complete sequence of 3′-untranslated region of Tau from rat central nervous system. Implications for mRNA heterogeneity. *J. Mol. Biol.* **241**, 325–331.

Sanes, J. R., Apel, E. D., Burgess, R. W. et al. (1998). Development of the neuromuscular junction: genetic analysis in mice. *J. Physiol. (Paris)* **92**, 167–172.

Schaller, K. L., Krzemien, D. M., McKenna, N. M. and Caldwell, J. H. (1992). Alternatively spliced sodium channel transcripts in brain and muscle. *J. Neurosci.* **12**, 1370–1381.

Schul, W., de Jong, L. and van Driel, R. (1998). Nuclear neighbours: the spatial and functional organization of genes and nuclear domains. *J. Cell. Biochem.* **70**, 159–171.

Sellers, J. R., Goodson, H. V. and Wang, F. (1996). A myosin family reunion. *J. Musc. Res. Cell Motil.* **17**, 7–22.

Sharp, N. J. H., Kornegay, J. N., van Camp, S. D. et al. (1992). An error in dystrophin mRNA processing in Golden Retriever muscular dystrophy, an animal homologue of Duchenne muscular dystrophy. *Genomics* **13**, 115–121.

Silman, I. and Futerman, A. H. (1987). Posttranslational modification as a means of anchoring acetylcholinesterase to the cell surface. *Biopolymers* **26**, S241–S253.

Sonenberg, N. (1996). mRNA translation: influence of the 5′ and 3′ untranslated regions. *Curr. Opin. Genet. Devel.* **4**, 310–315.

Spirin, A. S. (1986). *Ribosome Structure and Protein Biosynthesis.* Menlo Park, CA: Benjamin/Cummings.

Stein, G. S., van Wijnen, A. J., Stein, J. L., Lian, J. B., Pockwinse, S. and McNeil, S. (1998). Interrelationships of nuclear structure and transcriptional control: functional consequences of being in the right place at the right time. *J. Cell. Biochem.* **70**, 200–212.

Strachan, T. and Read, A. P. (1996). *Human Molecular Genetics.* Oxford: BIOS Scientific.

Straub, V. and Campbell, K. P. (1997). Muscular dystrophies and the dystrophin–glycoprotein complex. *Curr. Opin. Neurol. Neurosurg.* **10**, 168–175.

Tawil, R., Figlewicz, D. A., Griggs, R. C. et al. (1998). Facioscapulohumeral dystrophy: a distinct regional myopathy with a novel molecular pathogenesis. *Ann. Neurol.* **43**, 279–282.

Tinsley, J. M. and Davies, K. E. (1993). Utrophin: a potential replacement for dystrophin? *Neuromusc. Disord.* **3**, 537–539.

Tinsley, J. M., Blake, D. J. and Davies, K. E. (1993). Apo-dystrophin-3: a 2.2kb transcript from the DMD locus encoding the dystrophin glycoprotein binding site. *Hum. Mol. Genet.* **2**, 521–524.

Tong, B. D., Auer, D. E., Jaye, M. et al. (1987). cDNA clones reveal differences between human glial and endothelial cell platelet-derived growth factor A-chains. *Nature* **328**, 619–621.

Tromp, G. and Prockop, D. J. (1988). Single base mutation in the proα2(I) collagen gene that causes efficient splicing of RNA from exon 27 to exon 29 and synthesis of a shortened but in-frame proα2(I) chain. *Proc. Natl. Acad. Sci. USA* **85**, 5254–5258.

Walling, H. W., Baldassare, J. J. and Westfall, T. C. (1998). Molecular aspects of Huntington's disease. *J. Neurosci. Res.* **54**, 301–308.

Walsh, F. S. and Doherty, P. (1991). Structure and function of the gene for neural cell adhesion molecule. *Semin. Neurosci.* **3**, 271–284.

Walsh, F. S., Parekh, R. B., Moore, S. E. et al. (1989). Tissuespecific O-linked gycosylation of the neural cell adhesion molecule (NCAM). *Development.* **105**, 803–811.

Wasserman, W. W. and Fickett, J. W. (1998). Identification of regulatory regions which confer muscle-specific gene expression. *J. Mol. Biol.* **278**, 167–181.

Weil, D., Küssel, P., Blanchard, S. et al. (1997). The autosomal recessive isolated deafness, DFNB2, and the Usher 1B syndrome are allelic defects of the myosin-VIIA gene. *Nat. Genet.* **16**, 191–193.

Winkelmann, J. C., Costa, F. F., Linzie, B. L. and Forget, B. G. (1990). β Spectrin in human skeletal muscle: tissue-specific differential processing of 3′ β spectrin pre-mRNA generates a β spectrin isoform with a unique carboxyl terminus. *J. Biol. Chem.* **265**, 20449–20454.

Winkler, J., Thal, L. J., Gage, F. H. and Fisher, L. J. (1998). Cholinergic strategies for Alzheimer's disease. *J. Mol. Med.* **76**, 555–567.

Yang, L., Lochmuller, H., Luo, J. et al. (1998). Adenovirus-mediated dystrophin minigene transfer improves muscle strength in adult dystrophic (MDX) mice. *Gene Ther.* **5**, 369–379.

Yuasa, K., Miyagoe, Y., Yamamoto, K., Nabeshima, Y., Dickson, G. and Takeda, S. (1998). Effective restoration of dystrophin-associated proteins in vivo by adenovirus-mediated transfer of truncated dystrophin cDNAs. *FEBS Lett.* **425**, 329–336.

Zhang, J. S. and Longo, F. M. (1995). LAR tyrosine phosphatase receptor: alternative splicing is preferential to the nervous system, coordinated with cell growth and generates novel isoforms containing extensive CAG repeats. *J. Cell Biol.* **128**, 415–431.

Zhidkova, N. I., Belkin, A. M. and Mayne, R. (1995). Novel isoform of β1 integrin expressed in skeletal and cardiac muscle. *Biochem. Biophys. Res. Commun.* **214**, 279–285.

5

Mitochondria

Eric A. Shoubridge

Introduction

The primary function of mitochondria is to provide the cell with aerobic energy in the form of ATP, by a process called oxidative phosphorylation. All nucleated cells in the body rely on this energy source for normal physiological function. Skeletal muscle is particularly vulnerable to shortfalls in the production of mitochondrial ATP because of the high metabolic demands of muscle work. A large number of neuromuscular disorders have been described in which the molecular basis can be traced to a defect in supplying metabolic fuels to mitochondria or a defect in the process of oxidative phosphorylation itself. Mitochondria are the only cellular organelles outside the nucleus that contain their own DNA (mtDNA); consequently, deficiencies in aerobic energy production can be caused by gene defects in either the nuclear or the mitochondrial genomes. This chapter deals with the basic structure, biochemistry, molecular biology and genetics of mitochondria.

Mitochondrial structure and morphology

Mitochondria are cytoplasmic organelles approximately $0.5–1.0\,\mu m$ in diameter, similar in size to the bacteria from which they are thought to have been derived by endosymbiosis more than 1 billion years ago. They are enclosed by a double membrane system: an outer membrane that is permeable to most small molecules less than $10\,kDa$, and an impermeable inner membrane across which an electrochemical gradient is formed to drive ATP synthesis. The outer membrane contains a number of proteins, including porin, monoamine oxidase, enzymes of phospholipid biosynthesis and part of the protein import system. Its lipid composition is similar to that of other microsomal membranes. The inner membrane is a highly specialized struc-

ture containing the protein complexes of the electron transport system and numerous carriers involved in moving metabolites into and out of the matrix compartment. It is rich in cardiolipin and highly convoluted into foldings called cristae, which greatly increase its surface area. The shape and pattern of the cristae are cell-type specific; muscle fibres typically have a large number of flattened cristae, which are necessary to support the high metabolic demands of muscle. The matrix space enclosed by the inner membrane contains the pyruvate dehydrogenase complex and enzymes for the tricarboxylic acid cycle, β-oxidation of fatty acids, haem biosynthesis, the urea cycle, ketone metabolism and amino acid metabolism. It also contains the chaperonins and peptidases for processing and assembly of the respiratory chain components and mtDNA (Fig. 5.1) and the enzymatic machinery necessary for its replication and expression. (See Chapter 8 for a more detailed discussion of mitochondrial biochemistry.)

Although mitochondria are often depicted in textbooks as small spherical bodies, the reality is often much more complex. Mitochondria take on a variety of shapes ranging from simple spheres to large interconnected reticular networks. The mechanisms controlling mitochondrial morphology are largely unknown; however, recent work suggests that a family of high-molecular-weight GTPases may play an important role (Yaffe, 1999).

Mitochondria in skeletal muscle are conventionally classified as either subsarcolemmal or intermyofibrillar, indicating the locations in the myofibre where they are found. Mitochondrial volume fraction varies from approximately 2% to 5% in human skeletal muscle, a difference that is associated with different fibre types and energy requirements. Type I (slow-twitch oxidative) muscle fibres, which are designed for continuous low power work, have more mitochondria than type IIB (fast glycolytic) fibres, which are tailored for high-power burst work that is fueled largely

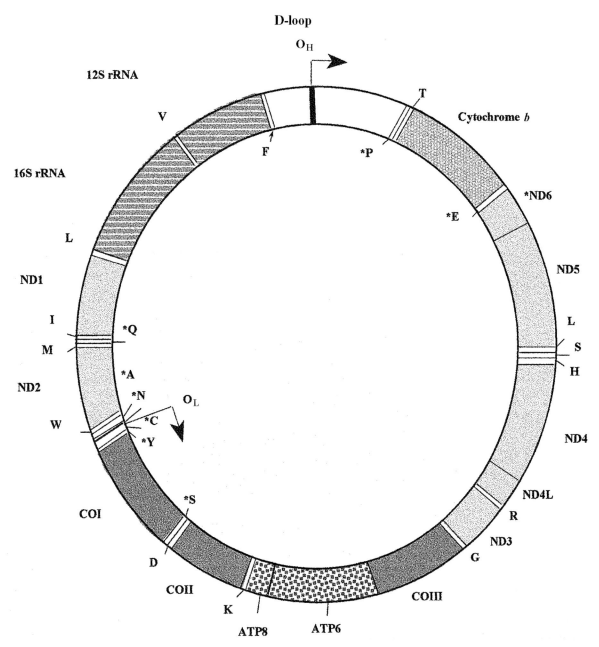

Fig. 5.1. Human mitochondrial DNA. Locations of polypeptide genes encoding complex I subunits (ND1, ND2, ND3, ND4, ND4L, ND5, ND6), the complex III subunit (cytochrome *b*), the complex IV subunits (COI, COII, COIII) and the complex V subunits (ATP6, ATP8), the intervening transfer RNAs, and the ribosomal RNA genes (12S rRNA and 16S rRNA). Abbreviations: CO, cytochrome *c* oxidase; ND, NADH CoQ reductase; ATP, ATP synthase; Q, coenzyme Q_{10}; O_L, origin of light strand replication; O_H, origin of heavy strand replication. Asterisks indicate genes coded on the L-strand. Transfer RNAs: A, alanine; R, arginine; N, asparagine; D, aspartate; C, cysteine; E, glutamate; Q, glutamine; G, glycine; H, histidine; I, isoleucine; L, leucine; K, lysine; M, methionine; F, phenylalanine; P, proline; S, serine; T, threonine; W, tryptophan; Y, tyrosine; V, valine.

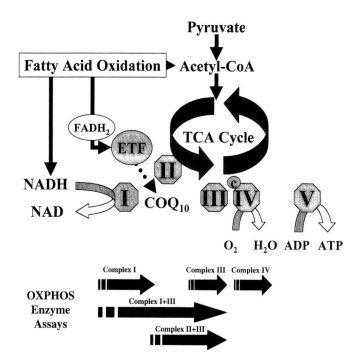

Fig. 5.2. Oxidative phosphorylation, tricarboxylic acid cycle and fatty acid oxidation. Because of the close inter-relationship among these pathways, primary abnormalities in oxidative phosphorylation (OXPHOS) may cause a variety of metabolic abnormalities. Common enzyme assays used to assess OXPHOS are shown. Arrows indicate the enzyme (complex I, complex III, complex IV) or enzymes (complex I + III, complex II + III) tested with each assay.

by anaerobic pathways. Mitochondrial volume in type IIA (fast oxidative glycolytic) fibres, which rely on both aerobic and glycolytic pathways of energy delivery, is similar to that in type I fibres. In human muscle, the volume fraction of mitochondria usually varies by a factor of two or three between fibre types, while in rodents, with muscles that are more specialized than humans, the differences can be larger. There is an inverse relationship between mass-specific oxygen consumption and body mass in mammals; consequently, homologous muscle groups generally have much higher mitochondrial densities in small than in large mammals.

The ultrastructural pattern of organization of mitochondria in normal muscle is very ordered. The subsarcolemmal population consists of what appear to be independent organelles clustered between the myofibrils and the plasma membrane. Intermyofibrillar mitochondria are interspersed between myofibres; on cross-section they appear as pairs in the half I bands adjacent to the Z line. In three dimensions there are, in fact, bracelets that encircle the myofibre.

Mitochondrial biochemistry

Mitochondria contain a broad spectrum of enzymatic activities including the enzymatic machinery for fatty acid oxidation, oxidative phosphorylation, haem biosynthesis and part of the urea cycle. The most important functions, as far as muscle disease is concerned, are oxidative phosphorylation and fatty acid oxidation.

Electron transport and oxidative phosphorylation

The electron transport–oxidative phosphorylation system is located in the inner mitochondrial membrane (Fig. 5.2). Functionally the system is composed of five enzyme complexes: NADH CoQ reductase (I), succinate CoQ reductase (II), ubiquinol cytochrome c reductase (III), cytochrome c oxidase (COX) (IV) and ATP synthase (V). These complexes are large oligomers composed of more than 80 polypeptides in total, 13 of which are encoded in the mitochondrial genome (Fig. 5.1). Complexes I–IV make up the respiratory chain; coenzyme Q and cytochrome c act as shuttle molecules to move electrons between the complexes. Electrons derived from the oxidation of glucose or fatty acids enter the chain as the reduced forms of nicotinamide or flavin adenine dinucleotides (NADH or $FADH_2$) at complex I or II and are passed to carriers of progressively greater electron affinity and ultimately accepted by molecular oxygen to form water. Complex I transfers electrons through a series of redox groups that includes flavin mononucleotide (FMN) and six iron–sulphur clusters. It is composed of about 43 subunits, seven of which are encoded in mtDNA (Fig. 5.1). Complex II performs a key reaction in the tricarboxylic acid cycle in which succinate is dehydrogenated to fumarate and the electrons are donated to CoQ. It is located on the matrix side of the membrane and its four subunits are encoded by nuclear genes. Complex III transfers electrons between the two shuttle molecules, CoQ and cytochrome c. It is composed of 11 subunits, only one of which (cytochrome b) is encoded in mtDNA (Fig. 5.1). Complex IV accepts electrons from cytochrome c and donates them molecular oxygen. Three of its thirteen subunits are encoded in mtDNA (Fig. 5.1). At three stages along this chain (complexes I, III and IV), energy is conserved by pumping protons across the inner mitochondrial membrane from the matrix space, which establishes an electrochemical gradient for protons across this membrane. The energy conserved in this gradient is then used to synthesize ATP in the ATP synthase (V) reaction, functionally coupling electron transport along the respiratory chain to oxidative phosphorylation. Complex V is composed of two parts, an F_1 segment that catalyses the synthesis of ATP, and

F_o component that translocates protons into the mitochondrial matrix. It consists of 12 or 13 subunits, two of which are mitochondrially encoded (Fig. 5.1).

Fatty acid oxidation

Lipids are an important source of metabolic energy for sustained work in skeletal muscle, and mitochondria are the major site for their oxidation. Long-chain free fatty acids are taken up by the muscle cell and activated to their coenzyme A (CoA) esters in the cytosol by acyl-CoA synthetase. These are then esterified to their carnitine esters by carnitine palmitoyl transferase (CPT) I and translocated into the mitochondrial matrix on a specific transporter. Once inside the matrix, the carnitine esters are reconverted to fatty acyl-CoAs by CPT II. Short- and medium-chain fatty acids can cross the mitochondrial membranes directly and are activated in the matrix. The fatty acyl-CoAs are oxidized in a series of four reactions in the β-oxidation pathway, resulting in the removal of two carbons for each turn of the β-oxidation spiral and the production of $FADH_2$ and NADH.

Mitochondrial molecular biology

Mitochondrial DNA

Structure, genetic code and organization

mtDNA is a double-stranded circular DNA molecule of ~16.5kb in all mammals (Fig. 5.1). The two stands are referred to as heavy (H) and light (L), reflecting their behaviour in caesium chloride density gradients. Mammalian mtDNA codes for 13 polypeptides, all of which are subunits of the enzyme complexes in the respiratory chain, and the 22 transfer RNAs (tRNAs) and two ribosomal RNAs (rRNAs) necessary for their translation. The genetic code of mammalian mtDNA is different to the 'universal' genetic code: UGA, the universal STOP, is Trp, AUA is Met and AGA, AGG (universal Arg) are STOP codons. Consequently, genes encoded in mtDNA cannot be translated on cytosolic ribosomes.

The mitochondrial genome is exceedingly compact, containing no introns and only one noncoding region of ~1kb, the D-loop. This is a triple-stranded region that contains one of the replication origins (O_H) and the promoters for transcription of the H and L strands. The genome copy number of mtDNA is 10^3–10^4 in most cells, organized as approximately five copies (range 2–10) per organelle (Nass, 1969; Satoh and Kuroiwa, 1991). Gametes are a notable exception to this generalization: mature oocytes have approximately 10^5 mtDNAs (Piko and Taylor, 1987) and sperm about 10^2 (Hecht et al., 1984).

Replication

Replication of mtDNA occurs asynchronously from two origins; one for the H strand in the D-loop and a second for the L strand about two-thirds of the way around the molecule (Clayton, 1982). It is catalysed by a distinct polymerase, the γ-DNA polmerase, and leading strand synthesis at O_H is primed by a short piece of RNA generated by transcription from the L-strand promoter. Thus, replication of the genome is linked in some way to the transcription of mtDNA genes. Transcription initiation of mtDNA (and, therefore, priming of mtDNA replication) requires the presence of the only known mitochondrial transcription factor Tfam (formerly referred to as mtTFA) (Shadel and Clayton, 1997: Larsson et al., 1998). In contrast to nuclear DNA, replication of mtDNA is not linked to the cell cycle (Clayton, 1982). This 'relaxed' form of replication allows some templates to replicate more than once during the cell cycle, others not at all. Thus, while mtDNA copy number is tightly regulated in a cell- and tissue-specific manner (by largely unknown mechanisms), sequence variants can segregate during mitosis owing to unequal replication from templates in the parent cell and random sampling of mtDNAs at cytokinesis (Birky, 1994). In a postmitotic cell, sequence variants segregate as mitochondria turnover. In the absence of selection, the rate of segregation of mtDNA sequence variants depends primarily on two parameters: mtDNA copy number and the turnover rate of mtDNA.

Transcription

mtDNA is transcribed as polycistronic RNAs in three different transcription units: the H-strand rDNA region, the entire H strand and the entire L strand (Shadel and Clayton, 1997). These must then be processed into mature rRNAs, tRNAs and mRNAs. Transcription requires Tfam which binds to sequences near the promoter elements. Maturation of these transcripts requires different types of (nuclear encoded) RNA-processing enzyme. The rRNAs are transcribed about 25 times more frequently than the whole H-strand transcription unit. Differential rRNA transcription is determined by a termination site contained in the coding sequence for tRNA[Leu], which binds a specific nuclear-encoded factor mTERF (Christianson and Clayton, 1986; Kruse et al., 1989; Fernandez-Silva et al., 1997). The rate of transcription of mitochondrial rRNAs and mRNAs is low in proportion to mtDNA copy number (compared with nuclear-encoded genes); however, it is thought that transcription is not rate limiting for mitochondrial gene expression (Attardi and Schatz, 1988).

Post-transcriptional mechanisms such as differential stability and/or translation efficiency of mRNAs are thought to be important in the regulation of the expression of mtDNA-encoded genes (Attardi et al., 1990). Additionally, although tRNAs are transcribed at vastly different rates in the three transcription units, steady-state concentrations of all tRNAs are remarkably similar (Attardi et al., 1990). It has been suggested that tRNA levels may be in some way determined by the activity of the individual tRNA aminoacyl synthetases.

Translation

The mitochondrial translation system is unique in many respects, although functionally it is most similar to that in prokaryotes. Mitochondrial ribosomes have a similar mass to bacterial ribosomes, but a much high protein:RNA ratio, and similar antibiotic sensitivity (Denslow et al., 1989). Mitochondrial mRNAs are not capped at their $5'$ ends and translation initiation begins with formyl-tRNA^{Met}. However, mitochondrial mRNAs lack a $5'$ leader sequence, and interaction of the small ribosomal subunit appears to be sequence independent. Binding of mRNA to the small subunit appears to prevent association with other ribosomes, and this may account for the rarity or absence of polysomes (Liao and Spremulli, 1990).

Mitochondrial biogenesis

At least several hundred proteins are necessary for mitochondria to perform their diverse biochemical activities. As only a handful are encoded in the mitochondria themselves, the vast majority, which are synthesized on cytosolic ribosomes, must be transported to the mitochondrion and inserted into the correct location in the mitochondrion. In the case of the respiratory chain enzymes, this must be coordinated with the expression of the mtDNA-encoded polypeptides. The protein import system in mitochondria has been the object of intense investigation since the 1980s, particularly in model organisms (Schatz, 1996; Kaldi and Neupert, 1998; Pfanner, 1998). Most targeted polypeptides have N-terminal leader sequences that are rich in basic amino acid residues and capable of forming an amphipathic α-helical structure. Polypeptides are transported in the unfolded state complexed with cytoplasmic chaperones like HSP70 (heat shock protein 70) and this complex interacts with the outer membrane receptor (TOM) complex. The polypeptide is then ratcheted in through the inner membrane transport (TIM) complex by the action of chaperones in the matrix, where it is processed by proteases and inserted into the

correct location. Not all mitochondrial proteins have N-terminal leaders, and recently a completely parallel import system for carrier proteins such as the ATP/ADP translocase has been identified (Koehler et al., 1998; Pfanner, 1998; Endres et al., 1999).

The process by which new mitochondrial membranes are elaborated is much less well understood than the protein import pathways. Cardiolipin, a phospholipid unique to mitochondria, is synthesized in mitochondria. The other major phospholipids in mitochondrial membranes (phosphatidylserine, phosphatidylethanolamine, phosphatidylcholine and phosphatidylinositol) are transferred from their site of synthesis in the endoplasmic reticulum via regions of membrane continuity (Vance and Shiao, 1996).

Control of mitochondrial volume fraction in muscle

Although the mature muscle fibre is a postmitotic, multinuclear syncytium, it is very plastic, being able to adapt to changing demands of work dictated by input from the motor nerve. Endurance training has long been known to increase mitochondrial number and aerobic capacity, while strength training is either without effect or decreases mitochondrial volume fraction. Numerous studies involving cross-re-innervation of fast muscles with a slow motor neuron, or chronic stimulation of a fast motor neuron by a electrode with the input characteristic of a slow motor neuron, have shown a severalfold upregulation of mitochondrial volume in response to the increasing aerobic demand associated with the transformation of the contractile properties of the muscle (Salmons and Henriksson, 1981; Pette and Vrbova, 1985). From this large body of information it is clear that input from the motor nerve has a major influence on mitochondrial biogenesis. The signalling cascade that controls this process is, however, not well understood.

Intracellular calcium has been suggested to play a role in the response of mitochondria to cellular stress, mediated by a reduction in mtDNA copy number or respiratory chain inhibitors (Biswas et al., 1999), and in the conversion of fibre type, a process that may be mediated by the activity of calcineurin (Chin et al., 1998). Calcineurin is a serine/threonine protein phosphatase that is regulated by calcium-calmodulin. Its function has been well studied in lymphocytes, where it regulates the cytoplasmic to nuclear movement of a transcription factor (NFAT). Calcineurin activity is modulated by the steady-state intracellular calcium level, but it is insensitive to large transient changes in intracellular calcium such as those created by input from a fast motor neuron. In skeletal muscle, calcineurin specifically activates the promoters of the slow isoforms of muscle proteins through an interaction with another muscle transcription factor (MEF2). Inhibition of its activity by cyclosporin A (cyclosporine) was shown to effect a fast to slow conversion of fibre type in vivo. Whether this pathway might also be directly involved in signalling changes in the number of mitochondria and the copy number of mtDNA is not known.

Mitochondrial genetics

Transmission of mtDNA

Inheritance of mtDNA is strictly maternally in mammals (Giles et al., 1980; Kaneda et al., 1995); new sequence variants are transmitted along maternal lineages without the benefit of recombination with male mtDNA. Most individuals have a single sequence variant of mtDNA in all of their cells (mtDNA homoplasmy). There is, however, a great deal of sequence variability between individuals. In human populations, individuals typically differ by 0.3%, or about 50 nucleotides in the mtDNA sequence. The rarity of mtDNA heteroplasmy and the high degree of population polymorphism suggest that new mtDNA sequence variants are rapidly segregated in maternal lineages. This is paradoxical given the high genome copy number in mature oocytes ($\sim 10^5$ copies of mtDNA) and the relatively small number of cell divisions in oogenesis.

These considerations led Hauswirth and Laipis (Hauswirth and Laipis, 1982; Laipis et al., 1988) to hypothesize the existence of a genetic bottleneck for mtDNA in oogenesis or early embryogenesis. This concept was based largely on observations of a heteroplasmic D-loop sequence variant in Holstein cows, which was observed to segregate rapidly in a few generations (Laipis et al., 1988; Ashley et al., 1989). Rapid segregation of mtDNA sequence variants has also been observed in human pedigrees segregating pathogenic or silent mtDNA mutations (Howell et al., 1991, 1992, 1994; Larsson et al., 1992; Zhu et al., 1992; Santorelli et al., 1994; Uziel et al., 1997).

The number of mitochondria and the mtDNA copy number change dramatically during oogenesis and early embryogenesis. Ultrastructural analyses of human primordial germ cells indicate that they contain about 10 mitochondria; this number increases to about 200 in an oogonium and to several thousand in the oocyte in a primordial follicle (Jansen and de Boer, 1998). Measurements of mtDNA copy number in immature oocytes of the mouse suggest that there are approximately 10^3 copies (Piko and Taylor, 1987), increasing by 100-fold to approximately 10^5 in the mature oocyte. The mtDNA copy number is not known in either primordial germ cells or in oogonia but if

it is similar to that in somatic cells (approximately five per organelle), it is clear that there is greater than a 1000-fold increase in mtDNA copy number during oogenesis, from perhaps as few as 50 in the primordial germ cells to 100 000 in the preovulatory oocyte. After fertilization, cell division of the early embryo proceeds without mtDNA replication (Piko and Taylor, 1987). By the time the cells of the inner cell mass are set aside in the blastocyst (~ 100 cells), mtDNA copy number is reduced to about 10^3, in the same range as in most somatic cells.

Two different hypotheses were proposed to explain the bottleneck for transmission of mtDNA: amplification of a limited number of mtDNA templates during oocyte maturation (Hauswirth and Laipis, 1982) or nonrandom sampling of mtDNAs in the cells of the inner cell mass of the blastocyst (Ashley et al., 1989). These have recently been tested in heteroplasmic mice constructed from two different *Mus musculus domesticus* strains, NZB and BALB/c, using single-cell polymerase chain reaction (Jenuth et al., 1996). Little intercellular variation was observed in the degree of mtDNA heteroplasmy in the primordial germ cell population, suggesting that they were a more or less random sample of the mtDNA population in the zygote. However, analysis of primary oocytes revealed that the rapid segregation of the two mtDNA sequences observed in the offspring of heteroplasmic females had already occurred by the time this population was differentiated in fetal life. Segregation of mtDNA between the primary and mature oocytes was quantitatively unimportant, as was segregation between the mature oocytes and neonates.

These results indicate that most of the segregation of mtDNA occurs during mitosis in the migratory primordial germ cells and oogonia, supporting the concept of a single bottleneck for the transmission of mtDNA. Studies of D-loop length variants in humans are consistent with the mouse studies, showing that segregation has occurred by the time oocytes are mature (Marchington et al., 1997, 1998). Using a population genetic model, the effective number of segregating units of mtDNA has been estimated at about 200 in the mouse (Jenuth et al., 1996). This is in broad agreement with estimates obtained from human pedigrees segregating pathogenic point mutations, suggesting that the process may be similar in humans.

Segregation of mtDNA in somatic cells

Although it is very likely that the expression of mtDNA is required during fetal life, and there is abundant opportunity for mitotic segregation of mutant mtDNAs during this period, studies of fetal tissues in individuals carrying pathogenic mtDNA mutations show little tissue-to-tissue variation in the proportion of mutant and wild-type mtDNAs (Harding et al., 1992; Matthews et al., 1994). This suggests that selection for respiratory chain function is not strong during fetal life and that the proportion of mutant mtDNAs at birth is largely determined by the proportion in the oocyte. Similar observations have been made in heteroplasmic mice, in which there is little variation in heteroplasmy among tissues at birth but strong, tissue-specific selection for alternative mtDNA genotypes as the animal ages (Jenuth et al., 1997). Additional evidence for the proposition that selection against pathogenic mutations is weak until postnatal life comes from pedigree analysis of patients segregating mtDNA mutations. Although rapid shifts in the proportions of mutant mtDNAs can occur between generations, the shift appears just as likely to occur in the direction of wild-type mtDNA as mutant mtDNA in most pedigrees, and in some pedigrees to favour the mutant.

In contrast to the situation during development, mitotic segregation of pathogenic mtDNA sequence variants occurs throughout postnatal life. The load of mtDNA mutations inherited at birth undoubtedly plays an important role in the clinical phenotype of patients with pathogenic mtDNA mutations, but tissue-specific segregation can modify the proportions of mutant and wild-type mtDNAs significantly; this is often associated with a worsening clinical course. There is good evidence for increases in the proportions of some pathogenic mtDNA mutations with age in the skeletal muscle of patients with mitochondral encephalomyopathies (Larsson et al., 1990; Poulton and Morten, 1993; Weber et al., 1997) in whom mutant mtDNAs are often undetectable in actively dividing cells in the same individuals. This had led to the suggestion that there may be feedback mechanisms that promote the replication of mutant mtDNAs in postmitotic cells, reflecting a futile attempt to restore oxidative phophorylation function, and selection against cells with a growth disadvantage because of the presence of the mutants in actively mitotic cells. It is interesting to note that the most dramatic segregation patterns are observed in sporadic cases, where mutant mtDNAs are often only detectable in skeletal muscle (Holt et al., 1988; Moraes et al., 1993; Fu et al., 1996).

References

Ashley, M. V., Laipis, P. J. and Hauswirth, W. W. (1989). Rapid segregation of heteroplasmic bovine mitochondria. *Nucl. Acids Res.* **17**, 7325–7331.

Attardi, G. and Schatz, G. (1988). Biogenesis of mitochondria. *Annu. Rev. Cell Biol.* **4**, 289–333.

Attardi, G., Chomyn, A., King, M. P., Kruse, B., Polosa, P. L. and Murdter, N. N. (1990). Regulation of mitochondrial gene expression in mammalian cells. *Biochem. Soc. Trans.* **18**, 509–513.

Birky, C. W., Jr (1994). Relaxed and stringent genomes: why cytoplasmic genes don't obey Mendel's laws. *J. Hered.* **85**, 355–365.

Biswas, G., Adebanjo, O. A., Freedman, B. D. et al. (1999). Retrograde Ca^{2+} signalling in C2C12 skeletal myocytes in response to mitochondrial genetic and metabolic stress: a novel mode of inter-organelle crosstalk. *EMBO J.* **18**, 522–533.

Chin, E. R., Olson, E. N., Richardson, J. A., Yang, Q. et al. (1998). A calcineurin-dependent transcriptional pathway controls skeletal muscle fiber type. *Genes Dev.* **12**, 2499–2509.

Christianson, T. W. and Clayton, D. A. (1986). In vitro transcription of human mitochondrial DNA: accurate termination requires a region of DNA sequence that can function bidirectionally. *Proc. Natl. Acad. Sci. USA* **83**, 6277–6281.

Clayton, D. A. (1982). Replication of animal mitochondrial DNA. *Cell* **28**, 693–705.

Denslow, N. D., Michaels, G. S., Montoya, J., Attardi, G. and O'Brien, T. W. (1989). Mechanism of mRNA binding to bovine mitochondrial ribosomes. *J. Biol. Chem.* **264**, 8328–8338.

Endres, M., Neupert, W. and Brunner, M. (1999). Transport of the ADP/ATP carrier of mitochondria from the TOM complex to the TIM22.54 complex. *EMBO J.* **18**, 3214–3221.

Fernandez-Silva, P., Martinez-Azorin, F., Micol, V. and Attardi, G. (1997). The human mitochondrial transcription termination factor (mTERF) is a multizipper protein but binds to DNA as a monomer, with evidence pointing to intramolecular leucine zipper interactions. *EMBO J.* **16**, 1066–1079.

Fu, K., Hartlen, R., Johns, T., Genge, A., Karpati, G. and Shoubridge, E. A. (1996). A novel heteroplasmic tRNAleu(CUN) mtDNA point mutation in a sporadic patient with mitochondrial encephalomyopathy segregates rapidly in skeletal muscle and suggests an approach to therapy. *Hum. Mol. Genet.* **5**, 1835–1840.

Giles, R. E., Blanc, H., Cann, H. M. and Wallace, D. C. (1980). Maternal inheritance of human mitochondrial DNA. *Proc. Natl. Acad. Sci. USA* **77**, 6715–6719.

Harding, A. E., Holt, I. J., Sweeney, M. G., Brockington, M. and Davis, M. B. (1992). Prenatal diagnosis of mitochondrial DNA8993 T–G disease. *Am. J. Hum. Genet.* **50**, 629–633.

Hauswirth, W. W. and Laipis, P. J. (1982). Mitochondrial DNA polymorphism in a maternal lineage of Holstein cows. *Proc. Natl. Acad. Sci. USA* **79**, 4686–4690.

Hecht, N. B., Liem, H., Kleene, K. C., Distel, R. J. and Ho, S. M. (1984). Maternal inheritance of the mouse mitochondrial genome is not mediated by a loss or gross alteration of the paternal mitochondrial DNA or by methylation of the oocyte mitochondrial DNA. *Dev. Biol.* **102**, 452–461.

Holt, I. J., Harding, A. E. and Morgan-Hughes, J. A. (1988). Deletions of muscle mitochondrial DNA in patients with mitochondrial myopathies. *Nature* **331**, 717–719.

Howell, N., Bindoff, L. A., McCullough, D. A. et al. (1991). Leber hereditary optic neuropathy: identification of the same mitochondrial ND1 mutation in six pedigrees. *Am. J. Hum. Genet.* **49**, 939–950.

Howell, N., Halvorson, S., Kubacka, I., McCullough, D. A., Bindoff, L. A. and Turnbull, D. M. (1992). Mitochondrial gene segregation in mammals: is the bottleneck always narrow? *Hum. Genet.* **90**, 117–120.

Howell, N., Xu, M., Halvorson, S., Bodis-Wollner, I. and Sherman, J. (1994). A heteroplasmic LHON family: tissue distribution and transmission of the 11778 mutation. [Letter] *Am. J. Hum. Genet.* **55**, 203–206.

Jansen, R. P. and de Boer, K. (1998). The bottleneck: mitochondrial imperatives in oogenesis and ovarian follicular fate. *Mol. Cell. Endocrinol.* **145**, 81–88.

Jenuth, J. P., Peterson, A. C., Fu, K. and Shoubridge, E. A. (1996). Random genetic drift in the female germline explains the rapid segregation of mammalian mitochondrial DNA. [See comments]. *Nat. Genet.* **14**, 146–151.

Jenuth, J. P., Peterson, A. C. and Shoubridge, E. A. (1997). Tissue-specific selection for different mtDNA genotypes in heteroplasmic mice. *Nat. Genet.* **16**, 93–95.

Kaldi, K. and Neupert, W. (1998). Protein translocation into mito-chondria. *Biofactors* **8**, 221–224.

Kaneda, H., Hayashi, J., Takahama, S., Taya, C., Lindahl, K. F. and Yonekawa, H. (1995). Elimination of paternal mitochondrial DNA in intraspecific crosses during early mouse embryogenesis. *Proc. Natl. Acad. Sci. USA* **92**, 4542–4546.

Koehler, C. M., Jarosch, E., Tokatlidis, K., Schmid, K., Schweyen, R. J. and Schatz, G. (1998). Import of mitochondrial carriers mediated by essential proteins of the intermembrane space. *Science* **279**, 369–373.

Kruse, B., Narasimhan, N. and Attardi, G. (1989). Termination of transcription in human mitochondria: identification and purifi-cation of a DNA binding protein factor that promotes termina-tion. *Cell* **58**, 391–397.

Laipis, P. J., Van de Walle, M. J. and Hauswirth, W. W. (1988). Unequal partitioning of bovine mitochondrial genotypes among siblings. *Proc. Natl. Acad. Sci. USA* **85**, 8107–8110.

Larsson, N. G., Holme, E., Kristiansson, B., Oldfors, A. and Tulinius, M. (1990). Progressive increase of the mutated mitochondrial DNA fraction in Kearns–Sayre syndrome. *Pediatr. Res.* **28**, 131–136.

Larsson, N. G., Tulinius, M. H., Holme, E. et al. (1992). Segregation and manifestations of the mtDNA tRNA(Lys) A→G(8344) muta-tion of myoclonus epilepsy and ragged-red fibers (MERRF) syn-drome. *Am. J. Hum. Genet.* **51**, 1201–1212.

Larsson, N. G., Wang, J., Wilhelmsson, H. et al. (1998). Mitochondrial transcription factor A is necessary for mtDNA maintenance and embryogenesis in mice. [See comments] *Nat. Genet.* **18**, 231–236.

Liao, H. X. and Spremulli, L. L. (1990). Identification and initial characterization of translational initiation factor 2 from bovine mitochondria. *J. Biol. Chem.* **265**, 13618–13622.

Marchington, D. R., Hartshorne, G. M., Barlow, D. and Poulton, J. (1997). Homopolymeric tract heteroplasmy in mtDNA from tissues and single oocytes: support for a genetic bottleneck. *Am. J. Hum. Genet.* **60**, 408–416.

Marchington, D. R., Macaulay, V., Hartshorne, G. M., Barlow, D. and Poulton, J. (1998). Evidence from human oocytes for a genetic bottleneck in an mtDNA disease. *Am. J. Hum. Genet.* **63**, 769–775.

Matthews, P. M., Hopkin, J., Brown, R. M., Stephenson, J. B., Hilton-Jones, D. and Brown, G. K. (1994). Comparison of the relative levels of the 3243 (A→G) mtDNA mutation in heteroplasmic adult and fetal tissues. *J. Med. Genet.* **31**, 41–44.

Moraes, C. T., Ciacci, F., Bonilla, E., Ionasescu, V., Schon, E. A. and DiMauro, S. (1993). A mitochondrial tRNA anticodon swap asso-ciated with a muscle disease. *Nat. Genet.* **4**, 284–288.

Nass, M. M. (1969). Mitochondrial DNA. I. Intramitochondrial dis-tribution and structural relations of single- and double-length circular DNA. *J. Mol. Biol.* **42**, 521–528.

Pette, D. and Vrbova, G. (1985). Neural control of phenotypic expres-sion in mammalian muscle fibers. *Muscle Nerve* **8**, 676–689.

Pfanner, N. (1998). Mitochondrial import: crossing the aqueous intermembrane space. *Curr. Biol.* **8**, R262–R265.

Piko, L. and Taylor, K. D. (1987). Amounts of mitochondrial DNA and abundance of some mitochondrial gene transcripts in early mouse embryos. *Dev. Biol.* **123**, 364–374.

Poulton, J. and Morten, K. (1993). Noninvasive diagnosis of the MELAS syndrome from blood DNA. [Letter] *Ann. Neurol.* **34**, 116.

Salmons, S. and Henriksson, J. (1981). The adaptive response of skeletal muscle to increased use. *Muscle Nerve* **4**, 94–105.

Santorelli, F. M., Shanske, S., Jain, K. D., Tick, D., Schon, E. A. and DiMauro, S. (1994). A T→C mutation at nt 8993 of mitochondrial DNA in a child with Leigh syndrome. *Neurology* **44**, 972–974.

Satoh, M. and Kuroiwa, T. (1991). Organization of multiple nucle-oids and DNA molecules in mitochondria of a human cell. *Exp. Cell. Res.* **196**, 137–140.

Schatz, G. (1996). The protein import system of mitochondria. *J. Biol. Chem.* **271**, 31763–31766.

Shadel, G. S. and Clayton, D. A. (1997). Mitochondrial DNA main-tenance in vertebrates. *Annu. Rev. Biochem.* **66**, 409–435.

Uziel, G., Moroni, I., Lamantea, E., et al. (1997). Mitochondrial disease associated with the T8993G mutation of the mitochon-drial ATPase 6 gene: a clinical, biochemical and molecular study in six families. *J. Neurol. Neurosurg. Psychiatry* **63**, 16–22.

Vance, J. E. and Shiao, Y. J. (1996). Intracellular trafficking of phos-pholipids: import of phosphatidylserine into mitochondria. *Anticancer. Res.* **16**, 1333–1339.

Weber, K., Wilson, J. N., Taylor, L., Brierley, E. et al. (1997). A new mtDNA mutation showing accumulation with time and restric-tion to skeletal muscle. *Am. J. Hum. Genet.* **60**, 373–380.

Yaffe, M. P. (1999). The machinery of mitochondrial inheritance and behaviour. *Science* **283**, 1493–1497.

Zhu, D. P., Economou, E. P., Antonarakis, S. E. and Maumenee, I. H. (1992). Mitochondrial DNA mutation and heteroplasmy in type I Leber hereditary optic neuropathy. *Am. J. Med. Genet.* **42**, 173–179.

6

The sarcotubular system

Kimby N. Barton and David H. MacLennan

Structure and function of the sarcotubular system

Muscle contraction and relaxation are regulated by the concentration of free Ca^{2+} in the sarcoplasm. Calcium concentrations, in turn, are regulated by the interplay between proteins in two elaborate membranous structures, the organelle referred to as the sarcoplasmic reticulum and invaginations of the sarcolemma, referred to as transverse tubules or T-tubules (Franzini-Armstrong, 1970). The sarcoplasmic reticulum in skeletal muscle is an extensive intracellular muscle membrane system that surrounds each myofibril like a water jacket. The T-tubules criss-cross muscle cells at defined intervals, facilitating movement of specific ions between the sarcoplasm and the extracellular space. This is possible because the T-tubular membrane is highly enriched in Ca^{2+}, Na^+ and K^+ channels and because the 'lumen' of the T-tubule is continuous with the extracellular space.

The periodicity of entry of T-tubules into the muscle cell and the segmentation of sarcoplasmic reticular structure and function are both defined by the transverse periodicity of structure and function in myofibrils. Myofibrils are segmented longitudinally into short, repeating contractile elements referred to as sarcomeres (Huxley, 1969). Prominent features of sarcomere structure are the transverse Z lines, which mark the boundaries of the sarcomere; the I bands, which are made up solely of thin filaments that protrude longitudinally on both sides of each Z line; the A bands, which are made up of longitudinal thick filaments with or without interdigitating thin filaments; an H zone near the centre of the A band, which represents a region of variable length where thin filaments do not interdigitate; and an M line, which defines the middle of the sarcomere (Fig. 6.1). Each half of the sarcomere is a mirror image of the other.

Contractile force is generated by ATP-activated motors in myosin molecules in the thick filaments, which interact with actin molecules in the thin filaments (Rayment and Holden, 1994). The interaction between actin and myosin molecules, oriented in a bipolar manner, results in shortening of the sarcomere as the thin filaments are drawn toward the centre of the sarcomere. In skeletal and cardiac muscle, the physical interactions between actin and myosin are possible only when Ca^{2+} is bound to a low-molecular-weight, high-affinity Ca^{2+}-binding protein called troponin C (Ebashi et al., 1969). Troponin C is located within a heterotrimeric, globular troponin complex, which forms a regulatory structure within the thin filament by attaching to filamentous tropomyosin. Muscle relaxes when cytoplasmic Ca^{2+} concentrations are lowered, resulting in dissociation of Ca^{2+} from troponin C and release of the interaction between the actin- and myosin-containing filaments (Zot and Potter, 1987).

T-tubules invaginate from the sarcolemma at the level of the A–I band junction in mammalian skeletal muscle; as a result two layers of tubules form transverse bypasses across each sarcomere (Fig. 6.1). The sarcoplasmic reticulum is located between these two layers of T-tubules (Eisenberg et al., 1974). The sarcoplasmic reticulum is also segmented, with terminal cisternae at either end separated by anastomosing tubules of longitudinal reticulum. The terminal cisternae form an inflated collar around the myofibril, which contains a high density of lumenal proteins; the longitudinal reticulum contains relatively little lumenal structure. The Ca^{2+} release channels are highly concentrated on the faces of the terminal cisternae that apposes the T-tubule (the junctional face).

The T-tubule carries an action potential into the interior of the muscle cell; depolarization of the T-tubule membrane is transduced into Ca^{2+} release from the lumen of the sarcoplasmic reticulum, resulting in muscle contraction.

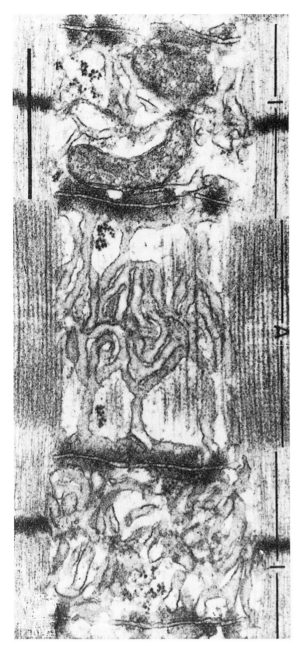

Fig. 6.1. A longitudinal section of the extensor digitorum longus muscle from a 30-day-old mouse from (Luff and Atwood, 1971). Thick filaments are seen in the centre of the A band region; thin filaments are seen in the I band. The transverse tubular system and the sarcoplasmic reticulum are in the centre of the picture. Transverse tubules running perpendicular to the fibres can be seen near the A–I junction. The sarcoplasmic reticulum consists, in part, of convoluted tubules overlying the A and I band regions; at the A–I junction, it is thickened to terminal cisternae, which abut the transverse tubular system. The matrix in the terminal cisternae is believed to consist of calsequestrin. (Reproduced from **The Journal of Cell Biology**, 1971, **51**, 369–383, by copyright permission of the Rockefeller University Press.)

Subsequently, Ca^{2+} is pumped back into the lumen of the sarcoplasmic reticulum, resulting in relaxation. Since cytoplasmic Ca^{2+} concentrations are so critical to muscle contraction and relaxation, the sarcotubular system of Ca^{2+} pumps and channels must be carefully regulated in a process referred to as excitation/contraction (E–C) coupling.

There are a number of key functional proteins in the sarcotubular system: Ca^{2+} channels, Ca^{2+} pumps, integral proteins of the membranes and luminal proteins. These will be discussed in more detail in this chapter.

Calcium channels

Calcium-release channel/ryanodine receptor

A major component in the junctional terminal cisternae of the sarcoplasmic reticulum is the Ca^{2+} release channel commonly referred to as the ryanodine receptor (RYR) (Fig. 6.2). The 15 nm gap between the junctional terminal cisternae of the sarcoplasmic reticulum and the T-tubule is filled with this huge, tetrameric sarcoplasmic reticular protein, which provides the primary channel for the release of Ca^{2+} stored in the terminal cisternae of the sarcoplasmic reticulum into the sarcoplasm, where it initiates muscle contraction (Fleischer and Inui, 1989).

The genes for the Ca^{2+}-release channels have been cloned from skeletal (*RYR1*), cardiac (*RYR2*) and non-muscle sources (*RYR3*) (Takeshima et al., 1989; Otsu et al., 1990; Zorzato et al., 1990; Giannini et al., 1992). The proteins encoded by these genes contain from 4872 to 5037 amino acid residues and have masses between 550 and 565 kDa. Predicted transmembrane sequences are found in the C-terminal fifth of each molecule, the minimum number being four (Takeshima et al., 1989) and the maximum number being 12 (Zorzato et al., 1990). The cytoplasmic component, bridging the gap between T-tubular and sarcoplasmic reticular membranes, therefore, lies between residues 1 and about 4500. The Ca^{2+}-release channels form tetrameric complexes with masses of approximately 2300 kDa (Wagenknecht et al., 1989).

The low-resolution, three-dimensional architecture of the tetrameric complexes has been deduced by reconstruction from cryoelectron microscopy (Radermacher et al., 1994; Serysheva et al., 1995). RYR consists of a large cytoplasmic assembly attached to a smaller transmembrane domain. The cytoplasmic assembly has large peripheral cavities connected to a central cavity by radial channels and has large lobes at each of its corners. It appears to be formed by the loose packing of 10 or more

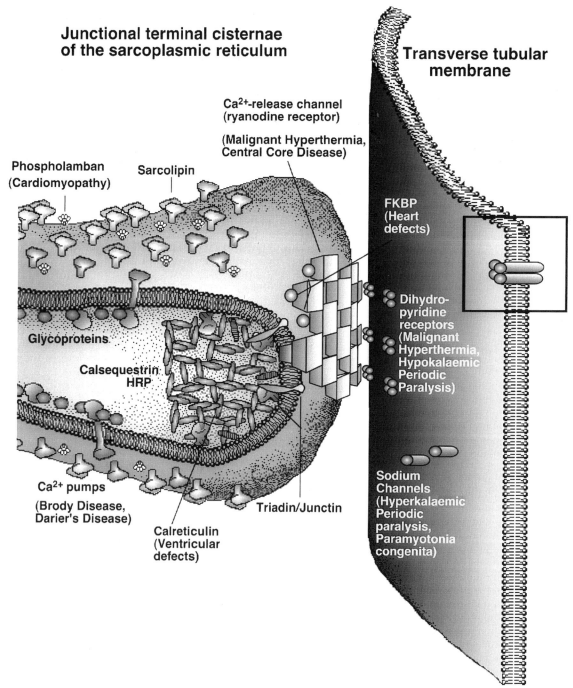

Fig. 6.2. A proposed arrangement of proteins in the sarcoplasmic reticulum and transverse (T) tubular membranes. A junctional terminal cisterna and its contiguous longitudinal sarcoplasmic reticulum are shown abutting the T tubule membrane. Four dihydropyridine receptor (DHPR) molecules in the T-tubule membrane are shown to be clustered to form a tetrad. The Ca^{2+}-release channel (ryanodine receptor or RYR) is shown as a square pyramidal structure in the junctional face membrane of the terminal cisterna of the sarcoplasmic reticulum, but RYR is a homotetrameric molecule with fourfold symmetry. The topography of the two membranes shows that each DHPR molecule in a DHPR tetrad can interact with a RYR monomer within the RYR homotetramer, but only in every other RYR homotetramer, since half of the homotetrameric RYR molecules are not apposed to DHPR tetrad clusters. Triadin (and junctin) are located in the junctional terminal cisternae membranes. These transmembrane molecules interact with both RYR and calsequestrin, assuring a high, buffered concentration of Ca^{2+} at the release site. Other Ca^{2+}-binding proteins are found in the lumen of both longitudinal and junctional sarcoplasmic reticulum. The Ca^{2+} pump (SERCA) molecules are the major transmembrane proteins in the longitudinal reticulum. The pumps associate with small regulatory proteins, phospholamban (cardiac) and sarcolipin (fast-twitch skeletal muscle), in the longitudinal reticulum membrane. The T-tubule is enriched in ion channels: Ca^{2+} (DHPR), Na^+, K^+ and Cl^- channels. Muscle diseases associated with a number of these proteins are indicated.

domains and its most striking feature is the large amount of solvent-occupied volume contained within various channels, holes and grooves. A channel-like feature can be resolved at the distal end of the transmembrane assembly, probably corresponding to the mouth of the ion-conducting channel. Four cavities appear on the sides of the transmembrane assembly near its junction with the cytoplasmic assembly. They may represent the exit site for Ca^{2+} when the channel is open. The volume occupied by the transmembrane and lumenal regions is in good agreement with 10 transmembrane sequences per monomer. The overall structure of the tetrameric complex is suggestive of a scaffold and seems well adapted to maintain the structural integrity of the triad junction, while allowing ions to diffuse freely from the transmembrane domain.

The Ca^{2+}-release channel has high single-channel conductance of 80 to 100 pS for Ca^{2+} and 400 to 800 pS for monovalent cations. In isolation, it is activated by micromolar Ca^{2+} and millimolar adenine nucleotides but is inhibited by millimolar Ca^{2+} or Mg^{2+} and by calmodulin, all of which are potential cellular regulators (Coronado et al., 1994; Meissner, 1994). Caffeine, ryanodine and dantrolene are pharmacological agents with high specificity for the channel. Caffeine, which activates the channel at millimolar concentrations, is often used in functional studies, while dantrolene closes the channel. It is the specific antidote for the excess Ca^{2+} release that initiates an episode of malignant hyperthermia (Britt, 1984). Ryanodine binds to the open channel with high affinity and converts the channel to an open subconductance state at low concentration but inhibits at high concentration (Coronado et al., 1994; Meissner, 1994).

Proteins modulating calcium release channels

FK506-binding protein
FK506-binding protein (FKBP) is a *cis-trans*-peptidyl-prolyl isomerase that binds the immunosuppressant drugs FK506 (tacrolimus) and rapamycin (Harding et al., 1989). FKBP12 is a 12 kDa protein that copurifies with the skeletal RYR (RYR1) in a stoichiometric ratio of four FKBP12 per RYR tetramer (Qi et al., 1998). In vitro studies have shown that dissociation of FKBP12 from RYR1 alters RYR1 gating properties by stabilizing the closed state of the channel and decreasing the frequency of subconductance states (Timerman et al., 1993). It appears to improve cooperativity among the four RYR subunits, resulting in stable full conductance channels (Marx et al., 1998). FKBP, directly visualized by cryoelectron microscopy, is located along the edge of the square-shaped cytoplasmic domain of RYR, at a distance of approximately 12 nm from the channel-forming domain. In this position, it may modulate channel

gating (Wagenknecht et al., 1997). Treatment of skinned muscle fibres with FK506, which dissociates FKBP12 from RYR, disrupts E–C coupling (Lamb and Stephenson, 1996). Mice in which the gene encoding FKBP12 was disrupted were found to have normal skeletal muscle but to have severe dilated cardiomyopathy and ventricular defects, demonstrating a phenotype for FKBP12 deficiency (Shou et al., 1998).

Calmodulin
Calmodulin is a cytoplasmic, Ca^{2+}-dependent enzyme regulator and a modulatory ligand of the RYR. In vitro studies have shown that calmodulin binds to RYR with nanomolar affinity and modulates its Ca^{2+} channel activity by direct protein–protein interactions without involvement of Ca^{2+}-dependent kinases (Meissner, 1994). The effect of calmodulin on the channel is dependent on Ca^{2+} concentration. At nanomolar levels, an increase in calmodulin increases the open probability of the channel, thereby increasing Ca^{2+} release severalfold; at higher Ca^{2+} concentrations, it has the opposite effect. Cryoelectron microscopy shows that calmodulin binds to the cytoplasmic assembly at a site within a cleft that faces the junctional sarcoplasmic reticular membrane, about 10 nm from the entrance to the transmembrane ion channel (Wagenknecht et al., 1994, 1997). It binds to a domain connected directly to a cytoplasmic extension of the transmembrane assembly and, therefore, might cause structural changes in the domain that, in turn, might modulate channel gating.

Slow or L-type calcium channel/dihydropyridine receptor

A major component of the T-tubule is the five subunit L-type Ca^{2+} channel protein (DHPR) that is the receptor for Ca^{2+} channel blockers such as dihydropyridine. The α_1-subunit of 212 kDa forms the Ca^{2+} channel and binds dihydropyridines (Tanabe et al., 1987). It consists of four repeat domains, I to IV, each domain containing six transmembrane sequences, S1 to S6. In each domain, transmembrane sequence S4 is positively charged; about every fourth residue in the otherwise hydrophobic sequence is either Lys or Arg. This results in stacking of positive charges with limited mobility across the membrane. A relatively hydrophilic loop on the extracellular surface between S5 and S6 in domains III and IV is involved in pore formation (Nakayama et al., 1991). A cytoplasmic loop between domains II and III forms a functional connection with RYR (Tanabe et al., 1990). A cytoplasmic loop between domains III and IV contains the first *DHPR* mutation associated with malignant hyperthermia (Monnier et al., 1997).

The α_1-subunit is both a voltage sensor and a Ca^{2+}

Table 6.1. Genetic diseases of voluntary muscle and their chromosomal locations

Disease	OMIM No.[a]	Gene and chromosomal location	Involved protein[b]
Brody disease	601003	*ATP2A1*, 16p12	SERCA1
Darier's disease	124200	*ATP2A2*, 12q23-q24.1	SERCA2b
Hyperkalaemic periodic paralysis	170500	*SCN4A*, 17q23.1-q25.3	Na^+ channel α_1-subunit
Hypokalaemic periodic paralysis	170400	*CACNL1A3*, 1q32	DHPR α_1-subunit
Malignant hyperthermia	145600	*RYR1*, 19q13.1	RYR1
Paramyotonia congenita		*SCN4A*, 17q23.1-q25.3	Na^+ channel α_1-subunit

Note:

[a] For further information on genetic diseases the OMIM website, *Online Mendelian Inheritance in Man*, can be accessed at http://www.ncbi.nlm.nih.gov/omim

[b] See text for description of these proteins.

channel (Tanabe et al., 1987). During depolarization a 'charge movement', which precedes Ca^{2+} release from internal stores, can be detected in the transverse tubular membrane (Schneider and Chandler, 1973). Modulation of this charge movement by dihydropyridines suggests that it originates in the DHPR (Rios et al., 1992). The stacked charges in the S4 domain of the DHPR provides the structural basis for a charge movement in response to depolarization of the transverse tubular membrane. Since Ca^{2+} entry through the DHPR is a late event in E–C coupling and skeletal muscle (but not cardiac muscle) can be stimulated to contract and relax repeatedly in the Ca^{2+}-free medium, Ca^{2+}-channel function is not critical to E–C coupling (Bers, 1991). These observations lead to the conclusion that the voltage sensor is the key component of DHPR involvement in E–C coupling in skeletal muscle.

The other subunits of the DHPR complex are considered to be regulatory. They are the integral α_2/δ-subunits, which are cleaved post-translationally from a single transcript, the peripheral β-subunit, which has clear regulatory properties (Lacerda et al., 1991) and the integral γ-subunit.

Interactions of calcium channel receptors

Structural analysis shows that four DHPR molecules in the T-tubular membrane are normally tightly clustered in direct apposition to one tetrameric RYR molecule in the junctional terminal cisternae of the sarcoplasmic reticulum; consequently one DHPR molecule can potentially interact with one RYR subunit (Block et al., 1994) (see Fig. 6.2). Only one in two RYR tetramers is apposed to the DHPR cluster, however; as a result the mechanism of opening of alternative Ca^{2+}-release channels may be indirect. The apposition of the two proteins is sufficiently close that protein–protein interactions can occur between the two receptors, in line with the suggestion

that physical interactions open the Ca^{2+}-release channel. The charge movement in the DHPR, which is the probable response to voltage change, precedes Ca^{2+} release, and its block by dihydropyridines also blocks Ca^{2+} release (Rios et al., 1992). These observations are viewed as evidence that a conformational or positional change in the DHPR is transmitted directly to the RYR, leading to its activation.

Diseases resulting from mutations in the ryanodine receptor

Defects in Ca^{2+} regulatory systems involved with E–C coupling have been shown to be fatal or to lead to disease (Table 6.1). Knock-out of *RYR1* (Takeshima et al., 1994) is fatal, but knock-out of *RYR3* (Takeshima et al., 1996) is relatively benign. Point mutations in *RYR1*, however, can lead to muscle disease. Malignant hyperthermia (MH) is an inherited, autosomal dominant abnormality that can result in an adverse response to potent inhalational anaesthetics and depolarizing skeletal muscle relaxants. The major features of this reaction are skeletal muscle contracture, hypermetabolism and elevated temperature. All of these features can be linked directly to elevated Ca^{2+} in skeletal muscle: contracture and glycogenolysis are triggered directly by elevated Ca^{2+}, while hypermetabolic events and rising temperature result from excess ATP utilization and resynthesis (MacLennan and Phillips, 1992). Inheritance of the abnormality has been linked in about 50% of patients to *RYR1* encoding the skeletal muscle RYR (Loke and MacLennan, 1998). Mutations are clustered in areas giving rise to two regions in the cytoplasmic domain that are not involved in channel formation but are likely to be involved in channel regulation.

Central core disease (CCD) is a rare, nonprogressive myopathy presenting in infancy and characterized by hypotonia and proximal muscle weakness. MH is a common symptom for many patients with CCD. Inheritance of CCD has also been linked to *RYR1* in virtually all cases where it has been investigated (Brownell, 1988). Mutations giving rise to CCD are interspersed with those linked with MH in two 'hotspots' (Loke and MacLennan, 1998), but a mutation giving rise to CCD has been found in a third region, the channel-forming domain (Lynch et al., 1999). CCD and MH appear to be differentiated on the basis of the severity of the Ca^{2+} leak that characterizes these abnormal channel (Tong et al., 1999).

Diseases resulting from mutations affecting the dihydropyridine receptor

Malignant hyperthermia
A functional knock-out of the gene encoding the skeletal muscle DHPR (*CACNL1A3*) is the basis for muscular dysgenesis in the mouse (Tanabe et al., 1988). This animal model, bearing specific mutations in an E–C coupling component, has played a key role in unravelling the functions of, and the interactions between, DHPR and RYR proteins (Protasi et al., 1998). The homozygous mutation results in the loss of the α_1-subunit of the DHPR, leading to loss of charge movement, Ca^{2+} currents and E–C coupling. Function is restored by transfection of cultured dysgenic mouse myoblasts with cDNA encoding the α_1-subunit of the DHPR.

Mutations in the DHPR have also been linked to MH. In the only case published to date (Monnier et al., 1997), the mutation occurs in the DHPR III–IV loop, which may form a site of physical interaction between the skeletal muscle DHPR and RYR proteins (Leong and MacLennan, 1998). These observations highlight the fact that proteins in the two membrane systems, the sarcoplasmic reticulum and the T-tubule, interact closely to regulate Ca^{2+} concentrations in skeletal muscle.

Diseases that affect muscle membrane excitability
There are two groups of diseases that affect muscle membrane excitability: those in which the sarcolemma is hyperexcitable, responding to normal depolarizations with long trains of action potentials (myotonic discharges), and those in which the membrane is intermittently hypoexcitable, leading to muscle weakness or paralysis (Barchi, 1993). Hypokalaemic periodic paralysis (hypoKPP), an autosomal dominant skeletal muscle disorder, manifests as episodic weakness or paralysis associated with low serum K^+. Episodes are precipitated by a variety of conditions that cause an efflux of K^+ from serum into cells.

A related disease, hyperkalaemic periodic paralysis (hyperKPP) is also autosomal dominant with complete penetrance. A hallmark of this disease is a rise in serum K^+ during an attack, often dramatically. Paramyotonia congenita is an autosomal dominant disease characterized by myotonic symptoms made worse by exposure to cold. Sodium channel myotonias are characterized by diffuse myotonic discharges in skeletal muscle and slowed relaxation after voluntary muscle contraction. In these diseases, myotonia improves with exercise.

These disease have been linked to mutations in the Na^+, Ca^{2+} and Cl^- channels located in the T-tubules. Mutations in *CACNL1A3* encoding the α_1-subunit of the skeletal muscle DHPR (the slow Ca^{2+} channel) have been linked to hypoKPP (Jurkat-Rott et al., 1994). It is unclear how mutations located in the S4 segments of domains II and IV result in hypokalaemia and paralysis. HyperKPP is associated with missense mutations in the α_1-subunit of the skeletal muscle Na^+ channel (Ptáček et al., 1991). Other mutations in the same gene can result in paramyotonia congenita and sodium channel myotonia (Koch et al., 1992), which are also caused by defects in Cl^- channels (Lerche et al., 1993). These mutations impair fast inactivation of skeletal muscle or shift activation toward hyperpolarized potentials, causing muscle depolarization, myotonia and onset of weakness.

Calcium pumps

Calcium ATPase

Calcium released to the cytoplasm is transported back to the lumen of the sarcoplasmic reticulum by the sarco(endo)plasmic reticular Ca^{2+}-ATPase (SERCA) (Martonosi, 1995) located throughout all regions of the sarcoplasmic reticular membrane with the exception of the junctional terminal cisternae (Saito et al., 1984). SERCA and plasma membrane Ca^{2+} ATPases (PMCAs) have the highest affinity for Ca^{2+} removal from the cytoplasm and, together, set resting cytoplasmic Ca^{2+} concentrations. The Ca^{2+}-ATPase of fast-twitch skeletal muscle sarcoplasmic reticulum (SERCA1) is a 110 kDa, P-type ATPase that transports 2 mol Ca^{2+} per 1 mol protein at the expense of 1 mol ATP hydrolysis. Three differentially expressed genes referred to as *SERCA1*, *SERCA2* (expressed in cardiac muscle and, in alternatively spliced form, ubiquitously) and *SERCA3* encode at least six isoforms (Poch et al., 1998).

More than half of the protein forms a cytoplasmic globular headpiece, which is connected to a 10-transmembrane helix membrane domain via a cluster of four α-helices forming a stalk (MacLennan et al., 1985; Zhang et al., 1998). The headpiece is likely to resemble the structure of haloacid dehalogenase (Hisano et al., 1996; Aravind et al., 1998). The catalytic events of nucleotide binding and phosphorylation of Asp-351 occur in the cytoplasmic domain between helices M4 and M5. Calcium ions are bound to two sites in the transmembrane domain made up from transmembrane helices M4, M5 and M6, which associate as a right-handed coiled coil (Rice et al., 1997). The wide separation of the phosphorylation and Ca^{2+}-binding sites within the ATPase molecule implies long-distance transmission of conformational effects, and the rigid domains and long helices provide a plausible medium for this (MacLennan et al., 1997).

SERCA enzymes are typical of the class of P-type ATPases that form a phosphoprotein intermediate and undergo conformational changes during the course of ATP hydrolysis (MacLennan et al., 1997). Some of the conformational states can be stabilized, either by adjustment of reaction conditions or through mutagenesis, and these can be characterized as intermediates in the overall reaction cycle. The phosphorylated intermediate $E_1P(Ca)_2$ can phosphorylate ADP, while E_2P can only react with water. The formation of E_1P requires that both high-affinity Ca^{2+}-binding sites be occupied. The enzyme is then phosphorylated by ATP and, concomitantly, the two Ca^{2+} are occluded and can no longer exchange with unlabelled Ca^{2+}. The rate-limiting transition to E_2P is accompanied by loss of Ca^{2+} into the lumen, the affinity having fallen by three orders of magnitude. Hydrolysis of E_2P and regeneration of the high-affinity Ca^{2+}-binding sites $(E_1P(Ca)_2)$ complete the reversible cycle.

The mechanism of Ca^{2+} transport must take into account the characteristics of the transport process and the structure of the pump. The Ca^{2+}-binding and Ca^{2+} translocation sites are located in a cavity between M4, M5 and M6, where they are formed by the precise juxtaposition of Ca^{2+}-binding residues located in the three helices (MacLennan et al., 1997; Zhang et al., 1998). Access to the cavity is controlled by interactions between the larger residues near the cytoplasmic ends of the helices. The phosphorylation-induced domain movements that close off the cytoplasmic access to the cavity will initiate occlusion. Further long-range, phosphorylation-induced domain movements will open the exit gate, permitting release of weakly bound Ca^{2+} to the lumen. Later conformation changes will result in dephosphorylation of the low-energy, phosphorylated conformation of the enzyme (E_2P) and reformation of the high-energy Ca^{2+}-bound form of the enzyme $(E_1P(Ca)_2)$, completing the Ca^{2+} transport cycle.

Proteins modulating calcium pumps

Phospholamban

Phospholamban is a pentameric protein made up of 6 kDa subunits. It is located in the sarcoplasmic reticulum of cardiac, smooth and slow-twitch skeletal muscles, where it associates with and regulates the activity of the SERCA2a pump (Simmerman and Jones, 1998). In this role, it is a major regulator of the kinetics of cardiac contractility (Luo et al., 1994). Phospholambin contains 52 amino acid residues organized into a cytoplasmic sector of 30 residues, which contains a site for phosphorylation by protein kinase A and calmodulin kinase, and a transmembrane domain, made up solely of uncharged residues, probably in an α-helical conformation (Fujii et al., 1987). Desphosphorylated phospholamban is an inhibitor of Ca^{2+} transport and phosphorylation of phospholamban is associated with an increase in the affinity of the Ca^{2+} pump for Ca^{2+}, leading to the stimulation of the rate of Ca^{2+} uptake at low Ca^{2+} concentrations. The major effects of phosphorylation of phospholamban are an increase in the rate of cardiac relaxation and an increase in cardiac contractility. Increased contractility is an outcome of increased Ca^{2+} uptake and storage during the relaxation phase, setting the stage for enhanced Ca^{2+} release in the contractile phase (Bers, 1991).

Cytoplasmic interaction sites are formed by charged and hydrophobic amino acids in phospholamban domain I and by amino acids Lys-Asp-Asp-Lys-Pro-Val402 in SERCA2a (Toyofuku et al., 1994a,b). Transmembrane interactions occur through amino acids on one face of the the transmembrane helix of phospholamban (Kimura et al., 1997) and transmembrane helix six of SERCA2a (Asahi et al., 1999). Cytoplasmic and transmembrane interaction sites appear to form a regulatory circuit through long-range interactions (Kimura et al., 1997). The inhibitory interactions are disrupted by phosphorylation of the cytoplasmic domain of phospholamban or by binding of Ca^{2+} to the transmembrane domain of SERCA2a.

Mutations in either the transmembrane or the cytoplasmic domains of phospholamban can increase its inhibitory function dramatically (Kimura et al., 1997). If these mutations occurred naturally, they could lead to cardiomyopathy. Indeed transgenic mice expressing these dominant, highly inhibitory mutations do express signs of cardiomyopathy related to altered Ca^{2+} regulation.

Sarcolipin

Sarcolipin is a homologue of phospholamban that is expressed in fast-twitch skeletal muscle fibres, the same fibres that express SERCA1a (Odermatt et al., 1996, 1997). Like phospholamban, sarcolipin is an inhibitor of

SERCA1a activity at low Ca^{2+} concentrations; however, unlike phospholamban, it activates Ca^{2+} pump activity by about 40% at high Ca^{2+} concentrations (Odermatt et al., 1998). Thus sarcolipin might act as a 'turbo charger' to remove Ca^{2+} from the myoplasm at high Ca^{2+} concentrations, thereby enhancing the overall rate of relaxation of fast-twitch fibres. Insight into the importance of sarcolipin in fast-twitch fibre kinetics has been gained from studies of conversion of fast- to slow-twitch fibres by chronic low-frequency stimulation. Within 3 to 4 days, the maximal activity of Ca^{2+} pumps is reduced by about 40%, a first step in the process that leads to a reduction in the rate of relaxation in slow-twitch fibres (Leberer et al., 1987). This early loss of ATPase activity is not associated with any loss of SERCA1 protein (Leberer et al., 1987) but is coincident with a 40% loss in sarcolipin protein (Odermatt et al., 1998). Consequently, the early loss in ATPase activity may result from the loss of the regulatory sarcolipin protein.

Diseases involving calcium ATPases

Brody disease is a rare, inherited disorder of skeletal muscle relaxation, resulting in exercise-induced impairment of skeletal muscle relaxation, stiffness and cramps (Brody, 1969). Calcium uptake and Ca^{2+}-ATPase activities are reduced in the sarcoplasmic reticulum (Brody, 1969; Karpati et al., 1986; Danon et al., 1988; Wevers et al., 1992), leading to the prediction that Brody disease results from defects in *ATP2A1*, which encodes SERCA1. Sequencing of *ATP2A1* DNA from families with Brody disease has revealed several mutations that result in truncation of SERCA1, resulting in loss of function (Odermatt et al., 1996). Even though SERCA1 is believed to account for over 99% of the Ca^{2+} pumps in fast-twitch skeletal muscle, patients with Brody disease are able to relax their fast-twitch skeletal muscles, although at a significantly reduced rate. Several compensatory mechanisms have been proposed, including compensatory Ca^{2+} removal by PMCA pumps or by Na^+/Ca^{2+} exchangers in the plasma membrane, mitochondrial Ca^{2+} uptake, or proliferation of the sarcoplasmic reticulum containing compensating levels of SERCA2 or SERCA3. Of these possible compensatory processes, only the last would be predicted to result in Ca^{2+} loading of the sarcoplasmic reticulum, a process necessary for subsequent muscle contraction.

Defects in SERCA1 are not the only cause of Brody disease, however, since about half of the families studied have no mutations in *ATP2A1* (Odermatt et al., 1996). One possibility is that that the enhanced effectiveness of a SERCA1 inhibitor might result in Brody disease. Since sarcolipin can be converted to more highly inhibitory forms by mutation, particularly at its C-terminus, attempts were made to find such highly inhibitory forms of sarcolipin in non-*ATP2A1*-linked Brody families. Sequencing of the gene encoding sarcolipin in several individuals from families with Brody disease, however, did not reveal any mutations that might cause the disease (Odermatt et al., 1997).

Darier's disease is an autosomal dominant skin disorder characterized by loss of adhesion between epidermal cells and by abnormal keratinization. Mutations in *ATP2A2* encoding SERCA2b, the ubiquitously expressed non-muscle isoform of the Ca^{2+} pump, have been linked to Darier's disease in a large number of families (Sakuntabhai et al., 1999). Most of the mutations that have been identified in these patients disrupt mRNA splicing, create truncations or occur in regions encoding domains that are highly conserved and are likely to be critical for normal function of SERCA2b. This suggests that SERCA2b has a role in a Ca^{2+}-signalling pathway regulating cell–cell adhesion and differentiation of the epidermis, but it is unclear why expression of both alleles is essential in skin. The disease is sometimes associated with neuropsychiatric problems, but not with muscle disease.

Integral membrane proteins of the sarcoplasmic reticulum

Triadin

Triadin is a 95 kDa protein in skeletal and cardiac muscle junctional sarcoplasmic reticulum (Knudson et al., 1993; Guo et al., 1996). One skeletal muscle and three cardiac muscle isoforms have been cloned, all of which share identical sequences from residues 1 to 264. The protein contains a single hydrophobic segment of sufficient length to cross the membrane as an α-helix and the rest of the molecule is heavily charged with a preponderance of positively charged Lys. Triadin may serve as a functional link between RYR in the membrane of the terminal cisternae and calsequestrin in the lumen of the sarcoplasmic reticulum. Two types of binding may occur between triadin and RYR. The first is a low-affinity ionic interaction between lumenal portions of triadin and RYR and the second is a specific high-affinity binding of a short, relatively hydrophobic segment (Guo et al., 1996). The long, highly charged C-terminal tail, predicted to lie on the lumenal side, is considered optimal for possible interactions with calsequestrin. Triadin has been reported to bind to calsequestrin and RYR in a Ca^{2+}-dependent manner, through amino acid sequences located in the lumenal domain of the molecule. The Ca^{2+} dependence of calsequestrin binding to triadin was demonstrated by passing calsequestrin over an affinity column constructed from triadin. The presence of calsequestrin prevents the formation of triadin oligomers.

Junctin

Junctin was first identified as a 26 kDa calsequestrin-binding protein in cardiac and skeletal muscle, but it is the major calsequestrin-binding protein in cardiac sarcoplasmic reticular vesicles (Zhang et al., 1997). Although junctin and triadin are the products of different genes, the two molecules exhibit structural and functional homology. The 210 amino acid residue sequence is predicted to form a short N-terminal domain, a transmembrane sequence and a highly charged lumenal domain. Junctin appears to bind directly to calsequestrin, triadin and RYR. The binding interaction is localized to the lumenal domain of junctin that is highly enriched in charged amino acids organized into Lys-Glu-Lys-Glu motifs. Junctin and triadin may interact directly in the junctional sarcoplasmic reticular membrane and stabilize a complex that anchors calsequestrin to RYR. These results suggest that junctin, triadin, calsequestrin and RYR form a quaternary complex that may be required for normal regulation of Ca^{2+} release.

Mitsugumin

Mitsugumin 72 is a 72 kDa protein found in the junctional terminal cisternae (Nagaraj et al., 1999). It is 661 amino acid residues long and comprises a large cytoplasmic region and a C-terminal membrane-spanning sequence (Nagaraj et al., 1999). The cytoplasmic region bears homology with proteins that associate with cell-surface membrane and exhibit selective affinity for phospholipids. A 14 amino acid residue motif, designated a SMAP (surface membrane association profile) motif, appears eight times in the cytoplasmic region. Expression of mitsugumin in RYR1/RYR3-deficient myoblasts results in the formation of the triad junction by generating a junctional complex of the cell surface with endoplasmic reticular membranes. The association of mitsugumin with other proteins at the junctional face of the terminal cisternae has not yet been evaluated.

Calmodulin-dependent protein kinase

A 60 000 kDa Ca^{2+}-calmodulin-dependent protein kinase has been associated with the teminal cisternae of the sarcoplasmic reticulum (Campbell and MacLennan, 1982; Chu et al., 1990; Leddy et al., 1993). This kinase phosphorylates a series of proteins in the sarcoplasmic reticulum

membrane and may regulate the function of these proteins.

Motonin kinase

Myotonin kinase, the protein disrupted in myotonic dystrophy, has been associated with the sarcoplasmic reticulum (Shimokawa et al., 1997; Kameda et al., 1998; Ueda et al., 1998). Neither the functional/regulatory role of the kinase in the sarcoplasmic reticulum nor its role in the pathogenesis of myotonic dystrophy has yet been determined.

Lumenal proteins of the sarcoplasmic reticulum

Calsequestrin

Calsequestrin is a major Ca^{2+}-binding protein in the lumen of the sarcoplasmic reticulum (MacLennan and Wong, 1971). It is located at the junctional face of the terminal cisternae where it acts as a Ca^{2+} buffer, lowering the free Ca^{2+} concentration inside the sarcoplasmic reticulum and lowering the gradient against which the ATPase must pump Ca^{2+}. Two *CASQ* genes encode a fast-twitch skeletal muscle isoform and a cardiac/slow-twitch isoform (Fliegel et al., 1987; Scott et al., 1988). The mature rabbit skeletal muscle isoform has a mass of 42 435 Da. It binds 40–50 mol Ca^{2+}/mol of protein with a high capacity and moderate (approximately 1 mol/l) affinity. Electron microscopy has shown that crystal-like arrays of calsequestrin molecules can form from a nucleation site that begins in the junctional face membrane (Franzini-Armstrong, 1980). The sites of nucleation are almost certainly formed from triadin and junctin. These associations create a physical linkage of calsequestrin to the junctional face membrane and to RYR. Transgenic mice with 10-fold overexpression of cardiac calsequestrin develop a serious cardiomyopathy (Jones et al., 1998).

Several studies have indicated that calsequestrin undergoes Ca^{2+}-induced changes in conformation (Aaron et al., 1984; Cozens and Reithmeier, 1984; Ohnishi and Reithmeier, 1987; Slupsky et al., 1987). Transient increases in free lumenal Ca^{2+} concentration are observed when Ca^{2+} release is triggered by caffeine in isolated sarcoplasmic reticular vesicles containing calsequestrin, but not in those where calsequestrin was extracted, suggesting that Ca^{2+} release channel activity affects calsequestrin affinity for Ca^{2+} (Ikemoto et al., 1989). A loss in responsiveness to Ca^{2+} of heavy sarcoplasmic reticular vesicles that have been deprived of calsequestrin by treatment with ethylenediamine tetraacetic acid (EDTA) has been interpreted as evidence of calsequestrin interaction with RYR. Calsequestrin potentiated [^{3}H]-ryanodine binding to solubilized, heavy sarcoplasmic reticular vesicles (Ohkura et al., 1998) and the Ca^{2+} dependence of this binding was enhanced by calsequestrin.

The crystal structure of calsequestrin suggests a mechanism by which it may attain its high-capacity Ca^{2+} binding (MacLennan and Reithmeier, 1998; Wang et al., 1998). Three negative thioredoxin-like domains surround a hydrophilic centre. At low cation concentration, the three domains are stable, probably because of electrostatic repulsion between acidic amino acids on the surface of the individual domains. Trace amounts of cations are able to promote the collapse of the three domains into a compact structure, by lowering electrostatic repulsion and by forming intermolecular bridges between the acidic, carboxyl tails. Polymer formation is furthered by an increase in Ca^{2+} concentration. The N-terminal segment of one monomer crosses the dimer interface and wraps itself around the other monomer, leading to a 'domain swapping' or 'arm exchange' configuration. In between the two dimer interfaces are dense populations of acidic residues, forming electronegative pockets. Calcium ions are coordinated by the acidic residues, filling the cavities inside the dimers. The loose association of Ca^{2+} with the surface of the calsequestrin crystal creates conditions for rapid release of Ca^{2+} from the Ca^{2+}–calsequestrin complex.

Calreticulin

Calreticulin is another Ca^{2+}-binding protein, first identified in sarcoplasmic reticular membranes (MacLennan et al., 1972). It is a minor component of skeletal muscle and cardiac muscle sarcoplasmic reticular membranes and, therefore, probably plays only a minor role in Ca^{2+} storage in these muscle membrane systems. It may play a more prominent role in the endoplasmic reticulum of tissues where protein synthesis is high. Like calsequestrin, calreticulin binds 25 mol Ca^{2+}/mol protein with low affinity, but, unlike calsequestrin, it also has a single high-affinity Ca^{2+}-binding site (Ostwald and MacLennan, 1974; Ostwald et al., 1974). Calcium-binding sites are not evident in the primary sequence and may form conformationally. Structural analysis of the amino acid sequence indicates that the protein can be divided into three domains (Nash et al., 1994). The third domain, containing 37 acidic amino acid residues, is the most likely to bind Ca^{2+} with high capacity and low affinity. The protein contains an endoplasmic reticular retention signal sequence, Lys-Asp-Glu-

Leu (Fliegel et al., 1989). An intrinsic chaperone protein in the endoplasmic reticular membrane, calnexin, shares sequence identity with calreticulin (Wada et al., 1991). This homology suggests that calreticulin has a chaperone function.

Calreticulin is only a minor component in the adult heart but is highly expressed in the cardiovascular system during early embryogenesis. It is essential for cardiac development, since disruption of the gene for calreticulin in homozygous mice resulted in embryonic death (Mesaeli et al., 1999). The major features of the disruption are failure of absorption of the umbilical hernia, marked decrease in ventricular wall thickness and deep intertrabecular recesses in the ventricular walls. Impairment of Ca^{2+} release dependent on inositol 1,4,5,-trisphosphate and of nuclear import of the NFAT3 transcription factor critical for cardiac development have been demonstrated in cells isolated from the knock-out mice. These data confirm that calreticulin plays a key role in Ca^{2+} regulatory systems.

Sarcalumenin

Sarcalumenin exists as two alternatively spliced products of the same gene, an acidic 160 kDa glycoprotein and a 53 kDa glycoprotein, which occur in a ratio of about 10 to 1 (Leberer et al., 1989a,b). These proteins are located in the lumen of the longitudinal reticulum and may be associated with the lumenal surface of the membrane (Leberer et al., 1990). The mature 53 kDa glycoprotein is made up of 453 amino acid residues and 2 mol [(GlcNAc)$_2$(Man)$_9$]. The cDNA encoding the 160 kDa glycoprotein is identical to that encoding the 53 kDa glycoprotein except that it contains an in-frame insertion of 1308 nucleotides near the 5′ end. Consequently, the two glycoproteins have the same 19 residue signal sequence, but a highly acidic amino acid sequence of 436 residues is inserted after the signal sequence in the 160 kDa form.

The function of the two glycoproteins is not clear. The 160 kDa form of sarcalumenin has low-affinity, high-capacity Ca^{2+}-binding properties similar to calsequestrin and calreticulin. This may be a generalized and essential property of all proteins that reside in the lumen of sarco(endo)plasmic reticulum, where the free Ca^{2+} concentration is higher than that of the cytoplasm but lower than that of the extracellular space (MacLennan and Reithmeier, 1998). Like calsequestrin, the expression of these glycoproteins is restricted to striated muscle. Their location in the longitudinal reticulum suggests that their function may be to reduce the free Ca^{2+} concentration at the site of Ca^{2+} ejection into the sarcoplasmic reticular lumen, thereby assisting in the overall process of Ca^{2+} pumping.

Histidine-rich calcium-binding protein

In a search for low density lipoprotein (LDL) receptors, a sarcoplasmic reticular protein was found, unexpectedly, to bind LDL (Hofmann et al., 1989a,b). Subsequent staining with $^{45}Ca^{2+}$ and Stains-All revealed that this protein, with an apparent mass of 165 kDa, is a lumenal, acidic Ca^{2+}-binding protein. It is possible that LDL binding is not a biologically relevant property of this molecule. Purification and cloning of this protein showed that it is four times as rich in histidine as most proteins (13%) and very rich in acidic amino acids (31%). On this basis, the protein was named the histidine-rich Ca^{2+}-binding protein (HCP). The middle segment of the protein is composed of nine tandem repeats of a 29 amino acid residue sequence, which begins with a His-rich tetramer and is followed by 11 acidic amino acid residues. These acidic repeats are believed to form all or part of the Ca^{2+}-binding domain. A polyglutamate stretch, followed by a region rich in Cys, is found toward the C-terminus of the protein. This sequence is likely to be involved in LDL binding. HCP co-localizes with RYR on the junctional face of the terminal cisternae and is a substrate for the 60 kDa calmodulin-dependent protein kinase, which is also located in the junctional terminal cisternae of rabbit sarcoplasmic reticulum (Damiani et al., 1995).

Conclusion

The sarcotubular network in skeletal and cardiac muscle constitutes an elaborate Ca^{2+} regulatory system made up of a number of integral and peripheral membrane proteins. Research since the 1960s has led to the characterization of many of these proteins, but several more remain unidentified and uncharacterized. Interactions among these proteins lead to Ca^{2+} release, triggering muscle contraction, while other interactions regulate Ca^{2+} reuptake, initiating muscle relaxation. Inherited muscle diseases have been associated with a variety of channels, pumps and regulatory proteins in this system. As we understand more about this Ca^{2+} regulatory system, our knowledge of diseases such as malignant hyperthermia, central core disease, Brody disease, hyper- and hypokalaemic periodic paralysis, myotonias and other poorly characterized muscle diseases will result.

Acknowledgements

We thank our many colleagues for advice and discussion in the preparation of this review. Research grants to D.H.M., supporting original work from our laboratory, were from the Medical Research Council of Canada (MRCC), the Muscular Dystrophy Association of Canada, the Heart and Stroke Foundation of Ontario and the Canadian Genetic Diseases Network of Centers of Excellence. K. B is a predoctoral fellow of the MRCC.

References

Aaron, B. M., Oikawa, K., Reithmeier, R. A. and Sykes, B. D. (1984). Characterization of skeletal muscle calsequestrin by ^{1}H NMR spectroscopy. *J. Biol. Chem.* **259**, 11876–11881.

Aravind, L., Galperin, M. Y. and Koonin, E. V. (1998). The catalytic domain of the P-type ATPase has the haloacid dehalogenase fold. [See comments] *Trends Biochem. Sci.* **23**, 127–129.

Asahi, M., Kimura, Y., Kurzydlowski, K., Tada, M. and MacLennan, D. H. (1999). Transmembrane helix M6 in sarco(endo)plasmic reticulum Ca(2+)-ATPase forms a functional interaction site with phospholamban. Evidence for physical interactions at other sites. *J. Biol. Chem.* **274**, 32855–32862.

Barchi, R. L. (1993). Ion channels and disorders of excitation in skeletal muscle. *Curr. Opin. Neurol. Neurosurg.* **6**, 40–47.

Bers, D. M. (1991). *Developments in Cardiovascular Medicine.* Dordrecht: Kluwer Academic.

Block, B. A., O'Brien, J. and Meissner, G. (1994). Characterization of the sarcoplasmic reticulum proteins in the thermogenic muscles of fish. *J. Cell Biol.* **127**, 1275–1287.

Britt, B. A. (1984). Dantrolene, *Can. Anaesth. Soc. J.* **31**, 61–75.

Brody, I. A. (1969). Muscle contracture induced by exercise. A syndrome attributable to decreased relaxing factor. *N. Engl. J. Med.* **281**, 187–192.

Brownell, A. K. (1988). Malignant hyperthermia: relationship to other diseases. *Br. J. Anaesth.* **60**, 303–308.

Campbell, K. P. and MacLennan, D. H. (1982). A calmodulin-dependent protein kinase system from skeletal muscle sarcoplasmic reticulum. Phosphorylation of a 60000-dalton protein. *J. Biol. Chem.* **257**, 1238–1246.

Chu, A., Sumbilla, C., Inesi, G., Jay, S. D. and Campbell, K. P. (1990). Specific association of calmodulin-dependent protein kinase and related substrates with the junctional sarcoplasmic reticulum of skeletal muscle. *Biochemistry* **29**, 5899–58905.

Coronado, R., Morrissette, J., Sukhareva, M. and Vaughan, D. M. (1994). Structure and function of ryanodine receptors. *Am. J. Physiol.* **266**, C1485–C1504.

Cozens, B. and Reithmeier, R. A. (1984). Size and shape of rabbit skeletal muscle calsequestrin. *J. Biol. Chem.* **259**, 6248–6252.

Damiani, E., Picello, E., Saggin, L. and Margreth, A. (1995). Identification of triadin and of histidine-rich Ca(2+)-binding protein as substrates of 60kDa calmodulin-dependent protein kinase in junctional terminal cisternae of sarcoplasmic reticulum of rabbit fast muscle. *Biochem. Biophys. Res. Commun.* **209**, 457–465.

Danon, M. J., Karpati, G., Charuk, J. and Holland, P. (1988). Sarcoplasmic reticulum adenosine triphosphatase deficiency with probable autosomal dominant inheritance. *Neurology* **38**, 812–815.

Ebashi, S., Endo, M. and Otsuki, I. (1969). Control of muscle contraction. *Q. Rev. Biophys.* **2**, 351–384.

Eisenberg, B. R., Kuda, A. M. and Peter, J. B. (1974). Stereological analysis of mammalian skeletal muscle. I. Soleus muscle of the adult guinea pig. *J. Cell Biol.* **60**, 732–754.

Fleischer, S. and Inui, M. (1989). Biochemistry and biophysics of excitation–contraction coupling. *Annu. Rev. Biophys. Biophys. Chem,* **18**, 333–364.

Fliegel, L., Ohnishi, M., Carpenter, M. R., Khanna, V. K., Reithmeier, R. A. and MacLennan, D. H. (1987). Amino acid sequence of rabbit fast-twitch skeletal muscle calsequestrin deduced from cDNA and peptide sequencing. *Proc. Natl. Acad. Sci. USA* **84**, 1167–1171.

Fliegel, L., Burns, K., MacLennan, D. H., Reithmeier, R. A. and Michalak, M. (1989). Molecular cloning of the high affinity calcium-binding protein (calreticulin) of skeletal muscle sarcoplasmic reticulum. *J. Biol. Chem.* **264**, 21522–21528.

Franzini-Armstrong, C. (1970). Studies of the triad. I. Structure of the junction in frog twitch fibres. *J. Cell Biol.* **47**, 488–499.

Franzini-Armstrong, C. (1980). Structure of sarcoplasmic reticulum. *Fed. Proc.* **39**, 2403–2409.

Fujii, J., Ueno, A., Kitano, K., Tanaka, S., Kadoma, M. and Tada, M. (1987). Complete complementary DNA-derived amino acid sequence of canine cardiac phospholamban. *J. Clin. Invest.* **79**, 301–304.

Giannini, G., Clementi, E., Ceci, R., Marziali, G. and Sorrentino, V., 1992, Expression of a ryanodine receptor-Ca^{2+} channel that is regulated by TGF-beta. *Science* **257**, 91–94.

Guo, W., Jorgensen, A. O. and Campbell, K. P. (1996). Triadin, a linker for calsequestrin and the ryanodine receptor. *Soc. Gen. Physiol. Ser.* **51**, 19–28.

Harding, M. W., Galat, A., Uehling, D. E. and Schreiber, S. L. (1989). A receptor for the immunosuppressant FK506 is a *cis-trans* peptidyl-prolyl isomerase. *Nature* **341**, 758–760.

Hisano, T., Hata, Y., Fujii, T. et al. (1996). Crystal structure of L-2-haloacid dehalogenase from *Pseudomonas* sp. YL. An alpha/beta hydrolase structure that is different from the alpha/beta hydrolase fold. *J. Biol. Chem.* **271**, 20322–20330.

Hofmann, S. L., Brown, M. S., Lee, E., Pathak, R. K., Anderson, R. G. and Goldstein, J. L. (1989a). Purification of a sarcoplasmic reticulum protein that binds Ca^{2+} and plasma lipoproteins. *J. Biol. Chem.* **264**, 8260–8270.

Hofmann, S. L., Goldstein, J. L., Orth, K., Moomaw, C. R., Slaughter, C. A. and Brown, M. S. (1989b). Molecular cloning of a histidine-rich Ca^{2+}-binding protein of sarcoplasmic reticulum that contains highly conserved repeated elements. *J. Biol. Chem.* **264**, 18083–18090.

Huxley, H. E. (1969). The mechanism of muscular contraction. *Science* **164**, 1356–1365.

Ikemoto, N., Ronjat, M., Meszaros, L. G. and Koshita, M. (1989). Postulated role of calsequestrin in the regulation of calcium release from sarcoplasmic reticulum. *Biochemistry* **28**, 6764–6771.

Jones, L. R., Suzuki, Y. J., Wang, W. et al. (1998). Regulation of Ca^{2+} signalling in transgenic mouse cardiac myocytes overexpressing calsequestrin. *J. Clin. Invest.* **101**, 1385–1393.

Jurkat-Rott, K., Lehmann-Horn, F., Elbaz, A. et al. (1994). A calcium channel mutation causing hypokalemic periodic paralysis, *Hum. Mol. Genet.* **3**, 1415–1419.

Kameda, N., Ueda, H., Ohno, S. et al. (1998). Developmental regulation of myotonic dystrophy protein kinase in human muscle cells in vitro. *Neuroscience* **85**, 311–322.

Karpati, G., Charuk, J., Carpenter, S., Jablecki, C. and Holland, P. (1986). Myopathy caused by a deficiency of Ca^{2+}-adenosine triphosphatase in sarcoplasmic reticulum (Brody's disease). *Ann. Neurol. Ann. Neurol.* **20**, 38–49.

Kimura, Y., Kurzydlowski, K., Tada, M. and MacLennan, D. H. (1997). Phospholamban inhibitory function is activated by depolymerization. *J. Biol. Chem.* **272**, 15061–15064.

Knudson, C. M., Stang, K. K., Jorgensen, A. O. and Campbell, K. P. (1993). Biochemical characterization of ultrastructural localization of a major junctional sarcoplasmic reticulum glycoprotein (triadin). *J. Biol. Chem.* **268**, 12637–12645.

Koch, M. C., Steinmeyer, K., Lorenz, C., et al. (1992). The skeletal muscle chloride channel in dominant and recessive human myotonia. *Science* **257**, 797–800.

Lacerda, A. E., Kim, H. S., Ruth, P. et al. (1991). Normalization of current kinetics by interaction between the alpha 1 and beta subunits of the skeletal muscle dihydropyridine-sensitive Ca^{2+} channel. *Nature* **352**, 527–530.

Lamb, G. D. and Stephenson, D. G. (1996). Effects of FK506 and rapamycin on excitation–contraction coupling in skeletal muscle fibres of the rat. *J. Physiol. (Lond.)* **494**, 569–576.

Leberer, E., Hartner, K. T. and Pette, D. (1987). Reversible inhibition of sarcoplasmic reticulum Ca-ATPase by altered neuromuscular activity in rabbit fast-twitch muscle. *Eur. J. Biochem.* **162**, 555–561.

Leberer, E., Charuk, J. H., Clarke, D. M., Green, N. M., Zubrzycka-Gaarn, E. and MacLennan, D. H. (1989a). Molecular cloning and expression of cDNA encoding the 53 000-dalton glycoprotein of rabbit skeletal muscle sarcoplasmic reticulum. *J. Biol. Chem.* **264**, 3484–3493.

Leberer, E., Charuk, J. H., Green, N. M. and MacLennan, D. H. (1989b). Molecular cloning and expression of cDNA encoding a lumenal calcium binding glycoprotein from sarcoplasmic reticulum. *Proc. Natl. Acad. Sci. USA* **86**, 6047–6051.

Leberer, E., Timms, B. G., Campbell, K. P. and MacLennan, D. H. (1990). Purification, calcium binding properties and ultrastructural localization of the 53 000- and 160 000 (sarcalumenin)-dalton glycoproteins of the sarcoplasmic reticulum. *J. Biol. Chem.* **265**, 10118–10124.

Leddy, J. J., Murphy, B. J., Qu, Y., Doucet, J. P., Pratt, C. and Tuana, B. S. (1993). A 60 kDa polypeptide of skeletal-muscle sarcoplasmic reticulum is a calmodulin-dependent protein kinase that associates with and phosphorylates several membrane proteins. *Biochem. J.* **295**, 849–856.

Leong, P. and MacLennan, D. H. (1998). The cytoplasmic loops between domains II and III and domains III and IV in the skeletal muscle dihydropyridine receptor bind to a contiguous site in the skeletal muscle ryanodine receptor. *J. Biol. Chem.* **273**, 29958–29964.

Lerche, H., Heine, R., Pika, U. et al. (1993). Human sodium channel myotonia: slowed channel inactivation due to substitutions for a glycine within the III-IV linker. *J. Physiol. (Lond.)* **470**, 13–22.

Loke, J. and MacLennan, D. H. (1998). Malignant hyperthermia and central core disease: disorders of Ca^{2+} release channels. *Am. J. Med.* **104**, 470–486.

Luff, A. R. and Atwood, H. L. (1971). Changes in the sarcoplasmic reticulum and transverse tubular system of fast and slow skeletal muscles of the mouse during postnatal development. *J. Cell. Biol.* **51**, 369–383.

Luo, W., Grupp, I. L., Harrer, J. et al. (1994). Targeted ablation of the phospholamban gene is associated with markedly enhanced myocardial contractility and loss of beta-agonist stimulation. *Circ. Res.* **75**, 401–409.

Lynch, P. J., Tong, J., Lehane, M., Mallet, A. et al. (1999). A mutation in the transmembrane/luminal domain of the ryanodine receptor is associated with abnormal Ca^{2+} release channel function and severe central core disease. [In Process Citation] *Proc. Natl. Acad. Sci. USA* **96**, 4164–4169.

MacLennan, D. H. and Phillips, M. S. (1992). Malignant hyperthermia. *Science* **256**, 789–794.

MacLennan, D. H. and Reithmeier, R. A. (1998). Ion tamers. [News; comment] *Nat. Struct. Biol.* **5**, 409–411.

MacLennan, D. H. and Wong, P. T. (1971). Isolation of a calcium-sequestering protein from sarcoplasmic reticulum. *Proc. Natl. Acad. Sci. USA* **68**, 1231–1235.

MacLennan, D. H., Yip, C. C., Iles, G. H. and Seeman, P. (1972). Isolation of sarcoplasmic reticulum proteins. In: *The Mechanism of Muscle Contraction*, pp. 469–478. Cold Spring Harbor, New York: Cold Spring Harbor Laboratory Press.

MacLennan, D. H., Brandl, C. J., Korczak, B. and Green, N. M. (1985). Amino-acid sequence of a $Ca^{2+}+Mg^{2+}$-dependent ATPase from rabbit muscle sarcoplasmic reticulum, deduced from its complementary DNA sequence. *Nature* **316**, 696–700.

MacLennan, D. H., Rice, W. J. and Green, N. M. (1997). The mechanism of Ca^{2+} transport by sarco(endo)plasmic reticulum Ca^{2+}-ATPases. *J. Biol. Chem.* **272**, 28815–28818.

Martonosi, A. N. (1995). The structure and interactions of $Ca(2+)$-ATPase. *Biosci. Rep.* **15**, 263–281.

Marx, S. O., Ondrias, K. and Marks, A. R. (1998). Coupled gating between individual skeletal muscle Ca^{2+} release channels (ryanodine receptors). [See comments] *Science* **281**, 818–821.

Meissner, G. (1994). Ryanodine receptor/Ca^{2+} release channels and their regulation by endogenous effectors. *Annu. Rev. Physiol.* **56**, 485–508.

Mesaeli, N., Nakamura, K., Zvaritch, E. et al. (1999). Calreticulin is essential for cardiac development. *J. Cell Biol.* **144**, 857–868.

Monnier, N., Procaccio, V., Stieglitz, P. and Lunardi, J. (1997). Malignant-hyperthermia susceptibility is associated with a mutation of the alpha 1-subunit of the human dihydropyridine-sensitive L-type voltage-dependent calcium-channel receptor in skeletal muscle. [See comments] *Am. J. Hum. Genet.* **60**, 1316–1325.

Nagaraj, R. Y., Bhat, M. B., Nishi, M., Takeshima, H. and Ma, J. (1999). Co-expression of ryanodine receptor and MG29 (a novel triad junction protein) in CHO cells. *Biohys. J.* **76**, A470.

Nakayama, H., Taki, M., Striessnig, J., Glossmann, H., Catterall, W. A. and Kanaoka, Y. (1991). Identification of 1,4-dihydropyridine binding regions within the alpha 1 subunit of skeletal muscle Ca^{2+} channels by photoaffinity labelling with diazipine. *Proc. Natl. Acad. Sci. USA* **88**, 9203–9207.

Nash, P. D., Opas, M. and Michalak, M. (1994). Calreticulin: not just another calcium-binding protein. *Mol. Cell. Biochem.* **135**, 71–78.

Odermatt, A., Taschner, P. E., Khanna, V. K. et al. (1996). Mutations in the gene-encoding SERCA1, the fast-twitch skeletal muscle sarcoplasmic reticulum Ca^{2+} ATPase, are associated with Brody disease. *Nat. Genet.* **14**, 191–194.

Odermatt, A., Taschner, P. E., Scherer, S. W. et al. (1997). Characterization of the gene encoding human sarcolipin (SLN), a proteolipid associated with SERCA1: absence of structural mutations in five patients with Brody disease. *Genomics* **45**, 541–553.

Odermatt, A., Becker, S., Khanna, V. K. et al. (1998). Sarcolipin regulates the activity of SERCA1, the fast-twitch skeletal muscle sarcoplasmic reticulum Ca^{2+}-ATPase. *J. Biol. Chem.* **273**, 12360–13669.

Ohkura, M., Furukawa, K., Fujimori, H. et al. (1998). Dual regulation of the skeletal muscle ryanodine receptor by triadin and calsequestrin. *Biochemistry* **37**, 12987–12993.

Ohnishi, M. and Reithmeier, R. A. (1987). Terbium-binding properties of calsequestrin from skeletal muscle sarcoplasmic reticulum. *Biochim. Biophys. Acta* **915**, 180–187.

Ostwald, T. J. and MacLennan, D. H. (1974). Isolation of a high affinity calcium-binding protein from sarcoplasmic reticulum. *J. Biol. Chem.* **249**, 974–979.

Ostwald, T. J., MacLennan, D. H. and Dorrington, K. J. (1974). Effects of cation binding on the conformation of calsequestrin and the high affinity calcium-binding protein of sarcoplasmic reticulum. *J. Biol. Chem.* **249**, 5867–5871.

Otsu, K., Willard, H. F., Khanna, V. K., Zorzato, F., Green, N. M. and MacLennan, D. H. (1990). Molecular cloning of cDNA encoding the Ca^{2+} release channel (ryanodine receptor) of rabbit cardiac muscle sarcoplasmic reticulum. *J. Biol. Chem.* **265**, 13472–13483.

Poch, E., Leach, S., Snape, S., Cacic, T., MacLennan, D. H. and Lytton, J. (1998). Functional characterization of alternatively spliced human SERCA3 transcripts. *Am. J. Physiol.* **275**, C1449–C1458.

Protasi, F., Franzini-Armstrong, C. and Allen, P. D. (1998). Role of ryanodine receptors in the assembly of calcium release units in skeletal muscle. *J. Cell Biol.* **140**, 831–842.

Ptáček, L. J., George, A. L., Jr, Griggs, R. C. et al. (1991). Identification of a mutation in the gene causing hyperkalemic periodic paralysis. *Cell* **67**, 1021–1027.

Qi, Y., Ogunbunmi, E. M., Freund, E. A., Timerman, A. P. and Fleischer, S. (1998). FK-binding protein is associated with the ryanodine receptor of skeletal muscle in vertebrate animals. *J. Biol. Chem.* **273**, 34813–34819.

Radermacher, M., Rao, V., Grassucci, R., Frank, J. et al. (1994). Cryo-electron microscopy and three-dimensional reconstruction of the calcium release channel/ryanodine receptor from skeletal muscle. *J. Cell Biol.* **127**, 411–423.

Rayment, I. and Holden, H. M. (1994). The three-dimensional structure of a molecular motor. *Trends Biochem. Sci.* **19**, 129–134.

Rice, W. J., Green, N. M. and MacLennan, D. H. (1997). Site-directed disulfide mapping of helices M4 and M6 in the Ca^{2+} binding domain of SERCA1a, the Ca^{2+} ATPase of fast twitch skeletal muscle sarcoplasmic reticulum. *J. Biol. Chem.* **272**, 31412–31419.

Rios, E., Pizarro, G. and Stefani, E. (1992). Charge movement and the nature of signal transduction in skeletal muscle excitation-contraction coupling. *Annu. Rev. Physiol.* **54**, 109–133.

Saito, A., Seiler, S., Chu, A. and Fleischer, S. (1984). Preparation and morphology of sarcoplasmic reticulum terminal cisternae from rabbit skeletal muscle. *J. Cell Biol.* **99**, 875–885.

Sakuntabhai, A., Ruiz-Perez, V., Carter, S. et al. (1999). Mutations in ATP2A2, encoding a Ca^{2+} pump, cause Darier disease .[See comments] *Nat. Genet.* **21**, 271–277.

Schneider, M. F. and Chandler, W. K. (1973). Voltage dependent charge movement of skeletal muscle: a possible step in excitation–contraction coupling. *Nature* **242**, 244–246.

Scott, B. T., Simmerman, H. K., Collins, J. H., Nadal-Ginard, B. and Jones, L. R. (1988). Complete amino acid sequence of canine cardiac calsequestrin deduced by cDNA cloning. *J. Biol. Chem.* **263**, 8958–8964.

Serysheva, I. I., Orlova, E. V., Chiu, W., Sherman, M. B., Hamilton, S. L. and van Heel, M. (1995). Electron cryomicroscopy and angular reconstitution used to visualize the skeletal muscle calcium release channel. *Nat. Struct. Biol.* **2**, 18–24.

Shimokawa, M., Ishiura, S., Kameda, N. et al. (1997). Novel isoform of myotonin protein kinase: gene product of myotonic dystrophy is localized in the sarcoplasmic reticulum of skeletal muscle. *Am. J. Pathol.* **150**, 1285–1295.

Shou, W., Aghdasi, B., Armstrong, D. L. et al. (1998). Cardiac defects and altered ryanodine receptor function in mice lacking FKBP12. *Nature* **391**, 489–492.

Simmerman, H. K. and Jones, L. R. (1998). Phospholamban: protein structure, mechanism of action and role in cardiac function. *Physiol. Rev.* **78**, 921–947.

Slupsky, J. R., Ohnishi, M., Carpenter, M. R. and Reithmeier, R. A. (1987). Characterization of cardiac calsequestrin. *Biochemistry* **26**, 6539–6544.

Takeshima, H., Nishimura, S., Matsumoto, T. et al. (1989). Primary structure and expression from complementary DNA of skeletal muscle ryanodine receptor. *Nature* **339**, 439–445.

Takeshima, H., Iino, M., Takekura, H. et al. (1994). Excitation-contraction uncoupling and muscular degeneration in mice lacking functional skeletal muscle ryanodine-receptor gene. *Nature* **369**, 556–559.

Takeshima, H., Ikemoto, T., Nishi, M. et al. (1996). Generation and characterization of mutant mice lacking ryanodine receptor type 3. *J. Biol. Chem.* **271**, 19649–19652.

Tanabe, T., Takeshima, H., Mikami, A. et al. (1987). Primary structure of the receptor for calcium channel blockers from skeletal muscle. *Nature* **328**, 313–318.

Tanabe, T., Beam, K. G., Powell, J. A. and Numa, S. (1988). Restoration of excitation-contraction coupling and slow calcium current in dysgenic muscle by dihydropyridine receptor complementary DNA. *Nature* **336**, 134–139.

Tanabe, T., Beam, K. G., Adams, B. A., Niidome, T. and Numa, S. (1990). Regions of the skeletal muscle dihydropyridine receptor critical for excitation–contraction coupling. *Nature* **346**, 567–569.

Timerman, A. P., Ogunbumni, E., Freund, E., Wiederrecht, G., Marks, A. R. and Fleischer, S. (1993). The calcium release channel of sarcoplasmic reticulum is modulated by FK-506-binding protein. Dissociation and reconstitution of FKBP-12 to the calcium release channel of skeletal muscle sarcoplasmic reticulum. *J. Biol. Chem.* **268**, 22992–22999.

Tong, J., McCarthy, T. V. and MacLennan, D. H. (1999). Measurement of resting cytosolic Ca^{2+} concentrations and Ca^{2+} store size in HEK-293 cells transfected with malignant hyperthermia or central core disease mutant Ca^{2+} release channels. [In process citation] *J. Biol. Chem.* **274**, 693–702.

Toyofuku, T., Kurzydlowski, K., Tada, M. and MacLennan, D. H. (1994a). Amino acids Glu^2 to Ile^{18} in the cytoplasmic domain of phospholamban are essential for functional association with the Ca^{2+}-ATPase of sarcoplasmic reticulum. *J. Biol. Chem.* **269**, 3088–3094.

Toyofuku, T., Kurzydlowski, K., Tada, M. and MacLennan, D. H. (1994b). Amino acids Lys-Asp-Asp-Lys-Pro-Val^{402} in the Ca^{2+}-ATPase of cardiac sarcoplasmic reticulum are critical for functional association with phospholamban. *J. Biol. Chem.* **269**, 22929–22932.

Ueda, H., Kameda, N., Baba, T. et al. (1998). Immunolocalization of myotonic dystrophy protein kinase in corbular and junctional sarcoplasmic reticulum of human cardiac muscle. *Histochem. J.* **30**, 245–251.

Wada, I., Rindress, D., Cameron, P. H. et al. (1991). SSR alpha and associated calnexin are major calcium binding proteins of the endoplasmic reticulum membrane. *J. Biol. Chem.* **266**, 19599–19610.

Wagenknecht, T., Grassucci, R., Frank, J., Saito, A., Inui, M. and Fleischer, S. (1989). Three-dimensional architecture of the calcium channel/foot structure of sarcoplasmic reticulum. *Nature* **338**, 167–170.

Wagenknecht, T., Berkowitz, J., Grassucci, R., Timerman, A. P. and Fleischer, S. (1994). Localization of calmodulin binding sites on the ryanodine receptor from skeletal muscle by electron microscopy. *Biophys. J.* **67**, 2286–2295.

Wagenknecht, T., Radermacher, M., Grassucci, R., Berkowitz, J., Xin, H. B. and Fleischer, S. (1997). Locations of calmodulin and FK506-binding protein on the three-dimensional architecture of the skeletal muscle ryanodine receptor, *J. Biol. Chem.* **272**(51), 32463–32471.

Wang, S., Trumble, W. R., Liao, H., Wesson, C. R., Dunker, A. K. and Kang, C. H. (1998). Crystal structure of calsequestrin from rabbit skeletal muscle sarcoplasmic reticulum. [See comments] *Nat. Struct. Biol.* **5**, 476–483.

Wevers, R. A., Poels, P. J., Joosten, E. M., Steenbergen, G. G., Benders, A. A. and Veerkamp, J. H., 1992, Ischaemic forearm testing in a patient with Ca^{2+}-ATPase deficiency. *J. Inherit. Metab. Dis.* **15**, 423–425.

Zhang, L., Kelley, J., Schmeisser, G., Kobayashi, Y. M. and Jones, L. R. (1997). Complex formation between junctin, triadin, calsequestrin and the ryanodine receptor. Proteins of the cardiac junctional sarcoplasmic reticulum membrane. *J. Biol. Chem.* **272**, 23389–23397.

Zhang, P., Toyoshima, C., Yonekura, K., Green, N. M. and Stokes, D. L. (1998). Structure of the calcium pump from sarcoplasmic reticulum at 8–A resolution. [In process citation] *Nature* **392**, 835–839.

Zorzato, F., Fujii, J., Otsu, K. et al. (1990). Molecular cloning of cDNA encoding human and rabbit forms of the Ca^{2+} release channel (ryanodine receptor) of skeletal muscle sarcoplasmic reticulum. *J. Biol. Chem.* **265**, 2244–2256.

Zot, A. S. and Potter, J. D. (1987). Structural aspects of troponin–tropomyosin regulation of skeletal muscle contraction. *Annu. Rev. Biophys. Biophys. Chem.* **16**, 535–559.

7

The extracellular matrix of skeletal muscle

Paul C. Holland and Salvatore Carbonetto

Introduction

The extracellular matrix (ECM) of skeletal muscle is found within several discrete but interconnected layers produced by connective tissue, Schwann cells, nerve fibres and muscle itself. A collagenous layer, termed the epimysium, surrounds the entire muscle, while another predominantly collagenous membrane, termed the perimysium, subdivides the muscle into groups of muscle fibres (fascicles). Each individual muscle fibre is surrounded by a layer of complex molecular composition, termed the endomysium. The endomysium consists of an outer fibrillar layer and an inner basement membrane. The basement membrane itself also contains several discrete layers. The outermost layer of the basement membrane, the reticular lamina, is rich in collagen fibrils and is continuous with the fibrillar layer of the endomysium. Between the reticular lamina and the plasma membrane lies the basal lamina (BL), which contains a 10–15nm thick electron-opaque layer, the lamina densa, and an inner, 5–10nm thick, less opaque layer, the lamina rara. Between the lamina rara and the plasma membrane there is a carbohydrate-rich layer, termed the glycocalyx, which contains the glycosylated extracellular domains of plasma membrane proteins and certain of their immediate ligands.

Most obviously, the connective tissue and the ECM shape the muscle giving the contractile cells cohesiveness and elasticity. However the basement membrane has additional functions and is molecularly distinct at the neuromuscular junction (NMJ) and myotendinous junctions. The basement membrane consists largely of laminins and collagens, which together with entactin/nidogen, perlecan and other glycoproteins are its major structural elements. Laminin is a large multifunctional molecule with domains that mediate its polymerization into a meshwork within the extracellular space and other domains that anchor laminin to plasma membrane proteins. The latter are bound to proteins within the cytoskeleton, linking this network of intracellular proteins with those in the ECM. These two proteinaceous networks form a superstructure necessary for maintenance of muscle integrity, and disruptions of either network lead to a variety of muscular dystrophies. However, the basement membrane is more than a superstructure for mature muscle. Receptors in the ECM can span the membrane to signal intracellularly and activate pathways involved in cell differentiation, regeneration, division and motility. Also, embedded within the ECM are growth factors and ECM proteins that can activate receptor tyrosine kinases and profoundly affect the differentiation of the myofibre. Furthermore, the ECM at the NMJ mediates synaptogenesis between motor neuron and muscle and regulates gene transcription of those nuclei within the subsynaptic region apart from those within the rest of the myofibre. Trauma, which causes myofibres to degenerate, will leave behind a tube of basement membrane that can serve as a template for regeneration of a new muscle fibre, replete with postsynaptic specializations derived from satellite cells that reside and proliferate within the tube.

The following discussion will focus largely on the basement membrane of voluntary muscle and its composition, assembly, specializations and function. Of particular interest is the important role the basement membrane has in maintaining muscle integrity. In addition, the basement membrane is an essential organizer of the motor endplate and lessons learned from its function in synapse formation may well bear on our understanding of neuromuscular disorders and on its function in maintaining muscle integrity.

Components of the extracellular matrix

Because of their large size and relative insolubility, the purification and characterization of ECM proteins can be

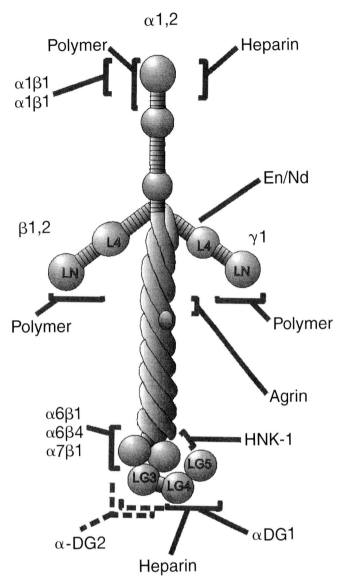

Fig. 7.1. Laminin structure and its sites of interaction with various integrins and extracellular matrix components. Features common to laminin-1 ($\alpha1\beta1\gamma1$), laminin-2 ($\alpha2\beta1\gamma1$), laminin-3 ($\alpha1\beta2\gamma1$) and laminin-4 ($\alpha2\beta2\gamma1$) are illustrated. HNK-1, the HNK-1 carbohydrate epitope on glycoproteins; LN, laminin N-terminal domain (domain VI); L4, laminin domain IV; LG, laminin G-domain (for a review of laminin domain structure see Timpl and Brown (1996). En/Nd, entactin/nidogen; α-DG, α-dystroglycan; polymer, sites involved in laminin self-polymerization into a network. Note that integrins $\alpha1\beta1$ and $\alpha2\beta1$ bind at the opposite end of the molecule from integrins $\alpha6\beta1$, $\alpha6\beta4$ and $\alpha7\beta1$. (From Colognato, H. and Yurchenco, P. D. (2000). *Dev. Dynam.* **218**, 213–234.)

difficult. Consequently, until recently, little was known of the structural and biochemical properties of many of these proteins. As an increasing numbers of genes or cDNAs encoding ECM proteins have been cloned and sequenced, it has become clear that the majority of ECM proteins are composed of various numbers and combinations of modules, defined by consensus sequences found in other extracellular proteins. For example, laminin, agrin and perlecan contain globular regions (G-domains) that are involved in binding to the dystrophin-associated protein (DAP) α-dystroglycan (α-DG). A standard nomenclature for the modules found in extracellular proteins has been proposed and widely adopted (Bork and Bairoch, 1995) and the structures of various basement membrane proteins have recently been reviewed according to this nomenclature (Timpl and Brown, 1996). The ability to express recombinant proteins containing one or more of these modules has led to considerable insight into the possible protein–protein interactions and other biochemical properties of many ECM proteins. However the functions of many of the modules found in ECM proteins are presently unknown (e.g. epidermal growth factor (EGF)-like motifs) and we know a great deal more about the predicted structure and sequence homologies of some of these proteins than we do about their precise role in the basement membrane.

Laminins

Laminin is a ubiquitous component of all developing and adult BL examined to date, and is present in the lamina densa of skeletal muscle BL (Sanes, 1982). Each laminin molecule is composed of three distinct but homologous subunits, which oligomerize to form a cruciform protein (Fig. 7.1). The subunits described to date are encoded by genes for five α-, three β- and two γ-chains. Laminin subunits were first characterized in the laminin-1 secreted by mouse sarcoma cells and were termed the A, B1 and B2 chains (400, 210 and 200 kDa, respectively). Several different forms of laminin are now known and the A, B1 and B2 chains of laminin-1 have been renamed $\alpha1$, $\beta1$, and $\gamma1$, respectively, to designate that each belongs to a subfamily of homologous polypeptides ($\alpha1$–5, $\beta1$–3, and $\gamma1$–2). Eleven distinct heterotrimers ($\alpha1$–5$\beta1\gamma1$, $\alpha1$–5$\beta2\gamma1$, $\alpha3\beta3\gamma2$) can assemble from these subunits (Miner et al., 1997). These different laminin forms are listed in Table 7.1. The extrasynaptic BL of adult muscle is rich in laminin-2 ($\alpha2\beta1\gamma1$) whereas the synaptic BL contains laminin-4 ($\alpha2\beta2\gamma1$), laminin-9 ($\alpha4\beta2\gamma1$) and laminin-11 ($\alpha5\beta2\gamma1$) (Patton et al., 1997). The $\alpha2$-chain is also known as the M chain or merosin. The heterotrimer laminin-2 is also sometimes

Table 7.1. Laminin heterotrimers

Trimer	Subunit composition
Laminin-1	$\alpha1\beta1\gamma1$
Laminin-2	$\alpha2\beta1\gamma1$
Laminin-3	$\alpha1\beta2\gamma1$
Laminin-4	$\alpha2\beta2\gamma1$
Laminin-5	$\alpha3\beta3\gamma2$
Laminin-6	$\alpha3\beta1\gamma1$
Laminin-7	$\alpha3\beta2\gamma1$
Laminin-8	$\alpha4\beta1\gamma1$
Laminin-9	$\alpha4\beta2\gamma1$
Laminin-10	$\alpha5\beta1\gamma1$
Laminin-11	$\alpha5\beta2\gamma1$

Source: Modified from Miner et al., 1997.

referred to as merosin. The $\beta2$-chain was originally identified in laminin found at the synaptic cleft, and termed S-laminin. Mutations that affect expression of the $\alpha2$-chain of laminin result in a form of congenital muscular dystrophy with little or no involvement of NMJs. Phenotypic abnormalities in mice with mutations that eliminate expression of the gene for the $\beta2$-subunit are much less apparent, with only minor disruptions of NMJ structure and function.

Collagens

Collagens typically consist of three polypeptide chains (α-chains) wound together to form a unique triple-helical structure (Kadler et al., 1996). The constituent polypeptide chains have glycine, the smallest of all the amino acids, at every third residue in the chain (i.e. a repeat motif Gly-X-Y, where X and Y can be any amino acid residue). Collagens can be broadly divided into two classes: fibrillar and non-fibrillar. The fibrillar collagens (types I, II, III, V and XI) self-assemble into cross-striated fibrils from soluble triple-helical procollagen molecules, which are converted to collagen monomers by proteolytic cleavage of their N- and C-terminal propeptides (the structure composed of three individual α-chains in triple-helical association is traditionally referred to as a collagen monomer, despite the fact it is a trimeric molecule). The fibrillar collagens are the most abundant collagens in vertebrates. Type I collagen is found in all tissues except cartilage, where type II collagen predominates. Type III collagen is usually found in association with type I collagen. Collagen fibrils may contain more than one collagen type, and type I and type II collagen frequently occur in the same fibril. Types V and

XI collagen are less abundant in most tissues than types I–III.

Of the nonfibrillar collagens, type IV collagen has been studied the most extensively, as it is a major component of basement membranes. In contrast to the fibrillar collagens, the N- and C-terminal domains of type IV collagen monomers are not removed by proteolysis but are critically involved in the mechanism of type IV collagen self-polymerization into a three-dimensional network (see below). The insoluble polymers formed by nonfibrillar collagens are termed filaments to distinguish them from the cross-striated fibrils formed by the fibrillar collagens.

As there are more than 20 known collagen types, the subunits of which are encoded by at least 33 distinct genes (Prockop and Kivirikko, 1995; Kadler et al., 1996) a full discussion of the structure and distribution of all members of this family is beyond the scope of this review. The subsequent discussion will focus on those collagens known to be prominent in skeletal muscle.

Types I, III and V collagen

Immunohistochemical staining of skeletal muscle sections (Duance et al., 1977; Foidart et al., 1981; Sanes, 1982; Lehto et al., 1988) and biochemical analysis of purified skeletal muscle epimysium, perimysium and endomysium (Light and Champion, 1984) show that type I collagen and type III collagen are the major components of the epimysium and the perimysium. Types I and III collagen are also present in the endomysium (Foidart et al., 1981; Light and Champion, 1984; Lehto et al., 1988; Nishimura et al., 1997). Type V collagen is present in endomysium, within the basement membrane, but only in extrasynaptic regions of the sarcolemma (Sanes, 1982) and in the perimysium (Light and Champion, 1984; Nishimura et al., 1997). It has been proposed that type V collagen plays a critical role in connecting type I/type III collagen fibrils to the lamina densa of various connective tissues (Adachi et al., 1997).

Type IV collagen

Type IV collagen is confined to the endomysium, where it is concentrated within the basal lamina (Foidart et al., 1981; Sanes, 1982; Lehto et al., 1988). Six distinct genes encode six different α-chains, belonging to the type IV collagen family (Sado et al., 1998). The most abundant form of type IV collagen in most basement membranes, including that of skeletal muscle, is a trimer consisting of two $\alpha1$(IV) chains and one $\alpha2$(IV) chain. As with laminin, type IV collagen is found in the lamina densa of skeletal muscle BL (Sanes, 1982). Laminin and type IV collagen therefore, provide two separate networks in the lamina rara to which other components of the ECM can attach (discussed below).

The $\alpha3$(IV) and $\alpha4$(IV) chains are concentrated at the NMJ in skeletal muscle, whereas the $\alpha1$(IV) and $\alpha2$(IV) chains are less abundant in this region. This switch in the predominant type IV collagen isoform at the NMJ (Sanes et al., 1990) may result from differential transcription by the subsynaptic nuclei (discussed below). In humans, the genes for type IV collagen are located head to head in pairwise arrangements on chromosome 13 (*COL4A1/COL4A2*), chromosome 2 (*COL4A3/COL4A4*) and the X chromosome (*COL4A5/COL4A6*) and are driven by bidirectional promoters (Sado et al., 1998). Mutations in the genes for the $\alpha3$–6(IV) collagen result in clinical phenotypes (Zhou et al., 1993; Sado et al., 1998) but no effects of these mutations on skeletal muscle function or pathophysiology have been described to date. Mutations involving *COL4A3/COL4A4* result in an autosomal recessive form of Alport syndrome, a progressive fibrosis of the kidney affecting the glomerular basement membrane (Torra et al., 1999). The most common form of Alport syndrome is, however, X-linked dominant and is associated with mutation of *COL4A5*. Interestingly, mutations involving large deletions affecting both *COL4A5* and *COL4A6* give rise to Alport syndrome associated with diffuse leiomyomatosis, a benign proliferation of smooth muscle. Consequently, it has been suggested that type IV collagen formed by oligomerization of the $\alpha5$(IV) and $\alpha6$(IV) chains may be involved in a pathway controlling smooth muscle proliferation and differentiation (Zhou et al., 1993).

Type VI collagen

Type VI collagen expression increases during myoblast differentiation (Piccolo et al., 1995) and this protein is a major component of the endomysium of mature muscle (Marvulli et al., 1996; Nishimura et al., 1997). Although particularly abundant in skeletal muscle, type VI collagen has been identified in a variety of basement membranes. Type VI collagen filaments are invariably associated with type I, II and III collagen fibrils. Type VI collagen has also been shown to interact with proteoglycans (Tillet et al., 1994) and with type IV collagen (Kuo et al., 1997). In skeletal muscle, type VI collagen filaments may, therefore, provide a link between the BL and the type I/III collagen fibrils of the perimysium and epimysium. The importance of these interactions in skeletal muscle is revealed by the fact that mutations which affect expression of any one of the three distinct α-chains of type VI collagen result in Bethlem myopathy, an autosomal dominant myopathy of the proximal musculature (Jobsis et al., 1996). Consistent with these findings, null mutation of the gene encoding the $\alpha1$(VI) chain also results in a myopathy in mice (Bonaldo et al., 1998).

Types XV and XVIII collagen

Type XV and XVIII collagens are structurally different from other known collagen types. They belong to a subfamily of ECM proteins, termed multiplexins, which are characterized by multiple triple-helical domains interrupted by noncollagenous domains (Oh et al., 1994). Type XVIII collagen has recently been identified as a heparan sulphate proteoglycan (HSPG) (Halfter et al., 1998) and the highly homologous type XV collagen α-subunit also contains multiple sites for the attachment of carbohydrate moieties (Myers et al., 1996). Both type XV and XVIII collagen are prominent in the basement membrane of skeletal muscle (Myers et al., 1996; Halfter et al., 1998). Although the precise role of these collagens in the basement membrane is not known, it is of interest that a C-terminal fragment of collagen XVIII (endostatin) has anti-angiogenic and tumour-suppressing activity. By analogy, these collagens may play an important role in the regulation of muscle development or regeneration.

Collagen Q

Acetylcholinesterase (AChE) is the product of a single gene. As a result of alternative splicing and homo- and hetero-oligomer formation, AChE exists in a variety of different forms, including one in which tetramers of catalytic subunits are linked by disulphide bonds to a collagenous tail. Collagen-tailed AChE (also known as asymmetric AChE) is a component of the basal lamina and is concentrated at the NMJ. Asymmetric AChE occurs in three distinct forms, termed A_4, A_8 and A_{12}, to denote whether one, two or three tetramers of catalytic subunits of AChE are linked to the collagen tail. The gene encoding the collagen tail of the asymmetric forms of AChE (*COLQ*) has been cloned in the rat (Krejci et al., 1997). *COLQ* encodes a 458 amino acid residue polypeptide termed collagen Q, which contains a proline-rich attachment domain (PRAD; Pro-Arg-Ala-Asp) close to its N-terminus. The PRAD of collagen Q interacts with a tryptophan-rich amphipathic tetramerization domain in type T AChE (AChE$_T$), the form of AChE expressed in mature mammalian muscle (Simon et al., 1998). Collagen Q also contains two putative binding sites for heparan sulphate (Krejci et al., 1997), which may be involved in association of collagen Q with HSPGs and the immobilization of asymmetric forms of AChE in the ECM (Rossi and Rotundo, 1996).

Inactivation of *COLQ* by homologous recombination results in the complete absence of asymmetric forms of AChE and loss of AChE at NMJs (Feng et al., 1999). *COLQ*$^{-/-}$ mice appear normal until postnatal day 5 when tremors are exhibited when they move. Approximately 50% of *COLQ*$^{-/-}$ mice die by postnatal day 21 and only 10–20%

live into adulthood. Structural abnormalities are apparent at the NMJ of $COLQ^{-/-}$ mice and these animals are severely myasthenic (Feng et al., 1999). Recently, defects in $COLQ$ have been shown to be the cause of congenital myasthenic syndrome with endplate AChE deficiency (CMS type Ic) in humans (Donger et al., 1998; Ohno et al., 1998).

Entactin

Entactin, also known as nidogen, is an elongated 150 kDa glycoprotein with globular N-terminal (G1), central (G2) and C-terminal (G3) domains. Entactin codistributes with laminin in skeletal muscle basement membranes (Martinez-Hernandez and Chung, 1984). The G3 domain of entactin binds with high affinity to the laminin $\gamma1$-chain in the centre of the laminin cross (k_d 0.5 nmol/l) and the G2 domain of entactin binds to type IV collagen with lower affinity ($k_d \sim 0.5$ nmol/l). Because of its ability to bind to both type IV collagen and laminin, entactin is thought to play a critical role in the assembly and maintenance of the basement membrane by cross-linking the self-polymerizing networks that are independently formed by these molecules within the lamina densa of the basal lamina (reviewed by Timpl and Brown, 1996). A synapse-specific, glycosylated form of entactin has also been identified (Chiu and Ko, 1994).

Fibronectin

Fibronectin is one of the earliest discovered and most studied ECM proteins; its structure and its roles in diverse biological processes, including matrix assembly, have recently been reviewed (Romberger, 1997). Fibronectin is a heterodimer with each monomer an elongated flexible glycoprotein approximately 250 kDa in size. Most of the fibronectin polypeptide chain consists of repeats of three distinct modules, called the fibronectin type I, II and III repeats. Sequences homologous to these repeats are present in several other extracellular and ECM proteins. The N-terminal domain of fibronectin consists predominantly of type I and type II repeats and contains sequences that mediate attachment to collagen, gelatin and fibrin. The central domain of fibronectin consists predominantly of type III repeats and contains the RGD (Arg-Gly-Asp) sequence that mediates binding to $\alpha_5\beta_1$-integrin and certain other members of the integrin superfamily of cell adhesion molecules (discussed below). The C-terminal domain of fibronectin contains type I and type III repeats, an additional fibrin-binding site and sites mediating attachment to heparin and $\alpha_4\beta_1$-integrin.

Alternative splicing of fibronectin can occur at three

distinct sites, giving rise to 12 different isoforms in the rat (Schwarzbauer, 1991). Marked differences in the expression of alternatively spliced isoforms of fibronectin have been observed during the development of certain tissues, but all isoforms appear to be co-expressed in muscle and their pattern of expression does not change dramatically during development (Peters and Hynes, 1996). Fibronectin is present both synaptically and extrasynaptically in the basal lamina and more distally in the reticular lamina of skeletal muscle (Sanes, 1982). Fibronectin expression increases markedly during muscle regeneration, and fibronectin together with type I and III collagen makes up the bulk of the increased connective tissue found in the muscle of patients with Duchenne and congenital muscular dystrophies (Hantai et al., 1985).

Perlecan, agrin and other proteoglycans

Proteoglycans are ubiquitous constituents of basement membranes and consist of a core protein with covalently attached glycosaminoglycans, which are highly charged, linear polymers comprising dimeric sugar repeats, one of which is an amino sugar. There are several different types of glycosaminoglycan; the most abundant are heparan sulphate, chondroitin sulphate and hyaluronic acid. In addition to possessing distinctive glycosaminoglycan chains, proteoglycans have a much greater carbohydrate content than other glycosylated proteins. Proteoglycans are commonly classified according to their glycosaminoglycan moiety, for example as HSPGs or chondroitin sulphate proteoglycans. The BL of skeletal muscle contains several proteoglycans, the best characterized of which are perlecan (or HSPG2), agrin and type XVIII collagen. Skeletal muscle expresses other proteoglycans that are not regarded as components of the ECM, for example syndecan-1, which is a transmembrane protein (Larrain et al., 1998).

Perlecan

The core protein of perlecan consists of a single polypeptide chain (approximately 450 kDa and 80 nm in contour length) that can be divided into five domains on the basis of sequence homology to other proteins (Murdoch et al., 1992). The N-terminal domain (domain I) is unique. Domains II, III, and IV have sequence homology to the low-density lipoprotein receptor, domain IV of the $\alpha1$-chain of laminin, and the immunoglobulin-like repeats of neural cell adhesion molecule (NCAM), respectively. Domain V contains sequences with homology to the EGF receptor and the N-terminal globular (G) domains of the $\alpha1$-chain of laminin. Glycosaminoglycans (usually heparan sulphate) are attached to domains I and V of perlecan (Ettner et al., 1998). Perlecan can directly interact with a wide variety of ECM and plasma membrane proteins, including β_1-integrins, α-DG, the collagen-tailed form of AChE, laminin, entactin/nidogen, fibronectin and tenascin-C (Brown et al., 1997; Chung and Erickson, 1997; Hopf et al., 1999).

Although it is detectable in adult skeletal muscle BL (Peng et al., 1999), perlecan expression declines during myogenesis in vitro (Larrain et al., 1997). The myogenic inhibitory factor, basic fibroblast growth factor (bFGF), binds to the heparan sulphate chains of perlecan (Aviezer et al., 1994). The developmental downregulation of perlecan expression during myogenesis is similar to that of the transmembrane proteoglycan syndecan-1, which also binds bFGF through its heparan sulphate chains and inhibits myoblast differentiation through a bFGF-dependent mechanism (Larrain et al., 1998). Since both syndecan and perlecan bind bFGF, they could both modulate myoblast differentiation by regulating growth factor receptor interactions. The situation may be more complex than this, however, since syndecan may also act via its C-terminal, intracellular domain as an accessory molecule in integrin-mediated signalling pathways (Woods and Couchman, 1998).

Perlecan co-localizes with acetylcholine receptors (AChRs) in newly forming synapses (Anderson and Fambrough, 1983). Since α-DG is also found in these nascent clusters and binds to perlecan, it has been suggested that perlecan is involved in attaching the collagen-tailed form of AChE at NMJs (Peng et al., 1999).

Agrin

The core protein of agrin consists of a single polypeptide chain of approximately 225 kDa. HSPGs and other carbohydrate moieties are attached to the core protein to yield a 400–600 kDa proteoglycan. The N-terminal 130 amino acid residues of agrin constitute a unique and highly conserved domain, termed the NtA domain (for N-terminal domain in agrin) which binds to laminin-1, laminin-2 and laminin-4, although this fragment binds more strongly to the synaptic laminin isoform laminin-4 than to the extrasynaptic form laminin-2 (Denzer et al., 1997). Accordingly, it has been suggested that preferential binding of agrin to laminin-4 may be the basis of the observed tight association of neural agrin with the synaptic basal lamina (Denzer et al., 1997). Agrin also binds to integrins (Martin and Sanes, 1997), NCAM (Storms et al., 1996) and α-DG (Bowe et al., 1994; Campanelli et al., 1994; Gee et al., 1994; Sugiyama et al., 1994); the last interaction appears important in NMJ formation (discussed below).

Agrin can be synthesized and secreted by neurons as well by skeletal muscle, which is surrounded by an agrin-rich basement membrane, but in solution only agrin produced by neurons effectively clusters AChRs on cultured myotubes. The sequences responsible for the AChR-clustering activity of agrin are contained within the C-terminal 75 kDa of agrin (Cornish et al., 1999). This area resembles domain V of perlecan in that it consists of three laminin G-like modules (G1 to G3) interspersed with EGF-like modules. Alternative splicing can occur at two sites in the C-terminal domain of agrin, one within G2 and the other adjacent to G3, to give variants with or without a four amino acid residue insert in G2 and with or without an eight amino acid residue insert in G3. The four residue insert enhances AChR clustering activity but the eight residue insert is essential for clustering (Ferns et al., 1993). Consistent with the fact that only agrin produced by neurons can cluster AChRs on cultured myotubes, only neuronal cells produce agrin variants with the eight residue insert in G3. Agrin-deficient mice have severely malformed NMJs and die at birth (Gautam et al., 1996; Burgess et al., 1999).

Tenascins

Tenascin, first identified as an antigen in the endomysium of chick skeletal muscle fibres, is found only in the endomysium of muscle close to the myotendinous junction (Chiquet and Fambrough, 1984). Because this protein was isolated independently by several different laboratories, it has a confusing variety of names (myotendinous antigen, cytotactin, J1, hexabrachion, neuronectin and glioma-mesenchymal extracellular matrix antigen). The tenascins are now known to represent a gene family with at least four members. The form of tenascin originally isolated from the myotendinous junction is now commonly termed tenascin-C. Other members of the family identified to date are tenascin-R, tenascin-X and tenascin-Y. The tenascins are very large proteins. Subunit molecular weights range from 220 kDa (tenascin-C) to ~500 kDa (tenascin-X) and these subunits oligomerize into larger structures via their N-terminal domains (Redick and Schwarzbauer, 1995). All tenascins have a similar general structure, consisting of a cysteine-rich N-terminal domain, followed by a series of EGF-like repeats, multiple fibronectin type III repeats and a C-terminal globular domain homologous to fibrinogen (Bristow et al., 1993; Mackie, 1997).

Tenascin-C is present in a large number of developing tissues and is highly expressed in tumours. Consistent with its expression in developing tissues, tenascin-C levels increase transiently during skeletal muscle regeneration (Ringelmann et al., 1999). The biological functions of the tenascins are unknown. Originally thought to be an important adhesion molecule, it is now recognized that tenascin-C is at best a weak adhesion molecule and may be antiadhesive under some conditions (Chiquet-Ehrismann, 1991). In mature muscle, tenascin-C is confined to the muscle spindle and the NMJ (Pedrosa-Domellof et al., 1995). Given its localization to the NMJ, it is of interest that a specific interaction between tenascin-C and agrin has recently been demonstrated (Cotman et al., 1999). Examination of the NMJ in tenascin-C-deficient mice suggests that this molecule is not required for NMJ formation or regeneration (Moscoso et al., 1998), although it may be involved in stabilization and plasticity of the NMJ (Cifuentes-Diaz et al., 1998).

Tenascin-Y has recently been identified as a novel tenascin predominantly expressed in chicken cardiac and skeletal muscle. Tenascin-Y is expressed by fibroblasts present within the muscle connective tissue, rather than by the myonuclei (Hagios et al., 1996). Tenascin-R is expressed selectively in the central and peripheral nervous system, but tenascin-X is expressed prominantly in skeletal and cardiac muscle (Matsumoto et al., 1994). The embryonic pattern of expression of tenascin-X suggested it might play a critical role in muscle development (Burch et al., 1995). Tenascin-X deficiency is not, however, associated with a severe muscle phenotype but with a connective tissue disorder, typical of Ehlers–Danlos syndrome (Burch et al., 1997)

Extracellular matrix receptors

Alpha-dystroglycan

Until relatively recently, integrins were viewed as the major family of ECM receptors. The discovery of α-DG as a laminin-binding protein (Douville et al., 1988; Ibraghimov-Beskrovnaya et al., 1992; Smalheiser and Schwartz, 1987) and a dystrophin-associated protein (DAP; Ibraghimov-Beskrovnaya et al., 1992) has focused attention on this novel laminin receptor and its function in voluntary muscle.

Alpha-dystroglycan is a sialyated, mucin-like peripheral membrane protein (Fig. 7.2) in the shape of a dumbell with the mucin, rod region connecting the two globular domains. The protein core of α-DG is only 72 kDa (Ibraghimov-Beskrovnaya et al., 1992) but it is heavily and variably glycosylated, resulting in forms with apparent molecular weights as large as 200 kDa in skeletal muscle and 120 kDa in nervous and other tissues. The primary sequence of α-DG has potential sites for N- and O-glycosylation as well as for glycosaminoglycan side chains.

Table 7.2. Examples of direct protein–protein interactions in the extracellular matrix

Protein	LN	FN	PN	AG	Tn-C	Col IV	Col VI	ND	DG
LN			✓	✓				✓	✓
FN			✓			✓			
PN	✓	✓		✓				✓	✓
AG	✓				✓				✓
Tn-C			✓	✓					
Col IV		✓					✓	✓	
Col VI						✓			
ND	✓		✓			✓			
DG	✓		✓	✓					

Notes:

Because of its prominence in skeletal muscle α-dystroglycan (DG) is also included in this table, although it is a plasma membrane protein. LN, laminin; FN, fibronectin; PN, perlecan; AG, agrin; Tn-C, tenascin-C; Col IV, type IV collagen; Col VI, type VI collagen; ND, nidogen/entactin. Direct interaction between different proteins is indicated by a tick at the point of intersection of the proteins in the table. Self-polymerization also occurs for certain of these proteins (e.g. laminin and type IV collagen) but is not shown here.

Binding of α-DG to laminin has a relatively high affinity kd in nanamolar levels and it interacts with the last two (LG4–LG5) of the five globular domains in the laminin α-chain (Gee et al., 1993). Proteolytic fragments from the G-domain of the laminin α2-chain bind DG with higher affinity than fragments from the G-domain of the laminin α1-chain (Talts et al., 1999). As the α2-chain is common to laminin-2 and laminin-4 (the major skeletal muscle laminins), interactions between DG and muscle laminins may be stronger than those between DG and the laminins containing the α1-chain. Binding of laminin-1 but not laminin-2 to muscle α-DG is inhibited by heparin in solution (Pall et al., 1996) possibly reflecting a regulation of this binding by ECM proteoglycans with similar GAG side chains. Indeed HSPG inhibits binding of laminin from skeletal muscle of the *dy/dy* mouse, which has little or no α2-chain isoforms and where the most abundant form is laminin-8 (α4β1γ1) (Patton et al., 1997). This may help to explain why upregulation of this form in the *dy/dy* mouse, a model of congenital muscular dystrophy, is unable to compensate for the loss of laminin-2. Binding of α-DG to laminin appears to be through carbohydrate side chains (Ervasti and Campbell, 1993), rather than through the DG protein core. No definitive description of the responsible carbohydrate sequence has been reported, although this is

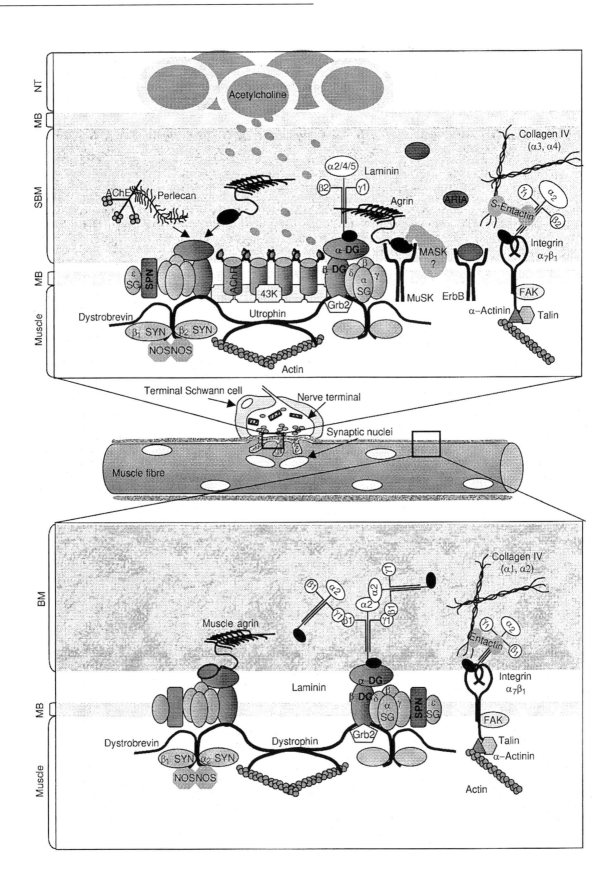

an active area of investigation in view of additional interactions of α-DG with agrin and perlecan as well as with several pathogens (discussed below).

The same gene encodes for α-DG and the 43 kDa transmembrane protein β-DG. The two proteins are apparently cleaved from a precursor during or soon after synthesis (Ibraghimov-Beskrovnaya et al., 1992). The α-DG is found on the membrane tightly bound to β-DG and the two form a subcomplex within a supermolecular complex of DAPs (reviewed in Brown, 1997; Straub and Campbell, 1997). The core of the DAP complex is formed by α- and β-DG binding to ECM proteins extracellularly through α-DG and to cytoskeletal proteins intracellularly through β-DG. The cytoplasmic tail of β-DG has proline-rich regions that bind to the cysteine-rich region of dystrophin (Jung et al., 1995; Rentschler et al., 1999) via an XPPXY consensus sequence in β-DG. In the vicinity of this region (amino acids 787–819) are three consensus sequences for binding to the SH3 domain of Grb2 (Yang et al., 1995), which is a signalling intermediate in the Ras pathway. Beta-dystroglycan can also associate with dystrophin isoforms DP 71 and DP 260 as well as with utrophin (Matsumura et al., 1992; Jung et al., 1995), an autosomal homologue of dystrophin. In addition, a site in β-DG close to the plasma membrane binds to rapsyn (Cartaud et al., 1998), an intracellular cytoskeletal accessory protein necessary for NMJ formation (discussed below). The DAP complex also includes six other membrane proteins, including the sarcoglycans (reviewed in Lim and Campbell, 1998), which are all (α–ε) single-pass transmembrane proteins and sarcospan. The α–δ-sarcoglycans form a tight complex that can be distinguished from other DAPs by their relative insolubility in detergents (Yoshida et al., 1994). The precise function of the sarcoglycans is unknown, though it has been suggested that they are required for stabilization of the α/β-DG complexes (Duclos et al., 1998; Araishi et al., 1999). Other data suggest that they may be involved in interaction of DAPs with integrins (Yoshida et al., 1998) or regulation of calcium influx

(Betto et al., 1999). Sarcospan, another transmembrane DAP, is a four-pass membrane protein that is a member of the tetraspanin family of membrane proteins, which participate in the formation of supramolecular protein complexes (Crosbie et al., 1997). Several tetraspanins interact with integrins, where they regulate cell differentiation and motility. In addition, a *Drosophila* tetraspanin has been implicated in nerve terminal differentiation during NMJ formation (Kopczynski et al., 1996).

Other DAPs include the syntrophins (α, β_1, β_2), nitric oxide synthase (NOS), dystrobrevin, and rapsyn (reviewed in Henry and Campbell, 1996). The syntrophins illustrate the difference in the composition of the DAP complex at junctional and extrajunctional regions of the muscle since β_2-syntrophin is localized mainly to NMJs (Peters et al., 1994) while α_1- and β_1-syntrophins are found extrajunctionally as well (Adams et al., 1993). The syntrophins contain one PDZ domain (Adams et al., 1993), a motif that has been implicated strongly in protein–protein interactions especially with regard to synapse formation in the CNS (Sheng, 1996; Torres et al., 1998). At NMJs, the syntrophin PDZ domain may bind neuronal NOS (nNOS) (Brenman et al, 1996) and to sodium channels via its N-terminal SXV sequence (Gee et al., 1998). The C-terminal region of syntrophin also contains a unique sequence that binds to dystrophin, utrophin and dystrobrevin (Ahn and Kunkel, 1995; Suzuki et al., 1995; Ahn et al., 1996; Peters et al., 1997). nNOS, like Grb 2, is a well-known signalling intermediate; however there is no evidence for intracellular signalling through DAPs.

The DAPs were identified as part of a series of elegant biochemical studies (Campbell and Kahl, 1989; Yoshida and Ozawa, 1990) in search of genes responsible for muscular dystrophy. As discussed elsewhere in this volume, subsequent cloning of these genes and genetic analysis have shown that mutations affecting DAPs lead to muscular dystrophies in humans, hamsters, and mice. For example, mutations in *LAMA2* lead to a form of congenital

Fig. 7.2. Molecules of the extracellular matrix (ECM), their receptors and interacting proteins at synaptic and extrasynaptic regions in skeletal muscle. A close up view of a synaptic region (*a*) and the extrasynaptic region (*b*) of skeletal muscle. The synaptic basement membrane (SBM) is enriched in the collagen IV chains $\alpha3$ and $\alpha4$ and contains laminin-4 ($\alpha2\beta2\gamma1$), laminin-9 ($\alpha4\beta2\gamma1$) and laminin-11 ($\alpha5\beta2\gamma1$), all of which can bind to α-dystroglycan (α-DG). Laminin-4 has also been shown to bind to $\alpha_7\beta_1$-integrin. In addition, laminins can self-assemble forming a complex meshwork in which other ECM molecules can be inserted via direct interactions with laminin or indirectly via cross-linking proteins. Proteins that directly interact with laminin include agrin and perlecan, while a synapse-specific glycoisoform of entactin (S-entactin) binds to both laminin and collagen IV providing a link between these two ECM molecules. The collagen-tailed form of acetylcholinesterase (AChE), which is localized to the neuromuscular junction (NMJ), is recruited by perlecan. ECM receptors found at the NMJ include α-DG, which binds laminin, agrin and perlecan, the laminin-binding $\alpha_7\beta_1$-integrin, the MASC/MuSK complex (see below), which binds neural agrin and initiates NMJ formation, and ErbB receptors, which bind ARIA and regulate acetylcholine receptor (AChR) gene expression in subsynaptic nuclei. Direct links with the actin cytoskeleton are ensured via the integrin β_1-subunit, which binds talin and α-actinin, and via α-DG, which interacts with utrophin. NT, nerve terminal; MB, plasma membrane; NOS, nitric oxide synthetase; SYN, syndecan; SPN, sarcospan; ε-SG, ε-sarcoglycan; FAK, focal adhesion kinase.

muscular dystrophy (Guicheney et al., 1997) and mutations in α-, β-, γ- and δ-sarcoglycans result in various types of limb girdle muscular dystrophy (types 2D, E, C, F respectively (Lim and Campbell, 1998)). DAPs are also greatly diminished on the muscle surface in patients with Duchenne muscular dystrophy or mice with dystrophin mutations (reviewed in Matsumura and Campbell, 1994). There are no reported naturally occurring mutations in the gene encoding α- and β-DG. Mice with targeted mutations in this gene die early in development, with disruptions in Reichert's basement membrane. This would suggest that humans with mutations in this gene may not survive early development (Williamson et al., 1997). However, chimaeric mice substantially deficient in DG develop a muscular dystrophy with severely disrupted NMJs (Côté et al., 1999). The precise functions of DAPs are still to be elucidated, although one popular notion is that they maintain the structural integrity of the cell surface since some, but not all, disruptions in the DAP complex lead to an increase in permeability to macromolecules, and dystrophic muscle is more fragile when subjected to controlled stress (Petrof, 1998).

Finally two intriguing observations suggest that α-DG is not only a receptor for ECM proteins but is also used as a 'receptor' for arena viruses, including the lymphocytic choriomeningitis virus and lassa fever virus (Cao et al., 1998), and for *Mycobacterium leprae* (Rambukkana et al., 1998). Infection of Schwann cells by *M. leprae* involves binding of bacteria complexed with laminin-2 to α-DG. In both these instances, binding of the infectious agent may involve carbohydrate side chains on α-DG, similar to its binding to laminin and other G-domain-containing proteins.

Integrins

Integrins are a superfamily of heterodimeric transmembrane proteins that mediate cell–matrix as well as cell–cell adhesion. The integrins identified in muscle to date belong to either the β_1 or the α_v subfamilies. Substrate specificity within the β_1 subfamily of integrins is dictated by the α-subunit. For example, the $\alpha_7\beta_1$-heterodimer is the major laminin-binding integrin in skeletal muscle while $\alpha_5\beta_1$-integrin, also expressed in muscle cells, recognizes a tripeptide (RGD) in fibronectin. Substrate specificity within the α_v subfamily is dictated by the β-subunit. For example, $\alpha_v\beta_3$-integrin recognizes a variety of ECM proteins including laminin, fibronectin and vitronectin, whereas $\alpha_v\beta_5$-integrin binds specifically to vitronectin and $\alpha_v\beta_1$-integrin binds agrin.

Although there has been no systematic analysis to identify all the integrins in skeletal muscle, the expression and localization of some integrins have been studied in detail. The involvement of integrins in muscle development and in the muscular dystrophies has been reviewed (Gullberg et al., 1998). Patterns of integrin expression change markedly during myogenesis, both as a result of altered gene expression and as a result of alternative splicing of certain α- and β-subunits. It is likely that integrins play important roles both during muscle development and in the maintenance of adult muscle fibres. Some, such as $\alpha_5\beta_1$- and $\alpha_v\beta_3$-integrins, are abundantly expressed by myoblasts but are downregulated as differentiation proceeds (Blaschuk and Holland, 1994; Gullberg et al., 1995; Blaschuk et al., 1997). Forced expression of these integrins can delay or prevent myogenesis, suggesting that they activate signal transduction pathways which maintain myoblasts in a proliferative state (Sastry et al., 1996, 1999; Blaschuk et al., 1997). Moreover, despite its markedly reduced expression in mature muscle, $\alpha_5\beta_1$-integrin may nevertheless play an important role as deficiency of the $\alpha5$-subunit causes a dystrophic type of myopathy in mice (Taverna et al., 1998).

In contrast to $\alpha_5\beta_1$- and $\alpha_v\beta_3$-integrin, $\alpha_7\beta_1$-integrin expression increases during myogenesis (Song et al., 1992). In adult muscle, $\alpha_7\beta_1$-integrin is localized at the NMJ. In the nonjunctional sarcolemma, $\alpha_7\beta_1$-integrin is concentrated at the myotendinous junction, where it is believed to play a role not only in the structural integrity of the junction but also in its embryonic development (Bao et al., 1993). It binds laminin-1, laminin-2 and laminin-4 (Yao et al., 1996; Crawley et al., 1997). The $\alpha_7\beta_1$-integrin-binding site in laminin has been mapped to the proteolytic fragment E8, which contains the LG1–LG3 modules of the C-terminal G domain of the laminin $\alpha1$-subunit (von der Mark et al., 1991). It has not yet been investigated whether laminin-2 and laminin-4 bind $\alpha_7\beta_1$-integrin via the corresponding laminin LG modules of the $\alpha2$-subunit. Other integrins can also bind laminin. For example $\alpha_1\beta_1$- and $\alpha_2\beta_1$-integrins bind to the N-terminal globular domain of the laminin $\alpha1$-chain, but these integrins show no affinity for laminins with $\alpha2$-chains (Pfaff et al., 1994) such as the 'muscle laminins' type 2 and 4.

The expression pattern of the integrin α_7-subunit is complex. The gene for the α_7-subunit undergoes alternative splicing affecting the intracellular, C-terminal domain to produce α_{7A}, α_{7B} and α_{7C} isoforms (Song et al., 1993), and affecting the extracellular domain to produce α_{7X1} and α_{7X2} splice variants, which have different affinities for laminin-1 than for laminin-2 or laminin-4 (Crawley et al., 1997). The α_{7A}- and α_{7B}-isoforms are confined to synaptic sites in adult muscle, while α_{7C}-isoform is present both synaptically and extrasynaptically (Martin et al., 1996). In $\beta2$-laminin-null mutant mice α_{7A}-isoform can still be detected at synaptic sites, whereas the α_{7B}-isoform cannot (Martin et al., 1996). Integrin variants with α_{7A} and α_{7B} cytoplasmic domain containing the α_{7X2} extracellular domain selectively co-cluster in culture within laminin-induced AChR clusters. Though the physiological significance of laminin in AChR aggregation in vivo is unclear, these data suggest that these isoforms may participate in the formation or maintenance of the NMJ. Also $\alpha_v\beta_1$-integrin has been reported to bind agrin and may regulate AChR aggregation (Martin and Sanes, 1997). A further level of complexity arises from the observation that the β_1-integrin subunit also undergoes alternative splicing. A cardiac and skeletal muscle specific isoform, β_{1D}, predominates in adult skeletal muscle in association with α_{7A} and α_{7B}-subunits (Belkin et al., 1996).

The relative function of integrins and α-DG in maintaining muscle integrity has been brought to the fore in studies of a subgroup of congenital muscular dystrophies caused by mutations in the gene encoding the laminin α2-chain (merosin-negative congenital muscular dystrophies). In these cases, the basement membrane is disrupted and DAPs are expressed at apparently normal levels (Vachon et al., 1997) but the $\alpha_7\beta_1$-integrin level is significantly reduced. Other data indicate that α-DG membrane interactions are disrupted and that apparently normal immunohistochemical localization may not reflect this disruption (Duclos et al., 1998). In culture, muscle cell lines selected for their deficiency in the laminin α2-isoforms have increased programmed cell death (Vachon et al., 1996), possibly reflecting the increased apoptosis in merosin-negative congenital muscular dystrophy and animal models of this disease (Vachon et al., 1996; Miyagoe et al., 1997). However, muscle cells engineered to express low levels of α-DG also have increased apoptosis (Montanaro et al., 1999). More importantly, mutations that affect the expression of all isoforms of the α_7-subunit of $\alpha_7\beta_1$-integrin give rise to congenital muscular dystrophy in humans (Hodges et al., 1997; Hayashi et al., 1998) and progressive muscular dystrophy in mice (Mayer et al., 1997). Therefore, these merosin-negative forms may be instances where disruptions in the ECM affect α-DG and integrins, with the latter responsible for the increased apoptosis (which is known to be regulated by integrins in other cells).

Integrins are involved in a wide variety of cellular processes including proliferation, motility, differentiation and apoptosis (Cary and Guan, 1999) and their expression in skeletal muscle along with α-DG raises many questions about the relative functions of these disparate ECM receptors. Several recent reports hint at interaction between DAPs and integrins. Both are concentrated at sites of cell matrix adhesion in cultured cells (Belkin and Smalheiser,

1996). Generally speaking, both α-DG and integrins mediate linkage to the cytoskeleton, though integrins are associated directly with α-actinin, talin and filamin and, ultimately, connect to actin, while α-DG is an extracellular protein and achieves its linkage to actin by its close association with β-DG. Integrins also mediate assembly of a fibronectin network on the surface of cells. However, α-DG seems the dominant receptor for the laminin network on muscle (Colognato et al., 1999). Integrins are associated with focal adhesion kinase and are well known to trigger second messengers following activation by their ligands (Cary and Guan, 1999). By comparison, α-DG is part of a complex that includes Grb2 and NOS (Yang et al., 1995; Brenman et al., 1996), but there is as yet no evidence that it activates these molecules. It seems likely that these two types of receptor collaborate on the muscle cell surface, and recent biochemical data suggesting the existence of bidirectional signalling between sarcoglycans and integrins in cultured myotubes support this notion (Yoshida et al., 1998).

Basement membrane assembly

Laminin and collagen IV form the infrastructure of the basement membrane. Collagen (IV) chains self-polymerize through their globular C-terminal domains and their N-terminal domains to form a three-dimensional network, stabilized by lateral associations of the triple helical domain and by disulphide and lysine aldehyde-derived cross-links. Laminin can reversibly self-polymerize through a calcium-dependent association of the N-termini of its subunits within the three short arms of laminins to form a hexagonal lattice with 30 nm links. Laminin isoforms 5–7, which have truncated short arms, are unable to form three-dimensional polymers like those formed by laminins-1–4. Laminin, and collagen type IV are found in the lamina densa of skeletal muscle BL (Sanes, 1982) and, therefore, provide two independent self-assembling matrices in the lamina rara to which other components of the ECM can attach.

At high concentrations, laminin polymerization occurs in solution but in vivo is localized to the muscle cell surface and its polymerization is mediated by binding to cell-surface receptors lower considerably the critical concentration for polymerization and allow formation of a well-defined laminin network (Colognato et al, 1999). Alpha-dystroglycan is expressed in many tissues including epithelia and has been directly implicated in basement membrane assembly. Targeted mutagenesis of the gene for DG results in embryonic death in mice, apparently as a result of disruptions in Reichert's basement membrane

(Williamson et al., 1997). Basement membranes formed by embryonic endoderm in vitro are defective in cells null for DG but can be rescued by viral injection of the DG gene (Henry and Campbell, 1998). In skeletal muscle cells in vitro, α-DG, and not integrins, mediates the assembly of a network of ECM on the cell surface (Colognato et al., 1999). Interestingly, this assembly involves activation of a tyrosine kinase, which may reflect signalling directly or indirectly by α/β-DG. Formation of this network, apart from binding of laminin and collagen to the cell surface, may be essential for maintaining muscle integrity since laminin from mice with a mutations in the laminin α2-chain (*dy/dy*) within the region of the short arm have a severe muscular dystrophy similar to that in many human congenital muscular dystrophies (Xu et al., 1994; Sunada et al., 1995). These mutated laminins are unable to assemble into a network on the surface of muscle cells in vitro (Colognato et al., 1999).

How does the basement membrane maintain muscle integrity? The most widely supported hypothesis is that it serves as a superstructure for the cell surface and is constructed of many relatively low-affinity protein–protein interactions between the ECM and the cell surface, which synergize to produce two tightly bound networks that buffer the cell against the stresses generated by its contractile apparatus (Campbell, 1995). Hence a proper meshwork formed by homophilic laminin interactions may be necessary to distribute these forces evenly over the cell. The DG complex may be important by interacting with dystrophin, which forms a network of its own with spacing of 125 nm beneath the plasma membrane. Once ECM assembly is initiated by DGs, other molecules in the ECM and the plasma membrane may be brought into play. Consider, for example, that integrins are well known to signal intracellularly and to regulate apoptosis, which has been implicated in muscular dystrophies (Tews and Goebel, 1997). Assembly of a laminin network in skeletal muscle may not require integrins (Colognato et al., 1999) but they may be activated once the α-DG triggers this process. Also the ECM harbours growth factors (Jo et al., 1995), which may be concentrated or brought into proximity with their receptors by incorporation within the basement membrane. No single growth factor responsible for muscle fibre viability has been identified, but a combination of several may function in this way. Both transforming growth factor-β and insulin-like growth factor (Florini et al., 1996) are potential candidates. In addition, the ECM contains at least one coreceptor, perlecan, which greatly enhances the interaction of fibroblast growth factor with its receptor (Aviezer et al., 1994). Furthermore, ECM proteins can directly activate receptor tyrosine kinases, as in the activation of the muscle-specific kinase (MuSK, discussed below) by agrin.

Agrin has no reported effect on muscle integrity but there may be new ECM receptors, like the recently discovered collagen receptor tyrosine kinase (Shrivastava et al., 1997), which participate in maintaining muscle integrity. Also, as noted above, DAPs may not be purely structural in their function, especially since α-DG is docked to β-DG and the latter is bound to the Grb2 (Yang et al., 1995) and is part of a complex associated with NOS (Brenman et al., 1996). Finally, several provocative experiments indicate that the conformation of the ECM, and not mere ECM–receptor interactions, regulate a host of fundamental cellular processes including cell replication and programmed cell death (Ingber, 1997).

Basement membrane remodelling

As mentioned above, the basement membrane is outside the normal degradative machinery of the cell, and myofibre degeneration leaves behind a basement membrane that can serve as a template for regeneration of a new muscle fibre. Despite its relative stability, turnover of individual basement membrane components does occur during myofibre degeneration and regeneration (Gulati et al., 1983). Early studies implicated secreted proteases (e.g. plasmin) produced locally through the action of muscle-derived plasminogen activator in the degradation of components of the myofibre basement membrane following denervation (Hantai and Festoff, 1987). More recently, attention has focused on the possible contribution of matrix-degrading metalloproteases (MMPs) to basement membrane turnover. The MMPs are a family of homologous proteins capable of degrading a variety of different components of the ECM (Matrisian, 1992). Human skeletal muscle satellite cells constitutively secrete MMP-2 (72 kDa gelatinase/type IV collagenase) and can be induced to secrete substantial amounts of MMP-9 (92 kDa gelatinase/type IV collagenase) and small amounts of MMP-1 (interstitial type I collagenase) (Guerin and Holland, 1995). Clearly these MMPs could mediate the degradation of selected ECM components during muscle regeneration. Consistent with this, recent studies in vivo indicate that MMP-2 activation is concomitant with the regeneration of new myofibres, whereas MMP-9 expression is associated with the inflammatory response (Kherif et al., 1999).

The extracellular matrix of the neuromuscular junction

The basement membrane of the NMJ appears ultrastructurally similar to that outside of the synapse but is molecularly specialized, containing isoforms of laminin, collagen, entactin and agrin as well as AChE (Carbonetto and Lindenbaum, 1995). The synaptic basement membrane regulates development and regeneration of the postsynaptic apparatus and innervating nerve terminal (McMahan, 1990). Damaged muscle fibres will regenerate normally within a tube of basement membrane and assemble a normal looking postsynaptic apparatus in the absence of a nerve terminal (Burden et al., 1979). Conversely, axons will grow into ghost myofibres consisting only of tubes of basement membrane from mature fibres, terminate their growth at the site of the old endplates and differentiate into a normal looking nerve terminal (Sanes et al., 1978). The primary signal for this instructive function of the basement membrane is agrin released by the nerve terminal and assembled within the subsynaptic ECM (reviewed in Sanes and Lichtman, 1999). The formation of a nascent ECM at the developing myoneural junction triggers the aggregation of AChRs beneath the nerve terminal. Agrin, with help from a putative coreceptor (MASC), activates a receptor tyrosine kinase MuSK to establish a molecular trap (Glass et al., 1996). This involves an as yet unidentified transmembrane protein (RATL) that links the extracellular region of MuSK to the intracellular protein rapsyn (Apel et al., 1995). Rapsyn can self-associate and initiate the formation of small clusters of AChR (Froehner et al., 1990; Phillips et al., 1991; Maimone and Merlie, 1993). Rapsyn also interacts with the cytoplasmic tail of β-DG (Cartaud et al., 1998) and DGs are found at the earliest and smallest clusters of AChRs forming under the nerve terminal (Cohen et al., 1995). Small aggregates of AChR clustered by rapsyn coalesce into larger postsynaptic densities possibly by binding to α/β-DG complexes (Jacobson et al., 1998) and associating with utrophin. Concomitantly agrin also stimulates a remodelling of the muscle ECM as reflected in the aggregation of laminin, perlecan and AChE within AChR aggregates (Anderson and Fambrough, 1983; Bayne et al., 1984; Nitkin and Rothschild, 1990; Cohen et al., 1997). With AChRs in place, a protosynapse is established that causes the first electrical impulses in the skeletal muscle in response to acetylcholine released by the nerve. This muscle activity inhibits the biosynthesis of AChRs over the entire myofibre (Goldman et al., 1988). In the face of this, the nerve terminal releases neuregulin (also called glial growth factor or ARIA; Jo and Burden, 1992; Jo et al., 1995), which stimulates the biosynthesis of AChRs (Jo et al., 1995) by binding to and activating Erb receptor tyrosine kinases. Importantly, the released neuregulin is incorporated into the subsynaptic basement membrane and helps to establish a stable compartment within the multi-

nucleate muscle fibre wherein the subsynaptic nuclei continue to synthesize AChRs subunits and other proteins while the extrajunctional nuclei do not (reviewed in Burden, 1998). This helps to localize the synaptic apparatus and the response of the muscle fibre to acetylcholine released by the nerve.

Consistent with the above scenario, mice null in genes encoding MuSK (DeChiara et al., 1996), agrins (Gautam et al., 1996; Burgess et al., 1999), rapsyn (Gautam et al., 1995), α-DG (Côté et al., 1999) and, to a lesser extent, utrophin and dystrophin (Deconinck et al., 1997; Grady et al., 1997) all have defective myoneural junctions. Most interestingly, mice with mutations affecting agrin or MuSK also have substantial defects in nerve terminals. In the latter, the nerve seems to wander over the muscle forming no mature endplates. Hence agrin in the ECM is essential for the transmission of signals from nerve to muscle and vice versa that leads to formation of a mature synapse.

Conclusion

Enormous progress has been made in understanding how the basement membrane maintains muscle integrity. It is widely thought that the ECM interacts with the cytoskeleton through α/β-DG to form a superstructure that links the basement membrane with dystrophin and actin in the cytoskeleton to sustain the integrity of highly contractile muscle cells. However, diseases that affect DAPs are rather heterogeneous mechanistically, suggesting that the functions of the ECM are manifold. At present, our limited knowledge of the function of the ECM makes it difficult to reconcile these differences. In this context, it is worth noting that ECM proteins can directly activate receptor tyrosine kinases and bind growth factors, as well as act as coreceptors for growth factors, and these will be important future issues in understanding the function of the muscle ECM and its dysfunction leading to neuromuscular disorders.

Acknowledgements

We thank Dr Peter Yurchenco for providing Figure 7.1 and Dr Federica Montanaro for help in constructing Figure 7.2 and for her comments on the manuscript. Work for this article was supported by grants to P. H. and to S. C. from the Medical Research Council of Canada and the Muscular Dystrophy Association (US).

References

Adachi, E., Hopkinson, I. and Hayashi, T. (1997). Basement-membrane stromal relationships: interactions between collagen fibrils and the lamina densa. [Review] *Int. Rev. Cytol.* **173**, 73–156.

Adams, M. E., Butler, M. H., Dwyer, T. M., Peters, M. F., Murnane, A. A. and Froehner, S. C. (1993). Two forms of mouse syntrophin, a 58 kDa dystrophin-associated protein, differ in primary structure and tissue distribution. *Neuron* **11**, 531–540.

Ahn, A. H. and Kunkel, L. M. (1995). Syntrophin binds to an alternatively spliced exon of dystrophin. *J. Cell Biol.* **128**, 363–371.

Ahn, A. H., Freener, C. A., Gussoni, E., Yoshida, M., Ozawa, E. and Kunkel, L. M. (1996). The three human syntrophin genes are expressed in diverse tissues, have distinct chromosomal locations and each bind to dystrophin and its relatives. *J. Biol. Chem.* **271**, 2724–2730.

Anderson, M. J. and Fambrough, D. M. (1983). Aggregates of acetylcholine receptors are associated with plaques of a basal lamina heparan sulphate proteoglycan on the surface of skeletal muscle fibres. *J. Cell Biol.* **97**, 1396–1411.

Apel, E. D., Roberds, S. L., Campbell, K. P. and Merlie, J. P. (1995). Rapsyn may function as a link between the acetylcholine receptor and the agrin-binding dystrophin-associated glycoprotein complex. *Neuron* **15**, 115–126.

Araishi, K., Sasaoka, T., Imamura, M. et al. (1999). Loss of the sarcoglycan complex and sarcospan leads to muscular dystrophy in β-sarcoglycan-deficient mice. *Hum. Mol. Genet.* **8**, 1589–1598.

Aviezer, D., Hecht, D., Safran, M., Eisinger, M., David, G. and Yayon, A. (1994). Perlecan, basal lamina proteoglycan, promotes basic fibroblast growth factor-receptor binding, mitogenesis and angiogenesis. *Cell* **79**, 1005–1013.

Bao, Z. Z., Lakonishok, M., Kaufman, S. and Horwitz, A. F. (1993). $\alpha_7\beta_1$ Integrin is a component of the myotendinous junction on skeletal muscle. *J. Cell. Sci.* **106**, 579–89.

Bayne, E. K., Anderson, M. J. and Fambrough, D. M. (1984). Extracellular matrix organization in developing muscle: correlation with acetylcholine receptor aggregates. *J. Cell Biol.* **99**, 1486–1501.

Belkin, A. M. and Smalheiser, N. R. (1996). Localization of cranin (dystroglycan) at sites of cell–matrix and cell–cell contact: recruitment to focal adhesions is dependent upon extracellular ligands. *Cell Adhes. Commun.* **4**, 281–296.

Belkin, A. M., Zhidkova, N. I., Balzac, F. et al. (1996). β_{1D} Integrin displaces the β_{1A} isoform in striated muscles: localization at junctional structures and signalling potential in nonmuscle cells. *J. Cell Biol.* **132**, 211–226.

Betto, R., Senter, L., Ceoldo, S., Tarricone, E., Biral, D. and Salviati, G. (1999). Ecto-ATPase activity of α-sarcoglycan (adhalin). *J. Biol. Chem.* **274**, 7907–7912.

Blaschuk, K. L. and Holland, P. C. (1994). The regulation of $\alpha_5\beta_1$ integrin expression in human muscle cells. *Dev. Biol.* **164**, 475–483.

Blaschuk, K. L., Guerin, C. and Holland, P. C. (1997). Myoblast $\alpha_v\beta_3$ integrin levels are controlled by transcriptional regulation of expression of the β_3 subunit and down-regulation of β_3 subunit expression is required for skeletal muscle cell differentiation. *Dev. Biol.* **184**, 266–277.

Bonaldo, P., Braghetta, P., Zanetti, M., Piccolo, S., Volpin, D. and Bressan, G. M. (1998). Collagen VI deficiency induces early onset myopathy in the mouse: an animal model for Bethlem myopathy. *Hum. Mol. Genet.* **7**, 2135–2140.

Bork, P. and Bairoch, A. (1995). Extracellular protein modules. *TIBS* **20**, Poster CO2.

Bowe, M. A., Deyst, K. A., Leszyk, J. D. and Fallon, J. R. (1994). Identification and purification of an agrin receptor from torpedo postsynaptic membranes: a heteromeric complex related to the dystroglycans. *Neuron* **12**, 1173–1180.

Brenman, J. E., Chao, D. S., Gee, S. H. et al.. (1996). Interaction of nitric oxide synthase with the postsynaptic density protein PSD-95 and α_1-syntrophin mediated by PDZ domains. *Cell* **84**, 757–767.

Bristow, J., Tee, M. K., Gitelman, S. E., Mellon, S. H. and Miller, W. L. (1993). Tenascin-X: a novel extracellular matrix protein encoded by the human XB gene overlapping P450c21B. *J. Cell Biol.* **122**, 265–278.

Brown, J. C., Sasaki, T., Gohring, W., Yamada, Y. and Timpl, R. (1997). The C-terminal domain V of perlecan promotes β_1 integrin-mediated cell adhesion, binds heparin, nidogen and fibulin-2 and can be modified by glycosaminoglycans. *Eur. J. Biochem.* **250**, 39–46.

Brown, R. H., Jr. (1997). Dystrophin-associated proteins and the muscular dystrophies. *Annu. Rev. Med.* **48**, 457–466.

Burch, G. H., Bedolli, M. A., McDonough, S., Rosenthal, S. M. and Bristow, J. (1995). Embryonic expression of tenascin-X suggests a role in limb, muscle and heart development. *Dev. Dynam.* **203**, 491–504.

Burch, G. H., Gong, Y., Liu, W. et al. (1997). Tenascin-X deficiency is associated with Ehlers-Danlos syndrome. *Nat. Genet.* **17**, 104–108.

Burden, S. J. (1998). The formation of neuromuscular synapses. *Genes Dev.* **12**, 133–148.

Burden, S. J., Sargent, P. B. and McMahan, U. J. (1979). Acetylcholine receptors in regenerating muscle accumulate at original synaptic sites in the absence of the nerve. *J. Cell Biol.* **82**, 412–425.

Burgess, R. W., Nguyen, Q. T., Son, Y. J., Lichtman, J. W. and Sanes, J. R. (1999). Alternatively spliced isoforms of nerve- and muscle-derived agrin: their roles at the neuromuscular junction. *Neuron* **23**, 33–44.

Campanelli, J. T., Roberds, S. L., Campbell, K. P. and Scheller, R. H. (1994). A role for dystrophin-associated glycoproteins and utrophin in agrin-induced AChR clustering. *Cell* **77**, 663–674.

Campbell, K. P. (1995). Three muscular dystrophies: loss of cytoskeleton–extracellular matrix linkage. *Cell* **80**, 675–679.

Campbell, K. P. and Kahl, S. D. (1989). Association of dystrophin and an integral membrane glycoprotein. *Nature* **338**, 259–262.

Cao, W., Henry, M. D., Borrow, P. et al. (1998). Identification of α-dystroglycan as a receptor for lymphocytic choriomeningitis virus and Lassa fever virus. *Science* **282**, 2079–2081.

Carbonetto, S. and Lindenbaum, M. (1995). The basement membrane at the neuromuscular junction: a synaptic mediatrix. *Curr. Opin. Neurobiol.* **5**, 596–605.

Cartaud, A., Coutant, S., Petrucci, T. C. and Cartaud, J. (1998). Evidence for in situ and in vitro association between β-dystroglycan and the subsynaptic 43K rapsyn protein. Consequence for acetylcholine receptor clustering at the synapse. *J. Biol. Chem.* **273**, 11321–11326.

Cary, L. A. and Guan, J. L. (1999). Focal adhesion kinase in integrin-mediated signalling. *Front. Biosci.* **4**, D102–D113.

Chiquet, M. and Fambrough, D. M. (1984). Chick myotendinous antigen. I. A monoclonal antibody as a marker for tendon and muscle morphogenesis. *J. Cell Biol.* **98**, 1926–1936.

Chiquet-Ehrismann, R. (1991). Anti-adhesive molecules of the extracellular matrix. *Curr. Opin. Cell. Biol.* **3**, 800–804.

Chiu, A. Y. and Ko, J. (1994). A novel epitope of entactin is present at the mammalian neuromuscular junction. *J. Neurosci.* **14**, 2809–2817.

Chung, C. Y. and Erickson, H. P. (1997). Glycosaminoglycans modulate fibronectin matrix assembly and are essential for matrix incorporation of tenascin-C. *J. Cell Sci.* **110**, 1413–1419.

Cifuentes-Diaz, C., Velasco, E., Meunier, F. A. et al (1998). The peripheral nerve and the neuromuscular junction are affected in the tenascin-C-deficient mouse. *Cell. Mol. Biol. (Noisy-le-grand)* **44**, 357–379.

Cohen, M. W., Jacobson, C., Godfrey, E. W., Campbell, K. P. and Carbonetto, S. (1995). Distribution of α-dystroglycan during embryonic nerve-muscle synaptogenesis. *J. Cell Biol.* **129**, 1093–1101.

Cohen, M. W., Jacobson, C., Yurchenco, P. D., Morris, G. E. and Carbonetto, S. (1997). Laminin-induced clustering of dystroglycan on embryonic muscle cells: comparison with agrin-induced clustering. *J. Cell Biol.* **136**, 1047–1058.

Colognato, H., Winkelmann, D. A. and Yurchenco, P. D. (1999). Laminin polymerization induces a receptor–cytoskeleton network. *J. Cell Biol.* **145**, 619–631.

Cornish, T., Chi, J., Johnson, S., Lu, Y. and Campanelli, J. T. (1999). Globular domains of agrin are functional units that collaborate to induce acetylcholine receptor clustering. *J. Cell. Sci.* **112**, 1213–1223.

Côté, P. D., Moukhles, H., Lindenbaum, M. and Carbonetto, S. (1999). Chimaeric mice deficient in dystroglycans develop muscular dystrophy and have disrupted myoneural synapses. *Nat. Genet.* **23**, 338–342.

Cotman, S. L., Halfter, W. and Cole, G. J. (1999). Identification of extracellular matrix ligands for the heparan sulfate proteoglycan agrin. *Exp. Cell. Res.* **249**, 54–64.

Crawley, S., Farrell, E. M., Wang, W. et al. (1997). The $\alpha_7\beta_1$ integrin mediates adhesion and migration of skeletal myoblasts on laminin. *Exp. Cell. Res.* **235**, 274–286.

Crosbie, R. H., Heighway, J., Venzke, D. P., Lee, J. C. and Campbell, K. P. (1997). Sarcospan, the 25-kDa transmembrane component of the dystrophin–glycoprotein complex. *J. Biol. Chem.* **272**, 31221–31224.

DeChiara, T. M., Bowen, D. C., Valenzuela, D. M. et al. (1996). The receptor tyrosine kinase MuSK is required for neuromuscular junction formation in vivo. *Cell* **85**, 501–512.

Deconinck, A. E., Rafael, J. A., Skinner, J. A. et al. (1997). Utrophin–dystrophin-deficient mice as a model for Duchenne muscular dystrophy. *Cell* **90**, 717–727.

Denzer, A. J., Brandenberger, R., Gesemann, M., Chiquet, M. and Ruegg, M. A. (1997). Agrin binds to the nerve-muscle basal lamina via laminin. *J. Cell Biol.* **137**, 671–683.

Donger, C., Krejci, E., Serradell, A. P. et al. (1998). Mutation in the human acetylcholinesterase-associated collagen gene, *COLQ*, is responsible for congenital myasthenic syndrome with end-plate acetylcholinesterase deficiency (Type Ic). *Am. J. Hum. Genet.* **63**, 967–975.

Douville, P. J., Harvey, W. J. and Carbonetto, S. (1988). Isolation and partial characterization of high affinity laminin receptors in neural cells. *J. Biol. Chem.* **263**, 14964–14969.

Duance, V. C., Restall, D. J., Beard, H., Bourne, F. J. and Bailey, A. J. (1977). The location of three collagen types in skeletal muscle. *FEBS Lett.* **79**, 248–252.

Duclos, F., Straub, V., Moore, S. A. et al. (1998). Progressive muscular dystrophy in α-sarcoglycan-deficient mice. *J. Cell Biol.* **142**, 1461–1471.

Ervasti, J. M. and Campbell, K. P. (1993). A role for the dystrophin–glycoprotein complex as a transmembrane linker between laminin and actin. *J. Cell Biol.* **122**, 809–823.

Ettner, N., Gohring, W., Sasaki, T., Mann, K. and Timpl, R. (1998). The N-terminal globular domain of the laminin α_1 chain binds to $\alpha_1\beta_1$ and $\alpha_2\beta_1$ integrins and to the heparan sulfate-containing domains of perlecan. *FEBS Lett.* **430**, 217–221.

Feng, G., Krejci, E., Molgo, J., Cunningham, J. M., Massoulie, J. and Sanes, J. R. (1999). Genetic analysis of collagen Q: roles in acetylcholinesterase and butyrylcholinesterase assembly and in synaptic structure and function. *J. Cell Biol.* **144**, 1349–1360.

Ferns, M. J., Campanelli, J. T., Hoch, W., Scheller, R. H. and Hall, Z. (1993). The ability of agrin to cluster AChRs depends on alternative splicing and on cell surface proteoglycans. *Neuron* **11**, 491–502.

Florini, J. R., Ewton, D. Z. and Coolican, S. A. (1996). Growth hormone and the insulin-like growth factor system in myogenesis. *Endocr. Rev.* **17**, 481–517.

Foidart, M., Foidart, J. M. and Engel, W. K. (1981). Collagen localization in normal and fibrotic human skeletal muscle. *Arch. Neurol.* **38**, 152–157.

Froehner, S. C., Luetje, C. W., Scotland, P. B. and Patrick, J. (1990). The postsynaptic 43K protein clusters muscle nicotinic acetylcholine receptors in *Xenopus* oocytes. *Neuron* **5**, 403–410.

Gautam, M., Noakes, P. G., Mudd, J. et al. (1995). Failure of postsynaptic specialization to develop at neuromuscular junctions of rapsyn-deficient mice. [See comments] *Nature* **377**, 232–236.

Gautam, M., Noakes, P. G., Moscoso, L. et al. (1996). Defective neuromuscular synaptogenesis in agrin-deficient mutant mice. *Cell* **85**, 525–535.

Gee, S. H., Blacher, R. W., Douville, P. J., Provost, P. R., Yurchenco, P. D. and Carbonetto, S. (1993). Laminin-binding protein 120 from brain is closely related to the dystrophin-associated glycoprotein, dystroglycan and binds with high affinity to the major heparin binding domain of laminin. *J. Biol. Chem.* **268**, 14972–14980.

Gee, S. H., Montanaro, F., Lindenbaum, M. H. and Carbonetto, S. (1994). Dystroglycan-α, a dystrophin-associated glycoprotein, is a functional agrin receptor. *Cell* **77**, 675–686.

Gee, S. H., Madhavan, R., Levinson, S. R., Caldwell, J. H., Sealock, R. and Froehner, S. C. (1998). Interaction of muscle and brain sodium channels with multiple members of the syntrophin family of dystrophin-associated proteins. *J. Neurosci.* **18**, 128–137.

Glass, D. J., Bowen, D. C., Stitt, T. N. et al. (1996). Agrin acts via a MuSK receptor complex. *Cell* **85**, 513–523.

Goldman, D., Brenner, H. R. and Heinemann, S. (1988). Acetylcholine receptor α-, β-, γ- and δ-subunit mRNA levels are regulated by muscle activity. *Neuron* **1**, 329–333.

Grady, R. M., Merlie, J. P. and Sanes, J. R. (1997). Subtle neuromuscular defects in utrophin-deficient mice. *J. Cell Biol.* **136**, 871–882.

Guerin, C. W. and Holland, P. C. (1995). Synthesis and secretion of matrix-degrading metalloproteases by human skeletal muscle satellite cells. *Dev. Dynam.* **202**, 91–99.

Guicheney, P., Vignier, N., Helbling-Leclerc, A. et al. (1997). Genetics of laminin α2 chain (or merosin) deficient congenital muscular dystrophy: from identification of mutations to prenatal diagnosis. *Neuromusc. Disord.* **7**, 180–186.

Gulati, A. K., Reddi, A. H. and Zalewski, A. A. (1983). Changes in the basement membrane zone components during skeletal muscle fibre degeneration and regeneration. *J. Cell Biol.* **97**, 957–962.

Gullberg, D., Sjoberg, G., Velling, T. and Sejersen, T. (1995). Analysis of fibronectin and vitronectin receptors on human fetal skeletal muscle cells upon differentiation. *Exp. Cell Res.* **220**, 112–123.

Gullberg, D., Velling, T., Lohikangas, L. and Tiger, C. F. (1998). Integrins during muscle development and in muscular dystrophies. *Front. Biosci.* **3**, D1039–D1050.

Hagios, C., Koch, M., Spring, J., Chiquet, M. and Chiquet-Ehrismann, R. (1996). Tenascin-Y: a protein of novel domain structure is secreted by differentiated fibroblasts of muscle connective tissue. *J. Cell Biol.* **134**, 1499–1512.

Halfter, W., Dong, S., Schurer, B. and Cole, G. J. (1998). Collagen XVIII is a basement membrane heparan sulfate proteoglycan. *J. Biol. Chem.* **273**, 25404–25012.

Hantai, D. and Festoff, B. W. (1987). Degradation of muscle basement membrane zone by locally generated plasmin. *Exp. Neurol.* **95**, 44–55.

Hantai, D., Labat-Robert, J., Grimaud, J. A. and Fardeau, M. (1985). Fibronectin, laminin, type I, III and IV collagens in Duchenne's muscular dystrophy, congenital muscular dystrophies and congenital myopathies: an immunocytochemical study. *Connect. Tissue Res.* **13**, 273–281.

Hayashi, Y. K., Chou, F. L., Engvall, E. et al. (1998). Mutations in the integrin α7 gene cause congenital myopathy. *Nat. Genet.* **19**, 94–97.

Henry, M. D. and Campbell, K. P. (1996). Dystroglycan: an extracellular matrix receptor linked to the cytoskeleton. *Curr. Opin. Cell. Biol.* **8**, 625–631.

Henry, M. D. and Campbell, K. P. (1998). A role for dystroglycan in basement membrane assembly. *Cell* **95**, 859–870.

Hodges, B. L., Hayashi, Y. K., Nonaka, I., Wang, W., Arahata, K. and Kaufman, S. J. (1997). Altered expression of the α7β1 integrin in human and murine muscular dystrophies. *J. Cell. Sci.* **110**, 2873–2881.

Hopf, M., Gohring, W., Kohfeldt, E., Yamada, Y. and Timpl, R. (1999). Recombinant domain IV of perlecan binds to nidogens, laminin-nidogen complex, fibronectin, fibulin-2 and heparin. *Eur. J. Biochem.* **259**, 917–925.

Ibraghimov-Beskrovnaya, O., Ervasti, J. M., Leveille, C. J., Slaughter, C. A., Sernett, S. W. and Campbell, K. P. (1992). Primary structure of dystrophin-associated glycoproteins linking dystrophin to the extracellular matrix. *Nature* **355**, 696–702.

Ingber, D. E. (1997). Tensegrity: the architectural basis of cellular mechanotransduction. *Annu. Rev. Physiol.* **59**, 575–599.

Jacobson, C., Montanaro, F., Lindenbaum, M., Carbonetto, S. and Ferns, M. (1998). α-Dystroglycan functions in acetylcholine receptor aggregation but is not a coreceptor for agrin-MuSK signalling. *J. Neurosci.* **18**, 6340–6348.

Jo, S. A. and Burden, S. J. (1992). Synaptic basal lamina contains a signal for synapse-specific transcription. *Development* **115**, 673–680.

Jo, S. A., Zhu, X., Marchionni, M. A. and Burden, S. J. (1995). Neuregulins are concentrated at nerve–muscle synapses and activate ACh-receptor gene expression. *Nature* **373**, 158–161.

Jobsis, G. J., Keizers, H., Vreijling, J. P. et al. (1996). Type VI collagen mutations in Bethlem myopathy, an autosomal dominant myopathy with contractures. *Nat. Genet.* **14**, 113–115.

Jung, D., Yang, B., Meyer, J., Chamberlain, J. S. and Campbell, K. P. (1995). Identification and characterization of the dystrophin anchoring site on β-dystroglycan. *J. Biol. Chem.* **270**, 27305–27310.

Kadler, K. E., Holmes, D. F., Trotter, J. A. and Chapman, J. A. (1996). Collagen fibril formation. *Biochem. J.* **316**, 1–11.

Kherif, S., Lafuma, C., Dehaupas, M. et al. (1999). Expression of matrix metalloproteinases 2 and 9 in regenerating skeletal muscle: a study in experimentally injured and mdx muscles. *Dev. Biol.* **205**, 158–170.

Kopczynski, C. C., Davis, G. W. and Goodman, C. S. (1996). A neural tetraspanin, encoded by late bloomer, that facilitates synapse formation. [See comments] *Science* **271**, 1867–1870.

Krejci, E., Thomine, S., Boschetti, N., Legay, C., Sketelj, J. and Massoulie, J. (1997). The mammalian gene of acetylcholinesterase-associated collagen. *J. Biol. Chem.* **272**, 22840–22847.

Kuo, H. J., Maslen, C. L., Keene, D. R. and Glanville, R. W. (1997). Type VI collagen anchors endothelial basement membranes by interacting with type IV collagen. *J. Biol. Chem.* **272**, 26522–26529.

Larrain, J., Alvarez, J., Hassell, J. R. and Brandan, E. (1997). Expression of perlecan, a proteoglycan that binds myogenic inhibitory basic fibroblast growth factor, is down regulated during skeletal muscle differentiation. *Exp. Cell Res.* **234**, 405–412.

Larrain, J., Carey, D. J. and Brandan, E. (1998). Syndecan-1 expression inhibits myoblast differentiation through a basic fibroblast growth factor-dependent mechanism. *J. Biol. Chem.* **273**, 32288–32296.

Lehto, M., Kvist, M., Vieno, T. and Jozsa, L. (1988). Macromolecular composition of the sarcolemma and endomysium in the rat. *Acta Anat.* **133**, 297–302.

Light, N. and Champion, A. E. (1984). Characterization of muscle epimysium, perimysium and endomysium collagens. *Biochem. J.* **219**, 1017–1026.

Lim, L. E. and Campbell, K. P. (1998). The sarcoglycan complex in limb-girdle muscular dystrophy. *Curr. Opin. Neurol.* **11**, 443–452.

Mackie, E. J. (1997). Molecules in focus: tenascin-C. *Int. J. Biochem. Cell. Biol.* **29**, 1133–1137.

Maimone, M. M. and Merlie, J. P. (1993). Interaction of the 43 kd postsynaptic protein with all subunits of the muscle nicotinic acetylcholine receptor. *Neuron* **11**, 53–66.

Martin, P. T. and Sanes, J. R. (1997). Integrins mediate adhesion to agrin and modulate agrin signaling. *Development* **124**, 3909–3917.

Martin, P. T., Kaufman, S. J., Kramer, R. H. and Sanes, J. R. (1996). Synaptic integrins in developing, adult and mutant muscle: selective association of α_1, α_{7A} and α_{7B} integrins with the neuromuscular junction. *Dev. Biol.* **174**, 125–139.

Martinez-Hernandez, A. and Chung, A. E. (1984). The ultrastructural localization of two basement membrane components: entactin and laminin in rat tissues. *J. Histochem. Cytochem.* **32**, 289–298.

Marvulli, D., Volpin, D. and Bressan, G. M. (1996). Spatial and temporal changes of type VI collagen expression during mouse development. *Dev. Dynam.* **206**, 447–454.

Matrisian, L. M. (1992). The matrix-degrading metalloproteinases. *Bioessays* **14**, 455–463.

Matsumoto, K., Saga, Y., Ikemura, T., Sakakura, T. and Chiquet-Ehrismann, R. (1994). The distribution of tenascin-X is distinct and often reciprocal to that of tenascin-C. *J. Cell Biol.* **125**, 483–493.

Matsumura, K. and Campbell, K. P. (1994). Dystrophin-glycoprotein complex: its role in the molecular pathogenesis of muscular dystrophies. *Muscle Nerve* **17**, 2–15.

Matsumura, K., Ervasti, J. M., Ohlendieck, K., Kahl, S. D. and Campbell, K. P. (1992). Association of dystrophin-related protein with dystrophin-associated proteins in mdx mouse muscle. *Nature* **360**, 588–591.

Mayer, U., Saher, G., Fassler, R. et al. (1997). Absence of integrin α_7 causes a novel form of muscular dystrophy. *Nat. Genet.* **17**, 318–323.

McMahan, U. J. (1990). The agrin hypothesis. *Cold Spring Harb. Symp. Quant. Biol.* **55**, 407–418.

Miner, J. H., Patton, B. L., Lentz, S. I., et al. (1997). The laminin α chains: expression, developmental transitions and chromosomal locations of α1–5, identification of heterotrimeric laminins 8–11 and cloning of a novel α_3 isoform. *J. Cell Biol.* **137**, 685–701.

Miyagoe, Y., Hanaoka, K., Nonaka, I. et al. (1997). Laminin α2 chain-null mutant mice by targeted disruption of the Lama2 gene: a new model of merosin (laminin 2)-deficient congenital muscular dystrophy. *FEBS Lett.* **415**, 33–39.

Montanaro, F., Lindenbaum, M. and Carbonetto, S. (1999). α-Dystroglycan is a laminin receptor involved in extracellular matrix assembly on myotubes and muscle cell viability. *J. Cell Biol.* **145**, 1325–1340.

Moscoso, L. M., Cremer, H. and Sanes, J. R. (1998). Organization and reorganization of neuromuscular junctions in mice lacking neural cell adhesion molecule, tenascin-C, or fibroblast growth factor-5. *J. Neurosci.* **18**, 1465–1477.

Murdoch, A. D., Dodge, G. R., Cohen, I., Tuan, R. S. and Iozzo, R. V. (1992). Primary structure of the human heparan sulfate proteoglycan from basement membrane (HSPG2/perlecan). A chimeric molecule with multiple domains homologous to the low density lipoprotein receptor, laminin, neural cell adhesion molecules and epidermal growth factor. *J. Biol. Chem.* **267**, 8544–8557.

Myers, J. C., Dion, A. S., Abraham, V. and Amenta, P. S. (1996). Type XV collagen exhibits a widespread distribution in human tissues but a distinct localization in basement membrane zones. *Cell. Tissue Res.* **286**, 493–505.

Nishimura, T., Ojima, K., Hattori, A. and Takahashi, K. (1997). Developmental expression of extracellular matrix components in intramuscular connective tissue of bovine semitendinosus muscle. *Histochem. Cell Biol.* **107**, 215–221.

Nitkin, R. M. and Rothschild, T. C. (1990). Agrin-induced reorganization of extracellular matrix components on cultured myotubes: relationship to AChR aggregation. *J. Cell Biol.* **111**, 1161–1170.

Oh, S. P., Kamagata, Y., Muragaki, Y., Timmons, S., Ooshima, A. and Olsen, B. R. (1994). Isolation and sequencing of cDNAs for proteins with multiple domains of Gly-Xaa-Yaa repeats identify a distinct family of collagenous proteins. *Proc. Natl. Acad. Sci. USA* **91**, 4229–4233.

Ohno, K., Brengman, J., Tsujino, A. and Engel, A. G. (1998). Human endplate acetylcholinesterase deficiency caused by mutations in the collagen-like tail subunit (ColQ) of the asymmetric enzyme. *Proc. Natl. Acad. Sci. USA* **95**, 9654–9659.

Pall, E. A., Bolton, K. M. and Ervasti, J. M. (1996). Differential heparin inhibition of skeletal muscle α-dystroglycan binding to laminins. *J. Biol. Chem.* **271**, 3817–3821.

Patton, B. L., Miner, J. H., Chiu, A. Y. and Sanes, J. R. (1997). Distribution and function of laminins in the neuromuscular system of developing, adult and mutant mice. *J. Cell Biol.* **139**, 1507–1521.

Pedrosa-Domellof, F., Virtanen, I. and Thornell, L. E. (1995). Tenascin is present in human muscle spindles and neuromuscular junctions. *Neurosci. Lett.* **198**, 173–176.

Peng, H. B., Xie, H., Rossi, S. G. and Rotundo, R. L. (1999). Acetylcholinesterase clustering at the neuromuscular junction involves perlecan and dystroglycan. *J. Cell Biol.* **145**, 911–921.

Peters, J. H. and Hynes, R. O. (1996). Fibronectin isoform distribution in the mouse. I. The alternatively spliced EIIIB, EIIIA and V segments show widespread codistribution in the developing mouse embryo. *Cell. Adhes. Commun.* **4**, 103–125.

Peters, M. F., Kramarcy, N. R., Sealock, R. and Froehner, S. C. (1994). β_2-Syntrophin: localization at the neuromuscular junction in skeletal muscle. *Neuroreport* **5**, 1577–1580.

Peters, M. F., Adams, M. E. and Froehner, S. C. (1997). Differential association of syntrophin pairs with the dystrophin complex. *J. Cell Biol.* **138**, 81–93.

Petrof, B. J. (1998). The molecular basis of activity-induced muscle injury in Duchenne muscular dystrophy. *Mol. Cell. Biochem.* **179**, 111–123.

Pfaff, M., Göhring, W., Brown, J. C. and Timpl, R. (1994). Binding of purified collagen receptors ($\alpha_1\beta_1$, $\alpha_2\beta_1$) and RGD-dependent integrins to laminins and laminin fragments. *Eur. J. Biochem.* **225**, 975–984.

Phillips, W. D., Kopta, C., Blount, P., Gardner, P. D., Steinbach, J. H. and Merlie, J. P. (1991). ACh receptor-rich membrane domains organized in fibroblasts by recombinant 43-kilodalton protein. *Science* **251**, 568–570.

Piccolo, S., Bonaldo, P., Vitale, P., Volpin, D. and Bressan, G. M. (1995). Transcriptional activation of the $\alpha 1$(VI) collagen gene during myoblast differentiation is mediated by multiple GA boxes. *J. Biol. Chem.* **270**, 19583–19590.

Prockop, D. J. and Kivirikko, K. I. (1995). Collagens: molecular biology, diseases and potentials for therapy. *Annu. Rev. Biochem.* **64**, 403–434.

Rambukkana, A., Yamada, H., Zanazzi, G. et al. (1998). Role of alpha-dystroglycan as a Schwann cell receptor for *Mycobacterium leprae. Science* **282**, 2076–2079.

Redick, S. D. and Schwarzbauer, J. E. (1995). Rapid intracellular assembly of tenascin hexabrachions suggests a novel cotranslational process. *J. Cell. Sci.* **108**, 1761–1769.

Rentschler, S., Linn, H., Deininger, K., Bedford, M. T., Espanel, X. and Sudol, M. (1999). The WW domain of dystrophin requires EF-hands region to interact with β-dystroglycan. *Biol. Chem.* **380**, 431–442.

Ringelmann, B., Roder, C., Hallmann, R. et al. (1999). Expression of laminin $\alpha 1$, $\alpha 2$, $\alpha 4$ and $\alpha 5$ chains, fibronectin and tenascin-C in skeletal muscle of dystrophic 129ReJ *dy/dy* mice. *Exp. Cell. Res.* *246, 165–182.*

Romberger, D. J. (1997). Fibronectin. *Int. J. Biochem. Cell. Biol.* **29**, 939–943.

Rossi, S. G. and Rotundo, R. L. (1996). Transient interactions between collagen-tailed acetylcholinesterase and sulfated proteoglycans prior to immobilization on the extracellular matrix. *J. Biol. Chem.* **271**, 1979–1987.

Sado, Y., Kagawa, M., Naito, I. et al. (1998). Organization and expression of basement membrane collagen IV genes and their roles in human disorders. *J. Biochem. (Tokyo)* **123**, 767–776.

Sanes, J. R. (1982). Laminin, fibronectin and collagen in synaptic and extrasynaptic portions of muscle fiber basement membrane. *J. Cell Biol.* **93**, 442–451.

Sanes, J. R. and Lichtman, J. W. (1999). Development of the vertebrate neuromuscular junction. *Annu. Rev. Neurosci.* **22**, 389–442.

Sanes, J. R., Marshall, L. M. and McMahan, U. J. (1978). Reinnervation of muscle fibre basal lamina after removal of myofibers. Differentiation of regenerating axons at original synaptic sites. *J. Cell Biol.* **78**, 176–198.

Sanes, J. R., Engvall, E., Butkowski, R. and Hunter, D. D. (1990). Molecular heterogeneity of basal laminae: isoforms of laminin and collagen IV at the neuromuscular junction and elsewhere. *J. Cell Biol.* **111**, 1685–1699.

Sastry, S. K., Lakonishok, M., Thomas, D. A., Muschler, J. and Horwitz, A. F. (1996). Integrin α subunit ratios, cytoplasmic domains and growth factor synergy regulate muscle proliferation and differentiation. *J. Cell Biol.* **133**, 169–184.

Sastry, S. K., Lakonishok, M., Wu, S. et al. (1999). Quantitative changes in integrin and focal adhesion signalling regulate myoblast cell cycle withdrawal. *J. Cell Biol.* **144**, 1295–1309.

Schwarzbauer, J. E. (1991). Alternative splicing of fibronectin: three variants, three functions. *Bioessays* **13**, 527–533.

Sheng, M. (1996). PDZs and receptor/channel clustering: rounding up the latest suspects. *Neuron* **17**, 575–578.

Shrivastava, A., Radziejewski, C., Campbell, E. et al. (1997). An orphan receptor tyrosine kinase family whose members serve as nonintegrin collagen receptors. *Mol. Cell.* **1**, 25–34.

Simon, S., Krejci, E. and Massoulie, J. (1998). A four-to-one association between peptide motifs: four C-terminal domains from cholinesterase assemble with one proline-rich attachment domain (PRAD) in the secretory pathway. *EMBO J.* **17**, 6178–6187.

Smalheiser, N. R. and Schwartz, N. B. (1987). Cranin: a laminin-binding protein of cell membranes. *Proc. Natl. Acad. Sci. USA* **84**, 6457–6461.

Song, W. K., Wang, W., Foster, R. F., Bielser, D. A. and Kaufman, S. J. (1992). H36-α7 is a novel integrin α chain that is developmentally regulated during skeletal myogenesis. [Published erratum appears in *J. Cell Biol.* (1992) **118**, 213.] *J. Cell Biol.* **117**, 643–657.

Song, W. K., Wang, W., Sato, H., Bielser, D. A. and Kaufman, S. J. (1993). Expression of α_7 integrin cytoplasmic domains during skeletal muscle development: alternate forms, conformational change and homologies with serine/threonine kinases and tyrosine phosphatases. *J. Cell. Sci.* **106**, 1139–1152.

Storms, S. D., Kim, A. C., Tran, B. H., Cole, G. J. and Murray, B. A. (1996). NCAM-mediated adhesion of transfected cells to agrin. *Cell. Adhes. Commun.* **3**, 497–509.

Straub, V. and Campbell, K. P. (1997). Muscular dystrophies and the dystrophin-glycoprotein complex. *Curr. Opin. Neurol.* **10**, 168–175.

Sugiyama, J., Bowen, D. C. and Hall, Z. W. (1994). Dystroglycan binds nerve and muscle agrin. *Neuron* **13**, 103–115.

Sunada, Y., Bernier, S. M., Utani, A., Yamada, Y. and Campbell, K. P. (1995). Identification of a novel mutant transcript of laminin $\alpha 2$ chain gene responsible for muscular dystrophy and dysmyelination in *dy*2J mice. *Hum. Mol. Genet.* **4**, 1055–1061.

Suzuki, A., Yoshida, M. and Ozawa, E. (1995). Mammalian α_1- and β_1-syntrophin bind to the alternative splice-prone region of the dystrophin COOH terminus. *J. Cell Biol.* **128**, 373–381.

Talts, J. F., Andac, Z., Gohring, W., Brancaccio, A. and Timpl, R. (1999). Binding of the G domains of laminin α1 and α2 chains and perlecan to heparin, sulfatides, α-dystroglycan and several extracellular matrix proteins. *EMBO J.* **18**, 863–870.

Taverna, D., Disatnik, M. H., Rayburn, H. et al. (1998). Dystrophic muscle in mice chimeric for expression of α_5 integrin. *J. Cell Biol.* **143**, 849–859.

Tews, D. S. and Goebel, H. H. (1997). DNA-fragmentation and expression of apoptosis-related proteins in muscular dystrophies. *Neuropathol. Appl. Neurobiol.* **23**, 331–338.

Tillet, E., Wiedemann, H., Golbik, R., Pan, T. C., Zhang, R. Z., Mann, K., Chu, M. L. and Timpl, R. (1994). Recombinant expression and structural and binding properties of α1(VI) and α2(VI) chains of human collagen type VI. [Published erratum appears in *Eur. J. Biochem.* (1994) **222**, 1064.] *Eur. J. Biochem.* **221**, 177–185.

Timpl, R. and Brown, J. C. (1996). Supramolecular assembly of basement membranes. *Bioessays* **18**, 123–132.

Torra, R., Badenas, C., Cofan, F., Callis, L., Perez-Oller, L. and Darnell, A. (1999). Autosomal recessive Alport syndrome: linkage analysis and clinical features in two families. *Nephrol. Dial. Transplant* **14**, 627–630.

Torres, R., Firestein, B. L., Dong, H. et al. (1998). PDZ proteins bind, cluster and synaptically colocalize with Eph receptors and their ephrin ligands. [See comments] *Neuron* **21**, 1453–1463.

Vachon, P. H., Loechel, F., Xu, H., Wewer, U. M. and Engvall, E. (1996). Merosin and laminin in myogenesis; specific requirement for merosin in myotube stability and survival. *J. Cell Biol.* **134**, 1483–1497.

Vachon, P. H., Xu, H., Liu, L. et al. (1997). Integrins ($\alpha_7\beta_1$) in muscle function and survival. Disrupted expression in merosin-deficient congenital muscular dystrophy. *J. Clin. Invest.* **100**, 1870–1881.

von der Mark, H., Durr, J., Sonnenberg, A., von der Mark, K., Deutzmann, R. and Goodman, S. L. (1991). Skeletal myoblasts utilize a novel β_1-series integrin and not $\alpha_6\beta_1$ for binding to the E8 and T8 fragments of laminin. *J. Biol. Chem.* **266**, 23593–23601.

Williamson, R. A., Henry, M. D., Daniels, K. J., Hrstka, R. F., Lee, J. C., Sunada, Y., Ibraghimov-Beskrovnaya, O. and Campbell, K. P. (1997). Dystroglycan is essential for early embryonic development: disruption of Reichert's membrane in Dag1-null mice. *Hum. Mol. Genet.* **6**, 831–841.

Woods, A. and Couchman, J. R. (1998). Syndecans: synergistic activators of cell adhesion. *Trends Cell. Biol.* **8**, 189–192.

Xu, H., Christmas, P., Wu, X. R., Wewer, U. M. and Engvall, E. (1994). Defective muscle basement membrane and lack of M-laminin in the dystrophic *dy/dy* mouse. *Proc. Natl. Acad. Sci. USA* **91**, 5572–5576.

Yang, B., Jung, D., Motto, D., Meyer, J., Koretzky, G. and Campbell, K. P. (1995). SH3 domain-mediated interaction of dystroglycan and Grb2. *J. Biol. Chem.* **270**, 11711–11714.

Yao, C. C., Ziober, B. L., Squillace, R. M. and Kramer, R. H. (1996). A7 integrin mediates cell adhesion and migration on specific laminin isoforms. *J. Biol. Chem.* **271**, 25598–25603.

Yoshida, M. and Ozawa, E. (1990). Glycoprotein complex anchoring dystrophin to sarcolemma. *J. Biochem. (Tokyo)* **108**, 748–752.

Yoshida, M., Suzuki, A., Yamamoto, H., Noguchi, S., Mizuno, Y. and Ozawa, E. (1994). Dissociation of the complex of dystrophin and its associated proteins into several unique groups by *n*-octyl β-D-glucoside. *Eur. J. Biochem.* **222**, 1055–1061.

Yoshida, T., Pan, Y., Hanada, H., Iwata, Y., and Shigekawa, M. (1998). Bidirectional signaling between sarcoglycans and the integrin adhesion system in cultured L6 myocytes. *J. Biol. Chem.* **273**, 1583–1590.

Zhou, J., Mochizuki, T., Smeets, H. et al. (1993). Deletion of the paired α 5(IV) and α 6(IV) collagen genes in inherited smooth muscle tumors. *Science* **261**, 1167–1169.

8

Aspects of skeletal muscle biochemistry in health and disease

John M. Land

Introduction

Skeletal muscle transforms chemical energy in the form of adenosine triphosphate (ATP) into useful mechanical energy. Carbohydrate, fat, and intramuscular creatine phosphate (CrP) generate the major amounts of ATP in human muscle cells. The relative proportions of each fuel used varies according to a series of factors, including age, diet, training and the intensity of exercise as well as its duration. In the human, skeletal muscle contributes approximately 40% of total body mass. Accordingly, it is not surprising that muscle metabolism influences and contributes to whole-body metabolic homeostasis and organ function. Examples of such interactions include the provision of substrates for hepatic gluconeogenesis and the release of glutamine for renal modulation of acid–base balance and immune cell activity. It is not surprising, therefore, that metabolic muscle diseases may affect systemic systems, while common conditions such as infection or heart failure can affect the metabolism and consequently the function of skeletal muscle.

This chapter will examine the metabolism of skeletal muscle, in particular those catabolic pathways that generate ATP. The effects of exercise and diet will be considered and the control mechanisms affecting muscle hypertrophy/atrophy will be examined. The fundamental role of muscle in amino acid metabolism will be explored, particularly how this relates to exercise and other tissues. Finally note will be made of those changes that occur to muscle during space travel.

Metabolic fuels

Carbohydrate, either as blood-borne glucose or intramuscular glycogen, and fat provide the majority of substrate for the production of ATP. Both carbohydrate and fat are catabolized oxidatively in type I (slow muscle) fibres. Fast-twitch fibres may be classified as oxidative (type IIA) or glycolytic (type IIB) (Brooke and Kaiser, 1970) and these latter fibres primarily use glucose anaerobically. A further source of ATP is CrP which is found in all skeletal muscle cells. However, CrP represents only a relatively minor source of ATP and it has been estimated that it could be depleted in a matter of a few seconds of exercise if it were the only source of ATP available (Newsholme, 1998).

Glucose

Glucose derived either directly from the portal circulation or synthesized and released from the liver is delivered to skeletal muscle by the bloodstream where it is taken up and stored as glycogen. Skeletal muscle, therefore, plays a significant role in glucose homeostasis. Clearly the role of blood flow is important in determining uptake, as is the blood concentration of glucose. However, equally important is the presence of glucose transport proteins within the muscle bulk. Three glucose transporter isoforms, GLUT 1, 3 and 4, are expressed in developing muscle, though a fourth, GLUT 5, which translocates fructose, is found in adult muscle (Hundal et al., 1998). As differentiation of myotubes occurs, GLUT 3 disappears completely while GLUT 1 represents only about 3% of the total amount of transporters. GLUT4 remains the predominant translocator. While GLUT 1 appears to be localized to the plasma membrane, GLUT 4 appears to be localized to both the plasma membrane and two intracellular locations (Guillet-Deniau, 1994). In the rat soleus muscle, the larger of the two subsarcolemmal pools appears to be associated with the *trans*-Golgi network and endosome. The exact location of the smaller pool remains unknown. In response to both muscle contraction and insulin, GLUT 4 appears to translocate to two locations: the plasma membrane and the T-tubules. The individual stimuli, insulin or contraction, appear to be able to produce additive and independent responses. For example, wortmannin, a phosphotidylinositol 3-kinase inhibitor, selectively inhibits insulin, but not contraction-stimulated glucose uptake (Lee et al., 1995). In contrast, the nitric oxide synthase (NOS) inhibitor L-NAME inhibits contraction-stimulated uptake of glucose and the translocation of GLUT 4 to the plasma membrane (Roberts et al., 1997), suggesting that nitric oxide mediates contraction-induced changes to GLUT 4. In this respect, it is noteworthy that NOS in skeletal muscle fibres appears to be an integral signalling component of the dystrophin–glycoprotein complex (Grozdenovic and Baumgarten, 1999). An ingenious model, the SNARE hypothesis, based on similarities between synaptosomes and muscle has been proposed. In this model for GLUT 4 translocation, specificity of targeting is generated by complexes that form between specific membrane transport vesicles and unique target membrane proteins (Hashimoto and James, 1998). Increasingly, it is becoming apparent that the majority of glucose uptake into muscle, particularly at times when requirements are high (i.e. during contraction), is facilitated by GLUT 4 T-tubule systems. The advantage to the muscle cell being that this system can deliver nutrients to the centre of the cell, as well as removing breakdown products from it (Dudek et al., 1994).

Once within the myocyte, glucose may either be stored as the glucose polymer glycogen, as in the postprandial period, or be metabolized to yield ATP. Glycogen is a large soluble molecule containing up to 30 000 glucose units joined primarily by linear (α1–4) glycoside bonds, but interspersed by occasional branching (α1–6) bonds. Thus, substantial glucose may be stored within the myocyte with minimal effect upon the intracellular osmotic pressure. Two enzymes are key to maintaining appropriate glucose levels in muscle. These are glycogen synthase and glycogen phosphorylase. Both are controlled in a coordinated way by hormones, particularly adrenaline (epinephrine), acting via signal transduction pathways. Central to these pathways is intracellular adenosine $3',5'$-monophosphate (cAMP), which is produced by the enzyme adenylate kinase when the hormone binds to the myocyte receptor. In turn, cAMP binds to an allosteric site on the regulatory subunit of protein kinase A, which then phosphorylates glycogen synthase, thus inactivating it. At the same time protein kinase A phosphorylates and, thus, activates phosphorylase kinase, an enzyme that acts to phosphorylate and activate glycogen phosphorylase. The net result is that glycogen synthesis is inhibited while its breakdown is

activated. This coordinated control allows glycogen synthesis and breakdown within muscle to meet the body's needs as signalled by changes in circulating hormone levels. More recently, it has been found that muscle glycogen synthesis may be modulated by appropriate changes in cell volumes (Low et al., 1997a), via a mechanism that involves integrin–extracellular matrix interactions and cytoskeletal proteins. In this way, alterations in extracellular osmotic pressure are capable of altering intracellular events, presumably by changes in the membrane architecture affecting the activity of adenylate cyclase.

The pathway of glucose utilization from glucose 6-phosphate to pyruvate, anaerobic glycolysis, is well documented and will not be discussed here, other than to point out some major points. For an excellent review the reader is referred to Matthews and van Holder (1995). Pyruvate may be considered the end-point of anaerobic glycolysis. In muscle, it has two potential fates. If the production rate is high and in excess of the capacity of the mitochondria to oxidize the molecule further then it may be reduced to lactate. Such a situation commonly occurs during bursts of extreme activity in which type IIB fibres, those with relatively sparse numbers of mitochondria, are primarily used. Equally, if a muscle contains mitochondria deficient in a subunit of the respiratory chain, the oxidative capacity of the muscle may well be significantly impaired and pyruvate will replace molecular oxygen as the terminal electron acceptor. This is the origin of the lactic acidaemia observed in many patients with mitochondrial myopathies.

More commonly, pyruvate is oxidized by both type I and type II fibres in someone undertaking moderate exercise. In part, this reflects the much more efficient nature of oxidative compared with anaerobic metabolism. The anaerobic utilization of glucose to lactate results in the production of 2 mol ATP. This compares very unfavourably with the 38 mol ATP that can be theoretically produced if glucose is fully oxidized to carbon dioxide and water.

The key enzyme for pyruvate if it is to be oxidized is pyruvate dehydrogenase (PDH). This multienzyme complex is found within the mitochondrial matrix and, as we will observe below, plays a significant role with carnitine palmitoyltransferase I (CPT I) in regulating whether skeletal muscle utilizes carbohydrate or fat. PDH is subject to regulation by both chemical modification (phosphorylation) and fine metabolic control (e.g. ratio of nicotinamide adenine dinucleotide to its reduced form ($NAD^+/NADH$) and the ratio of coenzyme A to acetyl-coenzyme A (acetyl-CoA)). When ATP levels are low, dephosphorylation of PDH to an active form is favoured. At this time it is most likely that intramitochondrial NAD^+ and coenzyme A levels will also be low. Therefore, the oxidative decarboxylation of pyruvate to acetyl-CoA is favoured. This can be observed if PDH activity is measured in biopsies from untrained subjects who are undertaking work representing increasing percentages of maximal oxygen uptake. Sequential increases in PDH activity are observed, with as great as a sixfold increase over the resting basal activity (Howlett et al., 1998). This most probably reflects increases in cellular free ADP and intracellular free phosphate (P_i) giving rise to increased intracellular Mg^{2+} and Ca^{2+} which stimulate PDH phosphatase, the enzyme that activates PDH. Interestingly, under these conditions, the level of glycogen phosphorylase in its active form appears constant across all but the most severe outputs despite increased glycogenolytic flux. This suggests that whereas the proportion of active PDH activity is directly related to the increasing power output this is not the case for glycogen phosphorylase. Rather its activity appears to be primarily matched to the demand for energy by alterations in free cellular concentrations of P_i and the purine nucleotides ADP and AMP. Only at the very highest levels of skeletal muscle power output is transformation of further glycogen phosphorylase enzyme to the active form required.

Following the PDH step the acetyl unit, produced as acetyl-CoA, is metabolized by the enzymes of the tricarboxylic acid (TCA) cycle to carbon dioxide and water. Skeletal muscle metabolite and flux studies (Gibala et al., 1998) in demand caused by exercise show a 100-fold increase in flux through the cycle with a concomitant increase of only two- or fourfold in TCA intermediates suggesting that there is considerable reserve in the capacity of the TCA cycle to respond to exercise. For a review of the enzymology of the TCA cycle the reader is referred to (Matthews and van Holder, 1995).

The reducing equivalents (electrons) released by the activity of the TCA cycle in the form of $NADH_2$ and $FADH_2$ (reduced flavin adenine dinucleotide) are reoxidized within the mitochondrion by the respiratory chain (Fig. 8.1). $NADH_2$ is oxidized by complex I of the chain utilizing an intermediate flavin mononucleotide (FMN) to reduce an iron–sulphur centre deep within its structure before reducing ubiquinone, which is present within the mitochondrial inner membrane. In a similar manner, the reducing equivalents from $FADH_2$ are the substrate for complex II to reduce further ubiquinone. Subsequently, reduced ubiquinone is oxidized by cytochrome b, which in turn reduces cytochrome c_1 of complex III. The final series of oxidoreduction reactions sees cytochrome c_1 being oxidized by the protein cytochrome c. Reduced cytochrome c is finally oxidized by cytochrome oxidase (complex IV), which contains the cytochromes a and a_3. This final reaction uses molecular oxygen derived from the bloodstream or myoglobin in muscle and results in the reduction of oxygen to water. In addition to this final step, as electrons have been passed along the respiratory chain protons have moved across the inner mitochondrial membrane to the cytosol. This establishes a proton gradient across the inner mitochondrial membrane, which manifests itself as a proton motive force with two components: a ΔpH and a membrane potential. The controlled movement of protons back through the mitochondrial ATPase, so-called complex V of the respiratory chain, provides the free energy for the formation of ATP from ADP and inorganic phosphate by a novel rotational catalytic mechanism (Boyer, 1997).

Fatty acids

Fatty acids are primarily utilized by the slow oxidative, type I fibres. Under normal circumstances, muscle cells store relatively small amounts of fatty acids. Even in some defects of fatty acid oxidation, accumulations of triacylglycerol are minimal unless the biopsy has been taken after a period of fasting. Therefore, fatty acids are primarily supplied to skeletal muscle from the bloodstream for oxidative purposes. Fats are transported in the bloodstream either bound to albumin or in the form of triacylglycerols in very low density lipoprotein or chylomicrons. The means by which fatty acids leave the vascular compartment in order to reach skeletal muscle cells is still the subject of debate. However, it is thought most likely that fatty acids actually pass through the endothelial cells, rather than diffusing through the interendothelial clefts. At the myocyte membrane, a group of specific fatty acid-binding proteins have been proposed to facilitate the uptake of fatty acids (Bonen et al., 1998a). There are four major proteins described: a plasma membrane fatty acid-binding protein ($FABP_{pm}$), a fatty acid translocase (FAT), a fatty acid transport protein (FATP) and a cytoplasmic fatty acid-binding protein ($FABP_c$). The last acts as an intracellular sink for fatty acids, thereby increasing their concentration in the cytoplasm of myocytes (Glatz et al., 1998). Bonen et al. (1998b) have provided the first evidence that $FABP_{pm}$ and FAT are involved in long-chain fatty acid uptake into skeletal muscle. In particular, they have demonstrated that $FABP_{pm}$ facilitates uptake of fatty acids into muscle vesicles, that the process observes Michaelis–Menton kinetics with a low physiological K_m (~ 6 nmol/l), and is inhibitable by a range of compounds including phloretin and sulfo-n-succinimidyl oleate. Furthermore, the group were able to demonstrate that maximal transport in red muscle vesicles is approximately twice that observed in white muscle vesicles,

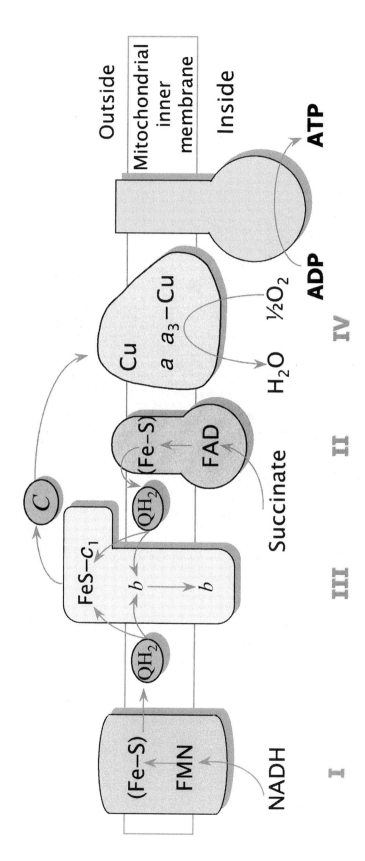

Fig. 8.1. The mitochondrial electron transport chain. a, a_3, b, c, and c_1 are all cytochromes; QH_2, ubiquinone; I–IV indicates complexes I–IV. See text for details.

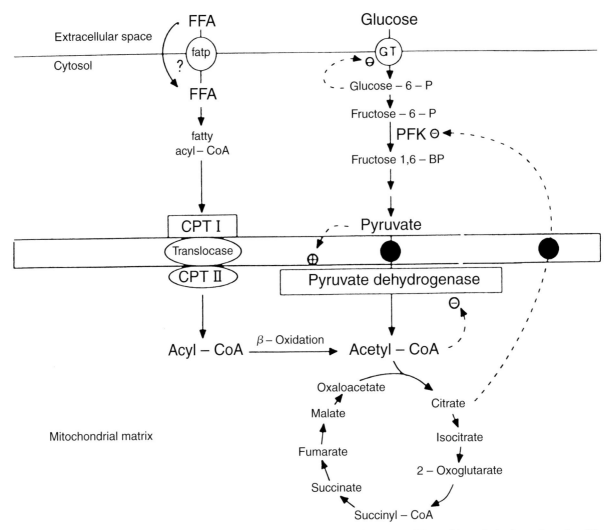

Fig. 8.2. The glucose–fatty acid cycle and relationship to the tricarboxylic acid cycle. CPT I and II, carnitine palmitoyl transferase I and II; Fatp, fatty acid transfer proteins; FFA, free fatty acid; GT, GLUT 4 translocator; PFK, phosphofructokinase; −, inhibition; +, activation.

reflecting the differing oxidative potential of fibre type (Bonen et al., 1998b). Furthermore, as the level of $FABP_{pm}$ in skeletal muscle can be increased by fasting (Turcotte et al., 1997), it is suggested that $FABP_{pm}$ may play a significant role in the regulation of free fatty acid uptake and utilization by skeletal muscle.

Once fatty acids have entered the muscle, it is believed that $FABP_c$ facilitates their intracellular transport to their site of oxidation or storage. Breakdown of triacylglycerol to its component parts is catalysed by a hormone-sensitive lipase, which is sensitive to both muscular contraction and circulating adrenaline. The latter works by increasing the activity of a cAMP-dependent protein kinase, similar to that used in the phosphorylase system. This phosphory-lates and thereby activates the lipase. The mechanism by which muscular contraction activates the hormone-sensitive lipase is not well understood. Breakdown of triacygly-cerol gives rise to glycerol and free fatty acid. Glycerol is returned to the bloodstream and subsequently to the liver, where it is a substrate for true gluconeogenesis. Fatty acids are oxidized within the mitochondrion. At rest, around 300 nmol fatty acids are oxidized per gram muscle/min. However, even with only moderate exercise this can rise to as much as 7500 nmol/min per g muscle. It is quite clear, therefore, that the flux of fatty acid oxidation needs to be carefully regulated. One major point at which this is achieved, in addition to control at the plasma membrane, is through CPT I, which is located on the inner aspect of the outer mitochondrial membrane (Fig. 8.2).

CPT I catalyses the synthesis of long-chain acylcarnitine

from carnitine and long-chain acyl-CoA. The carnitine derivative is then translocated to the inner aspect of the inner mitochondrial membrane by a specific translocase before being transformed back to the CoA ester by CPT II. This integrated process is regulated in skeletal muscle at the CPT I step. This enzyme has a regulatory binding site to which malonyl-CoA may bind and inhibit the enzyme. Malonyl-CoA is synthesized in muscle by an isoform of acetyl-CoA carboxylase. This isoform is distinct from those isoforms found in liver and adipose tissue but is subject to similar controls. Like PDH, it is subject to both fine metabolic control, being activated allosterically by citrate, and phosphorylative modification. The mechanism involves an AMP-dependent protein kinase that phosphorylates and thus inactivates acetyl-CoA carboxylase. In addition, cAMP also activates a second kinase, which itself activates an AMP-dependent kinase. This complicated system is shown schematically in Fig. 8.3. As we will note below, these mechanisms are appropriate for muscle since when tissue levels of ATP fall, such as during contraction, AMP levels rise as the tissue tries to enhance its ATP levels via the adenylate kinase reaction. Increased AMP levels then inactivates acetyl-CoA carboxylase, giving rise to a decrease in malonyl-CoA levels and, as a result, increased fatty acid β-oxidation and ATP production (Fig. 8.3).

Beta-oxidation occurs within the mitochondrial matrix and generates acetyl-CoA. It is characterized by repeated cycles of four sequential reactions. The steps include an initial flavin-dependent dehydrogenation, catalysed by three different isoforms of acyldehydrogenase, namely, very-long-chain, medium- and short-chain dehydrogenases. These act upon the appropriate chain length acyl-CoA to give FADH$_2$ and enoyl-CoA derivatives. The FADH$_2$ is reoxidized by the electron transport chain and the enoyl-CoA compounds are acted upon by the appropriate hydratase for the chain length of the acyl compound – long or short chain – to form 3-hydroxyacyl-CoA derivatives. The latter are then acted upon by the appropriate chain length hydroxyacyl dehydrogenases (again there are two, with long- and short-chain specificities) to yield 3-ketoacyl-CoA compounds. The cofactor for this step is NAD$^+$, which is subsequently reoxidized by the mitochondrial respiratory chain with concomitant production of ATP. The final step of β-oxidation is the production of acetyl-CoA by the action of two thiolase enzymes. One is specific for the four-carbon compound acetoacetyl-CoA, but all other thiolase steps are catalysed by a 3-ketoacyl-CoA thiolase with a broad chain length specificity. Acetyl-CoA produced from this reaction is incorporated into the TCA cycle as previously described. The remaining acyl-CoA moiety is now two carbon atoms shorter and the cycle of reactions is repeated.

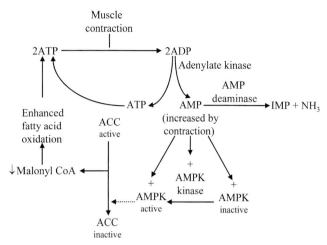

Fig. 8.3. Control of fatty acid oxidation: involvement of malonyl-CoA. AMP, adenosine monophosphate; ADP, adenosine diphosphate; ATP adenosine triphosphate; AMPK, AMP-dependent kinase; AMPK kinase, AMP-dependent-kinase kinase; ACC, acetyl-CoA carboxylase; IMP, inosine monophosphate.

In liver, fatty acid β-oxidation may be a prelude to ketone body production for subsequent export to and utilization by peripheral tissues, especially at times of systemic hypoglycaemia. The enzymes of ketogenesis however, are not found in muscle. Accordingly all fatty acid catabolism occurring in muscle is geared toward local energy production. This raises interesting metabolic control questions as we will see below, since in skeletal muscle glucose and fat may be utilized simultaneously.

Creatine phosphate

Although glucose (glycogen) and fat (triacylglycerol) provide the majority of ATP for normal skeletal muscle activity, a third compound, CrP, should not be overlooked. CrP is particularly important to fast-twitch, type II, fibres when the energy expenditure rate for muscular mechanical activity is in excess of that which can be provided by oxidative processes.

The intracellular biochemistry of CrP is interesting. It is synthesized adjacent to the mitochondria by a creatine kinase (mtCK) that is bound to the mitochondria and uses mitochondrially formed ATP and creatine. Once formed, the energy within the compound can be considered to be 'safe' since CK is the only enzyme within muscle that can utilize the compound. The CrP is then able to diffuse across the cell to locations of ATP usage such as the actinomysin ATPase and can buffer the ATP concentration at times of high usage that cannot be made good by glycolytic or

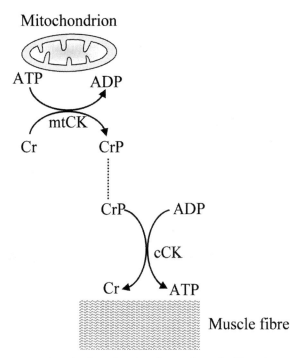

Fig. 8.4. The role of creatine phosphate and creatine kinase in delivering ATP to the muscle fibre. ADP, adenosine diphosphate; ATP, adenosine triphosphate; Cr, creatine; CrP, creatine phosphate; cCK, cytosolic creatine kinase; mtCK, mitochondrial creatine kinase.

oxidative means. This is achieved by a second CK in the cytoplasm (cCK). The intracellular sequestration of energy as CrP and its translocation are shown in outline in Fig. 8.4.

CrP is present in skeletal muscle in limited quantities. It has been calculated that the theoretical time for complete depletion of the compound is approximately 10 seconds. This compares with 2.5 minutes for glycogen being metabolized to lactate and 90 minutes for glycogen been fully oxidized to carbon dioxide and water. For fat (triacylgycerol), the corresponding figure for complete oxidation, for all body areas, is 5000 minutes (Newsholme, 1998).

Skeletal muscle: exercise and training

This section will outline how skeletal muscle deals metabolically with varying intensities and durations of activity. Particular attention will be paid the substrates used and the metabolic controls imposed. In addition, the adaptation of skeletal muscles in response to continued exercise (training) will be described.

Exercise

Exercise increases skeletal muscle glucose utilization (Kjaer et al., 1991). While local glycogenolysis contributes to muscles' need for glucose, two other physiological adaptations occur. These allow greater amounts of glucose to be extracted from the bloodstream. First, muscle blood flow increases linearly with increasing work load (Anderson and Saltin, 1985), by as much as 20-fold. Second, the subsarcolemmal glucose transport capacity of muscle increases (Kristiansen et al., 1997). Upon exercise or exposure of muscle to insulin, the facilitated diffusion carrier GLUT 4, which is normally sequestered in intracellular stores is transported to the T-tubular system of the muscle cell and to the sarcolemma (Watkins et al., 1997). Consequently, two- to fourfold increases in the arteriovenous differences for glucose are observed across skeletal muscle vascular beds. Clearly however, the markedly increased blood flow is proportionately more important in increasing skeletal muscle glucose uptake on exercise. The increased blood flow to the muscle vascular bed reflects increased insulin concentrations (Baron, 1994) and is believed to be mediated by nitric oxide produced by endothelial NOS (eNOS) in the vascular bed (Steinbert et al., 1994). Finally, it is possible to upregulate GLUT 4 activity. Kuo et al. (1999) studied rats following prolonged exercise that depleted muscle glycogen levels by 50%. On recovery, if glucose supplementation was given, marked increases in GLUT 4 protein could be seen within 90 minutes, by which time glycogen stores had been replenished. Furthermore, at 5 hours, GLUT 4 mRNA on polysomes was raised and glycogen continued to be synthesized. These results suggest that, under the correct metabolic conditions, hyper-recovery states for muscle glycogen mediated by increased GLUT 4 activity can occur and that these are influenced by pre- and posttranslational mechanisms.

Other studies have examined the relative contributions of plasma and intramuscular fuel sources at different exercise intensities. Romijn et al. (1993) used stable isotope techniques to study trained subjects exercising at 25, 65 and 80% of maximum oxygen consumption (Vo_2max). Their results are typical and show that the rate of oxidation of blood-borne substrates (glucose and free fatty acids) is relatively constant at all intensities of exercise. However, the proportion made up by blood-borne free fatty acid falls as exercise increases. Additionally, the contribution of intramuscular lipolysis also falls, particularly upon severe exercise, in contrast to the contribution of glycogen, which rises steeply (Fig. 8.5).

By combining isotopic measurements with arteriovenous difference assessments, it was possible to show that

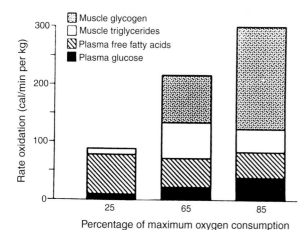

Fig. 8.5. Relative contributions of muscle fuels at different exercise levels. (Taken from Romijn et al., 1993.)

fatty acid oxidation equates to the fatty acid levels available when Vo$_2$max is 65% of maximum (Romijn et al., 1995). If plasma free fatty acid concentrations are then further increased by lipid infusion (plus heparin to stimulate lipase) at the highest rate of exercise, the contribution of fatty acids can be increased even further, although, in total, fatty acids were still responsible for less than 50% of the total oxidation rate, the remainder of oxidized substrate being primarily muscle glycogen. The conclusions drawn from these elegant experiments are that the availability of fatty acid from the adipose tissue can be limiting during exercise and that within skeletal muscle there is an upper limit to fatty acid oxidation, probably occurring at the mitochondrial level. Moreover, these results in humans are consistent with the glucose–fatty acid cycle hypothesis first put forward by Randle and others (Randle et al., 1963) using perfused, contracting heart muscle and resting diaphragm muscle. Coyle and co-workers (1997) undertook studies that further supported this view. They investigated whether increased glycolytic flux secondary to induced hyperglycaemia and hyperinsulinaemia reduced fatty acid oxidation during exercise. Their observations in six endurance-trained cyclists showed that glucose clamped at 6mmol/l caused a 34% reduction in total fat oxidation during exercise, which could all be accounted for by a reduction in plasma free fatty acid and intramuscular triglyceride turnover. They further went on to show, using radiolabelled substrates, that long-chain fatty acid oxidation (C$_{16}$ palmitate) fell in the presence of glycaemia, whereas medium-chain oxidation (C$_8$ octenoate) did not. They surmised therefore, that carbohydrate availability can directly regulate fat oxidation during exercise and that the CPT I probably regulates fatty acid utilization since oxi-

dation of octanoate (a medium-chain (C$_8$) fatty acid which does not need to utilize this system to gain entry to the mitochondria for subsequent catabolism) was unaffected. The metabolites believed to be central to this regulatory process are citrate and malonyl-CoA. These two are intimately related. Increased cytosolic citrate, an allosteric activator of acetyl-CoA carboxylase, leads to an increase in the concentration of malonyl-CoA in muscle perfused with glucose and insulin (Saha, 1997) and reduced fatty acid oxidation. This role for cytosolic citrate provides the metabolic link required for the glucose–fatty acid cycle (Randle et al., 1963). A second mechanism controlling the concentration of malonyl-CoA involves the phosphorylation of acetyl-CoA carboxylase, which is linked to changes in the ratios of ATP:AMP and/or CrP:Cr. Thus falls in ATP:AMP lead to phosphorylation of the enzyme and its inhibition, with subsequent falls in the concentration of intramuscular malonyl-CoA and enhanced fatty acid oxidation (Ruderman et al., 1999). These hypotheses are supported by further observations. Rasmussen and Winder (1997) have shown that quadriceps muscle shows a rise in AMP-dependent kinase activity upon treadmill exercise (see Fig. 8.3) which is mirrored by a fall in muscle acetyl-CoA carboxylase and malonyl-CoA levels and a corresponding increase in free fatty acid oxidation. Furthermore, in animals given a biologically active analogue of AMP (5-aminoimidazole-4-carboxamide), AMP-dependent kinase can be activated. This gives rise to a fall in acetyl-CoA carboxylase activity, a secondary fall in malonyl-CoA and markedly enhanced palmitate oxidation (Merrill et al., 1997). However, not all studies support a pivotal role for malonyl-CoA in the control of fatty acid oxidation during exercise. Odland and his colleagues (1996) measured malonyl-CoA in vastus lateralis muscle at rest and after 10 minutes cycling at 40% Vo$_2$max and 10 and 60 minutes at 65% Vo$_2$max. They observed marked increases in fatty acid oxidation, as assessed by the respiratory exchange ratio, but no changes in muscle malonyl-CoA content at any point compared with the resting state. Furthermore, the same group have gone on to suggest that the malonyl-CoA content of human skeletal muscle is generally unaffected whatever the degree of exercise (Odland et al., 1998).

When considering aerobic/anaerobic carbohydrate utilization in muscle, two enzymes are of prime importance, namely glycogen phosphorylase and PDH. In a study of these two enzymes at varying exercise power outputs (Howlett et al., 1998), it was shown that glycogen phosphorylase in the more active (a) form was not essentially different at any time point at moderate exercise (35 and 65% Vo$_2$max) although there was a small but significant fall in activity (15%) after 10 minutes at 90% Vo$_2$max in the untrained subjects studies. In contrast, the level of PDH in the active form rose successively at all work loads tested and at 90% Vo_2max it was nearly tenfold more active. Importantly, it was also noted that at the lower work loads there was no difference in muscle concentrations of lactate, pyruvate ADP, AMP or P_i; at higher work loads this was not the case. This suggests that increases in free P_i and AMP could stimulate glycogen phosphorylase, while the increase in ADP would augment rises in free Ca^{2+} levels brought about by muscular contraction. This last metabolic effect, acting in concert with the raised pyruvate concentration, would be expected to enhance the conversion of inactive to active PDH since Ca^{2+} is a required cofactor for PDH phosphatase (the enzyme which activates PDH) while pyruvate is a powerful inhibitor of PDH kinase (the enzyme which inhibits PDH) (Denton et al., 1972).

In a further study of the interaction between the pathways of fat and carbohydrate catabolism, Spriet's group (Odland et al., 1998) observed the effects of increased fat availability on muscle glycogen degradation and PDH activity during prolonged but relatively low activity. Infusion of fat, as Intralipid, caused significant increases in arterial free fatty acids, mean net leg fatty acid uptake and muscle citrate levels. It reduced respiratory exchange ratios (suggesting increased fat utilization) and net lactate efflux, although net leg glucose uptake was unaffected. The infusion of Intralipid reduced muscle glycogen degradation by a quarter, and there was a clear shift to fat rather than carbohydrate utilization. The reduction in glycogenolysis was probably accounted for by alterations to the fine metabolic control of glycogen phosphorylase (e.g. free P_i and AMP levels) and reduced flux through phosphofructokinase owing to its inhibition by increased muscle citrate. However, these would not affect carbohydrate flux through PDH. As expected, exercise in both the control and Intralipid study groups resulted in a rise in the amount of active PDH at all levels of exercise, though the levels were markedly lower at all time points in the Intralipid group. This illustrates that control by covalent modification (phosphorylation), for PDH at least, is important when muscle selects its metabolic fuel. The exact mechanism by which this is achieved remains uncertain, though enhanced PDH kinase activity secondary to an increased ratio of NADH:NAD in the presence of Intralipid appears to be the main candidate.

To confuse matters, the situation appears to be different at intense levels of exercise, at least in the nonathlete (Dyck et al., 1996). In these subjects receiving Intrapalid, near maximal exercise for 15 minutes did not result in downregulation of PDH even though a 45% reduction in muscle glycogenolysis was observed. The muscle levels of intermediary metabolites, for example citrate, acetyl-CoA, AMP and P_i were also unchanged. These results suggest that at high exercise intensities glycogen phosphorylase is downregulated if fatty acids are available, though the exact mechanism for this remains an enigma. This area of muscle exercise biochemistry remains a fruitful area for research.

Training

The effect upon skeletal muscle of training can be considered at the tissue and the cellular level of organization. At the tissue level, we all know that training, especially against force, leads to muscular hypertrophy. By comparison, immobilization, for example following a fracture of a long bone, results in atrophy. In muscle, it would appear that it is stretching of the myocytes which is the important mechanical signal for training of the muscle fibres. Moreover, it appears that, unless stretched, all muscle fibres would revert to being type II fast-twitch fibres. In other words, stretch and/or isometric force development enhance slow type I myosin expression and inhibit fast myosin expression (Gregory et al., 1986). How the mechanical signals are translated into cellular events has remained an enigma. However, recently, insights into understanding the process have been made. It is known that skeletal muscle expresses growth factors (for example fibroblast growth factor and insulin-like growth factor 1 (IGF1)) and that this expression is upregulated by exercise (Goldspink et al., 1995; Clarke and Feeback, 1996). Furthermore, it has now been shown that human muscle produces two isoforms of IGF (Yang et al., 1996; McKoy et al., 1999). One is termed muscle IGF1 (muscle L.IGF1) and is similar in structure to hepatic IGF1. It is also thought to have a systemic endocrine function like hepatic IGF1. However, the second isoform has been termed mechanogrowth factor or MGF. MGF is formed as a result of alternative splicing and has an altered 3′ exon sequence from that in liver IGF1. This isoform importantly is considered to have autocrine/paracrine functions (Goldspink, 1999). Its structure suits such a role since unlike hepatic IGF1 it is not glycosylated and is, therefore, likely to have only a very short half-life. Of particular interest is the observation that mRNA for MGF appears to be absent from the dystrophic muscles of *mdx* mice. It has, therefore, been postulated that muscle mass becomes increasingly dependent upon MGF as hepatic production of IGF1 falls with age and falling growth hormone levels (Rudman et al., 1981). In dystrophic muscle, the dystrophic process will be accelerated once an individual is past the pubertal growth spurt. This is a fascinating example of organ interplay in an area once considered to be a muscle-specific condition.

At the cellular level, it is agreed that training causes a shift from carbohydrate to fat in the preferred fuel selection for muscle during exercise. This corresponds with the propensity of MGF to upregulate those factors concerned in adapting fast-twitch to slow-twitch fibres and parallels the series of metabolic alterations that allow muscle to utilize fat in preference to carbohydrate. Nor need exercise be vigorous or prolonged before significant metabolic changes are seen. Chesley et al. (1996) subjected eight unfit men to a regimen consisting of cycling at 65% Vo_2max for just 2 hours per day. Thereafter, they were able to demonstrate a 42% reduction in muscle glycogenolysis during a 15 minute exercise challenge. In addition, they could demonstrate that, although the activity of the active phosphorylase was unchanged, there were marked reductions in the necessary allosteric activator AMP and substrate (P_i) for the enzyme. They concluded that post-transformational control of phosphorylase was responsible for the reduced glycogenolysis observed in their subjects. Furthermore, they observed a 20% increase in the citrate synthase activity of muscle biopsy samples taken from subjects. Citrate synthase is strictly a mitochondrial matrix enzyme and, therefore, may be taken as surrogate evidence for enhanced mitochondrial oxidative potential in the muscle. These results are consistent with previous studies (Hudlicka, 1990) where increases of other mitochondrial enzymes have been noted. In addition, moderate intensity training also leads to an increase in the muscle stores of lipid and glycogen and to what on first inspection appears to be a paradoxical decrease in myofibrillar content but in reality is only a relative decrease owing to the space taken up by the macromolecules (Hoppelar, 1986). Decreased activity results in a reversal of those biochemical and fibre changes described following exercise. Early studies used denervation atrophy as a model (Hudlicka, 1990) but, more recently, immobilization of skeletal muscle either by plaster casts or by pinning in a shortened position has been used. Upon immobilization, extensive atrophy occurs, with the type I fibres being particularly affected, as would be predicted by the loss of contraction-induced MGF available to the muscle (Goldspink, 1999) for autocrine functions. Changes in human muscle may be seen as early as one week after immobilization of vastus lateralis as a consequence of a long cast for a closed tibial fracture (Blakemore et al., 1996). At this time, the cross-sectional area of type I but not type II fibres, as well as the protein:DNA ratio, had started to fall. Large falls were also seen in cytochrome oxidase activity and GLUT 4 protein content of the immobilized muscle. Interestingly, there

were no changes in GLUT 5, the hexose translocator located exclusively in the sarcolemmal membrane. The authors suggest, therefore, that the expression of some nonmyofibrillar proteins is differentially regulated in response to muscle disease (Hundal et al., 1998).

The changes in fibre types, substrate and mitochondrial content are paralleled by changes in capillary and larger blood vessel supply to the muscle (reviewed by Hudlicka, 1985). Clearly one of the major roles of the enhanced vascular supply is to bring nutrients to and remove waste products from muscle during exercise. It is, therefore, perhaps surprising that although training causes a rise in the total amount GLUT 4 protein in muscle (Kristiansen et al., 1996; Richter et al., 1998), there is a training-induced decrease in carbohydrate utilization at submaximal power outputs. In addition to the lowered glycogenolysis described earlier, decreased muscle glucose uptake has been observed (Phillips et al., 1996) with a concomitant increase in uptake and oxidation of free fatty acids in trained compared with untrained humans (Hurley et al., 1986; Turcotte et al., 1992). These observations appear to be true both when made at the same absolute power output or when given as relative exercise intensity to correct for the higher absolute power outputs trained subjects can achieve. The exact mechanism for the reduced glucose uptake remains a matter of debate. Richter et al. (1998) studied subjects who had undergone intense endurance training of one thigh for three weeks and then undertook simultaneous two-legged dynamic knee extensions. Their data clearly showed that in the trained muscle there was a blunted exercise-induced movement of GLUT 4 translocator to the sarcolemma from the intracellular stores, despite the higher total GLUT 4 levels in the trained muscle (Richter et al., 1998). The reasons for the reduced movement of GLUT 4 in trained muscle may reflect the greater presence of fuel storage macromolecules, glycogen and lipid, since it is known that in trained muscle the glucose uptake rate is greater if the muscle has first been depleted of glycogen (Gollnick et al., 1981; Hespel and Richter, 1990). The simplest view would be that glycogen and/or fat simply physically impede the movement of GLUT 4 and its incorporation into the sarcolemma.

As we have noted, the effect of training is to increase muscle free fatty acid uptake at the expense of glucose uptake (Turcotte et al., 1992). We have also discussed that fatty acid uptake into muscle cells is a saturable facilitated diffusion process involving at least three binding proteins working in concert: $FABP_{pm}$, FATP and FAT (Bonen et al., 1998a). At lease one element of this system, $FABP_{pm}$, is rate limiting for fatty acid uptake into muscle but it is also of interest to note that the expression of $FABP_{pm}$ is greater in type I, slow-twitch oxidative fibres than in type II fibres. In parallel with upregulation of the transport system for free fatty acids, there is also evidence to suggest that training affects two other steps directly involved with fatty acid utilization. First, breakdown of triacylglycerol (lipolysis) at the sarcolemma by hormone-sensitive lipase is enhanced by training (Klein et al., 1994); as a result, more free fatty acid is made available to the transport system. This occurs despite the fact that only adipocyte hormone-sensitive lipase and not the muscle enzyme is increased by training. This might suggest that the muscle enzyme becomes more sensitive upon training to sympathetic stimulation acting via cAMP-dependent protein kinase. However, this sensitivity is enhanced for adipose tissue but not for muscle, at least in the rat. Clearly it is of importance to ascertain what the effect of contraction and free Ca^{2+} levels are on the hormone-sensitive lipase (Langfort et al., 1999). It must also be remembered that the rate of transportation of free fatty acids as the carnitine esters into the mitochondrial matrix, the site of fatty acid β-oxidation, is greater in trained than in untrained subjects (Sidossis et al., 1998).

Nitric oxide

In recent years, nitric oxide has been implicated in a rapidly expanding range of biological processes. Skeletal muscle biochemistry is no exception to the trend. Nitric oxide is now known to have two types of effect upon skeletal muscle (reviewed by Maréchal and Gailly, 1999). The first group, mediated by nitrosation of proteins, may give rise to impaired contractility and irreversible effects upon intermediary metabolism, especially mitochondrial function. The second type of effect reflects the novel cell signalling role of nitric oxide and is mediated by a cGMP-dependent pathway.

Balon and Nadler (1994) first showed that nitric oxide was released from incubated rat skeletal muscle preparations. Histochemical studies in animals showed all three major isoforms of NOS – neural (nNOS) inducible (iNOS) and endothelial (eNOS) – to be present in muscle (Lui et al., 1993; Kobzik et al., 1994). However, the expression of NOS in human tissue appears to be different from that seen in animals. Normally, human skeletal muscle expresses nNOS and eNOS: nNOS appears to be localized in all fibre types at the sarcolemma, associated as a signalling component of the dystrophin–α_1-syntrophin complex (Frandsen et al., 1996; Grozdanovic and Baumgerten, 1999) and eNOS is primarily found in the endothelium of the large vessels and the microvasculature. An early report that NOS is associated with mitochondria (Kobzik et al., 1995) has yet to be confirmed in humans. There is also an alternatively spliced isoform in muscle (nNOS-μ). This isoform has a 102 bp insert between exons 16 and 17 that codes for a 34 amino acid residue insert between the calmodulin- and FMN-binding sites. The significance of this isoform is uncertain (Silvagno et al., 1996). The inducible form of NOS is not normally seen in human muscle, though it may be expressed in patients with chronic heart failure (Riede et al., 1998; Hambrecht et al., 1999) and, presumably, those with infections (El Dwairi et al., 1998).

The role of nitric oxide in the contractile process depends on whether it acts directly or via a cGMP-mediated pathway. Direct effects upon isometric contraction and maximal velocity of shortening are complex. Its effects via the cGMP pathway improve the mechanical and metabolic efficiency of the muscle cell such that there appears to be a 'slow to fast' shift. Maréchal and Gailly (1999) have an excellent review of the situation.

Exercise-stimulated glucose transport in skeletal muscle is nitric oxide dependent as shown in rats (Roberts et al., 1997) and, in other animals (Etgen et al., 1997); definitive studies in humans are awaited. Balon and Nadler (1997) have presented further evidence that in situ stimulation induces increases in glucoses uptake in skeletal muscle of the rat hind limb that are inhibited by N-methyl methylarginine (NMMA), a potent inhibitor of NOS. These studies further support a role of nitric oxide in controlling increases in the activity of exercise-induced glucose transport.

There is also evidence to suggest that not only glucose but also pyruvate, palmitate and leucine oxidation can be increased by nitric oxide (Young and Leighton, 1998). Using the cGMP analogue 8-bromo-cGMP to mimic downstream effects of nitric oxide, it is possible to show that similar enhancements of glucose oxidation can be achieved as found with the nitric oxide donor sodium nitroprusside. Furthermore, removal of extracellular Ca^{2+} did not affect glucose oxidation stimulated by sodium nitroprusside, thereby eliminating increased intracellular Ca^{2+} as a mechanism for the changes. It was also noted that the guanylate cyclase inhibitor LY-83583 inhibited nitric oxide stimulated palmitate oxidation and activation of cGMP-dependent protein kinase. These results suggest that activation of the latter may override any direct inhibitory effects of nitric oxide, such as those on respiration (Cleeter et al., 1994), to stimulate substrate oxidation in skeletal muscle. This remains to be tested but is an interesting hypothesis.

Muscle and amino acid metabolism

In an average 70 kg human, skeletal muscle contains some 60% of the total body pool of 12 kg protein, and a similar percentage of the body's free amino acid pool (Wagenmakers, 1998). Early studies suggest that muscle protein degradation and biosynthesis were affected by a range of physiological conditions (Wolfe et al., 1982). However, it is now recognized that those early studies had methodological problems and, in fact, muscle proteins turn over only very slowly. In the main, this turnover appears to be unaffected by moderate exercise or diurnal rhythm. Accordingly, this area of muscle biochemistry will not be discussed further here; it is reviewed by Wagenmakers (1998). This section will deal primarily with the role of amino acids in facilitating energy metabolism in muscle and the interrelation of muscle to other tissues.

Of all the amino acids, only six are metabolized by muscle. They are the branched chain amino acids leucine, isoleucine and valine, plus aspartate, glutamate and asparagine. All play a fundamental role in energy metabolism in muscle.

Exercise

Only leucine and part of the isoleucine molecule can be oxidized to carbon dioxide and water by human muscle (Elia et al., 1989). The nitrogen atoms of leucine and isoleucine are lost from the muscle in the form of alanine and/or glutamine. To facilitate glutamine synthesis, glutamate (one nitrogen atom per molecule) is continuously taken up from the circulation and converted into glutamine, with two nitrogen atoms per molecule (Nurjham et al., 1995). Alanine, by contrast, appears to be synthesized from pyruvate in muscle. The pyruvate may be derived from glucose taken up from the bloodstream or produced by glycogen degradation (Chang and Goldberg, 1978), with each source probably contributing in equal proportions (Nurjham et al., 1995).

As leucine and isoleucine may be oxidized to provide energy, their role in muscle metabolism is clear. But what of the other four amino acids: valine, aspartate, asparagine and glutamate? To understand their role one must return to the fundamental role of muscle, namely producing mechanical work for exercise. Within minutes of starting moderate exercise, profound changes in the free pool concentrations of glutamate and alanine are observed. After 10 minutes, glutamate concentrations may fall by as much as 70%, while alanine levels rise by nearly as much (van Hall et al., 1995). At the same time, the total concentration of

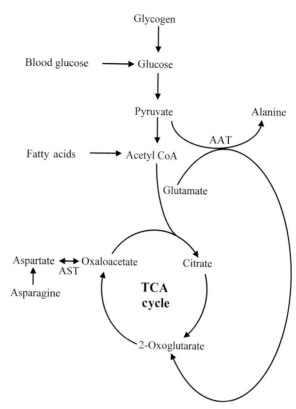

Fig. 8.6. Anaplerotic reactions and the tricarboxylic acid (TCA) cycle. AAT, alanine aminotransferase; AST, aspartate aminotransferase.

TCA cycle metabolites rises fourfold (Gibala et al., 1998). Taken together, these observations suggest that muscle utilizing flux through the alanine and other aminotransferase reactions (Fig. 8.6) is supplementing the TCA cycle with intermediates, primarily 2-oxoglutarate and oxaloacetate, to facilitate the oxidation of acetyl-CoA derived from pyruvate (glucose/glycogen) or fatty acids. Consistent with this view is the observation that, in addition to the release of alanine into the circulation during exercise, there is also increased uptake of glutamate from the bloodstream. This ensures that the muscle free pool of glutamate is not rapidly depleted and the potential for exercise reduced by substrate limitation. Moreover, following exercise, enhanced rates of glutamate uptake persist, presumably to replenish intramuscular pools (van Hall et al., 1995).

Anaplerosis in muscle

The metabolic pathways utilized to replenish metabolic pools, such as those of the TCA cycle, are termed anaplerotic. In brain, liver and adipose tissue, one of the most active pathways is that afforded by pyruvate carboxylase, an enzyme that carboxylates pyruvate to oxaloacetate. This enzyme is not present in muscle. As a result, alanine aminotransferase is of fundamental importance for muscle anaplerosis (Gibala et al., 1997). This is highlighted in two conditions where flux through the enzyme is severely curtailed. The first example is that of severe glycogen depletion, which is seen after prolonged exercise, for example marathon running. In this situation, no glycogen is available to supply pyruvate. Flux is reduced, restricting the production of TCA cycle intermediates including 2-oxoglutarate (Graham et al., 1995). The second example mimics the first. It is McArdle's disease, muscle glycogen phosphorylase deficiency. In this condition, patients are unable to produce pyruvate despite the presence of endogenous glycogen. Consequently, if pyruvate requirements exceed the capability of the bloodstream to supply glucose and hence pyruvate, the anaplerotic pathway via alanine aminotransferase is once again limited. These patients show no, or only minimal, changes in alanine and glutamate concentrations in blood or muscle, respectively, on exercise (Sahlin et al., 1995). In these situations, other less efficient anaplerotic pathways are thought to be used. These primarily utilize deamination reactions coupled with glutamine synthesis as a means of providing the TCA cycle intermediates 2-oxoglutarate and oxaloacetate:

Aspartate + Isoleucine → Oxaloacetate + Glutamine
2 Glutamate → Glutamine + 2-Oxoglutarate.

Unfortunately, the capacity of these is very limited and they cannot substitute entirely for a deficient alanine aminotransferase pathway. While it is clear that increased levels of TCA intermediates are required for exercise to occur, it should be noted that large increases in concentrations are not required. Gibala et al. (1998) showed quite clearly that 'a tremendous' (*sic*) (100-fold) increase in TCA flux is observable in skeletal muscle despite a modest (threefold) increase in TCA cycle intermediates. Thus the concentration of TCA cycle intermediates appears to exert a significant controlling influence upon energy metabolism in skeletal muscle.

Understanding the biochemical pathways for anaplerosis in muscle allows an understanding as to why branch-chain amino acid supplements do not enhance exercise capacity in patients with McArdle's disease. Clearly, if large quantities are administered they will tend to deplete the TCA cycle of 2-oxoglutarate and oxaloacetate via the respective branch-chain amino transferases, which are 'near equilibrium', enzymes. One would predict, therefore, that peak exercise capacity should be reduced. This is found to be the case (MacLean et al., 1998).

Glutamine

Glutamine is formed as an integral part of anaplerosis, namely nitrogen removal, which allows muscle to respond to the metabolic demands placed upon it by exercise. But glutamine is increasingly recognized as more than a molecule that facilitates the removal, to the liver, of nitrogen. It appears to be involved in the regulation of a range of physiological processes, which tempts one to think of the metabolite as a modulator of myocyte biochemical function.

Skeletal muscle has a range of amino acid transporters, the most active of which appears to be the N^m glutamine transporter (Rennie et al., 1998). This transporter is sensitive to sodium, pH, corticosteroids and insulin and it appears to play a crucial role in glutamine's physiological roles. Intramyocyte levels of glutamine are controlled by this transporter and by glutamine synthetase, the enzyme responsible for glutamine synthesis from glutamate. Glutamine synthetase is also responsive to corticosteroids and its activity rises in response to physiological stress (Labow et al., 1999). Moreover, glutamine affects the post-transcriptional processing of the enzyme by causing feedback destabilization of the protein. Thus, the combination of changes of transporter function and alterations in glutamine synthase activity regulates muscle cell glutamine levels and assures that the cell is highly responsive to physiological stress. During various catabolic states, such as trauma, surgery or prolonged and high intensity training, glutamine homeostasis is challenged and concentrations, especially in muscle, may not be maintained (Rowbottom et al., 1996).

Within the myocyte, glutamine is believed to influence several systems. Of particular importance are observations that it may modulate glycogen synthesis (Low et al., 1996) and alter the balance of protein metabolism by inhibiting catabolism and stimulating anabolism (MacLennon et al., 1988). The exact mechanism by which these changes may occur is unknown. However, it is believed that similarities may exist between myocytes and hepatocytes and in the latter it has been quite clearly shown that changes in cell volume are coupled to intracellular events (Haussinger, 1996). Swelling of myocytes in response to hypo-osmolality activates the N^m carrier. It has been proposed, therefore, that the myocyte N^m system acts as a component of a 'positive-feedback' mechanism amplifying anabolic effects (Rennie et al., 1996). One way in which this may be achieved involves the transmembrane integrin proteins. The integrins act as a mechanocoupling system (Ingber, 1997). Low and Taylor (1998) have shown that for the glutamine transporter there appears to be a requirement for an active phosphatidylinositol kinase possibly to maintain the integrins in an 'active' conformation thereby allowing muscle cells to modulate amino acid transport in the appropriate time frame (Low et al., 1997b). It should also be noted that this kinase is an enzyme common to a number of intracellular signalling pathways (Ingber, 1997), and as such could be expected to influence other aspects of carbohydrate and protein metabolism.

Muscle, glutamine and oxidative stress

Skeletal muscle is one of the body's major sites of glutamine synthesis. Glutamine may be considered as one of the precursors of glutathione, a molecule which is in the forefront of the human body's defence mechanisms against oxidative stress (Amores-Sanchez and Medina, 1999). Skeletal muscle is a tissue that may, upon exercise, be called upon to use large quantities of oxygen and, therefore, it is at risk of damage from reactive oxygen species. Upon training, athletes appear to upregulate their skeletal muscle glutathione redox cycle enzymes, but, interestingly, not their superoxide dismutase activity (Hellsten et al., 1996), to protect against this risk. It appears that mitochondrial DNA is particularly at risk (Sakai et al., 1999) as are older subjects (Liang et al., 1997). In the critically ill patient, there is a significant fall in the total free amino acid content to one-half of normal in the first few days; glutamine is even more severely affected, falling to 25% of its normal level (Gamrin et al., 1997). In contrast, the branched-chain amino acids are increased, suggesting that glutamate availability limits their contribution to anaplerosis (see earlier). These observations confirm a similar study (Hammarqvist et al., 1997) in which glutathione was measured in both muscle and blood of critically ill patients. In this study, glutathione was found to be significantly lower in the patients' muscle and furthermore to be mainly in the biologically inactive oxidized form. Similar findings were also found in patients undergoing surgical trauma (Luo et al., 1996). Of particular interest in this last study was the observation that the loss of glutathione was more marked in muscle than in plasma, and that the large changes observed (40% loss) occurred early, within 24 hours of surgery.

The consequences of the alterations in glutathione status are not yet fully understood. By analogy with the brain, another 'electrical tissue', one would predict that activity of complex I of the mitochondrial electron transport chain would be lost in the presence of oxidative stress (Bolaños et al., 1995; Stewart et al., 1998). This would be expected to impair the muscles' ability to produce ATP for contractile activity. Furthermore, by analogy with Parkinson's disease, a condition in which both complex I activity and cellular glutathione are low, one might expect

muscle to degenerate rapidly unless a therapeutic intervention such as refeeding occurred early. The degenerations would occur as a result of complex I impairment itself, giving rise to even greater oxidative stress (Heales et al., 1998). Data from patients in intensive care support this view (J. M. Land, S. J. R. Heales, I, Hargreaves and M. Singer, unpublished data).

If glutathione and glutamine are so fundamental to the well-being of critically ill patients, then supplementation ought perhaps to be beneficial. One such study of 84 patients with multiorgan failure has given rise to promising results, with a 71% improved six-month survival observed in the group supplemented with glutamine. Clearly this needs further investigation, but improved understanding of muscle biochemistry, glutamine and glutathione offers the prospect of simple therapeutic interventions for critically ill patients. Finally, a novel observation (Zable et al., 1997) is that reduced glutathione inhibited Ca^{2+}-stimulated ryanodine binding to the sarcoplasmic reticulum and the single channel gating activity of the reconstituted Ca^{2+}-release channel in a dose-dependent manner. In contrast, the oxidized form of glutathione is a potent agent in reversing these changes. Consequently, both absolute amounts and the redox status of glutathione may have significant effects upon the gating of the Ca^{2+}-release channel.

Muscle, glutamine, and other tissues

Quantitatively, muscle is the most important tissue for the synthesis and release of glutamine. The release of glutamine is highly controlled by a system including a carrier that is sensitive to Na^+, pH and hormones. A consequence of this tight control was that glutamine was originally thought of as a nonessential amino acid. It is now probably more accurate to term glutamine a 'conditionally essential' amino acid (Lacey and Wilmore, 1990). This view reflects the fact that muscle is not always able to maintain blood and body levels of glutamine, for example after severe exercise or trauma, and, as a result, function of organ tissues may be compromised. Table 8.1 lists those tissues that are dependent on glutamine and some of the processes supported by it.

It is not the brief of this chapter to discuss tissues other than muscle but some specific comments seem justified if only to reinforce the belief that muscle tissue and its biochemical activity are intimately related to activities in other distant tissues.

One aspect of the biochemistry of the gut that has remained an enigma for many years is 'why is there a partial urea cycle in enterocytes?' The answer to this may be that glutamine is an unconventional energetic

Table 8.1. Glutamine and some tissue activities

Tissue	Activity
Gut	Mucosal integrity, barrier function, acid–base function
Kidney	Acid–base balance, gluconeogenesis
Liver	Gluconeogenesis
Immune system	Purine/pyrimidine synthesis, antisepsis

substrate, supplying both carbon skeleton for oxidation and nitrogen to complex hydrogen as an ammonium ion. Any excess nitrogen may then be removed and detoxified by the urea cycle in the gut. The same situation is true of the kidney with respect to nitrogen, though here the carbon skeleton is primarily used for gluconeogenic purposes, supplying 20–25% of whole-body glucose production, albeit for local renal utilization (Stumvoll et al., 1999). It has long been known that lactate and alanine return to the liver, providing substrate for gluconeogenesis (Felig et al., 1970). Recent work in humans suggests that glutamine from muscle is also a major gluconeogenic precursor and is used to facilitate carbon skeleton transfer between muscle and the liver (Nurjham et al., 1995). Finally, it was originally believed that lymphocytes and macrophages of the immune system utilized glucose as their primary energy source. However, the observation that both these cell types have large glutaminase activities prompted studies which showed that glutamine may be as significant at providing energy as glucose (Ardawi and Newsholme, 1983). In addition, of course, glutamine provides nitrogen for purine and pyrimidine nucleotides for nucleic acid synthesis.

The plasma pool of glutamine is relatively large (600–800 μmol/l) but the pool concentration falls quickly to less than half normal values in response to both physiological and pathological stress. At this level of glutamine, the functional response of human and rat lymphocytes to mitogenic stimulation is markedly impaired (Parry-Billings et al., 1990). Findings such as these prompted studies with athletes which showed that those who suffered the 'overtraining syndrome' had low plasma glutamine and compromised immune function (Walsh et al., 1998). Moreover, athletes who have taken supplements of glutamine have been found to have lower reported incidences of infections following marathon runs (Castell et al., 1996), as well as less evidence of muscle tissue damage, which in itself would be expected to compromise their immune function for several days after racing. This has prompted some to speculate that glutamine is a potentially useful supplement for athletes, particularly those engaged in heavy exercise training and punishing racing schedules (Antonio and Street, 1999).

Skeletal muscle and chronic heart failure

In chronic heart failure (CHF), poor ventricular function gives rise to low cardiac output and, at the level of skeletal muscle, a relatively anaerobic situation with hypoxaemia and lactic acidaemia. However, in addition, intrinsic abnormalities of skeletal muscle are also observed that frequently limit exercise tolerance in patients with CHF (Adams et al., 1999). In a study of 43 patients (Schaufelberger et al., 1997), it was noted that all patients had higher lactate and lactate dehydrogenase levels and the expression of oxidative enzymes was decreased. Furthermore, the percentage of type I fibres and capillarization were decreased while the percentage of type IIB fibres was increased.

Advanced stages of CHF are known to be associated with the systemic activation of cytokines, some of which have been shown to be capable of inducing NOS. Using electron microscopy immunocytochemistry with specific anti-NOS antibodies, it has been possible to show that iNOS is expressed in myocyte cytoplasm from both normal individuals and those with CHF but is more marked in cells from the latter (Riede et al., 1998). These findings have been confirmed and extended (Hambrecht et al., 1999). These latter authors noted that mtCK was decreased in biopsies from patients and that there existed an inverse relationship between iNOS and mtCK levels. As nitrosylation of proteins was raised, the low mt-CK levels could reflect this or, more probably, reduced cellular glutathione levels, a molecule known to be required for CK activity (Gunst et al., 1998). Consequently, the changes in fibre type distribution, oxidative enzyme systems and mtCK, which would have a negative effect on the bioenergetic systems of skeletal muscle, plus the increased potential to produce nitric oxide, which could attenuate the contractile process (Maréchal and Gailly 1999), could result in the exercise intolerance seen in CHF (Adams et al., 1997).

Confirmation that oxidative bioenergetic systems are impaired in patients with CHF comes from an elegant nuclear magentic resonance study of 22 patients (van der Ent et al., 1998). The forearm flexor compartment was studied during three mild intermittent exercise episodes between 0 and 40% of maximum voluntary contraction. By avoiding local acidosis (tissue pH <6.9), type IIB fibre activation was avoided. At rest, there was higher P_i and lower CrP in the muscles of patients with CHF than in normal individuals. The phosphate potential and workload relationship could be extrapolated to show that the patients on exercise would exhaust their intracellular energy at much lower exercise levels than in the controls. Furthermore, maximum absolute workloads were lower in patients, and the recovery time to pre-test levels of CrP following a period of exercise was longer.

Apoptosis has been observed in diagnostic cardiac biopsy samples from patients with CHF, suggesting that cell death may account in part for the reduced cardiac output. Recently, similar observations have been made in skeletal muscle biopsies from patients with CHF (Adams et al., 1999). In a series of 34 patients with moderate CHF, apoptosis was detected in 47% of patients with CHF compared with none in controls (using terminal deoxynucleotidyl transferase-mediated deoxyuridine triphosphate nick-end labelling technique: the TUNEL technique). Furthermore, those patients with evidence of apoptosis showed increased iNOS expression, and a reduced level of the caspase inhibitor Bcl-2, supporting the hypothesis that intrinsic skeletal muscle dysfunction may well be a part of the pathology of CHF.

Despite the increased biochemical understanding of the peripheral events in CHF, diuretics, digoxin and angiotensin-converting enzyme inhibitors remain the mainstay of treatment. Undoubtedly peripheral muscle training has a valuable part to play (Cider et al., 1997; Maiorana et al., 2000) and dietary creatine supplementation may offer minor benefit (Andrews et al., 1998). The use of alternative substrates such as propionyl-L-carnitine is still debated (Ferrari and di Giuli, 1997). Recognition that skeletal muscle apoptosis is part of the pathology of CHF may suggest new therapeutic stratagems.

Skeletal muscle and space travel

It is well recognized that space travel rapidly causes marked muscle wasting, which reduces the travellers' capabilities (Vandenburgh et al., 1999); recovery after return to earth may be slow (Miyamoto et al., 1998). Evidence from animal models suggests that slow-twitch, type I fibres are most sensitive to atrophy, which is also accompanied by transformation of muscle from a slow to a fast myosin heavy chain (MHC) phenotype (Staron et al., 1998), including the expression of two fast MHC isoforms not found in control animals, namely MHCIId and MHCIIb. In addition to the altered MHC expression, atrophy of muscles appears to occur secondarily to an early decrease in protein synthetic rates, with no change in degradation rates. However, on longer flights, degradation

rates do appear to increase and are implicated in atrophy (Booth and Criswell, 1997). Return to a gravitational field reverses the changes observed. Of course, this may not always occur in future longer flights. Consequently, a number of countermeasures against atrophy have been tested to allow prolonged space flight. In animal models, resistance exercise plus growth hormone and IGF1 is effective. Whether in humans the provision of a gravitational field is essential for normal expression of skeletal protein mass and slow phenotype is not known. Given the recent observation of specific muscle splice variants of IGF1 (Goldspink, 1999), it may be possible to design therapies using recombinant MGF to prevent skeletal muscle atrophy, thereby allowing humans to journey and work beyond their current habitat. An intriguing thought as we start this new millennium.

Conclusion

I trust that this chapter has convinced you that the intermediary biochemistry of skeletal muscle is intriguing. The fundamentals of metabolic control were elucidated in the late 1960s, but we still do not fully understand how they apply to carbohydrate and fatty acid oxidation in muscle. Similarly, amino acid metabolism in muscle remains a productive area of research. The emerging role of glutamine in controlling and influencing many aspects of muscle metabolism, as well as its fundamental role as a preferred substrate for a range of other tissues (kidney, gut, and leukocytes), serves to remind us that dysfunction of muscle may have a knock-on effect in unexpected places. The reverse is also true, as we have noted in CHF, where intrinsic alterations to muscle metabolism may be observed. Finally the resurgence of interest in space travel issues a challenge particularly to those exploring the factors that control muscle growth and function.

References

Adams, C., Yu, J., Mobius-Winkler, S. et al. (1997). Increased inducible nitric oxide synthase in skeletal muscle biopsies from patients with chronic heart failure. *Biochem. Mol. Med.* **61**, 152–160.

Adams, V., Jiang, I. T., Yu, J. et al. (1999). Apoptosis in skeletal myocytes of patients with chronic heart failure associated with exercise tolerance. *J. Am. Coll. Cardiol.* **33**, 959–965.

Amores-Sanchez, M. I. and Medina, M. A. (1999). Glutamine, as a precursor of glutathione, and oxidative stress. *Mol. Genet. Metab.* **67**, 100–105.

Anderson, P. and Saltin, B. (1985). Maximal perfusion of skeletal muscle in man. *J. Physiol.* **366**, 233–249.

Andrews, A., Greenhaff, P., Curtis, S., Perry, A. and Cowley, A. J. (1998). The effect of dietary creatine supplementation on skeletal muscle metabolism in congestive heart failure. *Eur. Heart J.* **19**, 617–622.

Antonio, J. and Street, C. (1999). Glutamine: a potentially useful supplement for athletes. *Can. J. Appl. Physiol.* **24**, 1–14.

Ardawi, M. S. M. and Newsholme, E. A. (1983). Glutamine metabolism in lymphocytes of the rat. *Biochem. J.* **212**, 835–842.

Balon T. W. and Nadler J. L. (1994) Nitric oxide release is present from incubated skeletal muscle preparations. *J. Appl. Physiol* **77**: 2519–2521.

Balon, T. W. and Nadler, J. L. (1997). Evidence that nitric oxide increases glucose transport in skeletal muscle. *J. Appl. Physiol.* **82**, 359–363.

Baron, A. D. (1994). Haemodynamic actions of insulin. *Am. J. Physiol.* **267**, E187–E202.

Blakemore, S. J., Rickhuss, P. K., Watt, P. W., Rennie, M. J. and Hundal, H. S. (1996). Effects of limb immobilisation on cytochrome *c* oxidase activity and GLUT 4 and GLUT 5 protein expression in human skeletal muscle. *Clin. Sci.* **91**, 591–599.

Bolaños, J. P., Heales, S. J. R., Land, J. M. and Clark, J. B. (1995). Effect of peroxynitrite on the mitochondrial respiratory chain: differential susceptibility of neurones and astrocytes in primary culture. *J. Neurochem.* **64**, 1965–1972.

Bonen, A., Dyck, D. J. and Luiken, J. J. F. P. (1998a). Skeletal muscle fatty acid transport and transporters. In: *Skeletal Muscle Metabolism in Exercise and Diabetes*, eds. E. A. Richter, B. Kiens, H. Galbo and B. Saltin. pp. 193–206. New York: Plenum.

Bonen, A., Luiken, J. J., Liu, S. et al. (1998b). Palmitate transport and fatty acid transporters in red and white muscle. *Am. J. Physiol.* **275**, E471–E478.

Booth, F. W. and Criswell, D. S. (1997). Molecular events underlying skeletal muscle atrophy and the development of effective countermeasures. *Int. J. Sports Med.* **18**, S265–S269.

Boyer, P. D. (1997). The ATP synthase – a splendid molecular machine. *Ann. Rev. Biochem.* **66**, 717–749.

Brooke, M. H. and Kaiser, K. K. (1970). Muscle fibre types: how many and what kind? *Arch. Neurol.* **23**, 369–379.

Castell, L. M., Poortmans, J. R., Leclerq, R., Brasseur, M., Duchateau, J. and Newsholme, E. A. (1996). Some aspects of the acute phase response after a marathon race, and the effects of glutamine supplementation. *Eur. J. Appl. Physiol.* **75**, 47–53.

Chang, T. W. and Goldberg, A. L. (1978). The origin of alanine produced in skeletal muscle. *J. Biol. Chem.* **253**, 3677–3684.

Chesley, A., Heigenhauser, G. J. and Spriet, L. L. (1996). Regulation of muscle glycogen phosphorylase activity following short-term endurance training. *Am. J. Physiol.* **270**, E328–E335.

Cider, A., Tygesson, H., Hedberg, M., Seligman, L. Wennerblom, B. and Sunnerhagen, K. S. (1997). Peripheral muscle training in patients with clinical signs of heart failure. *Scand. J. Rehab. Med.* **29**, 121–127.

Clarke, M. S. and Feeback, D. L. (1996). Mechanical load induces sarcoplasmic wounding and FGF release in differentiated human skeletal muscle cultures. *FASEB J.* **10**, 502–509.

Cleeter, M. W., Cooper, J. M., Darley-Usmar, V. M., Concader, S. and Schapira, A. V. .H. (1994). Reversible inhibition of cytochrome *c* oxidase, the terminal enzyme of the mitochondrial respiratory chain by nitric oxide: implications for neurodegenerative diseases. *FEBS Letts.* **345**, 527–535.

Costill, D. K., Coyle, E. F., Dalsky, W., Evans, E., Fink, W. and Hoops, D. (1997). Effects of elevated plasma FFA and insulin on muscle glycogen usage during exercise. *J. Appl. Physiol.* **43**, 695–699.

Coyle, E. F., Jeukendrup, A. T., Wagenmakers, A. J. M. and Saris, W. H. (1997). Fatty acid oxidation is directly regulated by carbohydrate metabolism during exercise. *Am. J. Physiol.* **273**, E268–E275.

Denton, R. M., Randle, P. J. and Martin, B. R. (1972). Stimulation by calcium ions of pyruvate dehydrogenase phosphatase. *Biochem. J.* **128**, 161–163.

Dudek R. W., Dohm, G. L., Holman, G. D., Cushman, S. W. and Wilson, C. M. (1994). Glucose transporter localisation in rat skeletal muscle: autoradiographic study using ATB-(2–³H) BMPA photolabel. *FEBS Letts.* **339**, 205–208.

Dyck, D. J., Peters, S. A., Wendling. P. S., Chesley, A. and Hultman Spriet, L. L. (1996). Regulation of muscle glycogen phosphorylase activity during intense aerobic cycling with elevated FFA. *Am. J. Physiol.* **265**, E116–E125.

El Dwairi, Q., Comtois, A., Guo, Y. and Hussain, S. N. (1998). Endotoxin-induced skeletal muscle contractile dysfunction: contribution of nitric oxide syntheses. *Am. J. Physiol.* **274**, C770–C779.

Elia, M., Schlatmann, A., Goren, A. and Austin, S. (1989). Amino acid metabolism in muscle and in the whole body of man before and after ingestion of a single mixed meal. *Am. J. Clin. Nutr.* **49**, 1203–1210.

Etgen, G. J., Fryburg, D. A. and Gibbs, E. M. (1997). Nitric oxide stimulates skeletal muscle glucose transport through a calcium/contraction and phosphatidylinositol-3-kinase independent pathway. *Diabetes* **46**, 1915–1919.

Felig, P., Pozefsky, T., Marliss, E. and Cahill, G. F. (1970). Alanine: a key role in glyconeogenesis. *Science* **167**, 1003–1004.

Ferrari, R. and de Giuli, F. (1997). The propionyl-L-carnitine hypothesis: an alternative approach to treating heart failure. *J. Card. Fail.* **3**, 217–224.

Frandsen, U., Lopez-Figuera, M. and Hellston, Y. (1996). Localisation of nitric oxide synthase in human skeletal muscle. *Biochem. Biophys. Res. Commun.* **227**, 88–93.

Gamrin, L., Andersson, K., Hultmann, E., Nilsson, E., Essen, P. and Wernerman, J. (1997). Longitudinal changes of biochemical parameters in muscle during critical illness. *Metabolism* **46**, 756–762.

Gibala, M. J., MacLean, D. A., Graham, T. E. and Saltin, B. (1997). Anaplerotic processes in human skeletal muscle during brief dynamic exercise. *J. Physiol. (Lond.)* **502**, 703–713.

Gibala, M. J., Maclean, D. A., Graham, T. E. and Saltin, B. (1998). Tricarboxylic acid cycle intermediate pool size and estimated cycle flux in human muscle during exercise. *Am. J. Physiol.* **275**, E235–E242.

Glatz, J. F. C., van Breda, E. V. and van der Vusse, G. J. (1998). Intracellular transport of fatty acids in muscle. *Adv. Exp. Med. Biol.* **441**, 207–218.

Goldspink, D. F., Cox, V. M., Smith, S. K. et al. (1995). Muscle growth in response to mechanical stimuli. *Am J. Physiol.* **268**, E288–E297.

Goldspink, G. (1999). Changes in muscle mass and phenotype and the expression of autocrine and systemic growth factors by muscle in response to stretch and overload. *J. Anat.* **194**, 323–334.

Gollnick, P., Pernow, B., Essen, B., Jansson, E. and Saltin, B. (1981). Availability of glycogen and plasma FFA for substrate utilization in leg muscle of men during exercise. *Clin. Physiol.* **1**, 27–42.

Graham, T. E., Turcotte, L. P., Kiens, B. and Richter, E. A. (1995). Training and muscle ammonia and amino acid metabolism in humans during prolonged exercise. *J. Appl. Physiol.* **78**, 725–735.

Gregory, P., Low, R. and Stirewalt, W. S. (1986). Changes in skeletal muscle myosin isoenzymes with hypertrophy and exercise. *Biochem. J.* **238**, 55–63.

Grozdanovic, Z. and Baumgarten, H. G. (1999). Nitric oxide synthase in skeletal muscle fibres: a signalling component of the dystrophin-glycoprotein complex. *Histol. Histopathol.* **14**, 243–256.

Guillet-Deniau, I., Leturque, A. and Girard, J. (1994). Expression and cellular-localisation of glucose transporters (GLUT1, GLUT 3, GLUT 4) during differentiation of myogenic cells from rat foetuses. *J. Cell. Sci.* **107**, 487–496.

Gunst, J. J., Langlois, M. R., Delanghe, J. R., DeBuyzere, M. L. and Leroux-Roels, G. G. (1998). Serum creatine kinase activity is not a reliable marker for muscle damage in conditions associated with low extracellular glutathione concentration. *Clin. Chem.* **44**, 939–943.

Hambrecht, R., Adams, V., Gielen, S. et al. (1999). Exercise intolerance in patients with chronic heart failure and increased expression of inducible nitric oxide synthase in the skeletal muscle. *J. Am. Coll. Cardiol.* **33**, 174–179.

Hammarqvist, F., Luo, J. L., Cotgreave, I. A., Andersson, K. and Wernerman, J. (1997). Skeletal muscle glutathione is depleted in critically ill patients. *Crit. Care Med.* **25**, 78–84.

Hashimoto, M. and James, D. E. (1998). Snaring GLUT 4 at the plasma membrane in muscle and fat. *Adv. Exp. Med. Biol.* **441**, 47–61.

Haussinger, D. (1996). The role of cell hydration in the regulation of cell function. *Biochem. J.* **313**, 697–710.

Heales, S. J. R., Bolaños, J. P., Stewart, V. C., Brookes, P. S., Land, J. M. and Clark, J. B. (1998). Nitric oxide, mitochondria and neurological disease. *Biochim. Biophys. Acta* **1410**, 215–228.

Hellsten, Y., Apple, F. S. and Sjodin, B. (1996). Effect of sprint cycle training on activities of antioxidant enzymes in human skeletal muscle. *J. Appl. Physiol.* **81**, 1484–1487.

Hespel, P. and Richter, E. A. (1990). Glucose uptake and transport in contracting, perfused rat muscle with different pre-contraction glycogen concentrations. *J. Physiol.* **427**, 347–359.

Hoppelar, H. (1986). Exercise induce ultrastructural changes in skeletal muscle. *J. Sports Med.* **7**, 187–204.

Howlett, R. A., Parolin, M. L., Dyck, D. J. et al (1998). Regulation of skeletal muscle glycogen phosphorylase and PDH at varying exercise power outputs. *Am. J. Physiol.* **275**, R418–R425.

Hudlicka, O. (1985). Regulation of muscle blood flow. *Clin. Phys.* **5**, 201–229.

Hudlicka, O. (1990). The response of muscle to enhanced and reduced activity. *Clin. Endo. Metab.* **4**, 417–439.

Hundal, H. S., Darakhshan, F., Kristiansen, S., Blakemore, S. J. and Richter, E. A. (1998). GLUT 5 expression and fructose transport in human skeletal muscle. *Adv. Exp. Med. Biol.* **441**, 35–45.

Hurley, B. F., Nemeth, P. M., Martin, W. H., Gagbert, J. M., Dalsky, G. P. and Holloszy, J. O. (1986). Muscle triglyceride utilization during exercise: effect of training. *J. Appl. Physiol.* **60**, 562–567.

Ingber, D. (1997). Tensegrity: the architectural basis of cellular mechanotransduction. *Annu. Rev. Physiol.* **59**, 575–599.

Karb, G. (1999). *Cell and Molecular Biology*, 2nd edn. New York: Wiley.

Kjaer, M., Kiens, B., Hargreaves, M. and Richter, E. A. (1991). Influence of active muscle mass on glucose homeostasis during exercise in humans. *J. App. Physiol.* **71**, 552–557.

Klein, S., Coyle, E. F. and Wolfe, R. R. (1994). Fat metabolism during low-intensity exercise in endurance-trained and untrained men. *Am. J. Physiol.* **267**, E934–E940.

Kobzik, L., Reid, M. B., Bredt, D. S. and Stamler, J. S. (1994). Nitric oxide in skeletal muscle. *Nature* **372**, 546–548.

Kobzik, L., Stringer, B., Balligard, J., Reid, M. B. and Stamler, J. S. (1995). Endothelial type nitric oxide synthase in skeletal muscle fibres: mitochondrial relationships. *Biochem. Biophys. Res. Commun.* **21**, 375–381.

Kristiansen, S., Hargreaves, M. and Richter, E. A. (1996). Exercise-induced increase in glucose transport, GLUT 4 and VAMP-2 in plasma membranes from human muscle. *Am. J. Physiol.* **270**, E197–E201.

Kristiansen, S., Hargreaves, M. and Richter, E. A. (1997). Progressive increase in glucose transport and GLUT 4 in human sarcolemmal vesicles during moderate exercise. *Am. J. Physiol.* **272**, E385–E389.

Kuo, C. H., Browning, K. S. and Ivy, J. L. (1999). Regulation of GLUT 4 protein expression and glycogen storage after prolonged exercise. *Acta Physiol. Scand.* **165**, 193–201.

Labow, B. I., Souba, W. W. and Abcouwer, S. R. (1999). Glutamine synthase expression in muscle is regulated by transcriptional and posttranscriptional mechanisms. *Am. J. Physiol.* **276**, E1136–E1145.

Lacey, J. M. and Wilmore, D. W. (1990). Is glutamine a conditionally essential amino acid? *Nutr. Rev.* **48**, 297–309.

Langfort, J., Ploug, T., Ihlemann, J., Saldo, M., Holm, C. and Galbo, H. (1999). Expression of hormone sensitive lipase and its regulation by adrenaline in skeletal muscle. *Biochem. J.* **340**, 459–465.

Lee, A. D., Hansen, P. A. and Holloszy, J. O. (1995). Wortmannin inhibits insulin-stimulated but not contraction-stimulated glucose transport activity in skeletal muscle. *FEBS Lett.* **361**, 51–54.

Liang, P., Hughes, V. and Fukagawa, N. K. (1997). Increased prevalence of mitochondrial DNA deletions in skeletal muscle of older individuals with impaired glucose tolerance: possible marker of glycaemic stress. *Diabetes* **46**, 920–923.

Low, S. Y. and Taylor, P. M. (1998). Integrin and cytoskeletal involvement in signalling cell volume changes to glutamine transport in rat skeletal muscle. *J. Physiol.* **512**, 481–485.

Low, S. Y., Rennie, M. J. and Taylor, P. M. (1996). Modulation of glycogen synthesis in rat skeletal muscle by changes in cell volume. *J. Physiol.* **495**, 299–303.

Low, S. Y., Rennie, M. J. and Taylor, P. M. (1997a). Involvement of integrins and the cytoskeleton in modulation of muscle glycogen synthesis by changes in cell volume. *FEBS Lett.* **417**, 101–103.

Low, S. Y., Rennie, M. J. and Taylor, P. M. (1997b). Signalling elements involved in amino acid transport responses to altered muscle cell volume. *FASEB J.* **11**, 1111–1117.

Lui, S., Adcock, I. M., Old, R. W., Barnes, P. J. and Evans, T. W. (1993). Lipopolysaccharide treatment in vivo induces widespread tissue expression of inducible nitric oxide synthase mRNA. *Biochem. Biophys. Res. Commun.* **196**:,1208–1213.

Luo, J. L., Hammarqvist, F., Anderson, K. and Wernerman, J. (1996). Skeletal glutathione after surgical trauma. *Ann. Surg.* **223**, 420–427.

Maiorana, A., O'Driscoll, G., Cheetham, C. et al. (2000). Combined aerobic and resistance exercise training improves functional capacity and strength in CHF. *J. Appl. Physiol.* **88**, 1565–1570.

MacLean, D., Vissing, J., Vissing, S. F. and Haller, R. G. (1998). Oral branch-chain amino acids do not improve exercise capacity in McArdle's disease. *Neurology* **51**, 1456–1459.

MacLennon, P. A., Smith, K., Weryk, B., Watt, P. W. and Rennie, M. J. (1988). Inhibition of protein breakdown by glutamine in perfused rat skeletal muscle. *FEBS Lett.* **237**, 133–136.

Maréchal, G. and Gailly, P. (1999). Effects of nitric oxide on the contraction of skeletal muscle. *Cell Mol. Life Sci.* **55**, 1088–1102.

Matthews, C. K. and van Holder, K. E. (1995). *Biochemistry*, 2nd edn, pp. 445–516. California: Benjamin Cummings.

McKoy, G., Ashley, W., Mander, J. et al. (1999). Expression of insulin growth factor-1 splice variants and structural genes in rabbit skeletal muscle induced by stretch and stimulation. *J. Physiol.* **516**, 583–592.

Merrill, G. F., Kurth, E. J., Hardie, D. G. and Winder, W. W. (1997). AICA riboside increases AMP-activated protein kinase, fatty acid oxidation and glucose uptake in rat muscle. *Am. J. Physiol.* **273**, E1107–E1112.

Miyamoto, A., Shigematsu, T., Fukunaga, T., Kawakami, K., Mukai, C. and Sekiguchi, C. (1998). Medical baseline data collection on bone and muscle change with space flight. *Bone* **22**, 79S-82S

Newsholme, E. (1998). Fuels for athletic performance. *Biochemist* **20**, 14–17.

Nurjham, N., Bucci, A., Perriello, G. et al. (1995). Glutamine: a major gluconeogenic precursor and vehicle for interorgan carbon transport in man. *J. Clin. Invest.* **95**, 272–277.

Odland, L. M., Heigenhauser, G. J. F., Lopaschuk, E. D. and Spriet, L. L. (1996). Human skeletal muscle malonyl-CoA at rest and during prolonged submaximal exercise. *Am. J. Physiol.* **270**, E541–E545.

Odland, L. M., Howlett, R. A., Heigenhauser, G. J. F., Hultman, E. and Spriet, L. L. (1998). Skeletal muscle malonyl-CoA at the onset of exercise at varying power outputs in humans. *Am. J. Physiol.* **274**, E1080–E1085.

Parry-Billings, M., Evans, J., Calder, P. C. and Newsholme, E. A. (1990). Does glutamine contribute to immunosuppression after major burns. *Lancet* **336**, 523–526.

Phillips, S. M., Green, H. J., Tarnopolsky, M. A., Heigenhauser, G. J. F., Hill, R. E. and Grant, S. M. (1996). Effects of training duration on substrate turnover and oxidation during exercise. *J. Appl. Physiol.* **81**, 2182–2191.

Randle, P. J., Hales, C. N., Garland, P. B. and Newsholme, E. A. (1963). The glucose-fatty acid cycle. Its role in insulin sensitivity and the metabolic disturbances of diabetes mellitus. *Lancet* **i**, 785–789.

Rasmussen, B. B. and Winder, W. W. (1997). Effect of exercise intensity on skeletal muscle malonyl-CoA and acetyl-CoA carboxylase. *J. Appl. Physiol.* **83**, 1104–1109.

Rennie, M. J., Khogali, S. E. O., Low, S. Y. et al. (1996). Amino acid transport in heart and skeletal muscle and the functional consequences. *Biochem. Soc. Trans.* **24**, 869–873.

Rennie, M. J., Low, S. Y., Taylor, P. M., Khogali, S. E. O., Yao, P.-C. and Ahmed, A. (1998). Amino acid transport during muscle contraction and its relevance to exercise. *Adv. Exp. Med. Biol.* **441**, 299–305.

Richter, E. A., Jensen, P., Kiens, B. and Kristansen, S. (1998). Sarcolemmal glucose transport and GLUT 4 translocation during exercise is diminished by endurance training. *Am. J. Physiol.* **274**, E89–E95.

Riede, U. N., Forstermann, U. and Drexler, H. (1998). Inducible nitric oxide synthase in skeletal muscle of patients with chronic heart failure. *J. Am. Coll. Cardiol.* **32**, 964–969.

Roberts, C. K., Barnard, R. J., Scheck, S. H. and Balon, T. W. (1997). Exercise-stimulated glucose transport in skeletal muscle is nitric oxide dependent. *Am. J. Physiol.* **273**, E220–E225.

Romijn, J. A., Coyle, E. F., Sidossis, L. S., Gastaldelli, A., Horowitz, J. F., Endert, E. and Wolfe, R. R. (1993). Regulation of endogenous fat and carbohydrate metabolism in relation to exercise intensity and duration. *Am. J. Physiol.* **265**, E380–391.

Romijn, J. A., Coyle, E. F., Zhang, X.-J., Sidossis, L. S. and Wolfe, R. R. (1995). Relationship between fatty acid delivery and fatty acid oxidation during strenuous exercise. *J. Appl. Physiol.* **79**, 1939–1945.

Rowbottom, D. G., Keast, D. and Morton, A. R. (1996). The emerging role of glutamine as an indicator of exercise stress and overtraining. *Sports Med.* **21**, 90–97.

Ruderman, N. B., Saha, A. K., Vavvas, D. and Witters, L. A. (1999). Malonyl-CoA, fuel sensing and insulin resistance. *Am. J. Physiol.* **276**, E1–E18.

Rudman, D. M., Kutner, M. H., Rogers, C. M., Lubin, M. F., Fleming, G. A. and Brain, R. P. (1981). Impaired growth hormone secretion in the adult population. *J. Clin. Invest.* **67**, 1361.

Saha, A. K., Vavvas, D., Kurowski, T. G. et al. (1997). Malonyl-CoA regulation in skeletal muscle: its link to cell citrate and the glucose-fatty acid cycle. *Am. J. Physiol.* **272**, E641–E648.

Sahlin, K., Jorfeldt, L., Henriksson, K. G., Lewis, S. R. and Haller, R. G. (1995). Tricarboxylic acid cycle intermediates during incremental exercise in healthy subjects and in patients with McArdle's disease. *Clin. Sci.* **88**, 687–693.

Sakai, Y., Iwamura, Y., Hayashi, J.-I., Yamamoto, N., Ohkoshi, N. and Nagata, H. (1999). Acute exercise causes mitochondrial DNA deletion in rat skeletal muscle. *Muscle Nerve* **22**, 258–261.

Schaufelberger, M., Eriksson, B. O., Grimby, G., Held, P. and Swedberg, K. (1997). Skeletal muscle alterations in patients with chronic heart failure. *Eur. Heart J.* **18**, 971–980.

Sidossis, L. S., Wolfe, R. R. and Coggan, A. R. (1998). Regulation of fatty acid oxidation in untrained versus trained men during exercise. *Am. J. Physiol.* **274**, E510–E515.

Silvagno, F., Xia, H. and Bredt, D. S. (1996). Neuronal nitric oxide synthase-μ, an alternatively spliced isoform expressed in differentiated skeletal muscle. *J. Biol. Chem.* **271**, 11204–11208.

Staron, R. S., Kraemer, W. J., Hikida, R. S. et al. (1998). Comparison of soleus muscles from rats exposed to microgravity for 10 versus 14 days. *Histochem. Cell. Biol.* **110**, 73–80.

Steinbert, H. O., Brechtel, G., Johnson, A., Fineberg, N. and Baron, A. D. (1994). Insulin mediated skeletal muscle vasodilation is nitric oxide dependent: a novel action of insulin to increase nitric oxide release. *J. Clin. Invest.* **94**, 1172–1179.

Stewart, V. C., Land, J. M., Clark, J. B. and Heales, S. J. R. (1998). Astrocytic mitochondrial respiratory chain Complex I activity and cellular glutathione. *Biochem. Soc. Trans.* **26**, S345.

Stumvoll, M., Perriello, G., Meyer, C. and Gerich, J. (1999). Role of glutamine in human carbohydrate metabolism in kidney and other tissues. *Kidney Int.* **55**, 778–792.

Turcotte, L. P., Richter, E. A. and Kiens, B. (1992). Increased plasma FFA uptake and oxidation during prolonged exercise in trained *vs* untrained humans. *Am. J. Physiol.* **262**, E791–E799.

Turcotte, L. P., Srivastava, A. K. and Chiasson, J. L. (1997). Fasting increases plasma membrane fatty acid-binding protein (FABP(PM)) in red skeletal muscle. *Mol. Cell Biochem.* **166**, 153–158.

van der Ent, M., Jeneson, J. A., Rennie, W. J., Berger, R., Gampricotti, R. and Visser, F. (1998). A non-invasive selective assessment of type I mitochondrial function using ^{31}P NMR spectroscopy. Evidence for impaired oxidative phosphorylation rate in skeletal muscle in patients with chronic heart failure. *Eur. Heart J.* **19**, 124–131.

van Hall, G., Saltin, B., van der Vusse, G. J., Soderlund, K. and Wagenmakers, A. J. M. (1995). Deamination of amino acids as a source for ammonia production in human skeletal muscle during prolonged exercise. *J. Physiol.* **489**, 251–261.

Vandenburgh, H., Chromiak, J., Shansky, J., Del-Tatto, M. and Lemaire, J. (1999). Space travel directly induces skeletal muscle atrophy. *FASEB J.* **13**, 1031–1038.

Wagenmakers, A. J. M. (1998). Protein and amino acid metabolism in human muscle. *Adv. Exp. Med. Biol.* **441**, 307–319.

Walsh, N. P., Blannin, A. K., Robson, P. J. and Gleeson, M. (1998). Glutamine exercise and immune function. Links and possible mechanisms. *Sports Med.* **26**, 177–191.

Watkins, S. C., Fredericksen, A., Theriault, R., Korythowski, M., Turner, D. S. and Kelley, D. E. (1997). Insulin stimulated GLUT 4 translocation in human skeletal muscle: a quantitative confocal microscopical assessment. *Histochem. J.* **29**, 91–96.

Wolfe, R. R., Goodenenough, R. D., Wolfe, M. H., Royle, G. T. and Nadel, E. R. (1982). Isotopic analysis of leucine and urea metabolism in exercising humans. *J. Appl. Physiol.* **52**, 458–466.

Yang, S. Y., Alnaqeeb, M., Simpson, H. and Goldspink, G. (1996). Cloning and characterisation of an IGF-I isoform expressed in skeletal muscle subjected to stretch. *J. Musc. Res. Cell Met.* **17**, 487–495.

Young, M. E. and Leighton, B. (1998). Fuel oxidation in skeletal muscle is increased by nitric oxide/cGMP – evidence for involvement of cGMP-dependent protein kinase. *FEBS Lett.* **424**, 79–83.

Zable, A. C., Favero, T. G. and Abramson, J. J. (1997). Glutathione modulates ryanodine receptor from skeletal muscle reticulum. Evidence for redox regulation of the Ca^{2+} release mechanism. *J. Biol. Chem.* **272**, 7069–7077.

9

The neuromuscular junction and neuromuscular transmission

Angela Vincent

Introduction

Neuromuscular transmission is the process by which the action potential in a motor nerve axon leads to an action potential in the relevant twitch fibre of a vertebrate skeletal muscle. The neuromuscular junction (NMJ) is a chemical synapse and transmission depends on release of acetylcholine (ACh) from the motor nerve terminal and its interaction with acetylcholine receptors (AChRs) on the postsynaptic muscle surface. This results in the generation of a local potential change in the postsynaptic membrane, called an 'endplate' potential (EPP). The EPP itself is not large enough to cause more than a relatively local depolarization of the muscle fibre membrane, but it induces a regenerating action potential by activating voltage-gated sodium channels (VGSCs). When sufficient VGSCs are opened, the resulting depolarization leads to a regenerative action potential that can propagate along the muscle fibre.

Understanding neuromuscular transmission is of particular relevance to a range of different diseases. The autoimmune disease myasthenia gravis is the best known condition to affect the NMJ. This and other autoimmune and genetic disorders caused by mutations in the genes for the AChR are discussed in Chapter 32. In addition, the NMJ is the target for many neurotoxins, which are present in the venom of snakes, spiders, scorpions and other species of animals. In some parts of the world, envenomation is an important cause of neuromuscular failure and, because of their specificity for NMJ proteins, many of the toxins have been helpful in the study of neuromuscular transmission and its disorders. There are also many substances in plants that affect neuromuscular transmission. These have been used, or modified, to provide therapeutic compounds or to block neuromuscular transmission artificially during anaesthesia.

In this chapter, the structure and development of the NMJ will first be discussed, followed by the normal physiology and pharmacology of neuromuscular transmission. Since the physiology and pharmacology are covered by many excellent books (see Aidley, 1999), it will not be discussed in detail but there will be emphasis on the aspects that are relevant to human disease and the targets for various drugs and toxins. Finally, recent studies that show that modulation of neuromuscular transmission can occur both presynaptically and postsynaptically will be summarized. These findings are not yet clearly shown to be of relevance to normal function and are barely mentioned in textbooks, but they may turn out to be important in disease mechanisms and could throw light on possible therapeutic targets for the future.

Structure and development of the neuromuscular junction

Microscopic structure

An understanding of neuromuscular transmission depends on appreciation of the special structure of the nerve–muscle synapse. The motor nerve unit consists of the motor neuron cell body in the spinal cord and the motor nerve axon that arises from it. This branches when it reaches the surface of the muscle, and each branch loses its myelin sheath just before forming the motor nerve terminals that synapse on the surface of each muscle fibre. In mammals, the NMJ is oval in shape and about 30–50 μm in its largest dimension, which usually runs parallel to the length of the fibre. The NMJ can be easily demonstrated in muscle tissue by fixing and staining for acetylcholinesterase (AChE). Fig. 9.1a illustrates the very small size of the AChE-stained NMJs compared with the muscle fibres,

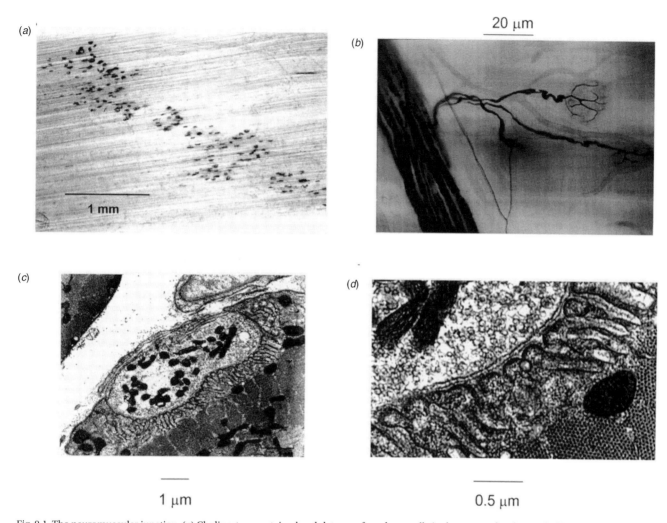

Fig. 9.1. The neuromuscular junction. (*a*) Cholinesterase-stained endplates are found generally in the centre of each muscle fibre. The endplates are very small compared with the length of the fibres (*b*) Combined cholinesterase and silver stain to show the motor nerves and their terminal branches. (*c,d*) Electron micrographs of a single nerve terminal at two magnifications showing the presynaptic vesicles and mitochondria, and the extent of postsynaptic folding with increased membrane density at the top of the folds. (Courtesy of Dr Clarke Slater, University of Newcastle.)

which can be up to several centimetres in length. When silver staining is used, the fine structure of the nerve terminal expansion can be seen (Fig. 9.1*b*). Further details are shown in electron micrographs. Each nerve terminal expansion (or 'bouton') is encased in a thin extension of a Schwann cell (Fig. 9.1*c*). These Schwann cell extensions express high levels of particular proteins such as neural cell adhesion molecule (NCAM) and S-100, which differ quantitatively from those found in the myelin sheath (Mirsky and Jessen, 1999). The muscle surface at the point of contact between the nerve and the muscle surface is often raised, but the terminal branches are sunk into synaptic depressions where the sarcolemma forms postsynaptic folds (Fig. 9.1*c,d*). In between the muscle and the nerve terminal, a distance of about 50 nm, the basal lamina can be seen (Fig. 9.1*d*). The basal lamina extends as a double layer into each of the folds (Hall and Sanes, 1993). The basal lamina appears to be rather amorphous but contains many essential molecules, including different forms of collagen IV, laminins and heparan sulphate proteoglycans. At the NMJ, the basal lamina forms a network or scaffold that anchors NMJ-specific proteins; these include AChE, S-laminin (synapse-specific laminin), agrin (AChR-aggregating molecule) and neuregulins, all of which are involved in development, maintenance and function of the NMJ (see below).

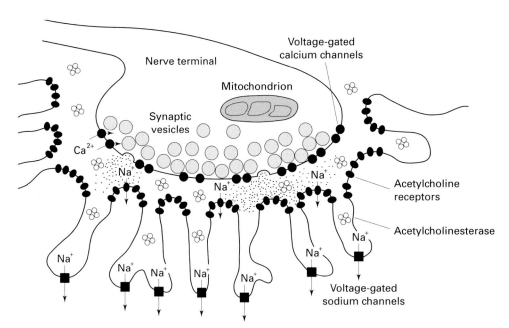

Fig. 9.2. Ion channels at the neuromuscular junction. A schematic representation of the nerve terminal shows the relative positions of the voltage-gated calcium and sodium channels, and the acetylcholine receptors.

The presynaptic nerve terminal contains mitochondria, which provide the energy for synthesis and release of ACh (Fig. 9.1c,d). There are large numbers of small synaptic vesicles, which are particularly concentrated near the membrane opposite the postsynaptic folds (Fig. 9.1d). At this point, there are cytoplasmic densities, called active zones, clustering at points along the nerve terminal opposite the entrance to the folds (not clearly visible in Fig. 9.1). These are where the voltage-gated calcium channels (VGCCs) are located and where the synaptic vesicles fuse with the plasma membrane to release their contents (Fig. 9.2); in tissue that has been quick frozen during high rates of ACh release, it is possible to observe 'omega' profiles that are thought to demonstrate the fusion of the synaptic vesicles with the motor nerve terminal (Fig. 9.2) (Heuser, 1989).

Under the electron microscope, the surface of the postsynaptic membrane opposing the motor nerve terminal is visibly denser than the extrasynaptic membrane or the membrane that forms the lower two-thirds of the postsynaptic folds (Figs. 9.1d and 9.2). Classical studies using the snake toxin α-bungarotoxin, which binds specifically and irreversibly to the AChRs, indicated that this increased density corresponds to the location of AChRs, present at $>10000/\mu m^2$ postsynaptic membrane (Salpeter et al., 1988). By contrast, the AChR density outside the NMJ in mature muscle falls to about $10/\mu m^2$ (Fambrough, 1979). The VGSCs and NCAM are located in the lower two-thirds of the postsynaptic folds (Fig. 9.2) (Wood and Slater, 1998).

Below the postsynaptic folds, within the cytoplasm of the myofibril, are several nuclei, which, in contrast to those present extrasynaptically, are responsible for producing the proteins that are involved in postsynaptic structure and function (see Hall and Sanes, 1993).

Molecular architecture of the presynaptic nerve terminal

Freeze fracture and etching studies show that the synaptic vesicles are attached to actin filaments, which form a scaffold throughout the nerve terminal (Hirokawa et al., 1989), but those at the active zones appear to be independent of an association with actin. On freeze fracture of the nerve terminal membrane at the active zones, active zone particles, which are thought to represent VGCCs, are found to be distributed in parallel arrays. Recent studies using electron tomography have begun to define the molecular structure of the active zones by reconstructing three-dimensional images from 50 nm thin sections (Harlow et al., 1998). The results suggest the presence of beams that extend perpendicular to the length of the nerve terminal and which are attached to ribs that arch towards and tether the synaptic vesicles (illustrated in Fig. 9.3a). The VGCCs, and probably calcium-activated potassium channels, are attached to the ribs localizing them close to the synaptic vesicles. The changes that occur in the arrangement of these structures when calcium entry through the VGCCs leads to fusion of the synaptic vesicles with the nerve terminal membrane, has not yet been explored by this technique. Other proteins, such as syntaxin and the α-latrotoxin receptor (see below), may also be part of this macromolecular structure (Fig. 9.3a).

Molecular architecture of the postynaptic membrane

One of the most exciting developments in the 1990s has been our growing understanding of the postsynaptic molecules that are essential for maintaining the density of AChRs and other molecules at the NMJ (Fig. 9.3b). Many earlier studies had shown that AChRs purified from the electric fish *Torpedo marmorata* were associated with a 43 kDa protein that was subsequently called RAPsyn (receptor-aggregating protein at the synapse). RAPsyn is a cytoplasmic protein of approximately 400 amino acid residues that appears to be essential for the localization of AChRs and many other NMJ-specific proteins (Froehner et al., 1990; Noakes et al., 1993); at the motor endplate, RAPsyn is highly concentrated at the tops of the folds, beneath the AChRs. Utrophin is a protein that shows extensive homology to dystrophin but which in normal muscle is highly concentrated at the NMJ at the tops of the junctional folds, with a similar distribution to the AChRs and RAPsyn (Bewick et al., 1996). Alpha-dystrobrevin 1 also co-localizes with AChRs, and utrophin is thought to link the AChR/α-dystrobrevin complex to actin filaments. By contrast, dystrophin is present at the base of the folds, as well as throughout the sarcolemma. At the NMJ, it associates with α-dystrobrevin 2, ankyrin and β-spectrin, co-localizing with VGSCs and NCAM (Wood and Slater, 1998). Alpha dystroglycan and the sarcoglycans are large macromolecular protein complexes that appear to interact with either utrophin or dystrophin. Consequently, utrophin or dystrophin appear to form the link between the dystroglycan/sarcoglycan complex and the cytoskeleton and at the same time, determine which functional membrane proteins are included in the complex. In addition, the neuronal form of nitric oxide synthase (nNOS) binds to syntrophins and is concentrated at the NMJ, as is a cGMP-dependent kinase that can be activated by NO. It is not known under which conditions nNOS is activated, nor by which membrane or other signals (Chao et al., 1997). Curiously, many of these proteins have also been identified in inclusion bodies in inclusion body myositis (Askanas et al., 1998).

The basal lamina between the nerve and the postsynaptic membrane, and within the postsynaptic folds, contains several synapse-specific proteins. AChE is tethered to the basal lamina at the NMJ by a covalent interaction involving its collagen tail, ColQ, and follows the distribution of the basal lamina into the postsynaptic folds. ColQ is not found outside the NMJ. The laminins are a family of collagen-like proteins that are important for cell–cell interactions. Laminin-β_2 contributes to a protein, s-laminin, that is synapse specific. Agrin and ARIA (AChR-inducing activity) are proteins released by the motor nerve that bind to the basal lamina at the NMJ, enabling them to interact with their postsynaptic receptors to regulate gene expression (see below).

Development of the neuromuscular junction

The accessibility of the NMJ has made it a useful model for developmental studies as well as for structural and functional ones. The motor neurons arise in the ventral portion of the neural tube and their axons run through the peripheral nerves to the muscles, branching many times to innervate 10–100 fibres. Schwann cells form from the neural crest and follow the motor axons to their destinations. Muscle originates from mesodermal cells that migrate to the appropriate sites and differentiate into myoblasts. The myoblasts fuse to form multinucleated myotubes, which mature into multinucleated muscle fibres. Because of the ease with which the distribution of AChRs can be followed using radioactive or fluorescent labelled neurotoxins such as α-bungarotoxin, many of the studies of this maturation process have related to the presence and characteristics of the AChRs, but clearly many other gene products are also involved.

The changes in AChR distribution over time in rodents is illustrated in Fig. 9.4. AChR expression is low during the myoblast stage but increases once the myotubes have fused (Fambrough, 1979; Sanes and Lichtman, 1999). At this stage, the AChRs form clusters with a density of around 1000/μm^2, but it appears that the NMJ begins to form at the initial point of contact of the incoming growth cone rather than at a convenient cluster of AChRs. Once this happens, the AChRs along other parts of the myotube surface begin to disappear, leaving a high density of receptors at the emergent NMJ. Over time, several days in the mouse or rat, these AChRs change their physiological characteristics from those of the fetal isoform, $\alpha_1(2)\beta\delta\varepsilon$, to the adult isoform, $\alpha_1(2)\beta\gamma\delta$, by substitution of a NMJ-specific ε-subunit for the γ-subunit (Missias et al., 1986). Eventually the surface of the muscle begins to form the characteristic postsynaptic folds. These changes occur postnatally in the mouse but prenatally in humans (Hesselmans et al., 1993). Thus the intense localization of the AChRs at the mature NMJ depends on a combination of increased junctional synthesis, particularly of the ε-subunit at the NMJ,

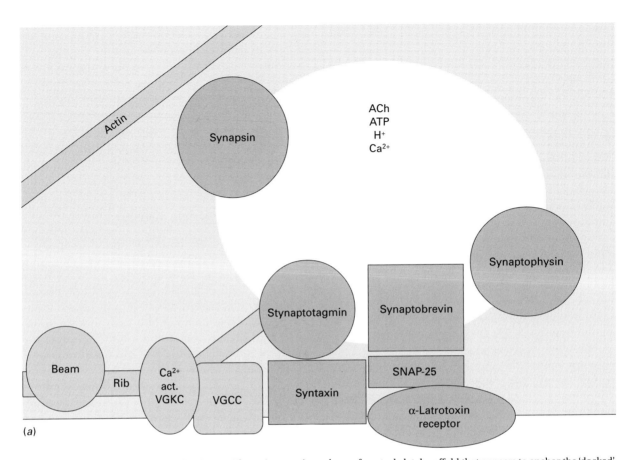

(a)

Fig. 9.3. Pre- and postsynaptic specialization. (a) The active zone is made up of a cytoskeletal scaffold that appears to anchor the 'docked' synaptic vesicle, via synaptotagmin, in close proximity to the voltage-gated calcium channel (VGCC) a calcium-activated voltage-gated potassium channel (VGKC) and syntaxin. Before docking, synapsins in the vesicular membrane attach the vesicles to actin filaments; release from this restraint is dependent on calcium-calmodulin kinase activation. (b) The tops of the postsynaptic folds contains muscle acetylcholine receptors (AChRs) (α_1, β, ε, δ) and many structural proteins such as the dystroglycans, dystrobrevins, syntrophins and utrophin. The lower parts of the folds contain the voltage-gated sodium channels (VGSC) tethered to ankyrin via dystrobrevin and dystrophin. In addition, there are other postsynaptic proteins that are involved in development and maintenance of the postsynaptic specialization (see Fig. 9.5). RAPsyn, receptor-aggregating protein at the synapse; AChE, acetylcholinesterase; MuSK, muscle-specific kinase; nNOS, neuronal nitric oxide synthetase; MASC, myotube-associated specificity component.

diffusion of extrajunctional AChRs within the membrane towards the forming NMJ and decreased extrajunctional synthesis of AChR (see Fig. 9.5). Another change characteristic of the mature NMJ is that the turnover of the AChRs is dramatically reduced from a half-life of around 16 hours to a half-life of many days, perhaps 10 or more, in the mature state (Fambrough, 1979; Salpeter and Loring, 1985). In contrast to AChRs, VGSCs cluster around the developing NMJ and only become concentrated in the postsynaptic folds after the NMJ has matured (Wood et al., 1998).

The nerve terminal also differentiates during formation of the NMJ, partly in response to muscle-derived factors. Neurotrophins are released from muscle cells, and there

are many trophic substances and cell adhesion molecules involved in trans-synaptic communication and stability. The changes have not been studied in such detail, but it appears that the active zones and their detailed infrastructure develop in parallel with, and partly in response to, the postsynaptic changes.

During development, the NMJ may be innervated by more than one motor axon (polyneuronal inervation), but as the NMJ matures only one motor axon survives at most NMJs. This phenomenon only occurs in twitch fibres; tonic fibres, as partly present in ocular and laryngeal muscles, do not conduct action potentials and have multiple endplate regions. Discussion of polyneuronal innervation and

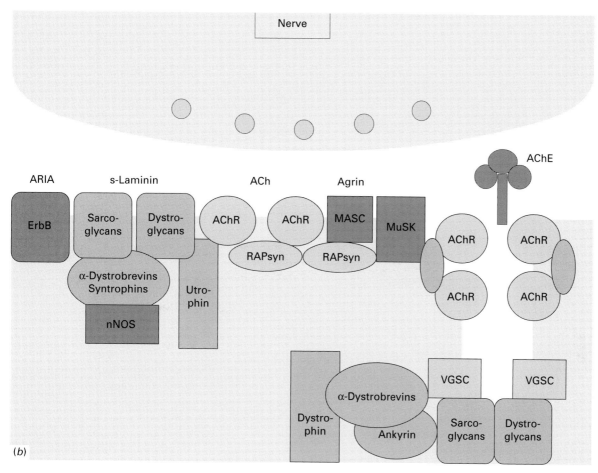

Fig. 9.3. (*cont.*)

synapse elimination is beyond the scope of this chapter (Sanes and Lichtman, 1999).

Muscle-specific development is dependent on a series of transcription factors such as MyoD, Myf5, MRF4 and myogenin. These act on E-boxes, which are regulatory elements in the promoter regions of the muscle-specific genes. After innervation, the expression of some of the genes becomes restricted to the NMJ. This occurs when nerve-induced muscle activity induces the local production of myogenic transcription factors that upregulate AChR expression at the NMJ via an N-box, which is found only in the promoter regions of NMJ-specific genes. When the nerve to a muscle is cut, AChRs are re-expressed throughout the muscle fibre. Lomo and Westgaard (1975) showed that this increase in extrajunctional AChR expression could be prevented by electrical stimulation of the muscle. From these and other observations, it is thought that calcium released from the sarcoplasmic reticulum during muscle contraction represses extrajunctional AChR expression by activating protein kinase C, which in turn leads to downregulation of

the myogenic factors MyoD, Myf5, MRF4 and myogenin. Thus during normal activity there is continuous calcium-dependent repression of synthesis of some extrajunctional proteins (Sanes and Lichtman, 1999). At the NMJ, by contrast, these effects are overcome by local production of myogenic factors.

When a muscle is denervated by disease or by artificially cutting the nerve, the total amount of AChR increases many fold. These changes can be seen in diabetic neuropathy and, to a lesser extent, when a muscle and its nerve supply are subject to chronic ischaemia. Nevertheless, the original NMJ survives for many weeks, continues to express a high concentration of AChR and AChE and can be easily reinnervated (Fambrough, 1979). This appears to be because the nerve-released factors that regulate protein expression at the NMJ are retained by the basal lamina. The importance of the basal lamina in maintenance of the NMJ was demonstrated by experiments by Sanes and his colleagues. They induced complete muscle fibre necrosis but found that the basal laminae remained intact around the

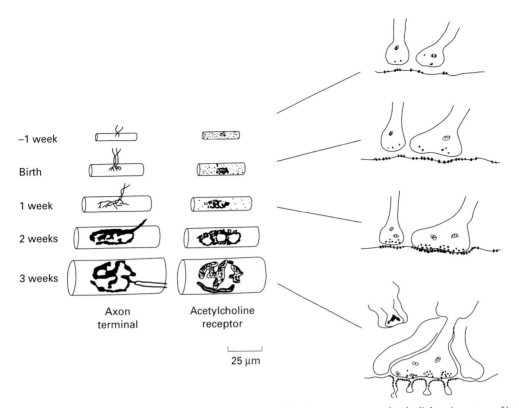

Fig. 9.4. Development of the neuromuscular junction. On the left, the appearance under the light microscope of junctions stained for acetylcholinesterase during development in the rodent. On the right, the distribution of acetylcholine receptors (AChR) is shown, and the development of the postsynaptic folds. The adult AChRs replace the fetal AChRs between 1 and 3 weeks. In humans, the processes are thought to occur before birth, probably after 30 weeks. (Adapted from Vincent and Wray (1992) courtesy of Dr Clarke Slater.)

degenerating muscle fibres, and that the high density of AChE remained at the former NMJ (Sanes et al., 1978). These and many other experiments (Sanes and Scheller, 1997) show that the NMJ is a remarkably stable synapse, ensuring that even when damage to nerve or muscle does occur, there is every chance of reinnervation and recovery of function.

The importance of individual molecules in development of the normal neuromuscular junction

Much work since the early 1980s has added molecular detail to the general description given above of the events that are responsible for the NMJ development. In particular, the use of mice that have had a particular gene 'knocked-out' has made it possible to study the role of individual molecules in the normal development process and is of potential relevance to the identification of candidate targets for the congenital myasthenic syndromes. Table 9.1 summarizes some of these findings for genes affecting the NMJ.

There are two molecules released from the motor nerves that are of particular importance in the normal development and maintenance of the NMJ. During the early stages of development, a protein called agrin is released from the incoming nerve and leads to AChR clustering. Agrin is a heparan sulphate proteoglycan of around 400 kDa that is synthesized by motoneurons, transported down the motor axon and released into the basal lamina (McMahan, 1990). Alternative splicing of the gene for agrin leads to different forms, some of which, collectively known as z-agrins, are essential for NMJ development. Z-agrins lead to phosphorylation of a membrane kinase called MuSK (muscle-specific kinase), which colocalizes with AChRs (Bowen et al., 1998). However, agrins cannot be shown to bind directly to MuSK and appear to act via another receptor that has not yet been clearly defined but is usually referred to as MASC (myotube-associated specificity component). MuSK can be cross-linked to agrin, suggesting that MASC and MuSK are intimately associated. The process of agrin binding and MuSK phosphorylation is responsible for activation of intracellular signalling

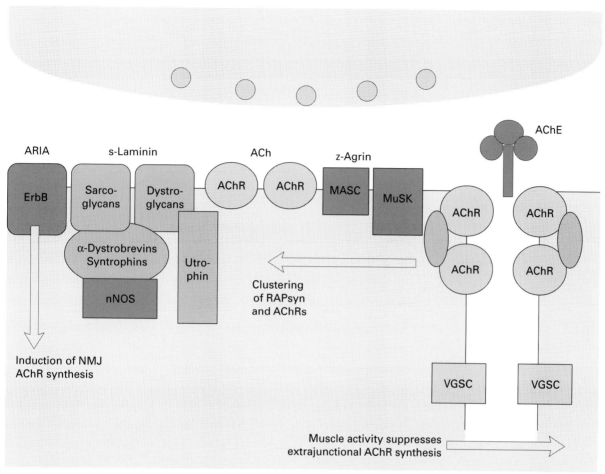

Fig. 9.5. Interactions involved in development and maintenance of the postsynaptic specialisation. Z-agrin released from the nerve interacts with the MASK/MuSK complex, leading to activation of intracellular signals that result in clustering of RAPsyn and AChRs. ARIA released from the nerve activates different intracellular signals that lead to increased expression of the AChR, particularly the ε-subunit, at the NMJ. Muscle activity suppresses extrajunctional synthesis of AChR and other proteins. Muscle forms of agrin, and laminin bound to dystroglycans, may act as retrograde signals to produce differentiation of the motor nerve terminal and stabilization of the presynaptic apparatus. Abbreviations as in Fig. 9.3.

pathways that result in AChR clustering (Fig. 9.5) (Sanes and Lichtman, 1999). Both agrin and MuSK have been knocked-out in experimental animals, leading to lethal phenotypes (DeChiara et al., 1996; Gautam et al., 1996). Mice homologous for deficient MuSK had no NMJs and little or no postsynaptic differentiation. Although AChR synthesis occurred, there were few AChR clusters or clusters of AChE, utrophin or RAPsyn. The phenotype expressed by agrin homologous knock-out mice was similar, though there were more RAPsyn clusters. Other splice forms of agrin are released by the muscle and play a less crucial role in development.

Another important molecule, ARIA, is one of a family of alternatively spliced proteins called neuregulins; these are involved in many aspects of development. ARIA is released from the motor nerve terminal and accumulates in the basal lamina, binds to its specific receptor, which is clustered on the NMJ postsynaptic membrane. The receptor is probably a dimer formed by ErbB2 and ErbB3 tyrosine kinases. This process also leads to activation of signalling pathways, resulting in stimulation of the transcription factors that bind to the N-boxes in the promoter regions of the genes for AChR and lead to transcription, particularly of the ε-subunit of the AChR (Koike et al., 1995). ARIA knock-out mice die in utero before NMJ development, but heterozygotes have NMJs that are similar to junctions in myasthenia gravis, with reduced AChRs and reduced EPP miniature (MEPP) amplitudes (Sandrock et al., 1997).

Table 9.1. Phenotypes of some of the knock-out mice with affected neuromuscular junctions

Targeted gene	Survival	During development	Presynaptic changes	Postsynaptic changes
Agrin: homozygote; MuSK homozygote very similar	Few hours only	No RAPsyn or AChR clustering	Axons simplified; nerve terminals simplified; reduced numbers of vesicles	No folds; markedly reduced clusters of AChR
RAPsyn: homozygote	Few hours only	MuSK and agrin normal; reduced AChR clusters	Reduced arborization of the motor nerve; nerve terminals simplified	No folds No AChR clusters
S-laminin: homozygote	2–3 weeks	Normal RAPsyn and AChR clustering	Reduced active zones; Schwann cell intrusions into the synaptic cleft	Reduced folds, otherwise fairly normal; AChRs normal
AChR ε-subunit: homozygote	6 weeks	Reduced clusters	Normal	Persistence of AChR γ-subunit for several weeks allows survival
ARIA: heterozygote homozygote, lethal in utero	Reduced	Not studied	Not marked	Reduced AChRs; myasthenia-like
Utrophin: homozygote	Normal	Normal MuSK, agrin and RAPsyn clusters	None	Reduced folds; slightly reduced AChRs

Notes:
AChR, acetylcholine receptor; RAPsyn, receptor-aggregating protein at the synapse; ARIA, acetylcholine receptor-inducing activity; MuSK, muscle-specific kinase.

This suggests that a heterozygous mutation in this neuregulin form could lead to a congenital myasthenic syndrome.

RAPsyn knock-out mice have very poor survival, with NMJs that fail to develop AChR clusters and cannot sustain life (Gautam et al., 1995). However, in RAPsyn-deficient mice, MuSK still responds to agrin and forms clusters on the muscle surface. Therefore, the agrin–MuSK interaction is independent of RAPsyn and may be an earlier step in NMJ differentiation. Interestingly, the laminin β2-chain and AChE are still clustered on the cell surface in RAPsyn-deficient mice, suggesting that they are also controlled by an earlier step in development or have independent targeting and localization at the NMJ (Gautam et al., 1995).

Although utrophin is clearly concentrated in the postsynaptic density, it is not essential for normal function, at least in mice (Deconinck et al., 1997). Utrophin knock-out mice appear normal and neuromuscular transmission is not compromised. However, there is a modest reduction in AChR numbers at the NMJ, which appears to be related to a reduction in the number and depth of postsynaptic folds. Although utrophin is thought to link the cytoskeleton to α_1-dystroglycans and RAPsyn, the distribution of AChRs is clearly not dependent on normal utrophin. Curiously, in muscle biopsies from patients with congenital myasthenic syndromes or with myasthenia gravis, a reduction in AChRs is usually accompanied by a reduction in utrophin (Slater et

al., 1997) suggesting that utrophin localization could be secondary to that of AChR rather than the reverse. Fig. 9.5 summarizes the main interactions that are involved in forming and maintaining the high density of AChRs at the NMJ.

The first knock-out mouse with an altered NMJ was deficient in laminin-β2 (Noakes et al., 1995). These mice survived for two or three weeks after birth, but the presynaptic nerve terminals were simplified, ACh release was reduced and there were few active zones. In addition, the postsynaptic folds were few in number (Table 9.1), and there was some sprouting of nerve terminals, but otherwise the postsynaptic membrane appeared normal. Since the phenotype of this knock-out mouse is more striking presynaptically than those involving RAPsyn or agrin, it may be that laminin-β2 acts as a retrograde signal. Alternatively, since it is thought to bind to the dystroglycan complex, it may be is responsible for interacting with the presynaptic membrane at the active zones and helping to direct the clustering of the presynaptic cytoskeletal components.

Physiology and pharmacology of neuromuscular transmission

Many of the standard textbooks describe synaptic transmission in the context of the NMJ in detail, including the key experiments that demonstrated its chemical nature (Vincent and Wray, 1992; Aidley, 1999). Here, only the most important features will be discussed, and the action of some of the pharmacological compounds that target the NMJ (Tables 9.2–9.4).

Acetylcholine storage and calcium-dependent release

ACh is synthesized in the cytoplasm of the nerve terminal from choline and acetyl-CoA by the enzyme acetylcholine choline transferase. ACh is taken up into the synaptic vesicles in exchange for protons via an ACh transporter (Usdin et al., 1995). That is sensitive to hemicholinium. ATP in the cytoplasm generates the energy required to transport the protons into the vesicles so that they can be exchanged for ACh. Interestingly, ATP is also present in the vesicle, is released with ACh and can act on both pre- and postsynaptic receptors to modulate neuromuscular transmission (see below). After ACh is released, about 50% of it binds to the AChRs, but any remaining, and the ACh that dissociates from the AChRs, is hydrolysed by AChE to acetate and choline. Choline is taken up into the nerve terminal by the choline transporter, which is sensitive to the drug vesamicol, and then becomes available for further synthesis of ACh.

The first step in successful transmission is the arrival of the action potential at the motor nerve terminal and the opening of the VGCC. The generation and propagation of the action potentials, in both nerve and muscle, is dependent on the membrane potential. This is maintained by the action of the Na^+/K^+ ATPase, which exchanges two potassium ions for three sodium ions, thus maintaining the chemical gradient. The action potential is carried by VGSC, sensitive to block by tetrodotoxin, which are densely localized in the nodes of Ranvier and at the final heminode. As the VGSCs close, voltage-gated potassium channels (VGKCs) open to help to restore the membrane potential to its resting level, which is closer to the equilibrium potential for potassium than for sodium.

The opening of the VGCC leads to a rapid, short-lived and highly localized increase in the cytoplasmic concentration of free calcium (Smith and Augustine, 1988). Until fairly recently, it was not possible to measure directly calcium entry into the nerve terminal in mammalian tissues because the motor nerve terminal is very small. The role of calcium was demonstrated by Miledi and his colleagues using a variety of approaches including direct injection of calcium into the nerve terminal of the squid giant motor axon (see Aidley, 1999). More recently, other workers such as Llinas et al. (1995) and Stanley (1993) have used calcium imaging and patch clamp techniques to demon-

strate the relationship between motor nerve depolarization, calcium entry and transmitter release. It has been calculated that the concentration of calcium inside the nerve terminal reaches around $100\,\mu mol/l$ but lasts only a few milliseconds, principally because of buffering by intracellular components and, more slowly, by extrusion through the Na^+/Ca^{2+} exchanger. The rise in intracellular calcium is sufficient to trigger exocytosis of the synaptic vesicles, at least those that are anchored at the active zones and which have been 'primed' for release. However, it appears that four molecules of calcium are required to bind in order to release one vesicle (Dodge and Rahaminoff, 1967), and there may be only a limited number of primed vesicles and a low probability of release at each active zone (see Cull-Candy et al., 1980).

The mechanisms by which docked vesicles containing ACh fuse with the presynaptic motor nerve membrane and release their contents is still unclear, but there is now a substantial literature detailing the different vesicular and nerve terminal membranes involved in release. The most popular hypotheses relate to the concept of docking of vesicles by binding of a V-SNARE protein on the synaptic vesicle to a T-SNARE protein on the nerve terminal membrane. The complex formed becomes somehow 'primed' for release; release then occurs when calcium entry through the VGCCs acts on the calcium-sensitive vesicular protein synaptotagmin.

Following fusion, the vesicle membrane forms part of the nerve terminal membrane, with the intravesicular surface facing extracellularly. Subsequently, in a process that is also calcium dependent, the vesicle is reformed into clathrin-coated vesicles. The vesicle is then refilled with ACh. ACh-containing vesicles are not free in the cytoplasm but are tethered to actin filaments via the vesicle protein synapsin. Calcium-activation of calcium-dependent calmodulin kinase leads to phosphorylation of synapsin, release of the actin attachment and allows the vesicle to localize to an active zone. The cascade of synaptic vesicle events is described in detail by Sudhof (1995) and by de Camilli and Takei (1996).

The details of these processes, most of which are, in principle, common to exocytosis in neurosecretory and endocrine tissues, are beyond the scope of this chapter, but a diagramatic representation of some of the proteins involved is shown in Fig. 9.6. Several of the components of the presynaptic nerve terminal have been knocked-out in experimental studies, and *Drosophila* mutants have been studied in detail: many show an altered calcium-dependency of release or complete calcium independence (Sudhof, 1995). A type of congenital myasthenic syndrome, called familial infantile myasthenia, is thought to involve

Table 9.2. Drugs and toxins affecting the presynaptic nerve terminal at the neuromuscular junction

Substance	Natural source	Effect on function	Physiological effects on neuromuscular transmission
VGSC (nerve)			
Tetrodotoxin	Puffer fish	Blocks VGSC activity	Paralysis
Saxitoxin	Dinoflagellates	Blocks VGSC activity	Parlaysis
Alkaloids	Mainly plants	Alter activation/inactivation	Hyperactivity with or without paralysis
Anatoxin α-, β- and γ-toxins	Sea anemone, scorpions	Slow inactivation or enhance activation or shift action potential	Increased activity and lowered threshold
VGKC			
Tetraethylammonium (TEA) 4-Aminopyridine or 3,4-diaminopyridine	Synthetic	Blocks many types	Increases transmitter release; repetitive activity
Dendrotoxins	Snake, e.g. *Dendroaspis viridis*	Blocks some types	Increased transmitter release; alters threshold; spontaneous or repetitive neuronal activity
VGCC N type			
ω-Conotoxin GVIA	Cone snail (*Conus geographus*)	Blocks channel	Reduces nerve-evoked acetylcholine release in some species; may be expressed at NMJ during development
VGCC P type			
ω-Conotoxin MVIIC	Cone snail (*Conus magus*)	Blocks channel	Reduces nerve-evoked acetylcholine release at mammalian NMJs
ω-Agatoxin	Funnel web spider (*Agenopsis aperta*)	Blocks channels	Reduces nerve-evoked acetylcholine release at mammalian NMJs
Acetylcholine release			
Botulinum toxins	*Clostridium botulinum*	Cleaves snare proteins	Massive reduction in quantal release of acetylcholine
α-Latrotoxin	Black widow spider	?Forms fusion pore	Massive noncalcium-dependent release of acetylcholine
Muscarinic AChR			
Acetylcholine	Synaptic vesicles	Not known; probably G-protein dependent; could act via VGCCs or via release mechanism	May help to prevent excessive acetylcholine release
ATP and adenosine receptors			
ATP	Synaptic vesicles	Not known; probably G-protein dependent; could act via VGCCs or via release mechanism	May help to prevent excessive acetylcholine release
CGRP receptor			
CGRP	Synaptic vesicles	Not known; probably G-protein dependent; could act via VGCCs or via release mechanism	May help to prevent excessive acetylcholine release
Adrenergic receptors			
Noradrenaline	Sympathetic system	Not known	Increases acetylcholine release
Neuronal AChRs			
Acetylcholine	Synaptic vesicles	Not known	Increases acetylcholine release at beginning of a train of impulses

Notes:
VGSC, voltage-gated sodium channels; VGKC, voltage-gated potassium channels; VGCC, voltage-gated calcium channels; AChR, acetylcholine receptor; CGRP, calcitonin gene-related peptide; NMJ, neuromuscular junction.

Table 9.3. Drugs and toxins affecting the synapse

Substance	Natural source	Effect of function	Physiological effects on neurotransmission
Acetylcholinesterase Physostigmine Organophosphate	Plants	Blocks acetylcholinesterase	Increased activity leading to decensitization or persistent depolarization with weakness

Table 9.4. Drugs and toxins affecting the postsynaptic membrane at the neuromuscular junction

Substance	Natural source	Effect on function	Physiological effects on neuromuscular transmission
AChR			
α-Bungarotoxin	Snake *Bungarus multicinctus*	Blocks AChR	Reduction in postsynaptic effect of ACh leading to weakness
d-Tubocurarine	Plant	Blocks AChR	Reduced effect of ACh leading to weakness
Suxamethonium (succinylcholine)		AChR agonist	Increased activity leading to desensitization or persistent depolarization with weakness
Neuronal AChR			
AChR	Synaptic vesicles	?Activates calcium release and protein kinase C	May help to prevent excessive postsynaptic activity
CGRP receptor			
CGRP	Synaptic vesicles	?Activates calcium release and protein kinase C	May help to prevent excessive postsynaptic activity
ATP receptor			
ATP	Synaptic vesicles	?Activates calcium release and protein kinase C	May help to prevent excessive postsynaptic activity
VGSC (muscle)			
Tetrodotoxin	Puffer fish	Blocks VGSC	Muscle paralysis
μ-Conotoxin	Cone snail *Conus*	Blocks muscle VGSC more than nerve VGSC	Muscle paralysis

Notes:
Abbreviations as in Table 9.2.

defects in ACh packaging or release (Chapter 32). The next few years may provide more information on the target for mutations in this disorder.

ACh can be measured by mass spectrometry in the bathing solution (if its breakdown is prevented by AChE inhibitors; see Molenaar, 1992). The amount of ACh released at rest, however, does not appear to correspond to the amount calculated from the known frequency of spontaneous release (see below), and the increase in release that occurs during nerve stimulation is far less than would be expected. It appears that there is a steady spontaneous, nonquantal release of ACh from the motor nerve terminal, and probably some made in the muscle

fibres as well; both of these add to the nerve-evoked release and make it difficult to perform accurate biochemical measurements.

Many toxins from different species of venomous animals act on the presynaptic release mechanism. In addition to those that target specific ion channels (see below), there are two types of neurotoxin of particular interest. Botulinum toxins are formed from two chains (similar to tetanus toxin and some other bacterial toxins). The heavy chains bind to the nerve terminal and translocate the light chains into the cytoplasm. The light chains are metalloproteinases, which, in the presence of zinc, cleave the relevant protein (see Fig. 9.6), resulting in complete loss of nerve-evoked ACh

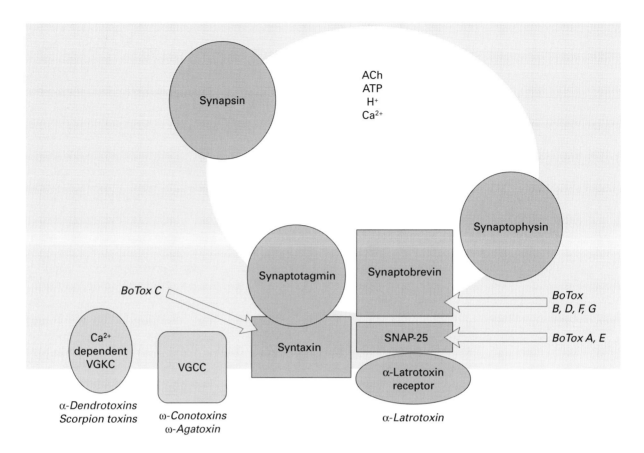

Fig. 9.6. Acetylcholine (ACh) release and neurotoxins. The release of ACh depends on complex interactions between many proteins, some of which are illustrated. Release of ACh is inhibited by ω-conotoxin and ω-agatoxin, which block VGCCs. Three of the cytoplasmic proteins are the targets for *Clostridium botulinum* toxins (BoTox), which cleave the proteins and effectively abolish nerve-evoked ACh release. By contrast, dendrotoxins and some scorpion toxins block the calcium-activated VGKCs and lead to prolonged depolarization with increased ACh release. Alpha-latrotoxin binds to neurexin and leads to a massive, calcium-independent release of ACh. Abbreviations as in Fig. 9.3.

release. Because the turnover of the nerve terminal is slow, perhaps reflecting the large distance from the motor neuron cell body, recovery from botulinum poisoning is also slow, but considerable nerve sprouting occurs. However, the slow recovery means that injection of botulinum toxin can be effective in the treatment of certain dystonias (Jankovic and Brin, 1997). By contrast, α-latrotoxin from the Black Widow spider (Hurlbut and Cecarrelli, 1979) causes massive quantal ACh release. The exact mechanism by which this toxin induces vesicle fusion is unknown, but it appears to be essentially calcium-independent, suggesting that the toxin somehow uncouples exocytosis from the normal calcium-dependent process. It binds to a specific receptor that is part of the macromolecular active zone complex (Fig. 9.6) and may form a channel in the presynaptic membrane that somehow induces fusion of synaptic vesicles.

Postsynaptic action of acetylcholine and measuring the quantal content

The easiest way to detect ACh release is by looking at the postsynaptic events that accompany it. These are of two kinds. Spontaneous release of (generally) single packets or 'quanta' of ACh are evident as MEPPs, around 0.5–1 mV in amplitude (Fig. 9.7a), that occur at rest with a frequency that shows a normal distribution. The MEPP amplitude, which depends on how many AChRs are activated, depends on postsynaptic factors such as the number of AChRs and the membrane potential. The frequency of the MEPPs can be dramatically increased by depolarization of the motor nerve terminal, for instance by increasing the external potassium concentration. MEPP frequency at rest is only partially calcium dependent, and even in the absence of extracellular calcium, MEPPs continue to occur. Van der Kloot and Molgo (1994) give a comprehensive

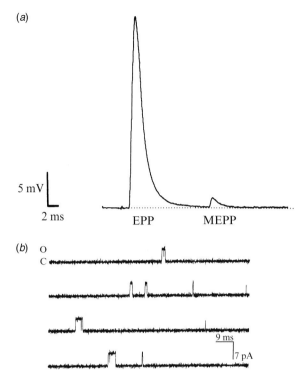

(a)

5 mV

2 ms

EPP   MEPP

(b) O
C

9 ms

7 pA

Fig. 9.7. Electrophysiological measurements at the neuromuscular junction. (*a*) Using μ-conotoxin to inhibit the muscle VGSCs, it is possible to measure endplate potentials and miniature endplate potentials simultaneously, allowing a direct comparison between their amplitudes and calculation of the quantal content. Mouse hemidiaphragm preparation (courtesy of Dr Mark Roberts). (*b*) Single acetylcholine receptor channel currents can be recorded in human muscle biopsies by patch clamp in the presence of 1 μmol/l acetylcholine. (From Milone et al. (1994) with permission.)

review of quantal ACh release. Marked increases in MEPP frequencies, similar to those found in the presence of α-latrotoxin (see above), are found in the presence of anti-GQ1b antibodies from patients with the Miller–Fisher syndrome (Plomp et al., 1999). These antibodies cause a complement-dependent increase in neurotransmitter release; it is not yet clear whether massive calcium influx follows binding of antibodies to the nerve terminal and complement-dependent lysis, or whether the antibodies and complement also somehow 'uncouple' release from its normal dependency on calcium.

When the motor nerve is stimulated, many quanta of AChR are released, and the EPP rapidly exceeds the threshold for generation of an action potential in the muscle-leading to muscle contraction. In order to measure the size of the EPP without interference from the action potential,

and from this to infer the number of quanta that make up the EPP, several approaches can be used. One is to cut the fibres on each side of the endplate region of the muscle. This leads to a slow decrease in the membrane potential that results in inactivation of some of the VGSCs that are responsible for the muscle action potential. When this occurs, it is possible to measure EPPs directly because the muscle no longer twitches in response to nerve stimulation. This has been used to measure the quantal content in human muscle biopsies (Plomp et al., 1995). An alternative is to add a drug that reduces the postsynaptic response to levels that are below the threshold for generation of the action potential. In 1 μmol/l d-tubocurarine, for instance, the EPP is reduced below the threshold; however, the individual MEPPs are barely detectable because d-tubocurarine reduces them too. The quantal content can, therefore, only be obtained from the variance of the EPP amplitude. If one wants to maintain detectable MEPPs, one can reduce the external calcium and increase magnesium concentration so that the number of packets released is decreased. When this is done, the size of the EPPs follows a Poisson distribution corresponding to the release of 0, 1, 2, 3, 4 etc. packets of ACh. Since the amplitude of the individual steps corresponds well to the average amplitude of the MEPPs, this provided the first evidence that the EPP was made up of the simultaneous release of single packets of ACh (Del Castillo and Katz, 1954; Aidley, 1999).

The conditions used to measure EPPs described above might alter the very processes that are being studied. An apparently better way by which to measure the quantal content is to use μ-conotoxin from *Conus geographus* (Hong and Chang, 1989). This toxin binds more strongly to the muscle VGSCs than to the nerve VGSCs. Consequently, if the toxin is applied until the preparation ceases to contract, and then washed off, the muscle VGSCs remain blocked for some time but the nerve VGSCs quickly recover. Under these conditions, a nerve-evoked EPP can be induced and measured, and the amplitude compared with that of the MEPPs in the same muscle fibre (Fig. 9.7). With appropriate correction for nonlinear summation (that is, as the postsynaptic depolarization approaches the equilibrium potential for sodium ions, the driving force for the current becomes smaller), the quantal content of rodent muscles can be determined with some accuracy. Whereas previous techniques using the variance method suggested that the quantal content was around 130 in the mouse (Wray, 1992), using μ-conotoxin, values of 30–50 are found (Plomp et al., 1995). However, further work is needed to make sure that these values are not reduced by a subtle presynaptic effect of μ-conotoxin.

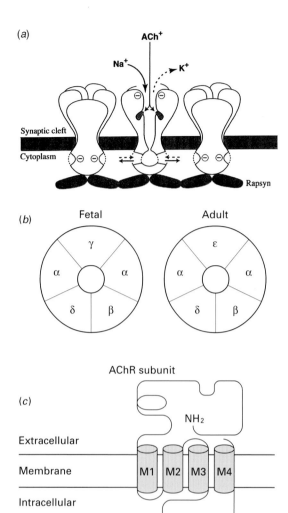

Fig. 9.8. The acetylcholine receptor. (*a*) The architecture of the receptor as determined by electron microscopy of tubular crystals of *Torpedo* sp. membranes. (From Miyazawa et al., 1999, with permission.) Binding of ACh to pockets at the interfaces of the α-subunits with their adjacent subunits leads to opening of the channel pore. After transit through the central pore, the cations flow through narrow openings in the cytoplasmic walls. (*b*) The adult and fetal receptors differ in that the former has a ε-subunit and the latter a γ-subunit. The acetylcholine-binding sites are located at the α/δ, α/ε or α/γ interfaces. (*c*) Each subunit consists of a large extracellular domain, containing a disulphide bond between cysteines at positions 128 and 144, four transmembrane domains and a large cytoplasmic loop.

Acetylcholine receptors at the neuromuscular junction

Many early studies (see Aidley, 1999) showed that MEPPs were inhibited by curare, and that this inhibition could be partly reversed by AChE inhibitors. Moreover, the existence of 'ACh sensitivity' of the postsynaptic membrane was demonstrated by showing that a short pulse of ACh applied by a pipette to the muscle surface caused a depolarization of the membrane similar to that in a single MEPP or EPP. In normal muscle, this ACh sensitivity was restricted to the NMJ region, whereas in preparations where the motor nerve had been cut some days before, the whole muscle surface became sensitive to ACh. Although it was clear that ACh was acting on the muscle membrane to produce a depolarization, it was not until the use of the snake α-neurotoxins that it was possible to demonstrate unequivocally that this ACh sensitivity resulted from the presence of a specific protein.

Following the demonstration that α-bungarotoxin bound specifically and irreversibly to the motor endplate of normal muscle, and also extrajunctionally in denervated muscle (Salpeter et al., 1988), the muscle proteins were solubilized in detergents and α-neurotoxins were used to purify the AChR 'protein' from *Torpedo* electric organ by the technique of affinity chromatography. The protein that was obtained bound the α-neurotoxins in solution and when reconstituted into artificial lipid membranes was able to demonstrate ACh-induced ion fluxes (Lindstrom, 1997).

Nowadays, no one questions the structure and function of the AChR because it is known to be one of a family of ligand-gated receptors that have very similar topologies and homologous genetic and protein sequences (Karlin and Akabas, 1995; Lindstrom, 1997). The exact conformation of the AChR is not known, since it has not been crystallized, but the availability of *Torpedo* electric organ membranes with very high densities of the AChR has made it possible to obtain very detailed reconstructions from image analysis (Fig. 9.8*a*) (Miyazawa et al., 1999). Each AChR consists of five subunits, of which the α-subunit is represented twice. Each subunit has a large extracellular domain of approximately 210 amino acid residues and includes a disulphide bond between residues 128 and 142. In addition, the α-subunits have cysteines at residues 191 and 192 and can exist in at least six isoforms. Each subunit has four transmembrane domains, a large cytoplasmic region between transmembrane domains 3 and 4 and a short C-terminal tail (Fig. 9.8*b*). Although the second transmembrane domain, which lines the channel pore, is thought to be α-helix, the other transmembrane domains are probably β-sheets (see Karlin and Akabas, 1995).

Little is known about the actual conformation of the extracellualr domains, but the ACh binding sites are thought to lie buried in clefts between the α- and adjacent subunits (Fig. 9.8*a*). When ACh binds to both these sites, the subunits rotate in such a way as to open the channel pore. Cations, mainly sodium but also potassium in the reverse direction, are conducted through the pore and emerge, not through a single pore as previously thought, but through exits between the subunits (Fig. 9.8*a*). The mean time for which the channel is open can be estimated either by 'noise analysis', as first shown by Katz and Miledi (1970), or by single channel recordings (Sackmann and Neher, 1995). The latter technique makes it possible to measure accurately the conductance, that is the current through the AChR, the frequency of AChR channel openings and the duration of open times. These measurements, which have been made in human muscle by Milone et al. (1994) (see Fig. 9.7*b*), have become particularly relevant to human disease mechanisms since several groups have shown that mutations in the AChR subunits, principally the α-, δ- and β-subunits, can result in a 'slow-channel syndrome' in which the channel stays open too long, or in a 'fast-channel syndrome' in which it closes prematurely. These syndromes are discussed in Chapter 32.

Adult and fetal acetylcholine receptors

The fetal or embryonic AChRs behave differently to those at the mature NMJ, with a longer open time and smaller conductance. Mishina et al. (1976) were the first to show clearly that the difference resulted from the change from a γ-subunit to an ε-subunit (Fig. 9.8*c*). Interestingly, the ε-subunit is the most frequent target for genetic mutations that cause AChR deficiency in humans. It would appear that similar mutations in the other subunits, which are expressed during development rather than after formation of the NMJ, would be lethal or cause a more severe phenotype. One possible result of nonlethal mutations in the subunits that make up the fetal isoform would be arthrogryposis. Maternal antibodies specifically able to block the function of the fetal isoform can cross the placenta and cause fetal paralysis, with consequent fixed joint contractures (Vincent et al., 1995). Any mutation affecting the AChR that substantially reduced normal muscle function in utero might be expected to have similar consequences.

Competitive block of acetylcholine receptors

Substances such as d-tubocurarine block ACh binding. This can be partly overcome by increasing the concentration of ACh or by inhibiting AChE. Drugs such as vecuronium and atracurinum act similarly but with faster on and off rates, making them suitable as muscle relaxants in clinical practice. However, d-tubocurarine, and indeed many other substances, can also block the open channel itself if present in high concentration and at hyperpolarized potentials (Colquhoun, 1992; Wray, 1992).

A potentially important example of 'channel block' is the effect of quinine and related compounds (Sieb et al., 1996). This is beginning to be used in the treatment of slow-channel syndrome, in which the AChR ion channels stay open too long, possibly leading to excess calcium entry and an 'endplate myopathy' (Harper and Engel, 1998). However, quinine-like compounds should be used with caution in patients with compromised neuromuscular transmission, since any channel-blocking action could exacerbate their muscle weakness.

Depolarizing block and desensitization

Drugs that act as agonists and are not hydrolysed by AChE, or any agonist in the presence of AChE inhibitors, can also cause neuromuscular failure by producing persistent depolarization. This causes inactivation of the VGSCs, resulting in absence of an action potential. In addition, during prolonged application of such agonists, the AChR itself can become inactivated owing to desensitization (Katz and Thesleff, 1957). At low concentrations of agonists, this occurs very slowly, and under normal conditions of ACh release in the presence of AChE, desensitization is unlikely to occur. However, in the slow-channel syndromes in which the mutant AChRs appear to desensitize more easily, or in congenital AChE deficiency, desensitization may well contribute to neuromuscular failure. For futher discussion of the involvement of desensitization during block induced by depolarizing drugs, see Wray (1981) and Colquhoun (1992).

An interesting use of desensitization is to isolate the channels for more detailed investigation. During desensitization, there are occasional clusters of channel openings that arise when a single channel escapes from desensitization and acts in a normal, nondesensitized manner. By analysis of these clusters, it has been possible to investigate the activity of single channels even at high agonist concentrations (Colquhoun, 1992).

Voltage-gated calcium channels at the neuromuscular junction

There are many different molecular types of VGCC, which can be distinguished by their sensitivity to different drugs and toxins and which are present at different sites in the nervous system (reviewed in Olivera et al., 1994). Each VGCC consists of an α-subunit, which contains the channel pore, in association with β-, γ- and $\alpha_2\delta$-subunits. At the mature NMJ the main type is the P/Q-type, which contains an α_{1A}-subunit. The spider toxin agatoxin and the snail toxin ω-conotoxin MVIIC block this calcium channel and can inhibit neurotransmitter release (Protti et al., 1996). Immunofluorescent antibodies to the toxins can be used to demonstrate the distribution of the channels (Day et al., 1997). During development of the NMJ – and possibly in the

Lambert–Eaton syndrome, and under conditions of persistent or high-frequency stimulation, calcium entry through other calcium channels may contribute to stimulated release (Protti et al., 1991; Smith et al., 1995; Katz et al., 1996).

The P/Q-type of VGCC is the target for antibodies in Lambert–Eaton myasthenic syndrome (Vincent et al., 1989). The α_{1A}-subunit is mutated in familial hemiplegic migraine (Ophoff et al., 1996). Curiously, no obvious changes in neuromuscular function have been detected in patients with the latter disease; it may be that reduced function of this channel during development results in persistence of the N type or some other VGCC type. This would be analagous to the persistence of the AChR γ-subunit, which probably contributes to neuromuscular transmission in adults with mutations in the AChR ε-subunit (see Chapter 32).

Voltage-gated potassium channels at the neuromuscular junction

VGKCs are even more diverse than calcium channels; there are many different genes coding for VGKCs and potentially many different splice variants. Moreover, since each VGKC is made up of four distinct subunits, rather than a single subunit of four repeating domains as in VGCCs, in theory there could be literally hundreds of different VGKC types. However, some information on their make up can be deduced by looking at the sensitivity of the channels to different drugs and toxins. Tetraethylammonium (TEA) blocks most VGKCs and is effective in reducing VGKC currents at the NMJ, with consequent prolongation in the calcium-induced release of ACh. 4-Aminopyridine, or its less lipid-soluble analogue 3,4-diaminopyridine, is more selective, and the effects on neuromuscular transmission are mainly to prolong the depolarization leading to increased ACh release. Alpha-dendrotoxin, a snake toxin, and scorpion toxins such as charybdotoxin inhibit a variety of voltage-gated and calcium-activated potassium channels. Harvey and his colleagues have shown that these toxins mainly increase the amplitude of the EPPs, presumably by prolonging the duration of the nerve impulse and increasing calcium entry, and/or cause repetitive EPPs (Vantanpour and Harvey, 1995). Since the repetitive EPPs were prevented by tetrodotoxin, they were probably a consequence of repetitive action potentials in the motor nerve terminal resulting from reopening of the VGSC at the heminode during the prolonged depolarization (Anderson and Harvey, 1988). Similar events are thought to underlie the repetitive muscle action potentials that are found in acquired neuromyotonia, in which there are antibodies to VGKC (see Chapter 32). The sensitivity of different potassium channels to toxins and other substances is reviewed in detail by van der Kloot and Molgo (1994).

Acetylcholinesterase at the neuromuscular junction

AChE is a hydrolytic enzyme responsible for terminating the action of ACh at the NMJ. It consists of a A_{12} form in which three globular tetramers are each linked by one strand of a collagen tail, called ColQ, to the basal lamina (Massoulie et al., 1993). The enzyme can be inhibited at two sites. The active site is blocked by the alkaloid anticholinesterases, which act competitively and are reversible. The organophosphates phosphorylate the active site and the inhibition is irreversible. Many compounds bind to the peripheral site at the mouth of the catalytic gorge and alter the conformation of the molecule or modify its properties.

Inhibition of AChE enhances the duration of ACh in the synaptic cleft, leading to EPPs and MEPPs that are larger in amplitude and show prolonged decay phases. As a result of the persistent ACh, however, desensitization occurs during repetitive activity and neuromuscular transmission can become compromised. The importance of normal AChE function, in general, is demonstrated by the lack of any known mutations in the enzyme itself (the knock-out in mouse is embryonic lethal), and its role in neuromuscular transmission is demonstrated by the NMJ disorder associated with mutations in the collagen tail. These patients have normal globular enzyme and lack only the A_{12} NMJ form (see Chapter 32).

Voltage-gated sodium channels in muscle

VGSCs are made up of a single ion pore-containing subunit (like the VGCCs), are located in the depth of the postsynaptic folds and are responsible for initiating the action potential in the muscle. Like all sodium channels they are subject to inactivation by persistent depolarization. Consequently, in order to function correctly, they must be opened by rapid pulses of depolarization with long enough in between to provide an inactivation phase followed by reactivation. Any drug or condition that alters VGSC inactivation, like some scorpion and anemone toxins, can lead either to increased activity or to persistent depolarization, with consequent muscle weakness.

Pre- and postsynaptic modulation of neuromuscular transmission

Modulation of presynaptic function

There have been many studies over the last few years that have shown subtle effects on the processes of neuromuscular transmission by substances that modulate the function of a protein without binding directly to it. The best example is the effect of ACh released from the presynaptic nerve terminal modulating its own release. ACh acts not only on the postsynaptic AChRs, which are made up of $\alpha_1(2)\beta\varepsilon\delta$-subunits (i.e. two of the α_1-subunit isoform), but also on the presynaptic nerve terminal via nicotinic and muscarinic AChRs. Wessler and his colleagues showed that nerve-evoked release of metabolically labelled [^{3}H]-ACh is increased by ACh or exogenous substances acting on presynaptic nicotinic AChR receptors (reviewed in Wessler, 1996). This neuronal nicotinic receptor is thought to be either $\alpha_2\beta_2$ or $\alpha_4\beta_2$, both of which are encoded by genes different from those that encode the α_1-subunit of muscle AChR (Lindstrom, 1997).

It is not clear by what mechanism the autostimulation of ACh release occurs. Calcium entry through the nicotinic AChRs could contribute to calcium in the nerve terminal, increasing nerve-evoked release. Alternatively, calcium may activate or alter a second messenger pathway that would otherwise reduce release. The presence of this autoreceptor on the nerve terminal explains the action of d-tubocurarine and the apparent decrease in EPP amplitude that occurs during a train of impulses in the presence of the nicotinic-blocking drug, since it would also block the release-enhancing effect of ACh (see also below).

There are also presynaptic muscarinic AChRs that are activated by nerve-evoked ACh and lead to a reduction in ACh release and, conversely, muscarinic AChRs that become active over longer periods of nerve stimulation, when their activation increases release. Muscarinic AChRs are a family of receptors with seven transmembrane domains and are linked to G-proteins. Their effects are probably determined by G-protein stimulation of an intracellular kinase followed by phosphorylation of components of the release mechanism or of the VGCCs themselves.

ACh release is also increased by stimulation of adrenergic receptors on the nerve terminal. These probably act via α_1-adrenoceptors and may cause stimulation of calcium entry through L-type calcium channels, since nifedipine, which acts on these channels, inhibits the effects of phenylephrine. Beta-adrenoceptors may be linked to activation of N-type calcium channels. Ephedrine-like drugs have been used to treat patients with myasthenic syndromes, presumably because they increase ACh release, but it should be noted that they can also block AChRs (Milone and Engel, 1996).

ATP is co-released with ACh from the synaptic vesicles and can act on two different presynaptic receptors. In one case, ATP itself is thought to act via purinergic receptors. In the other, adenosine produced from ATP by adenosine deaminase, acts on its own receptors. Both ATP and adenosine reduce ACh release, but the exact pathways involved are not known (Redman and Silensky, 1994).

Finally, calcitonin-gene related peptide (CGRP) is released from dense-cored vesicles that are present at the NMJ and activates CGRP receptors on the nerve terminal. It is thought that CGRP release only occurs during sustained or high-frequency stimulations, perhaps because under these conditions N- or L-type VGCCs are opened, leading to a more persistent, and less local, release of vesicles.

The relevance of these autoregulatory mechanisms (summarized in Fig. 9.9a) is not entirely clear, although it does appear that ACh seeks to modify its own release and prevent excessive postsynaptic activation. Since too much ACh can cause postsynaptic desensitization or depolarization block, this may be important. However, in myasthenic conditions it would be helpful for ACh release to be increased. In myasthenia gravis, or a pharmacological experimental myasthenia gravis induced by chronic administration of α-bungarotoxin, there is an increase in ACh release (Cull-Candy et al., 1980; Plomp et al., 1995). The increase in release was greatest at the endplates that had the smallest MEPPs, suggesting a compensatory mechanism (Plomp et al., 1995). Plomp and Molenaar (1996) found that tyrosine kinase inhibitors decreased the frequency and amplitude of MEPPs in mice treated with α-bungarotoxin, suggesting that tyrosine kinases modify the membrane properties both presynaptically (increasing MEPP frequency) and postsynaptically (increasing MEPP amplitudes). Upregulation of quantal release from the presynaptic nerve appeared to be dependent on calcium-calmodulin-dependent protein kinase II, since inhibitors of the kinase reduced release at those endplates where the compensatory mechanism was operating. This kinase is known to be involved in the mobilization of vesicles from their association with actin (see above), and increased activity should provide increased availability of transmitter.

An important question, in these and other related studies, is how does the presynaptic nerve terminal know that the postsynaptic efficacy of ACh is reduced? It is likely that there are retrograde signals from the muscle to the nerve that continually provide feedback information, both during development and during adult life (see van der Kloot and Molgo, 1994). Nitric oxide made in the postsynaptic cytoplasm at the NMJ, and diffusing to the presynaptic nerve terminal, is one possible retrograde signal; there are undoubtedly many others.

Modulation of postsynaptic function

ACh acts on the nicotinic AChR ($\alpha_1(2)\beta\delta\varepsilon$-subunits) at the NMJ to induce EPPs and the muscle action potentials. However, there is increasing evidence for other receptors postsynaptically. CGRP released from the motor nerve acts

(a)

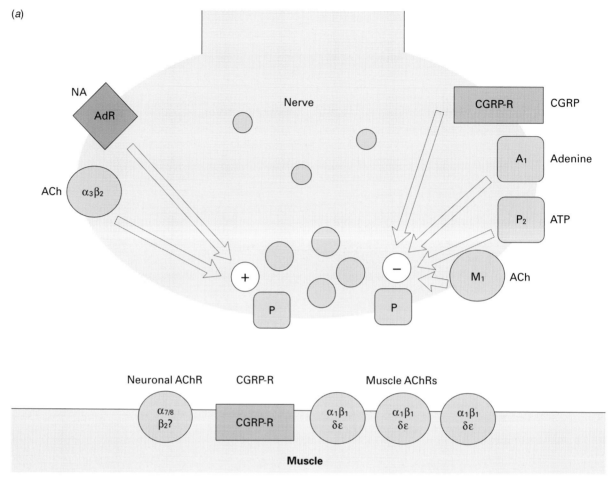

Fig. 9.9. Pre- and postsynaptic modulation of the function of the neuromuscular junction. (a) The nerve terminal contains receptors (R) for acetylcholine (ACh), ATP (which is co-released with ACh), adenosine (Ad) (resulting from breakdown of ATP), calcitonin gene-related peptide (CGRP) (released from dense-core vesicles) and adrenaline (NA). These probably modulate ACh release, either positively or negatively, by activating second messengers and altering VGCC function, by changing the availability of the synaptic vesicles or by the calcium sensitivity of the release process. (b) CGRP may also activate protein kinase A (PKA) postsynaptically, leading to priming of neuronal AChRs. ACh can bind to these neuronal receptors (possibly $\alpha_{7/8}\beta_2$), leading to calcium influx, which causes release of calcium from internal stores. Calcium activates protein kinase C (PKC), which can phosphorylate the AChRs, leading to desensitization and decreased postsynaptic sensitivity to ACh. Thus ACh and CGRP probably act in concert to reduce AChR sensitivity (Kimura et al., 1998).

on postsynaptic receptors to increase AChR synthesis (New and Mudge, 1986; Mule at al., 1988). This pathway involves a protein kinase linked through a G-protein and should also lead to AChR phosphorylation. AChR phosphorylation generally leads to increased desensitization and reduced function (Huganir and Greengard, 1990). In a series of papers, Kimura and his colleagues have produced evidence for a postsynaptic neuronal type AChR, perhaps utliizing an α_7- or α_8-subunit isoform, acting in concert with other receptors to modulate postsynaptic activity (Fig. 9.9b). The existence of these pathways is of potential clinical relevance because of their possible involvement in seronegative myasthenia gravis. In this condition, in which no antibodies to the postsynaptic AChR can be found, it is thought that there are other antibodies to a membrane target that indirectly affect AChR function (Vincent et al., 1998). Although the CGRP receptor would be a prime candidate target for these antibodies, the antibodies in seronegative myasthenia gravis do not appear to work via this pathway, and other potential membrane receptors are being sought. The neuronal postsynaptic AChR depicted in Fig. 9.9, or even the MuSK or the ErbB receptors involved in NMJ development and maintenance (Fig. 9.5b), are other possible candidates.

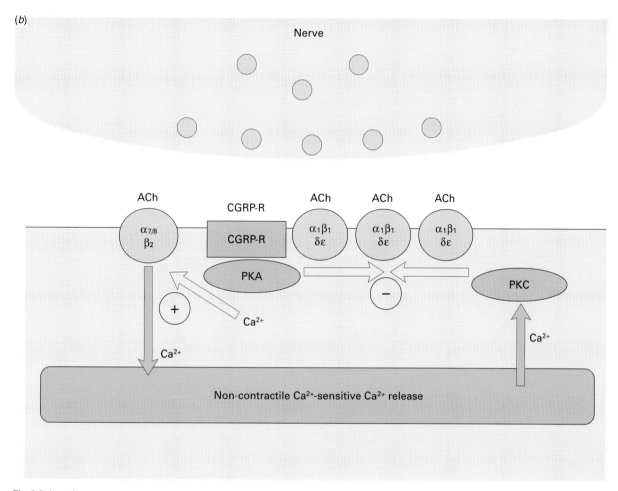

(b)

Fig. 9.9. (*cont.*)

Facilitation and depression

During or after trains of nerve stimuli, the amplitudes of the EPPs do not necessarily remain the same but can increase or decrease depending on various factors. Under normal conditions, when the nerve is stimulated at high frequency there is a decrease in amplitude of successive EPPs. This is not caused by a postsynaptic effect (such as desensitization) because the amplitude of the MEPPs remains the same. There may be depletion of ACh during high stimulation frequencies. However, most early experiments were done in the presence of d-tubocurarine, and it is now clear that there are subtle effects of d-tubocurarine on ACh release, caused by blocking of autoreceptors on the nerve terminal that are activated by released ACh (see above). Thus the depression is probably caused by inhibition by d-tubocurarine of a normal action of ACh on the presynaptic terminal that would seek to keep the quantal content constant during repetitive firing (Ferry and Kelly, 1988; Hong and Chang, 1991).

Facilitation, an increase in the EPPs during a train of stimuli, occurs principally when the EPP is small to begin with and results from accumulation of calcium within the nerve terminal during successive stimuli. It decays very rapidly and is not seen if the stimulus frequency is low because free calcium is rapidly cleared from the cytoplasm. Augmentation and post-tetanic potentiation are two other phenomena that are characterized by increased transmitter release. Augmentation lasts about 10 seconds, while potentiation lasts for several minutes. Since these can occur in calcium-free solutions, they are probably not related to influx of calcium but perhaps to some change in the number of quanta available for release together with changes in cytoplasmic calcium released from intracellular stores.

Neuromuscular transmission in health and disease

Successful neuromuscular transmission depends on release from the motor nerve terminal of sufficient ACh to induce an EPP that will open enough VGSCs to initiate a muscle action potential. The threshold for neuromuscular transmission is the membrane potential at which sufficient VGSCs open, and the safety factor for neuromuscular transmission is defined as the extent to which the amplitude of the EPP exceeds the threshold. Disorders of neuromuscular transmission can be identified by the physiological changes that occur; the main findings in a number of disorders are summarized in Table 9.5.

The EPP amplitude is determined principally by the number of packets of ACh released, the quantal content and by the postsynaptic response to each packet. The threshold probably varies between species, depending on the number, distribution and properties of the VGSCs. Consequently, there are three major determinants of successful transmission: the quantal content or number of packets of ACh released, the postsynaptic response to ACh and the density and voltage-dependency of the VGSCs. It is worth noting that, in addition to situations that directly affect these processes, ACh release will also be influenced by the nerve terminal membrane potential and the ACh sensitivity. The activity of the VGSCs will be influenced by the muscle resting membrane potential. These in turn can be affected by changes in external ions, VGSC, VGKC or chloride channel activity or in the Na^+/K^+ exchange, which underlies the electrochemical gradient that determines the membrane potential (see Aidley, 1999).

The quantal content can be altered by many factors (van der Kloot and Molgo, 1994) particularly conditions that reduce calcium entry. For instance, the quantal content will be reduced if there are fewer calcium channels, if their distribution at the active zones is disrupted, as occurs in the Lambert–Eaton myasthenic syndrome, or if there are changes in the release mechanisms, as in botulinum poisoning. Moreover, although the nerve action potential is usually considered to be an 'all-or-none' phenomenon, during application of tetrodotoxin, the quantal content decreases slowly rather than in an all-or-none fashion, indicating that a reduction in nerve depolarization during nerve stimulation can also reduce quantal release (M. Busby and A. Vincent unpublished observations, 1998).

If the postsynaptic membrane or the AChRs are reduced in number, the EPP may be too small to exceed the threshold. In myasthenia gravis, where there are antibodies to the AChRs, or in the inherited AChR deficiency syndrome, the number of AChRs is reduced and the postsynaptic effect of

each packet will be reduced, leading to small MEPPs. Similar results are found in individuals bitten by snakes or other venomous species that make postsynaptic neurotoxins.

Altered geometry of the NMJ will contribute to changes in the threshold for activation of the muscle action potential because of changes in the number or density of VGSCs. Slater et al. (1992) have discussed this particularly in relation to human neuromuscular transmission and its disorders. The ACh-induced depolarization of the motor endplate is retained, rather than dispersed, by the postsynaptic folds, channelling the depolarization towards the VGSCs that are located at the bottom of the folds. The folds not only retain the depolarization but, by virtue of their increased membrane area, are able to contain a large number of VGSCs (Wood and Slater, 1997). The threshold for activation of an action potential is lower at the NMJ than outside it, such that the EPP in mouse, at least, only has to depolarize the postsynaptic membrane to around $-60\,mV$ (from a resting potential of around $-80\,mV$) for an action potential to occur (Wood and Slater, 1995). Therefore, neuromuscular transmission should be particularly efficient in those species that have a great deal of postsynaptic folds and may be less efficient, or require larger quantal contents, in those in which postsynaptic folds are few. In human muscle, with very marked folds, the NMJ is probably very efficient, requiring only 20 or so packets of ACh. Nevertheless, it is not yet clear exactly what the threshold for activation of the VGSCs is in humans, and why the folding is so much greater than in other species. There are congenital myasthenic syndromes in which the folding is specifically reduced, and in many others reduced folds seems to be a secondary event (perhaps related to decreased utrophin, see Deconinck et al., 1997); these changes alone may be sufficient to compromise neuromuscular transmission.

In myasthenia gravis and its experimental model, the EPPs are reduced in amplitude because of the reduced numbers of AChRs. However, it has been reported that the quantal content is raised (Cull-Candy et al., 1980; Plomp et al., 1995), probably as a compensatory process. Therefore, it is not altogether clear why the patients are weak. One possibility is that the loss of postsynaptic folds decreases the efficiency by which the EPP activates VGSCs. Ruff and Lennon (1998) found that activation of VGSCs was reduced in muscle from patients with myasthenia gravis, leading to an increase in the amount of postsynaptic depolarization required to initiate an action potential. This provides an explanation for the patients' weakness despite the compensatory increase in ACh release. It seems possible that treatment of neuromuscular transmission disorders

Table 9.5. Neuromuscular transmission in disease

Disease	Pathological mechanism	Physiological hallmark	Functional effects	Consequence	Modifiers and pharmacological treatments
Autoantibody-mediated disorders					
Lambert–Eaton myasthenic syndrome	Antibodies to P-type VGCCs	Reduced EPPs; normal MEPP amplitudes	Reduced ACh release	Weakness	Improves following tetanus or sustained voluntary contraction; improves with anticholinesterases and 3,4-diaminopyridine
Myasthenia gravis	Antibodies to AChRs	Reduced EPP and MEPP amplitudes	Reduced AChR sensitivity of postsynaptic membrane	Weakness	Deteriorates during sustained contraction; improves with anticholinesterases and 3,4-diaminopyridine
Acquired neuromyotonia	Antibodies to VGKCs	Not yet studied in humans	Increased neuronal activity Repetitive EPPs	Muscle cramps and pseudomyotonia, also weakness	Improved by antiepileptic treatments
Genetic disorders					
AChR deficiency	Mutations in AChRs: mostly ε-subunit deficiency	Reduced EPP and MEPP amplitudes	Reduced postsynaptic activity	Weakness	Deteriorates during sustained contraction; improves with anticholinesterases and 3,4-diaminopyridine
Slow-channel syndrome	Mutations in AChRs α-, β- or δ-subunits causing prolonged openings	Prolonged EPP and MEPP time courses; very long AChR channel openings	Increased postsynaptic activity	Weakness and wasting, probably owing to desensitization, depolarization block and endplate myopathy	Made worse by anticholinesterases; quinine-like drugs may be helpful
Fast-channel syndrome	Mutations in AChRs	Reduced MEPP amplitudes and very short AChR channel openings	Reduced postsynaptic activity	Weakness	Improves with anticholinesterases and 3,4-diaminopyridine

Notes:
EPP, endplate potential; MEPP, miniature EPP; other abbreviations as in Table 9.2.

could be aimed at increasing VGSC function, as well as increasing the EPP size.

A complication is introduced when there is overactivity of neuromuscular transmission. In conditions such as the slow-channel syndrome, AChE deficiency or acquired neuromyotonia, in each of which one expects excessive or prolonged AChR activity, weakness is often a predominant symptom. The explanation for this must depend on one or a combination of different phenomena. In the case of acquired neuromyotonia, the changes are thought to be the result of reduced numbers of VGKCs, with consequent prolonged depolarization of the motor nerve terminal and excessive ACh release. In AChE deficiency, or in anti-AChE intoxication, there will be persistence of ACh after its release. In each of these situations, densensitization of the AChR may occur and lead to reduced postsynaptic activity. This is even more likely to occur in patients with the slow-channel syndrome, since these mutant AChRs show increased desensitization. Alternatively, and perhaps in parallel, excessive action of ACh on normally functioning AChRs will lead to persistent depolarization with inactivation of the VGSCs, similar to that which occurs with depolarizing blockers such as suxamethonium. A third pathogenic mechanism by which increased AChR activity can lead to muscle weakness is that excess entry of calcium through the AChR can lead to changes in cellular activity, with endplate damage. This route to an 'endplate myopathy' is thought to be responsible for weakness and wasting in the slow-channel syndrome, and probably also in congenital AChE deficiency (see Chapter 32).

Neuromuscular transmission in critically ill patients

Muscle wasting and weakness is, not surprisingly, common in patients in intensive care units and is usually attributed to immobilization with myofibrillar degeneration, use of specific drugs such as steroids and muscle relaxants or the development of a neuropathy. However, patients with burns and endotoxicosis show decreased rather than increased sensitivity to nondepolarizing relaxants such as d-tubocurarine and increased sensitivity to depolarizing relaxants such as succinylcholine. These phenomena appear in some patients to result from upregulation of AChR numbers at the NMJ, as shown in animal models (Hogue et al.,1990; Martyn et al., 1992). Strangely, antibodies to AChR have been reported in an experimental model of sepsis (Tzukagoshi et al., 1999), so the relationship between critical illness, sepsis and neuromuscular function is not yet clear (Martyn and Vincent, 1999). It should be interesting to compare the results in experimental animals with the effects of acute phase proteins or other substances that might be able to modulate neuromuscular transmission.

Acknowledgement

I am grateful to Dr Y. Liyanage for critical reading of the manuscript.

References

Aidley, D. J. (1999). *The Physiology of Excitable Cells.* Cambridge: Cambridge University Press.

Anderson, A. J. and Harvey, A. I. (1988). Effects of the potassium channel blocking dendrotoxins on acetylcholine release and motor nerve terminal activity. *Br. J. Pharmacol.* **93**, 215–221.

Askanas, V., King Engel, W. and Alvarez, R. B. (1998). Fourteen newly recognised proteins at the human neuromuscular junctions – and their nonjunctional accumulation in inclusion-body myositis. *Ann. N. Y. Acad. Sci. USA* **841**, 28–56.

Bewick, G. S., Young, C. and Slater, C. R. (1996). Spatial relationships of utrophin, dystrophin, β-dystroglycan and β-spectrin to acetylcholine receptor clusters during postnatal maturation of the rat neuromuscular junction. *J. Neurocytol.* **25**, 267–279.

Bowen, D. C., Park, J. S., Bodine, S. et al. (1998). Localization and regulation of MuSK at the neuromuscular junction. *Dev. Biol.* **199**, 309–319.

Chao, D. S., Silvagno, F., Xia, H., Cornwell, T. L., Lincoln, T. M. and Bredt, D. S. (1997). Nitric oxide synthase and cyclic GMP-dependent protein kinase concentrated at the neuromuscular endplate. *Neuroscience* **76**, 665–72

Colquhoun, D. (1992). Agonists, antagonists and synaptic transmission at the neuromuscular junction. In: *Neuromuscular Transmission: Basic and Applied Aspects*, eds. A. Vincent and D. Wray, p. 132. Oxford: Pergamon.

Cull-Candy, S. C., Miledi, R., Trautmann, A. and Uchitel, O. D. (1980). On the release of transmitter at normal, myasthenia gravis and myasthenic syndrome affected human end-plates. *J. Physiol.* **299**, 621.

Day, N. C., Wood, S. J., Ince, P. G. et al. (1997). Differential localization of voltage dependent calcium channel alpha 1 subunits at the human and rat neuromuscular junction. *J. Neurosci.* **17**, 6226–6235.

De Camilli, P. and Takei, K. (1996). Molecular mechanisms in synaptic vesicle endocytosis and recycling. *Neuron* **16**, 481–486

De Chiara, T. M., Bowen, D. C., Valenzuela, D. M. et al. (1996). The receptor tyrosine kinase MuSK is required for neuromuscular junction formation in vivo. *Cell* **85**, 501–512.

Deconinck, A. E., Potter, A. C., Tinsley, J. M. et al. (1997). Postsynaptic abnormalities at the neuromuscular junctions of utrophin-deficient mice. *J. Cell Biol.* **136**, 883–894.

Del Castillo, J. and Katz, B. (1954). Quantal components of the endplate potential. *J. Physiol.* **124**, 560–575.

Dodge, F. A. and Rahaminoff, R. (1967). On the relationship between calcium concentration and the amplitude of the end-plate potential. *J. Physiol.* **189**, 90P–92P.

Fambrough, D. M. (1979). Control of acetylcholine receptors in skeletal muscle. *Physiolog. Rev.* **59**, 165–227.

Ferry, C. B. and Kelly, S. S. (1988). The nature of the presynaptic effects of +-tubocurarine at the mouse neuromuscular junction. *J. Physiol.* **403**, 425–437.

Froehner, S. C., Luetje, C. W., Scotland, P. B. and Patrick, J. (1990). The postsynaptic 43K protein clusters muscle nicotinic acetylcholine receptors in *Xenopus* oocytes. *Neuron* **5**, 403–410.

Gautam, M., Noakes, P. G., Mudd, J. et al. (1995). Failure of postsynaptic specialisation to develop at neuromuscular junctions of rapsyn-deficient mice. *Nature* **377**, 232–236.

Gautam, M., Noakes, P. G., Moscoso, L., et al. (1996). Defective neuromuscular synaptogenesis in agrin-deficient mutant mice. *Cell* **85**, 525–535.

Hall, Z. W. and Sanes, J. R. (1993). Synaptic structure and development: the neuromuscular junction. *Cell* **72**, 99–121.

Harlow, M., Ress, D., Koster, A., Marshall, R. M., Schwarz, M. and McMahan, U. J. (1998). Dissection of active zones at the neuromuscular junction by EM tomography. *J. Physiol. (Paris)* **92**, 75–78.

Harper, C. M. and Engel, A. G. (1998). Quinidine sulfate therapy for the slow-channel congenital myasthenic syndrome. *Ann. Neurol.* **43**, 480–184.

Hesselmans, L. F. G. M., Jennekens, F. G. I., van den Oord, C. J. M., Veldman, H. and Vincent, A. (1993). Development of innervation of skeletal muscle fibres in man: relation to acetylcholine receptors. *Anat. Rec.* **236**, 553–562.

Heuser, J. E. (1989). Review of electron microscopic evidence favouring vesicle exocytosis as the structural basis for quantal release during synaptic transmission. *Q. J. Exp. Physiol.* **74**, 1051–1069.

Hirokawa, N., Sobue, K., Kanda, K., Harada, A. and Yorifuji, H. (1989). The cytoskeletal architecture of the presynaptic terminal and molecular structure of synapsin 1. *J. Cell Biol.* **108**, 111–126.

Hogue, C. H., Itani, M. and Martyn, J. A. J. (1990). Resistance to d-tubocurarine in lower motor neuron injury is related to increased acetylcholine receptors at the neuromuscular junction. *Anaesthesiology* **73**, 703–709.

Hong, S. J. and Chang, C. C. (1989). Use of geographutoxin II (μ-conotoxin) for the study of neuromuscular transmission in mouse. *Br. J. Pharmacol.* **97**, 934–940.

Hong, S. J. and Chang, C. C. (1991). Run-down of neuromuscular transmission during repetitive nerve activity by nicotinic antagonists is not due to desensitization of the postsynaptic receptor. *Br. J. Pharmacol.* **102**, 817–822.

Huganir, R. L. and Greengard, P. (1990). Regulation of neurotransmitter receptor desensitization by phosphorylation. *Neuron* **5**, 555–567.

Hurlbut, W. P. and Ceccarelli, B. (1979). Use of black widow spider venom to study the release of neurotransmitters. In: *Advances in Cytopharmacology*, pp. 87–115. New York: Raven.

Hurlbut, W. P., Iezzi, M., Fresce, R. and Ceccarelli, B. (1990). Correlation between quantal secretion and vesicle loss at the frog neuromuscular junction. *J. Physiol.* **425**, 501–526

Jankovic, J. and Brin, M. F. (1997). Botulinum toxin: historical prospective and potential new indications. *Muscle Nerve Suppl.* **6**, S129–S145.

Karlin, A. and Akabas, M. H. (1995). Toward a structural basis for the function of nicotinic acetylcholine receptors and their cousins. *Neuron* **15**, 1231–1244

Katz, B. and Miledi, R. (1970). Membrane noise produced by acetylcholine. *Nature* **226**, 962–963.

Katz, B. and Thesleff, S. (1957). A study of the desensitisation produced by cetylcholine at the motor endplate. *J. Physiol.* **138**, 63–80.

Katz, E., Ferro, P. A., Weisz, G. and Uchitel, O. D. (1996). Calcium channels involved in synaptic transmission at the mature and regenerating mouse neuromuscular junction. *J. Physiol.* **497**, 687–697.

Kimura, I. (1998). Calcium-dependent desensitising function of the postsynaptic neuronal-type nicotinic acetylcholine receptors at the neuromuscular junction. *Pharmacol. Therapeut.* **77**, 183–202.

Koike, S., Schaeffer, L. and Changeux, J. P. (1995). Identification of DNA element determining synaptic expression of the mouse acetylcholine receptor alpha-subunit gene. *Proc. Natl. Acad. Sci. USA* **92**, 10624–10628.

Lindstrom, J. (1997). Nicotinic acetylcholine receptors in health and disease. *Mol. Neurobiol.* **15**, 193–222.

Llinas, R., Sugimori, M. and Silver, R. B. (1995). The concept of calcium-concentration microdomains in synaptic transmission. *Neuropharmacology* **34**, 1443–1451

Lomo, T. and Westgaard, R. H. (1975). Control of ACh sensitivity in rat muscle fibres *Cold Spring Harb. Symp. Quant. Biol.* **40**, 263–274.

Martyn, J. A. and Vincent, A. (1999). A new twist to myopathy of critical illness. *Anaesthesiology* **91**, 337–339.

Martyn, J. A. J., White, D. A., Gronert, G. A., Jaffe, R. and Ward, J. M. (1992). Up and down regulation of acetylcholine receptors: effects on neuromuscular blockers. *Anaesthesiology* **76**, 822–843.

Massoulie, J., Pezzementi, L., Bon, S., Krejci, E. and Vallette, F. M. (1993). Molecular and cellular biology of cholinesterase. *Prog. Neurobiol.* **43**, 31–93.

McMahan, U. K. (1990). The agrin hypothesis. *Cold Spring Harb. Symp. Quant. Biol.* **55**, 407–418.

Milone, M. and Engel, A. G. (1996). Block of the endplate acetylcholine receptor channel by the sympathomimetic agents ephedrine, pseudoephedrine and albuterol. *Brain Res.* **740**, 346–352.

Milone, M., Hutchinson, D. O. and Engel, A. G. (1994). Patch clamp analysis of the properties of acetylcholine receptor channels at the normal human endplate. *Muscle Nerve* **17**, 1364–1369.

Mirsky, R. and Jessen, K. R. (1999). The neurobiology of Schwann cells. *Brain Res.* **9**, 293–311.

Mishina, M., Takai, T., Imoto, K. et al. (1976). Molecular distinction between fetal and adult forms of muscle acetylcholine receptor. *Nature* **321**, 406–411.

Missias, A. C., Chu, G. C., Klocke, B., Sanes, J. R. and Merlie, J. P. (1986). Maturation of the acetylcholine receptor in developing skeletal muscle: regulation of the AChR γ to ε switch. *Dev. Biol.* **179**, 223–238.

Miyazawa, A., Fujiyoshi, Y., Stowell, M. and Unwin, N. (1999). Nicotinic acetylcholine receptor at 4.6 A resolution: transverse funnels in the channel wall. *J. Mol. Biol.* **288**, 765–786.

Molenaar, P. C. (1992). Synthesis, storage and release of acetylcholine. In *The Neuromuscular Junction*, eds. A. Vincent and D. Wray, pp. 62–81. Oxford: Pergamon Press.

Mulle, C., Benoit, P., Pinset, C., Roa, M. and Changeux, J.-P. (1988). Calcitonin gene-related peptide enhances the rate of desensitisation of the nicotinic acetylcholine receptor in cultured mouse muscle cells. *Proc. Natl. Acad. Sci. USA* **85**, 5728–5732.

New, H. V. and Mudge, A. W. (1986). Calcitonin gene related peptide regulates muscle acetylcholine receptor synthesis. *Nature* **323**, 809–811.

Noakes, P. G., Philips, W. E., Hanley, T. A., Sanes, J. R. and Merlie, J. P. (1993). 43K protein and acetylcholine receptors colocalize during the initial stages of neuromuscular synapse formation in vivo. *Dev. Biol.* **155**, 275–280.

Noakes, P. G., Gautam, M., Mudd, J., Sanes, J. R. and Merlie, J. P. (1995). Aberrant differentiation of neuromuscular junction in mice lacking S-laminin/laminin β2. *Nature* **374**, 258–262.

Olivera, B. M., Miljanich, G. P., Ramachandran, J. and Adams, M. E. (1994). Calcium channel diversity and neurotransmitter release. *Annu. Rev. Biochem.* **63**, 823–867.

Ophoff, R. A., Terwindt, G. M., Vergouwe, M. N. et al. (1996). Familial hemiplegic migraine and episodic ataxia types are caused by mutations in the Ca^{2+} channel gene, CACNL1A4. *Cell* **87**, 543–552.

Plomp, J. J. and Molenaar, P. C. (1996). Involvement of protein kinases in the upregulation of acetylcholine release at endplates of α-bungarotoxin-treated rats. *J. Physiol.* **493**, 175–186.

Plomp, J. J., Van-Kempen, G. T. H., De Baets, M., Graus, Y. M. F., Kuks, J. B. M. and Molenaar, P. C. (1995). Acetylcholine release in myasthenia gravis: regulation at single end-plate level. *Ann. Neurol.* **37**, 627–636.

Plomp, J. L., Molenaar, P. C., O'Hanlon, G. M. et al. (1999). Miller Fisher anti-GQ1b antibodies: α-latrotoxin like effects on motor end plates. *Ann. Neurol.* **45**, 189–199.

Protti, D. A., Szczupak, L., Scornik, F. S. and Uchitel, O. D. (1991). Effect of ω-conotoxin GVIA on neurotransmitter release at the mouse neuromuscular junction. *Brain Res.* **557**, 336–339.

Protti, D. A., Reisin, R., Mackinley, T. A. and Uchitel, O. D. (1996). Calcium channel blockers and transmitter release at the normal human neuromuscular junction. *Neurology* **46**, 1391–1396.

Redman, R. S. and Silinsky, E. M. (1994). ATP released together with acetylcholine as the mediator of neuromuscular depression at frog motor nerve endings. *J. Physiol.* **477**, 117–127.

Ruff, R. L. and Lennon, V. A. (1998). End-plate voltage-gated sodium channels are lost in clinical and experimental myasthenia gravis. *Ann. Neurol.* **43**, 370–379.

Sackmann, B. and Neher, E. (eds.) (1995). *Single Channel Recording*, 2nd edn, New York: Plenum Press.

Salpeter, M. M. and Loring, R. H. (1985). Nicotinic acetylcholine receptors in vertebrate muscle: properties, distribution and neural control. *Prog. Neurobiol.* **25**, 297–325.

Salpeter, M. M., Marchaterre, M. and Harris, R. (1988). Distribution of extrajunctional acetylcholine receptors on a vertebrate muscle: evaluated by using a scanning electron microscope autoradiographic procedure. *J. Cell Biol.* **106**, 2087–2093.

Sandrock, A. W., Dryer, S. E., Rosen, K. M. et al. (1997). Maintenance of acetylcholine receptor number by neuregulins. *Science* **276**, 599–603.

Sanes, J. R. and Lichtman, J. W. (1999). Development of the vertebrate neuromuscular junction *Annu. Rev. Neurosci.* **22**, 389–442.

Sanes, J. R. and Scheller, R. H. (1997). Synapse formation: a molecular prospective. In: *Developmental Neurobiology*, eds. W. M. Cowan, S. L. Zipursky and T. H. Jessel, pp. 179–219. New York: Oxford University Press.

Sanes, J. R., Marshall, L. M. and McMahan, U. J. (1978). Reinnervation of muscle fibre basal lamina after removal of myofibres. *J. Cell Biol.* **78**, 176–(198.

Sieb, J. P., Milone, M. and Engel, A. G. (1996). Effects of the quinoline derivatives quinine, quinidine, and chloroquine on neuromuscular transmission. *Brain Res.* **712**, 179–189.

Slater, C. R., Lyons, P. R., Walls, T. H., Fawcett, P. R. W. and Young, C. (1992). Structure and function of neuromuscular junctions in the vastus lateralis of man. *Brain* **115**, 451–478.

Slater, C. R., Young, C., Wood, S. J. et al. (1997). Utrophin abundance is reduced at neuromuscular junctions of patients with both inherited and acquired acetylcholine receptor deficiencies. *Brain* **120**, 1513–1531.

Smith, D. O., Conklin, M. W., Jensen, P. H. and Atchison, W. D. (1995). Decreased calcium currents in motor nerve terminals of mice with Lambert–Eaton myasthenic syndrome. *J. Physiol.* **487**, 115–123.

Smith, S. J. and Augustine, G. J. (1988). Calcium ions, active zones and synaptic transmitter release. *Trends Neurosci.* **11**, 458–464.

Stanley, E. F. (1993). Single calcium channels and acetylcholine release at a presynaptic nerve terminal. *Neuron* **11**, 585–591

Sudhof, T. C. (1995). The synaptic vesicle cycle: a cascade of protein-protein interactions. *Nature* **375**, 645–653.

Tzukagoshi, H., Morita, J., Takahashi, K., Kunimoto, K. and Goto, F. (1999). A cecal ligation and puncture peritonitis model shows decreased nicotinic acetylcholine receptor numbers in rat muscle: immunopathologic mechanisms? *Anaesthesiology* **91**, 448–460.

Usdin, T. B., Eiden, L. E., Bonner, T. I. and Erickson, J. D. (1995). Molecular biology of the ACh transporter. *Trends Neurosci.* **18**, 218–224.

van der Kloot, W. and Molgo, J. (1994). Quantal acetylcholine release at the vertebrate neuromuscular junction. *Physiol. Rev.* **74**, 899–991.

Vantanpour, H. and Harvey, A. L. (1995). Modulation of acetylcholine release at mouse neuromuscular junctions by interaction of three homologous scorpion toxins with K^+ channels. *Br. J. Pharmacol.* **114**, 1502–1506.

Vincent, A. and Wray, D. (eds.) (1992). *Neuromuscular Transmission: Basic and Applied Aspects.* Oxford: Pergamon.

Vincent, A., Lang, B. and Newsom-Davis, J. (1989). Autoimmunity to the voltage-gated calcium channel underlies the Lambert–Eaton myasthenic syndrome, a paraneoplastic disorder. *Trends Neurosci.* **12**, 496–502.

Vincent, A., Newland, C., Brueton, L. et al. (1995). Arthrogryposis multiplex congenita with maternal autoantibodies specific for a fetal antigen. *Lancet* **346**, 24–25.

Vincent, A., Jacobson, L., Plested, P. et al. (1998). Antibodies affecting ion channel function in acquired neuromyotonia, in seropositive and seronegative myasthenia gravis, and in antibody-mediated artrhogryposis multiplex congenita. *Ann. N. Y. Acad. Sci. USA* **841**, 482–496.

Wessler, I. (1996). Acetylcholine release at motor endplates and autonomic neuroeffector junctions: a comparison. *Pharmacol. Res.* **33**, 81–94.

Wood, S. J. and Slater, C. R. (1995). Action potential generation in rat slow- and fast-twitch muscles. *J. Physiol.* **486**, 401–410.

Wood, S. J. and Slater, C. R. (1997). The contribution of postsynaptic folds to the safety factor for neuromuscular transmission in rat fast-and slow-twitch muscles. *J. Physiol.* **500**, 165–176.

Wood, S. J. and Slater, C. R. (1998). β-Spectrin is colocalized with both voltage-gated sodium channels and ankyrin G at the adult rat neuromuscular junction. *J. Cell Biol.* **140**, 675–684.

Wood, S. J., Shewry, K., Young, C. and Slater, C. R. (1998). An early stage in sodium channel clustering at developing rat neuromuscular junctions. *NeuroReport* **9**, 1991–1995.

Wray, D. (1981). Prolonged exposure to acetylcholine:noise analysis and channel inactivation in cat tenuissimus muscle. *J. Physiol.* **310**, 37

Wray, D. (1992). Neuromuscular transmission. In: *Disorders of Voluntary Muscle*, eds. I. Walton, G. Karpati and D. Hilton-Jones, pp. 139–178. Edinburgh: Churchill Livingstone.

10

The pathophysiology of excitation in skeletal muscle

Robert L. Barchi

Introduction

Although the generation of force in skeletal muscle ultimately reflects the chemical interaction of actin and myosin, useful muscular activity can only occur when this chemical interaction is faithfully coupled to the electrical activity of a motor neuron. This coupling is provided by the propagation of regenerative spikes or action potentials along the muscle sarcolemma; these impulses originate in the region of the endplate and subsequently spread across the entire muscle surface, eventually penetrating into the fibre interior along the elements of the T-tubular network. At membrane specializations known as triads, the T-tubular elements interact closely with the terminal cisternae of the sarcoplasmic reticulum (SR). When depolarization occurs at this point, through a transduction process involving direct protein–protein interaction between a calcium channel in the T-tubular membrane and the ryanodin receptor calcium release channel in the SR membrane, it results in the release of Ca^{2+} from the SR in the excitation–contraction (EC) coupling process. If the surface membrane of a muscle fibre fails to generate an action potential in response to endplate depolarization, contraction will not take place in spite of normal functioning at the neuromuscular junction and normal properties for the contractile proteins themselves; unexcitable surface membranes result in muscle paralysis. Conversely, if the surface membrane generates multiple, uncontrolled action potentials in response to a normal stimulus at the neuromuscular junction, sustained contractions can result where only a brief twitch was intended; hyperexcitable surface membranes are one cause of delayed relaxation in neuromuscular disease. Failure of EC coupling owing to molecular defects in either of the channel components can also result in weakness or paralysis of an otherwise normal muscle. This chapter will deal with the processes that

control the action potential in normal skeletal muscle, and with membrane defects that can produce hypo- and hyperexcitable states. The relationship between these factors and the pathogenesis of the myotonic disorders and of the periodic paralyses will then be considered.

Normal membrane excitation in skeletal muscle

The resting membrane potential

A microelectrode inserted into a normal skeletal muscle fibre will record a potential of -70 to $-90\,mV$ relative to the extracellular space. This potential is developed across the thin barrier (5–$7.5\,nm$) of the surface membrane. This membrane also marks the interface across which concentration gradients are established for monovalent and divalent anions and cations between the cytoplasm and the external environment. It is the interrelationship between these concentration gradients and the selective permeability of the surface membrane to these ions that controls the sign and the magnitude of the membrane potential. This potential can be altered either through modification of the concentration gradients themselves or through the modulation of the membrane's ionic conductance.

The interaction between membrane potential, ionic concentration gradients and membrane conductance can best be understood by first considering the simple case of a semipermeable membrane separating two chambers that contain different concentrations of a simple salt solution. Suppose such a membrane (Fig. 10.1), separating a $100\,mmol/l$ solution of KCl on the left-hand side from one of $5\,mmol/l$ on the right, is suddenly made selectively permeable to K^+ only. These ions will move down their concentration gradient from the side with the highest concentration (the left) to the side with the lowest (the right). However, since the membrane is not permeable to the counterion chloride (Cl$^-$), any movement of K$^+$ will produce an imbalance of charge, with more positive ions on the right side of the membrane and more negative ions on the left. This charge imbalance creates a membrane potential with an electrical gradient that will retard the further movements of K$^+$ along its chemical gradient. Eventually an equilibrium will be reached where the driving force on a single K$^+$ owing to the electrical field exactly balances the opposing drive of the concentration gradient and no further net movement of ions occurs. This potential (V_m), known as the Nernst potential after the 19th century physiologist who first described it, is given by the simple equation:

$$V_{\mathrm{m}} = -\frac{RT}{nF} \ln \left\{ \frac{[K^+]_i}{[K^+]_o} \right\} \tag{10.1}$$

Where V_m is the membrane potential, [K$^+$] is concentration of K$^+$ on inside (i) and outside (o), n is the charge on each ion (in this case, +1) and R, T, and F are physical constants. The equation predicts that increasing the concentration gradient increases the potential while decreasing the concentration gradient has the opposite effect.

Unfortunately, things are not as simple as this in the case of the muscle membrane. While the sarcolemma is very permeable to K$^+$, and the response of the membrane potential to changes in K$^+$ concentration does approximate to that predicted by the Nernst potential, the membrane is also measurably permeable to other ions as well, especially to Na$^+$ and to Cl$^-$. In normal muscle, both the concentration gradient and the relative membrane permeability for each of these ions play a role in determining the actual membrane potential across the sarcolemma. Although the derivation of the equation describing this situation is complicated, the final result resembles in its general form the simple Nernst relationship:

$$V_{\mathrm{m}} = -\frac{RT}{nF} \ln \left\{ \frac{P_K[K^+]_1 + P_{Na}[Na^+]_1 + P_{cl}[Cl^-]_2}{P_K[K^+]_2 + P_{Na}[Na^+]_2 + P_{cl}[Cl^-]_1} \right\} \tag{10.2}$$

Where 1 and 2 indicate the two compartments separated by the membrane. A new term must be introduced that indicates the membrane's relative permeability to each ionic species. This equation, known as the Goldman–Hodgkin–Katz (GHK) relationship, predicts that the membrane potential will reflect both the concentration gradient of each of the permeant ion species and the relative permeability (P) of the membrane to that ion. The dependence on relative permeability introduced by this equation is extremely important since it predicts that modulating membrane permeability alone, without any

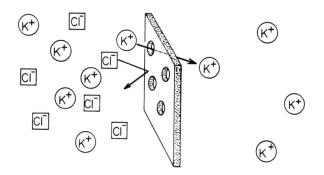

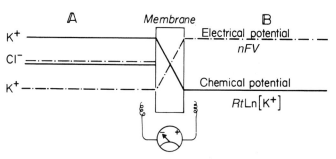

Fig. 10.1. A transmembrane potential develops when a semipermeable membrane separates two solutions with differing concentrations of a permeant ion. In this illustration, the membrane is permeable only to K$^+$. The electrical potential that results when K$^+$ attempts to move down its concentration gradient will exactly balance the chemical potential produced by that concentration gradient, and the net force acting on a single K$^+$ moving through the membrane will be zero. The membrane potential under these conditions, given by the Nernst equation, will vary as a function of the K$^+$ concentration gradient. (Reproduced from Barchi 1980 with permission.)

change in the concentration gradients themselves, can alter the membrane potential. With the typical concentration gradients for Na$^+$, K$^+$ and Cl$^-$ found in mammalian skeletal muscle, the membrane potential can range between approximately $-90\,$mV when the permeability to K$^+$ predominates and $+50\,$mV when the membrane is made selectively permeable to Na$^+$. It is this relationship between permeability and potential that forms the basis for the generation of an action potential.

There is another fundamental difference between the situation described by the Nernst equation and that of the GHK equation. With a perfectly selective membrane, the potential predicted by the Nernst equation will persist indefinitely, that is, the equation describes an equilibrium. This is not the case for a membrane permeable to multiple ions as described by the GHK equation. Here, for example, movement of K$^+$ in one direction can be electrically balanced by the movement of Na^+ along its concentration gradient in the opposite direction. Eventually these gradients will dissipate and the potential itself will disappear. In order for the membrane potential described by Equation (10.2) to persist, there must be a mechanism for maintaining the underlying concentration gradients. Ideally, each ion that crosses the membrane passively must be pumped actively back across the membrane. If this is done, a steady state will result; the electrical potential and the concentration gradients will remain constant, but at the necessary cost of energy in the form of the ATP needed to run the pump.

In skeletal muscle, the major membrane transport protein is the Na^+/K^+ ATPase. This protein actively transports Na^+ against its concentration gradient from the inside of the cell to the extracellular space while simultaneously moving K^+ in the opposite direction (for a review, see Jorgenson, 1982). The coupling of Na^+ and K^+ in this energy-dependent pumping process is not 1:1, however; about three Na^+ move outward for each two K^+ transported inward. If negative counterions cannot keep up with the movement of their positive partners, this asymmetrical pumping will produce a small membrane potential of its own. In normal muscle, the activity of the Na^+/K^+ ATPase can generate 3 to 10 mV of hyperpolarization, depending on the level of activity of the enzyme.

Active membrane properties

In muscle, small depolarizing current pulses introduced through an intracellular microelectrode produce proportionate changes in the membrane potential as expected for a passive R-C circuit as long as the magnitude of the depolarization does not exceed 10 to 15 mV. Larger depolarization, however, triggers a unique all-or-none regenerative potential change that reflects highly nonlinear changes in the underlying properties of the membrane itself. This regenerative spike or action potential is stereotyped in its form, and at its peak the internal potential becomes transiently positive with respect to the extracellular space.

Some insight into the mechanism by which the action potential arises can be gained by studying the relationship between the membrane potential at the peak of the spike and the external concentration of various cations. While the resting potential in muscle is sensitive to changes in external $[K^+]$ but not to external $[Na^+]$, the peak of the action potential demonstrates the reverse relationship; it is altered little by variations in $[K^+]$ but varies with $[Na^+]$ in a manner resembling a membrane that is permeable only to Na^+.

Membrane currents during an action potential

The details of the conductance changes that underlie the action potential in skeletal muscle were defined mainly through the use of voltage clamp techniques. After its seminal application to the squid giant axon by Hodgkin and Huxley (1952), this technique was modified for single muscle fibres by Adrian and his colleagues (Adrian et al., 1970). Their early findings confirmed that the basic mechanism involved in producing action potentials in nerve and muscles was the same. The initial rising phase of the action potential is produced by a large, voltage-dependent increase in membrane conductance to Na^+. The greater the depolarization, the larger and more rapid is the conductance change; thus, once initiated, the action potential becomes its own stimulus. This increase in Na^+ conductance is transient, however, and reverts to its resting level within a few milliseconds. This conductance inactivation, in conjunction with a secondary delayed increase in membrane conductance to K^+, results in the return of the membrane potential to its normal resting value.

Using the voltage clamp, relationships between conductance, voltage and time have been detailed in muscle for both the Na^+ and K^+ systems (Adrian et al., 1970; Adrian and Marshall, 1977). Over the years, a number of points have become clear. First, the membrane proteins controlling these conductances represent two discrete populations of ion channels, each providing a separate time- and voltage-dependent aqueous pathway through the membrane for a selected cation. Second, the basic properties of these two channels differ little from comparable sodium and potassium channels involved in the production of action potentials in the nerves and muscles of virtually all multicellular organisms. Third, the action potential is mainly the result of changes in relative conductance of the membrane to these two cations; the actual net movement of cations that occurs is small and there is no significant change in the cation concentration gradients across the membrane during a single action potential.

Sodium channel inactivation

In skeletal muscle, the kinetics of current flow through the sodium and potassium channels differs in a very fundamental way. When potassium channels are opened with depolarization, they tend to stay in the opened state and K^+ currents flow throughout the period of depolarization, terminating only when the membrane repolarizes. Sodium channels, by comparison, open transiently in response to depolarization and then revert to a nonconducting or inactivated state in spite of persistent depolarization (for a review, see French and Horn, 1983). The process of inactivation in the sodium channel is an extremely important one, and channel inactivation plays a central role in the control of membrane excitability. This aspect of sodium channel function requires some additional comment.

The voltage-dependent sodium channel can exist in at least three states. In the normal closed state, which predominates at the resting potential, the channel does not allow the movement of cations but is available to be activated by depolarization. With rapid depolarization, a second, opened, state is seen where Na^+ moves freely through the channel pore. With continued depolarization, the channel enters a third conformation, in which the pore is closed but the channel is inactivated and is no longer able to be opened by depolarization (Fig. 10.2). All three states appear to be interconvertible, and the inactivated state can be restored to the closed but activatable state simply by repolarizing the membrane to its resting level. Under appropriate testing conditions, other channel states can also be identified. For example, depolarization lasting many seconds can induce a deeper inactivated state through a process termed slow interaction. Under certain circumstances, these less common kinetic states can significantly influence channel excitability.

In a population of sodium channels, the fraction that will be found in an inactivated state increases with depolarization. The relationship between steady-state inactivation and membrane potential is sigmoidal, with the midpoint in skeletal muscle at about $-50\,mV$. Prolonged depolarization can thus paradoxically lead to inactivation of sodium channels and loss of membrane excitability rather than the increased excitability often expected.

Although the actual kinetic interrelationships between the various conformations of the sodium channel are in fact very complex, this simple scheme is sufficient to explain many of the basic properties of channel behaviour.

Single channel properties

The early view of sodium and potassium channels as continuously modulated conductance pathways that open and close in a smooth, graded fashion in response to triggering stimuli was based on voltage clamp measurements that recorded the response of large areas of surface membrane containing many thousands of channel molecules. This view changed dramatically with the introduction of the patch clamp technique (Fig. 10.3a) (Neher and Sackmann, 1976). In this method, very small patches of membrane (less than $1\,\mu m^2$ in area) can be isolated at the tip of a fire-polished microelectrode and subjected to the same sort of analysis used with the traditional macroscopic voltage clamp. These patches are so small that they may contain only a single channel.

The response of these very small membrane patches to abrupt depolarization is quite different from that of whole muscle fibres or squid axons. Instead of smoothly modulated changes in membrane current with depolarization (Fig. 10.3b), sharp step-like transitions between discrete current levels are seen at a given driving voltage (Fig. 10.3c). The amplitude of these current steps is constant and the actual change in current occurs so rapidly that usually it cannot be accurately resolved. If the same depolarizing step is repeated over and over in the same patch, the characteristics of these current steps remain constant; only their duration and the time of their occurrence during the pulse varies, each in a statistically definable manner. When thousands of such records are averaged, the smooth current increase and self-terminating inactivation characteristic of a traditional voltage clamp record is reproduced.

These small current pulses represent the opening and closing of individual ion channels. Each channel opens very rapidly to a characteristic conductance level, remains opened for a period of time and then closes again. The interval between the initiation of membrane depolarization and channel opening varies in a statistical manner for a single channel on multiple trials. Following an abrupt depolarization, the probability that a given single channel will be opened increases dramatically for a few milliseconds and then decreases again with time, reflecting the time-dependent onset of inactivation. For skeletal muscle, single sodium channels have a conductance of about $20\,pS$, resulting in a current flow of several thousand ions through each channel during an average opened interval of $1\,ms$.

At the level of individual ion channels, the response of the muscle membrane is not a smooth graded process; the currents recorded with macroscopic techniques such as the traditional voltage clamp actually represent the statistical average of the responses of many thousands of individual channels, each behaving in a stochastic manner in switching between closed and opened states. The relationship between parameters such as the probability of channel opening and the duration of each opening event on the one hand, and the membrane potential and time after depolarization on the other, define the response characteristics of the channel in the membrane in a manner analogous to the time- and voltage-dependent rate constants of the classical Hodgkin–Huxley formulation.

Molecular characteristics of muscle ion channels

Sodium channels

Along with an appreciation of single ion channel events at the biophysical level has come a greater understanding of

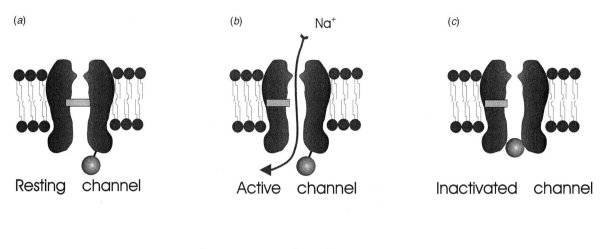

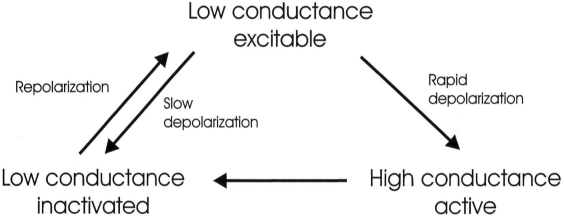

Fig. 10.2. Muscle action potentials are produced largely by transient changes in membrane conductance to Na^+. Membrane Na^+ conductance is controlled by a voltage-sensitive sodium channel which provides a water-filled pathway across the muscle surface membrane. In the channel, ion movement is controlled by several 'gates', which switch open or closed as a function of membrane potential and time. (*a*) At the normal membrane resting potential the channel is closed. (*b*) Rapid depolarization results in transient channel opening; during this interval, a Na^+ current can flow. (*c*) Prolonged depolarization causes a separate 'inactivation' gate to close; the channel no longer conducts Na^+ and cannot be opened again by further depolarization. Repolarization of the membrane restores the channel to its original closed but activatable state.

the molecular properties of the channel proteins themselves. Proteins making up the voltage-dependent sodium channel have been purified, cloned and sequenced from rat and human skeletal and cardiac muscle as well as from mammalian brain and from a variety of other species (for review, see Kallen et al., 1993). All of these sodium channel proteins are remarkably similar.

All voltage-dependent sodium channels contain one very large polypeptide of approximately 260 000 molecular weight designated the α-subunit. This subunit is a glycoprotein, with carbohydrate contributing about 24% by weight in skeletal muscle. The α-subunit has within its structure all the elements necessary for a functioning voltage-dependent ion channel. While the α-subunit is the

only protein present in the eel sodium channel, the channel in mammalian skeletal muscle and brain is associated with one or two additional small subunits of approximately 38 000 molecular weight that are also heavily glycosylated (Hartshorne and Catterall, 1984; Roberts and Barchi, 1987). These β-subunits are capable of modifying the kinetics of channel activation and inactivation (Isom et al., 1992).

The complete amino acid sequence for the α-subunit of many brain and muscle sodium channels have now been deduced from their cloned cDNA (reviewed in Kallen et al., 1993). A number of interesting conclusions can be drawn from a comparison of these sequences. These channels are highly homologous, with more than 60% sequence identity at the amino acid level between channels in species as

(a) Patch clamp single channel recording

(b) Traditional voltage clamp: large membrane area

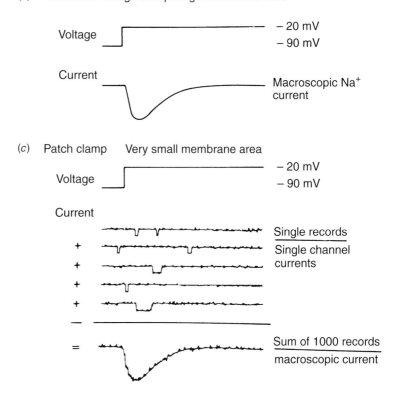

(a) Patch clamp single channel recording

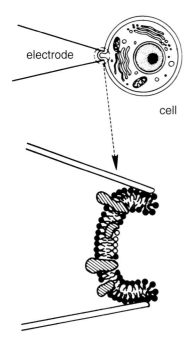

electrode

cell

Fig. 10.3. Voltage and patch clamp measurement of conductance. (*a*) With the technique of patch clamping, a small area of membrane can be sealed so tightly to the tip of a blunt glass microelectrode that it can be removed intact from the cell. The high resistance of the membrane-to-glass seal (usually tens of gigaohms) allows the investigator to resolve the tiny currents flowing through single ion channels in the membrane patch. (*b*) Classic macroscopic techniques for measuring membrane currents, such as voltage clamp, record the response of thousands of ion channels at a time. The current records often suggest a smoothly graded opening and closing of these channels with time, as shown in the record of membrane Na^+ currents flowing through the voltage-sensitive sodium channel. (*c*) Using patch clamp technology, the behaviour of single ion channels can be resolved. At this level, sodium channels are seen to open and close abruptly, moving rapidly between a zero conductance state and a characteristic open-channel conductance state. The smooth currents observed with macroscopic techniques represent the statistical average of the stochastic behaviour of individual channels with probabilities of opening and closing that vary with voltage and time.

divergent as eel and rat. Each α-subunit contains between 1800 and 2000 amino acid residues. Within this linear sequence are four large regions of internal homology, each encompassing 225 to 300 residues; sequence comparison indicates that these regions arose from duplication of a common primitive ancestral channel element. Within each of these regions are at least six areas predicted to be trans-membrane α-helices, and these regions are the most highly conserved areas when the domains are compared (Guy and Conti, 1990). The fourth helix in each domain (S4) is particularly interesting in that it exhibits a very highly conserved pattern of a positively charged arginine or lysine residue at every third position, separated by two nonpolar amino acids.

Cloned sodium channels can be transiently expressed in frog oocytes or mammalian cells, where they can be studied electrophysiologically. By modifying the cDNA, specific mutations can be introduced into the channel structure, and their effect on channel function assessed. Using this general approach, a considerable amount has been learned about the relationship between channel structure and function. For example, it is now clear that the positively charged S4 helix in each domain acts as part of the voltage-sensing elements of the channel (Stühmer et al., 1989; Auld et al., 1990). The region connecting repeat domains III and IV contributes to the inactivation of channel conductance after depolarization (Vassilev et al., 1989). The ion channel itself is formed by elements contributed from each of the four repeat domains, with the regions between the S5 and S6 helices forming part of the channel lining and controlling the specification of cation selectivity (Heinemann et al., 1992).

Calcium channels

Voltage-gated calcium channels control the movement of this important divalent cation across the surface and interior membranes of a variety of cells. In early studies, calcium channels were grouped into a number of related families on the basis of their pharmacological interactions with various drugs and ligands. These groups are now known to represent closely related gene families that are all members of a larger channel superfamily. Voltage-gated calcium channels are formed from one α_1-subunit of approximately 212 000 molecular weight that contains the ion channel, the voltage sensor and the other elements that control ion movement, and three associated peripheral subunits, α_2–δ, β and γ. The α_1-subunit is homologous to the α-subunit of the voltage-gated sodium channel and contains the same four internal repeat domains, each with six transmembrane helices. The S4 helix in each domain exhibits the characteristic pattern of a positive arginine or lysine at every third position, and the S5–S6 interhelical loop again forms the critical outer portion of the channel pore.

The predominant form of calcium channel in skeletal muscle is a member of the L-type dihydropyridine receptor family. In muscle, these channels are concentrated at the junction of the T-tubulules and the terminal SR (the triad). In this location, their primary function is not to gate an ionic current. Instead, the conformational change associated with voltage-dependent activation of this calcium channel is transmitted through direct protein–protein interaction, mediated by the interdomain II–III loop of the α_1-subunit, to the underlying ryanodine receptor calcium release channel of the SR (see Chapters 9 and 30). This allows depolarization of the T-tubular membrane to initiate the release of Ca^{2+} from the SR during the process of EC coupling.

Potassium channels

The delayed rectifier potassium channel that facilitates the repolarization of the nerve and muscle membrane after activation has also been characterized at the molecular level (reviewed in Kolb, 1990). These channels are members of a larger superfamily of potassium channels that includes the A-current potassium channel in *Drosophila* (Papazian et al., 1987; Butler et al., 1990) and related potassium channels in mammalian brain and muscle (Chandy et al., 1990; Roberds and Tankum, 1991).

Many members of this family have been cloned. The predicted molecular weight of these cloned proteins is smaller and more variable than that found for sodium channels, ranging between 60 000 and 75 000.

Initially, potassium channel proteins appeared to be unrelated to sodium channels because of their much smaller size. However, when analysed at the level of their primary sequence, these two types of voltage-dependent ion channel are clearly related. The structure of each potassium channel protein resembles one repeat domain of the larger sodium channel α-subunit. Each potassium channel gene product includes a single region containing the familiar six transmembrane helices and the characteristic positive S4 helix that are found in each of the four sodium channel repeat domains.

In the membrane, potassium channels are formed by tetramers of these smaller subunits (MacKinnon, 1991) and, in their functional state, these tetramers are comparable in organization to the sodium channel α-subunit. The individual subunits of the potassium channel play the same role as the repeat domains in the sodium channel. Virtually all the key functional elements documented by site-directed mutagenesis in potassium channels have been confirmed in analogous locations in the sodium channel. The S4 helix confers voltage dependence. The S5–S6 interhelical loop contributes to the formation of the ion pore and controls selectivity. The C-terminal cytoplasm tail each subunit can act as the inactivation 'gate' in a manner analogous to the cytoplasmic interdomain III–IV loop of the sodium channel. Some potassium channels are associated with β-subunits; interaction of the α-subunit tetramers with one or more β-subunits (three) can significantly alter channel kinetics.

Work with a voltage-independent bacterial form of potassium channel (which contains only the equivalent of the S5 and S6 transmembrane helices and the pore-forming linker between them) has recently provided remarkable new structural information on this entire class of ion channel. The crystal structure of this mini-channel has been determined by MacKinnon and his collaborators, providing high-resolution information on the channel pore and ion selectivity filter region (Doyle et al., 1998). The structure visualized by X-ray diffraction is remarkably similar to that inferred from previous biochemical and site-directed mutagenesis studies. The S5–S6 interhelical loop dips into the membrane to form the pore lining, while the S5 helices form an inverted tepee in the membrane that surrounds, and supports, the pore. The S6 helices are disposed more peripherally in the complex at the protein–lipid interface.

The structure of the pore does contain a few surprises.

The narrow outer region of the pore that provides the selectivity function is lined by the carbonyl oxygen residues of the peptide backbone, rather than by the polar elements of each amino acid side chain. The dimensions of the pore are such that ions probably move through this filter region in a partially dehydrated state. Beyond this constriction, which occupies the outer third of the pore, the channel diameter widens, eventually forming a funnel-shaped internal vestibule. The S5 helices come closest together about two-thirds of the way through the membrane. This may be the site at which conformational changes in helix positioning actually gate the channel open or closed.

Given the strong evolutionary and structural relationship between sodium, potassium and calcium channels, it is likely that the structure of this potassium mini-channel closely resembles that of the core region of the larger voltage-dependent channels.

Chloride channels

The Cl^- conductance in muscle is the dominant resting conductance in the sarcolemma. The channel protein that controls this conductance has also been cloned, sequenced and functionally expressed from eel electroplax and from rat skeletal muscle (Jentsch et al., 1990; Steinmeyer et al., 1991).

In rat skeletal muscle, the cDNA encoding this chloride channel contains a single open reading frame encoding a protein of 994 amino acid residues that is identical in more than half of its residues with the comparable protein cloned from the eel electroplax. Structural analysis of the primary sequence predicts up to 13 potential transmembrane helices (designated D1–D13 in the literature) in the central portion of the molecule but shows no evidence of the internal organizational features characteristic of the voltage-dependent cation channels discussed above. The chloride channel sequences exhibit no homology to the sequence of any other known ion channel or transporter molecule, and do not contain the positively charged helix motif that is the hallmark of the voltage-dependent cation channels (Steinmeyer et al., 1991). Rather, the skeletal chloride channel is a member of a unique but extended gene family, ClC, members of which are ubiquitously expressed in organisms from bacteria to humans. ClC proteins are classified according to their primary site of expression. ClC-0, the first member of the family to be identified, is found in *Torpedo* electroplax. ClC-1 is expressed in skeletal muscle. ClC-2 is found in many different cell types and may be involved in volume regulation.

When expressed in vitro, cRNA from these clones produce functional chloride channels with the anion selectivity, voltage dependence and kinetics characteristic of the major chloride conductance pathway previously described in mammalian skeletal muscle. Although the stoichiometry of the functional muscle channel has been controversial, current evidence suggests that ClC-1 exists as a dimer in the membrane. While details of tertiary structure remain to be resolved, it appears that the predicted D4 helix does not span the membrane but rather lies on the extracellular surface (Schmidt-Rose and Jentsch, 1997). Predicted helix D13 is located completely on the cytoplamic surface of the protein. Deletion of this helix does not affect channel expression or function (Gründer et al, 1992).

Membranes and muscle weakness in periodic paralysis

The periodic paralyses are disorders of skeletal muscle characterized by transient episodes of muscle weakness or paralysis. During these episodes there are often profound shifts in the serum K^+ concentration. These disorders usually occur as familial syndromes with autosomal dominant inheritance, although clinically indistinguishable sporadic cases do occur (Chapter 30). The periodic paralyses have traditionally been classified according to the characteristic changes in serum K^+ associated with the attacks of weakness. Hypokalaemic, normokalaemic and hyperkalaemic varieties have been described in the classical literature. The details of the clinical presentation of the various forms of periodic paralysis are considered in Chapter 30. Some of the common aspects of the membrane events that lead to the development of muscle weakness will be discussed here.

Membrane potential and membrane excitability

Between attacks of paralysis, the resting membrane potential in skeletal muscle of patients with periodic paralysis is usually normal or only slightly lower than normal, but EC coupling proceeds without difficulty (Shy et al., 1961; Creutzfeldt et al., 1963; Riecker and Bolte, 1976; McComas et al., 1968). During the onset of an attack of weakness, muscle strength declines in direct proportion to the loss of muscle membrane excitability as evidenced by the amplitude of the compound muscle action potential (Gordon et al., 1970). At the peak of paralysis, individual muscle fibres exhibit abnormally low resting membrane potentials (Creutzfeldt et al., 1963; Hofman and Smith, 1970) and an action potential cannot be produced by the usual depolarizing current stimulus. At the same time, motor nerve action potentials appear normal, processes at the endplate are intact and the underlying contractile apparatus responds normally to the direct application of calcium (Engel and Lambert, 1969).

Although the details of this scenario vary from one type of periodic paralysis to another, the basic story line is the same. Muscle paralysis is associated with failure of action potential generation in the fibre sarcolemma, and this in turn is correlated with a persistent depolarization of the membrane resting potential. How can these facts be reconciled with our understanding of the molecular basis for action potential generation? We have seen that prolonged depolarization will shift the membrane voltage-sensitive sodium channels into an inactivated state. The fraction of sodium channels in the membrane available for activation varies steeply with voltage near the resting potential. Since an action potential can only be generated when the net inward Na$^+$ current through these channels exceeds the total outward current carried through all other channels in the membrane, the number of sodium channels available to be opened is a critical factor in determining membrane excitability.

At normal muscle resting potentials, about 70% of the membrane sodium channels are available for activation. With this number of channels, the inward Na$^+$ current needed for an action potential is easily achieved. A persistent depolarization of only 10 to 20 mV, however, will increase the fraction of inactivated channels to nearly 50%, and the remaining channels will barely be able to generate the inward current density needed for an action potential. A further small depolarization renders the membrane totally incapable of generating an action potential even though the sodium channels themselves may be normal in number and in their molecular properties.

If the membrane is once again repolarized to its normal resting level, the equilibrium between closed but activatable channels and inactivated channels shifts back, the fraction of channels available for activation increases and normal excitability is restored. When action potentials once again couple depolarization of the neuromuscular junction to Ca^{2+} release from the SR, normal muscle function and strength return.

Pathophysiology of membrane depolarization

The sequence of events described above appears to be shared by most if not all of the periodic paralyses during episodes of muscle weakness. The triggering factors that lead to the underlying membrane depolarization, however, may be quite different in the various forms of this disease. Equation 10.2 predicts that depolarization can result from several factors. These include an increase in external K$^+$ concentration, a decrease in external Na$^+$ concentration or an increase in membrane permeability to Na$^+$ relative to that for K$^+$. Decreasing the contribution to the membrane potential from the electrogenic activity of the Na$^+$/K$^+$ ATPase will also depolarize the membrane. In the periodic paralyses, membrane depolarization results from an increase in the membrane permeability to Na$^+$ (reviewed by Rüdel and Ricker, 1985). In the toxic paralysis produced by barium ingestion or by experimental K$^+$ deficiency in animals, depolarization may be the result of a primary decrease in K$^+$ conductance, again with the ultimate effect of shifting the balance of membrane conductance to favour Na$^+$ (Kao and Gordon, 1975; Gallant, 1983). External factors such as insulin exposure or cooling, which lead to a further transient increase in Na$^+$ conductance, or a decrease in electrogenic pump activity can contribute to this depolarized state, resulting in further inactivation of the voltage-sensitive sodium channel, failure of excitation and paralysis.

In hyperkalaemic periodic paralysis and paramyotonia congenita, the increased Na$^+$ conductance is mediated by the voltage-gated sodium channel itself and can be prevented or reversed by the specific sodium channel blocker tetrodotoxin (TTX) (Lehmann-Horn et al., 1981, 1983). In hypokalaemic periodic paralysis, the increased resting membrane Na$^+$ conductance does not involve the voltage-dependent sodium channel, but rather another Na$^+$ pathway that may be coupled in some way to a defective calcium channel.

Microelectrode measurements on isolated muscle fibres from patients with hyperkalaemic periodic paralysis have identified a noninactivating, TTX-sensitive Na$^+$ current that is present only when the muscle fibre is exposed to elevated extracellular K$^+$ (Lehmann-Horn et al., 1987). This current represents a small percentage of the total membrane Na$^+$ current and is not present at normal K$^+$ concentrations. Single-channel recordings on myotubes formed from cultured muscle biopsy tissue obtained from patients with hyperkalaemic periodic paralysis demonstrate a class of sodium channel that undergoes persistent re-openings during prolonged depolarization, consistent with a failure of the inactivation process (Cannon et al., 1991). Abnormal inactivation of this type was not seen in control muscle and may be the molecular counterpart of the noninactivating Na$^+$ current seen earlier with whole cell recording.

Sodium channel defects in periodic paralysis

The molecular cloning of the various mammalian skeletal muscle sodium channels (Trimmer et al., 1989; Kallen et al.,

1990; George et al., 1992) opened the way for the characterization of defects in this channel protein in the periodic paralyses. Using information from the cloned human channel, the gene encoding the adult muscle channel, designated *SCN4A*, was determined to be at chromosome 17q23.1–25.5 (George et al., 1991). Using restriction fragment length polymorphisms defined within this gene, a number of laboratories confirmed linkage between the phenotypic expression of various forms of periodic paralysis and the skeletal sodium channel (Fontaine et al., 1990; Ebers et al., 1991; Koch et al., 1991; Ptáček et al., 1991, 1992). *SCN4A* was also found to be tightly linked to the expression of atypical forms of myotonia.

Using information about the gene structure of *SCN4A* to generate polymerase chain reaction probes for the exon regions of this channel gene, several laboratories subsequently identified point mutations in the gene for the skeletal muscle sodium channel in families with hyperkalaemic periodic paralysis, paramyotonia congenita and atypical myotonia (see Chapter 30 and Barchi (1995, 1997) for reviews). Most of these mutations are concentrated in domains III and IV, and in the cytoplasmic linking region between these domains. A smaller number of mutations occur in domain II while only a single mutation has been identified in domain I. All mutations identified to-date result in the substitution of a single amino acid in the channel primary sequence but are compatible with expression of full-length protein.

Many of these mutations have been recreated in the normal skeletal muscle channel background, and the effects of the mutation on channel kinetics studied directly after expression of the modified channel in oocytes or in cultured cells. Each mutation affects channel inactivation. Many slow the kinetics of channel inactivation and increase the rate of recovery from inactivation, resulting at the single-channel level in multiple channel re-openings and prolonged channel open times during a depolarization (reviewed in Barchi, 1995, 1997). At the macroscopic level, these factors produce slowly inactivating Na$^+$ currents after depolarization. Other mutations affect channel modal gating, increasing the percentage of time that mutant channels spend in a rare but naturally occurring slowly inactivating channel conformation. This produces a small noninactivating Na$^+$ current that remains after the normal Na$^+$ current induced by depolarization inactivates. Variable effects on the voltage dependence of channel inactivation are also seen. Most of the mutations have little or no effect on the kinetics of channel activation.

The concentration of identified mutations in the area of the gene coding for the interdomain III–IV linker is not surprising in light of the evidence that this region of the protein forms a key part of the inactivation gate. Other mutations affecting areas near the cytoplasmic ends of helices in the repeat domains may alter the cytoplasmic binding site for the interdomain III–IV linker as it moves inward to occlude the channel inner mouth, thereby altering inactivation kinetics. Several mutations that are more difficult to reconcile with current concepts of channel function involve residues on the outer surface of the protein. Presumably these mutations modify the conformational transitions of transmembrane helices that are linked to the movements of elements on the cytoplasmic surface involved in inactivation.

Mutations that slow the process of channel inactivation, or produce a significant population of noninactivating channels, will result in persistent membrane Na$^+$ currents after an action potential. This persistent inward current can prolong membrane depolarization. If this persistent depolarization is of sufficient length and magnitude, normal Na$^+$ channels will inactivate, available Na$^+$ current will decline, the action potential will fail and paralysis will ensue.

It is now clear that abnormalities of sodium channel inactivation that produce the phenotype of periodic paralysis can result from a variety of mutations at sites scattered throughout the channel structure. It is likely that more of these mutations will come to light as other families with these disorders are studied in detail. Some of these mutations may affect the specific portion of the channel involved directly in channel gating, but other more distant mutations that affect channel tertiary structure slightly have the real potential to alter the conformational energy of activated and inactivated states, thus shifting the state distribution toward an abnormal kinetic mode. Like the multiple mutations that can cause the various haemoglobinopathies, it is probable that many allelic mutations affecting sodium channel structure will lead to disorders with similar phenotypes.

Other channel defects

While many mutations in the voltage-gated sodium channel have been found in families with the periodic paralysis phenotype, not all forms of this syndrome are caused by sodium channel defects. Hypokalaemic periodic paralysis is associated with point mutations in the gene encoding the skeletal muscle L-type calcium channel. This protein links depolarization in the T-tubular membrane to Ca^{2+} release from the SR by direct protein–protein interaction with the ryanodine receptor calcium release channel of the terminal SR membrane. Mutant mice that fail to produce this L-type muscle calcium channel die immediately after birth was a result of muscular paralysis, and muscle cells in culture with this defective channel fail to contract in response to membrane depolarization. Transient expressions of the L-type calcium channel in these cultured cells restores their ability to contract.

Although the critical role of the L-type calcium channel in EC coupling is clear, the mechanism by which mutations interfere with this process remains to be determined. It is also puzzling that such mutations can produce the membrane depolarization previously reported in hypokalaemic periodic paralysis during an ictal event.

Serum potassium levels, membrane potential and paralysis

Although the details of the interplay between serum K^+, membrane potential and paralysis in each of the periodic paralyses remains to be clarified, shifts in serum K^+ probably reflect coupling to Na^+ movements through the Na^+/K^+ ATPase system rather than primary events that are directly responsible for paralysis. This coupling can result clinically in either hypokalaemia or hyperkalaemia depending upon the functional state of the Na^+/K^+ ATPase itself. For example, the increased inward Na^+ movement that would be associated with an abnormally large membrane Na^+ conductance will be a potent stimulus for pump activity. A sudden increase in Na^+ conductance from any specific triggering event will further stimulate this pump. Since the Na^+/K^+ ATPase exchanges extracellular K^+ for intracellular Na^+, pumping activity can rapidly reduce the K^+ concentration in the small volume of the extracellular space and produce hypokalaemia. This type of coupling accounts for the net K^+ movement into the cells of normal individuals that follows the administration of glucose and insulin.

In another setting, the Na^+/K^+ ATPase may not be able to increase its activity sufficiently to keep pace with an increased Na^+ leakage. In this case, progressive depolarization will result, with inward Na^+ movement coupled electrically to outward movement of K^+, leading to secondary hyperkalaemia. It is important to realize that either hyperkalaemia or hypokalaemia can result from the same fundamental defect in membrane Na^+ conductance depending on the magnitude of the conductance change and capacity of the Na^+/K^+ ATPase to respond to the additional sodium load.

The Na^+/K^+ ATPase may play a pivotal role in the onset of depolarization as well. A muscle membrane in delicate balance as the result of an increased inward Na^+ leak that is just compensated by a maximally activated pump could be thrown out of balance by the selective slowing of pump activity. This can easily occur with cooling, since the change in activity of energy-dependent pumping with temperature is nearly threefold greater than that for ion movement through an aqueous membrane channel.

Hyperexcitable states of the muscle membrane: myotonia

The myotonic syndromes are easily identified among the disorders of the neuromuscular system by their characteristic mechanical and electrical features. Myotonia is expressed clinically as the delayed relaxation of skeletal muscle after a voluntary contraction or a contraction induced by an electrical or mechanical stimulus. This delayed relaxation is a cardinal finding in a number of diseases that vary widely in their inheritance, pathology and prognosis (Chapter 27); these include myotonia congenita, myotonic dystrophy, paramyotonia congenita, chondrodystrophic myotonia and even some forms of hyperkalaemic periodic paralysis. Myotonia indistinguishable from that found in these natural disorders is also seen as a reaction to several classes of drug and chemicals and can be reproduced in laboratory animals.

When examined by electromyography, patients with myotonia exhibit a common picture of increased insertional activity and prolonged, repetitive discharges of motor unit potentials that wax and wane in frequency and amplitude (Fig. 10.4). This prolonged electrical activity correlates with the delay in muscular relaxation and, in most of the myotonias, is directly responsible for the abnormality of contraction. The waxing and waning frequency of these discharges produces the crescendo–decrescendo sound patterns on an audio monitor that early investigators referred to as 'dive bomber potentials'.

The remarkable similarity of the clinical and electrical appearance of myotonia in different muscle diseases initially suggested that a common underlying pathogenetic mechanism might explain this phenomenon at the membrane level in all diseases. This has not proved to be the case (Rüdel and Lehmann-Horn, 1985). Although one major group of myotonic disorders does share a common molecular mechanism, clinical myotonia is a phenotype shared by a number of otherwise unrelated defects affecting the behaviour of membrane ion channels.

Myotonia resulting from abnormal chloride conductance

Much of our early understanding of the pathophysiology of myotonia resulted from the detailed electrophysiological

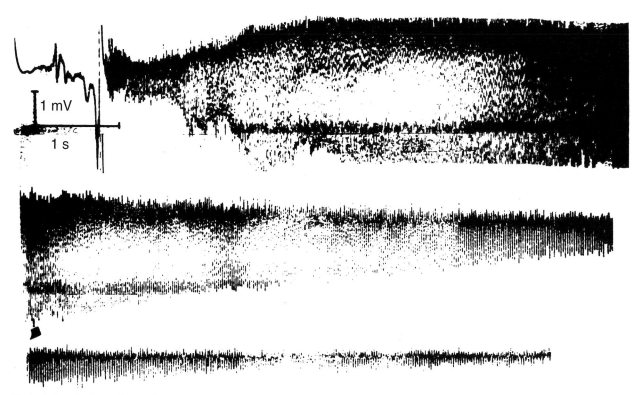

Fig. 10.4. Sustained membrane electrical activity that follows muscle activation or irritation is the electrical correlate of the delayed relaxation seen in myotonic skeletal muscle. In this example, a myotonic discharge was recorded in response to diazacholesterol, an agent that produces a toxic myotonic syndrome. (Reproduced with permission from Furman and Barchi, 1981.)

and biophysical studies of a naturally occurring congenital myotonia in goats (Bryant, 1979), which resembles myotonia congenita in humans. Classical experiments with nerve section and neuromuscular blockade localized the origin of the abnormal electrical activity in this disorder to the muscle membrane itself (Brown and Harvey, 1939). Subsequent measurements on single isolated intercostal muscle fibres demonstrated at the cellular level the correlate of the persistent electrical activity recorded by electromyogram (Adrian and Bryant, 1974). When the surface membrane of a myotonic fibre is depolarized by a constant current, a repetitive series of driven action potentials is seen that is followed by a long, depolarizing after-potential (Fig. 10.5). The amplitude of this depolarizing after-potential is proportional to the number of action potentials produced during the current pulse. When the after-potential becomes large enough, trains of self-sustaining, spontaneous action potentials are triggered. These events are not seen in normal fibres where depolarization generates only a few action potentials, much smaller after-depolarizations and no spontaneous activity. The delayed relaxation of myotonic fibre is the direct

consequence of this persistent spontaneous electrical activity. Measurement of membrane conductance in myotonic muscles reveals a remarkable increase in membrane resistance that is caused by the nearly complete absence of the normal membrane conductance to Cl^- (Bryant and Morales-Aguilera, 1971). In myotonic goats, this results from a reduced density of chloride channels rather than a normal number of channels having modified conductance properties; it probably represents the primary defect in this disorder (Bryant and Owenburg, 1980).

The mouse mutants designated *mto* or *adr* provide another model of human myotonia (Rüdel, 1990). When animals homozygous for the *adr* mutation start to walk, the hind legs become stiffly extended. The spasms of the hind limbs are especially prominent when the animal is startled. This stiffness causes problems in righting after an animal is placed on its back and accounts for the name originally given to the mutant: arrested development of righting response (*adr*). Animals homozygous for either the *adr* or the *mto* allele show delayed relaxation and myotonic discharges (Entriken et al., 1987; Reininghaus et al., 1988). The electrical responses recorded intracellularly in

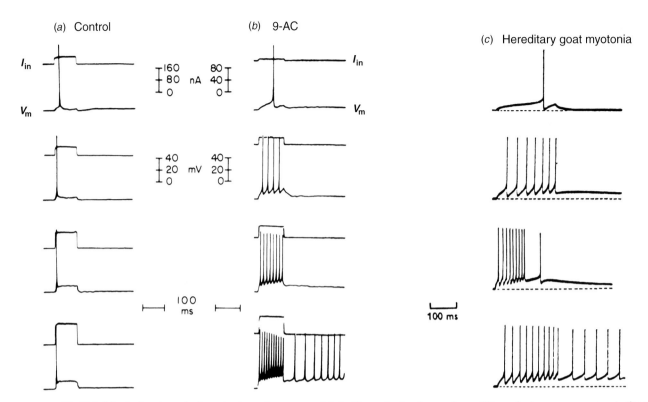

Fig. 10.5. Inherited and acquired myotonic syndromes associated with a reduction in membrane Cl^- conductance appear very similar at the single cell level. (*a*) Normal myotonic activity. (*b*) Myotonic activity induced by anthracine 9-carborylic acid (5×10^{-5} mol/l. (*c*) Myotonic activity in hereditary goat myotonia (Adrian and Bryant, 1974). In normal muscle fibres, an intracellar microelectrode will record one or two rapidly accommodating action potentials in response to a depolarizing current pulse. In hereditary goat myotonia, or experimental myotonia produced with inhibitors of membrane Cl^- conductance, depolarization produces multiple driven action potentials and a prolonged after-depolarization. If this after-depolarization exceeds a critical level, continuous self-sustaining action potentials will continue after the depolarizing pulse is stopped; this represents myotonia at a single-cell level. All recordings at 30 °C with 2 mmol/l Ca^{2+}. (Reproduced with permission from Furman and Barchi, 1978.)

these mutants are identical to those found in goat myotonia or myotonia produced by aromatic carboxylic acids (Mehrke et al., 1988). The membrane Cl^- conductance in skeletal muscle fibres of affected mice is markedly reduced (Mehrke et al., 1988). The *adr* and *mto* mutants, and three other related mutants with similar phenotypes, are allelic at a single gene that encodes the principal skeletal muscle chloride channel on mouse chromosome 6 (Heller et al., 1982; Watkins and Watts, 1984; Davisson et al., 1989).

Myotonia congenita in humans closely resembles the hereditary myotonia of goats. Myotonia congenita occurs in both an autosomal dominant and a recessive form (Chapter 27). Generalized myotonia is often noted in childhood and persists throughout life. Membrane studies with human myotonia congenita indicate that here, too, the primary pathophysiological defect is a marked reduction in muscle membrane resting conductance. A specific reduction in sarcolemmal Cl^- conductance was documented in intercostal muscle biopsies from these patients

through direct measurements using intracellular microelectrodes (Lipicky et al., 1971; Lipicky and Bryant, 1973).

A number of acquired myotonias are also directly caused by reduced Cl^- conductance in the sarcolemma. For example, carboxylic acids such as the herbicide 2,4 dichlorophenoxyacetic acid (2,4–D) have long been known to induce myotonia. This and related carboxylic acids produce myotonia by specific block of Cl^- conductance pathways (Palade and Barchi, 1977b; Furman and Barchi, 1978). At the single cell level, the electrophysiological features of this myotonia are indistinguishable from those recorded in hereditary myotonia (Bryant, 1982).

The physiological basis of myotonia with reduced chloride conductance

The origin of repetitive electrical activity

The repetitive electrical discharges seen in many of the myotonic disorders can be explained on the basis of the marked reduction in membrane Cl$^-$ conductance that they share. At the resting potential, muscle membranes are three to five times more permeable to Cl$^-$ than to K$^+$, while Na$^+$ permeability accounts for less than 1% of the total membrane permeability (Hutter and Noble, 1960; Palade and Barchi, 1977a). As discussed above, the Na$^+$ and K$^+$ permeabilities undergo rapid time- and voltage-dependent changes in response to a depolarizing stimulus that result in the generation of an action potential, while Cl$^-$ permeability remains relatively constant during the action potential and Cl$^-$ fluxes passively follow cation movements.

During normal muscle activity, action potentials are propagated both longitudinally along the surface sarcolemma and radially into the fibre interior along elements of the T-tubular system. With each action potential, small amounts of K$^+$ move out of the cell while small amounts of Na$^+$ move inward. The K$^+$ released into the large volume of the extracellular space has little effect on the overall K$^+$ concentration, but the situation is different in the limited 'extracellular' volume of the T-tubular system. Measurements indicate that the efflux of K$^+$ associated with a single action potential can increase its luminal concentration by 0.3 mmol/l; this change could depolarize the T-tubular membrane by as much as 1.7 mV if the major conductance in the T-tubule were to K$^+$ (Adrian and Bryant, 1974). With multiple action potentials, the cumulative effect of this intralumenal K$^+$ accumulation could be a membrane depolarization of 10 mV or more.

Under normal conditions, this depolarization is not reflected in the surface membrane potential because of the large stabilizing Cl$^-$ conductance that is present in the sarcolemma. In the absence of this Cl$^-$ shunt, however, the K$^+$ accumulation in the T-tubular lumen produced by a series of action potentials can locally depolarize the surface membrane sufficiently to initiate self-sustaining action potentials (Fig. 10.5). The observed increase in the after-potential of 1 mV per impulse seen in myotonic fibres is compatible with this mechanism (Adrian and Bryant, 1974). A study showing that K$^+$ diffuses from the T-tubule with a time constant of 0.4 s (Almers, 1972) compares favourably with the after-potential decay time of 0.5 s observed in intact muscle fibres.

The behaviour of myotonic fibres can be reproduced in normal skeletal muscle fibres by blocking Cl$^-$ conductance through substitution of an impermeant anion for Cl$^-$ (Rüdel and Senges, 1972) or by specific chloride channel-blocking compounds (Furman and Barchi, 1978). Disconnecting the T-tubular system from the surface membrane by glycerol shock abolishes the long lasting, depolarizing after-potential and sustained spontaneous activity produced by these compounds (Adrian and Bryant, 1974), underscoring the importance of the T-tubular system in the generation of this repetitive activity. Figure 10.6 summarizes several mechanisms that might lead to the reduced Cl$^-$ conductance observed in the membranes of the above myotonic diseases.

The sequence of events in the low Cl$^-$ conductance myotonias appears to be as follows. Voluntary contraction of a skeletal muscle produces multiple action potentials, which originate at the endplate, propagate along the muscle fibre and invade the T-tubular system. Each of these action potentials results in a small increase in the T-tubular K$^+$ concentration. Because of the markedly reduced Cl$^-$ conductance, the effect of this increase in extracellular K$^+$ is a slight depolarization. This depolarization is not large enough to force sodium channels into an inactivated state; rather, as they recover from the normal inactivation that occurs during the depolarization of the action potential itself, some channels will begin to reopen as a result of this slight depolarization. Since the sum of opposing currents is much reduced by the lack of a significant Cl$^-$ conductance, the resultant small inward Na$^+$ current can again initiate depolarization and recruitment of additional channels so that another action potential develops. The net result of this process is that each action potential creates a transient after-depolarization, which in turn acts as a stimulus for the triggering of the next action potential in the sequence. As long as no channel kinetic parameters are altered, a long train of spontaneous action potentials can result.

Termination of the myotonic discharge

Results of computer modelling with skeletal muscles confirm the plausibility of this Cl$^-$ hypothesis and indicate that repetitive activity can occur when the membrane Cl$^-$ conductance is reduced to about 15% of normal, a value near the residual conductance found in these myotonic syndromes (Bretag, 1973; Barchi, 1975; Adrian and Marshall, 1976). Modelling has also been useful in demonstrating the sensitivity of the repetitive activity to minor changes in sodium channel kinetic parameters; a slight reduction in the rate recovery from inactivation, for example, can completely abolish myotonic activity in spite of a very low Cl$^-$ conductance. An increase in sodium channel slow inactivation will also prevent repetitive activity. In addition, since the magnitude of the actual depolarization that occurs with T-tubular K$^+$ accumulation depends on K$^+$ equilibrium potential, small changes in the concentration of extracellular K$^+$ can prevent the appearance of repetitive activity. For example, a slight reduction in external K$^+$, of a magnitude expected with the activation of the Na$^+$/K$^+$ ATPase, will block repetitive firing, as will the slight hyperpolarization produced by the electrogenic activity of this pump.

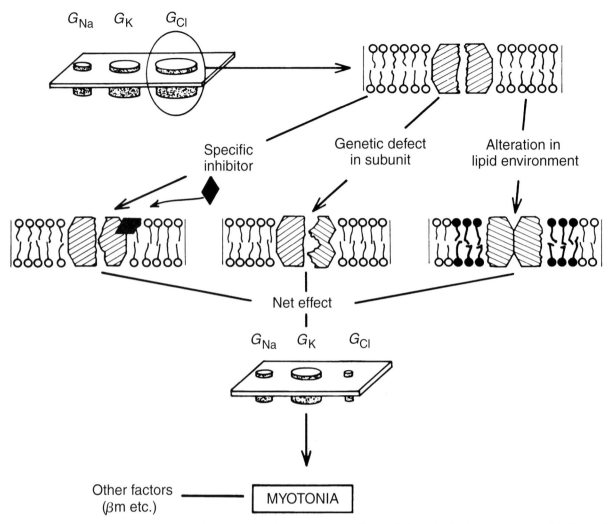

G_{Na} G_K G_{Cl}

Specific
inhibitor

Genetic defect
in subunit

Alteration in
lipid environment

Net effect

G_{Na} G_K G_{Cl}

Other factors ——— MYOTONIA
(βm etc.)

Fig. 10.6. The best-studied group of myotonic disorders is characterized by a pathological reduction in membrane chloride conductance. Even with this group, however, there are multiple mechanisms that can ultimately lead to the same membrane abnormality. Chloride channels may be genetically abnormal or may be specifically blocked by some exogenous or endogenous agent. Alternatively, normal channels might be induced to behave abnormally by an alteration in the membrane lipid environment in which they reside. In each case the end result is membrane hyperexcitability and clinical myotonia. (Reproduced with permission from Furman and Barchi, 1978.)

Although the precise factors that alter the frequency of a myotonic discharge and ultimately cause it to stop in a given fibre are unknown, it is easy to speculate on how one or more of these factors could be involved. Continued muscular activity will certainly result in the influx of sufficient Na^+ to activate the Na^+/K^+ ATPase. This activation will produce a hyperpolarizing electrogenic component and could as well result in the transient decline in local K^+ concentration outside the sarcolemma. Both factors will slow down the frequency of, or stop, a myotonic discharge. Furthermore, the kinetic parameters of normal sodium channels vary over a considerable range and are

probably modulated by cellular processes, such as phosphorylation, that remain to be completely elucidated. This sort of modulation could also play an important role in modifying myotonic activity.

Hyperactivity versus paralysis

Why does the depolarization following an action potential in a myotonic discharge produce hyperexcitability, while the depolarization associated with periodic paralysis results in the loss of all electrical excitability? Part of the answer lies in the magnitude of the depolarization. In myotonia, the depolarizations are small; they are sufficient to allow some channel activation yet not large enough to cause a significant increase in steady-state inactivation. Another modifying factor is the effect of a given mutation on other sodium channel kinetic parameters, such as activation. A third consideration is the time scale on which the depolarization takes place. The process of channel activation occurs much more rapidly than inactivation; if this were not so, sodium channels would never open during depolarization, and an action potential could not be produced. With brief depolarizations, activation initially predominates. Longer depolarizations will eventually lead to inactivation. In myotonia, these depolarizing after-potentials last only for tens of milliseconds. In the periodic paralyses, the magnitude of depolarization is greater and the duration is essentially indefinite. Here the steady-state effects predominate, and the influence of channel inactivation is the controlling factor. At the onset of membrane depolarization in periodic paralysis, one might expect transient hyperexcitibility if the critical criteria of rapidity and extent are satisfied. Indeed, in at least one form of hyperkalaemic periodic paralysis, hyperirritability and myotonic symptoms immediately precede the development of paralysis. In several other of the periodic paralyses, symptoms of myotonia can be seen in the intrictal state.

Other mechanisms producing membrane hyperexcitability

Low levels of membrane Cl^- conductance is a common factor that ties together a number of the myotonic disorders, but it certainly does not explain them all (Fig. 10.6). In myotonic dystrophy, the most common of the human muscle diseases in which myotonia is a major feature, membrane Cl^- conductance is normal or only slightly reduced (Lipicky, 1977). The primary genetic defect in this disease involves a muscle protein kinase, not an ion channel. In myotonia produced by 20,25-diazacholesterol, an inhibitor of cholesterol biosynthesis, repetitive electrical activity is again found although the chloride conductance is reduced only slightly (Furman and Barchi, 1981).

Although the exact mechanism that leads to the myotonic activity in these disorders remains to be elucidated, it is clear that there are other factors in addition to alterations in Cl^- conductance that can induce repetitive activity in skeletal muscle. One important mechanism by which repetitive activity can be produced is an alteration in the kinetics of the voltage-gated sodium channel. A number of polypeptide neurotoxins that kill by interacting with the sodium channel do so by reducing or eliminating channel

inactivation. These toxins characteristically produce repetitive action potentials in excitable membranes that are exposed to them. Similar repetitive activity follows the application of alkaloid toxins such as veratridine or batrachotoxin to muscle; again, the principal effect of these compounds is on sodium channel inactivation.

Under normal circumstances, the steady-state relationship between channel inactivation and voltage does not overlap with the similar curve relating fractional channel activation. At long times, inactivation of all channels will occur at voltages more negative than those at which activation begins. The direct consequence of this fact is the conduction failure that occurs in periodic paralysis. However, some channel mutations shift the voltage dependence of these steady-state channel voltage relationships in such a way that curves for inactivation and activation overlap in the voltage range around $-50\,mV$. At modest depolarizations, some channels can re-activate before entering the inactivated state, giving rise to 'window currents'. Window currents play an important role in repetitive activation of a variety of ion channels in various physiological settings.

In skeletal muscle, any factor that delays the rate or extent of channel inactivation under conditions where re-activation can occur, producing a window current, is a potential candidate for triggering repetitive electrical activity. With the failure of sodium channel inactivation, the repolarization produced by the activation of potassium channels is incomplete, closed sodium channels are immediately available for re-activation and opened non-inactivated channels can contribute directly to the initiation of a new depolarization phase. Factors causing this sequence could be exogenous, as with the neurotoxins, or could represent endogenous defects in the channel structure or its environment. In some forms of periodic paralysis, such window currents have been reported. This may explain the appearance of both activity and conduction failure in the phenotype of the same channel mutation. Factors involving channels other than the sodium or chloride channel may also be implicated in the generation of repetitive electrical activity. For example, a common mechanism for periodic bursting activity in neurons and for rhythmical electrical discharges in cardiac pacemaking cells involves the modulation of Ca^{2+}-dependent K^+ conductances. However, none of these potential mechanisms have yet been implicated in the production of human myotonic activity. Working out the mechanism by which a mutation in the gene encoding a muscle protein kinase produces repetitive electrical activity in myotonic dystrophy remains an elusive yet fertile area for future research.

The future

It is clear that a number of neuromuscular diseases involve either primary or secondary defects in membrane ion channels. In the past, these channels were difficult to study, especially in human skeletal muscle. Most observations were indirect and restricted to the electrophysiological measurements of the transmembrane currents that the channels control.

That situation has changed dramatically. Details of channel structure can now be derived through analysis of channel primary sequences, as deduced from the cloning of mRNA or from analysis of the genomic DNA. Patch clamp methods allow individual ion channels to be studied directly in the muscle membrane, and expression techniques make it possible to measure the single-channel electrophysiological properties of ion channels both in their natural conformation and after specific alterations have been made in their primary sequences.

The stage is now set for rapid advances in the study of disorders characterized by hyperexcitability or hypoexcitability of the muscle membrane and for direct analysis of the relationships between abnormal structure and function in the channel proteins themselves.

References

Adrian, R. H. and Bryant, S. H. (1974). On the repetitive discharge in myotonic muscle fibres. *J. Physiol. (Lond.)* **240**, 505–515

Adrian, R. H. and Marshall, M. W. (1976). Action potentials reconstructed in normal and myotonic muscle fibres. *J. Physiol. (Lond.)* **258**, 125–143.

Adrian, R. H. and Marshall, M. W. (1977). Sodium currents in mammalian muscle. *J. Physiol. (Lond.)* **268**, 233–250.

Adrian, R. H., Chandler, W. K., and Hodgkin, A. L. (1970). Voltage clamp experiments in striated muscle fibres. *J. Physiol.* **208**, 607–644.

Almers, W. (1972). Potassium conductance changes in skeletal muscle and the potassium concentration in the transverse tubules. *J. Physiol. (Lond.)* **225**, 33–56.

Auld, V. J., Goldin, A. L., Krafte, D. S., Catterall, W. A. et al. (1990). A neutral amino acid change in segment IIS4 dramatically alters the gating properties of the voltage-dependent sodium channel. *Proc. Natl. Acad. Sci. USA* **87**, 323

Barchi, R. L. (1975). Myotonia: an evaluation of the chloride hypothesis. *Arch. Neurol.* **32**, 175–180.

Barchi, R. L. (1995). Molecular pathology of the skeletal muscle sodium channel. *Annu. Rev. Physiol.* **57**, 355–85

Barchi, R. L. (1997). Mini Review: ion channel mutations and diseases of skeletal muscle. *Neurobiol. Dis.* **4**, 254–264

Bretag, A. H. (1973). Mathematical modeling of the myotonic action potential. In: *New Developments in Electromyography and Clinical Neurophysiology*, Vol. 1. ed. J. E. Desmedt. Basel: Karger.

Brown, G. L. and Harvey, A. M. (1939). Congenital myotonia in the goat. *Brain* **62**, 341–363.

Bryant, S. H. (1979). Myotonia in the goat. *Ann. N. Y. Acad. Sci.* **317**, 314–324.

Bryant, S. H. (1982). Abnormal repetitive impulse production in myotonic muscle. In: *Abnormal Nerves and Muscles as Impulse Generators*, eds. W. J. Culp and J. Ochoa, pp. 702–725. New York: Oxford University Press.

Bryant, S. H. and Morales-Aguilera, A. (1971). Chloride conductance in normal and myotonic muscle fibres and the action of monocarboxylic aromatic acids. *J. Physiol. (Lond.)* **219**, 367–383.

Bryant, S. H. and Owenburg, K. (1980). Characteristics of the chloride channel in skeletal-muscle fibers from myotonic and normal goats. *Fed. Proc.* **39**, 579–579.

Butler, A., Wei, A. and Salkoff, L. (1990). *Shal, Shab,* and *Shaw:* three genes encoding potassium channels in *Drosophila. Nucl. Acids Res.* **18**, 2173.

Cannon, S. C., Brown, R. H. and Corey, D. P. (1991). A sodium channel defect in hyperkalemic periodic paralysis: potassium induced failure of inactivation. *Neuron* **4**, 619–626.

Chandy, K. G., Williams, C. B., Spencer, R. H. et al. (1990). A family of three mouse potassium channel genes with intronless coding regions. *Science* **247**, 973–975.

Creutzfeldt, O. D., Abbott, B. C., Fowler, W. M. and Pearson, C. M. (1963). Muscle membrane potentials in episodic adynamia. *Electroencephalogr. Clin. Neurophysiol.* **15**, 508–516.

Davisson, M., Harris, B. and Lane, P. (1989). Chromosomal location of ADR. *Mouse Newslett.* **83**, 167–169.

Doyle, D. A., Morais Cabral, J., Pfuetzner, R. A. et al. (1998). The structure of the potassium channel: molecular basis of K^+ conduction and selectivity. *Science* **280**, 69–77.

Ebers, G., George, A. L., Barchi, R. L., Ting-Passador, S. S. et al. (1991). Paramyotonia congenita and hyperkalemic periodic paralysis are linked to the adult muscle sodium channel gene. *Ann. Neurol.* **30**, 810–816.

Engel, A. G. and Lambert, E. H. (1969). Calcium activation of electrically inexcitable muscle fibers in primary hypokalemic periodic paralysis. *Neurology* **19**, 851–858.

Entrikin, R., Abresch, R., Sharman, R., Larson, D. and Levine, N. (1987). Contractile and EMG studies of murine myotonia (*mto*) and muscular dystrophy (*dy/dy*). *Muscle Nerve* **10**, 293–298.

Fontaine, B., Khurana, T. S., Hoffman, E. P., Bruns, G. A. et al., (1990). Hyperkalemic periodic paralysis and the adult muscle sodium channel alpha-subunit gene. *Science* **250**, 1000–1002.

French, R. J. and Horn, R. (1983). Sodium channel gating: models, mimics and modifiers. *Annu. Rev. Biophys. Bioeng.* **12**, 319–356.

Furman, R. E. and Barchi, R. L. (1978). The pathophysiology of myotonia produced by aromatic carboxylic acids. *Ann. Neurol.* **4**, 357–365.

Furman, R. E. and Barchi, R. L. (1981). 20,25-Diazacholesterol myotonia: an electrophysiological study. *Ann. Neurol.* **10**, 251–260.

Gallant, E. M. (1983). Barium-treated mammalian skeletal muscle: similarities to hypokalaemic periodic paralysis. *J. Physiol. (Lond.)* **335**, 577–590.

George, A. L., Ledbetter, D. H., Kallen, R. G. and Barchi, R. L. (1991). Assignment of a human skeletal muscle sodium channel α-subunit gene (*SCN4A*) to 17q23.1–25.3. *Genomics* **9**, 555–556.

George, A. L., Komisarof, J., Kallen, R. G. and Barchi, R. L. (1992). Primary structure of the adult skeletal musle voltage-dependent sodium channel. *Ann. Neurol.* **31**, 131–137.

Gordon, A. M., Green, J. R. and Langunoff, D. (1970). Studies on a patient with hypokalemic familial periodic paralysis. *Am. J. Med.* **48**,. 185–195.

Gründer, S., Thiemann, A., Pusch, M. and Jentsch, T. J. (1992). Regions involved in the opening of ClC-2 chloride channel by voltage and cell volume. *Nature* **36**, 759–762.

Guy, H. R. and Conti, F. (1990). Pursing the structure and function of voltage-gated ion channels. *Trends Neurol. Sci.* **13**, 201–206.

Hartshorne, R. P. and Catterall, W. A. (1984). The sodium channel from rat brain: purification and subunit composition. *J. Biol. Chem.* **159**, 1667–1675.

Heinemann, S. H., Terlau, H., Strühmer, W., Imoto, K. and Numa, S. (1992). Calcium channel characteristics conferred on the sodium channel by single mutations. *Nature* **356**, 441–443.

Heller, A., Eicher, E., Hallett, M. and Sidman, R. (1982). Myotonia, a new inherited muscle disease in mice. *J. Neurosci.* **2**, 924–933.

Hodgkin, A. L. and Huxley, A. F. (1952). A quantitative description of membrane current and its application to conduction and excitation in nerve. *J. Physiol. (Lond.)* **117**, 500–544.

Hofman, W. W. and Smith, R. A. (1970). Hypokalemic periodic paralysis studied in vitro. *Brain* **93**, 445–474.

Hutter, O. F. and Noble, D. (1960). The chloride conductance of frog skeletal muscle. *J. Physiol. (Lond.)* **151**, 89–102.

Isom, L. L., de Jongh, K. S., Patton, D. E., Reber, B. F. X. et al. (1992). Primary structure and functional expression of the β_1-subunit of the rat brain sodium channel. *Science* **256**, 839–842.

Jentsch, T., Steinmeyer, K. and Schwarz, G. (1990). Primary structure of *Torpedo marmorata* chloride channel isolated by expression cloning in *Xenopus* oocytes. *Nature* **348**, 510–514.

Jorgensen, P. L. (1982). Mechanism of the Na^+K^+ pump. Protein structure and conformations of the pure Na^+K^+ ATPase. *Biochim. Biophys. Acta* **694**, 27–68.

Kallen, R. G., Sheng, Z. H., Yang, J., Chen, L., Rogart, R. B. and Barchi, R. L. (1990). Primary structure and expression of a sodium channel characteristic of denervated and immature rat skeletal muscle. *Neuron* **4**, 233–242.

Kallen, R. G., Cohen, S. A. and Barchi, R. L. (1993). Structure, function and expression of voltage-dependent sodium channels. *Mol. Neurobiol.* **7**, 383–428.

Kao, I. and Gordon, A. M. (1975). Mechanism of insulin produced paralysis of muscle from potassium-depleted rats. *Science* **188**, 740–741.

Koch, M. C., Ricker, K., Otto, M., Grimm, T. et al. (1991). Confirmation of linkage of hyperkalemic periodic paralysis to chromosome 17. *J. Med. Genet.* **28**, 583–586.

Kolb, H. A. (1990). Potassium channels in excitable and nonexcitable cells. *Rev. Physiol. Biochem. Pharmacol.* **115**, 51–91.

Lehmann-Horn, F., Rüdel, R., Dengler, R., Lorkovic, H., Haas, A. and Ricker, K. (1981). Membrane defects in paramytonia congenita with and without myotonia in a warm environment. *Muscle Nerve* **4**, 396–406.

Lehmann-Horn, F., Rüdel, R., Ricker, K., Lorkovic, H., Dengler, R. and Hopf, H. C. (1983). Two cases of adynamia episodica hereditaria: in vitro investigation of muscle cell membrane and contraction parameters. *Muscle Nerve* **6**, 113–121.

Lehmann-Horn, F., Küther, G., Ricker, K., Grafe, P., Ballanyi, K. and Rüdel, R. (1987). Adynamia episodica hereditaria with myotonia: a non-inactivating sodium current and the effect of extra cellular pH. *Muscle Nerve* **10**, 363–374.

Lipicky, R. J. (1977). Studies in human myotonic dystrophy. In: *Pathogenesis of Human Muscular Dystrophies*, ed. L. P. Rowland, Amsterdam: Excerpta Medica.

Lipicky, R. J. and Bryant, S. H. (1973). A biophysical study of human myotonias. In: *New Developments in Electromyography and Clinical Neurophysiology*, Vol. 1. ed. J. E. Desmedt. Basel: Karger.

Lipicky, R. J., Bryant, S. H. and Salmon, J. H. (1971). Cable parameters, sodium, potassium, chloride and water content, and potassium efflux in isolated external intercostal muscles of normal volunteers and patients with myotonia congenita. *J. Clin. Invest.* **50**, 2091–2103.

MacKinnon, R. (1991). Determination of the subunit stoichiometry of a voltage-activated potassum channel. *Nature* **350**, 232–235.

McComas, A. J., Mrozek, K. and Bradley, W. G. (1968). The nature of the electrophysiological disorder in adynamia episodica. *J. Neurol. Neurosurg. Psychiatry* **31**, 448–452.

Mehrke, G., Brinkmeier, H. and Jockusch, H. (1988). The myotonic mouse mutant *adr*: electrophysiology of the muscle fiber. *Muscle Nerve* **11**, 440–446.

Neher, E. and Sackmann, B. (1976). Single channel currents recorded from the membrane of denervated frog muscle fibers. *Nature* **260**, 799–802.

Palade, P. T. and Barchi, R. L. (1977a). Characteristics of the chloride conductance in muscle fibers of the rat diaphragm. *J. Gen. Physiol.* **69**, 325–342.

Palade, P. T. and Barchi, R. L. (1977b). On the inhibition of muscle membrane chloride conductances by aromatic carboxylic acids. *J. Gen. Physiol.* **69**, 875–896.

Papazian, D. M., Schwarz, T. L., Tempel, B. L., Jan, Y. N. and Jan, L. Y. (1987). Cloning of genomic and complementary DNA from *Shaker*, a putative potassium channel gene from *Drosphila*. *Science* **237**, 749–753.

Ptáček, L. J., Tyler, F., Trimmer, J. S., Agnew, W. S.and Leppert, M. (1991). Analysis in large hyperkalemic periodic paralysis pedigree supports tight linkage to a sodium channel locus. *Am. J. Hum. Genet.* **49**, 378–382.

Ptáček, L. J., Tawil, R., Griggs, R. C. et al. (1992). Linkage of atypical myotonia congenita to a sodium channel locus. *Neurology* **42**, 431–433.

Reininghaus, J., Füchtbaur, E.-M., Bertran, K. and Jockusch, H. (1988). The myotonic mouse mutant *adr*: physiological and histochemical properties of muscle. *Muscle Nerve* **11**, 433–439.

Riecker, G. and Bolte, J. D. (1976). Membranpotentiale einzelner skeletmuskelzellen bei hypokalamischer periodischer muskelparalyse. *Klin. Wochenschr.* **44**, 804–810.

Roberds, S. and Tankum, M. (1991). Cloning and tissue-specific expression of five voltage-gated potassium channel cDNAs expressed in rat heart. *Proc. Natl. Acad. Sci. USA* **88**, 1798.

Roberts, R. and Barchi, R. L. (1987). The voltage-sensitive sodium channel from rabbit skeletal muscle: chemical characterization of subunits. *J. Biol. Chem.* **262**, 2298–2303.

Rüdel, R. (1990). The myotonic mouse – a realistic model for the study of human recessive generalized myotonia. *Trends Neurosci.* **13**, 1–3.

Rüdel, R. and Lehmann-Horn, F. (1985). Membrane changes in cells from myotonia patients. *Physiol. Rev.* **65**, 310–346.

Rüdel, R. and Ricker, K. (1985). The primary periodic paralyses. *TINS* **8**, 467–470.

Rüdel, R. and Senges, J. (1972). Experimental myotonia in mammalian skeletal muscle. Changes in membrane properties. *Pflügers Arch.* **331**, 324–334.

Schmidt-Rose, T. and Jentsch, T. J. (1997). Transmembrane topology of a CLC chloride channel. *Proc. Natl. Acad. Sci. USA* **94**, 7633–7638.

Shy, G. M., Wanko, T., Rowley, P. T. and Engel, A. G. (1961). Studies in familial periodic paralysis. *Exp. Neurol.* **3**, 53–55.

Steinmeyer, K., Ortland, C. and Jentsch, T. (1991). Primary structure and functional expression of a developmentally regulated skeletal muscle chloride channel. *Nature* **354**, 301–304.

Stühmer, W., Conti, F., Suzuki, H., Wang, X. et al. (1989). Structural parts involved in activation and inactivation of the sodium channel. *Nature* **339**, 597–603.

Trimmer, J. S., Cooperman, S. S., Tomiko, S. A., Zhou, J. et al. (1989). Primary structure and functional expression of a mammalian skeletal muscle sodium channel. *Neuron* **3**, 33–49.

Vassilev, P., Scheuer, T. and Caterall, W. A. (1989). Inhibition of inactivation of single sodium channel by a site-directed antibody. *Proc. Natl. Acad. Sci. USA* **86**, 8147–8151.

Watkins, W. and Watts, D. (1984). Developmental changes in lactate dehydrogenase and aldolase activity of the A2D-adr mouse with abnormal muscle function: further comparison with the 129Redy mutant. *J. Neurosci.* **43**, 517–521.

11

Animal models of human muscle disease

Barry J. Cooper

Introduction

One approach to modelling human disease has been to study inherited diseases of animals that resemble those of humans. These diseases often had to be judged on the basis of phenotypic similarities without a confident basis for any similarity in pathogenetic mechanisms. The world of animal models, however, has been revolutionized by the advent of molecular genetics and transgenic technology. It is now possible to establish whether naturally occurring models truly correspond to a human inherited disease and, where they are lacking, to manufacture such models in the laboratory. The focus of this chapter will be on describing animal models with proven relevance to their human counterparts.

Animal models of muscular dystrophy

The *mdx* mouse

The *mdx* mouse was originally identified by Bulfield and coworkers (1984) in a colony of inbred C57BL/10ScSn mice. It was recognized because of increased levels of pyruvate kinase and creatine kinase. The mutation was found to be inherited as an X-linked trait, and it was proposed that the *mdx* mouse might serve as a model for Duchenne muscular dystrophy (DMD).

Clinical signs
Many investigators have studied this mutant, and there is general agreement that clinical signs are mild or absent (Dangain and Vrbova, 1984; Tanabe et al., 1986; Carnwath and Shotton, 1987; Torres and Duchen, 1987). The minimal nature of clinical signs and the nonprogressive lesions led to considerable controversy regarding the suitability of this

mutant as a model of DMD. Since the identification of the dystrophin gene, however, the *mdx* mouse has been shown to be a genetically accurate model of DMD.

A number of studies have been carried out in an attempt to document muscle weakness in the *mdx* mouse. Several investigators have found that *mdx* mice are heavier than controls, that their muscles are larger and that they are as strong or stronger than controls, except during the peak of muscle necrosis at 2–5 weeks of age (Dangain and Vrbova, 1984; Coulton et al., 1988a). However, when measurements are corrected for increased cross-sectional area of the muscle, weakness can be demonstrated. Several studies (Anderson et al., 1988; Sacco et al., 1992; Quinlan et al., 1992) have found that anterior tibial and soleus muscles of *mdx* mice are weaker than those of controls. Additionally, a technique designed to measure whole-body tension shows that *mdx* mice have muscle weakness throughout their life (Carlson and Makiejus, 1990). Therefore, although they demonstrate minimal signs on clinical examination, careful quantitative techniques can document muscle weakness.

Pathology
In the *mdx* mouse, extensive muscle necrosis occurs early in life. In most studies a dramatic onset of necrosis has been reported at about three weeks of age, with necrotic fibres occurring in clusters (Fig. 11.1) (Dangain and Vrbova, 1984; Tanabe et al., 1986; Carnwath and Shotton, 1987; Torres and Duchen, 1987; Coulton et al., 1988b). Hypercontracted fibres and fibres undergoing segmental necrosis and phagocytosis by macrophages are found, and calcification of fibres is sometimes reported (Coulton et al., 1988b). Prior to the onset of necrosis, muscle fibre nuclei are peripherally located (Tanabe et al., 1986). Following the wave of necrosis, regeneration occurs, which is recognized by the usual criteria of cytoplasmic basophilia and the

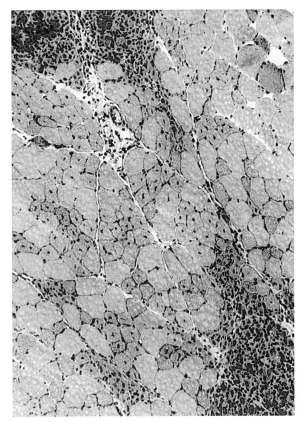

Fig. 11.1. Limb muscle from a 30-day-old *mdx* mouse showing locally extensive areas of necrosis and clusters of small regenerate fibres with centralized nuclei. (Frozen section, trichrome stain, ×80.)

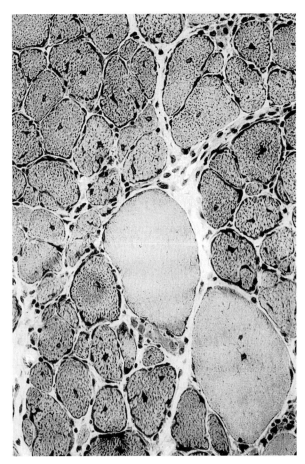

Fig. 11.2. Limb muscle from a 60-day-old *mdx* mouse showing evidence of regeneration. There is fibre size variation; most fibres have central nuclei and occasional fibres are markedly hypertrophied. There is mild endomysial fibrosis. (Frozen sections, trichrome stain, ×200.)

presence of centrally placed euchromatic nuclei. A peculiar feature of the mouse is that centrally placed nuclei persist and, in fact, can be used as a marker for regenerated fibres (Tanabe et al., 1986; Carnwath and Shotton, 1987; Torres and Duchen, 1987; Coulton et al., 1988b). In older mice, most muscle fibres have internalized nuclei and, therefore, have undergone at least one round of necrosis and regeneration (Fig. 11.2).

Torres and Duchen (1987) carried out a particularly detailed morphological study of the *mdx* mouse. They reported the occurrence of muscle lesions in younger animals than generally reported by other investigators. For example, they found scattered hyalinized fibres in 1-day-old animals, and full-fledged necrosis and phagocytosis by five days of age. These differences in age of onset of necrosis are most likely explained by the extensive sampling of several different muscles carried out by these authors, and they note that necrosis in very young animals was more common in the muscles of the head and shoulder girdle

than in the limb muscles. As discussed below, similar muscle-specific variation in the age of onset of muscle lesions has also been clearly documented in dystrophic dogs. This variation in susceptibility of different muscles to necrosis may result, in part, from differences in fibre size. It has been reported that small calibre dystrophic muscle fibres are relatively resistant to injury (Karpati, et al., 1982). Torres and Duchen (1987) also reported that there is no preferential involvement of either type I or type II fibres.

Although some early studies reported that regeneration in muscles of *mdx* mice was complete and that necrosis did not continue into later life (Dangain and Vrbova, 1984), subsequent studies by other investigators have shown that some level of necrosis and regeneration occurs at all ages (Carnwath and Shotton, 1987; Torres and Duchen, 1987; Coulton et al., 1988b). What is clear from these studies is that there is a peak incidence of muscle necrosis at around three weeks of age, followed by accumulation of centrally nucleated muscle fibres and a progressive decline in the incidence of necrotic fibres, which nevertheless persist in low numbers in animals one year of age or more. In one study, for example, soleus and plantaris muscles of three-week-old *mdx* mice contained more that 30% of fibres expressing the embryonic isoform of myosin heavy chain, a marker for regenerated fibres, while this number fell to 1–2% by one year of age (DiMario et al., 1991). Therefore, in limb muscles, regeneration seems to produce a population of centrally nucleated fibres that are relatively resistant to further bouts of necrosis. Autoradiographic studies have shown that muscle of *mdx* mice does not appear to have an inherently increased capacity for regeneration (Grounds and McGeachie, 1992) and is as capable of regeneration after experimental injury as normal muscle (Zacharias and Anderson, 1991).

The muscles of *mdx* mice also show consistently increased variation in fibre size (Torres and Duchen, 1987; Coulton et al., 1988b). This includes both abnormally large and abnormally small fibres. Hypertrophied fibres are detectable as early as a few weeks of age (Torres and Duchen, 1987) and become prominent in older mice (Fig. 11.2). Fibre hypertrophy, as discussed below, is also a feature of muscular dystrophy in the dog and the cat. A progressive increase in the proportion of type 1 fibres has also been reported in *mdx* muscles (Carnwath and Shotton, 1987; Stedman et al., 1991).

A unique feature of the *mdx* mouse is that the dystrophic process, in most muscles, does not produce the extensive fibrosis and loss of muscle fibres that characterizes DMD in humans (Coulton et al., 1988b). However, in a more recent study, it has been reported that extensive fibrosis occurs in the diaphragm and intercostal muscles of older animals (Stedman et al., 1991), the diaphragm showing an associated decrease in isometric strength and loss of tissue compliance (Stedman et al., 1991; Dupont-Versteegden and McCarter, 1992). The reasons for the discrepancies between limb muscles and diaphragm are unknown, but they may relate to differences in muscle work and to age. In a study of *mdx* mice allowed to live out their natural lifespan (Lefaucheur et al., 1995), significant fibrosis of hindlimb muscles, as well as diaphragm and intercostal muscles, was found in animals over 20 months of age. These findings correlated with reduced lifespan and apparent reduced activity in the older animals.

Ultrastructurally, necrosis in muscles of *mdx* mice is characterized by dilatation of the sarcoplasmic reticulum, hypercontraction, disorganization and lysis of myofibrils, and perforation of the sarcolemma. However, the last is associated with necrosis of muscle fibres, unlike in DMD, where it is reported to precede necrosis (Cullen and Jaros, 1988). Although disruption of the basal lamina was reported by Bulfield in his original description of the *mdx* mouse (Bulfield et al., 1984) this feature has not been observed in other studies (Torres and Duchen, 1987; Cullen and Jaros, 1988). The careful studies of Torres and Duchen (1987) failed to demonstrate lesions in the nervous system of *mdx* mice. A number of freeze-fracture studies using *mdx* mice have also been reported. To summarize, it appears that structural changes in the sarcolemma occur prior to the development of degenerative lesions, including reduction of P face intramembranous particles (IMPs), already apparent by three days of age, and of orthogonal arrays (OAs), which were similar in density in normal and *mdx* muscle at three days of age but were reduced at seven and 14 days (Shibuya and Wakayama, 1991).

Dystrophin is expressed in cardiac muscle fibres and cardiomyopathy is a consistent feature of both DMD and the canine model *xmd*. The literature regarding cardiac involvement in *mdx* is inconsistent. Some investigators have found no evidence of cardiomyopathy in *mdx* mice (Tanabe et al., 1986; Torres and Duchen, 1987) while others found cardiac lesions in at least some of the animals studied (Bridges, 1986; Carnwath and Shotton, 1987; Coulton et al., 1988b). The cause of these inconsistencies is not clear but may be related to the age of the animals studied. In the dog, for example, it is quite clear that the development of cardiac lesions is a relatively late event.

Molecular basis

The *mdx* mouse has been shown to lack dystrophin, the protein product of the Duchenne locus (Hoffman et al., 1987; Sugita et al., 1988). Mapping studies demonstrated that the responsible mutation lies within the murine homologue of the DMD locus (Cavanna et al., 1988; Ryder-Cook et al., 1988). Subsequently, the mutation responsible for the *mdx* mouse was shown to be a point mutation, substitution of a cytosine by thymine at nucleotide 3185 (Sicinski et al., 1989), introducing a termination codon. Subsequently, four additional strains of *mdx* have been identified in mutagen-treated mice (Chapman et al., 1989). The mutations responsible for all four of these have now been identified (Im et al., 1996). Although these strains vary in their pattern of transcript expression and in the expression of truncated dystrophin proteins, they have similar phenotypes. Some of these mutations are predicted to interfere with the expression of nonmuscle isoforms of dystrophin, which may prove useful in analysing their function. Yet another strain, dubbed *mdx-beta geo*, has been generated by insertion of a gene trap vector into the dystrophin gene 3′ of exon 63 (Wertz and Fuchtbauer, 1998) and a knock-out model has been created by targeting exon 52 (Araki et al., 1997). This knock-out lacks the dystrophin isoforms Dp140 and Dp260 but is phenotypically very similar to the *mdx*.

Paradoxically, immunostaining of *mdx* skeletal muscle shows occasional fibres, or small groups of fibres, that stain positively for dystrophin (Hoffman et al., 1990). The frequency of such fibres, although always low, varies between strains of *mdx* mice (Hoffman et al., 1990; Danko et al., 1992, Im et al., 1996) and tends to increase with age. Rare fibres staining for dystrophin have also been reported in muscle of humans with DMD (Nicholson et al., 1989) and in dystrophic dogs (see below). A recent study showed that alternative splicing produces transcripts that skip the mutation in exon 23 of the *mdx* mouse, allowing expression of truncated forms of dystrophin (Wilton et al., 1997).

Female mice heterozygous for the *mdx* mutation have been shown to express dystrophin in a mosaic pattern (Watkins et al., 1989; Karpati et al., 1990). However, the number of fibres negative for dystrophin, even in mice as young as 10 days, is considerably less than expected from the Lyon hypothesis, which would predict that 50% of myonuclei would be incompetent to synthesize dystrophin. Furthermore, the number of dystrophin-negative fibres progressively declines with age (Watkins et al., 1989; Karpati et al., 1990) such that by 60–90 days of age negative fibres are exceedingly rare. Inhibition of satellite cell proliferation by gamma-irradiation does not alter the rate at which dystrophin-negative fibre segments are replaced by segments expressing dystrophin, indicating that this phenomenon is a result of diffusion of dystrophin along the mosaic fibre rather than incorporation of competent satellite cells during growth or regeneration (Weller et al., 1991). Necrotic and regenerate fibres are very rare in such mosaic heterozygote muscle (Watkins et al., 1989; Karpati et al., 1990) and serum creatine kinase levels are normal (Tanaka et al., 1990), suggesting that expression of reduced levels of normal dystrophin is largely sufficient to protect the fibres from necrosis (Karpati et al., 1990). As would be expected, cardiac muscle of heterozygotes exhibits clear-cut mosaic staining for dystrophin (Karpati et al., 1990).

Pathogenesis

Despite the identification of defects in dystrophin and subsequently of disruption of the sarcolemmal dystrophin complex as the molecular basis for DMD, the events leading to muscle necrosis remain unclear. Nevertheless, the *mdx* mouse has proven useful in addressing a number of hypotheses.

The localization of dystrophin to the cytoplasmic face of the plasma membrane (Arahata et al., 1988; Zubrzycka-Gaarn et al., 1988) and its interaction with a complex of membrane glycoproteins, (Campbell and Kahl, 1989; Ervasti and Campbell, 1991; Ohlendieck et al., 1991) have led to speculation that dystrophin plays a role in stabilizing the sarcolemma, protecting it from injury associated with contraction. This hypothesis has been tested in the *mdx* mouse. It has been shown that isolated *mdx* muscle fibres are abnormally sensitive to osmotic lysis (Menke and Jockusch, 1991), suggesting that the dystrophic muscle membrane might be fragile. Similarly, exposure to hypoosmotic conditions results in increased influx of calcium ions in *mdx* myotubes compared with normal myotubes (Leijendekker et al., 1996), suggesting that dystrophic muscle cells might be abnormally permeable to calcium under stress conditions. More direct studies of sarcolemmal membrane of *mdx* mice using the patch clamp technique have shown small, but significant, differences in the tension required to rupture the membrane (Hutter et al., 1991).

If the lack of dystrophin does lead to contraction-associated injury, dystrophic muscle should be abnormally sensitive to exercise-induced injury. This question also has been addressed in the *mdx* mouse, with mixed results. In one study, it was found that both eccentric and concentric contractions produce more severe necrosis in *mdx* muscle than in controls (Weller et al., 1990). This result has been contradicted, however, in other studies. Sacco et al. (1992) found that eccentric exercise produced no more necrosis in anterior tibial muscle of *mdx* mice than in normal muscle. In more recent studies, the effects of eccentric exercise involving downhill running were studied in *mdx* mice expressing β-galactosidase in skeletal muscle (Vilquin et al., 1998). These studies clearly showed increased plasma levels of both creatine kinase and β-galactosidase within 1 hour of the exercise challenge and an increase in muscle uptake of intravenously injected Evans blue, indicating increased membrane damage compared with that seen in normal muscle (Brussee et al., 1997). Exercise in *mdx* mice has also been shown to result in increased levels of apoptosis, which may contribute to the initiation of dystrophic muscle cell injury (Sandri et al., 1997). The overall evidence, therefore, is that exercise, particularly eccentric exercise, exacerbates muscle injury in Duchenne-type dystrophy. Despite such studies, there is evidence from the study of aged *mdx* mice that non-weight-bearing exercise such as swimming or voluntary running can be beneficial (Hayes and Williams, 1998; Wineinger et al., 1998).

There has also been considerable interest in possible

abnormalities of calcium handling in dystrophic muscle, stemming from studies in humans in which increased intracellular calcium levels have been demonstrated in affected muscle (Bodensteiner and Engel, 1978). Total calcium content has been shown to be elevated in skeletal and cardiac muscle at all ages in the *mdx* mouse (Dunn and Radda, 1991). Using the fluorescent calcium chelator fura-2, Turner et al. (1988) demonstrated that resting intracellular calcium ion concentration ($[Ca^{2+}]_i$) is markedly increased in *mdx* muscle fibres compared with controls, and that calcium transients following stimulation were prolonged. Furthermore, these investigators showed that increased $[Ca^{2+}]_i$ was associated with increased rates of intracellular proteolysis. Increased rates of calcium-dependent proteolysis have also been implicated in *mdx* muscle by other investigators (MacLennan et al., 1991). Other studies have shown that similar increases in $[Ca^{2+}]_i$ are present in both cultured dystrophic myotubes from both humans and *mdx* mice (Fong et al., 1990) and that these dystrophic myotubes have impaired ability to regulate $[Ca^{2+}]_i$ in response to changes in extracellular calcium levels compared with control myotubes.

These alterations in calcium handling may be explained by increased activity of calcium-selective leak channels (Fong et al., 1990). Other studies have implicated additional mechanisms that could result in increases in $[Ca^{2+}]_i$. Stretch-activated channels have been described in both normal and *mdx* myotubes; in addition, stretch-inactivated calcium-permeable channels that are open for long periods of time have been identified in *mdx* myotubes but are rarely observed in controls (Franco and Lansman, 1990). Stretch-activated channels have also been demonstrated in freshly dissociated normal and *mdx* flexor digitorum brevis muscles, although stretch-inactivated channels were not present in these preparations (Haws and Lansman, 1991). Occasional patches from young *mdx* mice showed high levels of activity of stretch-activated channels.

Yet another potential mechanism of membrane damage that has been hypothesized to contribute to muscle necrosis in DMD is free radical injury (oxidative stress). Studies have found evidence of increased lipid peroxidation in dystrophin-deficient muscle (Ragusa et al., 1997), even before the onset of necrosis (Disatnik et al., 1998). These results suggest that oxidant injury is an early event in dystrophin-deficient muscle. Similarly, cultured myotubes from *mdx* mice have been shown to have increased susceptibility to oxidative injury (Rando et al., 1998). These findings were of considerable interest given the finding that neuronal nitric oxide synthase (nNOS) is associated with the dystrophin complex at the membrane of normal muscle and is redistributed in *mdx* muscle (Brenman et al., 1995; Chang et al., 1996). However, no evidence of free radical injury involving NO· has been found (Disatnik et al., 1998), results that are in agreement with experiments using knock-out mice (see below).

The *mdx* mouse is also proving to be useful in studies of the molecular pathogenesis of dystrophinopathies. Studies by Campbell and his co-workers have identified a membrane complex of glycoproteins and nonglycosylated proteins that interacts with dystrophin (Campbell and Kahl, 1989; Ervasti and Campbell, 1991). In *mdx* muscle, the components of this complex are greatly reduced (Ohlendieck and Campbell, 1991). These findings suggest that these proteins cannot be maintained in the membrane in the absence of dystrophin and that their reduction may be important in the pathogenesis of the disease. The fact that defects in other components of the complex cause forms of muscular dystrophy and that *mdx* and DMD myotubes cannot adhere effectively to laminin-$\alpha2$ (Angoli et al., 1997) supports the hypothesis that disruption of the dystrophin complex interferes with linkage between the cytoskeleton and the extracellular matrix. Campbell's group has shown that the autosomally encoded dystrophin analogue utrophin also can bind to components of this complex (Matsumura et al., 1992). These investigators have suggested that the expression of utrophin in skeletal and cardiac myocytes may be responsible for the resistance of the *mdx* to myonecrosis. The possibility that upregulation of utrophin might alleviate the clinical severity of DMD is an intriguing one, which has been addressed using transgenic and knock-out mice, discussed below.

Therapeutic studies

The *mdx* mouse has already been useful in studying two approaches to therapy, namely myoblast transfer and gene therapy. In the first, normal myoblasts are injected into the muscle of the dystrophic patient or animal. These cells are predicted to fuse with host muscle during the cycle of degeneration and regeneration, thus incorporating nuclei competent to synthesize dystrophin into regenerated muscle fibres. The end result of such therapy should be to produce muscle fibres that are mosaic in their capacity to produce dystrophin. Observations in carrier muscle, described above, suggest that dystrophin might become disseminated throughout such mosaicized fibres.

Studies by Partridge and his colleagues (1989) have indicated that injection of enzymatically dissociated myoblasts can indeed result in the formation of mosaicized fibres and the expression of dystrophin in dystrophic muscle. Muscles injected with normal myoblasts were found to contain many fibres expressing dystrophin at the sarcolemma. The injection of normal human myoblasts into *mdx* muscle has also been reported to result in the expression of dystrophin in a small percentage of fibres (Karpati et al., 1989). In subsequent experiments, Partridge et al. have shown that even more effective restoration of dystrophin-positive fibres occurs when normal myoblasts are injected into previously irradiated *mdx* muscle, in which endogenous satellite cell activity is inhibited (Morgan et al., 1990). In those experiments, up to 80% of muscle fibres expressed dystrophin, and the bulk and architecture of the treated muscle was restored to normal. Furthermore, injected myoblasts seemed to be able to migrate from the injection site throughout the treated tibialis anterior and extensor digitorum longus (EDL) muscles, and even into the nearby, but uninjected, peroneus muscle. Other experiments have shown that injection of myoblasts into nonirradiated recipients results in fusion of donor and host cells, while injection into irradiated muscle results in a high proportion of fibres formed by donor–donor fusion (Kinoshita et al., 1996). It also has been shown that muscle precursor cells, injected into irradiated muscle, can adopt the role of resting myoblasts (i.e. satellite cells) and participate in regenerative responses after multiple bouts of muscle injury (Gross and Morgan, 1999). In contrast to the *mdx* mouse, experiments in the canine model and trials in human patients have not resulted in significant expression of dystrophin-positive fibres. This may be explained by rapid death of injected myoblasts, as has been shown using Y-chromosome-specific probes to follow the fate of male-derived myoblasts injected into female *mdx* mice (Fan et al., 1996). In summary, therefore, although myoblast transfer itself may not become clinically applicable, these results offer considerable encouragement for any form of therapy, including gene therapy, where expression of dystrophin can be induced.

Studies of gene therapy in the *mdx* mouse have allowed important basic questions to be addressed. Several studies have shown beneficial effects of gene therapy using recombinant adenoviral vectors (rAdV). Injection of an rAdV – *dystrophin* minigene into the muscles of neonatal *mdx* mice resulted in expression of dystrophin and protection from mechanical damage (Deconinck et al., 1996). A similar study showed a high degree of short-term expression in neonates but less in older animals (Acsadi et al., 1996). These investigators also found histological improvement in transduced fibres; however, dystrophin-positive fibres were greatly reduced, even in neonatally injected animals, after 60 days, apparently reflecting the activity of $CD8^+$ cytotoxic lymphocytes. This problem can be at least reduced by immunosuppression (Lochmuller et al., 1996). Similarly, transfer of a dystrophin minigene using rAdV could be effected in adult *mdx* mice using FK506 (tacrolimus) immunosuppression (Yang et al., 1998). However, immunosuppression did not reduce the toxicity of the vector, which was dose dependent, and the therapeutic margin of safety was found to be narrow. Another approach to reducing immune responses is to delete as much of the viral genome as possible. Clemens et al. (1996) were able to construct an rAdV vector containing no viral genes that was able to accommodate the full-length dystrophin cDNA with a mCK promoter and a *lacZ* reporter gene. Intramuscular injection of this construct led to expression of full-length dystrophin and restoration of the dystrophin complex. The treated muscle showed a decrease in centrally nucleated fibres, suggesting that it protected against muscle degeneration.

Less has been published using retroviral vectors. In one study, retroviral producer cells releasing a vector carrying the dystrophin minigene were injected into immunoincompetent *mdx* mice (nude or immunosuppressed) (Fassati et al., 1997). Up to 18% of the fibres in the injected muscle expressed dystrophin, as well as α-sarcoglycan, as an indicator of restoration of the dystrophin complex.

Finally, a different approach, based on the idea that overexpression of utrophin can at least partially compensate for dystrophin deficiency, has been to use vectors expressing utrophin. One putative advantage of this approach is that the utrophin should not evoke an immune response, unlike dystrophin, which may be seen as a neo-antigen by dystrophic animals. In one such study, an rAdV vector expressing a truncated utrophin was injected into muscle of mice aged three to five days (Gilbert et al., 1999). The utrophin construct was stably expressed for at least 60 days. It restored the dystrophin complex and reduced the number of centrally nucleated fibres; the transduced fibres were impermeable to Evans blue. There was also evidence that the overexpression of utrophin conferred resistance to mechanical stress. Nevertheless, in older animals there was evidence of immune-mediated loss of expression.

Canine muscular dystrophy

In recent years, it has become apparent that muscular dystrophy occurs sporadically in the dog. Although the disease has been described in multiple breeds, the best-known canine model is the Golden Retriever strain known as the *xmd* (or GRMD) dog. The disease in the Golden Retriever was first recognized in the 1970s (de Lahunta, 1983) and later characterized as a model of DMD (Valentine et al., 1986; Kornegay et al., 1988).

Clinical signs

In contrast to the mouse, dogs with muscular dystrophy show a severe clinical phenotype, which is similar to that of humans with DMD (Kornegay et al., 1988; Valentine et al., 1989a). Typically, clinical signs first become obvious at six to nine weeks of age. However, serum creatine kinase is consistently elevated from birth and dystrophic pups can be identified on this basis. One of the earliest clinical signs noted in *xmd* dogs is an inability to open the jaw fully. Growth rate of dystrophic pups is depressed and affected pups tend to be less active than normal littermates, moving with a stiff 'bunny hopping' gait. By three months of age, affected dogs may develop abduction of the elbows and adduction of the hocks, with overflexion of the tarsi and overextension of the carpi (Fig. 11.3). Jaw mobility becomes further compromised, and the tongue is enlarged, particularly at its base. Muscle atrophy is apparent. The disease is progressive, but progression slows at about 6 months of age. By that age, there is marked muscle atrophy, particularly involving the muscles of the head, trunk and limbs, with proximal limb muscles tending to be less severely affected. In fact, Kornegay reported enlargement of the proximal limb muscles (Kornegay et al., 1988). Contracture associated with muscle fibrosis results in restricted extension of the shoulders and hips. Many of the affected muscles are firm to palpation. The base of the tongue is consistently enlarged, resulting in dysphagia and regurgitation. As the oesophagus of the dog contains skeletal muscle throughout its length, oesophageal dysfunction may contribute to dysphagia. Affected dogs tend to be reluctant to exercise and have difficulty in such tasks as rising from recumbency and climbing stairs. Respiration is usually rapid and characterized by increased abdominal movement. Older dogs eventually develop lordosis and medial deviation of the ventrocaudal edge of the costal arch. The latter deformity results from severe contracture of the diaphragm.

Dystrophic dogs also have dramatic electromyographic abnormalities (Kornegay et al., 1988; Valentine et al., 1989b). These consist of prominent spontaneous activity, predominantly complex repetitive discharges (pseudomyotonic discharges), which are found at all stages of the disease. Motor unit potentials are frequently brief and polyphasic. Nerve conduction velocities are normal.

Pathology

As in DMD, the essential lesion of muscular dystrophy in the *xmd* dog is necrosis (Valentine et al., 1990). In dogs showing early clinical signs, that is from about two to four months of age, the characteristic changes are the presence of numerous hypercontracted fibres (large dark fibres),

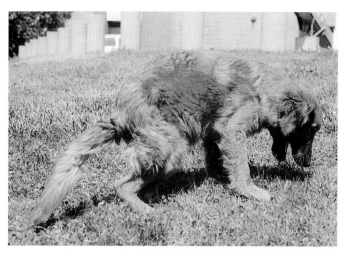

Fig. 11.3. A 6-month-old retriever dog showing typical signs of muscular dystrophy. Note the overflexion of the limbs and head-hanging stance, owing to muscle weakness, and the general loss of muscle mass. (Photograph courtesy of Dr Beth Valentine.)

active necrosis, infiltration by macrophages, and active muscle regeneration (Fig. 11.4). Necrotic and regenerating fibres tend to appear in clusters. Histochemical staining shows increased levels of calcium in necrotic and large dark fibres (Valentine et al., 1990). Furthermore, occasional fibres that are normal by conventional histological criteria show subsarcolemmal rims or crescents of calcium staining reminiscent of the 'delta' lesions described in human muscle (Bodensteiner and Engel, 1978). In young animals, particularly, the severity of lesions may vary from muscle to muscle, although the most severely involved muscles are predictable, as described below. In the *xmd* dog, muscle necrosis and regeneration continue throughout life, although the degree of activity in the muscle of older animals is less marked. As the disease progresses, muscle fibrosis becomes apparent (Fig. 11.5) and there may be a modest degree of infiltration of the dystrophic muscle by adipose tissue. There is marked fibre size variation, accounted for by the presence of both abnormally large and abnormally small fibres, and split fibres. Although in the dog the majority of nuclei in regenerating muscle fibres quickly become subsarcolemmal, many fibres in chronically affected dystrophic dogs contain a proportion of internalized nuclei, most commonly in hypertrophied fibres. Similar lesions also occur in the oesophagus of the dystrophic dog. There appears to be progressive emergence of type I fibre predominance in *xmd* muscle (Valentine et al., 1990), as is reported in both the *mdx* mouse and in patients with DMD (Carnwath and Shotton, 1987).

Studies of lesion development in very young *xmd* dogs

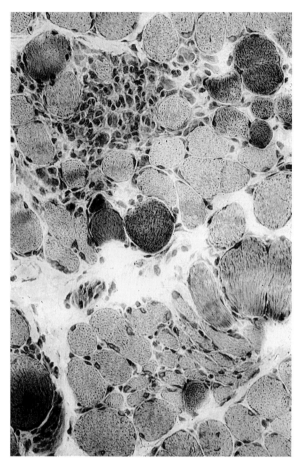

Fig. 11.4. Triceps muscle from a 4-month-old Golden Retriever dog with muscular dystrophy. There are large dark fibres, clusters of necrotic fibres and clusters of regenerating fibres. (Frozen section, trichrome stain, ×200.)

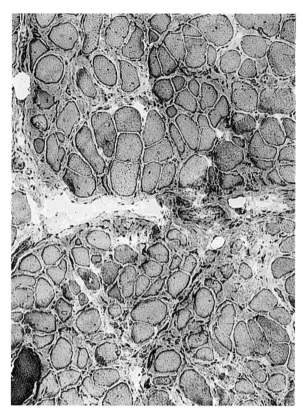

Fig. 11.5. Extensor carpi muscle from a 6-year-old Golden Retriever dog with muscular dystrophy. There is marked fibre size variation and extensive endomysial fibrosis. (Frozen section, trichrome stain, ×80.)

have revealed that the onset of necrosis is selective (Valentine and Cooper, 1991). Macroscopic and histological examination of a large number of muscles from affected pups (with typical progression of disease) from birth to eight weeks of age has demonstrated that the same muscles are always involved early and severely in the *xmd* dog. These are the tongue, the diaphragm and the trapezius, brachiocephalicus, omotransversarius, deltoideus, extensor carpi radialis and sartorius muscles. Occasionally the medial head of the triceps, the insertion of the biceps femoris, the rectus femoris and the cranial tibial muscle also have lesions. Other muscles do not develop significant lesions until six to eight weeks of age. In those muscles involved early in the disease, fibrosis develops by four weeks of age. In the tongue, regeneration is present even on the first day after birth, indicating that lesions develop in utero. A striking observation in these young animals is that

the average fibre diameter in those muscles developing early lesions is significantly larger than in normal muscles, or in muscles involved late in the disease. Such differences appear to result from marked hypertrophy of muscle fibres as an early component of the dystrophic disease process. This is reminiscent of the hypertrophy seen in the *mdx* mouse and in the dystrophic cat (see below) and suggests that fibre hypertrophy is a consistent abnormality in dystrophic muscle. The explanation of preferential susceptibility of these muscles is not entirely clear. It is apparent that those muscles that are susceptible at an early age are also developmentally advanced, having a more mature fibre typing pattern and being of somewhat larger size than other muscles (Valentine and Cooper, 1991). This suggests that fibre size may be a factor, as proposed by Karpati et al. (1990) for the *mdx* mouse. However, at the stage at which marked degenerative lesions develop the same muscles in control animals have fibre diameters considerably less than the 20–25 μm suggested to be the critical size. Another hypothesis is that development of lesions in these muscles is associated with early demands for work (or exercise). (Valentine and Cooper, 1991). Such an idea would be consistent with those discussed earlier for the *mdx* mouse. In fact, it has been shown in older *xmd* dogs that even mild exercise induces rapid, massive increases in serum creatine kinase levels, even though similar levels of exercise in controls produces little change (Valentine et al., 1989c). Only limited ultrastructural studies have been done in the *xmd* dog. The majority of the findings reflect those described at the light microscopic level (Valentine et al., 1990).

Like humans with DMD, *xmd* dogs also consistently develop cardiomyopathy, which can be the cause of death in dogs allowed to live their full lifespan. Clinically this is characterized by electrocardiographic alterations resembling those reported in humans (Moise et al., 1990). Echocardiography shows hyperechoic areas, which are first seen in affected dogs at about six months of age. These lesions correspond to the fibrosis and mineralization seen histologically. Echocardiography also reveals evidence of myocardial failure in older affected dogs.

Histological lesions, consisting of focal areas of mineralization with accompanying macrophages and giant cells, first become apparent in affected dogs at about six months of age (Valentine et al., 1989a). These changes are most obvious in the left ventricular papillary muscles and the apical left ventricular free wall and correlate well with the initial observation by echocardiography of hyperechoic areas at this age. In dogs over one year of age, the most commonly observed lesion is fibrosis, most obvious in the subepicardial left ventricular free wall, the left ventricular papillary muscles (Fig. 11.6), and in the right ventricular aspect of the interventricular septum. In occasional dogs, active necrosis of the myocardium may also be observed. The fibrotic myocardial lesions seen in older dogs are virtually identical to those described in humans dying of Duchenne muscular dystrophy (Perloff et al., 1966; Frankel and Rosser, 1976; Hunter, 1980). Studies in the dog suggest that cardiomyopathy develops as a consequence of myocardial necrosis with mineralization, clearance by macrophages and giant cells, and subsequent fibrosis. No explanation is yet available for the relatively late onset of lesions in the heart compared with skeletal muscle, or for the restricted distribution of such lesions.

In canine dystrophic muscle there is abundant evidence of regenerative activity, particularly in young animals with active lesions (Valentine et al., 1990). As in humans, however, the muscle eventually becomes fibrotic and regeneration fails in the sense that there is a net loss of muscle mass. Studies of necrotic lesions induced by the myotoxic venom notexin have shown that canine dystrophic muscle retains the capacity to mount a regenera-

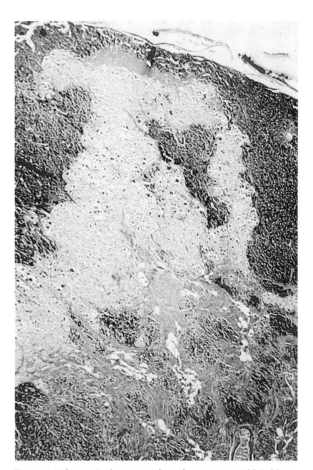

Fig. 11.6. Left ventricular myocardium from a 1-year-old Golden Retriever dog with muscular dystrophy. There is extensive loss of cardiac myocytes with fibrosis. The epicardium is at the top of the photograph. Collagen deposition is most severe towards the bottom. (Trichrome stain, ×30.)

tive response. Even in six-month-old dystrophic dogs, where advanced lesions of muscular dystrophy are already present, myotubes appeared three to four days after notexin injury and β-spectrin appeared by about seven days. These results are very similar to those for normal dogs (Sewry et al., 1992). The long-term loss of muscle mass in dystrophic animals, therefore, does not appear to result from the loss of the inherent capacity of satellite cells to respond. Interestingly, however, the maturation of newly formed muscle fibres appears to be delayed in canine dystrophic muscle, as judged by the prolonged expression of the neonatal isoform of myosin (Wilson et al., 1994). Very similar observations were made in dystrophin/utrophin double knock-out mice, suggesting that impaired differentiation is a consistent phenomenon in uncompensated dystrophin-deficient muscle.

Molecular basis

Early pedigree observations suggested that the canine disease was inherited as an X-linked recessive trait (de Lahunta, 1983; Valentine et al., 1986; Cooper et al., 1988a; Kornegay et al., 1988). Soon after it was shown that both dystrophin and its transcript were absent from *xmd* muscle (Cooper et al., 1988b). Subsequent studies have shown that the *xmd* dog (that is the original Golden Retriever strain) has a point mutation involving a single base change in the 3′ consensus splice site of intron 6 (Sharp et al., 1992). This results in skipping of exon 7 and termination of the dystrophin reading frame in exon 8. As in other models of DMD, the dystrophin complex is reduced in this canine model, with an apparent correlation between the loss of α-sarcoglycan, creatine kinase levels and function (Ervasti et al., 1994). Recently dystrophic German Shorthaired Pointers were described having a deletion of the entire dystrophin gene (Schatzberg et al., 1999). A mutation in Rottweilers has been identified in the author's laboratory as a point mutation in exon 57, resulting in the absence of truncated isoforms of dystrophin, other than Dp71. Interestingly, these large, heavily muscled dogs have an extremely severe phenotype, usually dying by four months of age. Utrophin is upregulated in canine muscular dystrophy (Lanfossi et al., 1999; Schatzberg et al., 1999) but its influence on the phenotype has not been fully analysed.

Canine carriers of the *xmd* trait have also been used to study the effects of X-inactivation on the expression and distribution of dystrophin (Cooper et al., 1990). In canine carriers, dystrophin is expressed in a mosaic pattern in skeletal muscle of very young animals, with about 10–12% of fibres in a particular cross-section being negative. Many other fibres stain weakly. Serial sectioning shows that individual fibres are mosaic, with both dystrophin-positive and dystrophin-negative areas appearing along their length. As the animals mature, dystrophin becomes more uniformly distributed and by 24 weeks of age less than 2% of fibres are negative. Therefore, in mosaic fibres of carrier dogs as in the *mdx* mouse, dystrophin appears to be progressively redistributed as the animals mature. Clinically manifesting carriers have not been recognized in the dog, but carriers do have modest elevations of serum creatine kinase, and degenerate or, rarely, regenerate fibres can be seen in skeletal muscle (Cooper et al., 1990).

In the heart, there is absolute mosaicism, with fibres being either positive or negative, and with none of the intermediate, or weakly staining, fibres seen in skeletal muscle (Cooper et al., 1990). This condition persists throughout the life of the carrier animal. Clinical studies of *xmd* carriers have shown that this persistent mosaicism results in the development of cardiomyopathy (Moise et al., 1990) characterized by electrocardiographic changes and the presence of hyperechoic areas similar to, but less severe than, those seen in affected animals. Histologically there is myocardial fibrosis.

Therapeutic studies

Given its phenotypic resemblance to DMD, the *xmd* dog is a potentially very useful model in which to investigate the pathogenesis of the disease and its treatment. Studies of gene therapy are in their early stages but expression of a dystrophin minigene has been obtained using rAdV vectors (Howell et al., 1998). However, as in other models, an immune response to the vector and transgene limited the duration of expression, which could be prolonged by immunosuppression with cyclosporin.

The dystrophic cat

Muscular dystrophy caused by defects in dystrophin has also been reported in the cat (Carpenter et al., 1989; Gaschen et al., 1992; Winand et al., 1994).

Clinical presentation

Interestingly, the major clinical manifestation of the disease in the cat is extreme muscle hypertrophy, including enlargement of the tongue and oesophagus. Other signs include adduction of the hocks and muscle stiffness, which results in difficulty in lying down, curling up and grooming. Serum levels of muscle-related enzymes are elevated. Cats tend not to be weak but tire easily and become dyspnoeic if stressed. They have abnormal high-frequency discharges on electromyography.

Pathology

All of the dystrophic cats studied have had similar histopathological lesions. These include hyalinized fibres and necrosis, with infiltration by macrophages, and regeneration. There is marked variation in muscle fibre size, with fibres ranging from very small to extremely large. Fibre splitting and internalized nuclei are common. There is mild endomysial fibrosis. Cardiomyopathy also occurs in dystrophic cats, with mineralization and fibrosis of the left ventricular free wall, papillary muscle and septum (Carpenter et al., 1989; Gaschen et al., 1999).

Molecular basis

All cats so far described have had dystrophin defects. The cats described by Carpenter et al. apparently completely lacked dystrophin (1989). Others have expressed dystrophin of apparently normal size at a greatly reduced level (about 5% of controls), with mosaic immunostaining of muscle fibres (Gaschen et al., 1992; Winand et al., 1994). The cat studied by Winand et al. (1994) is thought to be related to those studied by Gaschen et al. (1992) and was shown to have a deletion of the muscle and Purkinje promoters, while the cortical neuronal promoter was intact. It is thought that the low level of dystrophin present was accounted for by the expression of the cortical neuronal isoform.

The *dy* mouse

The dystrophia muscularis (*dy*) mouse has been studied as a potential model of muscular dystrophy for many years. However, it was supplanted by the *mdx* mouse when it was recognized that the *mdx* but not the *dy* mouse had a defect in the dystrophin gene. Interest in the *dy* mouse has been reawakened by the identification of a defect in merosin (the α_2-chain of laminin-2), making it a model for congenital muscular dystrophy.

The *dy* mouse was first described as an autosomal recessive trait in a colony of inbred strain 129 mice (Michelson, et al., 1955). Subsequently an allelic variant of the *dy* mouse, dubbed dy^{2J} was found (Meier and Southard, 1970). A third variant has been described in SM strain mice (Hayakawa and Tsuji, 1985).

Clinical signs

Affected mice are smaller that normal controls, with early onset of signs, including paresis of the hind limbs, spasmodic movements of the hind limb when the animal is suspended by the tail, and marked nodding movements of the head. They usually die between one and six months of age. Muscle atrophy develops, progressing from the hind limbs to the axial muscles and forelimbs, resulting in kyphosis. The dy^{2J} mice have a similar phenotype, but the disease is of later onset and progresses more slowly, allowing affected animals to be bred. In this discussion, the designation *dy* will be used to refer to the original mutation, while the other mutants will be referred to by their specific designations.

Pathology

Histologically, the original report described variation in muscle fibre size, central nucleation and interstitial scarring, all compatible with a dystrophic process (Fig. 11.7). There have been many subsequent studies of the development of muscle lesions and regeneration in the *dy* mouse (West and Murphy, 1960; Platzer and Chase, 1964; Banker, 1968; Ontell, 1981; Summers and Parsons, 1981; Ontell, 1986) but the essential feature of the myopathy of the *dy*

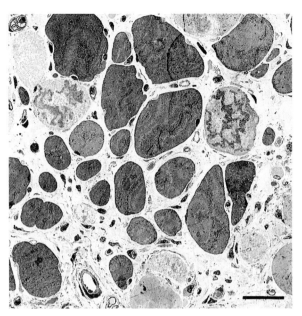

Fig. 11.7. Extensor digitorum longus muscle from a 17-week-old *dy* mouse showing marked fibre loss, fibre size variation and endomysial fibrosis (bar, 20 μm). (Reproduced, with permission, from Hermanson et al., 1988.)

mouse is muscle degeneration and necrosis, with evidence of regeneration, and, remarkably, subsequent fibrosis. In a comparison of the *dy* mouse and the *mdx* mouse, it was shown that the earliest lesions in both mutants are muscle fibre injury with hypercontracted fibres and subsequently necrotic fibres undergoing phagocytosis, with onset at 10–15 days of age (Woo et al., 1987). The striking difference between the two mutants was the development of interstitial fibrosis in the limb muscles of the *dy* mouse, which was associated with markedly increased fibre size variation and progressive loss of fibres. The loss of muscle mass in the *dy* mouse is apparently not the result of exhaustion of mitotic capacity because muscle of older *dy* mice subjected to trauma is still capable of regeneration (Bourke et al., 1988; Martin and Ontell, 1988). Freeze-fracture studies of the sarcolemma in *dy* mice have revealed reductions in intramembranous orthogonal arrays similar to those seen in *mdx* mice (Shibuya et al., 1997).

Interestingly, particularly in the light of the recent identification of defects in merosin, the *dy* mouse also has been documented to have abnormalities of peripheral nerves. The most striking of these are in the dorsal and ventral spinal roots where there is extensive failure of myelination (amyelination) of axons (Bradley and Jenkison, 1975; Stirling, 1975). Similar, but less obvious, abnormalities occur in the peripheral nerves (Stirling, 1975; Jaros and Bradley, 1979; Jaros and Jenkison, 1983). These lesions presumably account for the dramatic alterations in conduction that have been documented in the nerve roots and peripheral nerves of *dy* mice (Rasminsky et al., 1978). In addition, ephaptic transmission (cross-talk) has been demonstrated between nerve fibres in the roots (Rasminsky, 1980). Spontaneous electrical activity, apparently mostly neurally mediated, has also been demonstrated in muscle of *dy* mouse (Johnstone et al., 1986). These functional abnormalities very likely contribute to the clinical signs, particularly the dystonic movements, shown by *dy* mice. Abnormalities have also been reported in the neuromuscular junctions of these mice (Desaki et al., 1995).

Pathogenesis

A variety of studies in the *dy* mouse have attempted to understand the pathogenesis of muscular dystrophy. These are similar to those in the *mdx* mouse and often have similar results. For example, resting levels of calcium ions in muscle have been studied in the *dy* mouse, the results showing elevated resting levels, even in apparently intact fibres (Williams et al., 1990). How these findings relate to the fundamental defect and to the development of necrosis is, as in the *mdx* mouse, still unknown. Immobilization of hindleg muscles during the second postnatal week has also been shown to abrogate the dystrophic changes in muscle (Brocks et al., 1992). By comparison, mechanosensitive ion channels, which have been reported to be abnormal in *mdx* mice, are apparently not abnormal in *dy* mice (Franco-Obregon and Lansman, 1994). It will be potentially very useful to compare results of pathogenetic studies in the various models having defects in different components of the dystrophin complex. It would seem that the fundamental pathophysiological abnormalities important in the genesis of several forms of muscular dystrophy should be common to these models.

Molecular basis

As the components of the dystrophin complex have been characterized, they have become candidate genes for other forms of muscular dystrophy, both in humans and in animals. The recognition that α-dystroglycan binds laminin prompted investigation of possible laminin defects in muscular dystrophies. In humans, defects in merosin have been shown to be responsible for some forms of congenital muscular dystrophy (Helbling-Leclerc et al., 1995). In the *dy* mouse, it was shown that merosin, the predominant isoform of laminin in striated muscle and peripheral nerve, is a specific ligand for α-dystroglycan, that the mouse M chain (α2-chain of laminin-2) gene

mapped close to the *dy* locus on chromosome 10, and that merosin was markedly reduced in *dy* skeletal muscle, myocardium and peripheral nerve (Xu et al., 1994a; Sunada et al., 1994). In the dy^{2J} strain, immunofluorescence staining showed the expression of merosin in muscle and nerve, but the protein is truncated because of a point mutation in a splice site consensus sequence in the gene for the α2-chain of laminin (Xu et al., 1994b). Other studies of the *dy* mouse using immunofluorescence techniques have indicated that some laminin α2-chain is expressed in skeletal and cardiac muscle of *dy* mice, while it is lost in other tissues, including peripheral nerve and blood vessels of the brain (Sewry et al., 1998; Ringelmann et al., 1999). These results suggest that particular antibodies may, or may not, detect the α2-chain in muscle of *dy* mice and that there are differences between muscle and nonmuscle tissue. This may result from the expression of isoforms or splice variants. The expression of some laminin, with some degree of function, would be consistent with the findings in knockout mice null for the laminin α2-chain, in which the dystrophic syndrome is very severe, with onset of muscle necrosis by postnatal day nine and death by five weeks of age (Miyagoe et al., 1997). In summary, the *dy* mouse and its variants are useful models for merosin-deficient forms of congenital muscular dystrophy in humans.

The dystrophic hamster

Several strains of dystrophic hamster have been derived from the original mutants, which were first described in 1962 (Homburger and Bajusz, 1970; Homburger, 1979). All of these strains have a similar disease and will be reviewed here as a group.

Clinical signs

The dystrophic hamster is characterized by signs of muscular weakness and cardiac failure (Homburger et al., 1966). Onset of weakness can be detected at 60 days of age, or earlier. The longevity of the animals is reduced, depending to some degree on the strain studied (Homburger and Bajusz, 1970; Homburger, 1979). Serum creatine kinase levels are increased as early as two weeks of age (Homburger et al., 1966; Bhattacharya et al., 1987). The disease is inherited as an autosomal recessive trait (Homburger et al., 1966).

Pathology

Although a variety of early morphological changes have been described (Homburger, 1979; Mendell et al., 1979), the essential lesion in muscle of the dystrophic hamster appears to be necrosis (Fig. 11.8) (Homburger et al., 1966;

Homburger, 1979; Mendell et al., 1979). Degenerative changes can be detected as early as 11 days of age (Mendell et al., 1979). In well-developed lesions there is muscle necrosis, phagocytosis, marked variation in fibre diameter, fibre splitting, central nucleation and basophilia (Homburger and Bajusz, 1970; Bhattacharya et al., 1987). Calcification of muscle fibres can be demonstrated histochemically (Homburger et al., 1966; Mendell et al., 1979), and calcium content of both skeletal and cardiac muscle is increased (Bhattacharya et al., 1987). Lesions have been reported to be most severe in the musculature of the shoulder and to be exacerbated by exercise (Homburger et al., 1966). There is disagreement as to the degree to which fibrosis develops, with some investigators reporting none (Mendell et al., 1979), while others report significant fibrosis and fatty infiltration (Homburger and Bajusz, 1970; Bhattacharya et al., 1987). These differences may depend on the strain and age of animals studied. Ultrastructural studies have shown early changes in dystrophic hamster muscle to consist of dilatation of the sarcotubular system, increase in lipid, cell swelling, destruction of myofibrils and sarcolemmal defects (Caulfield, 1966).

Cardiomyopathy is a prominent feature of muscular dystrophy in the hamster, to the degree that the animal is often used as a primary model of cardiac disease and referred to as the cardiomyopathic hamster. Affected animals show electrocardiographic changes suggestive of cardiac hypertrophy from an early age (20–25 days). (Bhattacharya et al., 1987). Histological changes in the myocardium include hyalinization, necrosis and fragmentation of myocytes, calcification, phagocytosis and fibrosis (Bhattacharya et al., 1987). Cardiac lesions are evident by 30 to 40 days of age (Jasmin and Eu, 1979; Burbach, 1987) and are essentially necrotizing in nature. Early ultrastructural changes include cell swelling, hypercontraction of cardiac myocytes with contraction bands, dilatation of the sarcotubular network, mitochondrial calcification, myofibrillar lysis, the presence of perinuclear lysosomal bodies and activation of perivascular fibroblasts (Jasmin and Eu, 1979; Burbach, 1987).

There is an extensive literature describing studies of the pathogenesis of the defect in the dystrophic hamster. These studies will have to be re-evaluated in the light of recent findings of a defect in the dystrophin complex in this mutant and are, therefore, not reviewed in detail here. However, some similarities to other models exist. For example, as in the *mdx* mouse, denervation of dystrophic hamster muscle largely prevents the expression of necrosis (Karpati et al., 1982). Whether such effects are a consequence of reduced fibre size, reduced usage or other reasons remains to be proven.

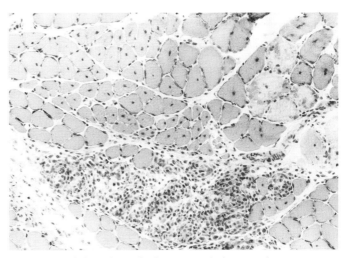

Fig. 11.8. Muscle from dystrophic hamster. At the bottom, a large cluster of necrotic fibres undergo phagocytosis. In the upper right corner, a few fibres are in the prephagocytic phase of necrosis. The majority of viable fibres are centronucleated and variably atrophic. (UMX 7.1 strain of dystrophic hamster, age 45 days, ×350; photograph courtesy of Dr George Karpati.)

Molecular basis

Early studies of the dystrophin complex in the dystrophic hamster revealed reduced dystrophin content (Iwata et al., 1993) and a deficiency of adhalin (Roberds et al., 1993). Subsequent studies have identified a deletion in the gene for δ-sarcoglycan (Nigro et al., 1997; Sakamoto et al., 1997, 1999) leading to a failure to synthesize the protein. This failure, in turn, leads to loss of other components of the dystrophin complex. Specifically, α-, β- and γ-sarcoglycans are lost (Mizuno et al., 1995; Straub et al., 1998). In addition, the expression of α-dystroglycan is reduced, although to a variable extent in different animals. Therefore, this is another example of disruption of one component of the dystrophin complex leading to loss of other components, loss of function of the complex and sarcolemmal instability. Based on these findings, the dystrophic hamster is a model for limb girdle muscular dystrophy (LGMD) type 2F (see Chapter 20).

Therapeutic studies

Recognition of the gene defect in the dystrophic hamster was quickly followed by attempts to correct it using gene therapy, with promising results. In one study, an rAdV vector was used (Holt et al., 1998), resulting in extensive expression of δ-sarcoglycan and concomitant restoration of the sarcoglycan complex and of α-dystroglycan. In addition, the integrity of the sarcolemma was restored and there was evidence of reduced fibre injury. The relatively small size of the δ-sarcoglycan cDNA also provides the opportunity to explore the use of alternative vectors. In a second study, adeno-associated virus (AAV), a nonimmunogenic vector, was used (Greelish et al., 1999). Administration of this construct intramuscularly produced long-term (up to 13 weeks) expression of δ-sarcoglycan, restored other members of the complex and conferred protection from membrane injury following exercise challenge. There was no evidence of an inflammatory response to the vector. Administration of the vector into the femoral artery after treatment with papaverine and histamine to permeabilize the vasculature resulted in widespread expression of δ-sarcoglycan 20–25 weeks after treatment. These results offer encouragement for gene therapy of patients with LGMD.

Transgenic and knock-out models

The study of pathogenetic mechanisms and treatment of the muscular dystrophies has been greatly facilitated in recent years by the development of transgenic and knock-out models. Transgenic animals can be used, for example, to manipulate the level of expression of gene products, to express different forms of the product and to restore the expression of a deleted product, such as dystrophin. They can be used to ask fundamental questions about restoring a missing gene product, while avoiding some of the difficulties of gene therapy, such as stability of expression, immune responses and the extent of expression.

Knock-out models will be of extraordinary use in analysing the function of genes, and the nature and mechanisms of diseases in which identified genes are defective. Until recently, we were dependent on nature to provide mutants that correspond to human diseases. Although such models will still be valuable, often they are simply not available. Now such models can be made in the laboratory. Many different knock-outs have already been developed to study the function of particular genes expressed in muscle. Here the discussion will be limited to those knock-outs and transgenics that are relevant to understanding the pathogenesis of, and therapy for, muscular dystrophy.

Knock-out models

Utrophin knock-outs
Given its similarity to dystrophin, its hypothesized ability to partially compensate for the absence of dystrophin, and its widespread distribution, including the neuromuscular junction and the myotendinous junction in muscle, there was great interest in analysing the role of utrophin through knock-out technology. Two such knock-outs have now

been generated, one targeting the C-terminus (Grady et al., 1997a) and the second the N-terminus (Deconinck et al., 1997a). Both mutants lack utrophin.

The consequences of the absence of utrophin are surprisingly mild and similar in the two models. The mice show no abnormalities in non-neuromuscular tissues. However, in both there are subtle abnormalities of the neuromuscular junction. There is a reduction in the number of postjunctional folds, a decrease in the number of acetylcholine receptors (AChR) and a concomitant subtle reduction in the amplitude of miniature endplate currents, without clinically apparent neuromuscular dysfunction. By analogy with dystrophin deficiency, an effect on putative utrophin-binding proteins might have been expected, but no such effect was found, at least as measured by expression of β-dystroglycan and α-sarcoglycan, which were normal at the neuromuscular junction and in extrajunctional muscle membranes. The deficiency of AChR in these animals appears postnatally during the period when postsynaptic folds appear, implying that utrophin might play some role in that process. Nevertheless, despite the precise co-localization of utrophin with AChR, utrophin does not appear to be essential to the formation or function of the neuromuscular junction.

Utrophin–dystrophin double knock-outs
By crossing *mdx* mice with utrophin knock-out mice, animals null for both dystrophin and utrophin have been generated, with the aim of analysing the ability of utrophin to compensate for lack of dystrophin and, conversely, the ability of dystrophin to compensate for lack of utrophin at the neuromuscular junction. As would be predicted if utrophin can functionally replace dystrophin, these utrophin–dystrophin deficient mice (referred to here as *mdx:utrn*$^-$) have a severe phenotype (Deconinck et al., 1997b; Grady et al., 1997b). They show decreased growth rate and eventual weight loss, weakness, abnormal gait, joint contractures, kyphosis and early death. Muscle lesions develop earlier in the *mdx:utrn*$^-$ than in *mdx*. Although Deconinck et al. (1997b) found that, overall, the skeletal muscle and myocardial lesions in *mdx:utrn*$^-$ were not drastically worse than those of the *mdx* mice, Grady et al. (1997b) present convincing evidence that muscle necrosis persists in the *mdx:utrn*$^-$ in contrast to the *mdx*, where it peaks at four to five weeks. Based on immunostaining for embryonic and neonatal isoforms of myosin heavy chains, they showed that active regeneration follows closely the onset of necrosis, is similar in both models at 4–5 weeks but persists beyond eight weeks only in the *mdx:utrn*$^-$ mice. Deconinck et al. (1997b) found a failure of myosin switching, reminiscent of that in the *xmd* dog. Both groups agree

that the *mdx:utrn⁻* mice develop widespread muscle fibrosis, which is seen only in the diaphragm of *mdx* mice. These findings support the notion that in the *mdx* mouse utrophin does compensate for the absence of dystrophin, resulting in a short-lived wave of necrosis followed by stable regeneration, while in the absence of utrophin cycles of necrosis and regeneration continue. This suggests that overexpression of utrophin in human patients, if it can be achieved, could alleviate the severity of the disease. Similarly, utrophin, which is known to be expressed in the heart of *mdx* mice, appears to provide protection against the development of cardiomyopathy. Grady et al. (1997b) found that over 50% of the *mdx:utrn⁻* mice develop myocardial necrosis, most prominent in the subepicardial myocardium, while cardiac lesions were not found in *mdx* mice.

In terms of functional consequences, Grady et al. (1997b) found a marked reduction in twitch tension development in muscle from *mdx:utrn⁻* mice, while that of *mdx* was near normal. This was partly explained by loss of muscle mass and by the presence of injured fibres. Most interestingly, these investigators found a significant prolongation of relaxation time in muscle from the *mdx:utrn⁻* mice. Relaxation time is partly dependent on the time required to reduce free calcium levels in the sarcoplasm, which might imply an abnormality in calcium handling in these muscles. This finding is likely to stimulate interest in the role of calcium homeostasis in muscular dystrophy, and the *mdx:utrn⁻* mice may provide a more critical model in which to examine it.

In contrast, dystrophin does not appear to compensate for the loss of utrophin at the neuromuscular junction. In the *mdx:utrn⁻* mice, simplification of the postsynaptic folds at the neuromuscular junction is more striking than that reported for the utrophin knock-out, but no significant difference in development and function of the neuromuscular junction was found between *mdx* and *mdx:utrn⁻*. Of interest was that one group (Grady et al., 1997b) did find a reduction in β-dystroglycan and α-sarcoglycan, similar to that found in *mdx*, and almost complete loss of dystrobrevin and β_2-syntrophin from the neuromuscular junction. These results differ from those of Deconinck et al. (1997b). The differences in these two studies remain to be clarified.

Additional evidence that utrophin can compensate for the absence of dystrophin comes from a recent study of extraocular muscles in *mdx* and *mdx:utrn⁻* mice (Porter et al., 1998). The extraocular muscles are spared in muscular dystrophy in humans and in animal models. Utrophin is upregulated in extraocular muscle without the need for preceding necrosis and regeneration. In *mdx:utrn⁻* mice, the extraocular muscles develop severe myopathic change,

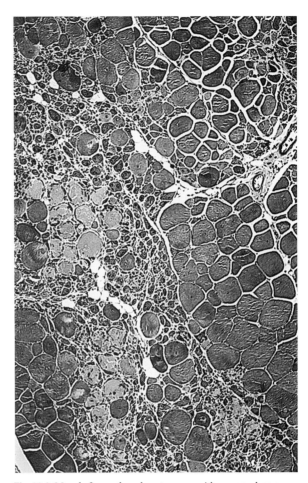

Fig. 11.9. Muscle from a knock-out mouse with γ-sarcoglycan deficiency showing extensive areas of muscle fibre necrosis. (Photomicrograph courtesy of Dr Elizabeth McNally.)

suggesting again that it is utrophin that provides the protection.

Sarcoglycan knock-outs

As previously discussed, a defect in the gene for δ-sarcoglycan in the dystrophic hamster established it as a model for LGMD type 2F. Models for other forms of LGMD with deficiency of γ- or α-sarcoglycan have been developed recently.

Knock-out mice with γ-sarcoglycan deficiency develop a severe, early-onset dystrophic phenotype, including cardiomyopathy (Hack et al., 1998). These mice display a stiff gait and wide-based stance. They have stunted growth and shortened lifespan. Serum creatine kinase is greatly elevated. Histological lesions include necrosis, infiltration by inflammatory cells, regeneration, calcification and fibrosis (Fig. 11.9). Abnormal muscle membrane permeability, particularly in the diaphragm, muscles of the shoulder girdle and pectoralis major muscle, is present as early as two weeks of age, and it can be seen in almost all muscle groups by four weeks. There is evidence of apoptosis in muscle, most commonly in degenerate fibres, but sometimes in apparently intact fibres, implying that apoptosis might play a role in early fibre injury. These animals also develop cardiomyopathy characterized by ventricular hypertrophy and fibrosis.

Gamma-sarcoglycan knock-outs also showed a rather specific secondary loss of β- and δ-sarcoglycans, with partial loss of α-sarcoglycan. However, dystrophin, ε-sarcoglycan, β-dystroglycan and the laminin α2-chain staining were all intact. Utrophin staining was also comparable to that in controls. The results in this knock-out model suggest that loss of the sarcoglycan complex is sufficient to cause a severe dystrophic phenotype. Mice lacking γ-sarcoglycan will serve as useful models of LGMD type 2C.

Knock-out mice deficient in α-sarcoglycan have also been developed (Duclos et al., 1998). They too develop a severe progressive dystrophic phenotype and serve as a model for LGMD type 2D. Lesions are progressive and present by eight days of age. They are characterized by necrosis, regeneration with central nucleation, atrophic and hypertrophied fibres, fibre splitting and fibrosis. Development of lesions is accompanied by increased serum enzymes, including creatine kinase. Older mice show calcification and fatty infiltration of muscle. Again, sarcolemmal injury was demonstrated, most obviously in muscles of the shoulder and pelvic girdles. Interestingly, no dye uptake was demonstrated in cardiac muscle and no cardiomyopathy developed in these mice.

The effect of α-sarcoglycan deficiency on other components of the dystrophin complex is apparently somewhat different from that of γ-sarcoglycan deficiency. In this study, severe loss of the sarcoglycan complex, including sarcospan, and a disruption of the association of α-dystroglycan and dystrophin with the sarcolemma were found. The expression of ε-sarcoglycan was normal, and utrophin was upregulated, probably as a result of the regenerative activity (Duclos et al., 1998).

In the same study, an adenovirus vector was used to restore the expression of α-sarcoglycan in neonatal mice. High levels of α-sarcoglycan were expressed for as long as 60 days and resulted in the restoration of the complete dystrophin complex. It also resulted in a reduction of central nucleation, implying a reduction in susceptibility to injury.

One puzzling question that arises from the study of these models of sarcoglycan deficiency relates to the development of cardiomyopathy. In the hamster lacking δ-sarco-

glycan, cardiomyopathy is a major abnormality. It is present in mice lacking γ-sarcoglycan yet appears to be absent in mice lacking α-sarcoglycan. Further studies, perhaps over longer periods of time, will be required to clarify this question. In the meantime, the generation of these models will provide additional opportunities to study pathogenetic mechanisms and therapy of the muscular dystrophies. The early success with gene therapy in the α-sarcoglycan knock-out model, as well as in the hamster, is encouraging.

Transgenic models

Transgenic models have been useful in two main areas of inquiry. First, to address whether restoration of dystrophin, or a truncated version of dystrophin, in dystrophic muscle (of the Duchenne type) will halt or reverse the progression of the disease. Second, to address what domains of dystrophin are important to its function, with a view to understanding the function of dystrophin and the phenotypes expressed in various mutations in humans.

A number of studies on the effects of expressing dystrophin in transgenic *mdx* mice have been published (Wells et al., 1992; Cox et al., 1993; Rafael et al., 1994; Phelps et al., 1995). To summarize these studies, it has been shown that either truncated ('minigenes' with deletions in the rod domain) or full-length forms of dystrophin can be expressed, that they localize to the sarcolemma and restore the expression of components of the dystrophin complex, and that they ameliorate the phenotype. These benefits have been apparent in mice overexpressing the construct or weakly expressing it. It appears from these studies that excess dystrophin is not toxic but that even modest expression is beneficial.

These studies of transgenic *mdx* mice, along with the current realization that loss of one component of the dystrophin complex leads to loss of other components, has suggested that the restoration of the complex should restore function and, therefore, should be the goal of therapy. However, this assumption may be an oversimplification. Transgenic mice have been produced that overexpress Dp71, a short isoform of dystrophin sharing its C-terminal and cysteine-rich domains, in skeletal muscle (Cox et al., 1994; Greenberg et al., 1994). Although the Dp71 protein localizes to the sarcolemma and restores at least some members of the dystrophin complex, it does not alleviate the severity of lesions. Indeed in both of these studies the severity of lesions appeared to be transiently increased. The failure to alleviate lesions was attributed to the inability of Dp71 to link the membrane complex to actin, as Dp71 lacks the N-terminal actin-binding domain. However, it would be interesting, in retrospect, to know whether the sarcoglycan complex is restored in this model and whether the presence of Dp71 interferes with the complementary function of utrophin.

Transgenic *mdx* mice have also been useful in studying the function of various regions of the dystrophin molecule and have supplemented data from patients in analysing genotype–phenotype relationships. For example, Rafael et al. (1996) demonstrated that the cysteine-rich domain of dystrophin is essential for interaction with the dystrophin complex and that loss of this interaction leads to a severe phenotype. Deletion of the extreme C-terminus has no obvious effect when the truncated dystrophin is expressed at normal levels. Similarly, deletion of the N-terminal actin-binding domain leads to a relatively mild phenotype, again as long as the truncated dystrophin is expressed at relatively high levels (Corrado et al., 1996). These studies have been very useful in understanding the various phenotypes expressed by patients and have helped to define the objectives of gene replacement therapy.

The ability of utrophin to substitute for the function of dystrophin and to ameliorate the dystrophic phenotype has also been addressed using transgenic models. It has been shown that expression of either truncated or full-length utrophin in transgenic *mdx* mice leads to substantial improvement in phenotype (Tinsley et al., 1996; Deconinck et al., 1997c; Tinsley et al., 1998). The expressed utrophin localizes to the sarcolemma, members of the dystroglycan and sarcoglycan complexes are restored and there is improvement of both structure and function. The effect was shown to be dependent on the level of utrophin expression, but the amount required for essentially full protection was no more than is normally expressed in non-muscle tissues (Tinsley et al., 1998). The ability of the truncated utrophin transgene to prevent the severe phenotype associated with *mdx:utrn$^-$* mice, discussed earlier, was tested by cross-breeding the two types of animal to produce *mdx:utrn$^-$* mice that expressed truncated utrophin but not endogenous full-length utrophin (Rafael et al., 1998). Again these mice were rescued, with major improvement in clinical signs and muscle lesions. Consequently, ways to upregulate the expression of utrophin may be an important therapeutic goal, and the use of models, including large animal models, will be important in evaluation of such protocols.

Myotonic disorders

Several potential models of myotonic diseases have been described. Some, like myotonia congenita of humans (Thomsen's disease), are transmitted as autosomal domi-

nant traits, while others resemble recessive generalized myotonia (Becker type) in being autosomal recessive traits.

Caprine myotonia

Myotonia in the goat is one of the oldest recognized models of human muscle disease (Bryant, 1979) and it has been extraordinarily useful in understanding the pathophysiological basis for myotonia. Onset of myotonia is at about two weeks of age. Affected goats show classical signs of myotonia and develop severe muscle spasms in response to sudden voluntary effort, particularly if startled. After recovery, the animals move with a stiff gait but become normal with continued movement. Affected goats also dimple in response to muscle percussion. It seems clear that caprine myotonia is inherited as an autosomal dominant trait, and the disease is, therefore, a model for congenital myotonia of humans (Harris and Mrak, 1985).

Muscle from myotonic goats shows little in the way of morphological changes. Apart from moderate hypertrophy and a diffuse increase in staining for calcium, routine histological and histochemical methods show few changes (Bryant, 1969; Atkinson et al., 1981). Ultrastructurally, proliferation and dilatation of the T-tubules and sarcoplasmic reticulum, as well as abnormalities of mitochondria, have been reported, although the significance of these changes is unclear (Atkinson et al., 1981).

Historically, the myotonic goat provided the first insights into the physiological abnormalities responsible for myotonia. Early studies showed that the major abnormality in myotonic muscle fibres was increased resting membrane resistance, other cable properties being normal (Lipicky and Bryant, 1966; Bryant, 1969). Subsequent studies implicated decreased chloride conductance (Bryant and Morales-Aguilera, 1971). The basis for repetitive firing of myotonic fibres has also been elucidated in the goat. It has been shown that myotonic fibres have a reduced rheobasic current (the minimum depolarizing current required to produce an action potential) and a prolonged latency at rheobase (Adrian and Bryant, 1974). This is associated with a prolonged after-depolarization following a brief train of stimuli, which can become large enough to cause repetitive activity. This activity depends on the integrity of the T-tubular system. These observations have led to the hypothesis that sustained activity in myotonic fibres results from the accumulation of potassium ions in the T-tubules following normal activity. In normal muscle the majority of the surface membrane conductivity is attributable to chloride ions, which counters the depolarizing action of the T-tubular potassium ions. Because myotonic fibres lack this conductance, accumulated potassium ions lead to sustained trains of action potentials and myotonic activity (Adrian and Bryant, 1974). Adrian and Marshall (1976), using computer modelling techniques, have shown that the absence of surface chloride conductance alone is sufficient to account for myotonic behaviour. Recent studies have identified a point mutation in the ClC-1 type of Cl⁻ channel, thus confirming that this model, like the murine and canine models discussed below, is an analogue of human myotonia congenita (Beck et al., 1996).

Murine models of myotonia: *adr* and *mto*

Three strains of myotonic mice, *adr*, *mto* and *adr*ᵏ have been described. All are inherited as autosomal recessive traits (Watkins and Watts, 1984) and all have been shown to be allelic. Thus the *mto* mouse is now generally designated as *adr*ᵐᵗᵒ. Clinical signs are similar in all strains, with onset at 10–12 days of age (Heller et al., 1982; Watkins and Watts, 1984). Signs are characterized by myotonic muscle contractions, resulting in the inability of affected animals to right themselves when placed on their backs. Causing the animals to move results in myotonia-like muscle contractions, the hind limbs being held in extension until the muscles again relax. Signs are exacerbated by cold, and percussion of muscles can elicit sustained local contractions. Older animals have difficulty moving and they exhibit thickening of the neck and forelimbs. Growth rate in affected animals is also decreased, and at maturity *adr* mice are considerably smaller than controls. Muscles of *adr* mice have been noted to be shorter, thicker and more red than those of controls (Watkins and Watts, 1984).

Electrophysiological findings are characteristic of myotonia. In the *adr* mouse, stimulation of muscle leads to runs of action potentials and prolonged after-contractions. In the *adr*ᵐᵗᵒ mouse, electromyography reveals characteristic 'dive bomber' myotonic discharges, with recurrent variation in frequency and amplitude (Heller et al., 1982; Entrikin et al., 1987). These effects are prolonged by cooling (Mehrke et al., 1988; Reininghaus et al., 1988). Based on measurements of muscle membrane time constants, chloride conductance in normal murine muscle accounts for more than 70% of the resting conductance, whereas in muscle of the *adr* mouse it represents less than 30%. Consequently, myotonia in this mutant also can be accounted for by reduced chloride conductance.

In both the *adr* and the *adr*ᵐᵗᵒ mutant there is apparently minimal necrosis of the muscle, and creatine kinase levels are normal (Heller et al., 1982; Schimmelpfeng et al., 1987; Jockusch et al., 1990). However, a number of biochemical and histochemical alterations of the muscle have been described. These reflect a change to a red muscle phenotype (Watkins and Watts, 1984). These changes can be partially reversed by long-term treatment with tocainide, a drug that can also reverse the electrophysiological features of myotonia in the *adr* mouse (Jockusch et al., 1988; Mehrke et al., 1988; Reininghaus et al., 1988). They are, therefore, considered to be secondary changes associated with the myotonic activity of the muscle.

Congenital myotonia in these murine models has been shown to be caused by a specific defect in the major muscle chloride channel, ClC-1 (Steinmeyer et al., 1991a). It has been shown that in the *adr* mutant, a transposon of the ETn family has been inserted into *ClC-1* destroying its ability to encode several membrane-spanning domains (Steinmeyer et al., 1991b). Immunohistochemical and biochemical studies have confirmed the absence of the channel from the sarcolemma (Gurnett et al., 1995). Southern blotting using probes for the ClC-1 channel also revealed aberrant fragments with one restriction enzyme site in the *adr*ᵐᵗᵒ mouse (Steinmeyer et al., 1991b). This and the fact that *adr*, *adr*ᵐᵗᵒ and *adr*ᵏ are allelic suggest that defects in the ClC-1 chloride channel are responsible for myotonia in all three mutants.

Canine and feline myotonia

Canine congenital myotonia has been most intensively studied in the Chow Chow breed, with the most complete clinical description being that of Farrow and Malik (1981). The disease is characterized by stiffness in the first movements after a period of rest, with the hind limbs being most noticeably affected. Onset of signs in affected Chows is as early as six weeks of age. However, signs become more severe as the animals grow older. Affected animals move with splayed, stiff forelimbs and often with a 'bunny hopping' gait of the hind limbs. Stiffness may become so severe that animals fall over, being unable to right themselves for as long as 30 seconds. These signs may be accompanied by dyspnoea. With exercise, signs become much less severe, although the gait may still be somewhat stiff. All voluntary muscles become dramatically hypertrophied. Percussion of the muscles produces a typical myotonic dimple lasting several seconds. Histologically, there is marked variation in fibre size with occasional atrophic fibres, and there may be mild muscle necrosis. Serum levels of creatine kinase are mildly elevated. Myotonic Chows show typical runs of myotonic discharges on electromyography. These are precipitated by insertion or movement of the needle electrode, or percussion of the muscle, and accompanied by the characteristic dive-bomber sounds on the loudspeaker. Cooling the muscle prolongs the myotonic discharges. Nerve conduction is normal.

Myotonia in the Chow Chow is clearly an inherited disease (Wentink et al., 1974; Farrow and Malik, 1981) but the mode of inheritance has not been firmly established. Analysis of the cases in the literature, however, suggests that the disease is inherited as an autosomal recessive trait. A similar autosomal recessive form of congenital myotonia in Miniature Schnauzer dogs has recently been reported to result from defects in the ClC-1 channel, resulting in reduced open probability at voltages near the resting membrane potential of skeletal muscle (Rhodes et al., 1999).

Hyperkalaemic periodic paralysis

In recent years, a condition resembling hyperkalaemic periodic paralysis (hyperKPP) has been recognized in American Quarterhorses. The syndrome is characterized by intermittent episodes of muscle fasciculation, weakness and, often, recumbency. It is usually recognized in young horses one to five years of age. Clinical signs typically begin with transient muscle fasciculations or spasms, which initially involve muscles of the neck and trunk and then spread to involve most muscle groups (Cox, 1986; Steiss and Naylor, 1986; Spier et al., 1990). Severe weakness develops. Muscle tone may be slightly increased and, during an attack, a percussion dimple may be elicited. Attacks typically last 15 to 90 minutes, but may be as long as 7 hours and may sometimes be fatal (Cox, 1986). Between attacks, affected horses appear normal, although they are characteristically very heavily muscled. Factors precipitating clinical episodes cannot always be identified (Cox, 1986; Spier et al., 1990), but stress or feeding material high in potassium may be predisposing factors (Steiss and Naylor, 1986). For diagnostic purposes, attacks may be precipitated by oral administration of potassium chloride (Cox, 1986; Spier et al., 1990).

Attacks are typically accompanied by haemoconcentration and hyperkalaemia (Cox, 1986; Steiss and Naylor, 1986; Spier et al., 1990) but these return to normal as the animal recovers. Electromyographically, even during periods of clinical normalcy, affected horses show spontaneous activity, including complex repetitive discharges and myotonic discharges, which produce typical dive bomber sounds (Steiss and Naylor, 1986; Robinson et al., 1990; Spier et al., 1990). In many cases, muscle from affected horses is histopathologically normal (Steiss and Naylor, 1986), but in some there may be central vacuoles in type IIB fibres (Spier et al., 1990). Ultrastructurally, dilata-tion of the terminal cisternae of the sarcoplasmic reticulum has been reported (Spier et al., 1990).

As in humans, muscle from affected horses shows lower than normal resting membrane potentials (Pickar et al., 1991). Muscle cell volume is increased and potassium content is decreased in equine hyperKPP muscle. Furthermore, the relative membrane permeability to sodium and potassium ions is increased. This is thought to result from an increase in sodium permeability, since tetrodotoxin hyperpolarizes the membrane of this hyperKPP muscle, bringing the resting membrane potential closer to that of normal muscle. Recent studies have shown that the defect involves impairment of sodium channel inactivation (Cannon et al., 1995).

It is clear that hyperKPP in the horse is an inherited condition (Steiss and Naylor, 1986; Spier et al., 1990; Naylor et al., 1992) and it is known that all affected horses originate from a single sire, whose popularity stemmed from the heavy musculature of his progeny. The weight of evidence supports autosomal dominant inheritance (Naylor et al., 1992). A mutation resulting in a C to G change in domain IV, transmembrane region S3, has been identified in the skeletal muscle sodium channel α-subunit (Rudolph et al., 1992). This results in the substitution of a leucine residue for a highly conserved phenylalanine, which is thought to lie in a transmembrane domain close to the cytoplasmic face of the membrane. Interestingly, amino acid substitutions in human hyperKPP also lie close to the cytoplasmic face of the membrane, although in different domains, suggesting that these domains are very important to the function of the channel.

In summary, hyperKPP in the horse is genetically analogous to hyperKPP of humans and it should provide an useful model in which to study functional alterations of the altered sodium channel. At present, the horse provides the only model of this disease.

Malignant hyperthermia

Malignant hyperthermia (MH) occurs in a number of domestic animal species, but undoubtedly it is of most importance in the pig, which serves as a very important model of the human disease. There is a very large literature on the disease in this species, but in recent years considerable progress has been made in understanding the pathophysiology and the molecular genetic basis of MH, much information being derived from the porcine model. MH occurs in several breeds of pigs, susceptibility varying between breeds and between locations. In certain breeds in Europe the incidence approaches 100%. The high incidence of the disease is thought to be associated with selection for heavily muscled, lean carcasses. Porcine MH may be manifested as three different syndromes. These are classical malignant hyperthermia following exposure to halothane and/or depolarizing muscle relaxants such as suxamethonium (succinylcholine); so-called porcine stress syndrome (PSS), in which environmental stresses precipitate signs similar to those of MH; and pale soft exudative pork (PSE), a problem of meat production.

Clinically, porcine MH resembles the human disease, in that precipitating factors, whether they be related to anaesthesia or to stress, result in a fulminant syndrome usually involving muscle rigidity, a hypermetabolic state and hyperthermia. These signs are accompanied by initial muscle fasciculation, lactic acidaemia, hypercapnia, hyperkalaemia, tachycardia, and elevated creatine kinase levels (Jones et al., 1973; Richter et al., 1992). Body temperature can reach 45°C, with the source of heat apparently being increased metabolic rate in skeletal muscle (Williams et al., 1978). Attacks are commonly fatal.

Morphologically, most studies report little in the way of abnormalities in skeletal muscle prior to the onset of an MH episode (Venable, 1973). In some cases, isolated necrotic fibres and some variation in fibre size and an increase in internal nuclei have been reported (Palmer et al., 1977, 1978). However, there appear to be no consistent alterations in fibre size or fibre type distribution (Gallant, 1980; Heffron et al., 1982). Immediately following attacks, the essential lesion is acute necrosis characterized by hypercontraction of muscle fibres, which is consistent with the rise in creatine kinase levels associated with an MH episode.

There is an extensive literature pertaining to the pathophysiological basis of MH in the pig. The sensitivity of porcine MH muscle to contractures caused by halothane or caffeine in vitro has been used as a method to detect susceptible animals and has focused attention on the potential role of calcium in the pathogenesis of the disease. This work has been reviewed by others (O'Brien, 1987; Marvasti and Williams, 1988) and it is now generally accepted that MH in the pig is associated with abnormal calcium homeostasis. López et al. (1988), using calcium-sensitive microelectrodes in intact muscle, have shown that the resting levels of calcium ions are raised about fourfold in muscle fibres of MH-susceptible pigs. During an MH episode, there is a large increase in calcium levels to about 20 times the resting levels. Treatment with dantrolene reduces calcium levels to near normal and aborts the MH episode. Using the calcium-sensitive dye Fura-2 to study intracellular calcium levels in MH muscle fibres in vitro, Iaizzo et al. (1988) found no difference between normal and MH-susceptible pigs, but intracellular calcium levels did rise following treatment with halothane. Moreover, studies using isolated sarcoplasmic reticulum preparations have shown that calcium-induced calcium release is hypersensitive, requiring lower concentrations of calcium ions, ATP or caffeine than normal preparations (O'Brien, 1986). Mickelson et al. (1986), using a preparation highly enriched for the calcium-sensitive calcium channel, showed enhanced release of calcium ions from MH sarcoplasmic reticulum following exposure to calcium ions, ATP or caffeine. Similar results were obtained using skinned muscle fibres from MH-susceptible pigs (Ohta et al., 1989). Taken together, these results suggest that MH involves a defect in the calcium-induced calcium release mechanism of the sarcoplasmic reticulum. Further evidence is provided by the finding that the calcium-sensitive calcium channel shows higher than normal affinity for ryanodine. As ryanodine is thought to bind when the channel is open, this suggests that there is an increased open-state probability in porcine MH muscle (Mickelson et al., 1990). Finally, ryanodine receptor (i.e. the calcium channel) from MH-susceptible pigs reconstituted in lipid bilayers shows increased open probability, prolonged mean open times and shortened mean closed times compared with normal receptor. In addition, although the calcium dependence of channel opening is essentially normal, the calcium concentration required for channel closure is increased (Shomer et al., 1993). These results confirm that the function of the ryanodine receptor is abnormal and provide a rational explanation for the pathogenesis of porcine MH.

There has been some confusion in the literature about the mode of inheritance of MH in pigs. However, recent studies have suggested that it is inherited as an autosomal recessive trait (Andresen and Jensen, 1977; Smith and Bampton, 1977). This is in contrast to the human syndrome, which is inherited as an autosomal dominant trait (MacLennan and Phillips, 1992). These differences are explained by the fact that the clinical porcine stress syndromes, including classical MH, are fully expressed only in pigs homozygous for the trait, whereas human heterozygotes are susceptible to the expression of MH when anaesthetized with halothane and suxamethonium. Nevertheless, abnormalities can be detected in vitro in heterozygous pigs (O'Brien, 1986; Mickelson et al., 1989) and there is evidence that heterozygotes can express clinical signs on exposure to halothane (Gallant et al., 1989). In pigs, the halothane susceptibility locus has been shown to be part of a linkage group on chromosome 6 (Doizé et al., 1990; Andresen and Jensen, 1977; Davies et al., 1988). The gene for the ryanodine receptor has also been mapped to chromosome 6 (Harbitz et al., 1990). Finally, a point mutation has been identified in the gene for the skeletal muscle ryanodine receptor (*ryr-1*) of MH-susceptible pigs. The mutation is C1843T, which results in substitution of a cysteine for arginine at residue 615 (Fujii et al., 1991). This mutation is extremely tightly linked to the MH phenotype, providing convincing evidence that it is indeed the mutation responsible for MH in the pig (Otsu et al., 1991). It is present in all breeds of MH-susceptible pigs that have been examined, and all preserve a common haplotype, based on the analysis of polymorphic sites in *ryr-1*. These data suggest that the MH mutation in all breeds of pigs originated in a common founder animal (Fujii et al., 1991). The gene *ryr-1* has been implicated in MH in at least some human families (MacLennan and Phillips, 1992). MH in the pig is, therefore, an excellent model of the human disease, both genetically and phenotypically, and it should continue to be useful for study of the pathogenesis of the disease. The identification of a common mutation in affected pigs will allow normal, heterozygous, and homozygous affected animals to be identified with certainty, allowing genetically defined animals to be used in experimental studies.

Myopathic glycogenoses

A number of glycogen storage diseases having the potential to serve as animal models of the corresponding human conditions have been described. This discussion will be limited to those that are well-characterized and available models, including glycogenosis types II, III, IV and VII.

Glycogenosis type II (Pompe's disease) has been studied in Shorthorn cattle by Howell et al. (1981). Two clinical syndromes have been described in this inbred herd in which calves die at a young age (three to seven months) or later (at 1–1.5 years of age). Animals with the early-onset form, which has been compared to the infantile onset disease in humans, develop respiratory distress and have evidence of heart failure. Those with the late-onset form, comparable to the human childhood form, develop signs predominated by muscle weakness. Both groups show cardiac conduction abnormalities (Robinson et al., 1983). There is lysosomal storage of glycogen in skeletal muscle, cardiac muscle and smooth muscle and in neurons of the central and autonomic nervous systems. There is evidence of muscle degeneration (Edwards and Richards, 1979; Howell et al., 1981); especially terminally, when creatine kinase levels may be markedly elevated. Breeding studies have indicated that the disease is inherited as an autosomal recessive trait (Howell et al., 1981). Tissue activity of acid α-glucosidase is markedly depressed in affected animals;

heterozygotes express intermediate levels of the enzyme (Howell et al., 1981).

A number of studies aimed at treatment of glycogenosis type II have used the Shorthorn model. Glycogen has been shown to accumulate in lysosomes in cultured muscle cells (Di Marco et al., 1984) and addition of purified acid α-glucosidase to the medium results in uptake of the enzyme and reduction of the levels of glycogen (Di Marco et al., 1985). Furthermore, lymphoreticular chimaerism, as occurs in twin calves, has been used as a model of naturally occurring bone marrow transplantation (Howell et al., 1991). This chimaerism results in increased levels of acid α-glucosidase in muscle and other tissues. In affected twin calves, glycogen levels were lowered in liver, spleen and lymph node, but not in muscle. Clinical signs and lesions in muscle were not altered. The authors concluded that bone marrow transplantation is unlikely to be useful in the treatment of Pompe's disease.

A model of glycogenosis type II has been described in Japanese quail (Matsui et al., 1983; Fujita et al., 1991). The disease is manifested clinically as muscle weakness. There is glycogen storage in skeletal, cardiac and smooth muscle as well as in neurons and other tissues. In skeletal muscle there is also myofibrillar disorganization (Higuchi et al., 1987). Acid α-glucosidase activity is reduced to about 10% of normal levels (Usuki et al., 1986). Because of this residual activity, the disease in quail has been compared to the adult-onset form in humans.

A knock-out mouse model in which the acid α-glucosidase gene is disrupted has been generated (Bijvoet et al., 1998). These animals completely lack enzyme activity and have lysosomal glycogen storage in skeletal muscle, heart and liver. At nine months of age they are clinically still normal, although they have cardiac enlargement and electrocardiographic abnormalities.

Glycogenosis type III has been reported in the German Shepherd dog. Clinical signs are apparently manifested from an early age and are dominated by muscle weakness and exercise intolerance (Rafiquzzaman et al., 1976). The mode of inheritance has not been clearly established. The disease results in severe hepatomegaly. There is glycogen storage in hepatocytes, in skeletal, cardiac and smooth muscle, and in neurons of the central nervous system. Ultrastructurally, the glycogen lies free in the cytoplasm. Biochemical studies have shown that the activity of debranching enzyme (amylo-1,6-glucosidase) is markedly reduced (Ceh et al., 1976). Furthermore, the stored glycogen has been shown to have abnormally short branches, as would be predicted.

Glycogenosis type IV has recently been reported in Norwegian Forest cats (Fyfe et al., 1992). Clinical signs are neuromuscular in nature, with muscle tremors, listlessness and a 'bunny hopping' gait. The disease is progressive, resulting in severe muscle atrophy and tetraplegia. Serum creatine kinase activity is increased. The electromyograph is abnormal, with high-frequency discharges and fibrillation potentials. Nerve conduction is normal. There is generalized storage of glycogen in many tissues and cells, including skeletal, cardiac and smooth muscle, hepatocytes, and neurons of the central and peripheral nervous systems. There is extensive atrophy and degeneration of skeletal muscle and axonal loss and demyelination in neural tissues. Ultrastructurally, stored glycogen is not membrane bound. Pedigree analysis is consistent with autosomal recessive inheritance. The activity of branching enzyme is markedly reduced in liver and muscle of affected cats and intermediate enzyme activity is present in heterozygotes. Spectral analysis of the stored glycogen has shown average chain lengths that are longer than normal, a finding consistent with a reduced number of branch points, as would be expected with a deficiency of branching enzyme. A colony of these cats has been established and they should be useful for further studies of the disease.

Summary

Many other interesting muscle diseases occur in animals that might be used as models for human disease. In this chapter, however, the discussion has been limited to those that are generally available and that have contributed already to our understanding of the corresponding muscle diseases in humans. Arguably the most significant of these are the models of the various forms of muscular dystrophy. Studies in these models have contributed to our understanding of the pathogenesis of these diseases, to adaptations that can influence the course of the disease and to approaches to therapy. As advances in techniques such as gene therapy are made, these models will be essential to the development of protocols that might be used in humans. Further developments will occur as additional models are created in the laboratory tailored to address specific questions related to gene function and disease phenotypes. It is likely that they will figure even more prominently in the next edition of this book.

References

Acsadi, G., Lochmuller, H., Janim, A. et al. (1996). Dystrophin expression in muscles of *mdx* mice after adenovirus-mediated *in vivo* gene transfer. *Hum. Gene Ther.* **7**, 129–40.

Adrian, R. H. and Bryant, S. H., (1974). On the repetitive discharge in myotonic muscle fibers. *J. Physiol.* **240**, 505–515.

Adrian, R. H and Marshall, M. W. (1976). Action potentials reconstructed in normal and myotonic muscle fibers. *J. Physiol.* **258**, 125–143.

Anderson, J. E., Bressler, B. H. and Ovalle, W. K. (1988). Functional regeneration in the hindlimb skeletal muscle of the *mdx* mouse. *J. Muscle Res. Cell Motil.* **9**, 499–515.

Andresen, E. and Jensen, P. (1977). Close linkage established between the HAL locus in pigs of the Danish Landrace breed. *Nord. Veterinaermedicin* **29**, 502–504.

Angoli, D., Corona, P., Baresi, R., Mora, M. and Wanke, E. (1997). Laminin alpha2 but not alpha1-mediated adhesion of human (Duchenne) and murine (*mdx*) dystrophic myotubes is seriously defective. *FEBS Lett.* **408**, 341–344.

Arahata, K., Ishiura, S., Ishiguro, T. et al. (1988). Immunostaining of skeletal and cardiac muscle surface membrane with antibody against Duchenne muscular dystrophy peptide. *Nature* **333**, 861–863.

Araki, E., Nakamura, K., Nakao, K. et al. (1997). Targeted disruption of exon 52 in the mouse dystrophin gene induced muscle degeneration similar to that observed in Duchenne muscular dystrophy. *Biochem. Biophys. Res. Commun.* **238**, 492–497.

Atkinson, J. B., Swift, L. L. and Lequire, V. S. (1981). Myotonia congenita. A histochemical and ultrastructural study in the goat: comparison with abnormalities found in human myotonia dystrophia. *Am. J. Pathol.* **102**, 324–335.

Banker, B. Q. (1968). A phase and electron microscopic study of dystrophic muslce: II. The pathological changes in the new born Bar Harbor 129 dystrophic mouse. *J. Neuropathol. Exp. Neurol.* **27**, 183–209.

Beck, C. L., Fahlke, C. and George, A. L., Jr (1996). Molecular basis for decreased muscle chloride conductance in the myotonic goat. *Proc. Natl. Acad. Sci. USA* **93**, 11248–11252.

Bhattacharya, S. K., Crawford, A. J. and Pate, J. W. (1987). Electrocardiographic, biochemical, and morphologic abnormalities in dystrophic hamster with cardiomyopathy. *Muscle Nerve* **10**, 168–767.

Bijvoet, A. G. A., van de Kamp, E. H. M., Kroos, M. A. et al. (1998). Generalized glycogen storage and cardiomyopathy in a knock out mouse model of Pompe disease. *Hum. Mol. Genet.* **7**, 53–62.

Bodensteiner, J. B. and Engel, A. G. (1978). Intracellular calcium accumulation in Duchenne dystrophy and other myopathies: a study of 567 000 muscle fibers in 114 biopsies. *Neurology* **28**, 439–446.

Bourke, D. L., Ontell, M. and Taylor, F. (1988). Spontaneous regeneration of older dystrophic muscle does not reflect its regenerative capacity. *Am. J. Anatomy* **181**, 1–11.

Bradley, W. G. and Jenkison, M. (1975). Neural abnormalities in the dystrophic mouse. *J. Neurol. Sci.* **25**, 249–255.

Brenman, J. E., Chao, D. S., Xia, H., Aldape, K. and Bredt, D. S. (1995). Nitric oxide synthase complexed with dystrophin and absent from skeletal muscle sarcolemma in Duchenne muscular dystrophy. *Cell* **82**, 743–752.

Bridges, L. R. (1986). The association of cardiac muscle necrosis and inflammation with the degenerative and persistent myopathy of *MDX* mice. *J. Neurol. Sci.* **72**, 147–157

Brocks, L., Wirtz, P., Loermans, H. and Binkhorst, R. (1992). Effects of early immobilization on the functional capacity of dystrophic (ReJ 129 *dy/dy*) mouse leg muscles. *Int. J. Exp. Pathol.* **73**, 223–229.

Brussee, V., Tardif, F. and Tremblay, J. P. (1997). Muscle fibres of *mdx* mice are more vulnerable to exercise than those of normal mice. *Neuromusc. Disord.* **7**, 487–492.

Bryant, S. H. (1969). Cable properties of external intercostal muscle fibres from myotonic and nonmyotonic goats. *J. Physiol.* **204**, 539–550.

Bryant, S. H. (1979). Myotonia in the goat. *Ann. N. Y. Acad. Sci.* **317**, 314–325.

Bryant, S. H. and Morales-Aguilera, A. (1971). Chloride conductance in normal and myotonic muscle fibres and the action of monocarboxylic aromatic acids. *J. Physiol.* **219**, 367–383.

Bulfield, G., Siller, W. G., Wight, P. A. and Moore, K. J. (1984). X chromosome-linked muscular dystrophy (*mdx*) in the mouse. *Proc. Natl. Acad. Sci. USA* **81**, 1189–92.

Burbach, J. A. (1987). Ultrastructure of cardiocyte degeneration and myocardial calcification in the dystrophic hamster. *Am. J. Anatomy* **179**, 291–307.

Campbell, K. P. and Kahl, S. D. (1989). Association of dystrophin and an integral membrane glycoprotein. *Nature* **338**, 259–262.

Cannon, S. C., Hayward, L. J., Beech, J. and Brown, R. H. Jr (1995). Sodium channel inactivation is impaired in equine hyperkalemic periodic paralysis. *J. Neurophysiol.* **73**, 1892–1899.

Carlson, C. G. and Makiejus, R. V. (1990). A noninvasive procedure to detect muscle weakness in the *mdx* mouse. *Muscle Nerve* **13**, 480–484.

Carnwath, J. W. and Shotton, D. M. (1987). Muscular dystrophy in the *mdx* mouse: histopathology of the soleus and extensor digitorum longus muscles. *J. Neurol. Sci.* **80**, 539–554

Carpenter, J. L., Hoffman, E. P., Romanul, F. C. A. et al. (1989). Feline muscular dystrophy with dystrophin deficiency. *Am. J. Pathol.* **135**, 909–919.

Caulfield, J. B. (1966). Electron microscopic observations on the dystrophic hamster muscle. *Ann. N. Y. Acad. Sci.* **138**, 151–159.

Cavanna, J. S., Coulton, G., Morgan, J. E. et al. (1988). Molecular and genetic mapping of the mouse *mdx* locus. *Genomics* **3**, 337–341.

Ceh, L., Hauge, J. G., Svenkerud, R. and Strande, A. (1976). Glycogenosis type III in the dog. *Acta Veterin. Scand.* **17**, 210–222.

Chang, W. J., Iannoccone, S. T., Lau, K. S. et al. (1996). Neuronal nitric oxide synthase and dystrophin-deficient muscular dystrophy. *Proc. Natl. Acad. Sci. USA* **93**, 9142–9147.

Chapman, V. M., Miller, D. R., Armstrong, D. and Caskey, C. T. (1989). Recovery of induced mutations for X chromosome-linked muscular dystrophy in mice. *Proc. Natl. Acad. Sci. USA* **86**, 1292–1296

Clemens, P. R., Kichanek, S., Sunada, Y. et al. (1996). In vivo muscle gene transfer of full-length dystrophin with an adenoviral vector that lacks all viral genes. *Gene Ther.* **3**, 965–972.

Cooper, B. J., Valentine, B. A., Wilson, S., Patterson, D. F. and Concannon, P. W. (1988a). Canine muscular dystrophy: confirmation of X-linked inheritance. *J. Hered.* **79**, 405–408.

Cooper, B. J., Winand, N. J., Stedman, H. et al. (1988b). The homologue of the Duchenne locus is defective in X-linked muscular dystrophy of dogs. *Nature* **334**, 154–156.

Cooper, B. J., Gallagher, E. A., Smith, C. A., Valentine, B. A. and Winand, N. J. (1990). Mosaic expression of dystrophin in carriers of canine X-linked muscular dystrophy. *Lab. Invest.* **62**, 171–178.

Corrado, K., Rafael, J. A., Mills, P. L. et al. (1996). Transgenic *mdx* mice expressing dystrophin with a deletion in the actin-binding domain display a 'mild Becker' phenotype. *J. Cell Biol.* **134**, 873–884.

Coulton, G. R., Curtin, N. A., Morgan, J. E. and Partridge, T. A. (1988a). The *mdx* mouse skeletal muscle myopathy: II. Contractile properties. *Neuropathol. Appl. Neurobiol.* **14**, 299–314.

Coulton, G. R., Morgan, J. E., Partridge, T. A. and Sloper, J. C. (1988b). The *mdx* mouse skeletal muscle myopathy: I. A histological, morphometric and biochemical investigation. *Neuropathol. Appl. Neurobiol.* **14**, 53–70.

Cox, G. A., Cole, N. M., Matsumura, K. et al. (1993). Overexpression of dystrophin in transgenic *mdx* mice eliminates dystrophic symptoms without toxicity. *Nature* **364**, 725–729.

Cox, G. A., Sunada, Y., Campbell, K. P. and Chamberlain, J. S. (1994). Dp71 can restore the dystrophin-associated glycoprotein complex in muscle but fails to prevent dystrophy. *Nat. Genet.* **8**, 333–339.

Cox, J. H, (1986). An episodic weakness in four horses associated with intermittent serum hyperkalemia and the similarity of the disease to hyperkalemic periodic paralysis in man. *Proc. Am. Ass. Equine Pract.* **92**, 299–304.

Cullen, M. J. and Jaros, E. (1988). Ultrastructure of the skeletal muscle in the X chromosome-linked dystrophic (*mdx*) mouse. Comparison with Duchenne muscular dystrophy. *Acta Neuropathol.* **77**, 69–81.

Dangain, J. and Vrbova, G. (1984). Muscle development in *mdx* mutant mice. *Muscle Nerve* **7**, 700–704.

Danko, I., Chapman, V. and Wolff, J. A. (1992). The frequency of revertants in *mdx* mouse genetic models for Duchenne muscular dystrophy. *Pediatr. Res.* **32**, 128–131.

Davies, W., Harbitz, I., Fries, R., Stranzinger, G. and Hauge, J. G. (1988). Porcine malignant hyperthermia carrier detection and chromosomal assignment using a linked probe. *Animal Genet.* **19**, 203–212.

Deconinck, N., Ragot, T., Marechal, G. and Perricaudet, M. and Gillis, J. M. (1996). Functional protection of dystrophic mouse (*mdx*) muscles after adenovirus-mediated transfer of a dystrophin minigene. *Proc. Natl. Acad. Sci. USA* **93**, 3570–3574.

Deconinck, A. E., Potter, A. C., Tinsley, J. M. et al. (1997a). Postsynaptic abnormalities at the neuromuscular junctions of utrophin-deficient mice. *J. Cell Biol.* **136**, 883–894.

Deconinck, A. E., Rafael, J. A., Skinner, J. A. et al. (1997b). Utrophin–dystrophin-deficient mice as a model for Duchenne muscular dystrophy. *Cell* **90**, 717–727.

Deconinck, N., Tinsley, J., De Backer, F. et al. (1997c). Expression of truncated utrophin leads to major functional improvements in dystrophin-deficient muscles of mice. *Nat. Med.* **3**, 1216–1221.

de Lahunta, A. (1983). *Veterinary Neuroanatomy and Clinical Neurology*, 2nd edn. Philadelphia, PA: Saunders.

Desaki, J., Matsuda, S. and Sakanaka, M. (1995). Morphological changes of neuromuscular junctions in the dystrophic mouse: a scanning and transmission electron microscopic study. *J. Electron Microsc.(Tokyo)* **44**, 59–65.

Di Marco, P. N., Howell, J. M. and Dorling, P. R. (1984). Bovine glycogenosis type II. Biochemical and morphological characteristics of skeletal muscle in culture *Neuropath. Appl. Neurobiol.* **10**, 379–395.

Di Marco, P. N., Howell, J. M. and Dorling, P. R. (1985). Bovine generalised glycogenosis type II. Uptake of lysosomal alpha-glucosidase by cultured skeletal muscle and reversal of glycogen accumulation. *FEBS Lett.***190**, 301–304.

DiMario, J. X., Uzman, A. and Strohman, R. C. (1991). Fiber regeneration is not persistent in dystrophic (*mdx*) mouse skeletal muscle. *Dev. Biol.* **148**, 314–321.

Disatnik, M-H., Dhawan, J., Yu, Y. et al. (1998). Evidence of oxidative stress in *mdx* mouse muscle: studies of the pre-necrotic state. *J. Neurol. Sci.* **161**, 77–84.

Doizé, F., Roux, I., Martineau-Doizé, B. and DeRoth, L. (1990). Prediction of the halothane (Hal) genotypes by means of linked marker loci (Phi, Po2, Pgd) in Quebec Landrace pigs. *Can. J. Vet. Res.* **54**, 397–399.

Duclos, F., Straub, V., Moore, S. A. et al. (1998). Progressive muscular dystrophy in α-sarcoglycan-deficient mice. *J. Cell Biol.* **142**, 1461–1471.

Dunn, J. F. and Radda, G. K. (1991). Total ion content of skeletal and cardiac muscle in the *mdx* mouse dystrophy: Ca^{2+} is elevated at all ages. *J. Neurol. Sci.* **103**, 226–231.

Dupont-Versteegden, E. E. and McCarter, R. J. (1992). Differential expression of muscular dystrophy in diaphragm versus hindlimb muscles of *mdx* mice. *Muscle Nerve* **15**, 1105–1110.

Edwards, J. R. and Richards, R. B. (1979). Bovine generalized glycogenosis type II. A clinicopathological study. *Br. Vet. J.* **135**, 338–348.

Entrikin, R. K., Abresch, R. T., Sharman, R. B., Larson, D. B. and Levine, N. A. (1987). Contractile and EMG studies of murine myotonia (*mto*) and muscular dystrophy (*dy/dy*). *Muscle Nerve* **10**, 293–298.

Ervasti, J. M. and Campbell, K. P. (1991). Membrane organization of the dystrophin–glycoprotein complex. *Cell* **66**, 1121–1131.

Ervasti, J. M., Roberds, S. L., Anderson, R. D., Sharp, N. J. Kornegay, J. N. and Campbell, K. P. (1994). α-Dystroglycan deficiency correlates with elevated serum creatine kinase and decreased muscle contraction tension in golden retriever muscular dystrophy. *FEBS Lett.* **350**, 173–176.

Fan, Y., Maley, M., Beilharz, M. and Grounds, M. (1996). Rapid death of injected myoblasts in myoblast transfer therapy. *Muscle Nerve* **19**, 853–860.

Farrow, B. R. H. and Malik, R. (1981). Hereditary myotonia in the Chow Chow. *J. Small Animal Pract.* **22**, 451–463.

Fassati, A., Wells, D. J., Sgro Serpent, P. A. et al. (1997). Genetic correction of dystrophin deficiency and skeletal muscle remodeling in adult *mdx* mouse via transplantation of retroviral producer cells. *J. Clin. Invest.* **100**, 620–628.

Fong, P., Turner, P. R., Denetclaw, W. F. and Steinhardt, R. A. (1990). Increased activity of calcium leak channels in myotubes of Duchenne human and *mdx* mouse origin. *Science* **250**, 673–676.

Franco, A. Jr. and Lansman, J. B. (1990). Calcium entry through stretch-inactivated ion channels in *mdx* myotubes. *Nature* **344**, 670–673.

Franco-Obregon, A. Jr and Lansman, J. B. (1994). Mechanosensitive ion channels in skeletal muscle from normal and dystrophic mice. *J. Physiol. (Lond.)* **481**, 299–309.

Frankel, K. A. and Rosser, R. J. (1976). The pathology of the heart in progressive muscular dystrophy: epimyocardial fibrosis. *Hum. Pathol.* **7**, 375–386.

Fujii, J., Otsu, K., Zorzato, F. et al. (1991). Identification of a mutation in porcine ryanodine receptor associated with malignant hyperthermia. *Science* **253**, 448–451.

Fujita, T., Nonaka, I. and Sugita, H.. (1991). Japanese quail and human acid maltase deficiency: a comparative study. *Brain Dev.* **13**, 247–255.

Fyfe, J. C., Giger, U., van Winkle, T. J. et al. (1992). Glycogen storage disease type IV: inherited deficiency of branching enzyme activity in cats. *Pediatr. Res.* **32**, 719–725.

Gallant, E. M. (1980). Histochemical observations on muscle from normal and malignant hyperthermia-susceptible swine. *Am. J. Vet. Res.* **41**, 1069–1071.

Gallant, E. M., Mickelson, J. R., Roggow, B. D., Donaldson, S. K., Louis, C. F. and Rempel, W. E. (1989). Halothane-sensitivity gene and muscle contractile properties in malignant hyperthermia. *Am. J. Physiol.* **257**, C781–C786.

Gaschen, F. P., Hoffman, E. P., Gorospe, J. R. M. et al. (1992). Dystrophin deficiency causes lethal muscle hypertrophy in cats. *J. Neurol. Sci.* **110**, 149–159.

Gaschen, L., Lang, J., Lin, S. et al. (1999). Cardiomyopathy in dystrophin-deficient hypertrophic feline muscular dystrophy. *J. Vet. Inter. Med.* **13**, 346.

Gilbert, R., Nalbantoglu, J., Petrof, B. J. et al. (1999). Adenovirus-mediated utrophin gene transfer mitigates the dystrophic phenotype of *mdx* mouse muscles. *Hum. Gene Ther.* **10**, 1299–1310.

Grady, R. M., Merlie, J. P. and Sanes, J. R. (1997a). Subtle neuromuscular defects in utrophin-deficient mice. *J. Cell Biol.* **136**, 871–882.

Grady, R. M., Teng, H., Nichol, M. C., Cunningham, J. C., Wilkinson, R. S. and Sanes, J. R. (1997b). Skeletal and cardiac myopathies in mice lacking utrophin and dystrophin: a model for Duchenne muscular dystrophy. *Cell* **90**, 729–738.

Greelish, J. P., Su, L. T., Lankford, E. B. et al.. (1999). Stable restoration of the sarcoglycan complex in dystrophic muscle perfused with histamine and a recombinant adeno-associated vector. *Nat. Med.* **5**, 439–443.

Greenberg, D. S., Sunada, Y., Campbell, K. P., Yaffe, D. and Nudel, U. (1994). Exogenous Dp71 restores the levels of dystrophin associated proteins but does not alleviate muscle damage in *mdx* mice. *Nat. Genet.* **8**, 340–344.

Gross, J. G. and Morgan, J. E. (1999). Muscle precursor cells injected into irradiated *mdx* mouse muscle persist after serial injury. *Muscle Nerve* **22**, 174–185.

Grounds, M. D. and McGeachie, J. K. (1992). Skeletal muscle regeneration after crush injury in dystrophic *mdx* mice: an autoradiographic study. *Muscle Nerve* **15**, 580–586.

Gurnett, C. A., Kahl, S. D., Anderson, R. D. and Campbell, K. P. (1995). Absence of the skeletal muscle sarcolemma chloride channel ClC-1 in myotonic mice. *J. Biol. Chem.* **270**, 9035–9038.

Hack, A. A., Ly, C. T., and Jiang, F. (1998). γ-Sarcoglycan deficiency leads to muscle membrane defects and apoptosis independent of dystrophin. *J. Cell Biol.* **142**, 1279–1287.

Harbitz, I., Chowdhary, B., Thomsen, P. D. et al. (1990). Assignment of the porcine calcium release channel gene, a candidate for the malignant hyperthermia locus, to the 6p11-q21 segment of chromosome 6. *Genomics* **8**, 243–248.

Harris, A. S. and Mrak, R. E. (1985). Myotonia congenita. In: *Muscle Membranes in Diseases of Muscle*, ed. R. E. Mrak, pp. 81–92. Boca Raton, FL: CRC Press.

Haws, C. M. and Lansman, J. B. (1991). Developmental regulation of mechanosensitive calcium channels in skeletal muscle from normal and *mdx* mice. *Proc. R. Soc. Lon. Ser. B: Biol. Sci.* **245**, 173–177.

Hayakawa, J. and Tsuji, S. (1985). A new mutant at the dystrophia muscularis (*dy*) locus in the SM strain of mice. *Lab. Animal* **19**, 1–2.

Hayes, A. and Williams, D. A. (1998). Contractile function and low-intensity exercise effects of old dystrophic (*mdx*) mice. *Am. J. Physiol.* **274**, C1138–C1144.

Heffron, J. J., Mitchell, G. and Dreyer, J. H. (1982). Muscle fibre type, fibre diameter and pH1 values of M. longissimus dorsi of normal, malignant hyperthermia- and PSE-susceptible pigs. *Br. Vet. J.* **138**, 45–50.

Helbling-Leclerc, A., Zhang, X., Topaloglu, et al. (1995). Mutations in the laminin α_2 chain gene (LAMA2) cause merosin-deficient congenital muscular dystrophy. *Nat. Genet.* **11**, 216–218.

Heller, A. H., Eicher, E. M., Hallet, M. and Sidman, R. L. (1982). Myotonia, a new inherited muscle disease in mice. *J. Neurosci.* **2**, 924–933.

Hermanson, J. W., Ontell, M. and Moschella, M. C. (1988). Effect of neonatal denervation-reinnervation on the functional capacity of a murine dystrophic muscle. *Exp. Neurol.* **102**, 210–216.

Higuchi, I., Nonaka, I. and Usuki, F. (1987). Acid maltase deficiency in the Japanese quail; early morphologic event in skeletal muscle. *Acta Neuropathol.* **73**, 32–37.

Hoffman, E. P., Brown, R. H., Jr and Kunkel, L. M. (1987). Dystrophin: the protein product of the Duchenne muscular dystrophy locus. *Cell* **51**, 919–928.

Hoffman, E. P., Morgan, J. E., Watkins, S. C. and Partridge, T. A. (1990). Somatic reversion/suppression of the mouse *mdx* phenotype in vivo. *J. Neurol. Sci.* **99**, 9–25.

Holt, K. H., Lim, L. E., Straub, V. et al. (1998). Functional rescue of the sarcoglycan complex in the BIO 14.6 hamster using delta-sarcoglycan gene transfer. *Mol. Cell* **1**, 841–848.

Homburger, F. (1979). Myopathy of hamster dystrophy: history and morphologic aspects. *Ann. N. Y. Acad. Sci.* **317**, 1–17.

Homburger, F. and Bajusz, E. (1970). New models of human disease in Syrian hamsters. *J. Am. Med. Assoc.* **212**, 604–610.

Homburger, F., Nixon, C. W., Eppenberger, M. and Baker, J. R. (1966). Hereditary myopathy in the Syrian hamster: studies on pathogenesis. *Ann. N. Y. Acad. Sci.* **138**, 14–27.

Howell, J. McM., Dorling, P. R., Cook, R. D. Robinson, W. F., Bradleym, S. and Gawthorne, J. M. (1981). Infantile and late onset form of generalised glycogenosis type II in cattle. *J. Pathol.* **134**, 266–277.

Howell, J. McM., Dorling, P. R., Shelton, J. N., Taylor, E. G., Palmer, D. G. and Di Marco, P. N. (1991). Natural bone marrow transplantation in cattle with Pompe's disease. *Neuromusc. Disord.* **1**, 449–454.

Howell, J. McM., Lochmuller, H., O'Hara, A. et al. (1998). High-level dystrophin expression after adenovirus-mediated dystrophin minigene transfer to skeletal muscle of dystrophic dogs: prolongation of expression with immunosuppression. *Hum. Gene Ther.* **9**, 629–634.

Hunter, S. (1980). The heart in muscular dystrophy. *Br. Med. Bull.* **36**, 133–134.

Hutter, O. F., Burton, F. L. and Bovel, D. L. (1991). Mechanical properties of normal and *mdx* mouse sarcolemma: bearing on function of dystrophin. *J. Muscle Res. Cell Motil.* **12**, 585–589.

Iaizzo, P. A., Klein, W. and Lehmann-Horn, F. (1988). Fura-2 detected myoplasmic calcium and its correlation with contracture force in skeletal muscle from normal and malignant hyperthermia susceptible pigs. *Pflugers Arch. Eur. J. Physiol.* **411**, 648–653.

Im, W. B., Phelps, S. F., Copen, E. H. Adams, E. G., Slightomm J. L. and Chamberlain, J. S. (1996). Differential expression of dystrophin isoforms in strains of *mdx* mice with different mutations. *Hum. Mol. Genet.* **5**, 1149–1153.

Iwata, Y., Nakamura, H., Fujiwara, K. and Shigekawa, M. (1993). Altered membrane-dystrophin association in the cardiomyopathic hamster heart muscle. *Biochem. Biophys. Res. Commun.* **190**, 589–595.

Jaros, E. and Bradley, W. G. (1979). Atypical axon-Schwann cell relationships in the common peroneal nerve of the dystrophic mouse: an ultrastructural study. *Neuropathol. Appl. Neurobiol.* **5**, 133–147.

Jaros, E. and Jenkison, M. (1983). Quantitative studies of the abnormal axon–Schwann cell relationship in the peripheral motor and sensory nerves of the dystrophic mouse. *Brain Res.* **258**, 181–196.

Jasmin, G. and Eu, H. Y. (1979). Cardiomyopathy of hamster dystrophy. *Ann. N. Y. Acad. Sci.* **317**, 46–58.

Jockusch, H., Reininghaus, J., Stuhlfauth, I. and Zippel, M. (1988). Reduction of myosin-light-chain phosphorylation and of parvalbumin content in myotonic mouse muscle and its reversal by tocainide. *Eur. J. Biochem.* **171**, 101–105.

Jockusch, H., Friedrich, G. and Zippel, M. (1990). Serum parvalbumin, an indicator of muscle disease in murine dystrophy and myotonia. *Muscle Nerve* **13**, 551–555.

Johnstone, D., Jaros, E. and Harris, J. B. (1986). Spontaneous electrical activity in muscles of dystrophic (*dy/dy*) mice. *J. Neurol. Sci.* **73**, 339–349.

Jones, E. W., Kerr, D. D. and Nelson, T. E. (1973). Malignant hyperthermia – observations in Poland China pigs. In: *International Symposium on Malignant Hyperthermia*, eds. R. A. Gordon, B. A. Britt and W. Kalow, pp. 198–205. Springfield: Charles C. Thomas.

Karpati, G., Carpenter, S. and Prescott, S. (1982). Prevention of skeletal muscle fiber necrosis in hamster dystrophy. *Muscle Nerve* **5**, 369–372.

Karpati, G., Pouliot, Y., Zubrzycka-Gaarn, E. et al. (1989). Dystrophin is expressed in *mdx* skeletal muscle fibers after normal myoblast implantation. *Am. J. Pathol.* **135**, 27–32.

Karpati, G., Zubrzycka-Gaarn, E. E., Carpenter, S., Bulman, D. E., Ray, P. N. and Worton, R. G. (1990). Age-related conversion of dystrophin-negative to -positive fiber segments of skeletal but not cardiac muscle fibers in heterozygote *mdx* mice. *J. Neuropathol. Exp. Neurol.* **49**, 96–105.

Kinoshita, I., Vilquin, J. T. and Tremblay, J. P. (1996). Mechanism of increasing dystrophin-positive myofibers by myoblast transplantation: study using *mdx*/beta-galactosidase transgenic mice. *Acta Neuropathol. (Berl.)* **91**, 489–493.

Kornegay, J. N., Tuler, S. M., Miller, D. M. and Levesque, D. C. (1988). Muscular dystrophy in a litter of golden retriever dogs. *Muscle Nerve* **11**, 1056–1064.

Lanfossi, M., Cozzi, F., Bugini, D. et al. (1999). Development of muscle pathology in canine X-linked muscular dystrophy. I. Delayed postnatal maturation of affected and normal muscle as revealed by myosin isoform analysis and utrophin expression. *Acta Neuropathol. (Berl.)* **97**, 127–138.

Lefaucheur, J. P., Pastoret, C. and Sebille, A. (1995). Phenotype of dystrophinopathy in old *mdx* mice. *Anat. Rec.* **242**, 70–76.

Leijendekker, W. J., Passaquin, A. C., Metzinger, L. and Ruegg, U. T. (1996). Regulation of cytosolic calcium in skeletal muscle cells of the *mdx* mouse under conditions of stress. *Br. J. Pharmacol.* **118**, 611–616.

Lipicky, R. J. and Bryant, S. H. (1966). Sodium, potassium, and chloride fluxes in intercostal muscle from normal goats and goats with hereditary myotonia. *J. Gen. Physiol.* **50**, 89–111.

Lochmuller, J., Petrof, B. J., Pari, G. et al. (1996). Transient immunosuppression by FK506 permits a sustained high-level dystrophin expression after adenovirus-mediated dystrophin minigene transfer to skeletal muscles of adult dystrophic (*mdx*) mice. *Gene Ther.* **3**, 706–716.

López, J. R., Allen, P. D., Alamo, L., Jones, D. and Sreter, F. A. (1988). Myoplasmic free $[Ca^{2+}]$ during a malignant hyperthermia episode in swine. *Muscle Nerve* **11**, 82–88.

MacLennan, D. H. and Phillips, M. S. (1992). Malignant hyperthermia. *Science* **256**, 789–794.

MacLennan, P. A., McArdle, A. and Edwards, R. H. T. (1991). Effects of calcium on protein turnover of incubated muscles from *mdx* mice. *Am. J. Physiol. Endocrinol. Metab.* **260**, E594–E598.

Martin, H. and Ontell, M. (1988). Regeneration of dystrophic muscle following multiple injections of bupivicaine. *Muscle Nerve* **11**, 588–596.

Marvasti, M. A. and Williams, C. H. (1988). Malignant hyperthermia and the sarcoplasmic reticulum: a review. In: *Experimental Malignant Hyperthermia*, ed. C. H. Williams, p. 57. New York: Springer-Verlag.

Matsui, T., Kuroda, S., Mizutani, M., Kiuchi, Y., Suzuki, K. and Ono T. (1983). Generalized glycogen storage disease in Japanese quail (*Coturnix coturnix japonica*). *Vet. Pathol.* **20**, 312–321.

Matsumura, K., Ervasti, J. M., Ohlendieck, K., Kahl, S. D. and Campbell, K. P. (1992). Association of dystrophin-related protein with dystrophin-associated proteins in *mdx* mouse muscle. *Nature* **360**, 588–591.

Mehrke, G., Brinkmeier, H. and Jockusch, H. (1988). The myotonic mouse mutant ADR: Electrophysiology of the muscle fiber. *Muscle Nerve* **11**, 440–446.

Meier, H. and Southard, J. L. (1970). Muscular dystrophy in the mouse caused by an allele at the *dy*-locus. *Life Sci.* **9**, 137–144.

Mendell, J. R., Higgins, R., Sahenk, Z. and Cosmos, E. (1979). Relevance of genetic animal models of muscular dystrophy to human muscular dystrophies. *Ann. N. Y. Acad. Sci.* **317**, 409–430.

Menke, A. and Jockusch, H. (1991). Decreased osmotic stability of dystrophin-less muscle cells from the *mdx* mouse. *Nature* **349**, 69–71.

Michelson, A. M., Russell, E. S. and Harman, P. J. (1955). Dystrophia muscularis: a hereditary primary myopathy in the house mouse. *Proc. Natl. Acad. Sci. USA* **41**, 1079–1083.

Mickelson, J. R., Ross, J. A., Reed, B. K. and Louis, C. F. (1986). Enhanced Ca^{2+}-induced calcium release by isolated sarcoplasmic reticulum vesicles from malignant hyperthermia susceptible pig muscle. *Biochim. Biophys. Acta* **862**, 318–328.

Mickelson, J. R., Gallant, E. M., Rempel, W. E. et al. (1989). Effects of the halothane-sensitivity gene on sarcoplasmic reticulum function. *Am. J. Physiol.* **257**, C787–C794.

Mickelson, J. R., Litterer, L. A., Jacobson, B. A. and Louis, C. F. (1990). Stimulation and inhibition of [^{3}H]ryanodine binding to sarcoplasmic reticulum from malignant hyperthermia susceptible pigs. *Arch. Biochem. Biophys.* **278**, 251–257.

Miyagoe, Y., Hanaoka, K., Nonaka, I. et al. (1997). Laminin alpha2 chain-null mutant mice by targeted disruption of the Lama2 gene: a new model of merosin (laminin 2)-deficient congenital muscular dystrophy. *FEBS Lett.* **415**, 33–39.

Mizuno, Y., Noguchi, S., Yamamoto, H. et al. (1995). Sarcoglycan complex is selectively lost in dystrophic hamster muscle. *Am. J. Pathol.* **146**, 530–536.

Moise, N. S., Valentine, B. A., Brown, C. A. et al. (1990). Duchenne cardiomyopathy in a canine model: electrocardiographic and echocardiographic studies. *J. Am. Coll. Cardiol.* **17**, 812–820.

Morgan, J. E., Hoffman, E. P. and Partridge, T. A. (1990). Normal myogenic cells from newborn mice restore normal histology to degenerating muscles of the *mdx* mouse. *J. Cell Biol.* **111**, 2437–2449.

Naylor, J. M., Robinson, J. A, and Bertone, J. (1992). Familial incidence of hyperkalemic periodic paralysis in quarter horses. *J. Am. Vet. Med. Assoc.* **200**, 340–343.

Nicholson, L. V. B., Davison, K., Johnson, M. A. et al. (1989). Dystrophin in skeletal muscle. II. Immunoreactivity in patients with Xp21 muscular dystrophy. *J. Neurol. Sci.* **94**, 137–146.

Nigro, V., Akazaki, Y., Belsito, A. et al. (1997). Identification of the Syrian hamster cardiomyopathy gene. *Hum. Mol. Genet.* **6**, 601–607.

O'Brien, P. J. (1986). Porcine malignant hyperthermia susceptibility: hypersensitive calcium-release mechanism of skeletal muscle sarcoplasmic reticulum. *Can. J. Vet. Res.* **50**, 318–328.

O'Brien, P. J. (1987). Etiopathogenetic defect of malignant hyperthermia: hypersensitive calcium-release channel of skeletal muscle sarcoplasmic reticulum. *Vet. Res. Commun.* **11**, 527–529.

Ohlendieck, K. and Campbell, K. P. (1991). Dystrophin-associated proteins are greatly reduced in skeletal muscle from *mdx* mice. *J. Cell Biol.* **115**, 1685–1694.

Ohlendieck, K., Ervasti, J. M., Snook, J. B. and Campbell, K. P. (1991). Dystrophin–glycoprotein complex is highly enriched in isolated skeletal muscle sarcolemma. *J. Cell Biol.* **112**, 135–148.

Ohta, T., Endo, M., Nakano, T. Morohoshi, Y., Wanikawa, K. and Ohga, A. (1989). Ca-induced Ca release in malignant hyperthermia-susceptible pig skeletal muscle. *Am. J. Physiol.* **256**, C358–C367.

Ontell, M. (1981). Muscle fiber necrosis in murine muscular dystrophy. *Muscle Nerve* **4**, 204–213.

Ontell, M. (1986). Muscular dystrophy and muscle regeneration. *Hum. Pathol.* **17**, 673–682.

Otsu, K., Khanna, V. K., Archibald, A. L. and MacLennan, D. H. (1991). Cosegregation of porcine malignant hyperthermia and probable causal mutation in the skeletal muscle ryanodine receptor gene in backcross families. *Genomics* **11**, 744–750.

Palmer, E. G., Topel, D. G. and Christian, L. L. (1977). Microscopic observations of muscle from swine susceptible to malignant hyperthermia. *J. Animal Sci.* **45**, 1032–1036.

Palmer, E. G., Topel, D. G. and Christian, L. L. (1978). Light and electron microscopy of skeletal muscle from malignant hyperthermia susceptible pigs. In: *Malignant Hyperthermia*, eds. J. A. Aldrete and B. A. Britt, pp. 103–112. New York: Grune and Stratton.

Partridge, T. A., Morgan, J. E., Coulton, G. R., Hoffman, E. P. and Kunkel, L. M. (1989). Conversion of *mdx* myofibers from dystrophin-negative to -positive by injection of normal myoblasts. *Nature* **337**, 176–179.

Perloff, J. K., de Leon, A. C. and O'Doherty, D. (1966). The cardiomyopathy of progressive muscular dystrophy. *Circulation* **33**, 625–648.

Phelps, S. F., Hauser, M. A. Cole, N. M. et al. (1995). Expression of full-length and truncated dystrophin mini-genes in transgenic *mdx* mice. *Hum. Mol. Genet.* **4**, 1251–1258.

Pickar, J. G., Spier, S. J., Snyder, J. R. and Carlsen, R. C. (1991). Altered ionic permeability in skeletal muscle from horses with hyperkalemic periodic paralysis. *Am. J. Physiol.* **260**, C926–C933.

Platzer, A. and Chase, W. (1964). Histological alterations in preclinical mouse muscular dystrophy. *Am. J. Pathol.* **44**, 931–943.

Porter, J. D., Rafael, J. A., Ragusa, R. J., Brueckner, J. K., Trickett, J. I. and Davies K. E. (1998). The sparing of extraocular muscle in dystrophinopathy is lost in mice lacking utrophin and dystrophin. *J. Cell Sci.* **111**, 1801–1811.

Quinlan, J. G., Johnson, S. R., McKee, M. K. and Lyden, S. P. (1992). Twitch and tetanus in *mdx* mouse muscle. *Muscle Nerve* **15**, 837–842.

Rafael, J. A., Sunada, Y., Cole, N. M. Campbell, K. P., Faulkner, J. A. and Chamberlain, J. S. (1994). Prevention of dystrophic pathology in *mdx* mice by a truncated dystrophin isoform. *Hum. Mol. Genet.* **3**, 1725–1733.

Rafael, J. A., Cox, G. A., Corrado, K. Jung, D., Campbell, K. P. and Chamberlain, J. S. (1996). Forced expression of dystrophin deletion constructs reveals structure–function correlations. *J. Cell Biol.* **134**, 93–102.

Rafael, J. A., Tinsley, J. M., Potter, A. C., Deconinck, A. E. and Davies, K. E. (1998). Skeletal muscle-specific expression of a utrophin transgene rescues utrophin–dystrophin deficient mice. *Nat. Genet.* **19**, 79–82.

Rafiquzzaman, M., Svenkerud, R., Strande, A. and Hauge, J. G. (1976). Glycogenosis in the dog. *Acta Vet. Scand.* **17**, 196–209.

Ragusa, R. J., Chow, C. K. and Poerter, J. D. (1997). Oxidative stress as a potential pathogenetic mechanism in an animal model of Duchenne muscular dystrophy. *Neuromusc. Disord.* **7**, 379–386.

Rando, T. A., Disatnik, M-H., Yu, Y. and Franco, A. (1998). Muscle cells from *mdx* mice have an increased susceptibility to oxidative stress. *Neuromusc. Disord.* **8**, 14–21.

Rasminsky, M. (1980). Ephaptic transmission between single nerve fibers in the spinal nerve roots of dystrophic mice. *J. Physiol.* **305**, 151–169.

Rasminsky, M., Kearney, R. E., Aguayo, A. J., and Bray, G. M. (1978). Conduction of nervous impulses in spinal roots and peripheral nerves of dystrophic mice. *Brain Res.* **143**, 71–85.

Reininghaus, J., Füchtbauer, E.-M., Bertram, K. and Jockusch, H. (1988). The myotonic mouse mutant ADR: physiological and histochemical properties of muscle. *Muscle Nerve* **11**, 433–439.

Rhodes, T. H., Vite, C. H., Giger, U., Patterson, D. F., Fahlke, C. and George, A. L. Jr (1999). A missense mutation in canine ClC-1 causes recessive myotonia congenita in the dog. *FEBS Lett.* **456**, 54–58.

Richter, A., Gerdes, C. and Löscher, W. (1992). Atypical reactions to halothane in a subgroup of homozygous malignant hyperthermia(MH)-susceptible pigs: indication of a heterogenous genetic basis for the porcine syndrome. *Deutsch. Tierarzt. Wochenschr.* **99**, 401–406.

Ringelmann, B., Roder, C., Hallmann, R. et al. (1999). Expression of laminin alpha1, alpha2, alpha4, and alpha5 chains, fibronectin, and tenascin-C in skeletal muscle of dystrophic 129ReJ *dy/dy* mice. *Exp. Cell Res.* **246**, 165–182.

Roberds, S. L., Ervasti, J. M., Anderson, R. D. et al. (1993). Disruption of the dystrophin–glycoprotein complex in the cardiomyopathic hamster. *J. Biol. Chem.* **268**, 11496–11499.

Robinson, J. A., Naylor, J. M. and Crichlow, E. C. (1990). Use of electromyography for the diagnosis of equine hyperkalemic periodic paresis. *Can. J. Vet. Res.* **54**, 495–500.

Robinson, W. F., Howell, J. M. and Dorling, P. R. (1983). Cardiomyopathy in generalised glycogenosis type II in cattle. *Cardiovasc. Res.* **17**, 238–242.

Rudolph, J. A., Spier, S. J., Byrns, G., Rojas, C. V., Bernoco, D. and Hoffman, E. P. (1992). Periodic paralysis in Quarter horses: a sodium channel mutation disseminated by selective breeding. *Nat. Genet.* **2**, 144–147.

Ryder-Cook, A. S., Sicinski, P., Thomas, K. et al. (1988). Localization of the *mdx* mutation within the mouse dystrophin gene. *EMBO J.* **7**, 3017–3021.

Sacco, P., Jones, D. A., Dick, J. R. T. and Vrbová, G. (1992). Contractile properties and susceptibility to exercise-induced damage of normal and *mdx* mouse tibialis anterior muscle. *Clin. Sci.* **82**, 227–236.

Sakamoto, A., Ono, K., Abe, M. et al. (1997). Both hypertrophic and dilated cardiomyopathies are caused by mutation of the same gene, delta-sarcoglycan, in hamster: an animal model of disrupted dystrophin-associated glycoprotein complex. *Proc. Natl. Acad. Sci. USA* **94**, 13873–13878.

Sakamoto, A., Abe, M. and Masaki, T. (1999). Delineation of genomic deletion in cardiomyopathic hamster. *FEBS Lett.* **447**, 124–128.

Sandri, M., Podhorska-Okolow, M., Geromel, V. et al. (1997). Exercise induces myonuclear ubiquitination and apoptosis in dystrophin-deficient muscle of mice. *J. Neuropathol. Exp. Neurol.* **56**, 45–57.

Schatzberg, C. F., Olby, N. J. Breen, M. et al. (1999). Molecular analysis of a spontaneous dystrophin 'knockout' dog. *Neuromusc. Dis.* **9**, 289–295.

Schimmelpfeng, J., Jockusch, H. and Heimann, P. (1987). Increased density of satellite cells in the absence of fiber degeneration in muscle if myotonic mice. *Cell Tissue Res.* **249**, 351–357.

Sewry, C. A., Wilson, L. A., Dux, L., Dubowitz. V. and Cooper, B. J. (1992). Experimental regeneration in canine muscular dystrophy-1. Immunocytochemical evaluation of dystrophin and beta-spectrin expression. *Neuromusc. Dis.* **2**, 331–342.

Sewry, C. A., Uziyel, Y., Torelli, S. et al. (1998). Differential labelling of laminin alpha 2 in muscle and neural tissue of *dy/dy* mice: are there isoforms of the laminin alpha 2 chain? *Neuropathol. Appl. Neurobiol.* **24**, 66–72.

Sharp, N. J. H., Kornegay, J. N., van Camp, S. D. et al. (1992). An error in dystrophin mRNA processing in golden retriever muscular dystrophy, an animal homologue of Duchenne muscular dystrophy. *Genomics* **13**, 115–121.

Shibuya, S. and Wakayama, Y. (1991). Changes in muscle plasma membranes in young mice with X chromosome-linked muscular dystrophy: a freeze-fracture study. *Neuropathol. Appl. Neurobiol.* **17**, 335–344.

Shibuya, S., Wakayama, Y., Oniki, H. et al. (1997). A comparative freeze-fracture study of plasma membrane of dystrophic skeletal muscles in *dy/dy* mice with merosin (laminin 2) deficiency and *mdx* mice with dystrophin deficiency. *Neuropathol. Appl. Neurobiol.* **23**, 123–131.

Shomer, N. H., Louis, C. F., Fill, M., Litterer, L. A. and Mickelson, J. R. (1993). Reconstitution of abnormalities in the malignant hyperthermia-susceptible pig ryanodine receptor. *Am. J. Physiol. Cell Physiol.* **264**, C125–C135.

Sicinski, P., Geng, Y., Ryder-Cook, A. S., Barnard, E. A., Darlison, M. G. and Barnard, P. J. (1989). The molecular basis of muscular dystrophy in the *mdx* mouse: a point mutation. *Science* **244**, 1578–1580.

Smith, C. and Bampton, P. R. (1977). Inheritance of reaction to halothane anaesthesia in pigs. *Genet. Res.* **29**, 287–292.

Spier, S. J., Carlson, G. P., Holliday, T. A. Cardinet, G. H. III and Pickar, J. G. (1990). Hyperkalemic periodic paralysis in horses. *J. Am. Vet. Med. Ass.* **197**, 1009–1017.

Stedman, H. H., Sweeney, H. L., Shrager, J. B. et al. (1991). The *mdx* mouse diaphragm reproduces the degenerative changes of Duchenne muscular dystrophy. *Nature* **352**, 536–539.

Steinmeyer, K., Klocke, R., Ortland, C. et al. (1991a). Inactivation of muscle chloride channel by transposon insertion in myotonic mice. *Nature* **354**, 304–308.

Steinmeyer, K., Ortland, C. and Jentsch, T. J. (1991b). Primary structure and functional expression of a developmentally regulated skeletal muscle chloride channel. *Nature* **354**, 301–4.

Steiss, J. E. and Naylor, J. M. (1986). Episodic muscle tremors in a Quarter horse: resemblance to hyperkalemic periodic paralysis. *Can. Vet. J.* **27**, 332–335.

Stirling, C. A. (1975). Abnormalities in Schwann cell sheaths in spinal nerve roots of dystrophic mice. *J. Anatomy* **119**, 169–180.

Straub, V., Duclos, F., Venzke, D. P. et al. (1998). Molecular pathogenesis of muscle degeneration in the δ-sarcoglycan-deficient hamster. *Am. J. Pathol.* **153**, 1623–1630.

Sugita, H., Arahata, K., Ishiguro, T. et al. (1988). Negative immunostaining of Duchenne muscular dystrophy (DMD) and *mdx* muscle surface membrane with antibody against synthetic peptide fragment predicted from DMD cDNA. *Proc. Jpn. Acad. Ser. B: Phys. Biol. Sci.* **64**, 37–41.

Summers, P. J. and Parsons, R. (1981). An electron microscopic study of satellite-cells and regeneration in dystrophic mouse muscle. *Neuropathol. Appl. Neurobiol.* **7**, 257–268.

Sunada, Y., Bernier, S. M., Kozak, C. A., Yamada, Y. and Campbell, K. P. (1994). Deficiency of merosin in dystrophic *dy* mice and genetic linkage of laminin M chain gene to *dy* locus. *J. Biol. Chem.* **269**, 13729–13732.

Tanabe, Y., Esaki, K. and Nomura, T. (1986). Skeletal muscle pathology in X chromosome-linked muscular dystrophy (*mdx*) mouse. *Acta Neuropathol.* **69**, 91–95.

Tanaka, H., Ikeya, K. and Ozawa, E. (1990). Difference in the expression pattern of dystrophin on the surface membrane between the skeletal and cardiac muscles of *mdx* carrier mice. *Histochemistry* **93**, 447–452.

Tinsley, J. M. Potter, A. C., Phelps, S. R., Fisher, R., Trickett, J. I. and Davies, K. E. (1996). Amelioration of the dystrophic phenotype of *mdx* mice using a truncated utrophin transgene. *Nature* **384**, 349–353.

Tinsley, J. M., Deconinck, N., Fisher, R. et al. (1998). Expression of full-length utrophin prevents muscular dystrophy in *mdx* mice. *Nat. Med.* **4**, 1441–1444.

Torres, L. F. B. and Duchen, L. W. (1987). The mutant *mdx*: inherited myopathy in the mouse. Morphological studies of nerves, muscles and end-plates. *Brain* **110**, 269–299.

Turner, P. R., Westwood, T., Regan, C. M. and Steinhardt, R. A. (1988). Increased protein degradation results from elevated free calcium levels found in muscle from *mdx* mice. *Nature* **335**, 735–738.

Usuki, F., Ishiura, S. and Sugita, H. (1986). Developmental study of α-glucosidases in Japanese quails with acid maltase deficiency. *Muscle Nerve* **9**, 537–543.

Valentine, B. A. and Cooper, B. J. (1991). Canine X-linked muscular dystrophy: selective involvement of muscles in neonatal dogs. *Neuromusc. Disord.* **1**, 31–38.

Valentine, B. A., Cooper, B. J., Cummings, J. F. and de Lahunta, A. (1986). Progressive muscular dystrophy in a golden retriever dog: light microscope and ultrastructural features at 4 and 8 months. *Acta Neuropathol.* **71**, 301–310.

Valentine, B. A., Cummings, J. F. and Cooper, B. J. (1989a). Development of Duchenne-type cardiomyopathy: morphologic studies in a canine model. *Am. J. Pathol.* **135**, 671–678.

Valentine, B. A., Kornegay, J. N. and Cooper, B. J. (1989b). Clinical electromyographic studies of canine X-linked muscular dystrophy. *Am. J. Vet. Res.* **50**, 2145–2147.

Valentine, B. A., Blue, J. T. and Cooper, B. J. (1989c). The effect of exercise on canine dystrophic muscle. *Ann. Neurol.* **26**, 588.

Valentine, B. A., Cooper, B. J., Cummings, J. F. and de Lahunta, A. (1990). Canine X-linked muscular dystrophy: morphologic lesions. *J. Neurol. Sci.* **97**, 1–23.

Venable, J. H. (1973). *International Symposium on Malignant Hyperthermia*. Springfield: Charles C. Thomas.

Vilquin, J.-T., Brussee, V., Asselin, I., Kinoshita, I., Gingras, M. and Tremblay, J. P. (1998). Evidence of *mdx* mouse skeletal muscle fragility in vivo by eccentric running exercise. *Muscle Nerve* **21**, 567–576.

Watkins, S. C., Hoffman, E. P., Slayter, H. S. and Kunkel, L. M. (1989). Dystrophin distribution in heterozygote *mdx* mice. *Muscle Nerve* **12**, 861–868.

Watkins, W. J. and Watts, D. C. (1984). Biological features of the new A2G-*adr* mouse mutant with abnormal muscle function. *Lab. Animals* **18**, 1–6.

Weller, B., Karpati, G. and Carpenter, S. (1990). Dystrophin-deficient *mdx* muscle fibers are preferentially vulnerable to necrosis induced by experimental lengthening contractions. *J. Neurol. Sci.* **100**, 9–13.

Weller, B., Karpati, G., Lehnert, S., Carpenter, S., Ajdukovic, B. and Holland, P. (1991). Inhibition of myosatellite cell proliferation by gamma irradiation does not prevent the age-related increase of the number of dystrophin-positive fibers in soleus muscles of *mdx* female heterozygote mice. *Am. J. Pathol.* **138**, 1497–1502.

Wells, D. J., Wells, K. E., Walsh, F. S. et al. (1992). Human dystrophin expression corrects the myopathic phenotype in transgenic *mdx* mice. *Hum. Mol. Genet.* **1**, 35–40.

Wentink, G. H., Hartman, W. and Koeman, J. P. (1974). Three cases of myotonia in a family of chows. *Tijdschr. Diergeneeskd.* **99**, 729–731.

Wertz, K. and Fuchtbauer, E. M. (1998). DMD (*mdx-beta geo*): a new allele for the mouse dystrophin gene. *Dev. Dynam.* **212**, 229–241.

West, W. and Murphy, E. (1960). Histopathology of hereditary, progressive muscular dystrophy in inbred strain 129 mice. *Anat. Rec.* **137**, 279–285.

Williams, C. H., Shanklin, M. D., Hedrick, H. B. et al. (1978). The fulminant hyperthermia-stress syndrome: genetic aspects, hemodynamic and metabolic measurements in susceptible and normal pigs. In: *Malignant Hyperthermia*, eds. J. Aldrete and B. A. Britt, pp. 113–40. New York: Grune and Stratton.

Williams, D. A., Head, S. I., Bakker, A. J. and Stephenson, D. G. (1990). Resting calcium concentrations in isolated skeletal muscle fibres of dystrophic mice. *J. Physiol. (Lond.)* **428**, 243–256.

Wilson, L. A., Dux, L., Cooper, B. J., Dubowitz, V. and Sewry, C. A. (1994). Experimental regeneration in canine muscular dystrophy; 2. Expression of myosin heavy chain isoforms. *Neuromusc. Disord.* **4**, 25–37.

Wilton, S. D., Dye, D. E., Blechynden, L. M. and Laing, N. G. (1997). Revertant fibers: a possible genetic therapy for Duchenne muscular dystrophy? *Neuromusc. Disord.* **7**, 329–335.

Winand, N. J., Edwards, M., Pradhan, D., Berian, C. A. and Cooper, B. J. (1994). Deletion of the dystrophin muscle promoter in feline muscular dystrophy. *Neuromusc. Disord.* **4**, 433–445.

Wineinger, M. A., Abresch, R. T., Walsh, S. A. and Carter, G. T. (1998). Effects of ageing and voluntary exercise on the function of dystrophic muscle from *mdx* mice. *Am. J. Phys. Med. Rehab.* **77**, 20–27.

Woo, M., Tanabe, Y., Ishii, H., Nonaka, I., Yokoyama, M. and Esaki, K. (1987). Muscle fibre growth and necrosis in dystrophic muscles: a comparative study between *dy* and *mdx* mice. *J. Neurol. Sci.* **82**, 111–122.

Xu, H., Christmas, P., We, X. R., Wewer, U. M. and Engvall, E. (1994a). Defective muscle basement membrane and lack of M-laminin in the dystrophic *dy/dy* mouse. *Proc. Natl. Acad. Sci. USA* **91**, 5572–5576.

Xu, H., Wu, X-R., Wewe, U. M. and Engvall, E. (1994b). Murine muscular dystrophy caused by a mutation in the laminin α2 (Lama2) gene. *Nat. Genet.* **8**, 297–302.

Yang, L., Lochmuller, H., Luo, J. et al. (1998). Adenovirus-mediated dystrophin minigene transfer improves muscle strength in adult dystrophic (*mdx*) mice. *Gene Ther.* **5**, 369–379.

Zacharias, J. M. and Anderson, J. E. (1991). Muscle regeneration after imposed injury is better in younger than older *mdx* dystrophic mice. *J. Neurol. Sci.* **104**, 190–196.

Zubrzycka-Gaarn, E. E., Bulman, D. E., Karpati, G. et al. (1988). The Duchenne muscular dystrophy gene product is localized in sarcolemma of human skeletal muscle. *Nature* **333**, 466–469.

Part II

Methods of investigation of muscle disease

12

Applied physiology of muscle

Eric L. Logigian and Richard L. Barbano

Introduction

The electrophysiologist is often consulted to help to evaluate patients with suspected muscle disease and symptoms of muscle weakness or fatigability. Less commonly, patients are referred with positive symptoms such as muscle 'cramps', twitching, stiffness or myoglobinuria. The main purposes of the electrophysiological study are to localize the lesion to nerve, muscle or neuromuscular junction; to determine its severity and spatial extent; and to shed light on the aetiology. Occasionally, the reason for referral is to help to select a muscle for biopsy and histological examination.

The first task in the electrophysiological evaluation of patients with possible muscle disease is to perform a directed neuromuscular examination. This is essential to establish one or more hypothetical diagnoses and to identify weak muscles for subsequent electrophysiological testing. The electrophysiological study is then planned around these two points. The major tools in the armamentarium of the electrophysiologist are nerve conduction studies, repetitive nerve stimulation, and concentric needle electromyography (EMG).

Typically, nerve conduction studies are performed first and help to exclude those peripheral neuropathies with prominent motor and little sensory fibre involvement, or with prominent proximal muscle weakness. If disorders of the neuromuscular junction are in the differential diagnosis, repetitive stimulation of nerves innervating symptomatic muscles are performed next to exclude abnormal decrement or increment in compound muscle action potential (CMAP) amplitude. The most difficult part of the electrodiagnostic work-up is needle EMG, which is usually performed last. Most laboratories perform qualitative EMG, in which the electrophysiologist samples several areas within several muscles, searching for particular abnormalities in spontaneous activity, motor unit morphology and recruitment. Occasionally, other techniques such as quantitative EMG or macro-EMG are used to define abnormalities of motor unit morphology more clearly, or single-fibre EMG (SFEMG) to demonstrate a more subtle disorder of neuromuscular transmission.

At the end of the study, the consultant synthesizes the clinical and electrophysiological data to reach a tentative neuromuscular diagnosis, syndrome or category of disease that best explains the symptoms, signs and electrophysiological abnormalities. This chapter will review the electrophysiological testing procedures, the abnormalities encountered and their significance. The electrodiagnostic signatures of the major muscle diseases are then reviewed.

Electrophysiological tests

Motor nerve conduction studies

A percutaneous electrical stimulus of a peripheral nerve depolarizes motor and sensory fibres resulting in a CMAP or a compound sensory nerve action potential (SNAP) that is recorded with surface electrodes over the target muscle or sensory nerve branch. For motor studies, the active electrode is typically placed over the motor point and the reference electrode over the more distal tendon (belly-tendon montage). The electrical stimulus is increased until it is supramaximal, that is, when the increasing CMAP amplitude plateaus. When supramaximal, the stimulus depolarizes all motor fibres innervating the muscle. The resultant CMAP is a population response: an electrical summation of action potentials from all muscle fibres of all motor units innervating the recorded muscle. The nerve is usually stimulated supramaximally at a distal site and at one or more proximal sites along the nerve. This allows

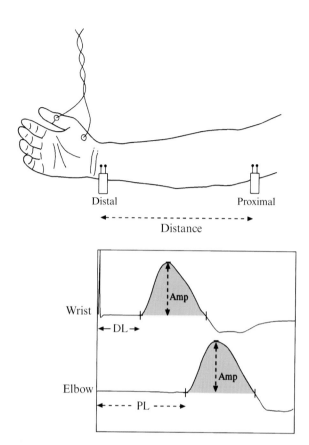

CV = Distance / PL−DL

Fig. 12.1. Compound muscle action potentials (CMAPs) evoked from the abductor pollicis brevis muscle after percutaneous, supramaximal median nerve stimulation at the wrist (distal site) and elbow (proximal site). The measurements of interest are the distal and proximal amplitude (Amp), distal motor latency (DL), proximal motor latency (PL), distance between the two stimulation sites, and calculated forearm conduction velocity (CV, formula shown). Also shown is the area of the negative phase of the CMAPs (shaded).

calculation of several measurements including distal and proximal motor latency, motor conduction velocity, CMAP amplitude and area evoked from distal and proximal sites (Fig. 12.1).

Diseases affecting motor nerve fibres may result in prolongation of distal latency and slowing of velocity, more so in demyelinative neuropathies than in those with predominant axon loss. CMAP amplitude and area may be reduced in axon loss neuropathies when re-innervation or nerve regeneration has not kept up with the denervation of muscle fibres. Amplitude and area may also decline in demyelinative neuropathies when a demyelinative lesion

is interposed between the stimulus and recording electrodes.

Disease of the neuromuscular junction or the muscle fibre itself does not significantly prolong distal latency or slow velocity. However, it may result in reduction of CMAP amplitude in proportion to the number of muscle fibre action potentials that are lost from neuromuscular junction blockade or from destruction of muscle fibres themselves.

Repetitive nerve stimulation

RNS results in a series of CMAPs recorded from a muscle innervated by the stimulated nerve. The measurement of interest is the change in amplitude or area of the successive supramaximal CMAPs compared with the initial baseline CMAP. Decline in amplitude or area is referred to as a decrement whereas an increase is an increment. The rate of stimulation is important; decrements are seen more often with low rates of stimulation, from 1–3 Hz whereas higher rates of 20–50 Hz are generally required to demonstrate increments. The reason for this obtains from an understanding of the kinetics of acetylcholine release at the neuromuscular junction.

After invasion of the nerve terminal by an action potential, the number of quanta of acetylcholine released from the terminal (m) is dependent on two major factors: the number of quanta in the immediately releasable pool (n) and the probability of release (p). An important determinant of p is the calcium concentration in the nerve terminal. The greater the value of n and p, the greater is m (Hubbard et al., 1969; Hubbard, 1973). The greater the value of m, the greater the endplate potential (EPP) and the greater the likelihood that the threshold for a muscle fibre action potential will be reached. In general, slow rates of stimulation of 1–3 Hz are not sufficient to allow calcium to accumulate in the nerve terminal, thus keeping p at stable levels. In contrast, n declines with each impulse since the immediately releasable pool of acetylcholine drops with each successive stimulus and attendant release of quanta. The net result is that m declines with each successive CMAP. The safety factor of neuromuscular transmission is such that, in normal subjects, the resultant drop in the EPP does not fall below the threshold for the muscle fibre action potential and, therefore, the CMAP does not drop in amplitude or area. However, in patients with pre- or postsynaptic disease of the neuromuscular junction, in whom the safety factor is reduced, the EPP for some muscle fibres may fall below the threshold, and a decrement in the CMAP during low-frequency stimulation may be seen. Typically, a reproducible decrement of at least 10% is considered

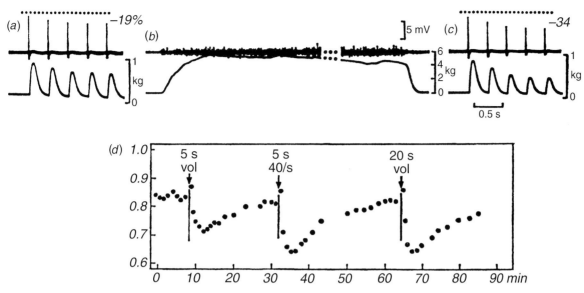

Fig. 12.2. Myasthenic decrement with repetitive nerve stimulation (RNS) of 3 Hz recording from adductor pollicis. Electrical (above) and mechanical twitch (below) responses before (*a*) and 3 minutes after (*c*) 20 seconds of fatiguing exercise. (*b*) The decrement in compound muscle action potential amplitude calculated between the first and the fifth response increases from 19% before exercise to 34% after exercise. (*d*) The decrement is plotted at various time points after different activation regimens: 5 seconds of voluntary (vol) exercise (left), 40 Hz repetitive nerve stimulation for 5 seconds (middle), and 20 seconds of voluntary exercise (right). (From Desmedt (1973) with permission from Karger, Basel.)

significant (Desmedt and Borenstein, 1976a). With each successive stimulus, the CMAP declines in amplitude and area and then plateaus. In myasthenia gravis (MG), the plateau is usually reached by the fourth or fifth potential (Fig. 12.2) (Ozdemir and Young, 1976). Thereafter, the CMAP may occasionally begin to increase, presumably because the immediately releasable pool of acetylcholine quanta is replenished by the intermediate store, and the value of *n* plateaus or begins to increase.

The physiology of high-frequency repetitive nerve stimulation of 20 to 50 Hz is different. The interstimulus interval (20 milliseconds for 50 Hz stimulation, and 50 milliseconds for 20 Hz stimulation) is shorter than the half-life of calcium in the nerve terminal, and therefore the value of *p* successively increases with each stimulus. The value of *n* declines initially but then plateaus, and the net effect is that *m* and the EPP successively increase. In patients with a disorder of neuromuscular transmission, this effect will minimize a decrement, but in patients in whom the initial CMAP amplitude is low, high-frequency RNS, and the resultant increased EPP, may 'unblock' enough junctions that there is a significant rise in CMAP amplitude and area. An alternative technique to high-frequency RNS is to compare a baseline CMAP with one evoked immediately after a maximal voluntary muscle contraction. The rationale here is that motor unit firing

frequencies during maximal voluntary contraction are in the range of high-frequency 20–50 Hz RNS. Since high-frequency RNS is painful, this alternative technique is preferable, but it requires that the patient be cooperative. Infants and cognitively impaired adults still require high-frequency RNS to demonstrate an increment.

Within the first few minutes after muscle activation from either voluntary muscle contraction or high-frequency RNS, several phenomena occur.

1. Pseudofacilitation. Immediately after exercise, CMAPs normally become more synchronized with increase in CMAP amplitude, and they decrease in duration. Amplitude may increase by as much as 40%, but CMAP area is little changed (Tim and Sanders, 1994). Pseudofacilitation is thought to be caused by an activation-induced increase in muscle fibre conduction velocity, rather than by improvement in neuromuscular junction transmission (Desmedt, 1958; Desmedt and Borenstein, 1976a).

2. True facilitation. Immediately after exercise, increments in CMAP amplitude of at least 50% accompanied by increments in CMAP area are most likely causesd by true facilitation rather than pseudofacilitation. Reversal of a baseline pre-exercise decrement may also be seen within the first few seconds after muscle activation and, like true facilitation of the initial CMAP, is probably a

result of an activation-induced increase in the calcium concentration in the terminal axon.

3. Postactivation or post-tetanic exhaustion. At 3 to 5 minutes after muscle activation, the baseline decrement seen with low-frequency RNS prior to muscle activation, may increase dramatically (Fig. 12.2) (Desmedt, 1973; Desmedt and Borenstein, 1976a). The pathophysiology of postactivation exhaustion is unclear, but it may result from receptor desensitization. This phenomenon is useful clinically in that it allows demonstration of a decrement in patients whose baseline RNS is normal or equivocal.

Obtaining meaningful data from RNS studies requires attention to a number of technical and physiological details.

1. The muscle should be immobilized if possible to avoid shifts in the baseline and changes in CMAP morphology that arise from movement of the recording relative to the reference electrodes.

2. The temperature of the recorded muscle should be measured and maintained at or above 34 °C. Lower temperatures may mask decrements or increments since the safety factor of neuromuscular transmission is higher for lower temperatures.

3. For suspected MG, the diagnostic yield of RNS increases when proximal limb or facial muscles are studied, and when RNS is performed after fatiguing exercise (or alternatively after high-frequency tetanic stimulation). One testing strategy includes 3 Hz RNS of ulnar, spinal accessory and facial nerves. If there is no significant decrement at rest, RNS is repeated immediately, and at 1, 2, 3, and 4 minutes after 30–45 seconds of exercise (or for uncooperative patients after tetanic stimulus for several seconds).

4. If the CMAP amplitude is low or borderline, an increment is specifically sought after a 15–30 second maximum voluntary contraction. If the patient cannot cooperate, high-frequency RNS at 20–50 Hz is performed. If there is an increment, the high-frequency train is continued until the increment plateaus.

5. It is important to perform a standard needle EMG examination to help to exclude neuromuscular diseases such as motor neuron disease or myotonic myopathy that do not primarily affect the neuromuscular junction but which may be associated with abnormal decrements on RNS.

In general, the decrements seen in primary disorders of neuromuscular transmission show the greatest decline from the first to the second CMAP, with the decrement maximal by about the fourth or fifth stimulus. This pattern is nonspecific, however. It may be seen occasionally in

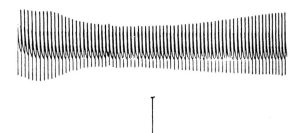

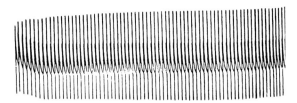

Fig. 12.3. Repetitive nerve stimulation study at 10 Hz recording from abductor digiti minimi in a patient with myotonia congenita demonstrates progressive decrement and then recovery (top trace). A subsequent study after recovery of the compound muscle action potential amplitude failed to reproduce the decrement (bottom trace). (With permission from Aminoff et al. (1977). The declining electrical response of muscle to repetitive nerve stimulation in myotonia. *Neurology* **27**, 812–816.)

patients with severe denervation such as active motor neuron disease (Denys and Norris, 1979; Berstein and Antel, 1981). In such patients, there are a significant number of immature neuromuscular junctions with reduced safety factor as a result of collateral sprouting and re-innervation of previously denervated muscle fibres. A decrement may also be seen in some myotonic myopathies, but the decrement in these disorders is generally progressive or continuous, does not plateau after 4–5 stimuli and may not be reproducible (Fig. 12.3) (Ozdemir and Young, 1976; Aminoff et al., 1977). Although such progressive *decrements* are unusual in primary disorders of the neuromuscular junction, patients with presynaptic disorders of neuromuscular transmission may show progressive *increments* with high-frequency RNS. Such patients may have a slow, continuous rise in CMAP amplitude that may not plateau for 10–100 stimuli (Fig. 12.4).

Needle electromyography

Spontaneous muscle activity and voluntary motor unit potentials (MUPs) can be recorded with various intramuscular, extracellular electrodes. For routine EMG, most electrodiagnostic laboratories use disposable concentric needle electrodes, but some still prefer monopolar

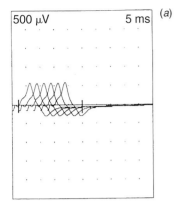

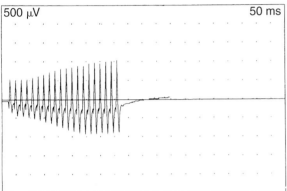

Fig. 12.4. Repetitive nerve stimulation (RNS) of the ulnar nerve recording from abductor digiti minimi (ADM) in an infant with culture-proven botulism. (*a*) Baseline amplitude of the ADM compound muscle action potential (CMAP) is low (580 μV), and there is no significant decrement or increment on 2 Hz RNS. (*b*) Progressive increment of the ADM CMAP after 50 Hz RNS. When the CMAP plateaus, the increment is 94% for amplitude and 61% for area.

needles. The differences between these two electrodes and their relative advantages have been recently reviewed (Joynt, 1998; Trojaborg, 1998). In the authors opinion, concentric needle electrodes have the advantages that there are more available normative reference data, there is less extraneous noise and there is greater consistency from needle to needle. The one disadvantage of concentric electrodes had been their larger diameter and, therefore, greater patient discomfort, but this is less an issue now given the availability of higher gauge, smaller diameter concentric electrodes. The concentric needle recording electrode is a small platinum wire surrounded by insulating material and a cannula of variable diameter. The tip of the electrode is bevelled at an angle of 15°. The wire serves as the recording electrode and the cannula as the reference electrode; each is connected to one of the two inputs to the differential amplifier.

For most primary disorders of muscle, needle EMG is the most sensitive electrodiagnostic procedure. The advantage of needle EMG over muscle biopsy is that numerous muscles can be easily sampled, and it is often necessary to examine a number of muscles to be sure of the findings. Symptomatic muscles should be targeted, which in most cases means the proximal girdle muscles of the upper and lower limbs along with the paraspinal muscles. Some proximal limb muscles are more informative than others. For example, in inflammatory myopathy, the spinati in the arms are more likely to yield abnormalities than are the deltoid or biceps, while in the legs, the iliaci and glutei may be more revealing than the quadriceps (Wilbourn, 1987). The routine needle EMG examination has three basic components: examination of insertional and spontaneous muscle activity, examination of motor unit morphology during submaximal voluntary muscle contraction, and examination of the EMG interference pattern during a maximum voluntary muscle contraction.

Insertional and spontaneous activity

In normal subjects, brief insertions of the needle electrode into relaxed muscle typically produce bursts of electrical activity lasting 50–100 milliseconds. In patients with muscle denervation, insertional bursts increase in duration. More severe denervation gives rise to runs of positive sharp waves and fibrillation potentials that persist with the needle stationary in the muscle (Fig. 12.5). Some forms of spontaneous activity are normal, namely endplate noise or endplate spikes, and the electromyographer must not confuse these normal waveforms with positive waves or fibrillation potentials. Although fibrillation potentials and sharp waves are most commonly observed in axon loss neuropathy, they also are seen in various muscle diseases (Table 12.1). In myopathy, the fibrillations result from segmental necrosis of muscle fibres with a portion of the fibre deprived of its endplate (Desmedt and Borenstein, 1975). By comparison, patients with severe muscle disease and replacement of skeletal muscle with fibrous and adipose tissue will have increased resistance to needle insertion and reduced insertional activity.

Chronic denervation of muscle may lead to groups of denervated muscle fibres in close proximity, each fibre being activated ephaptically by its neighbour in a fairly fixed sequence beginning with the fibre that serves as a pacemaker. This circus movement results in a spontaneous, complex repetitive discharge (Fig. 12.5), which tends to stop and start abruptly and is so regular that it sounds like a monotonous machine over the audio speaker. Because transmission occurs through ephapses rather than neuromuscular junctions, there is very little jitter (see

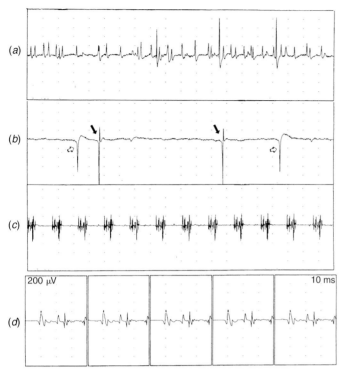

Fig. 12.5. Several kinds of spontaneous electromyographic activity can be seen in a patient with polymyositis. (*a*) Normal spontaneous activity has endplate spikes composed of biphasic, negative (upgoing), brief-duration (1–2 milliseconds) potentials. (*b*) Abnormal spontaneous activity involves brief duration triphasic fibrillation potentials (closed arrows) with an initial positive (downgoing) phase and longer duration, biphasic positive sharp waves (open arrows). (*c,d*) Complex, repetitive discharge (CRD) activity has regular *inter*-burst and *intra*-burst discharge frequencies. Sweep speeds (milliseconds/division); *a,b,d*, 10; *c*, 50. Sensitivity (μV/division); *a,b*, 100; *c,d*, 200.

below) between the various muscle fibres that participate in a complex repetitive discharge (Stålberg and Trontelj, 1979). Again, like fibrillations and positive sharp waves in active denervation, complex repetitive discharges can be seen as a manifestation of chronic denervation resulting from nerve or muscle disease.

Myotonic discharges (Fig. 12.6) are another important form of spontaneous activity. They consist of trains of low-amplitude, brief potentials that wax and wane in frequency and amplitude. They sound like old-fashioned dive bombers over the audio speaker or, in the modern era, like a decelerating and accelerating motorcycle. They are elicited either by needle movement, in which case their morphology is typically that of a positive sharp wave, or by voluntary muscle activation or muscle percussion, when they appear as triphasic or biphasic waves (Streib, 1987a).

These discharges most likely represent repetitive, spontaneous muscle fibre action potentials. They may be present in the absence of clinical myotonia. Detecting the presence of myotonia is a major diagnostic step, since it is far more common in muscle than nerve disease, and its presence narrows the differential diagnosis considerably (Table 12.1). Depending on the disease, some muscles are more likely to show electrical myotonia than others. In acid maltase deficiency or congenital myotonic dystrophy for example, myotonic discharges should be sought in paraspinal muscles.

Motor unit morphology

Just as the CMAP is an electrical summation of motor units, the MUP is an electrical summation of its constituent muscle fibre action potentials. Since the MUP is an extracellular recording made in a volume conductor, the shape of the MUP generally has two or three phases, as does the action potential of each muscle fibre. There is often an initial positive phase generated by approaching action potentials, a negative phase, the onset of which corresponds to action potentials in closest proximity to the recording surface of the electrode, and a terminal positive phase generated by the receding muscle fibre action potentials (Fig. 12.7*a*). The primary measurements of interest are: (i) the duration of the MUP, measured from onset of the intitial positive phase to the terminus of the final phase; (ii) the amplitude, measured from the lowest positive peak to the highest negative peak; and (iii) the total number of phases above and below the baseline (Fig. 12.7*b*). The number of turns, or serrations, in the MUP profile that do not cross the baseline is another quantifiable parameter related to and correlated with the number phases.

MUP duration is determined by muscle fibres within about 2.5 mm of the recording surface of the needle electrode (Nandedkar et al., 1988) and changes with the number and firing synchrony of its constituent muscle fibres within this zone. The number of phases and turns in a MUP is largely dependent on the firing synchrony of its muscle fibre action potentials. Firing synchrony increases with greater homogeneity in terminal axon length and conduction velocity, with neuromuscular junction delay and with muscle fibre size and propagation velocity (Buchthal et al., 1954a). The greater the synchrony, the shorter the MUP duration and the fewer the phases and turns. The MUP amplitude is dependent on a much smaller subset of muscle fibres than those determining MUP duration: those in closest proximity (about 0.5 mm) to the tip of the needle electrode (Rosenfalck and

Table 12.1. Myopathies with prominent abnormal spontaneous activity

Myopathy type	Fibrillation potentials or positive sharp waves	Myotonic discharges
Neuromuscular junction	Botulism	
Periodic paralysis		Paramyotonia congenita, hyperkalaemic periodic paralysis
Myotonic myopathy Nondystrophic		Myotonia congenita (dominant), myotonia congenita (recessive), paramyotonia congenita, hyperkalaemic periodic paralysis
Dystrophic		Myotonic dystrophy, proximal myotonic myopathy
Muscular dystrophy (nonmyotonic)	Duchenne muscular dystrophy, Becker muscular dystrophy	
Congenital	Centronuclear (myotubular) myopathy, Nemaline (rod) myopathy	Centronuclear (myotubular) myopathy[a]
Metabolic myopathy Glycogen	Acid maltase deficiency, debrancher deficiency, carnitine deficiency	Acid maltase deficiency[a], debrancher deficiency[a]
Endocrine	Hypothyroidism, high-dose corticosteroids	Hypothyroidism[a]
Toxic myopathy	Colchicine, D-penicillamine, alcohol, neuromuscular-blocking agents, zidovudine, Chloroquine	Colchicine[a], D-penicillamine[a] Cholesterol-lowering agents[a], Chloroquine[a]
Inflammatory myopathy	Polymyositis, dermatomyositis, inclusion body myopathy, sarcoidosis, trichinosis, HIV-associated myopathy	Polymyositis[a], dermatomyositis[a]

Notes:
[a] Electrical without clinical myotonia.
Source: Adapted from Wilbourn (1987) and Daube (1994).

Rosenfalck, 1975; Nandedkar et al., 1988). The amplitude and rise time of the negative phase of the MUP is, therefore, far more sensitive to slight movements of the electrode than is duration (Fig. 12.7*a*). The main difficulty in evaluating MUP morphology in a patient with neuromuscular symptoms is that the range of normal values is wide. For example, in the normal biceps brachii, MUP duration varies from about 3 to 17 milliseconds and amplitude from about 50 to 1000 μV (Buchthal et al., 1954a). Moreover, the ranges of these parameters are slightly different for different muscles, and all – MUP duration, amplitude and phases – slowly increase with age (Buchthal et al., 1954b).

It should be emphasized that there is no pathognomonic MUP morphological signature of muscle disease. In general, patients with acute or subacute myopathy show reduction in MUP duration (Fig. 12.8) and an increase in MUP phases and turns. Decrease in MUP amplitude is a later finding. MUP duration declines mainly because the disease process reduces the total number of muscle fibre action potentials. In contrast, the number of MUP phases and turns increases because the remaining muscle fibres fire less synchronously. (Muscle fibre conduction velocity, being proportional to fibre size, is more variable in muscle disease showing variation in fibre size. Increased variation in muscle fibre conduction velocity decreases fibre firing synchrony and thus increases the number of phases and turns.) It also follows that these abnormalities are not specific for diseases that target the muscle fibre or neuromuscular junction but will also be seen in those that affect the distal axon terminals (Engel, 1973). The other condition associated with brief-duration, low-amplitude MUPs is severe axon-loss neuropathy early in the recovery stage when nerve regeneration and muscle re-innervation has

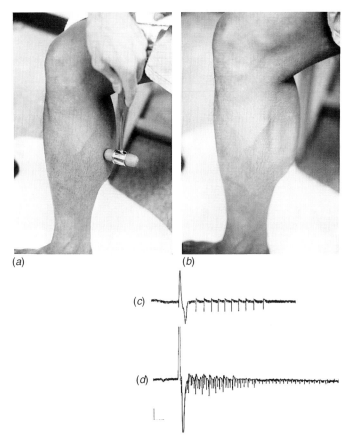

(a)   (b)

(c)

(d)

Fig. 12.6. Percussion myotonia in a patient with dominantly inherited myotonia congenita. Percussion of the hypertrophied medial gastrocnemius muscle (*a*) results in a large depression in the muscle. (*b*) Waning myotonic discharges are shown recorded from this muscle. A light tap produces a repetitive single muscle fibre discharge (*c*); a stronger tap results in a longer, repetitive discharge of several muscle fibres (*d*).

proceeded to a point where motor units consist of only a few muscle fibres (Weddell et al., 1944).

In more indolent myopathy, these MUP abnormalities may become less clear-cut, with an increasing number of MUPs with prolonged duration and even high amplitude. The explanation for these findings is that muscle disease results in split muscle fibres, denervated fibres, or regenerated fibres, which may over time become re-innervated by other motor units. The resultant remodelled motor units have decreased fibre firing synchrony, perhaps an increased complement of muscle fibres, and the MUPs are, therefore, of higher amplitude and longer duration than those of age-matched controls (Uncini et al., 1990). These morphological changes are not specific for chronic muscle disease and are also typical of chronic, partial motor axon or neuron loss, in which re-innervation of denervated

muscle fibres by remaining axons compensates for loss of other axons or neurons (Fig. 12.8*b*). In such patients, needle EMG distinguishes chronic myopathy from neuropathy either by the presence of two populations of MUPs, those with short and those with long duration, in the same muscle, or by the presence of some muscles with MUPs that are all clearly brief in duration.

Motor unit recruitment

The first concentric needle EMG studies of human skeletal muscle showed that muscle force increases as a result of increasing motor unit firing frequency and by recruitment of new motor units (Adrian and Bronk, 1929). In a slowly increasing ramp contraction of muscle, motor units are generally recruited according to the size principle (Henneman, 1957) with the smaller followed by the larger. When first recruited, motor units fire pseudo-regularly at about 4–6 Hz but then steadily increase firing rates to much higher values. At maximum voluntary force, firing frequencies vary with the muscle; they are approximately 30 Hz for the biceps brachii and adductor pollicis in the upper extremity and 11 Hz for the soleus in the lower extremity (Bellemare et al., 1983). The MUP spike density and amplitude of the interference pattern increase as force increases; as a result the pattern is fully developed at maximum force.

In myopathy, a so-called *early recruitment* pattern may be observed, in which the interference pattern is more full than would be expected for the level of force generated (Fig. 12.9) (Daube, 1991). The explanation offered for this phenomenon is that the force generated per motor unit is reduced in myopathy and, therefore, a greater number of motor unit discharges is required to maintain a given target force. Again, this finding is nonspecific in that it is also seen with disorders of the distal terminal axon or the neuromuscular junction. By contrast, in severe muscle disease, motor unit recruitment may be reduced; that is, the interference pattern shows a reduced number of rapidly firing motor units for the level of force generated. This *reduced recruitment* pattern is typical for patients with motor neuron or axon loss, but it can also be seen with severe muscle disease in which all constituent muscle fibres from a significant proportion of the motor unit population are destroyed, thus effectively reducing the number of motor units. In this situation, the nervous system cannot compensate for muscle weakness by early recruitment of motor units, so it compensates to some degree by an increasing firing frequency of the few remaining units. Inevitably though, throughout the range of force generated by the muscle, the motor unit spike interference pattern is less dense or full than normal.

Single-fibre electromyography

Using a needle with a small recording surface and a high-frequency, high-pass filter setting, SFEMG (Stålberg and Trontelj, 1979, 1994, Sanders and Stålberg, 1996) selectively records muscle fibre action potentials from a single motor unit. Only a small portion of the motor unit is observed with this technique, since the SFEMG electrode records electrical activity within about $300\,\mu M$ of the recording surface. The two parameters of interest are the determination of jitter, a measure of the safety factor of neuromuscular junction transmission, and of fibre density, a measurement of the spatial organization of the muscle fibres within the motor unit.

Jitter can be measured during voluntary activation of a muscle or during nerve stimulation. In the voluntary condition, the SFEMG needle electrode is positioned such that it optimally records from two or more fibres from the same motor unit. Using one fibre as the stable triggering potential, the variation in the time interval between the triggering potential and the second muscle fibre potential is measured over at least 50 motor unit discharges. The variation in intervals is a measure of jitter and is expressed statistically as the mean consecutive difference or mean sorted difference. This process is then repeated for a total of 20 separate muscle fibre pairs and a mean and range for these difference parameters are calculated. The results are interpreted using age-dependent normal values, which are available for a number of limb and cranial muscles (Gilchrist, 1992).

Disease of the neuromuscular junction is associated with increased jitter. When severe enough to produce muscle weakness, the neuromuscular junction disorder is associated with both increased jitter and blocking of the second potential (Fig. 12.10). The physiological explanation for increased jitter and blocking is as follows. The rate of rise of the muscle fibre EPP is proportional to its amplitude. The more severe the disorder of neuromuscular transmission, the more variable is the EPP amplitude from one motor unit discharge to the next. The more variable is the rate of rise of the EPP, the more variable is the synaptic delay, and the larger the jitter. In more severe disease, the EPP is not only quite variable but also intermittently subthreshold for generation of a muscle fibre action potential, and blocking is seen on SFEMG. Increased jitter and blocking are characteristic of neuromuscular junction disease, but they can also be seen in patients with neuropathy or motor neuronopathy, particularly during the early stages of re-innervation, and to a lesser extent with primary disorders of muscle. One interesting feature of myopathy is the presence of occasional fibre pairs with very low jitter;

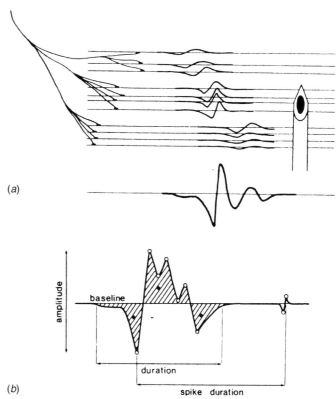

(a)

(b)

Fig. 12.7. The generation of a motor endplate potential (MUP) recorded with a concentric needle electrode. (*a*) The needle is placed in the fibres. Distant fibres contribute less to the spiky part. The initial slow wave is already recorded when the arriving depolarization is still far away, and the terminal slow wave still lasts for a while after the impulse has passed. At those two stages, the distance of the impulse to the recording electrode is similar for all fibres and, therefore, all of them contribute to a similar degree to the slow components. The spiky part, however, is generated when the depolarization is closest to the electrode tip, and now the distance and the contribution is very different for the adjacent and the remote fibres. (*b*) Definition of MUP parameters: ●, phase, ○, turn. The late component is called a satellite potential since it occurs outside of the limits for the duration (slow part). (Reprinted from Stålberg and Trontelj in: Vinken, P. et al. (eds.) *Handbook of Clinical Neurology*, copyright (1992), Vol. 62, pp. 49–84, with permission from Elsevier Science.)

this results from muscle fibre splitting, when both fragments are innervated by the same endplate.

Fibre density is the mean number of muscle fibre potentials seen by the SFEMG electrode on 20 separate insertions, each optimally positioned to record the first visible muscle fibre action potential. Fibre density increases with age and varies among muscles, but it is normally between 1.5 and 2.5 (Bromberg and Scott, 1994). Fibre density is

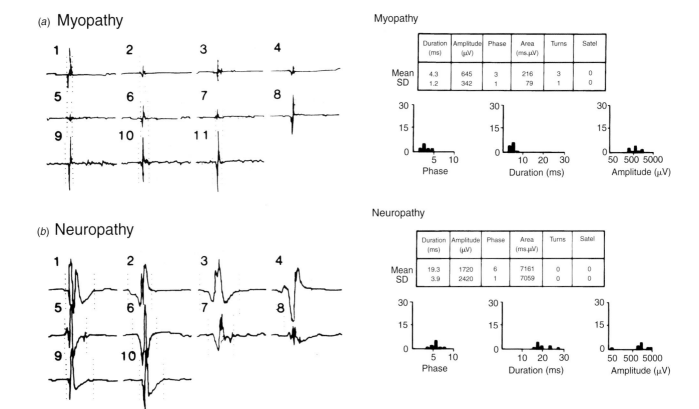

Fig. 12.8. Motor unit potentials (MUPs) from the vastus medialis in a patient with polymyositis (*a*) and in a patient with diabetic neuropathy (*b*). MUP duration is far briefer and on average lower in amplitude in the patient with myopathy than in the patient with neuropathy.

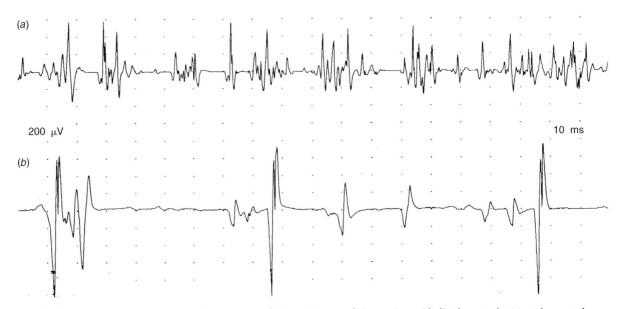

Fig. 12.9. Motor unit recruitment pattern in the extensor indicis proprius muscle in a patient with distal myopathy (*a*), and a normal subject (*b*). Each elevates the index finger against a 200 g weight. The recruitment is early in the patient with myopathy, for whom the interference pattern is nearly filled with brief duration motor units potentials compared with only a few units in the normal subject.

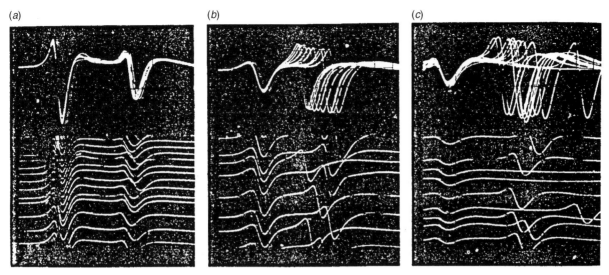

Fig. 12.10. Single fibre electromyographic study in a patient with myasthenia gravis. Muscle fibre pair with normal jitter (*a*), increased jitter (*b*) and increased jitter with blocking (*c*) in a patient with myasthenia gravis. (Reprinted from Stålberg and Trontelj (1976) with permission.)

particularly increased in neuropathy as a result of collateral sprouting of nerve fibres and re-innervation of denervated muscle fibres. Fibre density is increased in most myopathies as well, but usually to a lesser extent, and is caused by several mechanisms including muscle fibre splitting (Sanders and Stålberg, 1996).

Macro-electromyography

Macro-EMG uses a modified SFEMG electrode in which the recording surface is the distal 15 mm of the needle electrode cannula. In contrast to the concentric or monopolar EMG needle electrode, the large recording surface picks up electrical activity from all muscle fibres from a single motor unit that are distributed over a 5–15 mm region of muscle. This technique averages successive motor unit discharges using one of its fibres as a trigger, thereby recording the electrical activity of only the one motor unit with muscle fibres firing in a roughly time-locked fashion to the triggering potential. In general, macro-EMG MUP amplitude and area correlate with motor unit muscle fibre number (Stålberg, 1983), being low in myopathy because of muscle fibre drop out and high in neuropathy or neuronopathy because of re-innervation (Fig. 12.11). These macro-EMG findings suggest that the increased fibre density seen in neuropathy and myopathy have different explanations. In neuropathy, the process of re-innervation increases the total number of muscle fibres in the remaining motor units, whereas in myopathy, the total number of intact fibres per motor unit

is the same or less, but in places the fibres are split or grouped together (Stålberg, 1991).

Quantitative electromyography

Routine electromyography includes a qualitative assessment of spontaneous activity, motor unit morphology and the interference pattern. There are also quantitative methods that may be useful when the qualitative studies are not clearly diagnostic, or when serial studies are contemplated. Motor unit morphology can be quantified by analysing duration, amplitude, phases, turns, area, or area/amplitude ratio for 20 or more randomly selected simple motor units (e.g. less than five phases) from a given muscle and comparing the results with age-matched normative data. This kind of analysis can be performed manually (Rosenfalck and Rosenfalck, 1975), using spike-triggered averaging techniques (Stewart et al., 1989) or using various semi-automated computerized techniques (Dorfman et al., 1989; Nandedkar et al., 1995). The most sensitive parameters for myopathy seem to be MUP duration and the MUP area/amplitude ratio. Both parameters measure the thinness of the motor unit, which correlates with the loss of muscle fibre action potentials seen in many myopathies.

There are also computerized methods to analyse quantitatively the EMG interference pattern from a given muscle using age- and sex-matched normative data (Stålberg, 1983; Gilchrist et al., 1988). One parameter of interest is the turns/amplitude ratio, which can be measured at a single, standardized level of muscle force (Rose

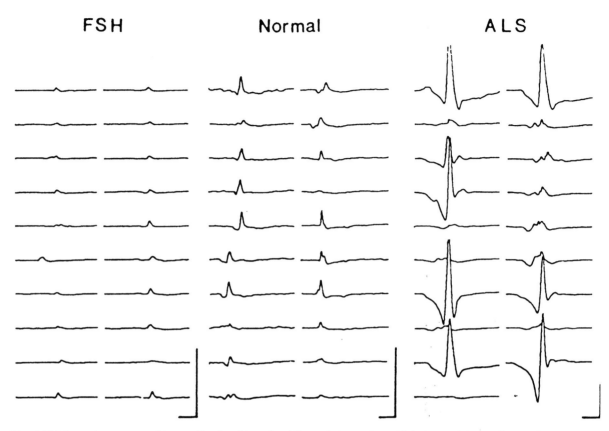

Fig. 12.11. Macro-electromyographic recording from biceps brachii muscle in a patient with facioscapulohumeral (FSH) dystrophy, in a normal subject, and in a patient with amyotrophic lateral sclerosis (ALS). Amplitude and area are reduced in the patient with myopathy, and increased in the patient with ALS. (Calibration 1 mV; 5 milliseconds.) (Reprinted from Stålberg and Trontelj, in: Vinken, P. et al. (eds.) *Handbook of Clinical Neurology*, copyight (1992), Vol. 62, pp. 49–84, with permission from Elsevier Science.)

and Willison, 1967) or over the range of forces generated by the muscle (Stålberg, 1983; Gilchrist et al., 1988). Patients with muscle disease have an elevated turns/amplitude ratio, while those with neuropathy have a reduced ratio (Stålberg, 1983; Gilchrist et al., 1988). Some studies have shown that quantitative analysis of the interference pattern is more sensitive for muscle disease than is quantitative analysis of motor unit morphology (Barkhaus et al., 1990).

There are clearly, on the one hand, some patients with evidence of myopathy on one or more of the quantitative techniques for whom a routine qualitative EMG study is normal. On the other hand, the overall sensitivity of the quantitative studies is not always higher than routine EMG (Gilchrist et al., 1988; Stewart et al., 1989). Whether quantitative techniques significantly increase the diagnostic sensitivity or specificity for myopathy is not yet clear. In any case, using histology as a gold standard, the diagnostic sensitivity of careful EMG in muscle disease in general is in the range

80–90% (Hausmanowa–Petrucewicz and Jedrezejowska, 1971; Buchthal and Kamieniecka, 1982).

Exercise testing: short and long exercise tests

The effect of exercise on neuromuscular junction physiology and its importance in the diagnosis of neuromuscular transmission defects has been described above. Exercise also produces characteristic changes in CMAP amplitude in patients with myotonic myopathy and periodic paralysis (McManis et al., 1986; Streib, 1987a). In patients with myotonic dystrophy and myotonia congenita (particularly the recessive form), brief exercise of 5–10 seconds will produce an immediate fall in the amplitude of the CMAP followed by prompt recovery within about 2 minutes. If the test is repeated, the fall in CMAP amplitude is reproducible in myotonia congenita but not in myotonic dystrophy. In one small series (Sander et al., 1997), the fall in postexercise CMAP amplitude and area was seen in myotonic

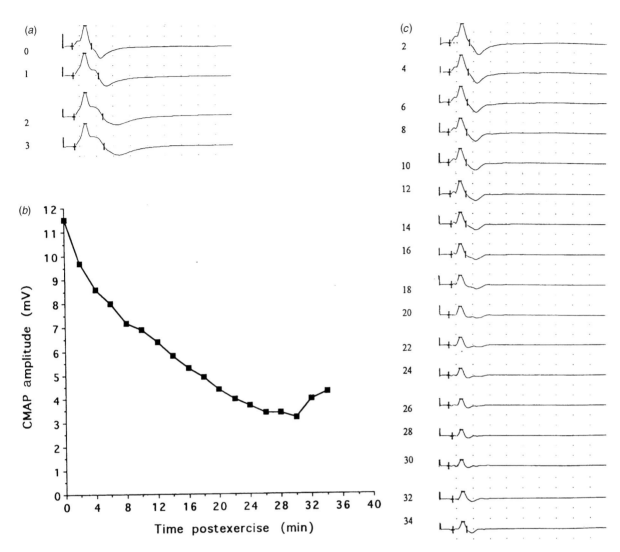

Fig. 12.12. Long exercise test in a patient with hypokalaemic periodic paralysis. (*a*) Compound motor action potentials (CMAPs) evoked (5 mV/division) from the abductor digiti minimi during brief pauses (1 minute) in a 3-minute exercise show a transient increase in amplitude (17%) and area (81%). (*b,c*) After exercise, there is gradual 70% decrease in CMAP amplitude (measured every 2 minutes), with the nadir at 30 minutes.

dystrophy, but not in proximal myotonic myopathy (PROMM), but whether these two disorders can be distinguished by exercise testing awaits confirmation.

A long exercise test of 2–5 minutes, with periodic breaks to prevent muscle ischaemia, is useful in the diagnosis of patients with periodic paralysis, in whom the short exercise test is usually negative. After an initial increment in amplitude, patients with acquired or inherited periodic paralysis show a progressive long-lasting fall in CMAP amplitude and area of about 50% at 20–40 minutes after exercise (Fig. 12.12). The CMAP slowly recovers over about 1 hour. This phenomenon can also be seen in some

patients with paramyotonia congenita, but typically, the postexercise decline in CMAP amplitude in patients with this disorder is more modest and reaches the nadir more quickly after completion of the exercise test (McManis et al., 1986).

Disorders of neuromuscular transmission

Disorders of neuromuscular transmission fall into two basic categories, those affecting postsynaptic function, such as MG, and those that are presynaptic, such as

Table 12.2. Disorders of neuromuscular transmission

Function affected	Disorder
Presynaptic	Lambert–Eaton myasthenic syndrome (LEMS)
	Botulism
	Familial infantile myasthenia
	Toxins/drugs (e.g. aminoglycosides)
Postsynaptic disease	Acetylcholine receptor (AChR) defect: myasthenia gravis, congenital AChR deficiency, toxins/drugs (e.g. curare, vecuronium)
	Acetylcholinesterase (AChE) defect: congenital endplate AChE deficiency, toxins (organophosphates)
	Slow-channel myasthenic syndrome

Lambert–Eaton myasthenic syndrome (LEMS) (Table 12.2). In general, both pre- and postsynaptic disorders demonstrate a decrement on low-frequency RNS, whereas presynaptic disorders more often show an increment on high-frequency RNS (or after maximum voluntary muscle contraction) than do postsynaptic disorders.

SFEMG is more sensitive than RNS; as a result, in milder disease of any type, RNS studies may be normal while SFEMG will be abnormal. In MG, the SFEMG abnormalities of jitter and blocking often increase with moderate increases in motor unit firing rate, while in presynaptic disorders such as LEMS, they tend to decrease (Trontelj and Stålberg, 1991).

Congenital myasthenia

The congenital myasthenic disorders are a group of rare disorders that usually present at birth or in infancy, and less commonly later in life (Engel, 1990; Harper, 1996a). Of the four major syndromes, two (classic slow-channel syndrome and congenital acetylcholinesterase deficiency) are associated with repetitive CMAPs after single-nerve stimuli (Fig. 12.13). The repetitive discharges are an important diagnostic clue, but the electromyographer must recognize that the subsequent discharges are of lower amplitude than the main response and are present only with slow (0.1–0.2 Hz) rates of stimuli. At faster rates of stimulation, the repetitive discharges decline in amplitude faster than does the main CMAP, and therefore these may go unnoticed. Both classic slow channel syndrome, and congenital acetylcholinesterase deficiency have a decrement on slow RNS.

The other two major syndromes (familial infantile myasthenia and congenital acetylcholine receptor deficiency) are not associated with repetitive discharges, but they do show significant decrements on low (2–3 Hz) rates of RNS of weak muscles at baseline, or after fatiguing exercise. Since both conditions respond somewhat to acetylcholinesterase inhibitors, adult patients can be confused with those with seronegative, autoimmune MG unless the history is probed for neuromuscular symptoms in infancy.

In all of the congenital myasthenic disorders, needle EMG often shows brief-duration, low-amplitude, polyphasic MUPs that may vary in amplitude from discharge to discharge. Insertional activity is usually normal. The few patients who have been studied with SFEMG have shown increased jitter and blocking.

Myasthenia gravis

The resting CMAP amplitude and area is in the normal range in the majority of patients with MG, and as a result there is little or no postactivation facilitation of the CMAP in most patients after rapid RNS or directly after maximum voluntary contraction. In contrast, low-frequency RNS often shows a significant decrement in CMAP amplitude and area.

The sensitivity of RNS in MG depends on disease severity, on the number of muscles tested and on various technical aspects of test performance (e.g. muscle temperature). Patients with ocular myasthenia are less likely than patients with generalized myasthenia to show a decrement (Ozdemir and Young, 1976; Sanders and Stålberg, 1996). In the largest series to date of 550 untreated patients with MG (Sanders and Stålberg, 1996) who underwent RNS of both a distal hand and a proximal shoulder muscle, 76% of patients with generalized MG and 48% of patients with ocular myasthenia had a significant decrement on RNS.

There are occasional patients with severe MG whose resting CMAP amplitude is low or in the low normal range. These patients often demonstrate significant facilitation of CMAP amplitude and area after a maximum voluntary contraction or rapid RNS (Mayer and Williams, 1974), and they will usually also have an abnormal decrement to low-frequency RNS. Because this is the pattern of RNS abnormalities seen in presynaptic disorders such as LEMS, patients with MG and this electrophysiological profile can be difficult to distinguish on electrodiagnostic grounds alone (Tim and Sanders, 1994). Clinical information and the acetylcholine receptor antibody titre may ultimately be required to reach a final diagnosis of MG.

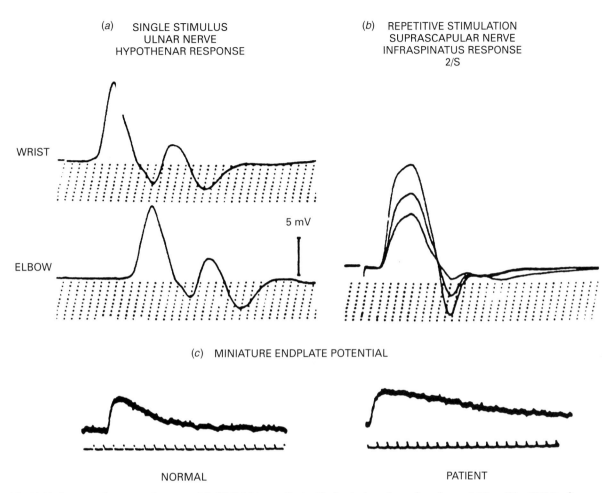

(a) SINGLE STIMULUS
ULNAR NERVE
HYPOTHENAR RESPONSE

(b) REPETITIVE STIMULATION
SUPRASCAPULAR NERVE
INFRASPINATUS RESPONSE
2/S

WRIST

ELBOW

5 mV

(c) MINIATURE ENDPLATE POTENTIAL

NORMAL

PATIENT

Fig. 12.13. Compound motor action potentials (CMAPs) in a patient with classic slow-channel syndrome. (a) Repetitive CMAPs after single nerve stimulation evoked by single stimulus applied to the ulnar nerve in a patient with classic slow channel syndrome. The two responses are separated by an interval of 8 milliseconds; the second response is smaller than the first. (b) Decremental response of infraspinatus CMAP during 2 Hz repetitive stimulation of the suprascapular nerve. (c) The duration and half-decay time of the miniature endplate potential are longer in the patient than in the normal control subject. (With permission from Engel et al. (1982). A newly recognized congenital myasthenic syndrome attributed to a prolonged open time of the acetylcholine-induced ion channel. *Ann. Neurol.* **11**, 553–569.)

The diagnostic yield of SFEMG is much higher than RNS, although it is a more labour intensive and more painful test for most patients. Increased jitter or blocking was found in the extensor digitorum communis muscle in 89% of patients with generalized MG, and 60% of patients with ocular MG (Sanders and Stålberg, 1996). If several muscles are tested, including the frontalis, the yield of SFEMG rises to 99% in generalized and 97% in ocular MG. The presence of blocking correlates with muscle weakness and is found in patients with more severe disease. For example, among 788 patients with MG who underwent SFEMG of the extensor digitorum communis, only 5% of patients with ocular MG (e.g. mild disease) showed block-

ing versus 28% of patients with generalized MG (Sanders and Stålberg, 1996).

In patients with more severe MG, and muscle weakness on examination, needle EMG typically discloses brief-duration, low-amplitude MUPs (Oosterhuis et al., 1972). In addition, variation in MUP amplitude from motor unit discharge to discharge may be observed (Fig. 12.14) (Lambert, 1966). This variation corresponds to intermittent blocking of neuromuscular transmission at the endplates of the muscle fibres constituting the motor unit. On occasion, fibrillation potentials may even be present and are more likely to be seen in paraspinal and bulbar muscles, particularly in the elderly (Barbieri et al., 1982).

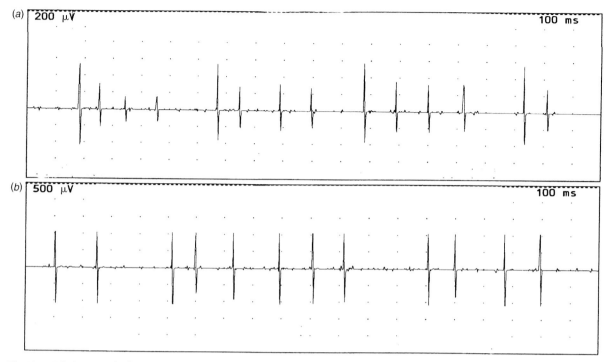

Fig. 12.14. Discharge to discharge variation in motor unit potential amplitude in a patient with severe generalized myasthenia gravis (*a*) and a normal subject (*b*) in whom there is minimal variation.

Lambert–Eaton myasthenic syndrome

The typical electrophysiological findings in LEMS were described by Lambert and colleagues (Lambert et al., 1956, 1961), and in a large series of 50 patients (O'Neill et al., 1988). In nearly all patients, the CMAP amplitude evoked from resting muscle is below the normal range; only 2 of 50 patients (4%) had normal CMAP amplitudes evoked from the abductor digiti minimi. Moreover, the resting CMAP is of low amplitude in virtually all muscles tested in a given patient, and the resting CMAP amplitude declines further with disease duration.

After 10–15 seconds of voluntary muscle contraction, or with rapid RNS at rates above 10 Hz, there is marked facilitation of CMAP amplitude and area (Fig. 12.15) (Lambert et al., 1956, 1961; O'Neill et al., 1988; Tim and Sanders, 1994). In the large series of 50 patients, a significant increment was found in 48 (96%). The mean increment in CMAP amplitude was 890%. RNS at 20 Hz produces a mean increment similar to that after voluntary contraction (O'Neill et al., 1988; Tim and Sanders, 1994) and may occasionally show an increment in the few patients who do not have one after voluntary activation (O'Neill et al., 1988). When rapid RNS is required for the diagnosis of LEMS, it is important to realize that the CMAP amplitude does not usually plateau by the end of a typical train of 5–10 stimuli, and

therefore longer trains may be needed. Low-frequency RNS at 2–3 Hz typically results in a significant decrement (Fig. 12.15). When the resting CMAP is very low, the decrement may not be measurable. In 47 patients with LEMS for whom decrement was measurable, the mean value was 27% (O'Neill et al., 1988).

Routine needle EMG examination shows brief duration, polyphasic MUPs in 90% of LEMS patients. There is often a gradual increase in MUP amplitude with sustained activation of muscle. On SFEMG, virtually all patients with LEMS have increased jitter and blocking (O'Neill et al., 1988), which tend to improve at higher MUP discharge rates (Trontelj and Stålberg, 1991). Fibrillations are not found in LEMS, an electrophysiological feature that may help to distinguish it from botulism (see below).

Botulism

Botulism is caused by a neurotoxin made by the anaerobic bacteria *Clostridium botulinum*. The toxin is the most potent known and results in presynaptic blockade of the neuromuscular junction. Botulism occurs in three major forms: infantile botulism resulting from colonization of the gut by *C. botulinum*, food-borne botulism from ingestion of the toxin in inadequately prepared food and wound botulism from wound contamination with *C. botulinum.* Electrophysiological studies often provide the earliest diagnostic clue to the disease.

A number of studies have helped to define the major electrophysiological features of botulism (Cherington, 1974, 1982; Guttmann and Pratt, 1976; Oh, 1977; Pickett et al., 1976; Cornblath et al., 1983). In the resting state, CMAPs evoked from weak muscles are of low amplitude. Facilitation after maximum voluntary contraction or after rapid RNS is seen less frequently in adults (about 60% of patients) than in infants (about 90% of patients); when present, the facilitation seen is generally more modest (often under 100%) (Fig. 12.4) than in LEMS (rarely less than 100%). To demonstrate true facilitation with rapid RNS at 20–50 Hz, long trains of stimuli over 10–30 seconds may be required, since CMAP amplitude does not usually plateau by the end of a short train of stimuli. While this is also the case with LEMS, it is of more importance in botulism, in which the presence of facilitation could be missed entirely with short trains of stimuli. The absence of post-activation facilitation in some patients with botulism despite good technique is likely related to the completeness of neuromuscular blockade or to the destruction of axon terminals in a large percentage of affected endplates. Although the degree of postactivation facilitation in botulism is less than in LEMS, it is also more long lasting (typically in excess of 5 minutes after activation) than that seen in LEMS (typically less than 1 minute) (Fig. 12.15). A decrement in resting CMAP amplitude with low-frequency RNS is also seen in botulism, but it too is less prominent than in LEMS (compare Figs. 12.4 and 12.15).

Needle EMG shows brief-duration, polyphasic MUPs in weak muscles. Active denervation is commonly seen in affected muscles within days to 2 weeks, appearing somewhat earlier in infantile than in adult botulism. SFEMG (Schiller and Stålberg, 1978) shows that jitter and blocking improve with higher discharge frequencies and that fibre density is reduced.

Drug- and toxin-induced disorders of neuromuscular transmission

There are a vast number of drugs and toxins that affect neuromuscular transmission (Swift, 1981; Rivner and Swift, 1993). Only the more common examples of this kind of myasthenia will be mentioned. Aminoglycoside antibiotics and magnesium intoxication act at the presynaptic site by interfering with the intracellular flow of calcium at the axon terminal, and therefore with release of acetylcholine. A presynaptic mechanism affecting acetylcholine release is also proposed in tick paralysis, caused by envenomation

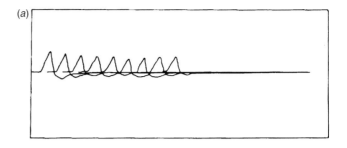

(a)

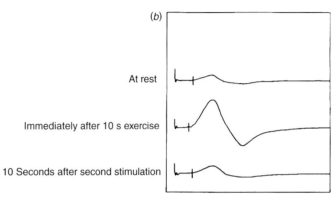

(b)

At rest

Immediately after 10 s exercise

10 Seconds after second stimulation

Fig. 12.15. Tests of the ulnar muscle in a patient with Lambert–Eaton myasthenic syndrome. (*a*) Decrement test shows a compound motor action potential (CMAP) of very low amplitude (1.2 mV). Repetitive nerve stimulation at 2 Hz results in a 27% decrement in CMAP amplitude. (*b*) Baseline CMAP is of very low amplitude (top trace); there is a 79-fold increment in CMAP amplitude within a few seconds of voluntary activation (middle trace). Ten seconds later, the CMAP has returned to the baseline low amplitude level (bottom trace).

by a feeding tick of several species. There are only a few electrophysiological studies in such patients. In all of these conditions, resting CMAP amplitude evoked from weak muscles is below the normal range. In magnesium intoxication, there is a decrement at low rates of stimulation, and a marked increment at high-frequency RNS (Swift, 1979). In human aminoglycoside toxicity (McQuillen et al., 1968), low CMAP amplitudes in resting muscle may not decrement at low-frequency RNS or increment at high-frequency RNS. The same is true for tick paralysis (Swift and Ignacio, 1975), although one study did show a decrement with high-frequency RNS (Morris, 1977).

A number of other drugs and toxins affect the neuromuscular junction postsynaptically, affecting the acetylcholine receptor itself. Polymyxin (polymixin) antibiotics, curare and many of the common anaesthetic agents (e.g. vecuronium and pancuronium) are in this category. When neuromuscular blockade by these agents is incomplete, single-nerve stimuli often evoke low-amplitude CMAPs in affected muscles at rest. RNS may result in further decrement in amplitude (McQuillen et al., 1968; McQuillen and Engbaek, 1975; Rivner and Swift, 1993).

Some drugs and chemicals owe their toxicity to interference with acetylcholinesterase. Organophosphate toxicity is an example. Its electrophysiological hallmark is the presence of repetitive CMAPs evoked by single-nerve stimulus in addition to a decrement on both high- and low-frequency RNS (Besser et al., 1989, 1990). These abnormalities are similar to those seen in other disorders characterized by excess or prolonged action of acetylcholine at the neuromuscular junction, such as two forms of congenital myasthenia: congenital endplate acetylcholinesterase deficiency and classic slow-channel syndrome (see above).

Periodic paralyses

Several diseases cause periodic failure in propagation of the muscle fibre action potentials from the region of the endplate to the remainder of the muscle fibre. The defect is at the level of the muscle membrane and results in intermittent weakness of skeletal muscle. The major causes of this syndrome are primary and secondary hypokalaemic periodic paralysis (hypoKPP), primary hyperkalaemic periodic paralysis (hyperKPP), and normokalaemic periodic paralysis. All forms of periodic paralysis have several electrophysiological features in common. During attacks of paralysis, there is reduction in CMAP amplitudes in approximate proportion to the degree of muscle weakness (Engel et al., 1965; Engel and Lambert, 1969; Gordon et al., 1970; Campa and Anders, 1974); in plegic muscles, CMAPs are unevokable. Similarly, needle EMG shows reduction in electrical activity with decreased insertional activity, decrease in MUP duration and amplitude and increase in the number of phases. As muscle weakness progresses, there is reduction in the number of recruitable motor units (Pozkanzer and Kerr, 1961; Brooks, 1969; Bradley et al., 1990).

Between attacks, CMAP amplitudes evoked from rested muscles are normal. However, the long exercise test is positive in about 70% of patients with primary or secondary periodic paralysis (McManis et al., 1986). After at least 2 minutes of intermittent strong voluntary contraction, the CMAP amplitude first increases by a mean of 37% and then slowly declines by a mean of 59%, reaching the nadir after a mean of 39 minutes. Control subjects have a maximum decrease in CMAP amplitude of 30%; therefore, CMAP

decrements of 40% or more are considered abnormal. Consequently, a positive long exercise test strongly supports the diagnosis of periodic paralysis, but a negative test does not exclude it. Moreover, the particular type of periodic paralysis cannot be determined from this test alone. It is also of interest that an initial postexercise increment of over 100% can be seen in patients with periodic paralysis (McManis et al., 1986). This finding is otherwise most commonly found in LEMS; the postexercise increment in these two groups of patients can be differentiated by the time it takes the CMAP to return to baseline. In LEMS this occurs within 1 minute; in periodic paralysis, it occurs more slowly, over 15–40 minutes, usually after a significant decrement.

Between attacks, insertional activity is normal in all forms of periodic paralysis except in some patients with the hyperKPP, in whom there may be myotonic discharges, runs of positive sharp waves and fibrillation potentials (Layzer et al., 1967; Brooks, 1969; Lehmann-Horn et al., 1987). MUP morphology is generally normal except in patients with fixed myopathy, in whom MUP duration, and amplitude may be reduced (Brooks, 1969; Dyken et al., 1969; Campa and Anders, 1974; Hoskins and Vroom, 1975). Finally, muscle fibre conduction velocity is reduced in hypoKPP (Zwarts et al., 1988), a finding that is consistent with a defect at the level of the muscle membrane.

Myotonic myopathies

The presence of clinical myotonia defines this group of diseases. The vast majority are hereditary. All have myotonic discharges on needle EMG. There are also several other diseases (Table 12.1) with electrical, but not clinical, myotonia that are not included in this group of disorders. The myotonic myopathies can be subdivided into the nondystrophic and dystrophic myotonias. The nondystrophic myotonias include autosomal dominant and recessive myotonia congenita, paramyotonia congenita, hyperKPP and several toxic or drug-induced myopathies. The dystrophic myotonias include myotonic dystrophy and PROMM.

Myotonia congenita

Both autosomal dominant and autosomal recessive myotonia congenita are caused by a defect in chloride conductance across the muscle membrane (Ptáček et al., 1993). In both forms, routine motor and sensory nerve conduction studies are normal. However, RNS may demonstrate a sizable decrement in CMAP amplitude and area, more so in the recessive than in the dominant form of the disease. The decrement differs from that in MG in that it is more evident at higher rates of stimulation (10 Hz) than at lower rates, and its onset is typically delayed for at least 10 stimuli for high-frequency RNS and for 50 stimuli at low-frequency RNS. The shape of the decrement also differs from that in MG in that there is a smooth, progressive decline in CMAP amplitude over numerous stimuli (Ozdemir and Young, 1976; Aminoff et al., 1977). Similarly, a decrement in CMAP amplitude can also be demonstrated after 5–10 seconds of maximal voluntary muscle contraction: the short exercise test (Streib et al., 1982). Again, the decrement after brief exercise is greater and is slower to recover in autosomal recessive than in dominant myotonia congenita.

Needle EMG reveals profuse myotonic discharges in proximal and distal muscles. MUP morphology is normal in the dominant form of myotonia congenita. In the recessive form, distal muscles may reveal brief-duration, low-amplitude, polyphasic MUPs (Sun and Streib, 1983).

Paramyotonia congenita and hyperkalaemic periodic paralysis

Paramyotonia congenita and hyperKPP, as well as a rare potassium-sensitive form of myotonia congenita, myotonia fluctuans, are caused by defects in the sodium channel of the muscle membrane (Ptáček et al., 1993). Routine motor and sensory nerve conduction studies are normal in patients with hyperKPP between attacks and in patients with paramyotonia congenita at normal temperature. In hyperKPP, the long exercise test often reveals an increment in the CMAP immediately after exercise, followed by a slow decline in CMAP amplitude reaching a nadir 30 minutes after completion of the test (McManis et al., 1986). By contrast, in paramyotonia congenita, the short (Streib, 1987b) or the long exercise test (McManis et al., 1986) may be abnormal in warm muscles as well, but there is no initial increment and the nadir of the decrement is reached virtually immediately, albeit with a prolonged recovery. With muscle cooling, all patients with paramyotonia congenita have a distinctive decrement in the CMAP of exercised muscles (Guttmann et al., 1986; Streib, 1987b)

Needle EMG examination shows generalized myotonia in paramyotonia congenita, more in distal than proximal muscles. Similarly, in most families with hyperKPP, myotonia is easily elicited in limb muscles (Streib, 1987a). Motor unit morphology is normal in patients with paramyotonia congenita whose muscles are warm. However, when cooled to 20 °C, patients with paramyotonia congenita exhibit inhibition of all electrical activity including myotonia, sometimes preceded by a burst of fibrillation potentials (Haas et al., 1979; Nielsen et al., 1982). As mentioned above, in some patients with hyperKPP, brief-duration, low-amplitude MUPs may be found (Brooks, 1969; Hoskins and Vroom, 1975).

Myotonic dystrophy and proximal myotonic myopathy

Myotonic dystrophy is a multi-system disease caused by an expansion of a CTG DNA repeat in a noncoding region just beyond the region coding for a cyclic AMP-dependent protein kinase (Ptáček et al., 1993) the function of which is phosphorylation of muscle membrane proteins. The number of triplet repeats correlates with the severity of the disease. Routine nerve conduction studies may disclose a mild sensorimotor polyneuropathy in diabetic or non-diabetic patients with myotonic dystrophy (Cros et al., 1988), with slightly slow distal sensory and motor nerve conduction velocity.

RNS at frequencies of 5–10 Hz may disclose a decrement of the CMAP similar to that seen in other myotonic disorders (Aminoff et al., 1977). Similarly, the short exercise test shows a substantial CMAP decrement with quick recovery (Streib et al., 1982; Streib, 1987a). If the test is repeated after rest of at least 5 minutes, the decrement becomes less reproducible in subsequent trials. By contrast, in myotonia congenita, the decrement remains demonstrable on repeated trials.

Needle EMG discloses prominent myotonic discharges even in muscles that do not manifest clinical myotonia. In adults with myotonic dystrophy, myotonic discharges are more likely to be found in distal upper extremity or facial muscles (Streib and Sun, 1983). In infants and children, they are more difficult to elicit and are more prominent in proximal or paraspinal muscles (Watters and Williams, 1967; Streib, 1987a). At least in some patients, cooling the muscle may help in eliciting electrical myotonia (Jablecki, 1993; Daube, 1994). Motor unit morphology is abnormal particularly in more severe disease. Brief-duration, low-amplitude, polyphasic MUPs can be observed in distal limb muscles, particularly in extensor muscles of the forearm and the tibialis anterior muscle (Streib and Sun, 1983; Streib, 1987a). These morphological abnormalities are not seen in autosomal dominant myotonia congenita but can be found in the autosomal recessive form. Finally, just as the CMAP decrements with RNS or after exercise, there is loss of stability of the MUP in myotonic dystrophy; as motor units repetitively discharge, they may slowly decline in MUP amplitude and recover with rest (Brown, 1974).

Similar to myotonic dystrophy, PROMM is also a multi-system disease associated with a myotonic myopathy, but without the CTG repeat or linkage to gene loci of other myotonic disorders (Ricker et al., 1994, 1995; Thornton et al., 1994). However, PROMM is clinically milder and less progressive than myotonic myopathy and the muscle weakness is proximal rather than distal, affecting hip and shoulder girdle musculature, and sparing facial muscles. It is sometimes associated with muscle hypertrophy rather than atrophy (as seen in myotonic dystrophy) and with an unusual, intermittent pain syndrome affecting proximal muscles.

The electrophysiology of PROMM has not been fully elucidated. Although some patients have been found to have evidence of a mild sensory neuropathy in the legs (Thornton et al., 1994; Sander et al., 1996), routine nerve conduction studies have been normal. RNS shows a decrement in proximal but not distal muscles (Sander et al., 1996). Neither is there a CMAP decrement in distal hand muscles after exercise (Sander et al., 1997), a finding that might distinguish patients with PROMM from those with myotonic dystrophy since in the latter the exercise test is typically positive.

On needle EMG, there are myotonic discharges, perhaps more in distal than in proximal limb muscles. In one report (Sander et al., 1996), myotonia was provoked with muscle warming and dampened with muscle cooling, another finding that could potentially distinguish PROMM from myotonic dystrophy, in which myotonia is often exacerbated by muscle cooling. MUP morphology appears to be slightly altered in PROMM. A few studies have shown brief-duration, polyphasic MUPs in proximal and distal limb muscles (Thornton et al., 1994; Sander et al., 1996).

Nonmyotonic muscular dystrophies

The nonmyotonic muscular dystrophies are generally hereditary, progressive myopathies (Table 12.3) without clinical myotonia and with nonspecific electrophysiological features. Motor nerve conduction studies are normal except when recording from an atrophic muscle, in which case the CMAP amplitude may be reduced. RNS does not show a significant decrement or increment; if these are present, they should prompt consideration of another disease. Sensory nerve conduction studies are usually normal, although a mild sensory neuropathy may be present in the distal myopathy of Welander.

As in most other myopathies, performance of needle EMG is the most important electrodiagnostic study. Kugelberg (1947) described most of the EMG abnormalities in muscular dystrophy, particularly the changes in motor unit morphology, over 50 years ago. The EMG

Table 12.3. The muscular dystrophies

Congenital muscular dystrophies
Duchenne muscular dystrophy
Becker muscular dystrophy
Emery–Dreifuss muscular dystrophy
Limb girdle muscular dystrophies
Facioscapulohumeral dystrophy
Myotonic dystrophy
Proximal myotonic myopathy
Oculopharyngeal dystrophy
Distal muscular dystrophies

abnormalities of each of the muscular dystrophies have recently been reviewed (Dumitriu, 1995). None of the nonmyotonic muscular dystrophies has distinctive EMG features.

The major EMG findings are as follows. There may be increased insertional activity or sustained fibrillations or positive waves, particularly early on in more severely affected muscles (Norris and Chatfield, 1955; Buchthal and Rosenfalck, 1966; Desmedt and Borenstein, 1975). In general, patients with Duchenne's and more severe Becker muscular dystrophy are more likely to have spontaneous activity than those with the other nonmyotonic dystrophies. Complex repetitive discharges may also be observed. Rare myotonic discharges may also be seen in some patients with these disorders, particularly in Duchenne or Becker dystrophy, but the myotonic discharges are briefer and sparser than in myotonic dystrophy. In the most severely affected muscles, the resistance to needle insertion may be increased, suggesting that the muscles have been replaced by connective tissue.

Motor unit morphology generally shows brief-duration, polyphasic MUPs with amplitudes that are normal to low (Kugelberg, 1947, 1949). In those dystrophies with more focal weakness, such as oculopharyngeal and the distal muscular dystrophies, the abnormalities are more easily demonstrable in weak muscles (Daube, 1994). As the disease progresses, prolonged duration, higher-amplitude polyphasic MUPs may occasionally be seen as well, along with increasing numbers of satellite potentials (Desmedt and Borenstein, 1976b). SFEMG typically shows increased fibre density and jitter (Sanders and Stålberg, 1996), and macro-EMG shows reduced or normal MUP amplitude (Fig. 12.11) (Hilton-Brown and Stålberg, 1983).

In the muscular dystrophies, as in other muscle disorders, abnormalities in motor unit recruitment depend on disease severity. In the initial stages of the disease, recruitment is normal in mildly weak muscles and may be appreciated as 'early' in moderately weak muscles. As the myopathy progresses, motor unit recruitment may be reduced in severely affected muscles, a finding explained by Eric Kugelberg (1949) as 'due to a process which more or less diffusely reduces the number of muscle fibres in the different units until they are put out of action'.

Congenital myopathies

Congenital myopathies have characteristic histological features on muscle biopsy, but in most cases minimal, nonspecific electrophysiological findings (Bodensteiner, 1994; Harper, 1996b). Indeed, of the various myopathies, patients with congenital myopathy are most likely to have a normal or at least minimally abnormal electrodiagnostic evaluation (Wilbourn, 1987).

Of the five best-characterized congenital myopathies – central core disease, nemaline (rod) myopathy, centro-nuclear (or myotubular) myopathy, congenital fibre type disproportion myopathy and multicore myopathy – centronuclear myopathy is the most distinctive electro-physiologically. The key findings in centronuclear myopathy include abnormal spontaneous activity, with fibrillation potentials and myotonic discharges (Hawkes and Absolon, 1975). Abnormal spontaneous activity is much less common in the other congenital myopathies. On occasion, patients with nemaline (Shy et al., 1963; Engel and Resnick, 1966; Karpati et al., 1972; Brownell et al., 1978), central core (Armstrong et al., 1971) and even congenital fibre type disproportion myopathy (Cavanaugh et al., 1979) have fibrillation potentials, but only patients with centronuclear myopathy have myo-tonic discharges.

Nonspecific EMG abnormalities such as brief, low-amplitude, or polyphasic MUPs have been described in all of the congenital myopathies (Mrozek et al., 1970; Hawkes and Absolon, 1975; Bodensteiner, 1994), particularly in more advanced disease. Increased fibre density has also been reported in central core disease (Cruz-Martinez et al., 1979). In nemaline myopathy, serial EMG studies (Karpati et al., 1972; Wallgren-Petersson et al., 1989) have demonstrated evolution of MUP abnormalities. MUP morphology was found to be normal early on. Subsequently, brief, low-amplitude, polyphasic MUPs were noted toward the end of the first decade, and long-duration, higher amplitude, polyphasic MUPs were seen normally in the second decade. This may explain why electrodiagnostic studies are normal or equivocal in many children with congenital myopathy, who typically undergo electrophysiological investigation once early in their illness.

Metabolic myopathies

Acid maltase deficiency (glycogenosis type II)

Acid maltase deficiency is an autosomal recessive glycogen storage disease that causes progressive proximal weakness. It is generally divided into infantile, childhood and adult forms.

Nerve conduction and RNS are normal (Engel et al., 1973). EMG is frequently abnormal. In adults, EMG abnormalities are most prominent proximally, including the respiratory muscles; in infants, they are more widespread. The salient EMG feature is the presence of myotonic discharges, without clinical myotonia, most often found in the trunk and paraspinal muscles in adults (Engel et al., 1973). Other spontaneous EMG activity includes fibrillation potentials, positive sharp waves and complex repetitive discharges. MUPs are usually of short duration and low amplitude, with increased polyphasia, again most prominent proximally. One patient has been reported with prolonged duration and high-amplitude MUPs (Karpati et al., 1977).

Myophosphorylase deficiency (glycogenosis type V)

Myophosphorylase deficiency, or McArdle's disease, is an autosomal recessive inherited disease characterized by exercise intolerance, with myalgia, easy fatigability and stiffness. Painful muscle contractures are also induced by exercise. About 30% of patients may have persistent muscle weakness.

Nerve conduction studies are normal. High-frequency (20 Hz) RNS produces a decremental response (Brandt et al., 1977). Decrement has also been reported at 5 Hz, albeit in an unusual case with late onset (Pourmand et al., 1983). EMG is normal between attacks in about half of patients; the other half show mild changes including occasional fibrillation potentials and short-duration, low-amplitude, polyphasic MUPs in proximal muscles. One patient with late-onset disease had profuse spontaneous potentials and complex repetitive discharges in proximal muscles (Pourmand et al., 1983). When attacks are induced by either ischaemic or vigorous isometric exercise, needle examination of the muscle contractures reveals electrical silence.

Debrancher deficiency (glycogenosis type III)

Debrancher deficiency is an autosomal recessive disorder that can present in either childhood or adulthood. In the childhood form, hepatomegaly accompanies weakness and hypotonia. Adults more often present with proximal weakness, although distal weakness and wasting of intrinsic hand muscles can also occur.

Sensory and motor nerve conduction velocities are usually normal but occasionally may be mildly reduced (Moses et al., 1986). In one study of four patients, no nerve conduction abnormalities were found (Sancho et al., 1990); in another study of eight patients, two had decreased motor nerve conduction velocity (Coleman et al., 1992). EMG is usually abnormal, although it has been reported as normal even in one patient with clinical weakness (Coleman et al., 1992). EMG shows prominent fibrillation potentials, positive sharp waves and complex repetitive discharges (DiMauro et al., 1979) in distal and proximal muscles. Myotonic discharges have also been reported (Sancho et al., 1990). Weak proximal muscles have brief, small, polyphasic MUPs with early recruitment (Sancho et al., 1990).

Branching enzyme deficiency (glycogenosis type IV)

Branching enzyme deficiency is a rapidly progressive disease of infancy with neuromuscular manifestations of hypotonia and muscle atrophy. When neuromuscular deficits predominate, the appearance may be similar to Werdig–Hoffmann disease; electrodiagnostic studies can usually distinguish them.

Nerve conduction studies are normal. EMG is normal (Daube, 1994) or may show short-duration, polyphasic MUPs with scattered fibrillation potentials (Jablecki, 1993). By contrast, fairly obvious acute and chronic denervation is the rule in Werdig–Hoffmann disease.

Phosphofructokinase deficiency (glycogenosis type VII)

Phosphofructokinase deficiency is a rare autosomal recessive disorder characterized by exercise intolerance, with muscle pain or contracture, and myoglobinuria. The clinical picture is similar to myophosphorylase deficiency, but without progressive weakness.

Nerve conduction studies are normal. RNS may show an abnormal decremental response to 20 Hz stimulation (Griggs et al., 1995). EMG may show occasional positive sharp waves or fibrillation potentials. MUPs may be normal, short duration or low amplitude (Agamanolis et al., 1980). During muscle contracture, there is electrical silence (DiMauro, 1979).

Carnitine palmityltransferase deficiency

Patients with carnitine palmityltransferase deficiency typically present with attacks of pain, stiffness and tightness of muscles after prolonged exercise or fasting, and in severe cases with myoglobinuria. Examination is typically normal between attacks, although fixed weakness has been reported (Kieval et al.,1989)

Nerve conduction studies are normal. One study reported a 28% decrement with repetitive stimulation at 5 Hz (Scarlato et al., 1977) that corrected after 4 months of carnitine supplementation. Needle EMG is usually normal although there are exceptions. No spontaneous activity is seen, but low-amplitude, short-duration MUPs have been reported (Bank et al., 1975; Kieval et al., 1989).

Carnitine deficiency

Carnitine deficiency has both a systemic and a myopathic form. The systemic form presents in childhood with progressive cardiomyopathy and acute attacks of hypoglycaemia. In the myopathic form, patients develop progressive painless proximal weakness with wasting of proximal muscles.

During acute attacks in systemic carnitine deficiency, nerve conduction studies are normal, but EMG shows short-duration, low-amplitude MUPs (Karpati et al., 1975). Fibrillation potentials may be seen. Fibrillation potentials and positive sharp waves may also be seen in the myopathic form; weak muscles show brief, small, polyphasic MUPs (Engel and Angelini, 1973).

Myoadenylate deaminase deficiency

Myoadenylate deaminase is involved in maintaining the supply of ATP during strenuous activity. Absence of the enzyme has been suggested as a cause of exertional and postexertional myalgias, although a cause-and-effect relationship has yet to be proved (Griggs et al., 1995).

Motor and sensory nerve conduction studies are normal. Needle EMG is most often normal as well. Minor EMG abnormalities have been reported in the form of occasional positive sharp waves and minimal MUP abnormalities (Keleman et al., 1982).

Mitochondrial myopathies

Patients with a number of different mitochondrial disorders have signs of a neuropathy or a myopathy. Little is written on the electrodiagnostic characteristics of individual members of this group of diseases; not surprisingly, the diagnosis of a mitochondrial myopathy rarely rests on electrodiagnostic testing.

If there is an associated peripheral neuropathy, as in some patients with the Kearns–Sayre syndrome, nerve conduction abnormalities may be found, including low-amplitude sensory responses accompanied by slightly pro-longed latencies (Yiannikas et al., 1986). On EMG, positive sharp waves and fibrillation potentials are rarely reported in mitochondrial myopathy, and when there are abnor-malities in MUP morphology, they are usually mild (Fowler et al., 1971). Short-duration, low-amplitude, polyphasic MUPs may be found in proximally weak muscles (Yiannikas et al., 1986). If there is a concomitant peripheral neuropathy, large-amplitude, polyphasic MUPs can be seen in distal muscles (Cohen et al., 1998). SFEMG is more often abnormal, with increased jitter in 77% (Krendel, et al., 1987) to 100% (Fawcett et al., 1982a) of patients with mitochondrial myopathy. SFEMG may not, therefore, dis-tinguish ocular myasthenia from mitochondrial myopathy (Ukchoke et al., 1994).

Endocrine myopathies

Corticosteroids

Myopathy occurs with elevated levels of corticosteroids from endogenous production, as in Cushing's disease, and more commonly from exogenous administration, as in the treatment of various inflammatory diseases.

Nerve conduction studies and RNS are normal. In typical steroid myopathy, EMG is usually normal, even in clinically weak muscles. Abnormal spontaneous activity is not seen, and MUP configuration is also normal except in severe myopathy, where short-duration, low-amplitude MUPs may be seen (Daube, 1994). This is in contrast to high-dose steroid therapy. In a recent study, four patients in intensive care who received high-dose steroids (without neuromuscular blocking agents) devel-oped flaccid quadriplegia (Hanson et al., 1997). Electro-physiological studies suggested acute myopathy with an associated axonal neuropathy. CMAP amplitudes were reduced in 12 of 12 motor nerves and SNAP amplitudes in 10 of 12 sensory nerves. Needle EMG showed positive sharp waves and fibrillation potentials in all muscles in the acute stage. Later, short-duration, low-amplitude and polyphasic MUPs were seen, with a tendency to early recruitment. Other reports of prominent EMG abnormalities in patients treated with high-dose corti-costeroids in the apparent absence of therapy with neuromuscular blocking agents (Hirano et al., 1992) also emphasizes the difference from the myopathy seen with chronic, lower dose steroid administration. Still, it seems unlikely that high-dose steroids alone commonly cause intensive-care setting acute quadriplegic myopathy (Rich et al., 1997).

Hypothyroidism

Hypothyroidism is associated with peripheral neuropathy, predisposition to entrapment neuropathies and myo-pathy. Nerve conduction studies are usually normal in patients with hypothyroid myopathy but may show mild-to-moderate prolongation of distal latencies and slowing of conduction velocities, indicating a concomitant neuropathy (Dyck and Lambert, 1970). F-wave latencies can be prolonged (Torres and Moxley, 1990); sensory responses may be unobtainable, but CMAP amplitudes are usually normal. Needle EMG findings are variable. Some studies report normal EMG findings, while others report abnormalities in 35% (Waldstein et al., 1958), to 70% (Rao et al., 1980) and 88% (Wilson and Walton, 1959) of patients. Increased insertional activity, fibrillation potentials and positive sharp waves (Torres and Moxley, 1990) may be seen together with myotonic discharges and complex repetitive discharges (Venables et al., 1978). In patients with severe hypothyroid myopathy, short-duration, low-amplitude, polyphasic MUPs can be demonstrated with early recruitment in proximal muscles (Rao et al., 1980; Khaleeli, et al., 1983). Myoedema, the mounding phenom-enon seen after percussion of a muscle in hypothyroid patients, is electrically silent (Mizusawa et al., 1984). Rarely, typical cramp potentials may be observed.

Hyperthyroidism

Chronic thyrotoxicosis is associated with several neuro-muscular abnormalities, including thyrotoxic periodic paralysis, concomitant autoimmune MG and thyrotoxic myopathy.

There is little written on the electrophysiology of thyro-toxic periodic paralysis. One study showed that EMG is abnormal during attacks and then normalizes with remis-sion (Puvanendran et al., 1977). During an attack, there was no abnormal spontaneous activity, but MUP morphol-ogy was abnormal in seven of eight patients, with decreased MUP duration in four, increased polyphasia in six and low-amplitude MUPs in three of the eight. Nerve conduction studies were normal.

In chronic thyrotoxic myopathy, motor nerve conduc-tion studies are normal, but sensory amplitudes and con-duction velocities may be mildly reduced (Sozay et al., 1994), and estimates of motor unit numbers may be reduced in distal hand and foot muscles (McComas et al., 1973). In the absence of concomitant MG, repetitive nerve stimulation is typically normal, although one study reported a significant decrement in 17% of patients (Puvanendran et al., 1979). On EMG, there is no abnormal spontaneous activity (Buchhal, 1970). In one study of 48 patients, only 68% of whom had clinical evidence of myo-pathy, all showed EMG abnormalities, mainly in proximal muscles (Puvanendran et al., 1979). Of the 48 patients, 47 showed short-duration MUPs, 44 had increased polypha-sia, six had fasciculations and three had myotonic-like dis-charges. In another study of 17 patients, abnormal MUPs were seen in the quadricep and extensor digitorum brevis muscles in about 50% of patients (Sozay et al., 1994).

Hypoparathyroid myopathy

Both hypoparathyroidism and pseudohypoparathyroidism are associated with hypocalcaemia and hypomagnesae-mia, and the neuromuscular manifestations of these syn-dromes may largely result from the hypolcalcaemia (Kruse et al., 1982). Their main clinical and electrodiagnostic man-ifestations are tetany and, rarely, a mild chronic myopathy.

Sensory and motor nerve conduction studies are normal (Kugelberg, 1940). In the absence of muscle spasms, EMG is usually normal, although some polyphasic MUPs with early recruitment may be seen (Wolf and Lusk, 1972). Fasciculations, as well as bursts of spontaneous MUPs in groups of variable number, are associated with hypocal-caemia (Snowdon et al., 1976). During spasms, rhythmic bursts of repetitive, grouped MUPs (tetanic discharges) occur spontaneously (Kugelberg, 1948). On voluntary acti-vation, MUPs may fire in doublets or triplets.

Hyperparathyroid myopathy

Most patients with hyperparathyroidism complain of gen-eralized weakness, fatigability and muscle stiffness. Proximal muscle weakness and atrophy may be found on examination.

In primary hyperparathyroidism, nerve conduction studies are usually normal (Patten et al., 1974). Secondary hyperparathyroidism is more frequently associated with a peripheral neuropathy with mild slowing of motor nerve conduction velocities (Skaria et al., 1975). On needle EMG examination, spontaneous activity is normal, but MUPs are often of short duration, low amplitude and are polyphasic (Karpati and Frame, 1964). Interestingly, large-amplitude, long-duration MUPs are also occasionally seen, possibly reflecting concomitant neuropathy (Patten et al., 1974).

Toxic myopathies

There are a number of drugs and toxins that are thought to cause various myopathies, including inflammatory, necro-tizing and mitochondrial myopathy. Electrodiagnostic fea-tures of the more common toxic myopathies are discussed.

Colchicine

Colchicine is an anti-inflammatory agent that interferes with microtubule formation. It is frequently used to treat gout. It can cause both an axonal sensorimotor poly-neuropathy and a vacuolar myopathy (Kuncl et al., 1989). The electrophysiological manifestations of colchicine neuropathy include reduction in motor and sensory response amplitude, slight prolongation of distal sensory and motor latencies, as well as F-wave latencies, and slight reduction in conduction velocities (Kuncl et al., 1987). Colchicine myopathy is associated with prominent EMG findings in proximal muscles, namely, short-duration, low-amplitude MUPs with early recruitment. Fibrillation potentials and complex repetitive discharges are abundant (DeDeyn et al., 1995). Myotonic discharges have also been noted (Rutkove et al., 1996). Distal muscles may show mixed changes because of the concomitant neuropathy; these include long-duration, high-amplitude MUPs in addition to abnormal spontaneous activity (Riggs et al., 1986). Within four weeks of discontinuation of the drug, many of these changes remit (Kuncl et al., 1987).

D-Penicillamine

D-Penicillamine, an agent used to treat rheumatoid arthri-tis, Wilson's disease and systemic sclerosis, can cause a painful inflammatory myopathy as well as MG (Fawcett et al., 1982b). Since muscle enzymes may be normal, electro-diagnostic studies can be useful to establish the diagnosis (Chappel and Willems, 1996).

Nerve conduction studies are normal. Proximal muscles show abundant fibrillation potentials and positive sharp waves. Voluntary activity recruits short-duration, poly-phasic MUPs (Chappel and Willems, 1996). Other less common EMG findings include myotonic discharges (Torres et al., 1980) and fasciculation potentials (Pinals, 1983). MUP changes persist for over a year after drug ces-sation (Cucher and Goldman, 1977).

Neuromuscular junction dysfunction should also be considered in patients with muscle weakness, since peni-cillamine may bind to the acetylcholine receptor and induce production of antibodies to the receptor. In such patients, RNS shows a decremental response similar to that seen in idiopathic MG.

Alcohol

Ingestion of alcohol has multiple effects on both the central and peripheral nervous systems. Acute alcohol ingestion can produce both painful and focal myopa-thies; chronic ingestion can contribute to a peripheral neuropathy and a relatively painless myopathy (Perkoff, 1971).

The electrophysiological findings in alcoholic myopathy are variable and dependent on whether there is a coexistent peripheral neuropathy (Perkoff et al., 1967). In patients with acute alcohol-induced necrotizing or hypokalaemic myopathy, EMG of proximal muscles shows abundant fibrillation potentials and positive sharp waves; MUPs are of low amplitude and short duration, with early recruitment (Mayer et al., 1968). In chronic alcohol abuse, a concomitant peripheral neuropathy may be present. In such patients, nerve conduction studies show decreased motor or sensory amplitudes with or without mild reduction in conduction velocity. EMG changes include short-duration, low-amplitude MUPs in proximal muscles. However, distal muscles may exhibit long-duration, high-amplitude MUPs, likely reflecting the presence of an underlying polyneuropathy (Jablecki, 1993).

Neuromuscular-blocking agents

Neuromuscular-blocking agents, such as vecuronium or pancuronium, have been associated with prolonged paralysis and striking electrophysiological abnormalities (Gooch, 1995). Conduction velocities of both sensory and motor nerves are usually normal. Sensory amplitudes are usually normal as well; if not, a superimposed neuropathy, such as critical illness polyneuropathy, should be considered (Lacomis et al., 1996). Motor responses are often absent or decreased in amplitude. In one series, CMAP amplitudes were reduced in 36 of 41 nerves tested, in most cases by greater than 50% (Lacomis et al., 1996). RNS yields variable results. While most such studies are normal, significant decrements have been reported (Barohn et al., 1994). These findings may depend on the timing of the study. Needle EMG is almost always abnormal. Fibrillation potentials are seen in 60–80% of proximal and distal muscles (Lacomis et al., 1996). MUPs recruit early and are short duration, low amplitude and polyphasic in the majority of muscles. Severely weak patients may be unable actively to recruit motor units and may have decreased insertional activity. In general, resolution occurs over months (Road et al., 1997).

Zidovudine

Zidovudine is an antiretroviral agent used to treat HIV infection. Shortly after its introduction, it became clear that it can cause a progressive painful myopathy, via mitochondrial toxicity, and that this toxic myopathy can be difficult to distinguish from primary HIV myopathy (Simpson et al., 1997).

In early disease, when muscle fatigue, myalgia and elevated creatine kinase levels precede overt weakness, EMG is frequently normal. Even when mitochondrial abnormalities are evident on biopsy, one study showed that four of six patients had normal EMG (Cupler et al., 1995). The other two patients had increased insertional activity with short-duration, small-amplitude, polyphasic MUPs. Another study of 11 patients found a good correlation between 'myopathic changes on EMG' (not otherwise defined) and histological evidence of inflammatory change and/or necrosis (Manji et al., 1993). In a separate series that defined zidovudine myopathy as a necrotizing myopathy with little inflammation and no nemaline rods, 16 of 18 patients had EMG abnormalities, including early recruitment of brief, small polyphasic MUPs with mild-to-moderate abundance of fibrillation potentials and positive sharp waves (Chalmers et al., 1991).

Cholesterol-lowering agents

The 3-hydroxy-3-methylglutaryl coenzyme A (HMGCoA) reductase inhibitors (the statins and nicotinic acid (niacin)) as well as gemfibrozil and clofibrate have all been implicated as a cause of myopathy. None of the agents typically cause neuropathy and, therefore, nerve conduction studies are normal. EMG only rarely shows fibrillation potentials unless the myopathy is severe, but myotonic discharges are apparently not infrequent (London et al., 1991). Experimentally, myotonia appears more commonly with simvastatin than pravastatin (Nakahara et al., 1998). With use of clofibrate, short-duration, low-amplitude and polyphasic MUPs have been reported, but only in muscles with significant weakness (Rush et al., 1986). Similar motor unit abnormalities may be seen in myopathy associated with other cholesterol-lowering agents as well.

Inflammatory myopathies

The major inflammatory myopathies are polymyositis, dermatomyositis and inclusion body myopathy. Polymyositis and dermatomyositis sometimes occur in the setting of systemic connective tissue disease, and especially adult dermatomyositis may occur in association with occult malignancy.

Polymyositis and dermatomyositis

The electrophysiological findings in polymyositis and dermatomyositis are identical. Motor conduction studies are normal, with the caveat that amplitude may be reduced when recording from severely affected, atrophic muscles. RNS and sensory conduction studies are also normal. The needle EMG examination is crucial to the diagnosis, but because the disease is patchy and multifocal (Wilbourn, 1987; Jablecki, 1993; Daube, 1994), numerous proximal muscles should be sampled, including the paraspinal muscles, before concluding that the study is negative.

One of the EMG hallmarks is the presence of abnormal insertional activity, and spontaneous activity in the form of positive waves and fibrillation potentials (Fig. 12.5b). In more chronic disease, complex repetitive discharges may be seen as well, and on occasion myotonic discharges may also be present (Daube, 1994). Several points about the spontaneous activity seen in polymyositis and dermatomyositis should be emphasized. First, the fibrillation potentials may be of very low amplitude and high gains of $50\,\mu V/division$ may be required to observe them (Wilbourn, 1987). Second, the fibrillation potentials may begin after a needle insertion only after a delay, and they tend to fire more slowly than with neurogenic disorders, requiring the electromyographer to be patient and pause after each insertion before re-insertion (Wilbourn, 1987; Daube, 1994). Third, almost all untreated patients have positive waves and fibrillation potentials although an extensive search in proximal and paraspinal muscles may be required to demonstrate them (Streib et al., 1979). Fourth, the presence of positive waves and fibrillation potentials can be used as a rough index of disease activity; with successful treatment these potentials tend to wane (Bohan and Peter, 1974). The absence of sharp waves or fibrillations is a strong argument against the diagnosis of PM or DM in an untreated patient, and in favour of steroid myopathy rather than active myositis in a steroid-treated patient with known polymyositis or dermatomyositis whose muscle weakness is progressing.

Abnormalities of MUP morphology are common in PM and DM. In early disease, a large proportion of motor units have multiple phases and turns, brief duration and, to some extent, low amplitude (Buchthal and Pinelli, 1953; Lambert et al., 1954; Barkhaus, et al., 1990; Trojaborg, 1990). Shorter MUP duration and increased phases are more robust findings than is decreased amplitude. As the disease becomes more chronic, there is remodelling of the motor unit. Some MUPs may be prolonged in duration and have higher amplitude than normal; if a delay line is used, satellite potentials (Fig. 12.7b) may be seen (Mechler, 1974; Lang and Partanen, 1976; Partanen and Lang, 1982; Barkhaus et al., 1990; Uncini et al., 1990). Motor unit recruitment is normal or early, particularly in the initial phases of the disease. In chronic, severe inflammatory myopathy, motor unit recruitment may actually be reduced, as is the case in virtually any severe myopathy. This finding may be observed in conjunction with increased resistance to needle insertion as a result of the replacement of muscle with connective tissue elements, another indication of severe disease.

SFEMG studies of patients with long-standing disease also shows evidence of motor unit remodelling with increased fibre density (Foote et al., 1978; Henriksson and Stålberg, 1978), a finding that correlates to some degree with the presence of fibre type grouping on muscle biopsy. In early or more active disease, jitter is increased and blocking may also be noted (Foote et al., 1978).

Inclusion body myopathy

Inclusion body myopathy is a more chronic inflammatory myopathy, typically with involvement of both proximal and distal muscles, sometimes with prominent side-to-side asymmetry, and with characteristic cytoplasmic and nuclear inclusions on muscle biopsy. Since inclusion body myopathy does not respond well to steroid or other immunosuppressive regimens, it is important to distinguish it from PM.

Sensory and motor nerve conduction studies demonstrate a relatively mild generalized sensory or sensorimotor polyneuropathy in 18–33% of patients (Eisen et al., 1983; Lotz et al., 1989; Joy et al., 1990; Barkhaus et al., 1999). Qualitative needle EMG shows increased insertional activity, fibrillation potentials or sharp waves in one or more muscles in virtually all patients with inclusion body myopathy (Eisen et al., 1983; Lotz et al., 1989; Joy et al., 1990; Luciano and Dalakas, 1997). Complex repetitive discharges are seen in one or more muscles in about a third of patients. Motor unit morphology is abnormal in all patients with inclusion body myopathy. One or more muscles will show an increased incidence of brief-duration MUPs in nearly all patients (Lotz et al., 1989; Joy et al., 1990). In addition, many patients will also demonstrate an increased incidence of long-duration MUPs (Eisen et al., 1983; Lotz et al., 1989; Joy et al., 1990; Luciano and Dalakas, 1997), particularly in distal leg muscles or in long-standing disease (Lotz et al., 1989; Luciano and Dalakas, 1997). In rare patients with inclusion body myopathy, only long-duration units may be seen (Eisen et al., 1983; Joy et al., 1990). There is also a high incidence of polyphasic MUPs and linked or satellite potentials in the vast majority of patients with inclusion body myopathy. Motor unit recruitment may be early, normal or reduced. Finally, SFEMG has shown slightly increased jitter and fibre density (Eisen et al., 1983; Joy et al., 1990)

The presence of prolonged duration, complex motor

units combined with abnormalities of nerve conduction and increased fibre density has led to the speculation that inclusion body myopathy has a neurogenic cause (Eisen et al., 1983). Recent quantitative studies have refuted this hypothesis. A quantitative electrophysiological study of motor unit morphology in the biceps brachii of patients with inclusion body myopathy showed that mean MUP duration was reduced in 12 of 17 patients; none showed a prolonged mean MUP duration. Occasional high-amplitude MUPs were observed, but these were not increased in duration or area (Barkhaus et al., 1999). Similarly, a macro-EMG study of the tibialis anterior muscle showed that MUP amplitude and area were overall slightly lower than that in normal subjects (Luciano and Dalakas, 1997). Therefore, it appears that the high incidence of prolonged duration, complex MUPs seen in patients with IBM is the result of chronic motor unit remodelling in response to a primary disorder of muscle, as seen in patients with other chronic myopathies (Lotz et al., 1989).

References

Adrian, E. D. and Bronk, D. W. (1929). The discharge of impulses in motor nerve fibers. Part II. The frequency of discharge in reflex and voluntary contractions. *J. Physiol.* **67**, 119–151.

Agamanolis, D., Askari, D., DiMauro, S. et al. (1980). Muscle phosphofructokinase deficiency: two cases with unusual polysaccharide accumulation and immunologically active enzyme protein. *Muscle Nerve* **3**, 456–467.

Aminoff, M. J., Layzer, R. B., Satya-Murti, S. and Faden, A. I. (1977). The declining electrical response of muscle to repetitive nerve stimulation in myotonia. *Neurology* **27**, 812–816.

Armstrong, R. M., Koenigsberger, R., Mellinger, J. and Lovelace, R. E. (1971). Central core disease with congenital hip dislocation; study of two families. *Neurology* **21**, 369–376.

Bank, W., DiMauro, S., Bonilla, E., Capuzzi, D., and Rowland, L. (1975). A disorder of muscle lipid metabolism and myoglobinuria. *N. Engl. J. Med.* **292**, 443–449.

Barbieri, S., Weiss, G. M. and Daube, J. R. (1982). Fibrillation potentials in myasthenia gravis. *Muscle Nerve (Special Lambert Symp.)* **5**, 550.

Barkhaus, P. E., Nandedkar, S. D. and Sanders, D. B. (1990). Quantitative EMG in inflammatory myopathy. *Muscle Nerve* **13**, 247–253.

Barkhaus, P. E., Periquet, M. I. and Nandedkar, S. D. (1999). Quantitative electrophysiologic studies in sporadic inclusion body myositis. *Muscle Nerve* **22**, 480–487.

Barohn, R., Jackson, C., Rogers, S., Ridings, L. and McVex, A. (1994). Prolonged paralysis due to nondepolaizing neuromuscular blocking agents and corticosteroids. *Muscle Nerve* **17**, 647–654.

Bellemare, F., Woods, J. J., Johansson, R. and Bigland-Ritchie, B. (1983). Motor-unit discharge rates in maximal voluntary contractions of three human muscles. *J. Neurophysiol.* **50**, 1380–1392.

Berstein, L. P. and Antel, J. P. (1981). Motor neuron disease: decremental responses to repetitive nerve stimulation. *Neurology* **31**, 202–204.

Besser, R., Gutmann, L. and Weilemann, L. S. (1989). Inactivation of end-plate acetylcholinesterase during the course of organophosphate intoxication. *Arch. Toxicol.* **63**, 412–415.

Besser, R., Vogt, T. and Gutmann, L. (1990). Pancuronium improves the neuromuscular transmission defect of human organophosphate intoxication. *Neurology* **40**, 1275–1277.

Bodensteiner, J. D. (1994). Congenital myopathies. *Muscle Nerve* **17**, 131–44.

Bohan, A. and Peter, J. B. (1974). Polymyositis and dermatomyositis. *N. Engl. J. Med.* **292**, 344–447, 403–407.

Bradley, W. G., Taylor, R., Rice, D. R. et al. (1990). Progressive myopathy in hyperkalemic periodic paralysis. *Arch. Neurol.* **47**, 1013–1017.

Brandt, N., Buchtal, F., Ebbesen, F., Kamieniecka, Z. and Krarup, C. (1977). Post-tetanic mehanical tension and evoked action potentials in McArdle's disease. *J. Neurol. Neurosurg. Psychiatry* **40**, 920–925.

Bromberg, M. B. and Scott, D. M. (1994). Single fibre EMG reference values: reformatted in tabular form. *Muscle Nerve* **17**, 820–21.

Brooks, J. E. (1969). Hyperkalemic periodic paralysis. Intracellular electromyographic studies. *Arch. Neurol.* **20**, 13–18.

Brown, J. C. (1974). Muscle weakness after rest in myotonic disorders: an electrophysiological study. *J. Neurol. Neurosurg. Psychiatry* **37**, 1336–1342.

Brownell, A. K. W., Gilbert, J. J., Shaw, D. T., Garcia, B., Wenkebach, G. and Lam, A. (1978). Adult onset nemaline myopathy. *Neurology* **28**, 1306–1309.

Buchthal, F. (1970). Electrophysiological abnormaliies in metabolic myopathies and neuropathies. *Acta Neurol. Scand.* **46**, 129–174.

Buchthal, F. and Kamieniecka, Z. (1982). The diagnostic yield of quantified electromyography and quantified muscle biopsy in neuromuscular disorders. *Muscle Nerve* **5**, 265–280.

Buchthal, F. and Pinelli, P. (1953). Muscle action potentials in polymyositis. *Neurology* **3**, 424–436.

Buchthal, F., Rosenfalk, P. (1966). Spontaneous electrical activity of human muscle. *Electroencephalogr. Clin. Neurophysiol.* **20**, 321–326.

Buchthal, F. and Guld, C. and Rosenfalck, P. (1954a). Action potential parameters in normal human muscle and their dependence on physical variables. *Acta Physiol. Scand.* **32**, 200–218.

Buchthal, F., Pinelli, P. and Rosenfalck, P. (1954b). Action potential parameters in normal human muscle and their physiological determinants. *Acta Physiol. Scand.* **32**, 219–229.

Campa, J. F. and Anders, D. B. (1974). Familial hypokalemic periodic paralysis. *Arch. Neurol.* **31**, 110–115.

Cavanaugh, N. P. C., Lake, B. D. and McMenniman, P. (1979). Congenital fiber type disproportion myopathy: a histologic analysis with an uncertain clinical outlook. *Arch. Dis. Child.* **54**, 735–743.

Chalmers, A., Greco, C. and Miller, R. (1991). Prognosis in AZT myopathy. *Neurology* **41**, 1181–1184.

Chappel, R. and Willems, J. (1996). D-Penicillamine-induced myositis in rheumatoid arthritis. *Clin. Rhematol.* **15**, 86–87.

Cherington, M. (1974). Botulism: ten year experience. *Arch. Neurol.* **30**, 432–437.

Cherington, M. (1982). Electrophysiologic methods as an aid in diagnosis of botulism: a review. *Muscle Nerve* **5**, S28–S29.

Cohen, O., Steiner, I., Argov, Z. et al. (1998). Mitochondrial myopathy with atypical subacute presentation. [Letter] *J. Neurol. Neurosurg. Psychiatry* **64**, 410–411.

Coleman, R., Winter, H., Wolf, B., Gilchrist, J. and Chen, Y. (1992). Glycogen storage disease type III (glycogen debranching enzyme deficiency): correlation of biochemical defects with myopathy and cardiomyopathy. *Ann. Intern. Med.* **116**, 896–900.

Cornblath, D. R., Sladky, J. and Sumner, A. (1983). Clinical electrophysiology of infant botulism. *Muscle Nerve* **6**, 448–452.

Cros, D., Harnden, P., Pouget, J., Pellisier, J. F., Gastaut, J. L., Serratrice, G. (1988). Peripheral neuropathy in myotonic dystrophy: a nerve biopsy study. *Ann. Neurol.* **23**, 470–476.

Cruz-Martinez, A., Ferrer, M. T., Lopez-Terradas, J. M., Pascual-Castroviejo and I., Mingo, P. (1979). Single-fibre electromyography in central core disease. *J. Neurol. Neurosurg. Psychiatry* **42**, 662–667.

Cucher, G. and Goldman, A. (1977). D-Penicillamine induced polymyositis in rheumatoid arthritis. *Ann. Intern. Med.* **85**, 615–616.

Cupler, E., Danon, M., Jay, C., Hench, K., Ropka, M. and Dalakas, M. (1995). Early features of zidovudine-associated myopathy: histopathological findings and clinical correlations. *Acta Neuropathol.* **90**, 1–6.

Daube, J. R. (1991). AAEM Minimonograph No. 11: needle examination in clinical electromyography. *Muscle Nerve* **14**, 685-700.

Daube, J. R. (1994). Electrodiagnosis of muscle disorders. In: *Myology*, Vol. 1, eds. A. G. Engel and C. Franzini-Armstrong, pp. 764–794. New York: McGraw Hill.

DeDeyn, P., Ceuterick, C., Saxena, V., Crols, R., Chappel, R. and Martin, J. (1995). Chronic colchicine-inducd myopathy and neuropathy. *Acta Neurol. Belg.* **95**, 29–32.

Denys, E. H. and Norris, F. H. (1979). Amyotrophic lateral sclerosis: Impairment of neuromuscular transmission. *Arch. Neurol.* **36**, 202–205.

Desmedt, J. E. (1958). Methodes d'etude de la fonction neuromusculaire chez l'homme. Myogramme isometrique, electromyogramme d'excitation et topographie de l'innervation terminale. *Acta Neurol. Belg.* **58**, 977–1017.

Desmedt, J. E. (1973). The neuromuscular disorder in myasthenia gravis. I. Electrical and mechanical responses to nerve stimulation in hand muscles. In: *New Developments in Electromyography and Clinical Neurophysiology*, Vol. 1, ed. J. E. Desmedt, pp. 241–304 Basel: Karger.

Desmedt, J. E. and Borenstein, S. (1975). Relationship of spontaneous fibrillation potentials to muscle fibre segmentation in human muscular dystrophy. *Nature* **258**, 531–534.

Desmedt, J. E. and Borenstein, S. (1976a). Diagnosis of myasthenia gravis by nerve stimulation. *Ann. N. Y. Acad. Sci.* **274**, 174–188.

Desmedt, J. E. and Borenstein, S. (1976b). Regeneration in Duchenne muscular dystrophy: Electromyographic evidence. *Arch. Neurol.* **33**, 642–650.

DiMauro, S. (1979). Metabolic myopathies. In: *Handbook of Clinical Neurology*, eds. P. Vinken and G. Bruyn, pp. 175–234. Amsterdam: Elsevier Science.

DiMauro, S., Hartwig, G., Hays, A. et al. (1979). Debrancher deficiency: Neuromuscular disorder in 5 adults. *Ann. Neurol.* **5**, 422–436.

Dorfman, L., Howard, J. and McGill, K. (1989). Clinical studies using automatic decomposition electromyography (ADEMG) in needle and surface EMG. In: *Computer-Aided Electromyography and Expert Systems*, ed. J. Desmedt, pp. 189-204. New York: Elsevier.

Dumitru, D. (1995). *Electrodiagnostic Medicine*, pp. 1029–1129. Philadelphia: Hanley and Belfus.

Dyck, P. and Lambert, E. (1970). Polyneuropathy associated with hypothyroidism. *J. Neuropathol. Exp. Neurol.* **29**, 631–658.

Dyken, M., Zeman, W. and Rusche, T. (1969). Hypokalemic periodic paralysis. Children with permanent myopathis weakness. *Neurology* **19**, 691–699.

Eisen, A., Berry, K. and Gibson, G. (1983). Inclusion body myositis (IBM): myopathy or neuropathy. *Neurology* **33**, 1109–1114.

Engel, A. G. (1990). Congenital disorders of neuromuscular transmission. *Sem. Neurol.* **10**, 12–26.

Engel, A. G. and Angelini, C. (1973). Carnitine deficiency of human skeletal muscle with associated lipid storage myopathy: a new syndrome. *Science* **179**, 899–902.

Engel, A. G. and Lambert, E. H. (1969). Calcium activation of electrically inexcitable muscle fibers in primary hypokalemic periodic paralysis. *Neurology* **19**, 851–858.

Engel, A. G., Lambert, E. H., Rosevar, J. W. and Tauxe, W. N. (1965). Clinical and electromyographic studies in a patient with hypokalemic periodic paralysis. *Am. J. Med.* **38**, 626–640.

Engel, A. G., Gomez, M., Seybold, M. and Lambert, E. (1973). The spectrum and diagnosis of acid maltase deficiency. *Neurology* **23**, 95–106.

Engel, A. G., Lambert, E. H., Mulder, D. M. et al. (1982). A newly recognized congenital myasthenic syndrome attributed to a prolonged open time of the acetylcholine-induced ion channel. *Ann. Neurol.* **11**, 553–569.

Engel, W. K. (1973). 'Myopathic EMG' – nonesuch animal. *N. Engl. J. Med.* **289**, 485–486.

Engel, W. K. and Resnick, J.S. (1966). Late onset rod myopathy: a newly recognized, acquired and progressive disease. *Neurology* **16**, 308–309.

Fawcett, P., Mastaglia, F. and Mechler, F. (1982a). Electrophysiologic findings including single fiber EMG in a family with mitochondrial myopathy. *J. Neurol. Sci.* **53**, 397–410.

Fawcett, P., MacLachlan, S., Nicholson, L., Argov, Z. and Mastaglia, F. (1982b). D-Penicillamine associated myasthenia gravis: immunological and electrophysiological studies. *Muscle Nerve* **5**, 328–334.

Foote, R. A., O'Fallon, W. M. and Daube, J. R. (1978). A comparison of single fiber and routine EMG in normal subjects and patients with inflammatory myopathy. *Bull. Los Angeles Neurol. Soc.* **43**, 95–103.

Fowler, W., Taylor, R. and Munsat, T. (1971). Electromyographic characteristics of congenital and early onset motor unit diseases. *Arch. Phys. Med. Rehab.* **52**, 343–361.

Gilchrist, J. M., Nandedekar, S. D., Stewart, C. R., Massey, J. M., Sanders, D. B. and Barkhaus, P. E. (1988). Automatic analysis of the interference pattern using the turns: amplitude ratio. *Electroencephalogr. Clin. Neurophysiol.* **70**, 534–540.

Gilchrist, J. M. for the ad hoc committee (1992). Single fiber EMG reference values: a collaborative effort. *Muscle Nerve* **15**, 151–161.

Gooch, J. (1995). AAEM Case Report no. 29: prolonged paralysis after neuromuscular blockade. *Muscle Nerve* **18**, 937–942.

Gordon, A. M., Green, J. R. and Lagunoff, D. (1970). Studies on a patient with hypokalemic familial periodic paralysis. *Am. J. Med.* **48**, 185–195.

Griggs, R., Mendell, J. and Miller, R. (1995). Metabolic myopathies. In: *Evaluation and Treatment of Myopathies*, eds. R. Griggs, J. Mendell and R. Miller, pp. 247–293. Philadelphia, PA: Davis.

Guttmann, L. and Pratt, L. (1976). Pathophysiologic aspects of human botulism. *Arch. Neurol.* **33**, 175–179.

Guttmann, L., Riggs, J. E. and Brick, J. F. (1986). Exercise induced membrane failure in paramyotonia congenita. *Neurology* **36**, 130–132.

Haas, A., Ricker, K., Hertel, G. and Heene, R. (1979). Influence of temperature on isometric contraction and passive muscular tension in paramyotonia congenita. *J. Neurol.* **221**, 151–162.

Hanson, P., Dive, A., Brucher, J., Bisteau, M., Dangoisse, M. and Deltombe, T. (1997). Acute corticosteroid myopathy in intensive care patients. *Muscle Nerve* **20**, 1371–1380.

Harper, C. M. (1996a). Neuromuscular transmission disorders in childhood. In: *Pediatric Clinical Electromyography*, eds. H. R. Jones, C. F. Bolton and C. M. Harper, pp. 353–385. Philadelphia, PA: Lippincott-Raven.

Harper, C. M. (1996b). Myopathies. In: *Pediatric Clinical Electromyography*, eds. H. R. Jones, C. F. Bolton and C. M. Harper, pp. 397–402. Philadelphia, PA: Lippincott-Raven.

Hausmanowa-Petrucewicz, I. and Jedrezejowska, H. (1971). Correlation between electromyographic findings and muscle biopsy in cases of neuromuscular disease. *J. Neurol. Sci.* **13**, 85–106.

Hawkes, C. H. and Absolon, M. J. (1975). Myotubular myopathy associated with cataract and electrical myotonia. *J. Neurol. Neurosurg. Psychiatry* **38**, 761–764.

Henneman, E. (1957). Relation between size of neurones and their susceptibility to discharge. *Science* **126**, 1345–1347.

Henriksson, K.-G. and Stålberg, E. (1978). The terminal innervation pattern in polymyositis: a histological and SFEMG study. *Muscle Nerve* **1**, 3–13.

Hilton-Brown, P. and Stålberg, E. (1983). Motor unit size in muscular dystrophy: a macro EMG and scanning EMG study. *J. Neurol. Neurosurg. Psychiatry*, **46**, 996–1005.

Hirano, M., Ott, B., Raps, E. et al. (1992). Acute, quadriplegic myopathy: a complication of treatment with steroids, nondepolarizing blocking agents, or both. *Neurology* **42**, 2082–2087.

Hoskins, P. S. and Vroom, F. Q. (1975). Hyperkalemic periodic paralysis. *Arch. Neurol.* **32**, 519–523.

Hubbard, J. I. (1973). Microphysiology of vertebrate neuromuscular transmission. *Physiol. Rev.* **53**, 674–723.

Hubbard, J. I., Llinas, R. and Quastel, D. M. J. (1969). *Electrophysiologic Analysis of Synaptic Transmission*. Baltimore, MD: Williams & Wilkins.

Jablecki, C. K. (1993). Myopathies. In: *Clinical Electromyography*, 2nd edn, eds. W. F. Brown and C. F. Bolton, pp. 653–689. Boston, MA: Butterworth-Heinemann.

Joy, J. L., Oh, S. J. and Baysal, A. I. (1990). Electrophysiological spectrum of inclusion body myositis. *Muscle Nerve* **13**, 949–951.

Joynt, R. L. (1998). The case for monopolar needles. *Muscle Nerve* **21**, 1804–1806.

Karpati, G. and Frame, B. (1964). Neuropsychiatric disorders in primary hyperparathyroidism. *Arch. Neurol.* **10**, 387–397.

Karpati, G., Carpenter, S. and Andermann, F. (1972). A new concept of childhood nemaline myopathy. *Arch. Neurol.* **24**, 291–304.

Karpati, G., Carpenter, S., Engel, A. et al. (1975). The syndrome of systemic carnitine deficiency. *Neurology* **25**, 16–24.

Karpati, G., Carpenter, S., Eisen, A., Aube, M. and DiMauro, S. (1977). The adult form of acid maltase (α-1,4-glucosidase) deficiency. *Ann. Neurol.* **1**, 276–280.

Keleman, J., Rice, D., Bradley, W., Munsat, T., DiMauro, S. and Hogan, E. (1982). Familial myoadenylate deaminase and exertional myalgia. *Neurology* **32**, 857–863.

Khaleeli, A., Griffith, D. and Edwards, R. (1983). The clinical presentation of hypothyroid myopathy and its relationship to abnormalities in structure and function of skeletal muscle. *J. Clin. Endocrinol.* **19**, 365–376.

Kieval, R., Sotrel, A. and Weinblatt, M. (1989). Chronic myopathy with a partial deficiency of the carnitine palmityltransferase enzyme. *Arch. Neurol.* **46**, 575–576.

Krendel, D., Sanders, D. and Massey, J. (1987). Single fiber electromyography in chronic progressive external ophthalmoplegia. *Muscle Nerve* **10**, 299–302.

Kruse, K., Scheunemann, W., Beier, W. and Schaub, J. (1982). Hypocalcemic myopathy in idiopathic hypoparathyroidism. *Eur. J. Ped.* **138**, 280–282.

Kugelberg, E. (1940). Accommodation in human nerves and its significance in the symptoms of circulation disturbances and tetany. *Acta Physiol. Scand.* **8** (suppl. 24), 1–105.

Kugelberg, E. (1947). Electromyogram in muscular disorders. *J. Neurol. Neurosurg. Psychiatry*, **10**, 110–122.

Kugelberg, E. (1948). Activation of human nerves by ischemia. Trousseau's phenomenon in tetany. *Arch. Neurol. and Psychiatry* **60**, 140–152.

Kugelberg, E. (1949). Electromyogram in muscular dystrophies. *J. Neurol. Neurosurg. Psychiatry*, **12**, 129–136.

Kuncl, R., Duncan, G., Alderson, K., Rogawski, M. and Peper, M. (1987). Colchicine myopathy and neuropathy. *N. Engl. J. Med.* **316**, 1562–1568.

Kuncl, R., Cornblath, D., Avila, O. and Duncan, G. (1989). Electrodiagnosis of human colchicine myoneuropathy. *Muscle Nerve* **12**, 360–364.

Lacomis, D., Giuliani, M., van Cott, A. and Kramer, D. (1996). Acute myopathy of intensive care: clinical, electromyographic, and pathological aspects. *Ann. Neurol.* **40**, 645–654.

Lambert, E. H. (1966). Defects in neuromuscular transmission in syndromes other than myasthenia gravis. *Ann. N. Y. Acad. Sci.* **135**, 367–384.

Lambert, E. H., Sayre, G. P. and Eaton, L. M. (1954). Electrical activity of muscle in polymyositis. *Trans. Am. Neurol. Assoc.* **79**, 64–69.

Lambert, E. H., Eaton, L. M. and Rooke, E. D. (1956). Defect of neuromuscular conduction associated with malignant neoplasms. *American J. Physiol.* **187**, 612–613.

Lambert, E. H., Rooke, E. D., Eaton, L. M. and Hodgson, C. H. (1961). Myasthenic syndrome occasionally associated with bronchial neoplasm: neurophysiologic studies. In: *Myasthenia Gravis*, ed. H. R. Viets, pp. 362–410. Springfield, IL: Thomas.

Lang, A. H. and Partanen, V. S. J. (1976). 'Satellite' potentials and the duration of motor unit potentials in normal, neuropathic and myopathic muscles. *J. Neurol. Sci.* **27**, 513–524.

Layzer, R. B., Lovelace, R. E. and Rowland, L. P. (1967). Hyperkalemic periodic paralysis. *Arch. Neurol.* **16**, 455–472.

Lehmann-Horn, F., Kuther, G., Ricker, K, Grafe, P., Ballanyi, K. and Rudel, R. (1987). Adynamia episodica hereditaria with myotonia: a non-inactivating sodium current and the effect of extracellular pH. *Muscle Nerve* **10**, 363–374.

London, S., Gross, K. and Ringel, S. (1991). Cholesterol-lowering agent myopathy (CLAM). *Neurology* **41**, 1159

Lotz, B. P., Engel, A. G., Nishino, H., Stevens, J. C. and Litchy, W. J. (1989). Inclusion body myositis: observations in 40 patients. *Brain* **112**, 727–747.

Luciano, C. A. and Dalakas, M. C. (1997). Inclusion body myositis: no evidence for a neurogenic component. *Neurlogy* **48**, 29–33.

Manji, H., Harrison, M., Round, J. et al. (1993). Muscle disease, HIV and zidovudine: the spectrum of muscle disease in HIV-infected individuals treated with zidovudine. *J. Neurol.* **240**, 479–488.

Mayer, R., Garcia-Mullin, R. and Eckholdt, J. (1968). Acute 'alcoholic' myopathy. *Neurology* **18**, 275.

Mayer, R. F. and Williams, I. R. (1974). Incrementing responses in myasthenia gravis. *Arch. Neurol.* **31**, 24–26.

McComas, A., Sica, R., McNabb, A., Goldberg, W. and Apton, A. (1973). Neuropathy in thyrotoxicosis. *N. Engl. J. Med.* **289**, 219–220.

McManis, P. G., Lambert, E. H. and Daube, J. R. (1986). The exercise test in periodic paralysis. *Muscle Nerve* **9**, 704–710.

McQuillen, M. P. and Engbaek, L. (1975). Mechanism of colistin-induced neuromuscular depression. *Arch. Neurol.* **32**, 235–238.

McQuillen, M. P., Cantor, H. E. and O'Rourke, J. R. (1968). Myasthenic syndrome associated with antibiotics. *Arch. Neurol.* **18**, 402–414.

Mechler, F. (1974). Changing electromyographic findings induring the chronic course of polymyositis. *J. Neurol. Sci.* **23**, 237–242.

Mizusawa, H., Takagi, A., Nonaka, T. et al. (1984). Muscular abnormalities in experimental hypothyroidism of rats with special reference to mounding phenomenon. *Exp. Neurol.* **85**, 480–492.

Morris, H. (1977). Tick paralysis: electrophysiologic measurements. *S. Med. J.* **70**, 121–122.

Moses, S., Gadoth, N., Ben-David, E. et al. (1986). Neuromuscular involvement in glycogen storage disease type III. *Acta Paed. Scand.* **7**, 289–296.

Mrozek, K., Strugalska, M. and Fidzianska, A. (1970). A sporadic case of central core disease. *J. Neurol. Sci.* **10**, 339–348.

Nakahara, K., Kuriyama, M., Sonoda, Y. et al. (1998). Myopathy induced by HMG-CoA reductase inhibitors in rabbits: a pathological, electrophysiological, and biochemical study. *Toxicol. Appl. Pharmacol.* **152**, 99–106.

Nandedkar, S. D., Barkhaus, P. E., Sanders, D. B. and Stålberg, E. V. (1988). Analysis of amplitude and area of concentric needle EMG motor unit action potentials. *Electroencephalogr. Clin. Neurophysiol.* **69**, 561–567.

Nandedkar, S. D., Barkhaus, P. E. and Charles, C. (1995). Multi-motor unit action potential analysis (MMA). *Muscle Nerve* **18**, 1155–1166.

Nielsen, V. K., Friis, M. L. and Johnsen, T. (1982). Electromyographic distinction between paramyotonia congenita and myotonia congenita: effect of cold. *Neurology* **32**, 827–832.

Norris, F. H. and Chatfield, P. O. (1955). Some electrophysiological aspects of muscular dystrophy. *Electroencephalogr. Clin. Neurophysiol.* **7**, 391–397.

Oh, S. (1977). Botulism: electrophysiologic studies. *Ann. Neurol.* **1**, 481–485.

O'Neill, J. H., Murray, N. M. F. and Newsome-Davis, J. (1988). The Lambert-Eaton myasthenic syndrome, a review of 50 cases. *Brain* **111**, 577–596.

Oosterhuis, H. J. G. H., Hootsmans, W. J. M., Veenhuyzen, H. B. and van Zadelhoff, I. (1972). The mean duration of motor unit action potentials in patients with myasthenia gravis. *Electroencephalogr. Clin. Neurophysiol.* **32**, 697–700.

Ozdemir, C. and Young, R. R. (1976). The results to be expected from electrical testing in the diagnosis of myasthenia gravis. *Ann. N. Y. Acad. Sci.* **274**, 203–222.

Partanen, V. S. J. and Lang, A. H. (1982). EMG dynamics in polymyositis: a quantitative single motor unit study. *J. Neurol. Sci.* **57**, 221–234.

Patten, B., Bilezikian, J., Mallette, L., Prince, A., Engel, W. and Aurbach, G. (1974). Neuromuscular disease in primary hyperparathyroidism. *Ann. Intern. Med.* **80**, 182–193.

Perkoff, G. (1971). Alcoholic myopathy. *Annu. Rev. Med.* **22**, 125–132.

Perkoff, G., Dioso, M., Bleisch, V. and Klinkerfuss, G. (1967). A spectrum of myopathy associated with alcoholism. *Ann. Intern. Med.* **67**, 481–501.

Pinals, R. (1983). Diffuse fasciculations induced by D-penicillamine. *J. Rheumatol.* **10**, 809.

Pickett, J., Berg, B., Chaplin, E. and Brunstetter-Shafer, M. A. (1976). Syndrome of botulism in infancy: clinical and electrophysiologic study. *N. Engl. J. Med.* **295**, 770–772

Pourmand, R., Sanders, D. and Corwin, H. (1983). Late onset McArdle's disease with unusual electromyographic findings. *Arch. Neurol.* **40**, 374–377.

Pozkanzer, D. C. and Kerr, D. N. S. (1961). A third type of periodic paralysis with normokalemia and favorable response to sodium chloride. *Am. J. Med.* **31**, 328–342.

Ptáček, L. J., Johnson, K. J. and Griggs, R. C. (1993). Genetics and physiology of the myotonic muscle disorders. *N. Engl. J. Med.* **328**, 482–489.

Puvanendran, K., Cheah, J. and Wong, P. (1977). Electromyographic study in thyrotoic periodic paralysis. *Austr. N. Z. J. Med.* **7**, 507–510.

Puvanendran, K., Cheah, J., Naganathan, N., Yeo, P. and Wong, P. (1979). Neuromuscular transmission in thyrotoxicosis. *J. Neurol. Sci.* **43**, 47–57.

Rao, S., Katiyar, B., Nair, K. and Misra, S. (1980). Neuromuscular status in hypothyroidism. *Acta Neurol. Scand.* **61**, 167–177.

Rich, M., Bird, S., Raps, E., McCluskey, L. and Teener, J. (1997). Direct muscle stimulation in acute quadriplegic myopathy. *Muscle Nerve* **20**, 665–673

Ricker, K., Koch, M. C., Lehmann-Horn, F. et al. (1994). Proximal myotonic myopathy: a new dominant disorder with myotonia, muscle weakness, and cataracts. *Neurology* **44**, 1448–1452.

Ricker, K., Koch, M. C., Lehmann-Horn, F. et al. (1995). Proximal myotonic myopathy: clinical features of a multisystem disorder similar to myotonic dystrophy. *Arch. Neurol.* **52**, 25–31.

Riggs, J., Schochet, S., Gutmann, L., Crosby, T. and DiBartolomeo, A. (1986). Chronic human colchicine myopathy and neuropathy. *Arch. Neurol.* **43**, 521–523.

Rivner, M. H. and Swift, T. R. (1993). Electrical testing in disorders of neuromuscular transmission. In: *Clinical Electromyography*, 2nd edn, eds. W. F. Brown and C. F. Bolton, pp. 625–651. Boston: Butterworth-Heinemann.

Road, J., Mackie, G., Jiang, T., Stewart, H. and Eisen, A. (1997). Reversible paralysis with status ashmaticus, steroids, and pancuronium: clinical electrophysiological correlates. *Muscle Nerve* **20**, 1587–1590.

Rose, A. and Willison, R. (1967). Quantitative electromyography using automatic analysis: studies in healthy subjects and patients with primary muscle disease. *J. Neurol. Neurosurg. Psychiatry,* **30**, 403–410.

Rosenfalck, P. and Rosenfalck, A. (1975). *Electromyography and Sensory/Motor Conduction: Findings in Normal Subjects.* Copenhagen: Rigshospitalet, Laboratory of Clinical Neurophysiology.

Rush, P., Baron, M. and Kapusta, M. (1986). Clofibrate myopathy: a case report and review of the literature. *Semin. Arthritis Rheum.* **15**, 226–229.

Rutkove, S., De Girolami, U., Preston, D. et al. (1996). Myotonia in colchicine myoneuropathy. *Muscle Nerve* **19**, 870–875.

Sancho, S., Navarro, C., Fernandez, J. et al. (1990). Skin biopsy findings in glycogenosis III: clinical, biochemical and electrophysiological correlations. *Ann. Neurol.* **27**, 480–486.

Sander, H. W., Tavoulareas, G. P. and Chokroverty, S. (1996). Heat-sensitive myotonia in proximal myotonic myopathy. *Neurology* **47**, 956–962.

Sander, H. W., Tavoulareas, G. P., Quinto, C. M., Menkes, D. M. and Chokroverty, S. (1997). The exercise test distinguishes proximal myotonic myopathy from myotonic dystrophy. *Muscle Nerve* **20**, 235–237.

Sanders, D. B. and Stålberg, E. V. (1996). AAEM Minimonograph No. 25: single-fiber electromyography. *Muscle Nerve* **19**, 1069–1083.

Scarlato, G., Albizatti, M., Bassi, S., Cerri, C. and Frattola, L. (1977). A case of lipid storage myopathy with carnitine deficiency: biochemical and electromyographic correlations. *Eur. Neurol.* **16**, 222–229.

Schiller, H. H. and Stålberg, E. (1978). Human botulism studies with single-fiber electromyography. *Arch. Neurol.* **35**, 346–349.

Shy, G. M., Engel, W. K., Somers, J. E. and Wanko, T. (1963). Nemaline myopathy: a new congenital myopathy. *Brain* **86**, 793–810.

Simpson, D., Slasor, P., Dafni, U., Berger, J., Fischl, M. and Hall, C. (1997). Analysis of myopathy in a placebo-controlled zidovudine trial. *Muscle Nerve* **20**, 382–338.

Skaria, J., Katiyar, B., Srivastave, T., Dube, D. (1975). Myopathy and neuropathy associated with osteomalacia. *Acta Neurol. Scand.* **51**, 37–58.

Snowdon, J., Macfie, A. and Pearce, J. (1976). Hypocalcaemic myopathy with paranoid psychosis. *J. Neurol. Neurosurg. Psychiatry* **39**, 48–52.

Sozay, S., Gokce-Kutsal, Y., Celiker, R., Erbas, T. and Basgoze, O. (1994). Neuroelectrophysiological evaluation of untreated hyperthyroid patients. *Thyroidol. Clin. Exp.* **6**, 55–59.

Stålberg, E. (1983). Macro EMG. *Muscle Nerve* **6**, 619–630.

Stålberg, E. (1991). Invited review: electrodiagnostic assessment and monitoring of motor unit changes in disease. *Muscle Nerve* **14**, 293–303.

Stålberg, E. and Trontelj, J. V. (1976). Single muscle fiber recording of the jitter phenomenon in patients with myasthenia gravis and in members of their families. *Ann. N. Y. Acad. Sci.* **274**, 192.

Stålberg, E. and Trontelj, J. V. (1979). *Single Fibre Electromyography.* London: Mirvalle Press.

Stålberg, E. and Trontelj, J. V. (1992). Clinical neurophysiology: the motor unit in myopathy. In: *Handbook of Clinical Neurology,* Vol. 62, eds. P. Vinken, G. Bruyn, H. Klawans, L. Rowland and S. DiMauro, pp. 49–84. Amsterdam: Elsevier Science.

Stålberg, E. and Trontelj, J. V. (1994). *Single Fiber Electromyography. Studies in Healthy and Diseased Muscle,* 2nd edn. New York: Raven Press.

Stewart, C. R., Nandedekar, S. D., Massey, J. M. et al. (1989). Evaluation of an automatic method of measuring features of motor unit action potentials. *Muscle Nerve* **12**, 141–148.

Streib, E. W. (1987a). AAEE Minimonograph No. 27: differential diagnosis of myotonic syndromes. *Muscle Nerve* **10**, 603–615.

Streib, E. W. (1987b). Paramyotonia congenita: successful treatment with tocainide. Clinical and electrophysiologic findings in seven patients. *Muscle Nerve* **10**, 155–162.

Streib, E. W. and Sun, S. F. (1983). Distribution of electrical myotonia in myotonic muscular dystrophy. *Ann. Neurol.* **14**, 80–82.

Streib, E. W., Wilbourn, A. J. and Mitsumoto, H. (1979). Spontaneous electrical muscle fiber activity in polymyosisits and dermatomyositis. *Muscle Nerve* **2**, 14–18.

Streib, E. W., Sun, S. F. and Yarkowski, T. (1982). Transient paresis in myotonic syndromes: a simplified electrophysiologic approach. *Muscle Nerve* **5**, 719–723.

Sun, S. F. and Streib, E. W. (1983). Autosomal recessive generalized myotonia congenita. *Muscle Nerve* **6**, 143–148.

Swift, T. R. (1979). Weakness from magnesium containing cathartics: electrophysiologic studies. *Muscle Nerve* **2**, 295–298.

Swift, T. R. (1981). Disorders of neuromuscular transmission other than myasthenia gravis. *Muscle Nerve* **4**, 334–353.

Swift, T. R. and Ignacio, O. J. (1975). Tick paralysis: electrophysiologic studies. *Neurology* **25**, 1130–1133.

Thornton, C. A., Griggs, R. C. and Moxley, R. T. (1994). Myotonic dystrophy with no trinucleotide repeat expansion. *Ann. Neurol.* **35**, 269–272.

Tim, R. W. and Sanders, D. B. (1994). Repetitive nerve stimulation studies in the Lambert–Eaton myasthenic syndrome. *Muscle Nerve* **17**, 995–1001.

Torres, C. and Moxley, R. (1990). Hypothyroid neuropathy and myopathy. *J. Neurol.* **237**, 271–274.

Torres, C., Griggs, R., Baum, J. and Penn, A. (1980). Penicillamine induced myasthenia gravis in progressive systemic sclerosis. *Arthritis Rheum.* **23**, 505–508.

Trojaborg, W. (1990). Quantitative electromyography in polymyositis: a reappraisal. *Muscle Nerve* **13**, 964–971.

Trojaborg, W. (1998). The case for concentric needles. *Muscle Nerve* **21**, 1806–1808.

Trontelj, J. V. and Stålberg, E. (1991). Single motor end-plates in myasthenia gravis and LEMS at different firing rates. *Muscle Nerve* **14**, 226–232.

Ukchoke, C., Ashby, P., Basinski, A., Sharpe, J. (1994). Usefulness of single fiber EMG for distinguishing neuromuscular from other causes of ocular muscle weakness. *Can. J. Neurol. Sci.* **21**, 125–128.

Uncini, A., Lange, D. J., Lovelace, R. E., Solomon, M. and Hays, A. P. (1990). Long-duration polyphasic motor unit potentials in myopathies: a quantitative study with pathological correlation. *Muscle Nerve* **13**, 263–267.

Venables, G., Bates, D. and Shaw, D. (1978). Hypothyroidism with true myotonia. *J. Neurol. Neurosurg. Psychiatry,* **41**, 1013–1015.

Waldstein, S., Bronsky, D. and Schrifter, H. (1958). The electromyogram in myxedema. *Arch. Intern. Med.* **101**, 97–102.

Wallgren-Petersson, C., Sainio, K. and Salmi, T. (1989). Electromyography in congenital nemaline myopathy. *Muscle Nerve* **12**, 587–593.

Watters, G. V. and Williams, T. W. (1967). Early onset myotonic dystrophy: clinical and laboratory findings in five families and a review of the literature. *Arch. Neurol.* **17**, 137–152.

Weddell, G., Feinstein, B. and Pattle, R. E. (1944). The electrical activity of voluntary muscle in man under normal and pathological conditions. *Brain* **67**, 178–257.

Wilbourn, A. (1987). The EMG Examination with myopathies. *J. Clin. Neurophysiol.* **10**, 132–148..

Wilson, J. and Walton, J. (1959). Some muscular manifestations of hypothyroidism. *J. Neurol. Neurosurg. Psychiatry,* **22**, 320–324.

Wolf, S. and Lusk, W. (1972). Hypocalcemic myoathy. *Bull. Los Angeles Neurol. Soc.* **37**, 167–177.

Yiannikas, C., McLeod, J., Pollard, J. and Baverstock, J. (1986). Peripheral neuropathy associated with mitochondrial myopathy. *Ann. Neurol.* **20**, 249–257.

Zwarts, M. J., Weerden, T. W. V., Links, P. et al. (1988). The muscle fiber conduction velocity and power spectra in familial hypokalemic periodic paralysis. *Muscle Nerve* **11**, 166–173.

13

Histochemistry and immunocytochemistry of muscle in health and disease

Caroline A. Sewry and Victor Dubowitz

Introduction

Histochemistry combines the study of morphology and biochemistry. It provides precise localization of specific chemical moieties and aids the characterization of a cell. The application of histochemical techniques to the study of skeletal muscle has made a dramatic contribution since the early 1960s, and has provided an essential diagnostic and research role in the study of neuromuscular disorders.

Histochemistry of muscle reveals many properties not detected by routine histology. Its main contributions are in (i) the recognition of fibre types and their response to disease, and to neural, hormonal and other influences; (ii) the demonstration of structural defects in muscle fibres; (iii) the detection of enzyme deficiencies, and (iv) the demonstration of abnormal storage of metabolites. Histochemistry has not been made obsolete by recent advances in molecular biology, or the advent of immunocytochemistry, although the latter is now of equal, or greater, importance in the assessment of some recessive disorders.

Recent years have seen a dramatic increase in the characterization of genes responsible for a wide variety of neuromuscular disorders (see the gene tables in each issue of *Neuromuscular Disorders*), and in several cases antibodies are now available to the defective gene product. In addition, secondary alterations in the expression of proteins are proving useful in diagnosis, in broadening knowledge of pathological changes and in the development of therapeutic strategies.

This review aims to cover the application of the most important histochemical and immunocytochemical techniques to the diagnosis of neuromuscular disorders. The avalanche of immunocytochemical studies of muscle in recent years makes it impossible to cover all of them, but those selected have been chosen for their relevance to diagnosis and to the wider understanding of pathological changes in human muscle. With the developments in the field covering several decades, it is not practical to reference all original articles. Reference to some old work has, therefore, been omitted and, where possible, more recent studies, reviews and books have been selected.

Methods

Choice of biopsy material

Selection of the muscle for biopsy should be based on clinical assessment. It is important not to sample a muscle that is so severely involved that little muscle remains nor to choose a muscle that is unaffected pathologically. In proximal disorders, biopsies are typically taken from the quadriceps (the vastus lateralis or rectus femoris) or deltoid. Even within a muscle selective involvement can occur, for example between the vasti and rectus femoris (Dubowitz 1995). Muscle imaging by ultrasound or magnetic resonance imaging can be useful for screening of differential muscle involvement and can aid in the choice of biopsy site. Other muscles sometimes selected for sampling are the gastrocnemius and biceps, but it is important to be aware of the anatomical differences between muscles, particularly with regard to proportions of fibre types (Johnson et al., 1973). It is also necessary to be aware of age-related changes, both with regard to fibre size and to histochemical features, and to take account of any previous trauma to the muscle, such as a sports injury or damage caused by electromyography (EMG) needles.

Biopsy techniques

All muscle biopsies from children and adults can be performed under local anaesthesia. In some conditions, general anaesthesia may be hazardous because of poor respiratory function or the risk of malignant hyperthermia. Premedication of children is often helpful. To avoid artefact, it is essential that the local anaesthetic only infiltrates the skin and subcutaneous tissue and does not penetrate the muscle itself.

Adequate biopsies can be obtained using commercially available needles. The one we favour is based on that developed by Bergström and has been extensively used in adults and children (Edwards et al., 1983; Heckmatt et al., 1984; Dubowitz, 1995). The needles are 4–5 mm in diameter and the samples, obtained through a 5–6 mm incision, may contain up to 1000 fibres or more. Although small, these samples are adequate for histochemical, immunocytochemical, electron microscopical and biochemical studies and for tissue culture. It may, however, sometimes be necessary to take multiple samples through the same incision to obtain sufficient muscle for all studies. Good transverse orientation of the muscle fibres under a dissecting microscope is important for light microscopical techniques, and this is a skill readily acquired by technical staff.

Needle biopsy techniques have the advantage of providing adequate samples by simple and rapid methods that can be carried out in outpatient facilities and do not require elaborate theatre conditions. The risk of infection is low and, as the incision is only a few millimetres in length and requires no stitches, the residual scar is small and often becomes almost invisible. Multiple samples can be taken through the same incision; samples for biochemistry can be taken and frozen rapidly. Open biopsies provide larger samples and may produce an aesthetically better section; however, in our experience, for the majority of patients the same conclusions can be drawn from a needle biopsy, and open biopsies rarely offer any added advantage. The larger size of open biopsies does, however, provide more tissue for retrospective studies, which, with the rapid advances in genetics, are of increasing importance.

Fetal muscle biopsy

Although rarely performed, muscle can be obtained from fetuses in utero using a needle under ultrasound guidance (Kuller et al., 1992; Evans et al., 1994; Overton et al., 2000). In Duchenne muscular dystrophy (DMD), for example, expression of dystrophin can be assessed when DNA from the proband is not available or is noninformative. Theoretically, fetal muscle samples can be used in any situation where the expression of the relevant protein is sufficiently abnormal for it to be detected immunocytochemically, or a structural feature is likely to be present. In practice, DNA and/or protein assessment of chorionic villus samples is preferred. There is insufficient information on the presence of structural changes (such as nemaline rods) in utero for fetal sampling to be diagnostically reliable.

Immunocytochemistry of samples from aborted fetuses at risk for DMD are also useful for prenatal diagnosis of subsequent pregnancies, as dystrophin expression can be assessed and the DNA analysed. Dystrophin can be detected from at least nine weeks of gestation and a significant reduction, or absence, occurs in fetuses at high risk for DMD (Clerk et al., 1992a,b).

Use of tissues other than muscle

Some proteins relevant to neuromuscular disorders are expressed in tissues other than muscle and can be used diagnositically. For example, skin expresses many of the extracellular matrix proteins found in muscle, and skin biopsies are a useful alternative to muscle, particularly when muscle wasting is extensive, as in patients with congenital muscular dystrophy (CMD) (Sewry et al., 1996, 1997a). Similarly, emerin is expressed in the nuclei of many tissues, and expression can be easily assessed in skin and oral foliate cells (Manilal et al., 1997; Sabatelli et al., 1998). Prenatal diagnosis can also be aided by studies of the expression of proteins in chorionic villi, for example in CMD caused by a primary deficiency of the laminin α2-chain, often referred to as merosin-deficient CMD (Muntoni et al., 1995). Details of the use of these tissues are given in the sections on specific diseases. It should also be remembered that cultured fibroblasts from skin biopsies are useful for some studies, including collagen synthesis and some mitochondrial studies. Fibroblasts can be transfected with MyoD to convert them to muscle cells for the analysis of muscle-specific proteins. It is likely that the use of tissues other than muscle will increase in the future.

Specimen preparation

All muscle biopsies must be frozen rapidly, preferably in isopentane cooled in liquid nitrogen. Orientation for light microscopy should be transverse, whilst for electron microscopy longitudinal sections are often more informative. All histological, histochemical and immunocytochemical studies can be carried out on cryostat sections, and for some enzyme techniques, and some antibodies, this is essential. Ideally, samples should be frozen as soon as possible after removal, but it is possible to do meaningful studies on some postmortem samples. With the development of antigen-retrieval techniques, some immunocytochemical studies can also be performed on fixed, wax-embedded material. This may be useful when only archival material is available.

Antibodies are visualized by the use of conjugates to enzymes, such as peroxidase or alkaline phosphatase, to fluorochromes, such as fluorescein isothiocyanate (FITC), rhodamine, or Texas red, or to metals, such as gold (Sewry and Qui Lu, 2000). The use of fluorescent versus enzyme markers is often a matter of choice, but in the authors' experience it may be easier with fluorescent markers to identify small areas of antibody localization and low levels of expression because the positive labelling is more easily seen against a black background.

Histological features

Histochemical techniques are not performed in isolation and reference is always made to histological preparations. In particular, haematoxylin and eosin, the Verhoeff–van Gieson and the modified Gomori trichrome stains all clearly demonstrate the size and shape of the fibres, the position of nuclei, and the presence of interstitial cells, blood vessels, nerves, connective tissue and adipose tissue (Fig. 13.1).

Normal muscle

In transverse section, normal muscle is composed of polygonally shaped fibres (Fig. 13.1a) (Dubowitz, 1985), that are closely applied to each other and show only a little variation in size (approximately 40–80 μm for males, and 30–70 μm for females). The size of fibres is dependent on age, and adult size is usually achieved by puberty. In neonatal muscle, some larger rounded fibres, resembling Wohlfart B fibres, are often present and may give a false impression of fibre size variability. Nuclei are peripherally situated in normal fibres, but up to 3% of fibres with internal nuclei is considered within normal limits. In the authors' experience, the presence of internal nuclei is rare in normal muscle from children, and the figure of 3% is probably an overestimate. In normal adult muscle they are more common, particularly in those involved in sporting activities. Connective tissue is minimal in endomysial areas of normal muscle, but the width of perimysial bands varies with age and these are particularly wide in muscle from neonates and infants. The number of capillaries relates to fibre type and is also age dependent, with a smaller network of capillaries being apparent with most techniques in muscle from neonates and infants.

Diseased muscle

Histological stains reveal changes in fibre size, shape and distribution. In myopathies, the changes are diffuse but in denervation there is chararcteristic grouping of atrophic fibres (Fig. 13.1b–d). Varying degrees of endomysial fibrosis may be seen; in dystrophic muscle this can be severe (Fig. 13.1c). The number of internal nuclei can vary, but large centrally placed nuclei are a particular feature of myotubular myopathy and myotonic dystrophy. Some patients with minicore myopathy may also show centrally placed nuclei. Necrosis can be identified by pale staining of fibres and may be associated with phagocytes. Hypercontracted areas of fibres stain intensely with most stains and represent damaged or necrotic fibres (Fig. 13.1b). Regenerating fibres are distinguished by their basophilia but this only represents the early stages of regeneration, and antibodies to fetal myosin more accurately identify fibres at varying stages of maturity. Basophilia may also be apparent in abnormal granular fibres in some conditions.

Abnormal structures such as rods in nemaline myopathy (Fig. 13.2) and abnormal mitochondria can be demonstrated with the modified Gomori trichrome technique (Dubowitz, 1985). Other histological stains are useful in particular circumstances, such as periodic acid–Schiff (PAS) for glycogen and Sudan black B or Oil red 0 for lipids. The use of the PAS method, with and without diastase digestion, is not only useful for the demonstration of excess glycogen in specific metabolic disorders but may also help to clarify the nature of some inclusions. It also identifies fibres in the early stages of damage in that they appear negative and lack glycogen. The routine use of stains for lipid is a matter of choice; lipid accumulation in some fibres is a nonspecific feature, but excess lipid can occur in some metabolic disorders. This is often suspected from other histological stains and can be confirmed by specific stains for fat.

Histochemical features

Enzyme histochemistry adds an extra dimension to the study of muscle and still has an essential role despite the increasing use of immunocytochemistry. In the early days of histochemistry, many enzymes were examined in muscle biopsies (Dubowitz and Pearse, 1961), but now assessment is generally restricted to a few selected procedures (Table 13.1).

The most important routine techniques are the demonstration of nicotinamide adenine dinucleotide dehydrogenase tetrazolium reductase (NADH-TR), cytochrome

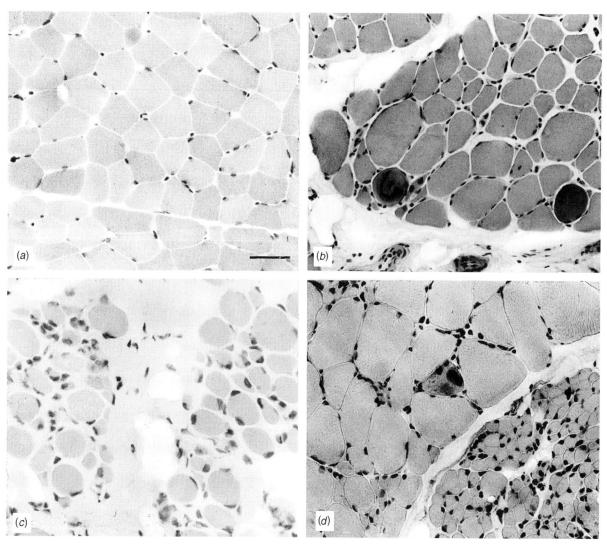

Fig. 13.1. Muscle biopsies stained with haematoxylin and eosin from (a) a normal child and children with (b) Duchenne muscular dystrophy, (c) congenital muscular dystrophy and (d) spinal muscular atrophy. Note the appearance of normal muscle in contrast to the diffuse variation in fibre size in dystrophic muscle (b,c) and the group atrophy and hypertrophy in denervated muscle (d). Note also the degree of connective tissue proliferation in (b) and (c). Bar = 50 μm.

oxidase (COX), succinate dehydrogenase (SDH) and adenosine trisphosphatase (ATPase) at varying pH. Other techniques are useful in specific disorders, for example phosphorylase or phosphofructokinase deficiency in glycogenoses. Acid phosphatase is useful in some storage disorders and in the study of biopsies with vacuoles; however, in the muscular dystrophies it is not essential and adds very little information not obtained with other techniques.

The major roles of enzyme histochemistry are in identifying muscle fibre types, revealing structural changes and identifying enzyme deficiencies. Defining fibre types is essential in the analysis of muscle and there is a reciprocal relationship between type I and type II fibres. Type I fibres,

with their greater mitochondrial content, have higher levels of oxidoreductases (NADH-TR, COX, SDH), but lower levels of transferases and hydrolases (ATPase, phosphorylase); type II fibres show the reverse pattern (Table 10.1). Type II fibres can be further subdivided histochemically into types IIA, IIB, IIC, according to the intensity of the histochemical end-product with the method for myosin ATPase at varying pH of the preincubating medium (Fig. 13.3). The main histochemical profiles of each fibre type are summarized in Table 13.1. Type IIC fibres usually represent less than 3% of the fibres in normal muscle but regenerating fibres are IIC fibres and their number increases in dystrophic muscle.

Table 13.1. Histochemical reactions of the different fibre types in human muscle

Method	Type I	Type IIA	Type IIB	Type IIC
ATPase				
pH 9.4	+	+++	+++	+++
Pre-incubated pH 4.6	+++	0	++	+++
Pre-incubated pH 4.3	+++	0	0	++ or +++
NADH tetrazolium reductase (NADH-TR)	+++	++	+	++ or +++
Cytochrome oxidase (COX)	+++	++	+	+
Succinate dehydrogenase (SDH)	+++	++	+	++
Phosphorylase	0 or +	+++	+++	+++
Periodic acid–Schiff base (PAS)	+ or ++	+++	++	++

Notes:

0, +, ++, +++: increasing intensity of stain.

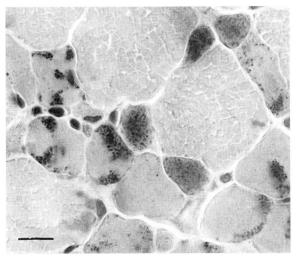

Fig. 13.2. Nemaline rods stained with the modified Gomori trichrome technique in tissue from a patient with nemaline myopathy. Bar = 10 μm.

Changes in the fibre type profile are common in neuro-muscular disorders. These may relate to specific fibre types, to the distribution of fibre types, or to fibre type proportions. In normal individuals, the proportion of fibre types not only varies between muscles but also within a muscle. In general, the proportion of type I fibres in normal quadriceps is less than 55%. If above this figure, type I fibres are considered to be predominant (Dubowitz, 1985).

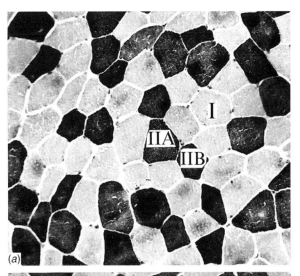

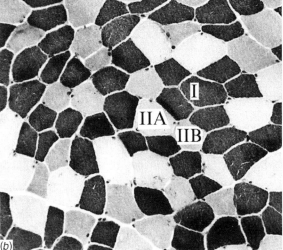

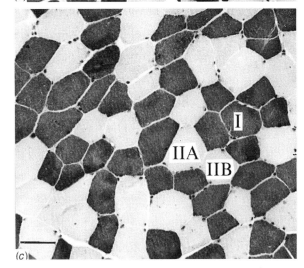

Fig. 13.3. Quadriceps muscle stained for myosin ATPase showing the three main fibre types (I, IIA, IIB). (*a*) ATPase pH 9.4, (*b*) preincubation at pH 4.6 and (*c*) preincubation at pH 4.3. Bar = 50 μm.

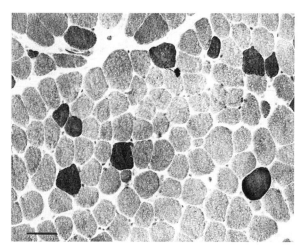

Fig. 13.4. Predominance of type I fibres in a patient with Duchenne muscular dystrophy (ATPase pH 9.4). Bar = 50 μm.

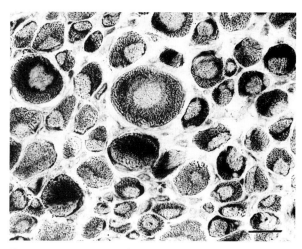

Fig. 13.6. Prominent central cores in most fibres in tissue from a patient with central core disease (NADH tetrazolium reductase). Bar = 50 μm.

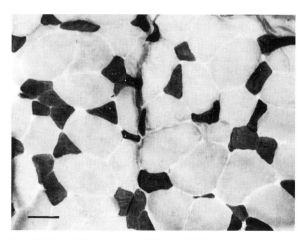

Fig. 13.5. Type II fibre atrophy (ATPase pH 9.4). Bar = 50 μm.

the defining feature of a disorder. Cores show a zone, usually central, that is devoid of enzyme activity (Fig. 13.6), while minicores appear as multiple small negative areas. Target fibres resemble cores but are characterized by three zones. The central area is devoid of stain and is circumscribed by a darkly stained zone; the third peripheral zone stains relatively normally. Target fibres are usually of type I and associated with denervating disorders. Core-like areas devoid of oxidative enzyme staining are common in several conditions, but the characteristic cores of central core disease are usually clearly delineated.

Type I predominance is a common, nonspecific myopathic feature but it is particularly pronounced in congenital myopathies (Fig. 13.4).

Selective involvement of one type of fibre is also common. Type II atrophy is nonspecific, and can be induced, for example by steroids and disuse (Fig. 13.5). It affects IIB fibres before IIA. Type I atrophy, in contrast, is less common and occurs in myotonic dystrophy and some congenital myopathies. It can also occur in some autosomal dominant myopathies, including Bethlem myopathy (Bethlem et al., 1969) and autosomal Emery–Dreifuss muscular dystrophy (EDMD). Grouping of fibre types is indicative of a neurogenic disorder and is thought to reflect re-innervation.

Enzyme histochemistry is essential for revealing structural changes, which are not apparent with routine histological stains. Some of these, such as cores and minicores, are

Disruption and disorientation of the myofibrillar network are common structural changes. These may give rise to whorled fibres, ring fibres or fibres with a 'moth-eaten' appearance. Alterations in the distribution of mitochondria are striking in lobulated fibres in which abnormal aggregation of oxidative enzymes is seen, particularly in triangular peripheral areas of fibres. These fibres rarely occur in biopsies from children and are a nonspecific feature (Guerard et al., 1985). They have recently been reported to be the predominant feature in one group of patients (Weller et al., 1999).

Mitochondrial abnormalities can be revealed by oxidative enzyme staining. Fibres with structurally abnormal mitochondria and large clusters of mitochondria appear 'ragged-red' with the Gomori trichrome method and stain intensely with oxidative techniques such as NADH-TR and SDH. Peripheral clusters of mitochondria also occur in normal muscle, particularly near capilliaries, and may appear as 'tramlines' and stain red with the trichrome method. Fibres devoid of COX activity occur in some mitochondrial myopathies, but they also occur in ageing muscle and sometimes in inflammatory myopathies.

Caution in interpreting the significance of COX-negative fibres is also required with regard to fibre typing. Type II fibres may sometimes appear to have very low activity, and careful comparisons with other methods is then needed.

Other structural defects can be revealed by histochemistry, such as cytoplasmic bodies, tubular aggregates, hyaline bodies and sarcoplasmic masses. These may be an abundant feature and they have given their name to some rare conditions (Dubowitz, 1985, 1995). It is not yet certain how many of these represent specific disease entities (Goebel and Anderson, 1999).

Immunocytochemical features

The number of immunocytochemical studies of human muscle has escalated dramatically in recent years, but not all are currently of diagnostic relevance. Antibodies to a wide variety of muscle proteins are now available, and most organelles and components of the fibre can be studied. Studies of secondary, as well as primary, abnormalities in protein expression are informative, both diagnostically and in widening our understanding of muscle pathology.

Immunocytochemistry also has a potential role in providing an alternative approach for fibre typing. Although ATPase histochemistry is the traditional method for distinguishing muscle fibre types, this can also be demonstrated with antibodies to myofibrillar proteins, in particular myosin isoforms. Immunocytochemistry of myosin isoforms has the additional advantage of revealing co-expression of different isoforms in the same fibre, which is relevant when immature isoforms may be present or when fibre type conversion is occurring. Antibodies to fetal myosin are also an easy way to distinguish immature fibres, particularly very small ones, and can give a useful indication of the degree of muscle regeneration, and by inference, of the muscle damage that preceded it (see Figs. 13.8–13.10, below). It is likely, however, that enzyme histochemistry will remain useful in situations where demonstrating the activity of an enzyme is more important than detecting its mere presence.

The immunocytochemical changes in specific neuromuscular disorders are discussed below together with the associated histochemical features, but initially, the following sections describe some properties that can be demonstrated in relation to the various components of muscle.

Extracellular matrix

The main components of the extracellular matrix are collagens, laminins and proteoglycans. There has been a long-standing interest in the extracellular matrix in neuromuscular disorders as an increase in fibrous tissue is a common feature. Early studies of collagen showed that the perimysium contains collagen types I and III, whereas the endomysium contains mainly type III, with relatively little type I (Duance et al., 1980; Stephens et al., 1982). The localization of fibronectin parallels that of collagen III. Collagen type IV and other basal lamina proteins, such as laminin, perlecan and nidogen, are seen around each fibre and round the vascular components (Bertolotto et al., 1983; Sewry et al., 1985, Brockington et al., 2000). Collagen VI is also localized around the fibre periphery. Architectural abnormalities such as splits and whorls may show extracellular matrix proteins associated with the abnormal membrane feature. Numerous collagen variants have now been identified but the localization of many of them has not been studied in human muscle. With the identification of gene defects in some components of the extracellular matrix, however, and a greater understanding of the multiple chains of each, interest in these families of proteins is increasing. For example, the involvement of the various chains of laminin in the CMDs, and of collagen VI in Bethlem myopathy (see below), has widened our understanding of the clinical spectrum in these conditions.

The basal lamina of muscle fibres seems to be relatively resilient and is often retained when plasma membrane proteins are lost. In postmortem samples, for example, labelling of the basal lamina can often be achieved, even though proteins such as dystrophin are not detectable. Similarly, necrotic fibres often, but not always, retain their basal lamina. In assessing pathological changes of basal lamina proteins, it is important to have a reliable control. Labelling of the laminin γ1-chain is useful for this, as expression is usually normal. It, therefore, provides a good method for judging preservation of the basement membrane.

Membrane-associated proteins

A large number of proteins associated with the plasma membrane of muscle fibres has been studied immunocytochemically. Those of interest include major histocompatibility complex (MHC) class I, immunoglobulins and complement, cell adhesion molecules, the glycoproteins associated with dystrophin, and integrins.

Major histocompatability proteins

Normal mature muscle fibres express minimal or no detectable class I or class II MHC or β_2-microglobulin, but all are detectable on endothelial cells of blood vessels, including capillaries (Appleyard et al., 1985; McDouall et al., 1989). MHC class I and β_2-microglobulin are expressed by regenerating fibres in a variety of disorders and by a proportion of mature fibres in inflammatory myopathies and Xp21 dystrophies. MHC class II, in contrast, is not expressed by muscle fibres in diseased muscle (Appleyard et al., 1985; McDouall et al., 1989), although there has been a report of MHC class II expression in some inflammatory situations (Zuk and Fletcher, 1988).

Immunoglobulin and complement

Immunoglobulin and complement deposition occurs nonspecifically in necrotic fibres and in inflammatory disorders, the muscular dystrophies and myasthenia gravis (Engel and Biesecker, 1982; Isenberg, 1983; Morgan et al., 1984). Complement has also been reported in an X-linked vacuolar myopathy (Villanova et al., 1995). Immunoglobins and complement have been localized to the sarcolemma, blood vessel endothelium and whole muscle fibres. Isenberg (1983) also suggested that immunoglobulin deposition can be used to distinguish myopathic from neuropathic disorders.

Studies of myasthenia gravis have shown immunoglobulin and complement (C3 and C9) at motor endplates (Engel et al., 1977), providing evidence for antibody-dependent complement-mediated injury at the postsynaptic membrane. Aspects of the neuromuscular junction and the acetylcholinesterase receptor are discussed in more detail elsewhere in this book.

Cell adhesion molecules

Antibodies to the neural cell adhesion molecule (NCAM) and its isoforms have been used to demonstrate that NCAM is confined to the neuromuscular junction in innervated fibres but is extrajunctional in denervated and immature fibres (Cashman et al., 1987; Figarella-Branger et al., 1990). Normal mature fibres therefore do not express NCAM, but it is detected on regenerating fibres, non-innervated fibres, satellite cells, myotubes in culture and denervated fibres in neurogenic disorders .

The glycoprotein complex associated with dystrophin

Dystrophin is associated with a complex of proteins, some of which are glycosylated and are transmembrane or extracellular; other proteins associated with dystrophin are intracellular (Straub and Campbell, 1997; Lim and Campbell, 1998; Ozawa et al., 1998). The dystrophin-associated complex is thought to provide a structural link between the subsarcolemmal cytoskeleton and the extracellular matrix. Membrane components of the dystrophin-associated glycoprotein complex identified to date are the dystroglycans (α and β), the sarcoglycans (α, β, γ, δ and ε), and a 25 kDa component called sarcospan (Lim and Campbell, 1998). The glycoproteins are also associated with intracellular proteins, the syntrophins, dystrobrevin and nitric oxide synthase (NOS). No neuromuscular diseases have yet been found to be caused by defects in the syntrophins, dystrobrevin, sarcospan, ε-sarcoglycan or NOS. Antibodies to the various components localize to the sarcolemma (see Fig. 13.15, below), and both primary and secondary abnormalities in their expression have been found, illustrating the importance of their role in the muscular dystrophies. The expression of all components at the light microscopic level shows uniform labelling of the sarcolemma in a variety of neuromuscular disorders where dystrophin is normal. The notable exceptions are the primary defects in some forms of autosomal recessive limb-girdle muscular dystrophy (LGMD), and the secondary changes in DMD and Becker muscular dystrophy (BMD) (see below).

Other membrane proteins of clinical importance are caveolin 3 and dysferlin, as mutations in the genes for these are responsible for different forms of LGMD. Mutations in caveolin 3 have been found in one dominant form of LGMD (Minetti et al., 1998a) but there are limited immunocytochemical reports (Minetti et al., 1998b). Expression of caveolin appears normal when there are mutations in dystrophin or the sarcoglycans (Crosbie et al., 1998).

Dysferlin is also located at the sarcolemma, and a reduction in labelling occurs in patients with mutations in the gene responsible for LGMD type 2B (LGMD2B) and Miyoshi myopathy (Bashir et al., 1998; Anderson et al., 1999). The protein is present early in muscle development and no secondary abnormalities in other neuromuscular disorders have yet been observed (Anderson et al., 1999).

Cytoskeleton

The cytoskeleton forms a filamentous network that links the myofibrils to each other and to the sarcolemma and nucleus. The number of proteins believed to be involved in the cytoskeleton is increasing and those that have been studied in diseased human muscle include β-spectrin, vinculin, desmin, vimentin and plectin. Dystrophin and utrophin, the protein structurally very similar to dystrophin, are also usually considered to be cytoskeletal proteins because of their structural homology to other cytoskeletal proteins and their localization. Alpha-actinin is part of the same family of cytoskeletal proteins but most studies in human muscle have been on the myofibrillar form. Several cytoskeletal proteins have been shown to have a periodic distribution at the sarcolemma and are prominent at areas termed costameres, overlying the Z line or I bands (Pardo

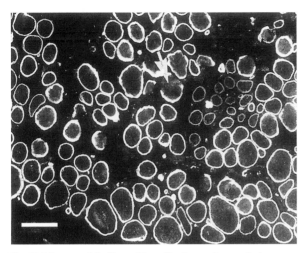

Fig. 13.7. Immunolabelling with antibodies to β-spectrin in muscle from a patient with muscular dystrophy. Note the weakly labelling regenerating fibres and the necrotic fibres with areas of unlabelled sarcolemma (arrow). Bar = 50 μm.

et al., 1983; Porter et al., 1992; Straub et al., 1992). Several cytoskeletal proteins are also concentrated at the neuromuscular junction.

Beta-spectrin

The sarcolemma of human skeletal muscle fibres expresses a β-spectrin-like protein (Appleyard et al., 1984) and the periphery of fibres is clearly delineated. Basophilic, regenerating fibres may show reduced labelling of β-spectrin (Fig. 13.7) and in DMD some basophilic fibres have no detectable labelling. Normal regenerating fibres gradually acquire β-spectrin (Sewry et al., 1992) and some fetal myotubes at early stages of development also have reduced expression (Clerk et al., 1992a). Necrotic fibres often do not label with antibodies to β-spectrin, or other cytoskeletal proteins, as they lose their plasma membrane. Similarly, focal regions where the plasma membrane is lost also appear negative (Fig. 13.7). Antibodies to β-spectrin are, therefore, a useful way of assessing the preservation of the plasma membrane and of avoiding false-negative results when assessing labelling of other sarcolemmal proteins such as dystrophin and the sarcoglycans.

Dystrophin

Considerable research has been devoted to dystrophin, the high-molecular-weight protein defective in DMD and BMD (see Brown and Lucy, 1997; Emery, 1993). It is now known that the dystrophin gene gives rise to at least eight different transcripts from different promoters. These different isoforms are differentially expressed in skeletal,

cardiac and smooth muscle, fetal muscle and neural tissue. In skeletal and cardiac muscle, the full-length transcripts from 5′ promotors are probably the most important; antibodies corresponding to various regions of the protein show uniform labelling of the sarcolemma of fibres in normal muscle and in non-Xp21 disorders (see Figs. 13.11 and 13.15, below). Immunolabelling of dystrophin is enhanced at the myotendinous junction and at the neuromuscular junction. Dystrophin expression in Xp21 dystrophies and in some carriers is abnormal (see section on the muscular dystrophies). Initial studies with antibodies to dystrophin indicated that abnormalites were only seen in Xp21 disorders, but it is now apparent that secondary changes in dystrophin expression can also occur. In particular, secondary abnormalities can occur when some sarcoglycans are abnormal (Vainzof et al., 1996), and changes have been reported in Fukuyama CMD (Arikawa et al., 1991) and in inflammatory myopathies (Sewry et al., 1991).

Utrophin

An autosomal protein, utrophin, coded by human chromosome 6, has considerable homology to dystrophin (see Brown and Lucy, 1997). Utrophin is ubiquitously expressed in a variety of tissues. In normal mature muscle, it is expressed on blood vessels, including capillaries, and peripheral nerves but is absent from muscle fibres, except at the neuromuscular junction (Nguyen thi Man et al., 1991; Ohlendieck et al., 1991; Tanaka et al., 1991). In regenerating fibres in a variety of disorders, however, it is expressed on the sarcolemma and internally (Helliwell et al., 1992b). Overexpression occurs in DMD and BMD (see Fig. 13.12, below) (Helliwell et al., 1992b), but this rarely occurs in LGMDs. Utrophin has also been reported on mature fibres in inflammatory myopathies but in our experience this is not a consistent finding. Occasionally traces may be detected on most fibres in some neonates (Sewry et al., 1994b); the reason is unknown.

Intermediate filaments

Intermediate filaments are a group of immunologically related proteins approximately 10 nm in diameter that have a characteristic, tissue-specific distribution. Those most extensively studied in muscle are desmin (skeletin) (Thornell et al., 1980) and vimentin (Lazarides, 1980).

Desmin occurs exclusively in muscle cells of all types and in skeletal muscle it forms a three-dimensional lattice linking the myofibrils to each other at the Z lines to maintain alignment (Lazarides and Hubbard, 1976). Desmin filaments are also involved in linking the myofibrils to the sarcolemma and to the nuclear membrane (Tokuyasu et al., 1983; Cullen et al., 1992). Desmin filaments are abundant in immature and regenerating muscle fibres and in rhabdomyosarcomas, but in normal mature muscle their concentration is low, except at the sarcolemma. Desmin persists in smooth muscle but is not detected in capillaries.

In diseased muscle, changes in desmin distribution accompany the myofibrillar disruption and disorientation seen in cores, minicores and ring fibres and with Z-line streaming (Thornell et al., 1980; Sewry, 1998). Abnormal structures and inclusions such as rods, cytoplasmic bodies, Mallory bodies and the 'caps' in cap disease have been shown to have desmin associated with them (Goebel and Anderson, 1999). Some disorders show increased levels in certain fibres, including X-linked myotubular myopathy, myotonic dystrophy, congenital fibre type disproportion, spinal muscular atrophy and neuropathies (Helliwell et al., 1989; Sewry, 1989; Sarnat, 1990). In necrotic fibres, the peripheral immunostaining for desmin is lost (Helliwell et al., 1989).

Several desmin-related myopathies are now known and involve cardiac, skeletal and smooth muscle (Abraham et al., 1998). The genetic basis for some cases of desmin-related myopathies is not known, but mutations in the gene for desmin have been shown to cause desmin accumulation in a myopathy with a cardiac involvement and in a severe skeletal myopathy (Goldfarb et al., 1998; Lobrinus et al., 1998; Munoz-Marmoi et al., 1998). Another desmin-related myopathy has been shown to result from a mutation in the gene for αB-crystallin on chromosome 11q21–23 (Vicart et al., 1998). This protein is a member of the heat shock protein family and has chaperone activity.

Vimentin is also highly expressed in developing and regenerating skeletal muscle fibres but it declines to an undetectable level in mature fibres (Bornemann and Schmalbruch, 1992). It persists, however, in the endothelial cells of capillaries. Abnormalities in the distribution of vimentin parallel those of desmin but no pronounced accumulation has been reported to be associated with a myopathy.

Myofibrillar proteins

The myofibrillar proteins are receiving increasing attention not only because their isoforms reflect the diversity and plasticity of muscle, and some are associated with specific structural changes, but also because mutations in some are now known to result in a neuromuscular disorder. The myofibrillar proteins studied immunocytochemically in normal and diseased human muscle include myosin heavy chain isoforms, actin, troponin isoforms, tropomyosin, α-actinin, titin and nebulin.

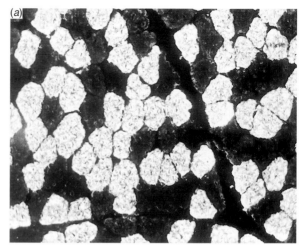

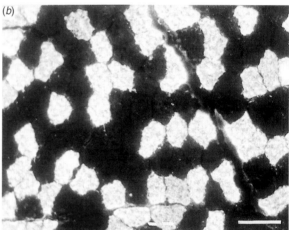

Fig. 13.8. Serial sections of normal muscle immunolabelled with antibodies to (*a*) slow myosin and (*b*) fast myosin, showing a reciprocal pattern. Bar = 50 μm.

Myosin heavy chains

Myosin heavy chains are encoded by a multigene family and exist in several isoforms, which are regulated in a tissue- and development-specific manner (Nguyen et al., 1982; Buckingham, 1985; Lzumo et al., 1986). In addition, hormones such thyroxine, activity and innervation can influence and induce isoform transitions (see Evered and Whealan, 1988). During development, embryonic and fetal (neonatal) isoforms are replaced by the adult fast and slow forms (Whalen et al., 1981; Butler-Browne et al., 1990). Most mature fibres express either the slow or fast isoform (Fig. 13.8), corresponding to the histochemical fibre types I and II, respectively, although occasional fibres may express both. In diseased muscle co-expression of one or more isoforms in the same fibre is common (see Fig. 13.10, below) and can be a useful indicator of abnormality.

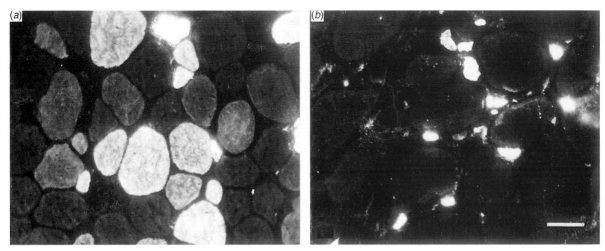

Fig. 13.9. Immunolabelling of fetal myosin in a muscle biopsy from a patient with (*a*) limb girdle muscular dystrophy and (*b*) mild congenital muscular dystrophy. Note the difference in the size, number and intensity of labelled fibres. Bar = 50 μm.

Embryonic and fetal myosin are rarely expressed in adult skeletal muscle and are an indicator of immaturity. The stage at which fetal myosin is no longer detected in normal human muscle has not been fully established. Muscles develop at different rates, and the normal controls used for many studies have either been premature babies or neonates biopsied because of a suspected neuromuscular problem. In practice, samples most likely to be assessed by a pathologist may contain a variable number of fibres with fetal myosin present in samples from children up to a year of age, but this indicator of immaturity may be for a variety of reasons and may be nonpathological. There have been few studies on the isoforms of fast myosin (IIA, IIB, IIX) in diseased human muscle, mainly because of the lack of specific antibodies.

Embryonic and fetal myosin are abundant in regenerating fibres. Fetal myosin is also expressed in an appreciable proportion of nonbasophilic fibres in the muscular dystrophies (Fig. 13.9). Small fibres in several disorders, including spinal muscular atrophy, CMD and many of the perifascicular fibres in dermatomyositis also express fetal myosin. Such fibres, therefore, may not be atrophic, as is commonly thought, but may be immature fibres. The size and number of fibres with fetal myosin in pathological muscle varies but, as they relate to regeneration, they can be a useful reflection of muscle damage (Fig. 13.9). Fetal myosin is frequently co-expressed with fast and/or slow isoforms in a variety of disorders. This co-expression accounts for the poor differentiation of fibre types that is sometimes seen in the muscular dystrophies with the myosin ATPase technique at pH 9.4, as the method cannot distinguish between the enzymes associated with each myosin isoform.

Actin

Actin, a major consituent of myofibrils, has recently received more attention in diseased muscle as pronounced accumulations have been reported in four patients with severe congenital myopathy (Goebel et al., 1997). Similar pathology has been described previously (Dubowitz, 1985), and recent molecular evidence has identified the actin gene as responsible (Nowak et al., 1999). It is also now apparent that there is considerable phenotypic variability in those with actin mutations. Mutations can give rise not only to actin accumulation but also to nemaline myopathy and to a cardiomyopathy (Olsen et al., 1998; Mogensen et al., 1999).

Tropomyosin

Extensive studies of tropomyosin isoforms in human muscle have not been reported, but a mutation in the gene for slow α-tropomyosin is responsible for one form of nemaline myopathy (Laing et al., 1995), in addition to a cardiomyopathy (Towbin, 1998).

Alpha-actinin

Isoforms of α-actinin have also been characterized and studied in relation to fibre typing. Alpha-actinin is a major constituent of Z lines and it is associated with rods in nemaline myopathy. Some antibodies are specific to certain fibre types; antibodies to α-actinin 2 label all muscle fibre types while antibodies to α-actinin 3 only label a subset of fast fibres (North and Beggs, 1996). Some biopsies may show an absence of α-actinin 3 and it was suggested that this might be of pathological significance in some CMDs (North and Beggs, 1996). This, however, is a nonspecific feature (Vainzof et al., 1997) and a common nonpathogenic polymorphism has recently been found in the gene to explain this (North et al., 1999).

Titin and nebulin

Titin and nebulin are two of the largest proteins described; both exist as multiple isoforms resulting from differential splicing (Millevoi et al., 1998; Gregorio et al., 1999). They are believed to have a role in maintaining myofibrillar alignment and contribute to the elasticity of the myofibrils. Interest in nebulin arose after Wood et al. (1987) found that nebulin was absent or reduced in DMD. Prior to the identification of the dystrophin gene, they suggested that nebulin was the defective gene product. Later, immunocytochemical studies showed that nebulin and titin are both expressed in DMD (Fürst et al., 1987; Bonilla et al., 1988) but that some degradation occurs (Patel et al., 1988; Matsumura et al., 1989; Cullen et al., 1992). The genes for both proteins are located on chromosome 2q and mutations in the nebulin gene have recently been detected in one form of nemaline myopathy (see below). Titin is a candidate protein for a distal form of muscular dystrophy (Udd et al., 1998). Nebulin, unlike titin, is not expressed in cardiac muscle, but a smaller homologue, nebulette, encoded by a gene on chromosome 12 (Millevoi et al., 1998), is an obvious candidate for disorders involving the heart.

Nuclear proteins

The nuclear proteins currently receiving most interest are those associated with the nuclear membrane. The gene encoding *emerin* is defective in the X-linked form and that for *lamin A/C* in an autsosomal dominant form of EDMD (Bione et al., 1994; Bonne et al., 1999). Other lamins, and nuclear membrane proteins such as the lamina-associated proteins (LAP1, LAP2) and the lamin B receptor, are obvious candidates for other neuromuscular disorders. Several isoforms of lamins have been identified, but two main groups, known as A and B, are classified according to their biochemical and structural properties (Stuurman et al., 1998). Lamin C is a spliced variant from the gene for lamin A. Nuclear lamins belong to the intermediate filament family of proteins and are a major constituent of the nuclear lamina underlying the inner nuclear membrane (Stuurman et al., 1998). They also localize inside the nucleus, either as discrete foci or diffusely.

Other nuclear proteins may also be abnormal in some disorders, such as those involved in myotonic dystrophy and spinal muscular atrophy; recent immunocytochemi-

cal data suggest that calpain 3, responsible for one form of LGMD, may localize to nuclei and be involved in nuclear function (Baghdiguian et al., 1999).

Histochemical and immunocytochemical changes in specific diseases

The muscular dystrophies

The muscular dystrophies have traditionally been defined as inherited disorders with progressive weakness and wasting of skeletal muscle. The most dramatic advances in our understanding of the pathological changes of muscle in recent years have undoubtedly been in the muscular dystrophies. Histopathological assessment of muscle, particularly with immunocytochemistry and molecular genetics, has led to a trend in classifying patients according to their protein defect (e.g. dystrophinopathies, sarcoglycanopathies; Dubowitz, 1998). Most histological or histochemical features are nonspecific and can occur in more than one clinical condition. Patterns, however, have long been known. Although some protein defects are specific, a variety of secondary changes have been identified that can both aid and confuse interpretation.

Duchenne muscular dystrophy

The pathology in DMD shows a diffuse pattern, with increased variability in fibre size, degeneration and regeneration of muscle fibres, and an increase in endomysial and perimysial fibrous tissue and of adipose tissue (Fig. 13.1*b*). There is sometimes an increase in cellularity, often near the regions of necrosis. Both major fibre types show a wide variation in fibre size, resulting from hypertrophy of some fibres and atrophy of others. Some of the variation observed transversely results from branching and splitting of fibres. Other features include an increase in internal nuclei, internal splits and varying degrees of myofibrillar disruption, such as that seen in whorled fibres. Unevenness of oxidative enzyme staining and moth-eaten fibres occur but are less common in DMD than in some other dystrophies. Hypercontracted fibres, necrotic fibres and phagocytosis are common features. Necrotic fibres may occur in clusters and appear pale with histological stains, but their histochemical fibre type properties with regard to myosin are often retained. Fibres that are unstained with PAS, and presumed to be damaged, are also frequent.

Predominance of type I fibres is common, and the differentiation into type I and II fibres with the ATPase technique at pH 9.4 is not always distinct, probably because of

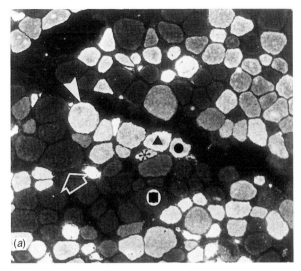

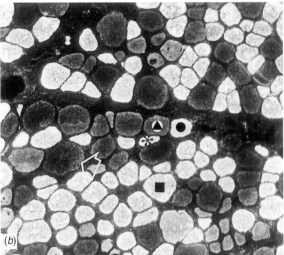

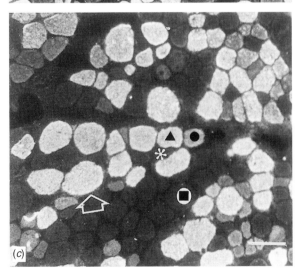

co-expression of myosin isoforms. With acid preincubation, fibre typing is often clearer; a deficiency of IIB fibres has been noted. Antibodies to isoforms of myosin show that slow myosin is often the predominant isoform and co-expression of more than one isoform in a fibre is common (Fig. 13.10); fast type IIB fibres may be preferentially affected (Webster et al., 1988, Marini et al., 1991). Fetal myosin is expressed not only in the basophilic regenerating fibres but also in nonbasophilic fibres of varying size and number (Fig. 13.10) (Marini et al., 1991). Basophilic fibres with expression of developmental isoforms of myosin commonly occur in clusters. They have a high RNA content, a prominent nucleolus in the nucleus, which is often central, and histochemically they stain as type IIC fibres. They also express other developmentally regulated proteins, including desmin, vimentin, NCAM, MHC class I antigens and utrophin. They may appear to have enhanced labelling of basal lamina proteins, probably resulting from duplication of the basal lamina (i.e. that of the original fibre and that of the regenerating fibre underneath).

Becker muscular dystrophy

The features of the muscle in BMD are similar to those seen in DMD but the degree of pathology is variable, and there is often no correlation with clinical severity. The variation in fibre size may be very wide, and very small fibres, either in clusters or diffusely spread throughout the muscle, may be present. The clusters of very small fibres led to the suggestion of neurogenic changes in BMD (Bradley et al., 1978). There is no physiological evidence to support this, and immunocytochemistry shows that these small fibres express fetal myosin, suggesting that they may be regenerating fibres. Fibre typing with enzyme histochemistry may be clearer than in DMD and type IIB deficiency does not occur.

Dystrophin expression in Duchenne and Becker muscular dystrophy

Localization of dystrophin to the sarcolemma and its identification as the defective gene product in DMD and BMD

Fig. 13.10. Serial sections of the quadriceps from a patient with Duchenne muscular dystrophy immunolabelled for (a) fetal myosin, (b) slow myosin and (c) fast myosin. Note the fetal myosin in several nonbasophilic fibres (a, arrowhead), co-expression of all isoforms in some fibres (●), and co-expression of fetal and fast (▲), or fetal and slow (*) in others. Some fibres only express slow myosin (■), and some only fast myosin (open arrow). Bar = 50 μm.

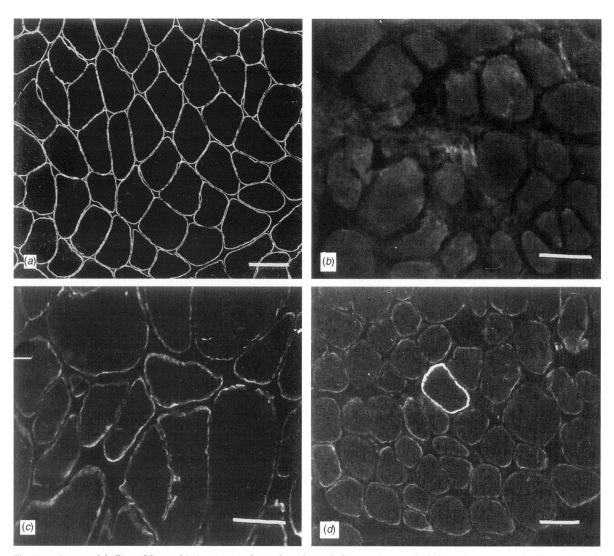

Fig. 13.11. Immunolabelling of dystrophin in (*a*) control muscle and muscle from patients with (*b,d*) Duchenne muscular dystrophy and (*c*) Becker muscular dystrophy. Note the uniform sarcolemmal labelling in control muscle, the absence of dystrophin in (*b*) and the reduced uneven labelling in (*c*). In (*d*) a revertant fibre is intensely labelled and low levels of dystrophin are detected on several other fibres. Bars = 50 μm.

led the way to the revolution in muscle pathology that has occurred during the 1990s (see Brown and Lucy, 1997). In most patients with DMD dystrophin is not detected on the majority of fibres. In contrast, those with BMD show reduced and/or uneven labelling of muscle fibres (Fig. 13.11). This difference is explained by deletions that disrupt the reading frame producing a severe Duchenne phenotype, while those that maintain it give rise to the milder BMD. Although about 95% of cases conform to this dogma there are several exceptions. Notable exceptions are patients who carry deletions of exons 3–7, which is a frameshift deletion and should result in no expression of

dystrophin and a severe phenoptype. These patients, however, show some expression of protein and often have a phenotype intermediate between DMD and BMD (Gangopadhyay et al., 1992). Other exceptions also involve changes in 5′ exons and around exon 3, and in very large deletions (Muntoni et al., 1994). In general, most patients with DMD show an absence of the C-terminus, while in most of those with BMD it is preserved. Exceptions, however, have been reported (Clemens et al., 1992; Helliwell et al., 1992a; see Brown and Lucy 1997).

Low levels of dystrophin expression can be detected in some patients with DMD, and dystrophin is particularly prominent on fibres known as 'revertant' fibres (Fig. 13.11*d*). The expression on these fibres is of normal intensity and arises from restoration of the reading frame. It is still a matter of debate whether the restoration is a genomic event or if it results from exon skipping. The number of revertant fibres in a biopsy is variable; some have none, others a few isolated ones and others have several in clusters. The number has been reported to show no correlation with severity (Fanin et al., 1992), but sampling is a problem that makes this difficult to address.

As the position and size of the mutations in the dystrophin gene vary, it is essential to use antibodies that correspond to more than one domain. In practice, it is important to use antibodies to an N-terminal, rod and C-terminal domain, and several commercial antibodies are now available. An important role of immunocytochemistry is in patients where the deletion cannot easily be detected by molecular techniques. In these cases the abnormality in protein expression, in particular an absence, is often easy to detect. The importance of using more than one antibody is illustrated in patients who have large deletions, as one antibody (to the deleted region) may show an absence while another reveals its presence, and in patients with point mutations when the epitope for an antibody is in the deleted region. Exon-specific antibodies can be useful in identifying the region of a point mutation (Thank et al., 1995).

Secondary abnormalities in protein expression in Duchenne and Becker dystrophy

Abnormal expression of dystrophin in Xp21 dystrophies is associated with secondary abnormalities in the expression of other proteins. The proteins associated with dystrophin in the sarcolemmal complex show reduced expression (Metzinger et al., 1997; Straub and Campbell, 1997; Lim and Campbell, 1998). In addition, the neuronal isoform of NOS has also been shown to be reduced (Brenman et al., 1995). Utrophin, in contrast, is overexpressed (Helliwell et al., 1992b, Taylor et al., 1997a) and is a useful diagnostic aid in BMD where dystrophin may show minimal reduction (Fig. 13.12).

Abnormal sarcolemmal utrophin expression is related to age, and patients with Xp21 dystrophies who are less than about two years of age show very little sarcolemmal expression, in contrast to older patients where it is usually abundant (Fig. 13.12) (Taylor et al., 1997a). Although many patients with BMD show overexpression of utrophin, it is not certain if this is a universal feature. As utrophin is also expressed on regenerating fibres, careful correlation with the expression of fetal myosin is often needed. Similarly, immaturity has to be taken into account in the assessment of MHC class I expression in patients with Xp21 dystrophy.

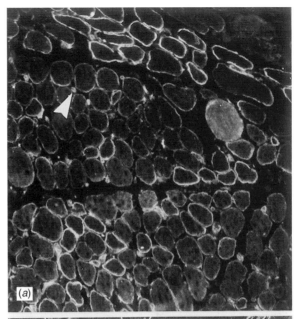

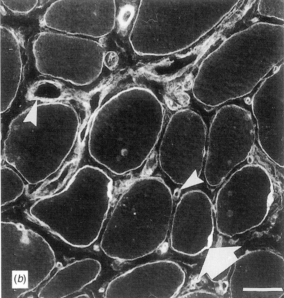

Fig. 13.12. Immunolabelling of utrophin in (*a*) a one-year-old and (*b*) an eight-year-old child with Duchenne muscular dystrophy. Note that not all fibres are labelled in the younger child but all fibres are labelled in the older one. The large arrow in (*b*) indicates a neuromuscular junction and the arrowheads indicate labelling of blood vessels, including capillaries. Bar = 50 μm.

Carriers of Duchenne and Becker muscular dystrophy

Muscle biopsies from some, but not all, carriers of DMD and BMD show morphological abnormalities (Dubowitz, 1985). In some carriers, these changes may be unequivocally abnormal but in others they may be minor and difficult to assess. Abnormalties can occur when serum creatine kinase activity is normal. Changes include variation in fibre size, increase in internal nuclei and patchiness or moth-eaten fibres with oxidative enzyme techniques. Quantitative assessment provided a basis for evaluating changes in the past, but molecular advances have tended to supersede this approach. Immunocytochemical studies of carriers of DMD and BMD have mainly been confined to studies of the expression of myosin (Marini et al., 1991), dystrophin (Dubowitz, 1995) and utrophin (Sewry et al., 1994a). Fibres expressing slow myosin are often predominant and patients with marked pathological changes have fibres that co-express the fast and slow, and/or fetal isoforms.

Dystrophin analysis has an essential role in differentiating between a manifesting carrier of DMD and autosomal forms of muscular dystrophy, in which dystrophin expression is often normal. Many manifesting carriers show a 'mosaic' pattern of dystrophin-positive and dystrophin-negative or dystrophin-deficient fibres (Fig. 13.13), although the pattern of dystrophin expression may vary along the length of the fibre. The degree of weakness is variable in symptomatic carriers and in some patients this has been reported to correlate with the number of dystrophin-negative fibres (Hoffman et al., 1992), while in others it does not (Sewry et al., 1993). If a biopsy from a young female is unequivocally dystrophic and dystrophin expression appears normal, it is unlikely that she is a manifesting carrier. This may not be the case in older females as the number of dystrophin-negative fibres may change, as in heterozygote mice and dogs (Cooper et al., 1990; Karpati et al., 1990). The number of dystrophin-negative fibres may also vary between muscles (Muntoni et al., 1992). Asymptomatic carriers usually show only minor changes in dystrophin immunolabelling and only occasional dystrophin-negative fibres; reduced abundance of dystrophin on immunoblots may be detected (Clerk et al., 1991). Utrophin can be expressed on both dystrophin-positive and dystrophin-negative fibres in carriers (Sewry et al., 1994a). In asymptomatic carriers with minimal alterations in dystrophin, utrophin can be a useful additional marker of abnormality (Sewry et al., 1994b).

X-linked Emery–Dreifuss muscular dystrophy

Although presentation is often in adolescence, patients with X-linked EDMD that present early without the typical clinical signs have been reported (Muntoni et al., 1998). Identification of the defective gene, and immunocytochemistry, have made accurate diagnosis possible, and the clinical and patholgical spectrum may broaden further.

Muscle biopsies usually show only mild changes with variation in fibre size, an increase in internal nuclei, occa-

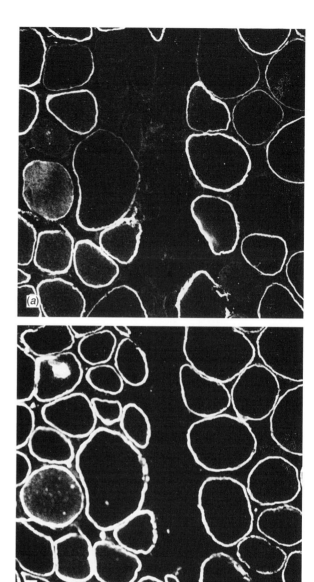

Fig. 13.13. Immunolabelling of (*a*) dystrophin and (*b*) β-spectrin in a manifesting carrier of Duchenne muscular dystrophy. Note the dystrophin-positive and dystrophin-deficient fibres but uniform spectrin labelling of all fibres. Bar = 50 μm.

sional necrotic fibres and focal proliferation of connective tissue. Whorled, split and moth-eaten fibres may also occur. The defective protein, emerin, is localized to the nuclear membrane and is found in all nuclei in normal muscle (Fig. 13.14). Most patients have mutations that result in an absence of emerin (Manilal et al., 1996; Nagano et al., 1996) but a few mutations result in detectable emerin (Manilal et al., 1998; Yates et al., 1999).

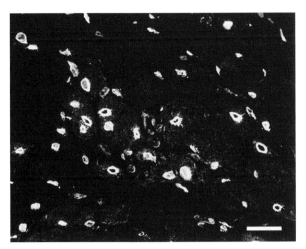

Fig. 13.14. Immunolabelling of the nuclear membrane with an antibody to emerin. Bar = 50 μm.

Skin and oral foliate cells can also be used to assess the presence or absence of emerin, and both tissues have been used to assess female carriers (Manilal et al., 1997; Sabatelli et al., 1998). Reduced expression detected immunocytochemically has not been reported and would probably be difficult to determine. Oral foliate cells are easy to obtain and can be used to assess presence or absence of emerin, but false-negative results may result if the antibodies do not penetrate all cells.

Autosomal dominant Emery–Dreifuss muscular dystrophy

The defective gene in autosomal dominant EDMD, on chromosome 1q11–q23, encodes the nuclear protein lamin A/C (Bonne et al., 1999). The muscle pathology in patients with known deletions is variable, and with the identification of more patients the spectrum will probably widen. Features include variation in fibre size, internal nuclei (which may be abundant), occasional small fibres with high oxidative enzyme content, and a tendency for the type I fibres to be smaller. Necrosis is not a prominent feature, but a small number of fibres with fetal myosin, indicative of regeneration, may be present. Emerin is present in all muscle nuclei, including those that are internal. Studies of the various nuclear lamins (A, A/C, B1, B2) have not yet revealed any obvious differences from controls, emphasizing the difficulty of assessing protein expression in dominant conditions. An interesting secondary protein abnormality, however, is the reduced expression of laminin-β1 on the muscle fibres (C. A. Sewry unpublished data). Expression on blood vessels is normal. This reduction is age related; it is seen in affected adults and adolescents but not in young children. Reduced laminin-β1 is not specific to autosomal dominant EDMD and occurs in some patients with Bethlem myopathy, and in others with a dominant myopathy and rigidity of the spine (Taylor et al., 1997b; Mian et al., 1997; Merlini et al., 1999). One of the families reported by Taylor et al. (1997b) is now known to have a mutation in the lamin A/C gene but this gene has been excluded in the other families (Brown et al., 2001), indicating further genetic heterogeneity in patients with reduced levels of laminin-β1.

Limb girdle muscular dystrophies

Recent advances illustrate the molecular and clinical heterogeneity in the LGMDs. Loci for four dominant (LGMD1A–D) and eight recessive (LGMD2A–H) forms have been identified, and several of the defective proteins are also known (Bushby, 1999; Speer et al., 1999). Some patients have defects that do not link to any of the known loci, indicating further heterogeneity in this group of disorders. With identification of these genes, the broad clinical and pathological spectrum of these disorders is now being appreciated.

Protein defects in dominant conditions are difficult to detect immunocytochemically. Caveolin 3, the defective protein in LGMD1C, is localized to the sarcolemma. Only a few mutations in the gene have been identified (Minetti et al., 1998a), and there are few published data on its expression in these patients; some may show reduced expression (Minetti et al., 1998b). The locus for LGMD1B on chromosome 1q includes the gene for the nuclear membrane protein lamin A/C and it is very likely that this is allelic to autosomal dominant EDMD (van der Kooi et al., 1997; Bonne et al., 1999).

Some morphological changes are more characteristic of this group of disorders than of the Xp21 dystrophies but the degree of 'dystrophic' change is variable. Fibre size variation may be extreme, with many very hypertrophied fibres, and the number of internal nuclei may be very high. The amount of necrosis, regeneration and fibrosis is variable. Fibre typing with the ATPase pH 9.4 technique is often more distinct than in DMD, and oxidative enzymes may show more moth-eaten or whorled fibres. Lobulated fibres and vacuoles also occur.

Dystrophin expression in the LGMDs is often normal (Fig. 13.15) but a secondary reduction can occur in some sarcoglycanopathies (LGMD2C–F) (Vainzof et al., 1996). In males with a deficiency of the sarcoglycans and dystrophin, studies of utrophin can be helpful in distinguishing between LGMD and BMD. The former usually have normal expression whereas those with BMD show overexpression.

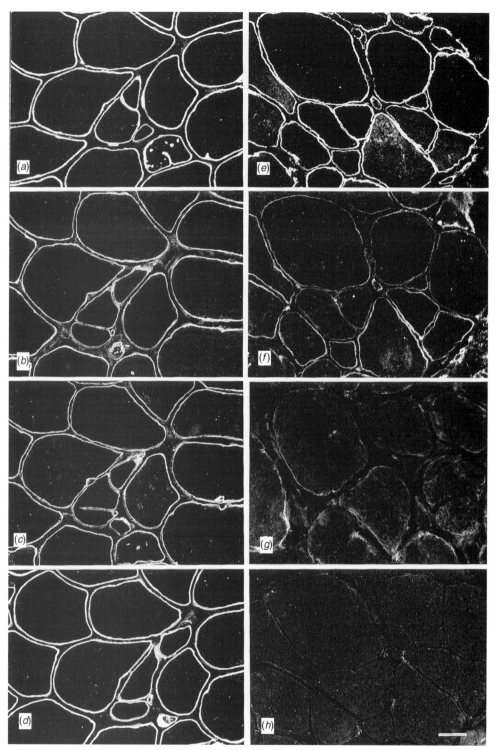

Fig. 13.15. Immunolabelling of (*a–d*) control muscle and (*e–h*) muscle from a patient with limb girdle muscular dystrophy. Antibodies used: (*a,e*) to dystrophin, (*b,f*) to α-sarcoglycan, (*c,g*) to β-sarcoglycan and (*d,h*) to γ-sarcoglycan. Note the uniform labelling of dystrophin in muscle from both sources and the uniform labelling of the sarcoglycans in control muscle. The muscle from the patient with limb girdle muscular dystrophy shows very reduced labelling of α- and β-sarcoglycan but no detectable γ-sarcoglycan. This patient was later found to have a mutation in the gene for γ-sarcoglycan. Bar = 25 μm.

Occasional patients with a sarcoglycanopathy, however, may have some utrophin (Sewry et al., 1994c).

Immunocyochemistry is particularly important in assessment of sarcoglycanopathies and it can help to direct molecular studies. The sarcoglycans (α, β, γ, δ), all encoded by different genes, act as a complex, so abnormal expression of one results in an alteration of all of them. The expression of each can vary from absence, to traces to a mild reduction (Fig. 13.15). Careful comparison with controls is sometimes needed to assess the degree of reduction. If an absence of one occurs, in the presence of reduced expression of the others, it is likely that the absence indicates the primary defect. Almost complete absence of all sarcoglycans can occur, sometimes in association with reduced expression of dystrophin. No muscular dystrophy has yet been found to be associated with ε-sarcoglycan.

LGMD2A is caused by mutations in the gene for the muscle-specific enzyme calpain 3 (Richard et al., 1995). Immunoblots have shown that abnormalities in expression can be detected in these patients (Anderson et al., 1998) but the antibodies used in this study were not suitable for immunocytochemistry. Recent immunocytochemical studies, however, have suggested that calpain 3 is localized to muscle nuclei and within the myofibrillar region, and that an absence can be detected in patients with LGMD2A (Baghdiguian et al., 1999). These studies also suggested a role for calpain 3 in apoptosis.

Studies of dysferlin, the defective protein in LGMD2B and the allelic Myoshi myopathy, are in progress following the identification of the gene (Bashir et al., 1998; Liu et al., 1998). Initial results suggest that immunocytochemistry will detect reduced expression of the protein (Anderson et al., 1999).

Facioscapulohumeral dystrophy

Pathology in facioscapulohumeral dystrophy, a slowly progressive disease is variable. Some biopsies show good retention of architecture and are characterized by scattered, very atrophic fibres and several hypertrophied fibres. Others are overtly dystrophic and may have moth-eaten and whorled fibres. An inflammatory response may be a predominant feature in some biopsies. Clusters of small fibres are seen in some cases and this has been put forward as evidence of neurogenic atrophy. Many of these, and the characteristic scattered small fibres, are type IIC fibres and express fetal myosin, suggesting that they are regenerating. MHC class I has also been observed in occasional patients (Tupler et al., 1998).

Congenital muscular dystrophies

The four main catergories of CMD are defined by the severity and involvement of the brain and eyes (Dubowitz, 1994, 1999). Muscle biopsies show proliferation of connective tissue, which may be extensive and disproportionate to the clinical severity (see Fig. 13.1c). Variation in fibre size is usually evident and type I fibres may be predominant. Necrosis is variable and regeneration apparent by the presence of basophilia and/or fibres with fetal myosin. Dystrophin expression is usually normal but occasional patients with the Japanese Fukuyama form of CMD have been reported to show abnormally labelled fibres (Arikawa et al., 1991). Similarly the dystrophin-associated proteins usually show normal expression but in the Fukuyama form a reduction of β-dystroglycan levels has been reported (Matsumura et al., 1993).

During recent years, the major role of the extracellular matrix in this group of disorders has become apparent (Muntoni and Sewry, 1998; Sewry and Muntoni, 1999). Approximately 40–50% of patients with the classical form of CMD have a primary deficiency of the laminin $\alpha2$-chain, caused by mutations in *LAMA2* on chromosome 6q22. Loci for other forms are known, but this is still the only primary protein defect that can be studied in muscle biopsies. The laminin $\alpha2$-chain, together with the $\beta1$- and $\gamma1$-chains, is a component of the laminin variant laminin-2 (merosin), and the chromosome 6q form of CMD is often referred to as 'merosin-deficient' CMD. The $\alpha2$-chain may be absent (Fig. 13.16), may show slight traces or may show partial expression. Laminin-$\alpha2$ is a large protein, and antibodies to more than one region may be required to assess the expression, particularly in those with partial expression (Sewry et al., 1997b). A secondary reduction of laminin occurs in Fukuyama CMD but localization studies of the recently identified gene product have not yet been reported. A secondary reduction of laminin $\alpha2$-chain also occurs in muscle–eye–brain disease and in an early onset form linked to chromosome 1q (Brockington et al., 2000). Secondary abnormalities in other laminin chains, in particular the $\alpha5$- and $\beta2$-chains, have also been reported in the various forms of CMD (Sewry and Muntoni, 1999).

As the laminin $\alpha2$-chain is expressed in tissues other than skeletal muscle, immunocytochemical studies of skin are useful for diagnosis (Fig. 13.16), and chorionic villus samples for prenatal diagnosis (Muntoni et al., 1995; Sewry et al., 1996, 1997a; Naom et al., 1997).

Myotonic dystrophy

Selective type I atrophy is a distinctive feature of myotonic dystrophy, and this may occur with type II hypertrophy, particularly in early stages of the disease. Moth-eaten fibres may be present and ring fibres and sarcoplasmic masses are common. Internal nuclei are often excessive

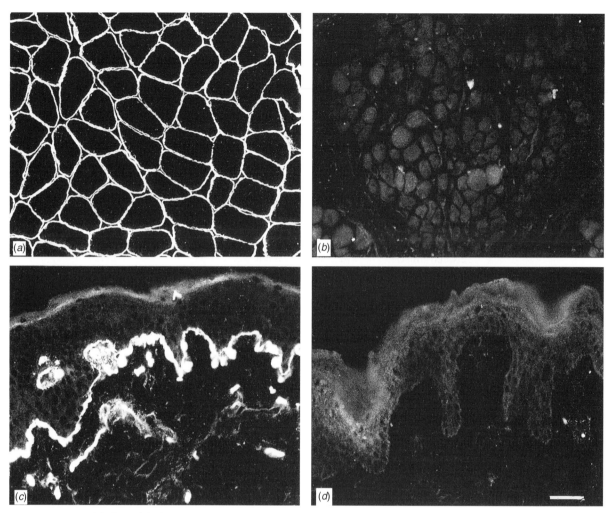

Fig. 13.16. Immunolabelling of the laminin α2-chain in muscle (*a*) and skin (*c*) from a normal individual and muscle (*b*) and skin (*d*) from a patient with congenital muscular dystrophy linked to chromosome 6q. Note the absence of laminin-α2 on the muscle fibres in (*b*) and its absence at the epidermal/dermal junction in (*d*). Bar = 50 μm.

and in young patients these may be central, causing confusion with myotubular myopathy. Genetic advances in both these disorders now make an accurate distinction easier, but studies of the defective gene product in myotonic dystrophy are not yet of diagnositic value.

Other muscular dystrophies

Studies of biopsies in other dystrophies, such as oculopharyngeal dystrophy and tibial muscular dystrophy, rely on conventional histological and histochemical studies, in particular, on the identification and localization of specific filamentous inclusions using the electron microscope (Griggs and Markesbury, 1994; Tomé and Fardeau, 1994). As more gene products are identified immunocytochemistry will have a greater role.

Congenital myopathies

The congenital myopathies are a heterogeneous group of disorders each of which is characterized by an abundance of a structural abnormality. Some of these abnormalities are not apparent with routine histological stains and are demonstrated by histochemical techniques. As more protein defects are identified, immunocytochemistry will have an increasing role, but it may be of less value in dominantly inherited disorders.

Nemaline myopathy

The characteristic feature in nemaline myopathy is the presence in many fibres of rod shaped structures that stain red with the modified Gomori trichrome technique. Clinically different forms with onset at birth, in infancy or in adulthood have been identified, and at least three different genes have been shown to be responsible (Wallgren-Pettersson et al., 1998). The gene for slow α-tropomyosin (chromosome 1q) is responsible for a rare dominant form, and a homozygous case has also been identified (Laing et al., 1995). Mutations in nebulin (chromosome 2q) occur in infantile cases (Pelin et al., 1999), and recently mutations in the actin gene have been found in both severe neonatal cases and milder cases with later onset (Nowak et al., 1999). Muscle biopsies may show no differentiation of fibre types, with all fibres staining as type I fibres, or there may be a bimodal distribution with atrophic type I fibres and larger type II fibres. In these latter patients the rods are often confined to the atrophic type I fibres. It is not yet clear if these patterns are associated with a specific genotype. The number of rods can vary between muscles and within a muscle. Rods label with antibodies to α-actinin. They are thought to be derived from Z lines, as they have a similar lattice structure and often show continuity with them. Immunocytochemical studies of patients with recessive disease with nebulin mutations do not show an absence of the protein, but differences in labelling can be seen. The data suggest different isoforms of this giant protein may be involved (Pelin et al., 1999). Desmin is located at the periphery of rods but not in them. The mutations in the actin gene that have so far been found are mainly dominant and several of the patients are severely affected, with some notable exceptions (Nowak et al., 1999). In patients who have nemaline rods, no significant abnormalities in actin localization has been observed, but actin accumulation occurred in the neonatal patients with severe disease identified by Goebel et al. (1997). Most rods are cytoplasmic but a few unusual cases with intranuclear rods have been reported; α-actinin and actin both localize to intranuclear rods (Goebel and Warlo, 1997; Goebel et al., 1997).

Central core disease

Central core disease is characterized by clearly delineated areas that lack oxidative enzyme staining in many fibres. They may also be apparent with histological stains such as the Gomori trichrome, when the absence of mitochondria in the cores is seen. The cores are usually central and single but they can also be eccentic, peripheral and multiple. They consistently affect type I fibres and in some patients the muscle appears undifferentiated, being composed entirely, or almost entirely, of type I fibres. ATPase staining and electron microscopy distinguish two types of core, according to the degree of myofibrillar disruption (Neville and Brooke, 1973; Sewry, 1985). 'Structured' cores retain their myofibrillar striations, although they may be very contracted, and ATPase activity is still present.

'Unstructured' cores show severe myofibrillar disruption and lack ATPase activity. In central core disease, the core area is extensive and runs most of the way down a fibre. This is in contrast to focal minicores (see below). Some patients have been found to have a mutation in the gene encoding the ryanodine receptor on chromosome 19q13, one of the genes responsible for malignant hyperthermia. Those with central core disease are, therefore, at risk for reaction to anaesthetics.

Immunocytochemical studies with antibodies to myofibrillar proteins often do not reveal the cores, probably because the myofibrils are present, albeit disrupted (Sewry, 1998). There are no reports on the expression of the ryanodine receptor in muscle biopsies from those with known mutations, but as inheritance is usually dominant and unlikely to result in an absence of protein, abnormalities may not be detected immunocytochemically.

Minicore disease (multicore disease)

Minicore disease is characterized by multifocal areas that are devoid of oxidative enzyme activity and have severely disrupted myofibrils. The size of the minicores is variable, but they do not run the length of the fibre. Variation in fibre size is often a feature, and internal nuclei, which may be central, are common. Type I fibre predominance is another frequent feature (Jungbluth et al., 1999).

Myotubular myopathy (centronuclear myopathy)

Myotubular myopathy takes it name from the resemblance of fibres with central nuclei to fetal myotubes. The more descriptive term of centronuclear myopathy was introduced as the fibres do not have all the properties of myotubes. There are clinically and genetically distinct forms, and the severe X-linked form has been shown to be caused by a defect in the gene for a protein kinase, myotubularin (Wallgren-Pettersson, 1998). There are no published reports on the localization of myotubularin in muscle biopsies. The common feature of all forms is the presence of central nuclei, although the number of affected fibres may vary between individuals, different muscles and with age (van der Ven et al., 1991; Helliwell et al., 1998). In longitudinal section, the central nuclei are regularly arranged down the length of the fibre and are interspersed with sarcoplasm. The number of central nuclei observed in transverse section is thus dependent on the plane of section. The central region shows aggregation of oxidative enzyme activity, often with a clear halo, and an absence of ATPase activity. Radial deposition of oxidative enzyme stain and glycogen may also be seen and type I fibre predominance is common.

Immunocytochemistry has shown accumulation of

desmin and vimentin and it has been suggested that this reflects a delay in maturation (Sarnat, 1990). There is no generalized arrest in development, however, and the expression of myofibrillar proteins and NCAM is normal (Soussi-Yanicostas et al., 1991; Figarella-Branger et al., 1992). In particular, the fibres with central nuclei do not express embryonic or fetal isoforms of myosin (Fig. 13.17) (van der Ven et al., 1991; Sewry, 1998). Fibres with slow myosin may be predominant, particularly in older patients (Sewry, 1998).

Centronuclear myopathy with type I hypotrophy

Engel et al. (1968) reported an 11-month-old child with severe and progressive weakness, whose muscle had profuse central nuclei, restricted to type I fibres, and also type I fibres that were small in diameter. They suggested that this might represent a maturational arrest, or 'hypotrophy' of the type I fibres rather than an atrophy (Fig. 13.18). Further patients with milder clinical involvement but a similar biopsy picture have been reported by Bethlem et al. (1969), Karpati et al. (1970) and Dubowitz (1985). It is not yet clear if these patients have a variant of myotubular myopathy, or if a different pathogenesis is involved.

Congenital fibre type disproportion

It is not clear if congenital fibre type disproportion represents a clinically distinct disorder or if it is merely a non-specific pathological feature. In normal muscle, type I and II fibres are of approximately equal diameter; however, patients have been described in which type I fibres were noted to be much smaller than type II. Brooke (1973) subsequently delineated a clinical picture associated with this that presented with hypotonia at birth, or in early infancy, and had a benign course. The only abnormality on biopsy is disproportion in size of the fibre types, with striking and uniform atrophy of the type I fibres and normal-sized or enlarged type II fibres. Type I fibres are frequently predominant. This condition has to be distinguished from myotonic dystrophy and myotubular myopathy with type I fibre atrophy, which also present with hypotonia and weakness in early infancy (Dubowitz, 1995), and from the early stage of infantile spinal muscular atrophy (Werdnig–Hoffmann disease) (Dubowitz, 1995).

Congenital myopathies with abnormal ultrastructural inclusions

Certain ultrastructural features have been shown to characterize other congenital myopathies (Goebel and Anderson, 1999). These include fingerprint body myopathy, sarcotubular myopathy, zebra body myopathy, reducing body myopathy, trilaminar muscle fibre disease and

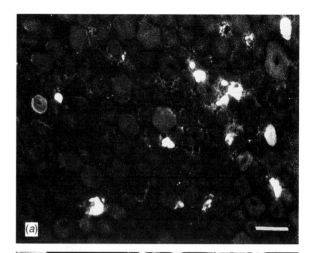

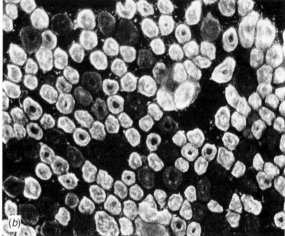

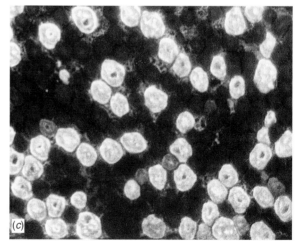

Fig. 13.17. Serial sections of muscle from a patient with X-linked myotubular myopathy immunolabelled with antibodies to (a) fetal myosin, (b) slow myosin and (c) fast myosin. Note the absence of fetal myosin from most fibres, even those with central nuclei (position of these corresponds to the central holes), and the predominance of fibres with slow myosin. Bar = 50 μm.

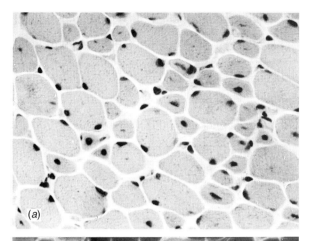

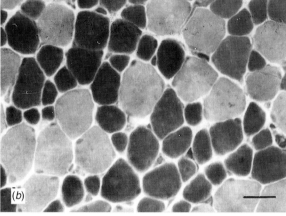

Fig. 13.18. Muscle from a female with type I hypotrophy/myotubular myopathy stained with (*a*) haematoxylin and eosin and (*b*) myosin ATPase pH 4.3. Note the central nuclei in the small fibres, which are mainly type I. Bar = 25 μm.

cap disease. Abnormalities are usually anticipated from routine histological stains, and histochemically may show disturbances in fibre size and fibre typing, in particular a predominance of type I fibres. Occasionally, more than one structural defect may occur, such as cytoplasmic bodies and reducing bodies, or tubular aggregates with central cores. A few immunocytochemical studies have been performed, including the association of desmin with some structural defects such as cytoplasmic bodies and Mallory-like bodies and the presence of some myofibrillar proteins such as tropomyosin and α-actinin (Goebel and Anderson, 1999).

Neurogenic disorders

Denervation and reinnervation is reflected in muscle biopsies by the presence of atrophic fibres associated with fibres of normal or enlarged size (see Fig. 13.1*d*) and by fibre type grouping, where large groups of fibres of one histochemical type occur alongside groups of the other type. The atrophic fibres may be present in large or small groups and are of both histochemical fibre types. The larger fibres are often uniform in type, which, like fibre type grouping, is thought to result from re-innervation of previously denervated fibres by surviving terminal axons that have sprouted. Small angulated fibres that are intensely stained with oxidative enzymes are also a feature of denervated muscle. These fibres vary in their ATPase activity and may be of either type.

Other pathological features of neurogenic disorders include split fibres, moth-eaten fibres and 'target' fibres or fibres with cores. In motor neuron disease, the degree of pathological change is variable and there is no correlation with age or severity. Froes et al. (1987) suggested that changes in females may be more severe. Studies of myosin heavy chain expression in chronic neuropathies and motor neuron disease have shown that fast and slow isoforms can occur together in some fibres. This was thought to be the result of neurally directed fibre type transformations, but there is no conclusive evidence for this and it is a common feature in most neuromuscular disorders. In addition, a small population of fibres that express fetal myosin may occur and may represent attempts at regeneration.

Spinal muscular atrophy

The most common form of spinal muscular atrophy maps to chromosome 5q11–q13. The most consistent defect is a deletion in the telomeric copy of the survival motor neuron (SMN) gene, although other genes in the locus have been implicated. Studies of the SMN protein are still at a developing stage. Three groups of patients are defined on the basis of clinical severity. The pathology in those with the severe infantile form (type I, Werdnig–Hoffmann disease) is similar to that in those with the intermediate type II, irrespective of the degree of weakness. It is usual to see large groups of atrophic fibres, although occasionally the grouping is not visible as all the fibres are atrophic. The small fibres are rounded and of both fibre types, although many often stain as type II fibres at pH 9.4 (Dubowitz, 1995). The larger fibres may occur singly or in groups and are often hypertrophic. They usually have uniform enzyme activity and stain as type I fibres, although occasional larger type II fibres may be present.

Immunocytochemistry shows that the larger fibres usually express exclusively slow myosin but that the small fibres co-express fast, slow and fetal myosin in various combinations (Fig. 13.19) (Sewry, 1989; Soussi-Yanicostas et al., 1992). Similar results are obtained with antibodies to

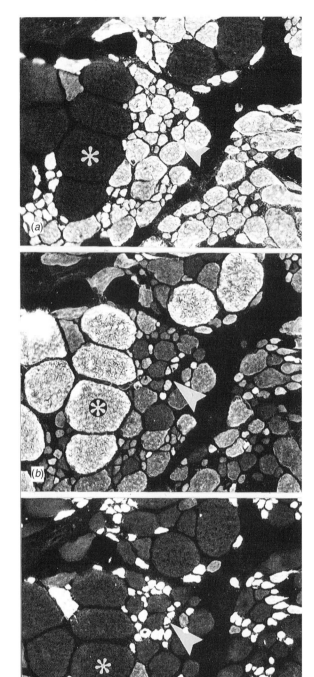

Fig. 13.19. Serial sections of muscle from a patient with spinal muscular atrophy. The sections are immunolabelled with antibodies to (a) fetal myosin, (b) slow myosin and (c) fast myosin. Note that the large fibres only express slow myosin (*) and many of the small fibres co-express all three isoforms (arrowheads). Bar = 50 μm.

troponin 1 isoforms (Dhoot and Pearce, 1984). The presence of fetal myosin in the atrophic fibres suggests that may be denervated before they are fully mature, but there does not seem to be a general arrest in maturation as other developmentally regulated proteins such as desmin, vimentin and titin are only detected in some atrophic fibres (Sewry, 1989; Soussi-Yanicostas et al., 1992). The expression of these proteins may be the result of regeneration. It is interesting to note that NCAM, which is usually extrajunctional on noninnervated fibres, is not uniformly expressed on all the atrophic fibres and is only observed on the fibres with higher levels of desmin (Sewry, 1989).

In patients with milder forms of spinal muscular atrophy (type III, Kugelberg–Welander disease), there may be less atrophy and grouping by fibre type. The extent of the atrophy varies and it is not possible to prognosticate on the basis of the findings in the muscle biopsy. In those with Kugelberg–Welander disease of longer duration, structural changes in the larger fibres may occur, such as whorled fibres or disruption of the myofibrillar network. Internal nuclei may also be a feature of the larger fibres; sometimes connective tissue may be increased. The similarity of these features to those in muscular dystrophies may be misleading when interpreting a biopsy.

Metabolic myopathies

Glycogenoses
Many enzyme defects in the pathway of glycogen synthesis and breakdown have been identified (DiMauro and Bruno, 1998) and a number of the genes responsible characterized (see the gene tables in every issue of *Neuromuscular Disorders*). They may affect skeletal muscle alone or be part of a multisystem disease.

Type II glycogenosis (Pompe's disease, acid maltase deficiency)
Childhood, infantile and adult forms of type II glycogenosis are recognized (Dubowitz, 1995; Hilton-Jones et al., 1995). Biopsies characteristically show vacuolation and excess glycogen, and this can also be demonstrated in lymphocytes. The vacuolated fibres also show high activity of acid phosphatase.

Type III glycogenosis (debranching enzyme deficiency)
Type III glycogenosis is characterized by an abnormal form of glycogen (amylopectin) in cardiac and skeletal muscle and in the liver, owing to the absence of amylo-1,6-glucosidase. Muscle biopsies may show few abnormalities (Dubowitz, 1995) but vacuolation and accumulation of glycogen can occur (Hilton-Jones et al., 1995). The PAS stain

shows a moderately strong reaction but differentiation of fibre types may be retained.

Type V glycogenosis (myophosphorylase deficiency)

Pathological changes in muscle biopsies are mild in type V glycogenosis although occasional necrotic fibres may be present. The consistent findings are an absence of phosphorylase enzyme activity and excess glycogen on PAS staining. The excess glycogen is often subsarcolemmal and may give a vacuolar appearance with histological stains. Three isoforms of phosphorylase exist and McArdle's disease is caused by mutations in the gene for the muscle form on chromosome 11q. Histochemical staining for phosphorylase, therefore, shows staining of the smooth muscle in blood vessels and staining of regenerating fibres, because of the presence of other isoforms.

Type VII glycogenosis (Tarui's disease)

The histological changes in type VII glycogenosis are similar to those of McArdle's disease, and the absence of phosphofructokinase can be demonstrated histochemically (Bonilla and Schotland, 1970). There have been rare cases in which phosphorylase or phosphofructokinase deficiency have been found together with another enzyme defect, that of myoadenylate deaminase (DiMauro and Bruno, 1998).

Other glycogenosis

Muscle biopsies in other glycogenoses show little, or no, abnormality and the enzyme defects cannot be demonstrated histochemically. Immunocytochemistry is of limited value in many metabolic disorders, particularly if an enzyme has inactive isoforms. Demonstration of the activity of the enzyme is then more important than detection of the presence of one or more isoforms.

Lipid storage myopathies

Excess lipid droplets in muscle fibres is a common feature of carnitine deficiency. Histological stains may also indicate where the lipid is located and give a 'vacuolated' appearance. Other disorders of lipid metabolism, such as deficiency of carnitine palmitiyltransferase and medium-chain acyl-CoA dehydrogenase may show some excess lipid in the muscle biopsy, but often no significant abnormality is seen. Lipid levels are higher in type I fibres in normal muscle, but the excess lipid in carnitine deficiency, which is often greater in type I fibres than type II, is clearly distinguishable. Excess lipid may also be seen in fibres in a variety of myopathies in which there is no evidence of a primary metabolic dysfunction.

Mitochondrial myopathies

Abnormal mitochondria in skeletal muscle are a feature of several multisystem disorders. The identification of causative deletions, depletions or duplications in the maternally inherited mitochondrial DNA, or in related nuclear-derived factors, has escalated in recent years (see the genes table in each issue of *Neuromuscular Disorders*). The ultrastructural changes in mitochondria are varied and not specific (Sewry, 1985), and no specific structural abnormality has been associated with a particular mitochondrial disorder. Mitochondrial abnormalities may be overlooked on routine histological staining, although some increased granularity may be seen with haematoxylin and eosin, and Verhoeff–van Gieson stains. Their presence becomes obvious when disrupted, red-staining fibres (ragged-red fibres) are seen with the Gomori trichrome stain and the oxidative enzyme preparations show strongly reactive fibres. Increased activity may be restricted to the periphery of the fibre but normal muscle fibres may show accumulations of peripheral mitochondria and should not be confused with ragged-red fibres. Electron microscopy confirms the presence of an abnormality in the number, size and structure of the mitochondria. Ragged-red fibres are not a consistent feature of mitochondrial myopathies, and ultrastructural abnormalities may also be absent. Absence of COX in some fibres and presence of ragged-red fibres occurs in most patients with mitochondrial DNA deletions, and mitochondrial encephalopathies, although this can occur in other situations (Johnson et al., 1988; Holt et al., 1989; Nonaka, 1992; Rifai et al., 1995). The fibres with no staining for COX have high SDH activity that often, but not always, corresponds to the ragged-red fibres.

Deficiencies in COX can be demonstrated immunocytochemically with antibodies to both the mitochondrial (I–III) and nuclear (IV–VIII) encoded subunits (Johnson et al., 1988). Antibodies can distinguish between the fatal, infantile form of COX deficiency and the benign, spontaneously remitting myopathy (Tritschler et al., 1992).

Inflammatory myopathies

The classic feature of the inflammatory myopathies (dermatomyositis, polymyositis and inclusion body myositis) is the marked inflammatory response, but this is not specific and can occur in other myopathies, including the muscular dystrophies. Inflammation may be absent in inflammatory myopathies, and the muscle biopsy may show little or no morphological change. Cathepsin D has been identified immunocytochemically in interstitial cells and in invading phagocytes (Whitaker et al., 1983) but most interest has centred around the distribution and proportion of T cell subsets, B cells and macrophages (Arahata and Engel, 1984, 1988a,b; Engel and Arahata, 1984). No differences have been found in the proportion of T cell subsets in peripheral blood (Iyer et al., 1983), but in muscle the proportion of suppressor/cytotoxic (CD8) and helper/inducer (CD4) phenotypes and B cells varies between endomysial and perivascular areas. T cells, particularly CD8+ T cells, are more prevalent in the endomysial than in perivascular areas, but the reverse occurs with B cells. In polymyositis and inclusion body myositis, but not in dermatomyositis, CD8+ T cells accompanied by macrophages invade apparently non-necrotic fibres and the cytotoxic phenotype predominants (Arahata and Engel, 1988a). This has been put forward as evidence of cell-mediated muscle fibre injury in polymyositis and inclusion body myositis. Many of the infiltrating cells are HLA-DR positive and, therefore, considered to be activated. Most CD8+ T cells use the α/β-receptor for antigen recognition but a second T-cell type that expresses a γ/δ-receptor has been identified. These two populations of T cells can be distinguished immunocytochemically but the γ/δ-type is rare (Hohlfeld et al., 1991).

Atrophy of both fibre types occurs, but hypertrophy is rare in inflammatory myopathies. In dermatomyositis, the atrophy may have a characteristic perifascicular distribution. These perifascicular fibres may have characteristics of regenerating fibres, staining as type IIC fibres, and express proteins associated with immaturity such as fetal myosin, desmin, utrophin, MHC class I (Helliwell et al., 1992b; Dubowitz, 1995). Oxidative enzyme staining may show dark-centred fibres, in addition to moth-eaten fibres (Dubowitz, 1985). Vacuoles may be present, particularly in inclusion body myositis. Endomysial connective tissue is often not excessive, and in dermatomyositis the connective tissue is reactive for alkaline phosphatase (Engel and Cunningham, 1970).

Expression of MHC class I on mature fibres is a common feature of all types of inflammatory myopathy (Appleyard et al., 1985) and in some cases this may be the only detectable abnormality (Fig. 13.20) (Topaloglu et al., 1996). It may not be a universal feature and some areas of a biopsy may not express class I, but when present it is a useful diagnostic marker (Fig. 13.20).

The characteristic feature of both the sporadic and hereditary forms of inclusion body myositis is rimmed vacuoles. Intracytoplasmic and intranuclear 16–18 nm filaments are visible with electron microscopy. Rimmed vacuoles, however, can occur in other myopathies (Tomé and Fardeau, 1998). The filaments in inclusion body myositis differ from the nuclear filaments in oculopharygeal muscular dystrophy. Sporadic cases of inclusion body

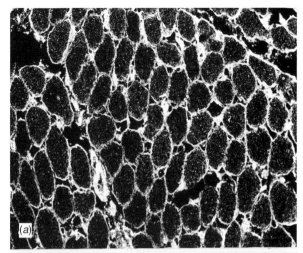
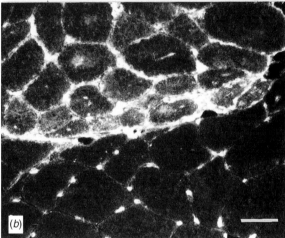

Fig. 13.20. Immunolabelling of MHC class I in muscle from two patients with dermatomyositis. Note the labelling of all fibres but minimal pathology in (a), but areas of labelled and unlabelled fibres in (b). Note also the normal labelling of capillaries in (b). Bar = 50 μm.

myositis usually involve inflammation and, therefore, differ pathologically from hereditary disease in which inflammation is rare (Tomé and Fardeau, 1998). Several proteins, many of which have also been found in the brain of patients with Alzheimer's disease, have been shown to be associated with the vacuoles (Askanas et al., 1998a). These include ubiquitin, β-amyloid, β-amyloid precursor protein, phosphorylated tau, prion protein, apolipoprotein E and presenilin 1 (Leclerc et al., 1993; Askanas et al., 1998a,b). Congophilia is also a feature of inclusion body myositis, particularly in sporadic disease. Fibres devoid of COX activity, ragged-red fibres and mitochondrial DNA deletions may occur and are more common in sporadic forms (Moslemi et al., 1997; Horvath et al., 1998).

Viruses have been implicated in the aetiology of poly-myositis, dermatomyositis (coxsackie virus B) and inclu-sion body myositis (paramyxovirus (mumps)) (Chou, 1986; Bowles et al., 1987), but results have been inconsistent and in situ hybridization studies have failed to localize these viruses in muscle biopsies of all patients.

Components of the complement pathway can be detected in necrotic muscle fibres (Engel and Biesecker, 1982) and on the surface of non-necrotic fibres (Sewry et al., 1987). In dermatomyositis, complement components are also observed in capillaries, and the number of capil-laries is reduced (Emslie-Smith and Engel, 1990).

Conclusions

Morphological studies of muscle have made a major contri-bution to the understanding of normal and diseased muscle. Histochemical techniques are essential for the eval-uation of muscle biopsies, and immunocytochemistry is proving to be of equal importance. The diagnositic role of immunocytochemistry, and the specificity that it offers, is rapidly increasing as more defective genes and their pro-teins are identified. Immunochemistry will continue to have a role in identifying primary protein defects and in unravell-ing the underlying cause of neuromuscular disorders.

References

Abraham, S. C., De Nofrio, D., Loh, E. et al. (1998). Desmin myopa-thy involving cardiac, skeletal, and vascular smooth muscle: report of a case with immunoelectron microscopy. *Hum. Pathol.* **29**, 876–882.

Anderson, L. V. B., Davidson, K., Moss, J. A. et al. (1998). Characterisation of monoclonal antibodies to calpain 3 and protein expression in muscle from patients with limb-girdle muscular dystrophy type 2A. *Am. J. Pathol.* **153**, 1169–1179.

Anderson, L. V. B., Davidson, K., Moss, J. A. et al. (1999). Dysferlin is a plasma membrane protein and is expressed early in human development. *Hum. Mol. Genet.* **8**, 855–861.

Appleyard, S. T., Dunn, M. J., Dubowitz, V., Scott, M. L., Pittman, S. J. and Shotton, D. M. (1984). Monoclonal antibodies detect a spectrin-like protein in normal and dystrophic human skeletal muscle. *Proc. Natl. Acad. Sci. USA* **81**, 776–780.

Appleyard, S. T., Dunn, M. J., Dubowitz, V. and Rose, M. L. (1985). Increased expression of HLA ABC class I antigens by muscle fibres in Duchenne muscular dystrophy, inflammatory myopa-thy and other neuromuscular disorders. *Lancet* **i**, 361–363.

Arahata, K. and Engel, A. G. (1984). Monoclonal antibody analysis of mononuclear cells in myopathies. I Quantitation of subsets according to diagnosis and sites of accumulation and demon-stration and counts of muscle fibers invaded by T cells. *Ann. Neurol.* **16**, 193–208.

Arahata, K. and Engel A. G. (1988a). Monoclonal antibody analysis of mononuclear cells in myopathies. IV: Cell-mediated cytotox-icity and muscle fiber necrosis. *Ann. Neurol.* **23**, 168–173.

Arahata, K. and Engel, A. G. (1988b). Monoclonal antibody analy-sis of mononuclear cells in myopathies. V: Identification and quantitation of T8$^+$ cytotoxic and T8$^+$ suppressor cells. *Ann. Neurol.* **23**, 493–499.

Arikawa, E., Ishihara, T., Nonaka, I., Sugita, H. and Arahata, K. (1991). Immunocytochemical analysis of dystrophin in congen-ital muscular dystrophy. *J. Neurol. Sci.* **105**, 79–87.

Askanas, V. A., Serratrice, G. and Engel, W. K. (1998a). *Inclusion Body Myositis and Myopathies.* Cambridge: Cambridge University Press.

Askanas, V., Engel, W. K., Yang, C. C., Alvarez, R. B., Lee, V. M. and Wisniewski, T. (1998b). Light and electron microscopic immu-nolocalisation of presenilin 1 in abnormal muscle fibers of patients with sporadic inclusion body myositis and autosomal-recessive inclusion-body myopathy. *Am. J. Pathol.* **152**, 889–895.

Baghdiguian, S., Martin, M., Richard, I. et al. (1999). Calpain 3 defi-ciency is associated with myonuclear apoptosis and profound pertubation of the IκBα/NF-κB pathway in limb-girdle muscu-lar dystrophy type 2A. *Nat. Med.* **5**, 503–511.

Bashir, R., Britton, S., Strachan, T. et al. (1998). A gene related to *Caenorhabditis elegans* spermatogenenesis factor fer-1 is mutated in limb-girdle muscular dystrophy type 2B. *Nat. Genet.* **20**, 37–42.

Bertolotto, A., Palmucci, L., Doriguzzi, C. et al. (1983). Laminin and fibronectin distribution in normal and pathological human muscle. *J. Neurol. Sci.* **60**, 377–382.

Bethlem, J., van Wijngaarden, G. K., Meijer, A. E. F. H. and Hülsmann, W. C. (1969). Neuromuscular disease with type 1 fiber atrophy, central nuclei, and myotube-like structures. *Neurology* **19**, 705–710.

Bione, S., Maestrini, E., Rivella, S. et al. (1994). Identification of a novel X-linked gene responsible for Emery–Dreifuss muscular dystrophy. *Nat. Genet.* **8**, 323–327.

Bonilla, E. and Schotland, D. L. (1970). Histochemical diagnosis of muscle phosphofructokinase deficiency. *Arch. Neurol. (Chicago)* **22**, 8–12.

Bonilla, E., Miranda, A. F., Prelle, A., et al. (1988). Immunocytochemical study of nebulin in Duchenne muscular dystrophy. *Neurology* **38**, 1600–1603.

Bonne, G., Di Barletta, M. R., Varnous, S. et al. (1999). Mutations in the gene encoding lamin A/C cause autosomal dominant Emery–Dreifuss muscular dystrophy. *Nat. Genet.* **21**, 285–288.

Bornemann, A. and Schmalbruch, H. (1992). Desmin and vimentin in regenerating fibers. *Muscle Nerve* **15**, 14–20.

Bowles, N. E., Dubowitz, V., Sewry, C. A. and Archard, L. C. (1987). Dermatomyositis, polymyositis, and coxsackie B virus infection. *Lancet* **i**, 1004–1007.

Bradley, W. G., Jones, M. Z., Mussini, J.-M. and Fawcett, P. R. (1978). Becker-type muscular dystrophy. *Muscle Nerve*, **1**, 111–132.

Brenman, J. E., Chao, D. S., Xia, H., Aldapa, K. and Bredt, D. S. (1995). Nitric oxide synthase complexed with dystrophin and absent from skeletal muscle sarcolemma in Duchenne muscular dystrophy. *Cell* **82**, 743–752.

Brockington, M., Sewry, C. A., Hermann, R., et al. (2000). Assignment of a form of congenital muscular dystrophy with secondary merosin deficiency to chromosome 1q42. *Am. J. Genet* **66**, 428–435.

Brown, S. C. and Lucy, J. A. (eds.) (1997). *Dystrophin: Gene, Protein and Cell Biology.* Cambridge: Cambridge University Press.

Brown, S. C., Muntoni, F. and Sewry, C. A. (2001). Sarcolemmal muscular dystrophies. *Brain Pathol.* **11**, 193–205.

Brooke, M. H. (1973). A neuromuscular disease characterized by fiber type disproportion. In: *Proceedings of 2nd International Congress on Muscle Disease*, ICS No. 237. ed. B. A. Kakulas. Amsterdam: Excerpta Medica.

Buckingham, M. E. (1985). Actin and myosin multigene family: their expression during the formation of skeletal muscle. *Essays Biochem.* **20**, 77–109.

Bushby, K. M. D. (1999). The limb-girdle muscular dystrophies (gene table). *Eur. J. Paed.Neurol.* **3**, 87–89.

Butler-Browne, G. S., Barbet, J. P. and Thornell, L. E. (1990). Myosin heavy and light chain expression during human skeletal muscle development and the precocious accumulation of the adult heavy chain isoforms by thyroid hormone. *Anat. Embryol.* **181**, 513–522.

Cashman, N. R., Covault, J., Wollman, R. L. and Sanes, J. R. (1987). Neural cell adhesion molecule in normal, denervated, and myopathic muscle. *Ann. Neurol.* **21**, 481–489.

Chou, S. M. (1986). Inclusion body myositis: a chronic persistent mumps myositis? *Hum. Pathol.* **17**, 765–777.

Clemens, P. R., Ward, P. A., Caskey, C. T., Bulman, D. E. and Fenwick, R. G. (1992). Premature chain termination causing Duchenne muscular dystrophy. *Neurology* **42**, 1755–1782.

Clerk, A., Rodillo, E., Heckmatt, J. Z., Dubowitz, V., Strong, P. N. and Sewry, C. A. (1991). Characterisation of dystrophin in carriers of Duchenne muscular dystrophy. *J. Neurol. Sci.* **102**, 197–205.

Clerk, A., Strong, P. N. and Sewry, C. A. (1992a). Characterisation of dystrophin during development of human skeletal muscle. *Development* **114**, 395–402.

Clerk, A., Dubowitz, V., Sewry, C. A. and Strong, P. N. (1992b). Characterisation of dystrophin in foetuses at risk for Duchenne muscular dystrophy. *J. Neurol. Sci.* **111**, 82–91.

Cooper, B. J., Gallagher, E. A., Smith, C. A., Valentine, B. A. and Winand, N. J. (1990). Mosaic expression of dystrophin in carriers of canine X-linked muscular dystrophy. *Lab. Invest.* **62**, 171–178.

Crosbie, R. H., Yanada, H., Venzke, D. P., Lisanti, M. and Campbell, K. P. (1998). Caveolin-3 is not an integral component of the dystrophin glycoprotein complex. *FEBS Lett.* **427**, 279–282.

Cullen, M. J., Fulthorpe, J. J. and Harris, J. B. (1992). The distribution of desmin and titin in normal and dystrophic human muscle. *Acta Neuropathol.* **83**, 158–169.

Dhoot, G. K. and Pearce, G. W. (1984). Changes in the distribution of fast and slow forms of troponin I in some neuromuscular disorders. *J. Neurol. Sci.* **65**, 1–15.

DiMauro, S. and Bruno C. (1998). Glycogen storage diseases of muscle. *Curr. Opin. Neurol.* **11**, 477–484.

Duance, V. C., Stephens, H. R., Dunn, M. J., Bailey, A. J. and Dubowitz, V. (1980). A role for collagen in the pathogenesis of muscular dystrophy? *Nature* **284**, 470–472.

Dubowitz, V. (1985). *Muscle Biopsy: A Practical Approach,* 2nd edn. London: Baillière Tindall.

Dubowitz, V. (1994). Workshop report: the 22nd ENMC sponsored workshop on congenital muscular dystrophy. *Neuromusc. Disord.* **4**, 75–81.

Dubowitz, V. (1995). *Muscle Disorders in Childhood*, 2nd edn. London: Saunders.

Dubowitz, V. (1998). What's in a name? Muscular dystrophy revisted. *Eur. J. Paed. Neurol.* **2**, 279–284.

Dubowitz, V. (1999). Workshop report: the 68th ENMC international workshop on congenital muscular dystrophy. *Neuromusc. Disord.* **9**, 446–454.

Dubowitz, V. and Pearse, A. G. E. (1961). Enzyme activity of normal and diseased human muscle: a histochemical study. *J. Pathol. Bacteriol.* **81**, 365–378.

Edwards, R. H. T., Round, J. M. and Jones, D. A. (1983). Needle biopsy of skeletal muscle: a review of 10 years' experience. *Muscle Nerve* **6**, 676–683.

Emery, A. E. H. (1993). *Duchenne Muscular Dystrophy*, 2nd edn. Oxford: Oxford University Press.

Emslie-Smith, A. M. and Engel, A. G. (1990). Microvascular changes in early and advanced dermatomyositis: a quantitative study. *Ann. Neurol.* **27**, 343–356.

Engel, A. G. and Arahata, K. (1984). Mononclonal antibody analysis of mononuclear cells in myopathies. II Phenotypes of autoinvasive cells in polymyositis and inclusion body myositis. *Ann. Neurol.* **16**, 209–215.

Engel, A. G. and Biesecker, G. (1982). Complement activation in muscle fiber necrosis: demonstration of the membrane attack complex of complement in necrotic fibers. *Ann. Neurol.* **12**, 289–296.

Engel, A. G., Lambert, E. H. and Howard, F. M. (1977). Immune complexes (IgG and C3) at the motor end-plate in myasthenia gravis. Ultrastructural and light microscopic localization and electrophysiologic correlations. *Mayo Clin. Proc.* **52**, 267–280.

Engel, W. K. and Cunningham, G. G. (1970). Alkaline phosphatase – positive abnormal muscle fibers of humans. *J. Histochem. Cytochem.* **18**, 55–57.

Engel, W. K., Gold, G. N. and Karpati, G. (1968). Type I fiber hypotrophy and central nuclei. A rare congenital muscle abnormality with a possible experimental model. *Arch. Neurol. (Chicago)* **18**, 435–444.

Evans, M. I., Hoffman, E. P., Cadrin, C., Johnson, M. P., Quintero, R. A. and Golbus, M. S. (1994). Fetal muscle biopsy: collaborative experience with varied indications. *Obstet. Gynecol.* **84**, 913–917.

Evered, D. and Whealan, J. (eds.) (1988). *Plasticity of the Neuromuscular System.* Ciba Foundation Symposium 138. Chichester: Wiley.

Fanin, M., Danieli, G. A., Vitiello, L., Senter, L. and Angelini, C. (1992). Prevalence of dystrophin positive fibers in 85 Duchenne muscular dystrophy patients. *Neuromusc. Disord.* **2**, 41–45.

Figarella-Branger, D., Nedelec, J., Pellisier, J. F., Boucraut, J., Bianco, N. and Rougon G. (1990). Expression of various isoforms of neural cell adhesive molecules and their highly polysialylated counterparts in diseased human muscles. *J. Neurol. Sci.* **98**, 21–36.

Figarella-Branger, D., Calore, E. E., Boucraut, J., Bianco, N., Rougon, G. and Pellissier, J. F. (1992). Expression of cell surface and cytoskeleton developmentally regulated proteins in adult centronuclear myopathies. *J. Neurol. Sci.* **109**, 69–76.

Froes, M. M. Q., Kristmundsdottir, F., Mahon, M. and Cumming, W. J. K. (1987). Muscle morphometry in motor neurone disease. *Neuropathol. Appl. Neurobiol.* **13**, 405–419.

Fürst, D., Nave, R., Osborn, M. et al (1987). Nebulin and titin expression in Duchenne muscular dystrophy appears normal. *FEBS Lett.* **224**, 49–53.

Gangopadhyay, S. B., Sherratt, T. G., Heckmatt, J. Z. et al. (1992). Dystrophin in frame shift deletion patients with Becker muscular dystrophy. *Am. J. Hum. Genet.* **51**, 562–570.

Goebel, H. H. and Anderson, J. R. (1999). Workshop report: the 56th ENMC sponsored international workshop on structural congenital myopathies (excluding nemaline myopathy, myotubular myopathy, and desminopathies). *Neuromusc. Disord.* **9**, 50–57.

Goebel, H. H. and Warlo, I. (1997). Nemaline myopathy with intranuclear rods – intranuclear rod myopathy. *Neuromusc. Disord.* **7**, 13–19.

Goebel, H. H., Anderson, J. R., Hubner, C., Oexle, K. and Warlo, I. (1997). Congenital myopathy with excess of thin filaments. *Neuromusc. Disord.* **7**, 160–168.

Goldfarb, L. G., Park, K. Y., Cervenakova, L. et al. (1998). Missense mutation in desmin associated with familial cardiac and skeletal myopathy. *Nat. Genet.* **19**, 402–403.

Gregorio, C. C., Granzier, H., Sorimachi, H. and Labiet, S. (1999). Muscle assembly: a titanic achievement? *Curr. Opin. Cell Biol.* **11**, 18–25.

Griggs, R. C. and Markesbery, W. R. (1994). Distal myopathies. In: *Myology*, 2nd edn, Vol. 2, eds. A. G. Engel and C. Franzi-Armstrong, pp. 1246–1257. New York: McGraw-Hill.

Guerard, M. J., Sewry, C. A. and Dubowitz, V. (1985). Lobulated fibres in neuromuscular diseases. *J. Neurol. Sci.* **69**, 345–356.

Heckmatt, J. Z., Moosa, A., Hutson, C., Maunder-Sewry, C. A. and Dubowitz, V. (1984). Diagnostic needle muscle biopsy: a practical and reliable alternative to open biopsy. *Arch. Dis. Child.* **59**, 528–532.

Helliwell, T. R., Gunhan, O. and Edwards, R. H. T. (1989). Lectin binding and desmin necrosis, regeneration, and neurogenic atrophy of human skeletal muscle. *J. Pathol.* **159**, 43–51.

Helliwell, T. R., Ellis, J. M., Mountford, R. C., Appleton, R. E. and Morris, G. E. (1992a). A truncated dystrophin lacking the C-terminal domain is localized at the muscle membrane. *Am. J. Hum. Genet.* **50**, 508–514

Helliwell, T. R., Nguyen thi Man, Morris, G. E. and Davies, K. E. (1992b). The dystrophin-related protein, utrophin, is expressed on the sarcolemma of regenerating human skeletal muscle fibres in dystrophies and inflammatory myopathies. *Neuromusc. Disord.* **2**, 177–184.

Helliwell, T. R., Ellis, I. H. and Appleton, R. E. (1998). Myotubular myopathy: morphological, immunocytochemical and clinical variation. *Neuromusc. Disord.* **8**, 152–161.

Hilton-Jones, D., Squier, M., Taylor, D. and Matthews, P. (1995). *Metabolic Myopathies.* London: Saunders

Hoffman, E. P., Arahata, K., Minetti, C., Bonilla, E. and Rowland, L. P. (1992). Dystrophinopathy in isolated cases of myopathy in females. *Neurology* **42**, 967–975.

Hohlfeld, R. and Engel, A. G. (1990). Induction of HLA-DR expression on human myoblasts with interferon-gamma. *Am. J. Pathol.* **136**, 503–508.

Hohlfeld, R., Engel, A. G., Ii, K. and Harper, M. C. (1991). polymyositis mediated by T lymphocytes that express the gamma/delta receptor. *N. Eng. J. Med.* **324**, 877–881.

Holt, I. J., Harding, A. E., Cooper, J. M. et al. (1989). Mitochondrial myopathies: clinical and biochemical features of 30 patients with major deletions of muscle mitochondrial DNA. *Ann. Neurol.* **26**, 699–708.

Horvath, R., Fu, K., Johns, T., Genge, A., Karpati, G. and Shoubridge, E. A. (1998). Characterization of the mitochondrial DNA abnormalities in the skeletal muscle of patients with inclusion body myositis. *J. Neuropathol. Exp. Neurol.* **57**, 396–403.

Isenberg, D. A. (1983). Immunoglobulin deposition in skeletal muscle in primary muscle disease. *Q. J. Med.* **207**, 297–310.

Iyer, V., Lawton, A. R. and Fenichel, G. M. (1983). T-cell subsets in polymyositis. *Ann. Neurol.* **13**, 452–453.

Izumo, S., Nadal-Ginard, B. and Mahdavi, V. (1986). All members of the MHC multigene family respond to thyroid hormone in a highly tissue-specific manner. *Science* **231**, 597–600.

Johnson, M. A., Polgar, J., Weightman, D. and Appleton, D. (1973). Data on the distribution of fibre types in 36 human muscles. An autopsy study. *J. Neurol. Sci.* **18**, 111–129.

Johnson, M. A., Kadenback, B., Droste, M., Old, S. L. and Turnbull, D. M. (1988). Immunocytochemical studies of cytochrome oxidase subunits in skeletal muscle of patients with partial cytochrome oxidase deficiency. *J. Neurol. Sci.* **87**, 75–90.

Jungbluth, H., Sewry, C. A., Brown, S. et al. (1999). Minicore myopathy in children; a clininal and histopathological study of 19 cases. *Neuromusc. Disord.* **10**, 264–273.

Karpati, G., Carpenter, S. and Nelson, R. F. (1970). Type I muscle fibre atrophy and central nuclei. A rare familial neuromuscular disease. *J. Neurol. Sci.* **10**, 489–500.

Karpati, G., Zubrzycka-Gaarn, E. E., Carpenter, S., Bulman, D. E., Ray, P. N. and Worton, R. G. (1990). Age-related conversion of dystrophin-negative to positive fiber segments of skeletal but not cardiac muscle fibres in heterozygote *mdx* mice. *J. Neuropathol. Exp. Neurol.* **49**, 96–105.

Kuller, J. A., Hoffman, E. P., Fries, M. H. and Globus, M. S. (1992). Prenatal diagnosis of Duchenne muscular dystrophy by fetal muscle biopsy. *Hum. Genet.* **90**, 34–40.

Laing, N. G., Wilton, S. D., Akkari, P. A. et al. (1995). A mutation in the alpha-tropomyosin gene TPM3 associated with autosomal dominant nemaline myopathy NEM1. *Nat. Genet.* **9**, 75–79.

Lazarides, E. (1980). Intermediate filaments as mechanical integrators of cellular space. *Nature* **283**, 249–256.

Lazarides, E. and Hubbard, R. D. (1976). Immunological characterization of the subunit of the 100 Å-filaments from muscle cells. *Proc. Natl. Acad. Sci. USA* **73**, 4344–4348.

Leclerc, A., Tomé, F. M. S. and Fardeau, F. (1993). Ubiquitin and *β*-amyloid protein in inclusion body myositis (IBM), familial IBM-like disorder and oculopharyngeal muscular dystrophy: an immunocytochemical study. *Neuromusc. Disord.* **3**, 283–292.

Lim, L. E. and Campbell, K. P. (1998). The sarcoglycan complex in limb-girdle muscular dystrophy. *Curr. Opin. Neurol.* **11**, 443–452.

Liu, J., Aoki, M., Illa, I. et al. (1998). Dysferlin, a novel skeletal muscular gene, is mutated in Miyoshi myopathy and limb-girdle muscular dystrophy. *Nat. Genet.* **21**, 31–36.

Lobrinus, J. A., Janzer, R. C., Kuntzer, T. et al. (1998). Familial cardiomyopathy and distal myopathy with abnormal desmin accumulation and migration. *Neuromusc. Disord.* **8**, 77–86.

Manilal, S., Nguyen thi Man, Sewry, C. and Morris, G. E. (1996). The Emery–Dreifuss muscular dystrophy protein, emerin, is a nuclear membrane protein. *Hum. Mol. Genet.* **5**, 801–808.

Manilal, S., Sewry, C. A., Nguyen thi Man, N., Muntoni, F. and Morris, G. E. (1997). Diagnosis of X-linked Emery–Dreifuss muscular dystrophy by protein analysis of leukocytes and skin. *Neuromusc. Disord.* **7**, 63–66.

Manilal, S., Recan, D., Sewry, C. A. et al. (1998). Mutations in Emery–Dreifuss muscular dystrophy and their effects on emerin protein expression. *Hum. Mol. Genet.* **7**, 855–864.

Marini, J.-F., Pons, F., Léger, J. et al. (1991). Expression of myosin heavy chain isoforms in Duchenne muscular dystrophy patients and carriers. *Neuromusc. Disord.* **1**, 397–409.

Matsumura, K., Shimizu, T., Nonaka, I. and Mannen, T. (1989). Immunocytochemical study of connectin (titin) in neuromuscular diseases using a monoclonal antibody: connectin is degraded extensively in Duchenne muscular dystrophy. *J. Neurol. Sci.* **93**, 147–156.

Matsumura, K., Nonaka, I. and Campbell, K. P. (1993). Abnormal expression of dystrophin-associated proteins in Fukuyama-type congenital muscular dystrophy. *Lancet* **341**, 521–522.

McDouall, R. M., Dunn, M. J. and Dubowitz, V. (1989). Expression of class I and II MHC antigens in neuromuscular diseases. *J. Neurol. Sci.* **89**, 213–226.

Merlini, L., Villanova, M., Sabatelli, P., Malandrini, A. and Maraldi, N. M. (1999). Decreased expression of laminin *β*1 in chromosome 21–linked Bethlem myopathy. *Neuromusc. Disord.* **9**, 326–329.

Metzinger, L., Blake, D. J., Squier, M. et al. (1997). Dystrobrevin deficiency at the sarcolemma of patients with muscular dystrophy. *Hum. Mol. Genet.* **6**, 1185–1191.

Mian, L., Dickson, D. W. and Spiro, A. J. (1997). Abnormal expression of laminin *β*1 chain in skeletal muscle of adult-onset limb-girdle muscular dystrophy. *Arch. Neurol.* **54**, 1457–1461.

Millevoi, S., Trombitas, K., Kolmerer, B. et al. (1998). Characterization of nebulette and nebulin and emerging concepts of their role for vertebrate Z-discs. *J. Mol. Biol.* **282**, 111–123.

Minetti, C., Sotgia, F., Bruno, C. et al. (1998a). Mutations in the caveolin-3 gene cause autosomal dominant limb-girdle muscular dystrophy. *Nat. Genet.* **18**, 365–368.

Minetti, C., Sotgia, F., Bruno, C. et al. (1998b). Autosomal dominant limn-girdle muscular dystrophy with caveolin-3 deficiency caused by mutation in the caveolin-3 gene. *Muscle Nerve* (Suppl. 7): S135.

Mogensen, J., Klausen, I. C., Pederson, A. K. et al. (1999). Alpha-cardiac actin is a novel disease gene in familial hypertrophic cardiomyopathy. *J. Clin. Invest.* **103**, R39–R43.

Morgan, B. P., Sewry, C. A., Siddle, K., Luzio, J. P. and Campbell, A. K. (1984). Immunolocalization of complement component C9 on necrotic and non-necrotic muscle fibres in myositis using monoclonal antibodies: a primary role of complement in auto-immune cell damage. *Immunology* **52**, 181–188.

Moslemi, A. R., Lindberg, C. and Oldfors, A. (1997). Analysis of multiple mitochondrial DNA deletions in inclusion body myositis. *Hum. Mutat.* **10**, 381–386.

Munoz-Marmoi, A. M., Strasser, G., Isamat, M. et al. (1998). A dysfunctional desmin mutation in a patient with severe generalized myopathy. *Proc. Natl. Acad. Sci. USA* **95**, 11312–11317.

Muntoni, F. and Sewry, C. A. (1998). From rags to riches. *Neurology* **51**, 14–16.

Muntoni, F., Mateddu, A., Marrosu, M. G. et al. 1992). Variable dystrophin expression in different muscles of a Duchenne muscular dystrophy carrier. *Clin. Genet.* **42**, 35–38.

Muntoni, F., Gobbi, P., Sewry, C. et al. (1994). Deletions in the 5′ region of dystrophin and resulting phenotypes. *J. Med. Genet.* **31**, 843–847.

Muntoni, F., Sewry, C., Wilson, L., Angelini, C., Trevisan, C. P., Brambati, B. and Dubowitz, V. (1995). Prenatal diagnosis in congenital muscular dystrophy. *Lancet* **345**, 591.

Muntoni, F., Lichtarowicz-Krynska, E. J., Sewry, C. A. et al. (1998). Early presentation of X-linked Emery–Dreifuss muscular dystrophy resembling limb-girdle muscular dystrophy. *Neuromusc. Disord.* **8**, 72–76.

Nagano, A., Koga, R., Ogawa, M. et al. (1996). Emerin deficiency at the nuclear membrane in patients with Emery–Dreifuss muscular dystrophy. *Nat. Genet.* **2**, 254–259.

Naom, I., Sewry, C., D'Alessandro, M. et al. (1997). Prenatal diagnosis of merosin deficient congenital muscular dystrophy: the role of linkage and immunocytochemical analysis. *Neuromusc. Disord.* **7**, 176–179.

Neville, H. E. and Brooke, M. H. (1973). Central core fibers: structured and unstructured. In: *Basic Research in Myology, Proceedings of International Congress on Muscle Diseases*, Part I, ICS No. 294, ed. B. Kakulas, pp. 497–511. Amsterdam: Excerpta Medica.

Nguyen, H. T., Gubis, R. M., Wydro, R. M. and Nadal-Ginard, B. (1982). Sarcomeric myosin heavy chain is coded by a highly conserved multigene family. *Proc. Natl. Acad. Sci. USA* **79**, 5230–5234.

Nguyen, thi Man, Ellis, J. M., Love, D. R. et al. (1991). Localisation of the DMDL gene-encoded dystrophin-related protein using a panel of nineteen monoclonal antibodies: presence at neuromuscular junctions, in the sarcolemma of dystrophic skeletal muscle, in vascular and other smooth muscles, and in proliferating brain cell lines. *J. Cell Biol.* **115**, 1695–1700.

Nonaka, I. (1992). Mitochondrial disease. *Curr. Opin. Neurol. Neurosurg.* **5**, 622–632.

North, K. N. and Beggs, A. H. (1996). Deficiency of a skeletal muscle isoform of alpha-actinin (alpha-actinin-3) in merosin-positive congenital muscular dystrophy. *Neuromusc. Disord.* **6**, 229–235.

North, K. N., Yang, N., Wattanasirichaigoon, D., Mills, M., Easteal, S. and Beggs, A. H. (1999). A common nonsense mutation results in α-actinin-3 deficiency in the general population. *Nat. Genet.* **21**, 353–354.

Nowak, K. J., Wattanasirichaigoon, D., Goebel, H. H. et al. (1999). Mutations in the skeletal muscle alpha actin gene in patients with actin myopathy and nemaline myopathy. *Nat. Genet.* **23**, 208–212.

Ohlendieck, K., Ervasti, J. M., Matsumara, K., Kahl, S. D., Leveille, C. J. and Campbell, K. P. (1991). Dystrophin-related protein is localised to neuromuscular junctions of adult skeletal muscle. *Neuron* **7**, 499–508.

Olsen, T. M., Michels, V. V., Thibodeau, S. N., Tai, Y.-S. and Keating, M. T. (1998). Actin mutations in dilated cardiomyopathies, a heritable form of heart failure. *Science* **280**, 750–752.

Overton, T., Smith, R., Sewry, C., Holder, S. E. and Fisk, N. M. (2000). Maternal contamination at fetal muscle biopsy. *Fetal Diagn. Ther.* **15**, 118–121.

Ozawa, E., Noguchi, S., Mizuno, Y., Hagiwara, Y. and Yoshida, M. (1998). From dystrophinopathy to sarcoglycanopathy: evolution of a concept of muscular dystyrophy. *Muscle Nerve* **21**, 421–438.

Pardo, J. V., D'Angelo Siliciano, J. and Craig, S. W. (1983). A vinculin-containing cortical lattice in skeletal muscle: transverse lattice elements ('costameres') mark sites of attachment between myofibrils and sarcolemma. *Proc. Natl. Acad. Sci. USA* **80**, 1008.

Patel, K., Voit, T., Dunn, M. J., Strong, P. N. and Dubowitz, V. (1988). Dystrophin and nebulin in muscular dystrophies. *J. Neurol. Sci.* **87**, 315–326.

Pelin, K., Hilpela, P., Donner, K. et al. (1999). Mutation in the nebulin gene associated with autosomal recessive nemaline myopathy. *Proc. Natl. Acad. Sci. USA* **96**, 2305–2310.

Porter, G. A., Dmytrenko, G. M., Winkelmann, J. C. and Bloch, R. J. (1992). Dystrophin co-localizes with β-spectrin in distinct sub-sarcolemma domains in mammalian skeletal muscle. *J. Cell Biol.* **117**, 997–1005.

Richard, I., Broux, O., Allamand, C. et al. (1995). Mutations in the proteolytic enzyme, calpain 3, cause limb-girdle muscular dystrophy 2A. *Cell* **81**, 27–40.

Rifai, Z., Welle, S., Kamp, C. and Thorton, C. A. (1995). Ragged red fibres in normal aging and inflammatory myopathy. *Ann. Neurol.* **37**, 24–29.

Sabatelli, P., Squarzoni, S., Petrini, S. et al. (1998). Oral exfoliative cytology for the non-invasive diagnosis in Emery–Dreifuss muscular dystrophy patients and carriers. *Neuromusc. Disord.* **8**, 67–71.

Sarnat, H. B. (1990). Myotubular myopathy: arrest of morphogenesis of myofibres associated with persistance of fetal vimentin and desmin. Four cases compared with fetal and neonatal muscle. *Can. J. Neurol.Sci.* **17**, 109–123.

Sewry, C. A. (1985). Ultrastructural changes in diseased muscle. In: *Muscle Biopsy: A Practical Approach*, 2nd edn, ed. V. Dubowitz, p. 129. London: Baillière Tindall.

Sewry, C. A. (1989). Contribution of immunocytochemistry to the pathogenesis of spinal muscular atrophy. In: *Current Concepts in*

Childhood Spinal Muscular Atrophy, ed. L. Merlini, L. C. Granata and V. Dubowitz, p. 57. New York: Springer-Verlag .

Sewry, C. A. (1998). The role of immunocytochemistry in congenital myopathies. *Neuromusc. Disord.* **8**, 394–400.

Sewry, C. A. and Muntoni, F. (1999). Inherited disorders of the extracellular matrix. *Curr. Opin. Neurol.* **12**, 519–526.

Sewry, C. A. and Qui Lu (2000). Immunological reagents and amplification systems. In: *Methods in Molecular Medicine – The Muscular Dystrophies*, ed. K. Bushby and L. V. B. Anderson. Totowa, NJ: Humana Press, in press.

Sewry, C. A., Appleyard, S. T., Dunn, M. J. and Capaldi, M. J. (1985). Immunocytochemistry of human skeletal muscle disease. In: *Immunocytochemistry*, 2nd edn, eds. J. Polak and S. van Noorden, p. 664. Bristol: Wright.

Sewry, C. A., Dubowitz, V., Abraha, A., Luzio P. and Campbell, A. K. (1987). Immunocytochemical localisation of complement components C8 and C9 in human diseased muscle; the role of complement in muscle fibre damage. *J. Neurol. Sci.* **81**, 141–153.

Sewry, C. A., Clerk, A., Heckmatt, J. Z., Vyse, T. and Dubowitz, V. (1991). Dystrophin abnormalities in polymyositis and dermatomyositis. *Neuromusc. Disord.* **1**, 333–339

Sewry, C. A., Wilson, L. A., Dux, L., Dubowitz, V. and Cooper, B. J. (1992). Experimental regeneration in canine musculr dystrophy. 1. Immunocytochemical evaluation of dystrophin and β-spectrin expression. *Neuromusc. Disord.* **2**, 331–342.

Sewry, C. A., Sansome, A., Clerk, A. et al. (1993). Manifesting carriers of Xp21 muscular dystrophy; lack of correlation between dystrophin expression and clinical weakness. *Neuromusc. Disord.* **3**, 141–148.

Sewry, C. A., Matsumura, K., Campbell, K. P. and Dubowitz, V. (1994a). Expression of dystrophin-associated glycoprotein and utrophin in carriers of Duchenne muscular dystrophy. *Neuromusc. Disord.* **4**, 401–409.

Sewry, C. A., Muntoni, F., Sansome, A., Philpot, J. and Dubowitz, V. (1994b). Sarcolemmal expression of utrophin in diverse neuromuscular disorders. *Muscle Nerve* (Suppl. 1), S103.

Sewry, C. A., Sansome, A., Matsumura, K., Campbell, K. P. and Dubowitz, V. (1994c). Deficiency of the 50 kDa dystrophin-associated glycoprotein and abnormal expression of utrophin in two South Asian cousins with variable expression of severe childhood autosomal recessive muscular dystrophy. *Neuromusc. Disord.* **4**, 121–129.

Sewry, C. A., Philpot, J., Sorokin, L. et al. (1996). Diagnosis of merosin (laminin α2)-deficient congenital muscular dystrophy by skin biopsy. *Lancet* **347**, 582–584.

Sewry, C. A., D'Alessandro, M., Wilson, L. A. et al. (1997a). Expression of laminin chains in skin in merosin-deficient congenital muscular dystrophy. *Neuropediatrics* **28**, 217–222.

Sewry, C. A., Naom, I., D'Alessandro, M. et al (1997b). Variable phenotype in merosin-deficient congenital muscular dystrophy and differential immunolabelling of two fragments of the laminin α2 chain. *Neuromusc. Disord.* **7**, 169–175.

Soussi-Yanicostas, N., Chevallay, M., Laurent-Winter, C., Tomé, F. M. S., Fardeau, M. and Butler-Browne, G. (1991). Distinct contractile protein profile in congenital myotonic dystrophy and X-linked myotubular myopathy. *Neuromusc. Disord.* **1**, 103–111.

Soussi-Yanicostas, N., Ben Hamida, C., Bejaoui, K., Hentati, F., Ben Hamida, M. and Butler-Browne, G. S. (1992). Evolution of muscle specific proteins in Werdnig–Hoffman disease. *J. Neurol. Sci.* **109**, 111–120.

Speer, M. C., Vance, J. M., Grubber, J. M., et al. (1999). Identification of a new autosomal dominant limb-girdle muscular dystrophy locus on chromosome 7. *Am. J. Hum. Genet.* **64**, 556–562.

Stephens, H. R., Duance, V. C., Dunn, M. J., Bailey, A. J. and Dubowitz, V. (1982). Collagen types in neuromuscular diseases. *J. Neurol. Sci.* **53**, 45–62.

Straub, V. and Campbell, K. P. (1997). Muscular dystrophies and the dystrophin-glycoprotein complex. *Curr. Opin. Neurol.* **10**, 168–175.

Straub, V., Bittner, R. E., Leger, J. J. and Voit, T. (1992). Direct visualisation of the dystrophin network on skeletal muscle fiber membrane. *J. Cell Biol.* **119**, 1183–1191.

Stuurman, N., Heins, S. and Aebi, U. (1998). Nuclear lamins: their structure, assembly and interactions. *J. Struct. Biol.* **122**, 42–66.

Tanaka, H., Ishiguro, T., Eguchi, C., Saito, K. and Ozawa, E. (1991). Expression of dystrophin-related protein associated with the skeletal muscle cell membrane. *Histochem. J.* **96**, 1–5

Taylor, J., Muntoni, F., Dubowitz, V. and Sewry, C. A. (1997a). Abnormal expression of utrophin in Duchenne and Becker muscular dystrophy is age-related. *Neuropathol. Appl. Neurobiol.* **23**, 399–405.

Taylor, J., Muntoni, F., Dubowitz, V. and Sewry, C. A. (1997b). Early onset autosomal dominant myopathy; a role for laminin β1? *Neuromusc. Disord.* **7**, 211–216.

Thank, L. T., Nguyen thi Man, Hori, S., Sewry, C. A., Dubowitz, V. and Morris, G. E. (1995). Characterization of internally-deleted dystrophins in Becker muscular dystrophy using a new panel of exon-specific mononclonal antibodies against a deletion-prone region of dystrophin. *Am. J. Med. Genet.* **58**, 177–186.

Thornell, L.-E., Edström, L., Eriksson, A., Henriksson, K.-G. and Angqvist, K. A. (1980). The distribution of intermediate filament protein (skeletin) in normal and diseased human skeletal muscle. *J. Neurol. Sci.* **47**, 153–170.

Tokuyasu, K. T., Dutton, A. H. and Singer, S. J. (1983). Immunoelectron microscopic studies of desmin (skeletin) localization and intermediate filament organization in chicken skeletal muscle. *J. Cell Biol.* **96**, 1736–1742.

Tomé, F. M. S. and Fardeau, M. (1994). Oculopharyngeal muscular dystrophy. In: *Myology*, 2nd edn, Vol. 2, eds. A. G. Engel and C. Franzi-Armstrong, pp. 1223–1235. New York: McGraw-Hill.

Tomé, F. M. S. and Fardeau, M. (1998). Hereditary inclusion body myositis. *Curr. Opin. Neurol.* **11**, 453–459.

Topaloglu, H., Muntoni, F., Dubowitz, V. and Sewry, C. (1996). Expression of HLA class I antigens in skeletal muscle is a diagnostic marker in juvenile dermatomyositis. *J. Child Neurol.* **12**, 60–63.

Towbin, J. A. (1998). The role of cytoskeletal proteins in cardiomyopathies. *Curr. Opin. Cell Biol.* **10**, 131–139.

Tritschler, H. J., Andretta, F. and Moraes, C. T. (1992). Mitochondrial myopathy of childhood associated with depletion of mitochondrial DNA. *Neurology* **42**, 209–217.

Tupler, R., Barbierato, L., Memmi, M., et al. (1998). Identical 'de novo' mutation at D4F104S1 locus in monozygotic male twins affected by facioscapulohumeral muscular dystrophy (FSHD) with different clinical expression. *J. Med. Genet.* **35**, 778–783.

Udd, B., Haravuori, H., Kalimo, H. et al. (1998). Tibial muscular dystrophy – from clinical description to linkage to chromosome 2q31. *Neuromusc. Disord.* **8**, 327–332.

Vainzof, M., Passos-Bueno, M. R., Canovas, M. et al. (1996). The sarcoglycan complex in the six autosomal recessive limb-girdle (AR-LGMD) muscular dystrophies. *Hum. Mol. Genet.* **5**, 1963–1969.

Vainzof, M., Costa, C. S., Marie, S. K. et al. (1997). Deficiency of alpha-actinin-3 (ACTN3) occurs in different forms of muscular dystrophy. *Neuropaediatrics* **28**, 223–228.

van der Kooi, A. J., van Meegan, M., Ledderhof, T. M., McNally, E. M., de Visser, M. and Bolhuis, P. A. (1997). Genetic localisation of a newly recognised autosomal dominant limb-girdle muscular dystrophy with cardiac involvement (LGMD1B) to chromosome 1q11–21. *Am. J. Hum. Genet.* **60**, 891–895.

van der Ven, P. F. M., Jap, P. H. K., Wetzels, R. H. W. et al (1991). Postnatal centralization of muscle fibre nuclei in centronuclear myopathy. *Neuromusc. Disord.* **1**, 211–220.

Vicart, P., Caron, A., Guicheney, P. et al. (1998). A missence mutation in the alphaB-crystallin gene causes a desmin-related myopathy. *Nat. Genet.* **20**, 92–95.

Villanova, M., Louboutin, J. P., Chateau, D. et al. (1995). X-linked vacuolated myopathy: complement membrane attack complex on surface membrane of injured muscle fibres. *Ann. Neurol.* **37**, 637–645.

Wallgren-Pettersson, C. (1998). Genetics of the nemaline myopathies and the myotubular myopathies. *Neuromusc. Disord.* **8**, 401–404.

Webster, C., Silberstein, L., Hays, A. P. and Blau, H. (1988). Fast muscle fibers are preferentially affected in Duchenne muscular dystrophy. *Cell* **52**, 503–513.

Weller, B., Carpenter, S., Lochmuller, H. and Karpati, G. (1999). Myopathy with trabecular fibres. *Neuromusc. Disord.* **9**, 208–214.

Whalen, R. G., Sell, S. M., Butler-Browne, G. S., Schwartz, K., Bouveret, P. and Pinset-Harstrom, I. (1981). Three myosin heavy chain isozymes appear sequentially in rat muscle development. *Nature* **292**, 805–809.

Whitaker, J. N., Bertorini, T. E. and Mendell, J. R. (1983). Immunocytochemical studies of cathepsin D in human skeletal muscle. *Ann. Neurol.* **13**, 133–142.

Wood, D. S., Zeviani, M., Prelle, A. et al. (1987). Is nebulin the defective gene product in Duchenne muscular dystrophy? *N. Eng. J. Med.* **316**, 107–108.

Yates, J. R. W., Bagshaw, J., Aksmanovic, V. M. et al. (1999). Genotype-phenotype analysis in X-linked Emery–Dreifuss muscular dystrophy and identification of a missense mutation associated with a milder phenotype. *Neuromusc. Disord.* **9**, 159–165.

Zuk, J. A. and Fletcher, A. (1988). Skeletal muscle expression of class II histocompatibility antigens (HLA-DR) in polymyositis and other muscle diseases with an inflammatory infiltrate. *J. Clin. Pathol.* **41**, 410–414.

14

Muscle pathology on semithin resin sections

Stirling Carpenter

Introduction

This chapter discusses skeletal muscle pathology on a light microscopic level with minimal reference to histochemistry and immunocytochemistry. This is an artificial situation, since much of our knowledge has come from correlation of methods, but as an exercise it can be stimulating. The discussion is based on semithin resin sections since they offer by far the best morphology. Despite this fact, they are often neglected, being considered only as a stage in processing for electron microscopy and not useful enough to send to a consultant along with the cryostat sections and electron micrographs. Nevertheless they offer a view analogous to very-low-power electron microscopy with the advantage of a much larger sampling area.

For good semithin sections, the muscle specimen should be fixed in a noncontracted state, preferably in an isometric clamp, and promptly placed, still clamped, in the fixative, preferably 2% buffered glutaraldehyde. After 2–6 hours of fixation in the refrigerator, the specimen is moved to refrigerated buffer without the clamp. Well oriented cross-sections and longitudinal sections can then be obtained as thin but comparatively wide slices. Both views are informative. The best resolution is obtained when sections are stained with paraphenylene diamine and viewed with phase optics, as in the illustrations here.

General reactions of muscle fibres

Necrosis and regeneration

Necrosis means the death of a cell: its inability to maintain homeostasis and its inevitable transition to debris. Since muscle cells are multinucleated and elongated, necrosis in them is often, and perhaps usually, segmental, although

this is seldom visualized (Fig. 14.1). Experimental studies have shown that necrosis, when initiated in one small segment of a muscle fibre, spreads in both directions along the fibre for a variable distance and for a time that is generally less than 6 hours, until the surviving stumps are covered by a protective membrane (Carpenter and Karpati, 1989).

Although several reports suggest that apoptosis can occur in skeletal muscle fibres, its status is not totally clear at present, and at least in the cytoplasmic changes that accompany segmental death of a mature skeletal muscle cell, no distinction can be made between apoptosis and necrosis.

Necrosis occurs in many but by no means all muscle diseases. Many reactions of muscle cells do not promote necrosis, and in many diseases, necrosis occurs at such a low rate that is rarely seen in biopsies. In Duchenne muscular dystrophy, it is usually prominent until late in the disease, when few fibres are left. Necrotic fibres often appear to be clustered in Duchenne dystrophy, while, by contrast, in polymyositis necrotic fibres appear to be single and apparently random. Necrosis is less commonly seen in dermatomyositis, where it may follow one of two patterns: occasional fibres at the periphery of fascicles or many adjacent fibres comprising the larger part of a fascicle (i.e. an infarct).

What are the changes that take place after necrosis is initiated and by which necrosis can be recognized through the microscope? Early stages of experimental necrosis, at the point where it begins, tend to show marked hypercontraction and tearing of myofibrils, giving a reticulated appearance (Fig. 14.1). A similar appearance is seen in dermatomyositis, although not in Duchenne dystrophy. It must be distinguished from the hypercontraction that occurs as a reaction to the biopsy procedure, in which relatively long segments tend to contract as a whole while on

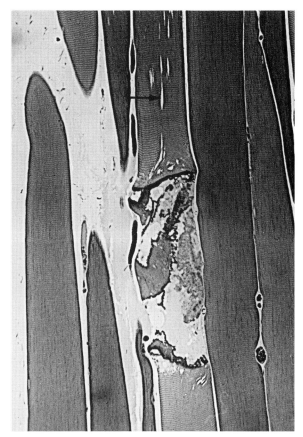

Fig. 14.1. The central fibre shows segmental necrosis 2 hours after it was punctured by a fine wire. The width of the necrotic segment may be exaggerated by retraction of the stumps. Elongated vacuoles (arrow) result from swelling of T-tubules. Experimental micropuncture in rat gastrocnemius (×500).

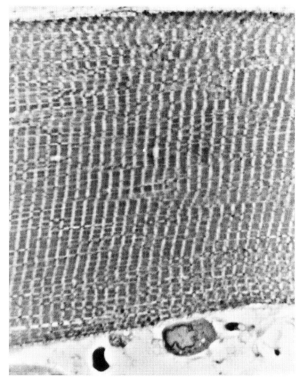

Fig. 14.2. In this necrotic fibre segment, the Z disc has disappeared although the A band is preserved and in good order. Section from a patient with acute ischaemic myopathy secondary to pitressin therapy for oesophageal varices (×1370).

their ends they stretch or tear the rest of the fibre. Fibres severed on the edges of the biopsy contract and, particularly in children's biopsies, isolated normal fibres in the centre of fascicles sometimes also contract excessively and tear themselves. Such fibres can be indistinguishable from the hypercontracted fibres that are particularly common in biopsies from patients with Duchenne dystrophy. This suggests that the Duchenne fibres are unusually fragile.

In early necrotic fibre segments where hypercontraction has not occurred, the Z disc can be seen to have disappeared within 2 hours (Fig. 14.2). The best examples of this tend to occur in ischaemic necrosis. In more contracted segments, only homogenization of the myofibrils is evident. Mitochondria lose their laterally elongated shape and become round and dark, often forming chains. While hypercontraction can cause the myofibrillar material of necrotic fibres to appear darker than normal, within hours the fibres lose density until they are paler than normal (Fig. 14.3). This happens without phagocytosis. The nuclei of necrotic fibres disappear rapidly. The nuclei seen within necrotic fibres are those of phagocytes or regenerative cells.

Invasion of necrotic fibres by mononuclear phagocytes is probably rare before 10 hours have passed. In Duchenne dystrophy, where monocytes are already present in the interstitial tissue, it may occur faster. Polymorphonuclear leukocytes are almost never a factor in human muscle biopsies, except in acute infections or infestation, such as trichinosis. Phagocytic invasion is dependent on blood supply (Hansen-Smith and Carlson, 1979); so is proliferation of regenerative cells, but less so. In conditions like dermatomyositis where blood supply is curtailed, phagocytosis is often delayed and regenerative cells may be seen forming a thick ring around necrotic debris (Fig. 14.4). In the centre of infarcts, necrotic fibres can persist for some time with neither phagocytosis nor regeneration.

Regeneration comes from the migration and proliferation of satellite cells as regenerative myoblasts (Bischoff, 1979) which appear first on sections as thin cells on the periphery of the old fibre. They divide, grow fatter, and fuse. Ribosomes make their cytoplasm bluish when the cells are stained with haematoxylin and eosin. After they

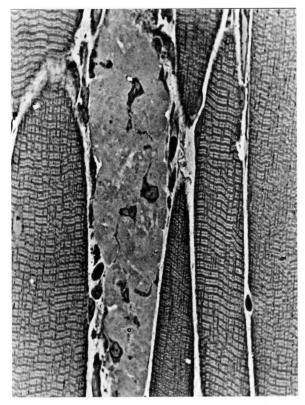

Fig. 14.3. The pale muscle fibre in the centre is in a stage of necrosis seen after several hours. The myofibrillar debris is featureless. Nucleated cells within the fibre are phagocytes. Sample from a patient with Duchenne dystrophy (×500).

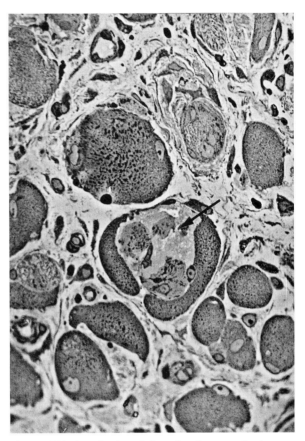

Fig. 14.4. This tissue has been infarcted, and regeneration has occurred in the site of one fibre before the necrotic material of the dead fibre was completely phagocytosed. The regenerating cells thus form a ring surrounding the necrotic debris (arrow). This phenomenon is characteristically seen in ischaemic lesions (×500).

have fused, myofibrils develop, at first separated by considerable cytoplasmic space. Partly because of this, a regenerated but not yet mature segment appears pale compared with mature fibres (Fig. 14.5). Glycogen is abundant and sometimes forms subsarcolemmal collections. Mitochondria are rounded or extended in the long axis of the fibre. Nuclei are large and pale with large nucleoli and are often at a distance from the sarcolemma.

Regeneration is not always a success. It may fail completely if satellite cells fail to proliferate; when proliferation is meagre, it will result in thin rounded fibres. Incomplete lateral fusion of myoblasts shows up as forked or split fibres. If myoblasts fail to proliferate adequately, fibres stay small and end prematurely. Myoblasts and regenerating fibres in many conditions appear to be immune, until they mature, to whatever has caused the original necrosis.

Small fibres

Fibres that are small may result from shrinkage or failure to grow, either primarily or after regeneration. Shrinkage is exemplified by the angular atrophic fibres of denervation, which tend to occur in groups. Bizarre spidery shapes are often seen at high power in resin sections. When denervation involves whole fascicles, as in juvenile spinal muscular atrophy, angularity is much less pronounced. As denervated fibres shrink, they retain most of their nuclei. A very atrophic denervated fibre will, therefore, often appear as a small bag of nuclei. These nuclear clump fibres usually appear rounded. In Werdnig–Hoffmann disease, atrophic fibres tend to be very numerous, and all tend to be round. Diagnosis is made easier by finding groups of hypertrophied fibres. Probably many of the small fibres are denervated before birth.

Atrophy of type II fibres, as seen in disuse, cachexia and chronic steroid treatment, obviously calls for histochemistry for its identification. Here the atrophic fibres, though angular, are scattered, and the atrophy does not go as far as when it results from denervation.

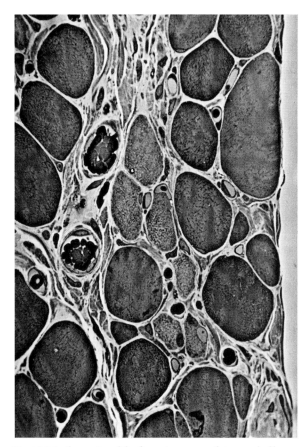

Fig. 14.5. In the centre of the figure is a group of six muscle fibres in a relatively late stage of regeneration. Their cytoplasm is slightly paler than that of the surrounding mature fibres, and most of their nuclei are pale. Section from a patient with Duchenne dystrophy (×500).

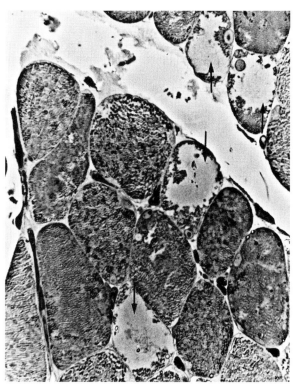

Fig. 14.6. In dermatomyositis, punched-out areas of myofibrillar loss may be found within muscle fibres (arrows). The space from which myofibrils have disappeared is filled with glycogen. Reduction in fibre volume is a subsequent step, which has not yet occurred here (×577).

A relatively acute form of atrophy is seen in acute quadriplegic myopathy, which usually follows high-dose steroid administration coupled with neuromuscular blockade. It can be identified by selective loss of myosin filaments.

Atrophic angular fibres, tending to occur in groups, are seen in most patients with inclusion body myositis. They have been interpreted as evidence that there is a component of denervation in the disease, although the fibres tend to be more miscellaneous in size than typical denervated fibres. They are probably injured fibres that have shrunk following loss of nuclei.

In diseases where necrosis is prevalent, as in Duchenne dystrophy, small rounded fibres represent regenerants that have not been able to grow larger because they do not have enough nuclei. There is no lack of satellite cells in Duchenne dystrophy, but with repeated cycles of necrosis and regeneration, their mitotic potential is progressively reduced (Webster and Blau, 1990). Fewer and fewer regenerative myoblasts are then available to fill long necrotic

segments. The resultant new fibre segments are slender and rounded and may end prematurely (Schmalbruch, 1984). They usually have surprisingly regular myofibrils. In congenital myopathies, small rounded fibres are often found (usually of histochemical type I), which for obscure reasons have never reached normal size.

Reactions and alterations of components of muscle fibres

Myofibrils

Loss of myofibrils may occur concurrently with loss of cell volume; as a result, myofibrillar loss per se is not evident. This occurs with atrophy of type II fibres and with denervation atrophy until its most advanced stages. In dermatomyositis, punched-out areas of myofibrillar loss are often seen in damaged fibres (Fig. 14.6). These areas tend to be filled with glycogen. Loss of cell volume is a subsequent event.

Selective loss of thick (myosin) filaments appears as loss

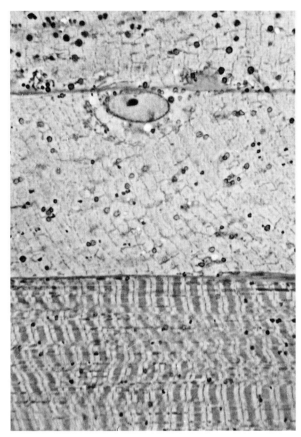

Fig. 14.7. This biopsy is from a patient who was paralysed with vecuronium while on a respirator and given high doses of corticosteroids. The bottom fibre has normal appearing myofibrils, while in the fibres above the A band density is absent, although Z discs are present. The nucleus appears reactive. The small dense dots, most prominent in the top fibre, are lipid globules, which are often in excess in fibres with A band loss (×1300).

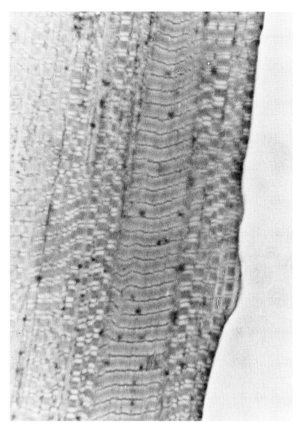

Fig. 14.8. A central core runs along the middle of this fibre. The A band is not quite as dense and its state of contraction is slightly different from that of the surrounding normal myofibrillar areas (×550).

of the A band and is best appreciated on longitudinal sections (Fig. 14.7). It is encountered in ischaemic conditions and also in a rather pure form in patients treated with high doses of steroids when they have been given a neuromuscular blocking agent to facilitate artificial respiration (Danon et al., 1976). When released from the respirator after a few days, the patient may be unable to walk and only recovers strength in weeks or months. Loss of the A band may be limited to the centre of fibres in a core-like pattern. Similar A band loss has been produced in rats by the combination of high-dose steroids and denervation (Massa et al., 1992). Myofibrils were promptly renewed when re-innervation was allowed. Occasional muscle fibres in other myopathies may show fairly selective myosin loss.

In central core disease, cytoplasmic organization is abnormal. A core is a circumscribed cytoplasmic area that extends from end to end of a muscle fibre and within which myofibrils are not distinct from one another, intramyofibrillar mitochondria are not present, Z discs are not quite straight and the degree of contraction is independent from that of the rest of the fibre (Fig. 14.8). Mutations of the gene for the sarcoplasmic reticulum calcium release channel (ryanodine receptor) are present in all patients with central core disease, and the mutant receptors are probably segregated into the cores.

Z disc reactions

Z disc streaming is a common pathological change in muscle fibres (Fig. 14.9). In very small lesions, streaming involves the area between two adjacent Z discs. It occurs particularly in zones where mitochondria are lacking. The targets and targetoids associated with denervation are circumscribed zones of mitochondrial lack within which there is Z disc streaming. This is probably a feature of re-innervation rather than of denervation per se. In one study, it was limited to re-innervated fibres (Massa et al., 1992). It

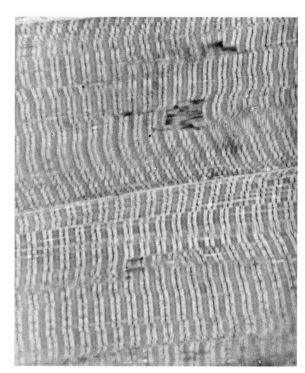

Fig. 14.9. Very small foci of Z disc streaming, some involving only a single sarcomere, are present in two fibres from a partially denervated muscle (×1350).

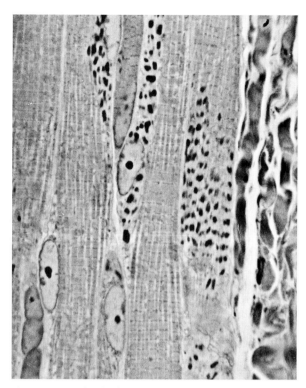

Fig. 14.10. Nemaline bodies are very dense on resin sections stained with paraphenylene diamine. They form within myofibrils from enlargement of the lattice of the Z disc. In early stages of their formation, their spacing approximates that of Z discs. When myofibrils break down, the nemaline bodies accumulate under the sarcolemma (×550).

tends to be rare in biopsies from those with motor neuron disease. Careful inspection of sections of normal muscle shows small mitochondria-free zones wherever vessels cross muscle fibres transversely. Within these zones there is occasionally Z disc streaming. Streaming is also common in ischaemia. This is probably why, of the inflammatory myopathies, it is by far the most common in dermatomyositis, where it tends to be multifocal within fibres. Patients considered to have multicore disease have small foci in their muscles that lack intermyofibrillar mitochondria and, therefore, often have Z disc streaming. Some of these are examples of desminopathy. These diseases are the most characteristic settings for Z disc streaming, but it does occur occasionally in others.

Nemaline bodies or rods appear as very black flecks within fibres. Their shape and the spacing that relates them to Z discs, from which they arise, is best seen in longitudinal sections (Fig. 14.10). They are easier to see in resin than in cryostat or paraffin sections. Apart from patients with nemaline myopathy, where rods seem to form in otherwise normal myofibrils, rods can probably occur as a secondary phenomenon. Tenotomy of the rat soleus, which produces zones of myofibrillar loss starting with the A bands, sometimes leads to formation of rods (Karpati et al., 1972). When

there is A band loss from any cause, some enlargement of the Z disc tends to occur, even reaching the size of small rods.

Cytoplasmic bodies appear as dense rounded structures with a clear halo (Fig. 14.11). Occasionally they are seen with tail-like connections to a line of Z discs. They are brightly eosinophilic on cryostat sections stained with haematoxylin and eosin. They are highly nonspecific, although a plethora might suggest a specific syndrome described as cytoplasmic body myopathy (Jerusalem et al., 1979)

Loss of Z discs is an early reaction in necrotic fibres. It can be seen 2 hours after the onset of experimental ischaemia (Karpati et al., 1974).

Mitochondria

Individual mitochondria can be seen on longitudinal sections of well-relaxed muscle fibres as small blips on either side of the Z discs. In transverse sections, they constitute the main density of the intermyofibrillar lattice in the I

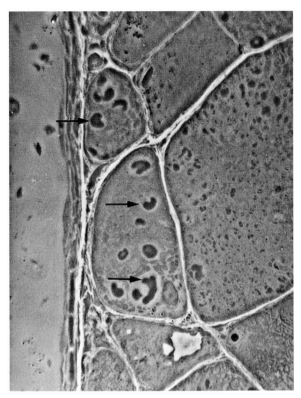

Fig. 14.11. Cytoplasmic bodies are dense oval to C-shaped structures within fibre (arrows). They are usually surrounded by a pale halo. They are nonspecific. This section is from a patient with desminopathy (×550).

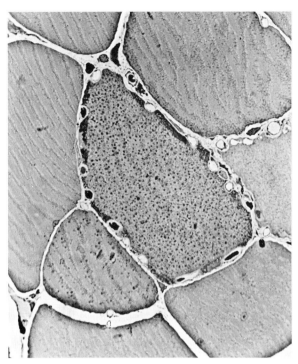

Fig. 14.12. In what corresponds to a ragged-red fibre, dark subsarcolemmal mitochondrial accumulations are present on all sides, as well as excess mitochondria between myofibrils. Small lipid globules are probably present, but they stain dark like the mitochondria. A large number of capillaries indent this fibre (×550).

band, reflecting the fact that they are elongated transversely to the myofibrillar axis. Normally, mitochondria do not project into the A band. When they do, it is a subtle, sensitive and nonspecific sign of abnormality. In good sections, one can detect the focal absence of mitochondria where a vessel transversely crosses a muscle fibre, as well as their absence in and around targets and multicores.

In muscle from children, subsarcolemmal dark collections of crowded mitochondria can occur normally around one or even two sides of several fibres. These crescents are much rarer in normal adult muscle. The point at which they become excessive may be difficult to decide. Fibres corresponding to ragged-red fibres show subsarcolemmal dark mitochondrial collections on all sides as well as a focal increase between myofibrils (Fig. 14.12). The tendency of such fibres to be wreathed by numerous capillaries is clearly seen on resin sections.

Vacuolation of mitochondria is a common artifact resulting from slowness of fixation. It tends to be most evident in the centre of specimens.

Nuclei

Displacement of nuclei from their normal subsarcolemmal position is the most common abnormality involving nuclei. Since semithin sections are much thinner than cryostat sections, they reveal far fewer central nuclei. In some patients with infantile centronuclear myopathy, this could make diagnosis difficult if only resin sections were used. In this disease the nuclei are in the precise geometric centre of the fibre, although some subsarcolemmal nuclei are also present. In late-onset centronuclear myopathy, tight clusters of nuclei may occur in the geometrical centre, as well as some that seem to be lifting away from the sarcolemma. In adult myotonic dystrophy, by contrast, the numerous central nuclei tend to be scattered randomly in the interior of fibres on cross-section.

Nuclei in regenerating fibres are pale and large with prominent nucleoli, but similar active nuclei can be seen in injured fibres in which repair processes are active, for example in dermatomyositis. Pyknotic nuclei are not often seen in muscle biopsies, aside from artifact. They occur in infantile polymyositis and reducing body myopathy, occasionally in myotonic dystrophy and in inclusion body myositis.

Intranuclear inclusions in inclusion body myositis are almost never apparent in resin sections, although egg-shaped spaces with a ground-glass density, a little larger than normal nuclei, may represent a stage of nuclear breakdown when almost all nuclear contents are replaced by filaments. In oculopharyngeal dystrophy, the relatively rare nuclei, which, by electron microscopy, contain the pathognomonic fine tubular inclusions, by light microscopy have a distinctive focal pallor (Tomé and Fardeau, 1980). Intranuclear nemaline bodies have been found in a small number of patients with nemaline myopathy, some with neonatal, others with adult-onset disease (Jenis et al., 1969; Engel and Oberc, 1975) In cryostat sections the nemaline bodies are red when stained with the modified trichrome and are surrounded by a halo.

Clumps of nuclei in markedly atrophic fibres are suggestive of denervation atrophy, but they also occur in inclusion body myositis and in some instances in limb girdle and myotonic dystrophy.

Vacuoles

Vacuoles in skeletal muscle fibres can be of many sorts. Division into clear vacuoles and those with visible contents may be helpful, although material such as glycogen can be carried artifactitiously into otherwise clear vacuoles.

An important source of clear vacuoles is the T-tubules, which can undergo marked acute focal swelling when there is massive ingress of sodium into a fibre. This was first shown by in vitro incubation of transected normal fibres in isotonic saline (Fig. 14.13) (Casademont et al., 1988). Dilatation of T-tubules extended with time progressively further and further from the cut end, as long as the incubation medium contained levels of sodium similar to those in the extracellular space. It has been postulated that the increased cytoplasmic sodium stimulates the Na^+/K^+ ATPase in the T-tubule walls, which expels three sodium ions while taking in two potassium ions. The increase ionic concentration in the T-tubular lumen draws water into it from the cytoplasm. Similar T-tubular swelling in the stumps of necrotic fibres was found in an in vivo model of focal necrosis (micropuncture; Carpenter and Karpati, 1989). When these vacuoles became large, their connection to T-tubules by electron microscopy was quite difficult to demonstrate. Similar vacuoles are seen in human muscle fibres in many conditions where focal necrosis has recently occurred. We call them 'stump vacuoles', since they occur in the stumps of necrotic fibres. The fact that they are not seen in Duchenne dystrophy, where necrosis is almost always present, is unexplained.

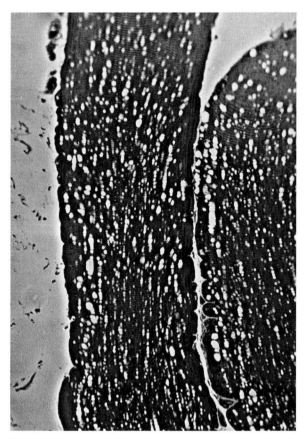

Fig. 14.13. These muscle fibres from a rat were cut and incubated for 20 minutes in oxygenated glucose-containing isotonic medium. The marked vacuolation seen here reflects T-tubule dilation. It was absent in fibre regions distant from the cut end, and in similar incubations it could be prevented by omitting sodium from the bathing medium ($\times$550).

Some biopsies from patients with Duchenne dystrophy show muscle fibres that, by electron microscopy, lack a plasma membrane but also lack other signs of necrosis. These fibres do show small rounded vacuoles of T-tubule origin. These can be seen by light microscopy, although they are difficult to distinguish from swollen mitochondria. They are not seen in stumps.

Some biopsies from patients with periodic paralysis have widely scattered vacuolated fibres. A fibre may contain a single gigantic vacuole or many small ones. They connect to the extracellular space through T-tubules. The mechanism of their formation may be related to that of stump vacuoles, although it has been suggested that they are the end-stage of autophagic vacuoles following breakdown of masses of dilated sarcoplasmic reticular vesicles (Engel, 1970).

Dilatation of sarcoplasmic reticulum to the point of forming vacuoles that can be seen by light microscopy is

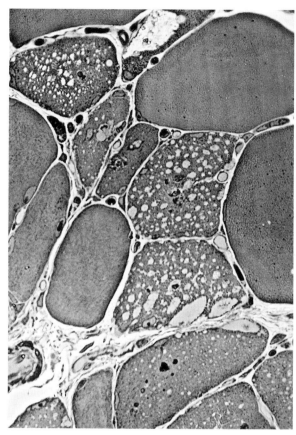

Fig. 14.14. In acid maltase deficiency, muscle fibres contain multiple small vacuoles from which glycogen may or may not be leached out. Dense material, representing lipofuscin is seen within some vacuoles. This biopsy is from a patient with the adult-onset variety, in which there may be sparing of many fibres or of many areas of some muscles (×550).

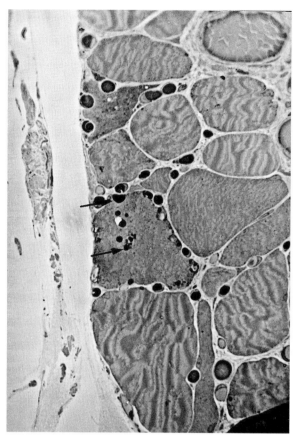

Fig. 14.15. In inclusion body myositis, dark granules (arrows) in scattered muscle fibres are membranous whorls. There is a focal increase in capillaries (×550).

probably rare. A single case reported as sarcotubular myopathy would be an example (Jerusalem et al., 1973). Mild degrees of sarcoplasmic reticular dilatation, where the somewhat dense content is not lost, are occasionally encountered, but the significance is uncertain.

Lysosomal vacuoles are the mark of acid maltase deficiency (Fig. 14.14). They may have the ground-glass density of glycogen, may appear empty (if glycogen has been leached out during fixation) or may contain lipofuscin-like material or membranous whorls. Nonmembrane-bound glycogen lakes, present in the infantile form, probably result from rupture of lysosomes. In the infantile form, storage also occurs in interstitial cells in the muscle. These rounded lysosomes, which are visible in resin sections, do not rupture and may be more characteristic.

Rimmed vacuoles are an expected finding in inclusion body myositis; the designation arises from their appear-

ance in cryostat sections (Fig. 14.15). With haematoxylin and eosin stain, they appear as collections of blue granules separated by an irregular fissure. Occasionally a red inclusion appears among the granules. In resin sections, the granules (which are membranous whorls) usually do not appear to be within vacuoles but free in the cytoplasm, which may retract slightly from them. In large accumulations, which may extend for inordinate lengths along muscle fibres, electron microscopy shows numerous vacuoles of various sizes accompanying the membranous whorls. The whorls are highly osmiophilic but tend to lack the refractility of lipofuscin granules. This distinction is inapparent in very thick sections. Membranous whorls are dissolved out of paraffin sections. If membranous whorls are not seen in the semithin resin sections, there is virtually no chance that electron microscopy on thin sections will show the characteristic filaments of inclusion body myositis.

Membranous whorls occur in some other situations. They may occur in autophagic vacuoles in acid maltase

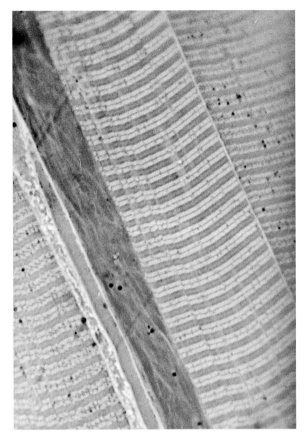

Fig. 14.16. Tubular aggregates form dense geographic masses inside muscle fibres, especially near the sarcolemma. On longitudinal sections like this they may be subdivided into blocks (×1350).

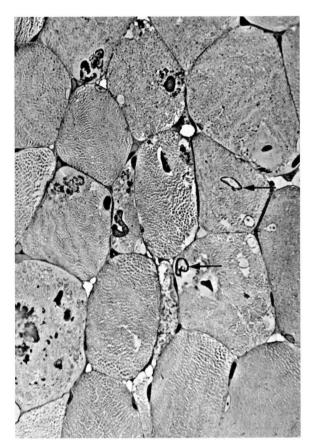

Fig. 14.17. Numerous very dense reducing bodies are present in this biopsy. Two nuclei are surrounded by thin layers of reducing body filaments (arrows) (×550).

deficiency, in rare fibres in periodic paralysis, in colchicine myopathy and in chloroquine myopathy. They are also seen in conditions where there is nuclear breakdown, such as Marinesco–Sjögren syndrome, reducing body myopathy and oculopharyngeal dystrophy.

Abnormal organelles

Tubular aggregates
Tubular aggregates are seen in some cramp syndromes but also occur nonspecifically in various myopathies, especially periodic paralysis (Engel et al., 1970). In resin sections, they are relatively dark, tending to fill geographical areas next to the sarcolemma (Fig. 14.16). In longitudinal sections, subdivisions may be visible within them, corresponding to blocks of parallel tubules.

Reducing bodies
Reducing bodies are virtually specific for the rare disease of reducing body myopathy, although reported cases are

clinically diverse (Carpenter et al., 1985). They are eosinophilic in cryostat or paraffin sections. In resin sections, they are very dark, especially on their periphery (Fig. 14.17). Often they have a characteristic shape like a broken egg. Sometimes the dark material can be seen to surround nuclei. Precise identification depends on histochemistry to show their reducing capacity. Electron microscopy shows their basic composition of tubular filaments, which may be so crowded that they are interpreted as granules.

Other structures than skeletal muscle cells

Connective tissue

Normally so little collagen is present between muscle fibres that it is only visible by electron microscopy. An exception is in the neighbourhood of neuromuscular junctions, where a small amount of collagen tends to encircle muscle fibres. Muscle that has been severely damaged

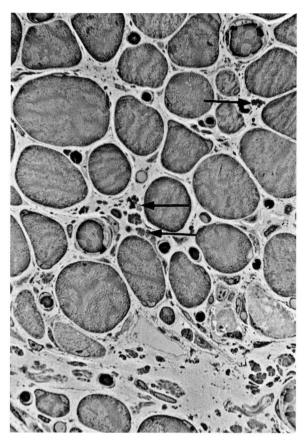

Fig. 14.18. Connective tissue proliferation in Duchenne dystrophy characteristically takes the form of dense discrete collagen bundles laid down parallel to the muscle fibres. On transverse sections, these bundles may have a somewhat cloverleaf-like shape (arrows) (×577).

from a variety of causes tends to show increased endomysial connective tissue, usually in the form of rather loose, randomly oriented collagen. This is seen particularly clearly in polymyositis and inclusion body myositis. Fibrosis in end-stage denervation tends to show proliferation of elastic fibres (black in resin sections, purple with the trichrome stain) along with the collagen.

In Duchenne and Becker dystrophy, the connective tissue proliferation, which begins to occur early, is distinctive, consisting of discrete dense bundles of collagen laid down parallel to the muscle fibres (Fig. 14.18). This pattern is also seen in some biopsies from patients without dystrophin deficiency but with a limb girdle syndrome. Fibrosis in other conditions, such as polymyositis and inclusion body myositis, is less discrete, less organized and more obviously related to cell loss.

When muscle cells have been lost and replaced by fat cells, no matter what the cause, collagen also tends to be lost.

Vessels

Paraffin sections, because of their relatively large sample size, find their greatest scope in the diagnosis of arteritis.

Capillaries are clearly seen in resin sections, provided that the muscle fibres have not been tightly squashed together. General tissue stains on cryostat or paraffin sections show only part of the capillary population, but good selective staining of all viable capillaries is provided by use of appropriate lectin or antibody staining.

In normal adult muscle, the lumen of a capillary is seen in most intersections of the interstitial space among muscle fibres. Roughly 1.5 capillary lumina accompany each muscle cell, and there are about 400–500 lumina/mm^2 of transverse muscle fibre area. In newborn infants, the number of capillaries per muscle fibre is far lower than in adults.

There is some lability in the capillary network. In denervation atrophy, as muscle fibres shrink, the capillaries surrounding them come closer together, causing an increase in the number of capillaries per unit of transverse muscle fibre area. The muscle appears overvascularized. At the same time, the endothelial cells of certain capillary lines undergo cell death (Carpenter and Karpati, 1982). In denervated muscle, one can often see an occasional capillary that is represented only by a basal lamina circle without endothelium.

Destruction and loss of capillaries is also seen in dermatomyositis, but the picture is very different (Fig. 14.19). It is cause of atrophy rather than a sequela (Emslie-Smith and Engel, 1990). The number of capillaries per unit of transverse muscle fibre area drops. Endothelial thickening and proliferation are usually seen, resulting in an increase of nuclei in surviving capillaries. Cells containing dark granules at the site of a capillary suggest active necrosis, as do single isolated red cells among the muscle fibres. Perifascicular areas are most often involved. Proliferation of thin-walled venules is sometimes present next to an area of capillary loss. Necrosis of larger vessels is seen in a few cases, where it is often associated with infarcts.

Thickening of the basal lamina of capillaries, appearing as a pale grey ground-glass density, is seen most commonly in diabetic patients. Occasionally it occurs without any obvious cause. In an extreme form ('pipe-stem capillaries') it has been reported with connective tissue disease (Emslie-Smith and Engel, 1991). Amyloid, which can be hard to distinguish from a thick basal lamina on resin sections, characteristically coats the surface of muscle fibres on the outside of fascicles.

An excess of capillaries is seen in some patients with inclusion body myositis and in those with marked histochemical type I fibre predominance. Ragged-red fibres

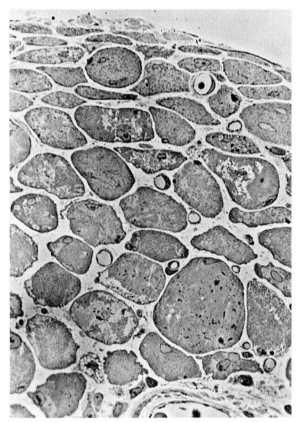

Fig. 14.19. In dermatomyositis, loss of capillaries leads to myofibrillar loss and shrinkage of muscle cells. Only a few dilated capillaries are left in this fascicle. Especially on the periphery of the fascicle, capillary loss is profound (×577).

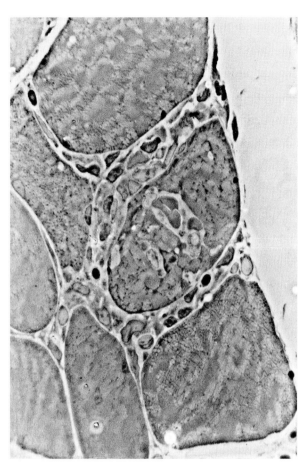

Fig. 14.20. In inclusion body myositis, seen here, and in polymyositis, lymphocytes and macrophages can be seen invading non-necrotic muscle fibres (×1350).

are often surrounded, and even indented, by an excess number of capillary lumina.

Inflammatory cells

In polymyositis, inflammatory infiltrates are conspicuous within muscle fascicles, where they are often associated with the phenomenon of partial invasion of non-necrotic muscle fibres by lymphocytes and macrophages (Fig. 14.20) (Engel and Arahata, 1984). Partial invasion is also commonly seen in inclusion body myositis, although sizeable inflammatory infiltrates are rare and may be absent from a biopsy. In dermatomyositis, infiltrates are confined to septa, although separate cells, in particular macrophages, may be found between muscle fibres in involved regions.

Intramuscular nerves

Specific changes in intramuscular nerves can rarely be seen. In denervating conditions, a decrease in myelinated axons is often seen if intramuscular nerves are found. Wallerian ovoids are much more infrequent. In Werdnig–Hoffmann disease, intramuscular nerves usually show extreme depletion of myelinated fibres. This can be diagnostically useful if the characteristic groups of hypertrophied fibres are not present among the sea of small round fibres. In chronic demyelinating disease, 'onion bulbs' are almost never seen in small intramuscular nerves. Polyglucosan bodies can occur nonspecifically in intramuscular axons of patients over the age of 40 years. If they are particularly numerous and the clinical data are suggestive, the possibility of adult polyglucosan disease must be considered, and the sural nerve, a more specific site, should be scrutinized (Robitaille et al., 1980). In giant axonal disease, focal distension of axons with neurofilaments occurs in intramuscular nerves, although the greater sample of the sural nerve is preferable for diagnosis (Carpenter et al., 1974). In infantile neuroaxonal dystrophy, changes occur predominantly in the most distal parts of axons, and abnormalities may be detectable, even before electron microcopy, in the large axons in muscle spindles, although electron microscopy on a skin sample is the optimal morphological procedure for diagnosis.

References

Bischoff, R. (1979). Tissue culture studies on the origin of myogenic cells during muscle regeneration in the rat. In: *Muscle Regeneration*, ed. A. Mauro, A., pp. 493–507. New York: Raven Press.

Carpenter, S. and Karpati, G. (1982). Necrosis of capillaries in denervation atrophy of human skeletal muscle. *Muscle Nerve* **5**, 250–254.

Carpenter, S. and Karpati, G. (1989). Segmental necrosis and its demarcation in experimental micropuncture injury of skeletal muscle fibers. *J. Neuropathol. Exp. Neurol.* **48**, 154–170.

Carpenter, S., Karpati, G., Andermann, F. et al.(1974). Giant axonal neuropathy: a clinically and morphologically distinct neurological disease. *Arch. Neurol.* **31**, 312–316.

Carpenter, S., Karpati, G. and Holland, P. (1985). New observations in reducing body myopathy. *Neurology* **35**, 818–827.

Casademont, J., Carpenter, S. and Karpati, G. (1988). Vacuolation of muscle fibres near sarcolemmal breaks represents T-tubule dilatation secondary to enhanced sodium pump activity. *J. Neuropathol. Exp. Neurol.* **47**, 618–628.

Danon, J. M., Karpati, G., and Carpenter, S. (1976). Subacute skeletal myopathy induced by 2,4-dichlorophenoxyacetate in rats and guinea pigs. *Muscle Nerve* **1**, 89–102.

Emslie-Smith, A. M. and Engel, A. G. (1990). Microvascular changes in early and advanced dermatomyositis: a quantitative study. *Ann. Neurol.* **27**, 343–356.

Emslie-Smith, A. M. and Engel, A. G. (1991). Necrotizing myopathy with pipestem capillaries, microvascular deposition of the complement membrane attack complex (MAC), and minimal cellular infiltration. *Neurology* **41**, 936–939.

Engel, A. G. (1970). Evolution and content of vacuoles in primary hypokalemic periodic paralysis. *Mayo Clin. Proc.* **45**, 774–814.

Engel, A. G. and Arahata, K. (1984). Mononuclear antibody analysis of mononuclear cells in myopathies. II: Phenotypes of autoinvasive cells in polymyositis and inclusion body myositis. *Ann. Neurol.* **16**, 209–215.

Engel, W. K. and Oberc, M. A. (1975). Abundant nuclear rods in adult-onset rod disease. *J. Neuropathol. Exp. Neurol.* **34**, 119–132.

Engel, W. K., Bishop, D. W. and Cunningham, G. G. (1970). Tubular aggregates in type II muscle fibers: ultrastructural and histochemical correlation. *J. Ultrastruct. Res.* **31**, 507–525.

Hansen-Smith, F. M. and Carlson, B. M. (1979). Cellular responses to free grafting of the extensor digitorum longus muscle of the rat. *J. Neurol. Sci.* **41**, 149–173.

Jenis, E. H., Lindquist, R. R. and Lister, R. C. (1969). New congenital myopathy with crystalline intranuclear inclusions. *Arch. Neurol.* **20**, 281–287.

Jerusalem, F., Engel, A. G. and Gomez, M. R. (1973). Sarcotubular myopathy: a newly recognized benign congenital, familial muscle disease. *Neurology* **23**, 897–906.

Jerusalem, F., Ludin, H., Bischoff, A. and Hartmann, G. (1979). Cytoplasmic body neuromyopathy presenting as respiratory failure and weight loss. *J. Neurol. Sci.* **41**, 1–9.

Karpati, G., Carpenter, S. and Eisen, A. A. (1972). Experimental core-like lesions and nemaline rods: a correlative morphological and physiological study. *Arch. Neurol.* **27**, 237–251.

Karpati, G., Carpenter, S., Melmed, C. and Eisen, A. A. (1974). Experimental ischemic myopathy. *J. Neurol. Sci.* **23**, 129–161.

Massa, R., Carpenter, S., Holland, P. and Karpati, G. (1992). Loss and renewal of thick myofilaments in glucocorticoid treated rat soleus after denervation and reinnervation. *Muscle Nerve* **15**, 1290–1298.

Robitaille, Y., Carpenter, S., Karpati, G. and DiMauro, S. (1980). A distinct form of adult polyglucosan body disease with massive involvement of central and peripheral neuronal processes and astrocytes: a report of four cases and a review of the occurrence of polyglucosan bodies in other conditions such as Lafora's disease. *Brain* **103**, 315–336.

Schmalbruch, H. (1984). Regenerated muscle fibres in Duchenne muscular dystrophy: a serial section study. *Neurology* **34**, 60–65.

Tomé, F. M. S. and Fardeau, M. (1980). Nuclear inclusions in oculopharyngeal dystrophy. *Acta Neuropath. (Berl.)* **49**, 85–87.

Webster, C. and Blau, H. M. (1990). Accelerated age-related decline in replicative life-span of Duchenne muscular dystrophy myoblasts: implications for cell and gene therapy. *Somat. Cell Mol. Genet.* **16**, 557–565.

15

Electron microscopy in the study of normal and diseased muscle

Stirling Carpenter

The material in this chapter is heavily weighted towards ultrastructural pathology, with normal ultrastructure referred to primarily as a background.

Myofibrils

Myofibrils form the contractile apparatus. By electron microscopy, they appear as bundles containing alternating bands of thick and thin filaments which form, respectively, the A and the I bands (Fig. 15.1). In the middle of the I band runs the Z disc, which appears dense because of its affinity for osmium tetroxide. A sarcomere is the distance between two Z discs. The thin filaments from two adjacent sarcomeres can be seen to insert into the Z disc in alternation, that is, they are not in direct continuity through the Z disc.

The thick filaments are $1.6\,\mu$m long and 15 to 18 nm thick (Harrington and Rodgers, 1984). They are formed of 360 or more molecules of myosin bundled together in a precise order (Fig. 15.2). Each myosin molecule is made up of two heavy chains and four light chains of two types. The heavy chains are coiled around each other to form the rod portion of the molecule and separate to form two globular heads where the light chains are attached. The myosin molecules in each half of a thick filament have reverse polarity, with the rod portions pointing towards the centre of the filament. Because of this, there is a zone (the pseudo-H zone) of decreased density in the middle of the A band where myosin heads are not present. The thick filaments are attached together in their centres by a structure called the M line, which appears on longitudinal sections as a combination of three to five lines crossing the myofibril. On cross-sections it appears as bars connecting the thick filaments, which have a rigid order, each being surrounded by six others at the corners of a hexagon. Structural proteins in the M line include M protein, myomesin and skelemin. Other proteins in the A band include H protein and C protein, the latter being localized to the head-bearing region of the A band, running in seven to nine transverse stripes (Gilbert, et al. 1996).

The thin filaments are 5 to 6 nm in diameter and 1 to 1.25 μm long (Walker and Schrodt, 1974). One end of the thin filaments interdigitates with the thick filaments to a variable degree. This is where the interaction of myosin heads with thin filaments, which is the basis of contraction, takes place (Rayment et al., 1993; Spudich et al., 1995). In a contracted myofibril, the I band almost disappears, since most of the length of the thin filaments is then between the thick filaments. The region of the A band into which the thin filaments have not penetrated is called the H zone and, like the I band, its thickness is variable.

On transverse sections of the zone of interdigitation, six actin filaments tend to surround each myosin filament, while in the middle of the I band the order of thin filaments appears random. As they approach the Z disc, each filament takes up position at the corner of a square. Within the Z discs, one square array is superimposed on another, the corners of which are in the centre of the squares of the first.

Each thin filament is made up of two spiralling chains of actin molecules, with elongated tropomyosin and globular troponin molecules in the grooves between the two chains. The Z disc is largely made up of α-actinin, an actin-binding protein, but it also contains Cap Z, zeugmatin and Z protein. Nebulin, a very large protein, is coextensive with the thin filaments, with which it makes side-to-side contacts, and is bound to the Z disc. It may have a role in regulating the length of the thin filaments. Titin, the largest known protein, runs from the M line to the Z disc (Keller, 1995). The part in the I band is elastic. It may have a role in centring the thick filaments in the sarcomere.

Intermediate filaments, 10 nm thick, which in normal adult muscle are made of desmin, form a net around myofibrils and link the Z discs of adjacent myofibrils to one another and to the subsarcolemmal cytoskeleton. In routine preparations of normal muscle they are difficult to visualize, although they are prominent in regenerating fibres and many fibres that have lost myofibrils.

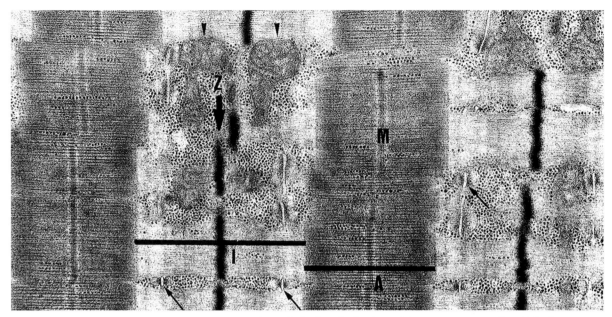

Fig. 15.1. This longitudinal electron micrograph of normal muscle displays the divisions of the sarcomeres, as well as triads (fine arrows) and mitochondria (arrowheads) in their normal para-Z disc position. The section grazes the I band (which is thinner than the A band), letting the intermyofibrillar space, where triads and mitochondria are situated, show itself in places. A, the A band; I, the I band; Z, the Z disc; M, the M line, which is within the clearing made by the pseudo-H zone. The small round granules in the intermyofibrillar space and focally between myofilaments are glycogen particles (×25 000).

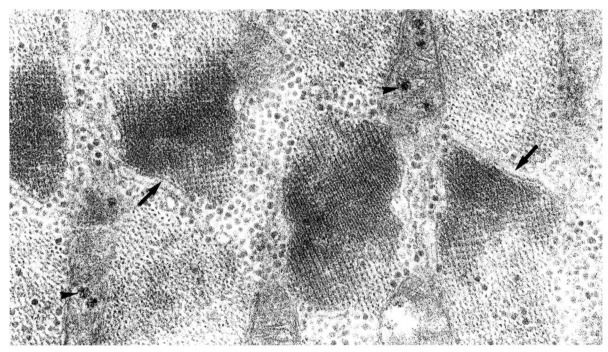

Fig. 15.2. This transverse section of normal muscle shows how the thin filaments line up at the four corners of hypothetical squares as they approach and insert into the Z discs. The section is slightly oblique so that, as it goes from top to bottom, it passes from one side of the Z discs to the other. The corners of the squares from one side become the centres of the squares from the other side. Tubules of the sarcoplasmic reticulum border the Z discs in places (arrows). Mitochondria are present and show prominent but normal matrix granules (arrowheads) (×100 000).

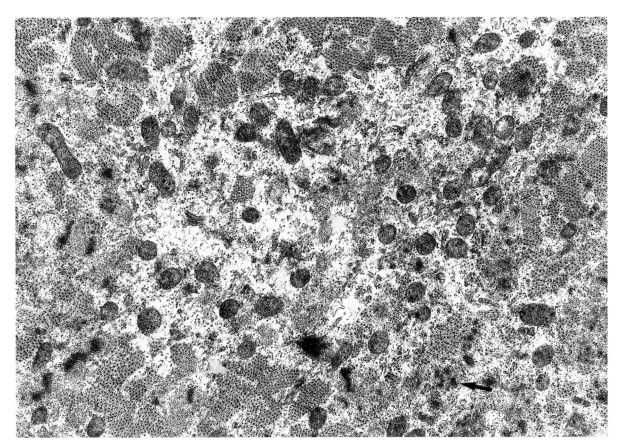

Fig. 15.3. A section of muscle from a patient with dermatomyositis. In the centre of this figure is an irregular area of myofibrillar loss. The myofibrils around it are small and there is occasional Z disc streaming (arrow). The area of loss contains mitochondria and intermediate filaments, which are poorly visible at this magnification (×17500).

Myofibrils in pathological states

Loss of myofibrils

Myofibrils are probably lost whenever there is significant atrophy of muscle fibres, but this not readily visible because the loss of cytoplasmic volume proceeds at the same rate as loss of myofibrils. In dermatomyositis, by contrast, focal myofibrillar loss can be studied (Fig. 15.3). At times, absence of individual thick filaments within myofibrils can be seen on transverse sections, and this may represent the initial stages of the process. The zone from which myofilaments are lost is filled in with glycogen and/or intermediate filaments.

Selective A band loss

Selective loss of the A band is reported in two situations. The first is the best documented and is in patients treated for status asthmaticus by high doses of steroids and concurrently given neuromuscular blockade to facilitate assisted respiration (Danon and Carpenter, 1991). Continuation of this treatment for five days or more results in widespread loss of myosin filaments in skeletal muscle. Clinical recovery ensues over weeks to months following cessation of treatment. Occasional patients have been reported with this loss of A bands who did not receive neuromuscular blockade or who did not have steroids, and rare patients who did not have either. The possible contributions of immobility and of endogenous steroids have not been evaluated. An experimental model has been studied in rats denervated and given high doses of steroids. Repair of myofibrils occurred rapidly after re-innervation (Massa et al., 1992).

The second situation is ischaemia. In certain patients with dermatomyositis, fibres with selective A band loss are found in the vicinity of infarcts (Fig. 15.4) (Carpenter et al., 1976). We have seen A band loss also in a patient with severe ischaemia from pitressin treatment of oesophageal varices and in a patient with thrombotic thrombocytopenia and extensive capillary necrosis in skeletal muscle.

The mechanism of selective myosin loss is not known. Dissolution of thick filaments into myosin monomers may

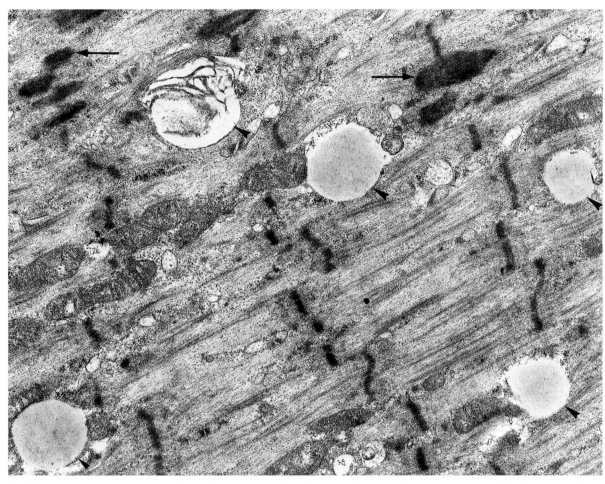

Fig. 15.4. A section of muscle from a patient with dermatomyositis. The myofibrils have suffered extensive loss of thick filaments, while thin filaments and Z discs are relatively well preserved. A few isolated thick filaments persist in most myofibrils. At the top of the picture can be seen small nemaline bodies (arrows), which can be produced when there is thick filament loss. Lipid droplets (arrowheads) often increase in number in such fibres, both in dermatomyositis and in the acute myopathy associated with steroids and neuromuscular blockade (×17500).

be a first step in the process. This can be brought about in vitro with salt solutions in high and unphysiological concentrations (Harrington and Rodgers, 1984). Possibly relevant is the model of soleus tenotomy in the rat, where a subset of myofibrils undergo total breakdown; the first stages of this process are characterized by selective A band loss.

Selective I band loss

We have seen selective I band loss only rarely, focally in a few fibres, and only in denervating conditions.

Z disc loss

Selective Z disc loss is characteristic of necrotic fibres (Fig. 15.5). It was seen in experimental ischaemia 2 hours after aortic ligation (Karpati et al., 1974). Activation by calcium of calpain in the Z disc is probably responsible.

Abnormal orientation of myofibrils: ring myofibrils

Rings are nonspecific, but they occur most frequently in myotonic dystrophy. Very small rings may not be visible on cryostat sections. Rings have been produced in experimental myotonia from dichlorophenoxyacetic acid (2,4-D) administration, where they were accompanied by evidence of a burst of synthetic activity of myofibrils.

Random disorientation of myofibrils

Myofibrils disposed in three perpendicular axes are seen in some fibres in denervating conditions.

Disorganization of myofibrils: Z disc streaming

Z disc streaming is a common lesion, seen in numerous situations. It combines a mild focal loss of myofilaments and loss of the Z disc lattice with streaming of the dense

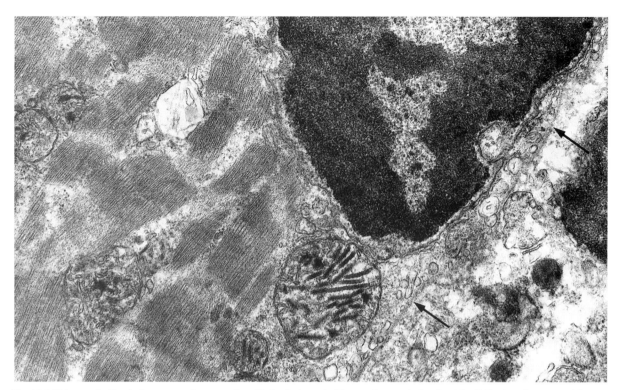

Fig. 15.5. This muscle fibre is from a rat soleus muscle suffering ischaemia 5 hours after aortic ligation. The Z disc has disappeared from the myofibrils. Mitochondria are rounded and show abnormal intracristal densities. The plasma membrane is absent, although the basal lamina (arrows) persists. All these features are typical of necrosis. The nucleus shows condensation of chromatin and a lucent band where the nuclear lamina should be visible on the inner side of the nuclear membrane (×20 000).

material of the Z disc along either thin or remaining thick filaments (Figs. 15.6 and 15.7). The appearance is relatively stereotyped, varying largely in the area covered. When Z disc streaming is confined to a single sarcomere, it is possible to see that it extends from one Z disc to the neighbouring one.

The target fibres found in denervating conditions show Z disc streaming occurring within areas that lack mitochondria. It may be actually a manifestation of re-innervation. The connection of Z disc streaming with areas that lack mitochondria is also seen in various multicore syndromes (some are examples of desminopathy, others of myosin heavy chain mutations (Fananapazir et al., 1993)) and in central core disease. Z disc streaming is very common in dermatomyositis, where it is multifocal within fibres rather than being concentrated in an area as in target fibres. These are the most common settings for Z disc streaming, but it can occur in many others. Two experimental models shed an interesting light. In experimental ischaemic myopathy (Karpati et al., 1974). and in 2,4-D intoxication (Danon et al., 1976), early lesions show loss of centring of thick filaments within the sarcomere, while lesions seen subsequently in a similar distribution within fibres show typical Z disc streaming.

Central cores

Central cores are areas extending over the whole length of muscle fibres in which mitochondria are absent, myofibrils are not distinct, the Z disc is not straight and the degree of contraction appears independent of that of the rest of the fibre (Fig. 15.8) Like any myofibrillar area that lacks mitochondria, central cores are prone to undergo Z disc streaming. Central core disease is caused by mutations in the gene for the calcium-release channel (ryanodine receptor) of the sarcoplasmic reticulum (MacLennan and Phillips, 1995). It is plausible that the mutant receptors are segregated into the cores.

Nemaline bodies

In the usual kind of autosomal dominant nemaline myopathy, the bodies or rods form within otherwise normal myofibrils. They comprise an extension of the lattice of the Z discs (Fig. 15.9). On longitudinal sections, they show both longitudinal and transverse periodicity (Engel and

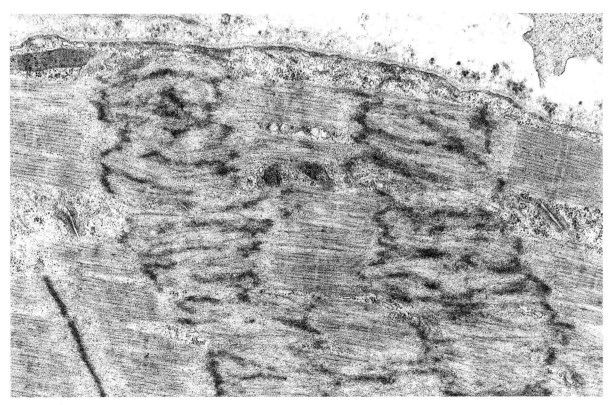

Fig. 15.6. This fibre, from a patient with dermatomyositis, shows Z disc streaming. Note that it can involve single sarcomeres (×25 000).

Gomez, 1967). With breakdown of myofibrils, they often accumulate beneath the sarcolemma. Very small nemaline bodies can be encountered in situations of A band loss. The experimental model of tenotomy in the rat can lead to formation of rods, probably because the initial stages of the lesion involve A band loss (Karpati et al., 1972).

Cytoplasmic bodies
Cytoplasmic bodies are formed from dense masses of randomly oriented thin filaments that individually have increased density; other thin filaments radiate from their surface, forming the clear halo usually seen around them. Cytoplasmic bodies in formation appear to arise from the Z disc, although they lack its lattice configuration (Fig. 15.10). Antibody studies have suggested that cytoplasmic bodies may vary considerably in the proportion of desmin associated with them (Baeta et al., 1996). Typical cytoplasmic bodies are nonspecific. Large numbers of cytoplasmic bodies can be associated with a syndrome of myopathy involving the respiratory muscles. Differentiation of this syndrome from desminopathy, as discussed below, is under review.

Spheroid bodies
Spheroid bodies are more complex than cytoplasmic bodies. They are made up of more or less spherical aggregates of fragments of myofibrils. When several are present in a fibre, they can increase its calibre. They may contain quantities of several proteins normally present only in trace amounts and be associated with Congo red-positive material. Because of this it has been proposed to group together numerous instances reported as spheroid body myopathy, cytoplasmic body myopathy, desminopathy, etc. under the new rubric of myofibrillary myopathy with desmin excess (de Bleeker et al., 1996; Nakano et al., 1996). Subsequently it has been demonstrated that some of these conditions are caused by mutations in the gene for desmin (Goldfarb et al., 1998) and others by mutations in the gene for β-spectrin, a chaperone protein that facilitates the polymerization of desmin (Vicart et al., 1998). These findings appear to justify the retention of the term of desminopathy for these cases. Other genes may be involved in other patients. (Wilhelmsen et al., 1996).

Diagnosis of desminopathy is facilitated by the electron microscopic demonstration of reticular strands of dense material between myofibrils (Fig. 15.11). This material has

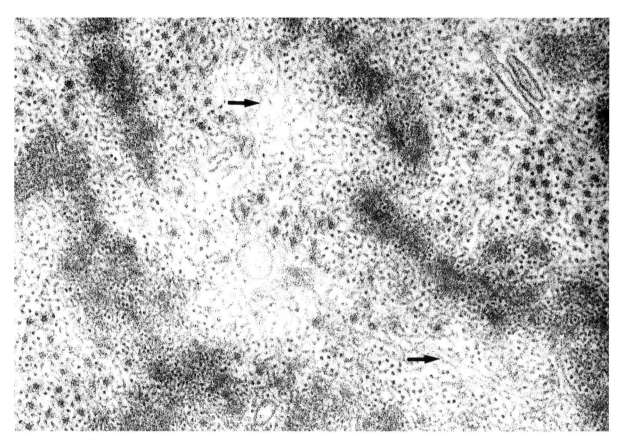

Fig. 15.7. This is a high-power transverse view of an area of Z disc streaming in a fibre from a patient with dermatomyositis. The Z disc lattice is absent. Electron-dense material is running among the thin filaments in discrete spots. Some groups of thick filaments interdigitated with thin filaments are present. Randomly oriented irregularly curving fine filaments (arrows) between aggregates of well-oriented actin filaments probably represent desmin (×100 000).

been interpreted as being derived from Z discs, since it may appear contiguous to them, but it is located between myofibrils and almost certainly is formed from abnormal desmin aggregates.

Sarcoplasmic reticulum

The sarcoplasmic reticulum takes up and stores calcium ions and releases them when activated by the voltage-gated calcium channel in the T-tubule membrane. Calcium uptake is dependent on the calcium-activated ATPase in the tubular component of the sarcoplasmic reticulum. Calcium release takes place through the ryanodine receptor, a large tetrameric molecule interposed between the terminal cisternae and the T-tubule membrane. The conjuncture of T-tubule and two flanking cisternae is known as a triad (Fig. 15.1). The ryanodine receptors are actually visible by electron microscopy as regular block-like densities connecting the two membranes. The lateral cisternae

tend to have finely granular contents of low to medium density.

Dilatation of the cisternae is relatively rare. They usually retain their finely granular contents. Two patients who had multiple clear vacuoles in the cisternae have been characterized as having sarcotubular myopathy. The sarcoplasmic reticulum is also the source of tubular aggregates and cylindrical spirals, which are discussed below.

T-tubules

The transverse or T-tubules communicate the action potential into the depths of the muscle fibre, where it activates the voltage-gated calcium channel, which in turn activates the calcium release channel of the sarcoplasmic reticulum. The T-tubular lumen is in continuity with the extracellular space, and the T-tubular membrane in continuity with the plasmalemma, although the two membranes differ in their protein composition.

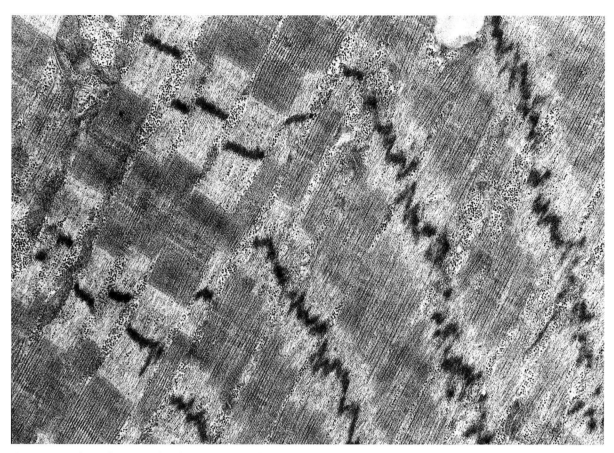

Fig. 15.8. Central core disease. To the left are normal myofibrils. To the right is the core, where the Z disc zigzags, mitochondria are absent and myofibrils are variable in size and not well defined. The degree of contraction of the core myofibrils is different from that of the normal myofibrils. This is most obvious comparing the I band widths (×17 500).

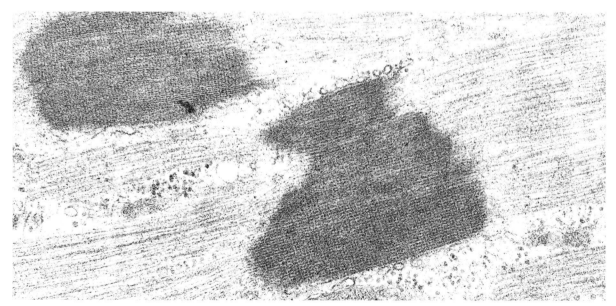

Fig. 15.9. Two nemaline bodies can be seen here in a biopsy from a patient with childhood-onset nemaline myopathy. Note that they appear to have formed in intact myofibrils. They have characteristic longitudinal and transverse periodicity (×50 000).

Fig. 15.10. This figure shows the edge of a cytoplasmic body that is probably in a stage of accretion. It is formed of a feltwork of fine filaments adjacent to the Z disc (×25 000).

T-tubules are most easily identified where they form triads with the sarcoplasmic reticulum, and this is most easily seen on longitudinal sections (Fig. 15.1). A small isolated segment of T-tubule, especially as seen on transverse sections, can be difficult to distinguish from a segment of tubular sarcoplasmic reticulum. Some longitudinally oriented segments of T-tubule occur. More positive identification is possible using a tracer substance such as lanthanum before fixation.

Proliferation of T-tubules in the form of focal honeycomb networks is a frequent reaction in chronically injured muscle fibres, for example in myotonic dystrophy or in any form of inflammatory myopathy. One case has been reported in which T-tubules gave rise to large aggregates of tubules and vacuoles, which eventually broke down and gave rise to intrusions of extracellular space (Carpenter et al., 1992).

Acute dilatation of T-tubules occurs frequently in the stumps of muscle fibres that have undergone focal necrosis (Fig. 15.12) (Carpenter and Karpati, 1989). This is caused by the massive ingress of sodium from the extracellular space into the necrotic segment. Until a protective membrane is established over the stump, sodium can diffuse freely into it and activate the Na^+/K^+ ATPase in the T-tubule wall. This enzyme moves three sodium ions into the T-tubule in exchange for two potassium ions, resulting in a build-up of osmotic pressure in the T-tubule, which draws water out of the fibre into its lumen. The swelling takes place between triads and usually results in vacuoles that are initially rounded but may become elongated in the long axis of the fibre. Identification of their connection to definite T-tubules in triads is extremely difficult after the initial phases. Experimental production and verification in vitro and in vivo has been possible (Casademont, et al., 1988). In human muscle, good examples of vacuolated stumps of necrotic fibres can be seen in dermatomyositis. An interesting difference is seen in Duchenne dystrophy, where small T-tubule vacuoles are seen within fibre segments that have focally lost their plasmalemma without showing other morphological signs of necrosis. In the stumps, by contrast, no vacuoles are found.

Mitochondria

A large proportion of the energy used by muscle cells is made available by mitochondria, where enzymes for

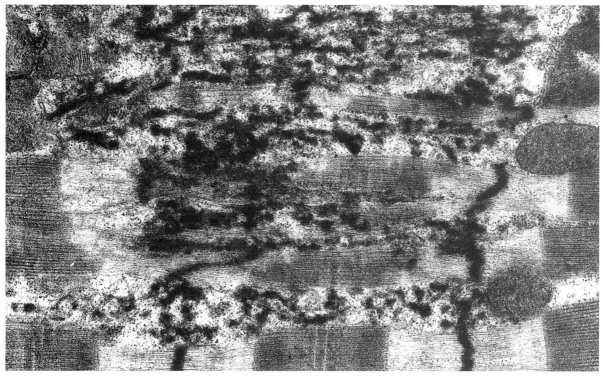

Fig. 15.11. Bands of electron-dense material extend between several myofibrils, some of which display Z disc streaming, in a section of muscle from a patient with desminopathy. The pattern is characteristic of the small lesions in desminopathy (×25 000).

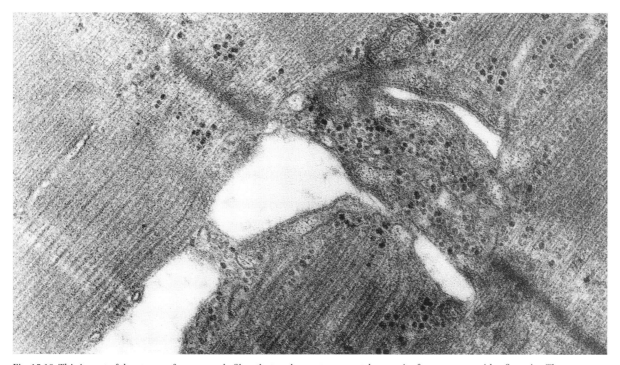

Fig. 15.12. This is part of the stump of a rat muscle fibre that underwent segmental necrosis after puncture with a fine wire. The elongated clear vacuoles that appeared in the stumps, as seen here, are derived from T-tubules. When the vacuoles become very large, their connection to T-tubules becomes more difficult to demonstrate (×50 000).

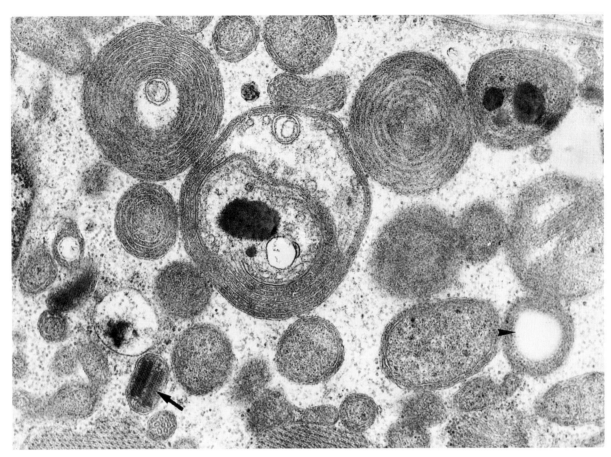

Fig. 15.13. This is a sample of the mitochondrial abnormalities that can be encountered in mitochondrial myopathy, including crystals (arrow), excess cristae, paucity of cristae, circumferential cristae, large matrix densities and a lipid vacuole indenting a mitochondrion (arrowhead). This biopsy is from a patient with Kearns–Sayre syndrome (×29 500).

β-oxidation of fatty acids, the tricarboxylic acid (Krebs) cycle, the respiratory chain and ATP synthase are located. Mitochondria are normally concentrated in four locations: between myofibrils at the I band level, under the sarcolemma, at the motor endplate and at the poles of myonuclei.

Mitochondria are easily recognizable by electron microscopy because of their double membranes. The outer membrane is relatively porous; consequently, the concentration of molecules in the outer compartment (the space between the two membranes) is rather similar to that of the cytosol. The inner membrane, which is extended by the cristae, is highly impermeable. The matrix normally contains a few distinct dense granules.

A very common artifact consists of watery swelling of the mitochondrial matrix. It is produced by slowness of fixation and is probably never a result of in vivo pathology.

Most mutations in the mitochondrial genome result in proliferation of the involved mitochondria, except in young children. This holds true in cases where a genetic mutation in the nucleus has resulted in secondary alterations in the mitochondrial genome. No abnormality is visible, however, in muscle mitochondria in Leber's optic atrophy, where all muscle mitochondria contain a mutation. The proliferated mitochondria usually show ultrastructural abnormalities, including abnormalities in size, abnormal distribution or numbers of cristae, excess matrix, large matrix densities and crystals in the intracristal space or external compartment (Fig. 15.13). These crystals are composed largely or totally of mitochondrial creatine kinase. The crystals that occur in type II fibres are rarer and somewhat different in ultrastructure from those in type I fibres, being more dense and more cubic. Some patients with mitochondrial myopathy only show an excess of ultrastructurally normal mitochondria, and most of the mutations of the nuclear genome that cause mitochondrial disease do not produce morphological changes in the muscle mitochondria.

Electron microscopy is not particularly useful in the routine work-up of a mitochondrial myopathy. Proliferation of mitochondria can be best appreciated with histochemistry (the modified succinate dehydrogenase reaction in particular). The crucial factor is the relative number of fibres affected, and this is not well determined from the small area of ultrathin sections. The ultrastructural changes offer no clues to identify the mutation.

A few instances of oligomitochondrial disease have been reported, in which the number of mitochondria in many type II fibres was reduced, especially in their centre. The residual mitochondria in these fibres were enlarged but otherwise morphologically normal (Nishino et al., 1998).

Mitochondria in necrotic fibres become rounded, tending to accumulate in rows between myofibrils, and take on increased electron density. Dense plates may appear within cristae and in the outer compartment. The mitochondria may lose their outer membranes before they are phagocytosed.

Nuclei

In normal adult muscle, myonuclei are apposed to the sarcolemma with no intervening myofibrils. Areas within the nucleus where chromatin is being actively transcribed are pale (euchromatin), while transcriptionally inactive areas are dark (heterochromatin). Communication between cytoplasm and nucleus takes place through the nuclear pores. The perinuclear cisterna is enclosed by the inner and outer nuclear membranes. Ribosomes may be attached to the outer nuclear membrane, suggesting that it is a part of the endoplastic reticulum. On the inner side of the inner nuclear membrane is a relatively uniform granular band known as the nuclear lamina. Fibrillar proteins called lamins, which may bind the ends of chromosomes to the lamina, are found in this region. The lamina is interrupted beneath the nuclear pores.

Nuclei that are impeded in their exchanges with the cytosol by surrounding organelles may exhibit an excess of heterochromatin and eventually lose their membranes. Examples are nuclei surrounded by tubular aggregates and nuclei surrounded by reducing bodies.

Accumulation of fine tubular filaments, 4 nm in external diameter, within myonuclei are pathognomonic of oculopharyngeal muscular dystrophy. They sometimes form palisades or knots. This disease has now been shown to result from expansion of a short GCG triplet repeat in a gene on chromosome 14q11, now called the polyadenylate binding protein-2 gene (Brais et al., 1998). The protein normally resides in nuclei and binds the polyadenylate tail of mRNA. GCG codes for alanine, and the tubular filaments may possibly be formed by polyalanine tracts in β-pleated form. Many patients with oculopharyngeal muscular dystrophy eventually develop pathological changes of inclusion body myositis in their muscles.

A variety of nuclear abnormalities can be seen in inclusion body myositis, including bizarre shapes, excess heterochromatin, accumulation of tubular filaments 120 to 150 nm in diameter and loss of nuclear membranes (Fig. 15.14). The filaments are more often seen in the cytoplasm in the vicinity of membranous whorls than in nuclei. They probably reach the cytoplasm through nuclear breakdown, which the membranous whorls reflect (Carpenter, 1996). The cytoplasmic filaments (and occasionally the nuclear ones) tend to have a slightly larger external diameter than the nuclear ones. On longitudinal views, they may show a vague periodicity. Incubation of frozen sections of muscle for 24 hours in phosphate-buffered saline before fixation gives a picture recalling paired helical filaments (Askanas and Engel, 1998), suggesting that the tubular centre of the filaments has been dissolved or rendered nonstaining. The ultimate nature of the filaments in inclusion body myositis still uncertain, although they may correspond to Congo red-staining material seen in muscle fibres in this disease.

The mutation that causes Emery–Dreifuss muscular dystrophy results in loss of a protein normally localized to the inner nuclear membrane. Electron microscopic abnormalities of nuclei have been reported, becoming more frequent with increasing age, including formation of regular tubules 300 to 350 nm in diameter, nuclear pyknosis and focal breakdown of the nuclear membranes (Fidzianska et al., 1998).

A great variety of nuclear abnormalities are seen in infantile polymyositis, including herniation of nucleoplasm through nuclear pores and various intranuclear inclusions, some of normal cytoplasmic organelles, like microtubules, others not seen outside of abnormal nuclei, like 22 nm filaments in a semicrystalline array (Sripathi et al., 1996).

In the Marinesco–Sjögren syndrome, nuclei become surrounded by a thick membrane, which may be derived from the outer nuclear membrane (Suzuki et al., 1997). This leads to increasing pyknosis of the nuclei and probably to apoptosis.

Accumulation in nuclei of masses of fine parallel 8 nm filaments, presumably representing actin, is a nonspecific reaction that probably reflects a burst of synthetic activity. In human muscle, it is seen most often in damaged fibres in dermatomyositis. It can be produced experimentally in guinea-pigs by administration of 2,4-D (Danon et al., 1976). In this model, the thin filaments in nuclei may be

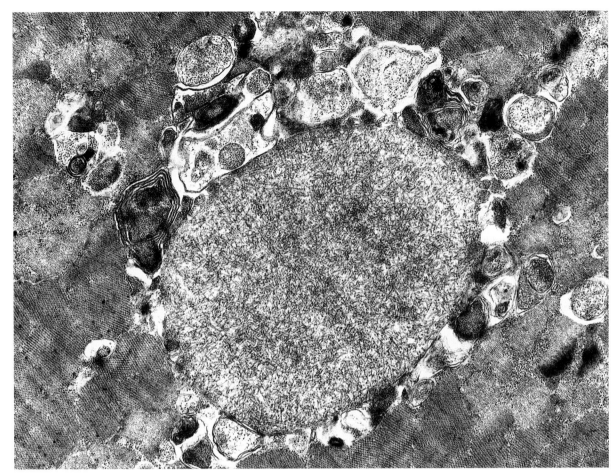

Fig. 15.14. This electron micrograph from a patient with inclusion body myositis shows an oval accumulation of abnormal filaments that is highly suggestive of the remains of a nucleus. It is surrounded by membranous whorls of various sizes ($\times14\,500$).

accompanied by Z disc. While proteins designed to be imported into nuclei are tagged by specific import sequences, small molecules can diffuse into nuclei through the nuclear pores. Globular actin in excess can apparently diffuse into nuclei, where it can be trapped if conditions favour its polymerization into filamentous actin. Nemaline bodies can also be encountered in nuclei in some cases of nemaline myopathy, especially of neonatal onset.

Breakdown of nuclei has been seen in inclusion body myositis (Carpenter et al., 1970). It is likely that formation of membranous whorls is a nonspecific consequence of nuclear breakdown. Aside from inclusion body myositis, they are encountered in the Marinesco–Sjögren syndrome and in reducing body myopathy, where nuclei also break down. In inclusion body myositis a so-far unidentified single-stranded DNA-binding protein can be detected by radioautography in some fibres, both in nuclei and in

rimmed vacuoles, suggesting that the former give rise to the latter.

The nuclei of muscle fibres in necrosis disappear rapidly; as a result, they are rarely encountered in necrotic human muscle. In experimental ischaemic myopathy produced by aortic ligation, nuclei were seen in which the lamina had dissolved within 2 hours (Karpati et al., 1974).

Sarcolemma

The sarcolemma is composed of the basal lamina and the plasma membrane, with which may be included the submembranous cytoskeleton. The plasma membrane is a lipid bilayer in which are embedded numerous proteins, the presence and distribution of which can only be determined by immunostaining. The basal lamina has two components by electron microscopy; the lamina lucida, which

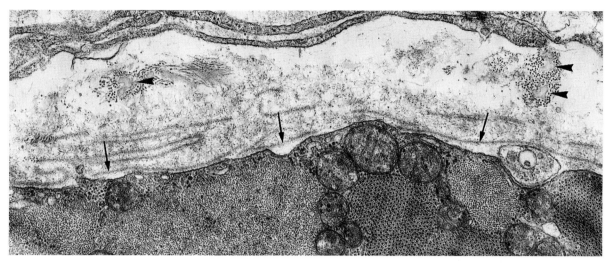

Fig. 15.15. In Duchenne dystrophy, many fibres show reduplication of broad stretches of basal lamina, as is seen here. In addition, focal absence of basal lamina can be seen in places next to the plasma membrane (arrows), suggesting that the basal lamina has a tendency to detach from the plasmalemma. This is a section from a relatively late stage of Duchenne dystrophy, which may explain the presence of some elastic fibres in the interstitial space (arrowheads) ($\times 25\,000$).

borders the plasmalemma, and the lamina densa. The pallor of the lamina lucida is crossed by vaguely seen strands, and it contrasts with the darkness of the lamina densa. The lamina lucida will not be seen if the sarcolemma is cut tangentially. Proteins in the lamina densa include type IV collagen and laminin-2 (merosin). Links between the basal lamina and the plasmalemma are normally formed by interaction of merosin with sarcoglycans and α-dystroglycan. The sarcoglycans and dystroglycans, in turn, are linked to dystrophin in the submembranous cytoskeleton, which is linked to cytoskeletal actin.

In Duchenne dystrophy, deficiency of dystrophin leads to paucity of sarcoglycans and dystroglycans. This is reflected by reduplication of many segments of basal lamina and occasional stretches of plasma membrane denuded of basal lamina (Fig. 15.15) (Carpenter and Karpati, 1979). The interior architecture of such fibres is usually surprisingly normal. In some cases of Duchenne dystrophy, fibres can be found in which stretches of plasma membrane are absent (Carpenter and Karpati, 1979). These fibres do not show the usual signs of necrosis, although they contain some vacuoles formed from T-tubules. Their myofibrils may be contracted or relaxed. This condition may be an initial stage of necrosis in Duchenne dystrophy.

Basal lamina abnormalities are characteristically seen in denervation atrophy, where sleeves of redundant basal lamina form long prolongations of the angular corners of fibres (Fig. 15.16). In polymyositis, focal reduplication of basal lamina occurs. It is often associated with small round

dense profiles, probably derived from fragments of the muscle fibre surface that are surrounded by a circle of basal lamina (Fig. 15.17). This is particularly striking when it is seen around a fibre that has undergone necrosis without regeneration.

Glycogen

Glycogen appears as rounded particles about 20 to 30 nm in diameter. It is seen under the sarcolemma and in relatively small amounts between myofibrils. Occasional particles may intrude between thin filaments. Decision as to when glycogen is significantly excessive may be difficult. Glycogen tends to fill areas of myofibrillar loss.

In sections stained only with uranyl acetate, glycogen particles have relatively little contrast, but they have strong contrast after staining with lead salts. It has been shown that lead actually stains the protein part of the glycogen particle (Rybicka, 1996). More specific staining is possible using the thiosemicarbazide method. Glycogen particles can also be lost from tissue during fixation and processing, leaving optically empty spaces.

An increase in glycogen particles of normal morphology is seen in some but not all glycogen storage diseases. In myophosphorylase deficiency (McArdle's disease) or phosphofructokinase deficiency (Tarui's disease), the excess of glycogen is relatively modest. Subsarcolemmal pockets are usually seen in scattered fibres. Necrosis and/or regeneration may also be present. Large cytoplasmic accumulations

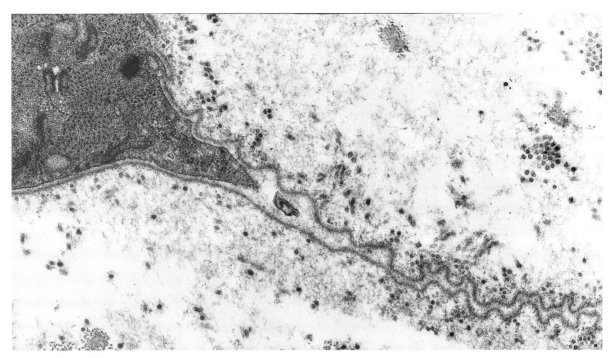

Fig. 15.16. In muscle fibres undergoing denervation atrophy, empty sleeves of basal lamina project from the surface of the fibre, usually starting, as here, from an angle of the surface. This redundant basal lamina retains its continuity with the part of basal lamina covering the plasmalemma (×30 000).

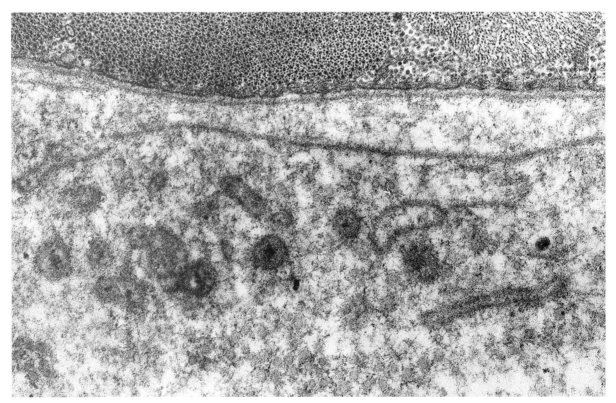

Fig. 15.17. In polymyositis, reduplication of basal lamina is seen over some fibres; it is often associated with small rounded masses of dense material surrounded by a sphere of basal lamina (×50 000).

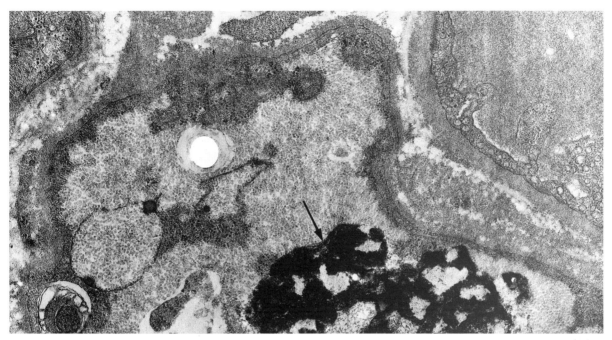

Fig. 15.18. In acid maltase deficiency, the masses of glycogen in muscle fibres may be in the cytosol as well as in lysosomes. This probably comes about by rupture of distended lysosomes. The glycogen particles liberated into the cytosol, though morphologically normal, probably are sufficiently altered in their composition that they cannot be metabolized. A large mass of lipofuscin-like material is also present in this muscle fibre (arrow) from a patient with adult-onset disease (×30 000).

are seen in deficiency of the debranching enzyme, with replacement of myofibrils. The glycogen particles appear normal by electron microscopy, although biochemically they can be shown to have short terminal chains.

In deficiency of acid maltase, a lysosomal enzyme, glycogen is found in membrane-bound vacuoles. In the infantile form there may also be extensive cytosolic glycogen, probably as a result of rupture of distended lysosomes (Fig. 15.18). Membranous whorls are also sometimes present in the lysosomes. In the adult-onset form, many muscle fibres can remain free of storage. The glycogen particles in acid maltase deficiency seems particularly prone to be dissolved in processing, leaving empty vacuoles. One must also remember that a little glycogen can be carried artifactitiously into any sort of clear vacuole that happens to occur in muscle fibres, and that a diagnosis of acid maltase deficiency is not made from finding a single glycogen-containing vacuole.

Instead of glycogen particles, a fibrillar polysaccharide is found by electron microscopy in deficiency of the branching enzyme (glycogenosis type IV or Anderson's disease) (Schröder et al., 1993). This type of deposit has been called polyglucosan. It is seen also in patients with later-onset cardioskeletal myopathy, in some of whom no abnormality of any isoform of the branching enzyme has been found. In some cases of phosphofructokinase deficiency,

along with cytoplasmic accumulation of morphologically normal glycogen, there may be glycogen particles linked like beads on a string and there may also be polyglucosan deposits (Agamanolis et al., 1980). This apparently happens because phosphofructokinase is a rate-limiting enzyme for glycolysis; when its activity is reduced, substrates may back up and the capacity of the branching enzyme may be exceeded by the pool of subunits. In hypothyroidism, polyglucosan bodies are found at the myotendinous junction.

Fibrillary polysaccharide also occurs in muscle fibres in Lafora's disease, but, unlike examples described above, it is present in membrane-bound spaces (Carpenter et al., 1974). These spaces have no activity of lysosomal enzymes. There is some evidence that they are derived from peroxisomes (Carpenter et al., 1974). Lafora's disease is caused by mutation in a tyrosine phosphatase in some families but not in others (Minassian et al., 1989).

Lysosomes

In normal muscle fibres, lysosomes are virtually absent, aside from lipofuscin bodies, which accumulate normally with ageing but are accentuated in denervated muscle. In vitamin E deficiency, which can be dietary or related to deficiency of the vitamin E transfer protein (Cavalier et al., 1998), lysosomal accumulation of ceroid occurs in skeletal muscle. It can be seen by electron microscopy as dense finely granular membrane-bound deposits, which tend to be present in the interior of fibres, unlike banal lipofuscin, which commonly is found under the sarcolemma.

Lysosomal structures that take the form of tubules with dense contents are present in muscle fibres in infantile myotonic dystrophy in the first few years of life. They are most easily found on the border of sarcoplasmic masses with more normally organized parts of the fibres. Their numbers on cryostat sections reacted for acid phosphatase are such as to suggest a storage disease. In many cases of polymyositis, a few fibres can be found in which numerous small autophagic vacuoles are present.

Four lysosomal storage diseases involve skeletal muscle fibres (Kawai et al., 1985; Carpenter and Karpati, 1986). Only one, acid maltase deficiency is symptomatic in muscle. In the others, characteristic deposits in muscle fibres can sometimes be useful for diagnosis. They are Batten's disease (ceroidlipofuscinosis), Fabry's disease and mannosidosis.

Abnormal organelles

Cylindrical spirals

Cylindrical spirals are complicated membranous structures only seen in type II fibres and are relatively rare. A number of the patients in whom they have been found suffer from a syndrome of cramps (Carpenter et al., 1979). In other patients, there is no consistent clinical reflection. A cylindrical spiral is formed by a flattened cisterna bent in several spiral turns around a small central core of nondescript cytoplasm. The cisterna is derived from sarcoplasmic reticular membranes, as emphasized by the occasional association of cylindrical spirals with tubular aggregates.

Fingerprint bodies

Fingerprint bodies are confined to type I fibres. By electron microscopy they present two main patterns, presumably depending on the angle at which they are cut. Most commonly, there are linear collections of small bar-like densities about 18 nm long, stacked with a periodicity of 15 to 20 nm. Three to ten lines of these bars may be formed. The second pattern is a quadrangular network with a periodicity of about 15 nm.

Fingerprint bodies are seen in some biopsies as an inci-

dental finding. They were so numerous in four patients with congenital myopathy that the name of fingerprint myopathy seemed justified. Three patients were children without any other marked abnormality in their muscle fibres (Engel et al., 1972; Fardeau et al., 1976). The other was a 55-year-old woman, weak from birth but still able to walk (Fardeau et al., 1976). The origin of fingerprint bodies remains unknown.

Reducing bodies

Reducing bodies are best identified by histochemistry, although their ultrastructure is relatively specific. They are seen essentially only in reducing body myopathy. By electron microscopy they are formed of osmiophilic tubular profiles which are so matted together that they appear to be granules (Fig. 15.19) (Carpenter et al., 1985). In some patients they envelop nuclei, causing nuclear breakdown, but they have never been reported within nuclei.

Tubular aggregates

Tubular aggregates are formed of masses of parallel tubules (Fig. 15.20). Their continuity with membranes of the sarcoplasmic reticulum has been demonstrated. An appearance of double-walled tubules is often encountered, but the inner tubules are probably not formed of true membranes. They occur only in type II fibres and only in males, except in some familial syndromes, where type I fibres and women are involved. They are most often seen in cramp syndromes.

Necrosis

It is important in composing pathological descriptions to be able to recognize cell death because it releases a chain of stereotyped pathological changes. Cell death in skeletal muscle fibres, given their length and plethora of nuclei, is usually segmental. It is possible that apoptosis occurs in skeletal muscle fibres in some situations (there are several reports to this effect using the TUNEL technique), but the cytoplasmic changes accompanying segmental death of a muscle fibre in any situation appear stereotyped and consistent with necrosis.

Necrosis implies that a cell has passed the point of no return in its maintenance of homeostasis. Morphological changes appear after this point has been passed. Early stages of necrosis can be best identified in skeletal muscle cells by a constellation of findings: loss of the Z disc, discontinuities in the plasma membrane and mitochondrial

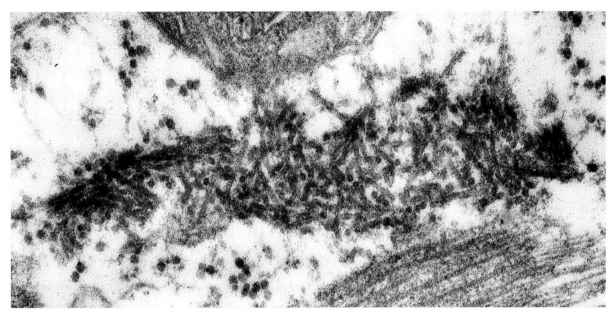

Fig. 15.19. A small collection of reducing body material is seen here between myofibrils. It is made up of filaments and round granules, which may be filaments in cross-section (×100 000).

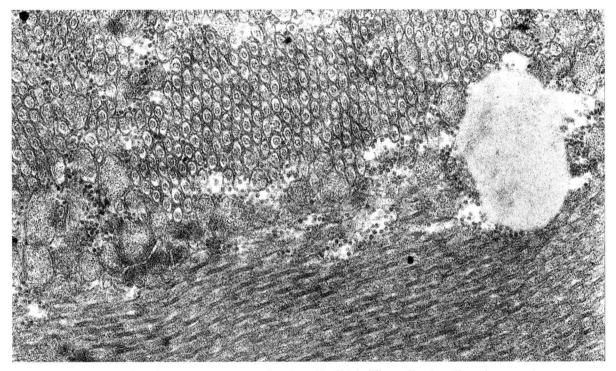

Fig. 15.20. Two subgroups of tubular aggregates are seen to be oriented in slightly different directions. Those that are cut in near cross-section appear to contain inner tubules. The patient had a subacute cramp syndrome (×50 000).

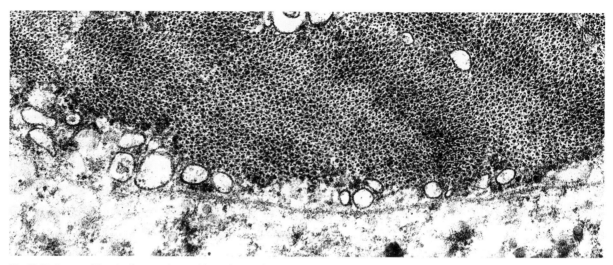

Fig. 15.21. In some biopsies from patients with Duchenne dystrophy, especially young ones with abundant necrosis, occasional fibres like this are found, in which the plasma membrane has disappeared although other signs of necrosis are not present. This may be the initial stage of necrosis in this disease. The myofibrils are not hypercontracted (×50000).

changes (mitochondria become round with dense intra-cristal densities and/or fluffy matrix densities (Fig. 15.5)). Of these changes, the most important is the status of the plasmalemma. In some biopsies from young patients with Duchenne dystrophy, fibres can be found that have breaches of variable size in their plasma membrane, without loss of Z discs or mitochondrial changes (Fig. 15.21). These fibres are probably irreversibly damaged, possibly depending on the size of the breaches, but this remains to be determined. An intact plasma membrane is necessary for cell survival.

When phagocytic invasion of necrotic muscle fibres has begun, cytoplasmic changes of necrosis are generally clear. One must remember that non-necrotic fibres can be invaded by lymphocytes and monocytes in polymyositis and inclusion body myositis. These fibres do not show the criteria mentioned above for necrosis, although they may show Z disc streaming and some alterations in the sarcoplasmic reticulum and T-tubules. In Duchenne dystrophy, necrosis is so prevalent that monocytes are present within the muscle tissue much of the time, and they may invade necrotic segments that have not yet been demarcated from surviving stumps. In this situation, therefore, intact Z discs can exist a few sarcomeres away from a macrophage.

The basal lamina of muscle fibres persists despite necrosis. At times it can be used in identifying muscle fibres where the cross-section has been replaced by inflammatory cells in the middle of an inflammatory infiltrate. The basal lamina will also persist for some weeks after necrosis even if regeneration has not taken place. Examples of this can most easily be found in Duchenne dystrophy and polymyositis.

Regeneration

Regeneration of skeletal muscle is brought about by the migration and proliferation of satellite cells. Normal satellite cells are present under the basal lamina of muscle fibres, making up about 5% of the nuclei in this position as seen by light microscopy (Fig. 15.22). In their proliferative stage, they can be called regenerative myoblasts, and they line up along the inner side of the basal lamina when they reach necrotic segments. Their outlines are relatively smooth and simple, in contrast to the ruffles of adjacent macrophages. They have abundant ribosomes and occasionally contain one or more prominent lysosomal bodies. They are sometimes seen in mitosis.

The proliferated myoblasts fuse with one another and with the stumps. Soon thereafter they begin to form myofibrils, although not all the myoblasts mature at the same rate. When the fused myoblasts have formed a fibre, it can be distinguished from normal fibres by the space between its myofibrils (which tends to contain intermediate filaments and microtubules), the occasional presence of organelles within the not fully compacted myofibrils and the presence of some stretches of the old basal lamina that are not in contact with the new plasma membrane (Fig. 15.23).

Regeneration, which replaces necrotic segments and is effected through proliferation and fusion of mononuclear

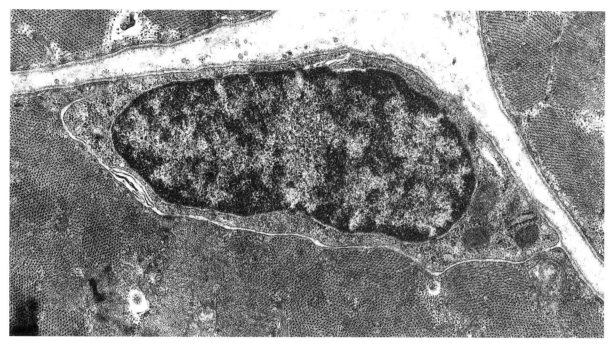

Fig. 15.22. A normal resting satellite cell is present under the basal lamina of this fibre (×25000).

myoblasts, should be clearly distinguished from repair, which occurs when a damaged fibre renews altered cytoplasmic components without dying. For example, in a patient treated with steroids and neuromuscular blockade, many fibres may undergo acute loss of thick filaments without becoming necrotic. In time they then generate thick filaments again, which are integrated into myofibrils. This process is an example of repair and not regeneration, even if the myosin heavy chains are not of the normal adult types.

Other cell types and structures

Vessels

Extensive changes in capillaries occur in dermatomyositis. Some endothelial cells will contain tubuloreticular structures in their smooth endoplasmic reticulum or perinuclear cisterna, as well as confronting cylindrical cisternae (Fidzianska and Goebel, 1989). These structures can be generated in lymphocytes in vitro by interferon treatment. They are seen in endothelial cells, lymphocytes and monocytes in viral infections and in collagen vascular disease (Fig. 15.24). In intramuscular capillaries, they are rare outside of dermatomyositis, lupus myositis and HIV infection. They are, therefore, diagnostically useful, especially as they are virtually never seen in polymyositis. Aside from these inclusions, capillaries in dermatomyositis often show hypertrophy and hyperplasia of endothelium, as well as necrosis.

Capillary death leaves the basal lamina behind as a marker of where the capillary had been. These basal lamina ghosts are not specific for any disease, because capillaries can be lost when muscle fibres atrophy. This is best demonstrated in denervation, but it occurs to some extent in disuse. In denervation, capillary channels move closer together as muscle fibres atrophy; as a result the muscle may appear overvascularized, although the number of capillaries per fibre drops (Carpenter and Karpati, 1982). Loss of these capillary lines probably occurs through apoptosis in the endothelium.

Connective tissue

An increase in interstitial connective tissue can be seen in many muscle diseases where there has been fibre loss. Normally there is almost no collagen between muscle fibres, although some groups of microfibrils may occur. The type of connective tissue proliferation in Duchenne dystrophy tends to be distinctive. It is largely in the form of discrete solid bundles of collagen laid down parallel to the muscle fibres (Fig. 15.25). Similar deposits are seen in many patients with limb girdle dystrophy. The connective

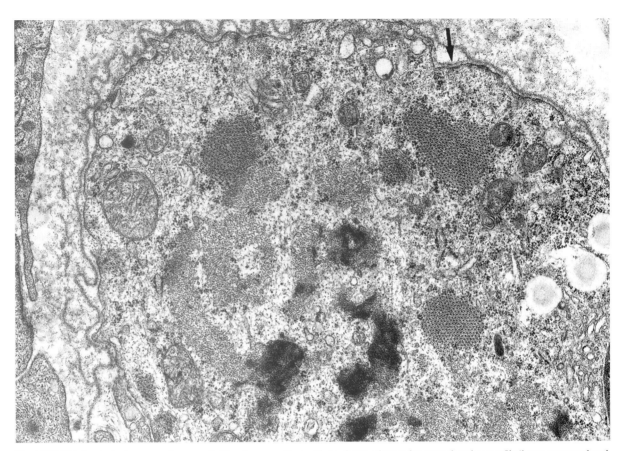

Fig. 15.23. This is a typical regenerating muscle fibre from a patient with Duchenne dystrophy. Note that the myofibrils are separated and irregular. The space between them contains intermediate filaments, which appear like dots and dashes at this magnification. The surface of the regenerating fibre is in contact with the pre-existing basal lamina in some places but not others. A small stretch of new basal lamina has formed (arrow) (×25 000).

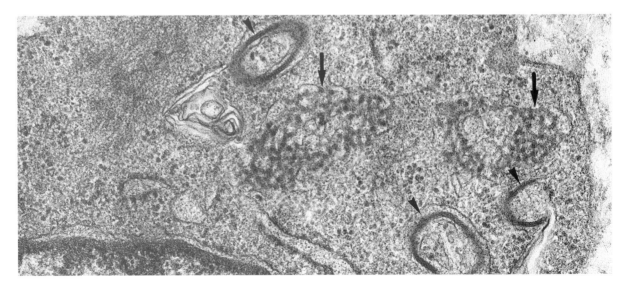

Fig. 15.24. This is part of a monocyte from the endomysium in a patient with dermatomyositis. Its cytoplasm contains both tubuloreticular structures (arrows) and cylindrical confronting cisternae (arrowheads). Both also occur in endothelium in this disease, although tubuloreticular structures are more common. The cylindrical confronting cisternae are sometimes seen in the necrotic debris of capillaries, where they have been called striated membranous structures (×50 000).

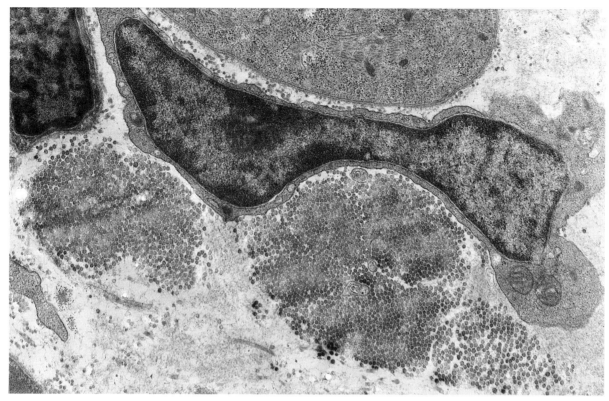

Fig. 15.25. In Duchenne dystrophy, collagen deposition particularly takes the form of dense bundles like these two laid down parallel to the muscle fibres. This may have some influence on the development of irreversible contractures in this disease (×25 000).

tissue in polymyositis and inclusion body myositis, in contrast, is looser and less precisely oriented. In the fibrosis encountered in some cases of denervation, elastic fibres are often present.

References

Agamanolis, D. P., Askari, A. D., DiMauro, S. et al. (1980). Muscle phosphofructokinase deficiency: two cases with unusual polysaccharide accumulation and immunologically active enzyme protein. *Muscle Nerve* **3**, 456–467.

Askanas, V. and Engel, W. K. (1998). Newest approaches to diagnosis and pathogenesis of sporadic inclusion-body myositis and hereditary inclusion-body myopathies, including molecular-pathologic similarities to Alzheimer disease. In *Inclusion-body Myositis and Myopathies*, eds. V. Askanas, G. Serratrice and W. K. Engel, pp. 3–78. Cambridge: Cambridge University Press.

Baeta, A. M., Figarella-Branger, D., Bille-Turc, F. et al. (1996). Familial desmin myopathies and cytoplasmic body myopathies. *Acta Neuropath. (Berl.)* **92**, 499–510.

Brais, B., Bouchard, J.-P., Xie, Y.-G. et al. (1998). Short GCG expansions in the PABP2 gene cause oculopharyngeal muscular dystrophy. *Nat. Genet.* **18**, 164–167.

Carpenter, S. (1996). Inclusion body myositis: a review. *J. Neuropathol. Exp. Neurol.* **55**, 1105–1114.

Carpenter, S. and Karpati, G. (1979). Duchenne muscular dystrophy: plasma membrane loss initiates necrosis unless it is repaired. *Brain* **102**, 147–161.

Carpenter, S. and Karpati, G. (1982). Necrosis of capillaries in denervation atrophy of human skeletal muscle. *Muscle Nerve* **5**, 250–254.

Carpenter, S. and Karpati, G. (1986). Lysosomal storage in human skeletal muscle. *Hum. Pathol.* **17**, 683–703.

Carpenter, S. and Karpati, G. (1989). Segmental necrosis and its demarcation in experimental micropuncture injury of skeletal muscle fibers. *J. Neuropathol. Exp. Neurol.* **48**, 154–70.

Carpenter, S., Karpati, G. and Wolfe, L. (1970). Virus-like filaments and phospholipid accumulation in skeletal muscle: study of a histochemically distinct chronic myopathy. *Neurology* **20**, 889–903.

Carpenter, S., Karpati, G., Andermann, F. et al. (1974). Lafora's disease: peroxisomal storage in skeletal muscle. *Neurology* **24**, 531–538.

Carpenter, S., Karpati, G., Rothman, S. and Watters, G. (1976). The childhood type of dermatomyositis. *Neurology* **26**, 952–962.

Carpenter, S., Karpati, G., Robitaille, Y. and Melmed, C. (1979). Cylindrical spirals in human skeletal muscle. *Muscle Nerve* **2**, 282–287.

Carpenter, S., Karpati, G. and Holland, P. (1985). New observations in reducing body myopathy. *Neurology* **35**, 818–827.

Carpenter, S., Karpati, G. and Holland, P. (1992). A chronic myopathy with coated vesicles and tubular masses. *Neuromusc. Disord.* **2**, 209–216.

Casademont, J., Carpenter, S. and Karpati, G. (1988). Vacuolation of muscle fibres near sarcolemmal breaks represents T-tubule dilatation secondary to enhanced sodium pump activity. *J. Neuropathol. Exp. Neurol.* **47**, 618–628.

Cavalier, L., Ouahchi, K., Kayden, H. J. et al. (1998). Ataxia with isolated vitamin E deficiency: heterogeneity of mutations and phenotypic variability in a large number of families. *Am. J. Hum. Genet.* **62**, 301–310.

Danon, J. M., Karpati, G. and Carpenter, S. (1976). Subacute skeletal myopathy induced by 2,4-dichlorophenoxyacetate in rats and guinea pigs. *Muscle Nerve* **1**, 89–102.

Danon, M. J. and Carpenter, S. (1991). Myopathy with thick filament (myosin) loss following prolonged paralysis with vecuronium during steroid treatment. *Muscle Nerve* **14**, 1131–1139.

de Bleeker, J. L., Engel, A. G. and Ertl, B. B. (1996). Myofibrillar myopathy with abnormal foci of desmin positivity: II. Immunocytochemical analysis reveals accumulation of multiple other proteins. *J. Neuropathol. Exp. Neurol.* **55**, 563–577.

Engel, A. G. and Gomez, M. R. (1967). Nemaline (Z disc) myopathy: observations of the origin, structure and solubility properties of the nemaline structures. *J. Neuropathol. Exp. Neurol.* **26**, 601–619.

Engel, A. G., Angelini, C. and Gomez, M. R. (1972). Fingerprint body myopathy: a newly recognized congenital muscle disease. *Mayo Clin. Proc.* **47**, 377–388.

Fananapazir, L., Dalakas, M. C., Cyran, F. et al. (1993). Missense mutations in the beta-myosin heavy-chain gene cause central core disease in hypertrophic cardiomyopathy. *Proc. Natl. Acad. Sci. USA* **90**, 3993–3997.

Fardeau, M., Tomé, F. M. S. and Derambure, S. (1976). Familial fingerprint body myopathy. *Arch. Neurol.* **724**, 725.

Fidzianska, A. and Goebel, H. H. (1989). Tubuloreticular structures (TRS) and cylindrical confronting cisternae (CCC) in childhood dermatomyositis. *Acta Neuropath. (Berl.)* **79**, 310–316.

Fidzianska, A., Toniolo, D. and Hausmanowa Petrusewicz, I. (1998). Ultrastructural abnormality of sarcolemmal nuclei in Emery–Dreifuss muscular dystrophy (EDMD). *J. Neurol. Sci.* **159**, 88–93.

Gilbert, R., Kelly, M. G., Mikawa, T. and Fischman, D. A. (1996). The carboxy terminus of myosin binding protein C (MyBP-C, C-protein) specifies incorporation into the A-band of striated muscle. *J. Cell Sci.* **109**, 101–111.

Goldfarb, L. G., Park, K.-Y., Cervenakova, L. et al. (1998). Missense mutations in desmin associated with familial cardiac and skeletal myopathy. *Nat. Genet.* **19**, 402–403.

Harrington, W. F. and Rodgers, M. E. (1984). Myosin. *Annu. Rev. Biochem.* **53**, 35–73.

Karpati, G., Carpenter, S. and Eisen, A. A. (1972). Experimental core-like lesions and nemaline rods: a correlative morphological and physiological study. *Arch. Neurol.* **27**, 237–251.

Karpati, G., Carpenter, S., Melmed, C. and Eisen, A. A. (1974). Experimental ischemic myopathy. *J. Neurol. Sci.* **23**, 129–161.

Kawai, H., Nishino, H., Nishida, Y. et al. (1985). Skeletal muscle pathology of mannosidosis in two siblings with spastic paraplegia. *Acta Neuropathol.* **68**, 201–204.

Keller, T. C. (1995). Structure and function of titin and nebulin. *Curr. Opin. Cell Biol.* **7**, 32–38.

MacLennan, D. H. and Phillips, M. S. (1995). The role of the skeletal muscle ryanodine receptor (RYR1) gene in malignant hyperthermia and central core disease. *Soc. Gen. Physiol.* **50**, 89–100.

Massa, R., Carpenter, S., Holland, P. and Karpati, G. (1992). Loss and renewal of thick myofilaments in glucocorticoid treated rat soleus after denervation and reinnervation. *Muscle Nerve* **15**, 1290–1298.

Minassian, B. A., Lee, J. R., Herbrick, J. A. et al. (1989). Mutations in a gene encoding a novel protein tyrosine phosphatase cause progressive myoclonus epilepsy. *Nat. Genet.* **20**, 171–174.

Nakano, S., Engel, A. G., Waclawik, A. J., Emslie-Smith, A. M. and Busis, N. (1996). Myofibrillar myopathy with abnormal foci of desmin positivity: I. Light and electron microscopy analysis of 10 cases. *J. Neuropathol. Exp. Neurol.* **55**, 549–562.

Nishino, I., Kobayashi, O., Goto, Y.-I. et al. (1998). A new congenital muscular dystrophy with mitochondrial structural abnormalities. *Muscle Nerve* **21**, 40–47.

Rayment, I., Holden, H. M., Whittaker, M. et al. (1993). Structure of the actin–myosin complex and its implications for muscle contraction. *Science* **261**, 58–65.

Rybicka, K. K. (1996). Glycosomes – the organelles of glycogen metabolism. *Tissue Cell* **28**, 253–265.

Schröder, J. M., May, R., Shin, Y. S. et al. (1993). Juvenile hereditary polyglucosan body disease with complete branching enzyme deficiency (type IV glycogenosis). *Acta Neuropathol. (Berl.)* **85**, 419–430.

Spudich, J. A., Finer, J., Simmons, B. et al. (1995). Myosin structure and function. *Cold Spring Harb. Symp. Quant. Biol.* **60**, 783–791.

Sripathi, N., Karpati, G. and Carpenter, S. (1996). A distinctive type of infantile inflammatory myopathy with abnormal myonuclei. *J. Neurol. Sci.* **136**, 47–53.

Suzuki, Y., Murakami, N., Goto, Y.-I. et al. (1997). Apoptotic nuclear degeneration in Marinesco-Sjögren syndrome. *Acta Neuropathol. (Berl.)* **94**, 410–415.

Vicart, P., Caron, A., Guicheney, P. et al. (1998). A missense mutation in the alpha-B-crystallin chaperone gene causes a desmin-related myopathy. *Nat. Genet.* **20**, 92–95.

Walker, S. M. and Schrodt, G. R. (1974). I segment lengths and thin filament periods in skeletal muscle fibres of the rhesus monkey and humans. *Anat. Rec.* **178**, 63–82.

Wilhelmsen, K. C., Blake, D. M., Lynch, T. J. et al. (1996). Chromosome 12-linked autosomal dominant scapuloperoneal muscular dystrophy. *Ann. Neurol.* **39**, 507–520.

16

Magnetic resonance imaging and spectroscopy of muscle

Doris J. Taylor, James L. Fleckenstein and Raffaele Lodi

Introduction

Many types of muscle disorder lead to changes in the chemical and physical properties of tissues that can be detected by nuclear magnetic resonance (NMR) through imaging (MRI) and spectroscopy (MRS). Safe, noninvasive and painless techniques based on the principles of NMR are used for imaging and for making biochemical measurements. The continuing development of instrumentation and complex pulse sequences has resulted in techniques that are increasingly versatile in their ability to measure a range of structural, physiological and biochemical parameters. This information assists not only in diagnosis and in monitoring treatment effects but also in revealing the basic pathophysiology that ultimately produces the clinical manifestations experienced by the patient and observed by the clinician.

There are two widely used NMR-based techniques, each providing a different kind of information (Andrew et al., 1990). MRI is used to examine patients' muscular anatomy and to distinguish which muscles are abnormal in size and shape. Muscle quality can be further characterized by discriminating between the mesenchymal alterations of muscle fat and oedema. This ability can be exploited to optimize the selection of muscle for biopsy, thereby improving the diagnostic yield of the procedure. Imaging can also be used to provide prognostic information and to monitor progression of muscle disease. These topics are reviewed by Fleckenstein and co-workers (1991c).

The second technique, MRS, is able to measure muscle metabolite concentrations and intracellular pH (pH_i) in vivo and follow the time course of biochemical changes during exercise, particularly those important to cellular energetics. Disease progression and response to therapy may be assessed by both MRS and MRI. There is an increasing trend to maximize the information available and

improve data interpretation by using these two complimentary techniques in combination with each other and with other methodologies such as electromyography and near-infrared spectroscopy.

Magnetic resonance methods

All MR signals are generated by the interaction of atomic nuclei with a strong magnetic field and energy pulses in the radiofrequency range. Only nuclei with the quantum mechanical property of spin one-half have magnetic characteristics. When placed in a magnetic field, these nuclei align themselves with the field and precess with an angular frequency of rotation (ω) that depends on the field strength (B_0) and a constant for each type of nucleus, known as the gyromagnetic ratio (γ): $\omega = \gamma B_0$. When radiofrequency pulses are applied, each nucleus absorbs energy at the frequency with which it is precessing. This energy is detected when the pulse is terminated and the nucleus relaxes back to its original energy state, inducing an electromotive force in a receiver coil. The time constant T_1 characterizes one of these exponential relaxation processes, the longitudinal relaxation time. A second relaxation process, transverse relaxation, is described by the time constant T_2. Because the magnetic field experienced by any individual nucleus is modified by its physicochemical environment, the same type of nucleus in different molecules (i.e. protons in fat and water) or in different parts of the same molecule (i.e. phosphorus in the α, β and γ phosphate groups of ATP) will have different resonant frequencies.

Magnetic resonance imaging

MR images are distribution maps of NMR-sensitive nuclei. Although it is theoretically possible to use any

NMR-sensitive nucleus to produce an image, practical constraints mean that most clinical studies exploit the properties of protons in water and fat. Radiofrequency pulses are used to excite the nuclei, which are then spatially encoded by applying magnetic field gradient pulses. Proton density or relaxation characteristics can be selectively emphasized by a careful choice of the pulse repetition time (TR) and the echo time (TE). Because fat has a short T_1, it is detected on T_1-weighted images (short TR/short TE) (Fig. 16.1). Because of its long T_2, fat also manifests high signal intensity (SI) on T_2-weighted images (long TR, long TE). Increased tissue water leads to increased spin density and elevated T_1 and T_2 relaxation times; hence, muscle oedema is detectable using MRI, particularly in T_2-weighted images (Fleckenstein et al., 1991a,c).

These principles are exemplified by oedema occurring in acute muscle trauma (Fig. 16.2). The appearance of oedema is nonspecific, however, and is shared by the 'oedema-like' changes of subacute denervation (Fig. 16.3 and 16.4) and many myopathies (see below). The long T_1 of oedema-like processes is frequently not apparent on T_1-weighted images (Fleckenstein et al., 1991c). Also, it can sometimes be difficult to differentiate coexisting intramuscular fat and oedema using conventional T_1- and T_2-weighted spin echo sequences. Multiple fat suppression sequences have been developed that improve detection of muscle oedema (Dwyer et al., 1988; Fleckenstein et al., 1991a,c). One of these employs an inversion pulse that nulls signal from tissue having a T_1 time equal to that of fat (short inversion time inversion recovery (STIR)). STIR has the additional advantage of producing heightened lesion conspicuity through additive effects to SI caused by oedema-associated increases in lesion spin density and T_1 and T_2 times (Dwyer et al., 1988). Other sequences employ frequency-selective pulses to null the fat signal. These techniques generally require a longer TE to achieve the same degree of lesion conspicuity as STIR sequences at the same TR. Important from a financial perspective, a variety of fat suppression sequences can be incorporated into fast scan techniques so that high sensitivity to muscle oedema can be realized with short scan times (Fleckenstein et al., 1991a). This makes muscle imaging an economically viable, as well as an informative application of MRI.

In addition to pulse sequences, operator-dependent choices that are important to image quality and interpretation are the coil size, imaging plane, number of excitations, voxel size, spatial resolution and photographic techniques. The added signal-to-noise afforded by a smaller coil gives images of high spatial resolution without an additional time cost. Such high resolution may be necessary to show fine detail in subtle lesions or in performing accurate volumetric studies (Roman et al., 1993). When tissue characterization is more important than fine anatomical detail, large voxels can be used to maximize signal to noise. The combination of small coils and large voxels reduces the number of excitations and phase-encoding steps. The end result is the potential for relatively fast and economical imaging for tissue characterization (Fleckenstein et al., 1991a). The axial plane provides most of the radiological information desired, although longitudinal planes are sometimes helpful in assessing the extent of disease and for assessing the relationship of muscle lesions with physical landmarks such as large joints. The plane chosen for encoding phase and frequency data is also of consequence since the specific artifacts related to those planes can be anticipated and directed away from the region of interest (Porter et al., 1987). The photographic technique used to display the data is also important.

Magnetic resonance spectroscopy

MRS is based on the same physical principles as MRI, but the signals are collected, amplified and then processed by Fourier transformation into a plot of frequency of nuclear rotation versus SI (Fig. 16.5). The variation in frequency, called chemical shift, is expressed in parts per million of the field strength, thus normalizing frequency with respect to the intensity of the magnet field. The requirement for magnetic field homogeneity generally dictates that the muscle to be examined must be positioned at magnet centre and remain in a fixed position during data collection. This geometric problem explains why most MRS studies, particularly those involving exercise, have been performed on forearm and calf muscles. In the most basic MRS experiment, a surface coil placed next to the muscle is used as both transmitter and receiver. Coil size and position as well as pulsing conditions determine the location and size of the volume of muscle interrogated. More complex coil arrangements and pulse sequences may be applied in order to obtain both MRS and MRI data from the same well-defined tissue volumes (Andrew et al., 1990). To increase the quality of the data, signals from a series of pulses are usually added together so that each spectrum is time averaged over a period ranging from a few seconds to many minutes, although in some cases a single pulse may produce useable data.

Tightly bound molecules such as membrane phospholipids, bone and ADP bound to myofibrils produce only very broad signals, which underlie the distinct spectral peaks arising from the freely tumbling molecules. Peak areas are proportional to metabolite concentrations.

(a)

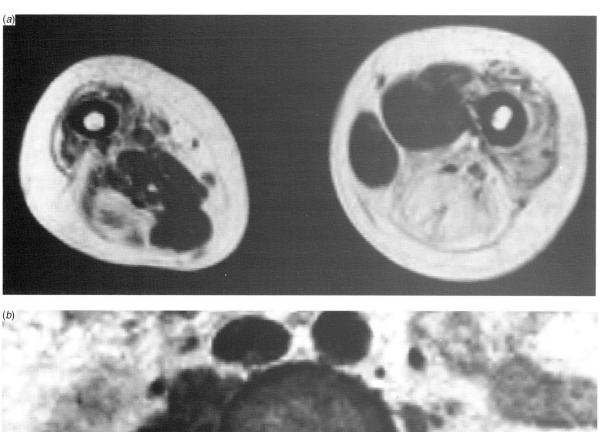

(b)

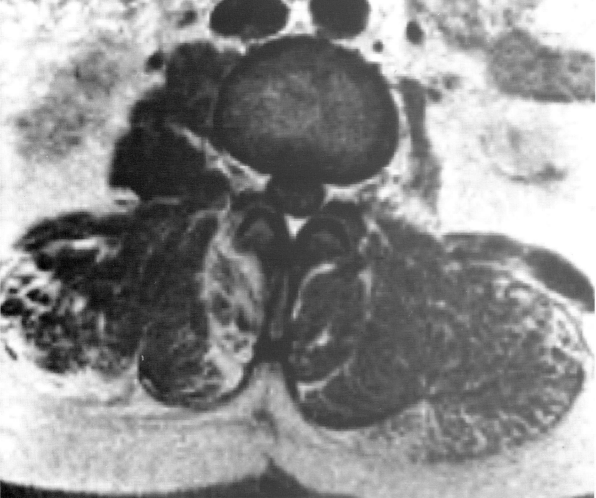

Fig. 16.1. Muscle mesenchymal alterations on MRI: fatty change. (*a*) In this patient with a remote history of poliomyelitis, T1-weighted image of the thighs shows typical asymmetric muscular atrophy. Note the increased volume of high signal intensity material (fat) in the regions of atrophy. Also, observe compensatory hypertrophy. (*b*) Similar features are apparent in a different patient in the paraspinal muscles. Note the irregularly marginated atrophic muscle bundles (moth-eaten appearance).

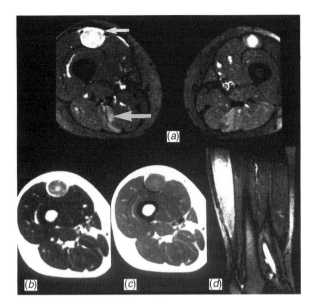

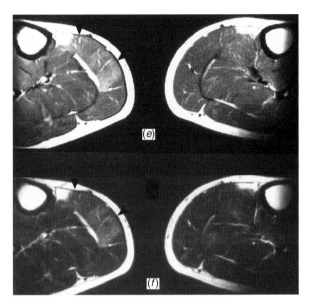

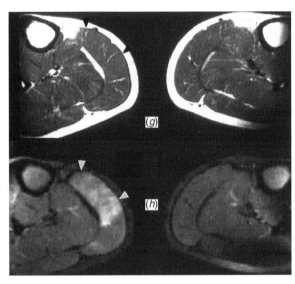

Fig. 16.2. Muscle mesenchymal alterations on MRI: oedema in acute and delayed muscle injuries. Although the mechanisms of the pain syndromes vary, the MRI appearances share the fundamental properties of oedema, i.e. high signal intensity on T_2-weighted (T_2W) images and little if any abnormality on T_1-weighted (T_1W) images. (a,b) A 'week-end athlete' with acute muscle strain while running for a ball, short inversion time inversion recovery (STIR) (a) and T_2W (b) MRI performed 36 hours after the event shows increased T_2 signal intensity in the rectus femoris muscle bilaterally with the right (short arrow) more severe than the left. Associated semitendinosus strains are less obvious (long arrow). (c) The T_1W image of the thigh shows the typical appearance of oedema by being inconspicuous. (d) A sagittal STIR image shows the longitudinal extent of the rectus femoris injury. (e–h) In a patient with painful calves 2 days after unaccustomed exercise, the typical pattern of oedema is again apparent, characterized by increased signal in the medial head of the right gastrocnemius muscle (arrowheads) on progressively T_2W images (e,f) but not on T_1W (g). The additive effect of long T_1 and T_2 and spin density accounts for the greater conspicuity on STIR (h). Serum creatine kinase was more than four times greater than normal, corroborating exertional myonecrosis.

Results are often expressed as concentration ratios or as changes in SI over time because absolute concentrations can only be derived if the true concentration of one of the MRS-visible metabolites is known. The most abundant naturally occurring isotope of phosphorus, ^{31}P, is the nucleus most frequently used in muscle studies. The few human muscle investigations using other nuclei have been largely confined to ^{1}H and ^{13}C, and there is wide scope for expanding their use. Proton MRS has been applied to problems such as quantifying the intracellular concentrations of creatine (Bottomley et al., 1997) and lactate (Pan et al., 1991a,b), quantitative and qualitative lipid analysis

(Barany et al., 1989; Boesch et al., 1997) and measuring tissue temperature (Morvan et al., 1992). The MR-detectable isotope of carbon, ^{13}C, occurs with a natural abundance of only 1.1%, so for many studies it would be necessary to administer ^{13}C-labelled compounds, usually [^{13}C]-glucose, to insure detection. Glycogen in muscle, however, is fully visible by natural abundance ^{13}C MRS (Avison et al., 1988).

MRS using ^{31}P detects the major phosphorus-containing

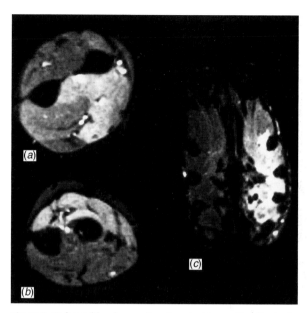

Fig. 16.3. Œdema-like changes in subacute denervation. Each of three patients sustained transection of a nerve near the elbow in the months prior to the MRI. The short inversion time inversion recovery (STIR) sequence shows to good advantage the distribution of oedema-like changes that characterizes subacute denervation. Median (*a*), radial (*b*), and ulnar (*c*) innervated muscles show typical hyperintensity in denervated muscles.

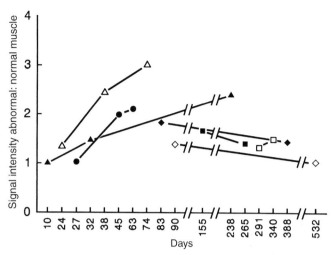

Fig. 16.4. Time course of short inversion time inversion recovery (STIR) signal intensity (SI) ratios in acute traumatic denervation. Note that the most prominent increases in SI ratio occur in the first several months of denervation. The return to normal of one patient (open diamonds) was observed more than a year after nerve grafting.

compounds and intracellular pH (pH$_i$) in the sarcoplasm of muscle (Fig. 16.5). Fat, fibrous tissue, blood and extracellular fluid contribute no significant signal, and mitochondrial volume in muscle is too small or mitochondrial metabolites are too tightly bound to interfere. In muscle the major compounds detectable are adenosine trisphosphate (ATP), phosphocreatine (PCr) and inorganic phosphate (Pi). The free (metabolically active) adenosine disphosphate (ADP) concentration can be calculated from the MRS data using the creatine kinase equilibrium reaction (Arnold et al., 1985):

$$[ADP] = \{([\text{total creatine}]/[PCr]) + 1\}[ATP]/(K[H^+])\quad (16.1)$$

where the total creatine is taken as 42.5 mmol/l cell water and K is the equilibrium constant $(1.66 \times 10^9 \text{ l/mol})$ (Harris et al., 1974; Veech et al., 1979).

Other visible compounds include phosphomonoesters (PME), which in muscle are largely the hexose phosphate intermediates of glycolysis plus any inosine monophosphate from the net breakdown of ATP. Phosphodiesters (PDE) such as glycerophosphocholine and glycerophosphoethanolamine are also seen as a small peak in normal muscle spectra and are indicative of membrane break-

down. Peak intensity of PDE increases with age and in disorders in which there is muscle necrosis or atrophy, such as dystrophy. Intracellular pH can be determined from the chemical shift difference between Pi and PCr because the chemical shift of Pi is pH sensitive in the physiological range. Similarly, the chemical shift of β-ATP is dependent on magnesium ion concentration (Gupta et al., 1983; Ward et al., 1996; Lodi et al., 1997b).

Much effort has been expended in developing quantitative methods of MRS data analysis to extract not only straightforward information about metabolite concentrations and pH$_i$ but also useful kinetic data on glycolytic ATP synthesis, oxidative ATP synthesis and intracellular pH regulation (Chance et al., 1986; Bendahan et al., 1990; Boska 1991; Argov et al., 1996; Kemp et al., 1993b; Lodi et al., 1997a). This topic has been well reviewed (Kemp and Radda, 1994). Care is needed in interpreting MRS data because some metabolite concentrations and pH$_i$ may be over- or underestimated in certain exercise conditions (Constantin-Teodosiu et al., 1997). Employing non-MR-based techniques simultaneously with MRS can aid in data interpretation and broaden the scope of the investigation. Near infrared spectroscopy provides data on state of tissue oxygenation (McCully et al., 1994; Chance and Bank, 1995), and electromyography can be used to study the correlation between metabolic and electrical changes (Vestergaard-Poulsen et al., 1994, 1995; Bendahan et al., 1996 1998a).

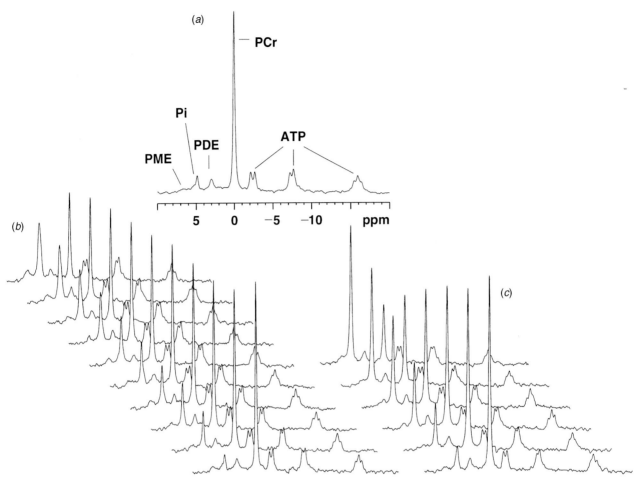

Fig. 16.5. Spectra of calf muscle using ^{31}P. (a) Resting muscle of a normal control, showing peak assignments. (b) Series of spectra collected from a normal control at rest (bottom spectrum) and throughout a period of aerobic, dynamic exercise, showing the progressive decrease in phosphocreatine (PCr) and increase in inorganic phosphate (Pi) during exercise. Each spectrum was collected over a period of 0.5 min. (c) A similar series of spectra to that in (b) collected from a patient with myophosphorylase deficiency; changes are more rapid than in the normal subject. See also Fig. 16.8. PDE, phosphodiesters; PME, phosphomonoesters.

Muscle anatomy, physiology and biochemistry

MRI and MRS complement clinical evaluation. In vivo testing using MRS as an adjunct to histological studies and to direct biochemical assay can add significantly to the understanding of the contribution of metabolism to phenotype. As helpful as in vitro measurements on muscle biopsies can be, they do not always accurately reflect in vivo activity (Taylor et al., 1997). Variability or inaccuracy may arise from small unrepresentative samples, site-specific differences, sample treatment and assay conditions; an abnormal gene product may have altered properties such as increased fragility, which invalidate the measurement. Measurements of in vitro enzyme activity,

the amount of gene product present or the proportion of abnormal mitochondrial DNA (mtDNA) may be misleading even if accurate, because lower-than-normal levels may be sufficient to allow normal muscle metabolism and function.

Magnetic resonance imaging

In addition to the capability of MRI to reveal data about muscle size and quality, it can also indicate muscle usage patterns because recently exercised muscle shows prolongation of T_2 times and increased signal on T_2-weighted images (Fig. 16.6) (Fleckenstein et al., 1988). This interesting phenomenon continues to defy satisfactory

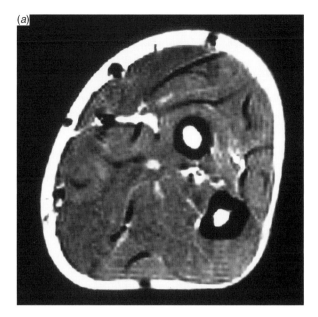

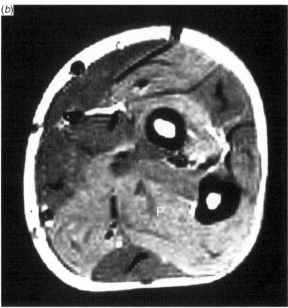

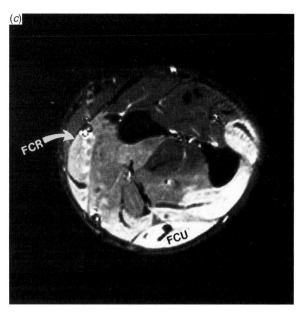

Fig. 16.6. Imaging of healthy muscle. (*a*) An axial T_2-weighted image of the forearm shows the typical low signal intensity of muscle circumscribed by a thin rim of high signal intensity fat, as well as fat within the bone marrow. Observe the absence of significant areas of fat within the muscle bulk and that the muscle volume could be quantified with simple software, if desired. (*b*) Following brief handgrip exercise, a normal physiological 'brightening' of muscle occurs transiently within stressed muscles (e.g. flexor digitorum profundus (P)) because of lengthening of the T_2 relaxation time; the precise mechanism by which this occurs is not known. (*c*) Using a short inversion time inversion recovery (STIR) sequence that is highly sensitive to muscle 'oedema', physiological exercise-related changes are more obvious. Note in this case, in which wrist flexion was performed, that different intensities of muscle activation are suggested by variable degrees of signal change, particularly in the finger flexors lying deep to wrist flexors; FCU, flexor carpi ulnaris; FCR, flexor carpi radialis. Such heterogeneity of muscle recruitment must be taken into account when performing 'blind' exercise tests, such as surface coil magnetic resonance spectroscopy (MRS).

explanation, but the fact that the effect is absent in patients with blocked glycogen breakdown (e.g. those with myophosphorylase deficiency) implies that lactate production may be important. Alternatively, acidosis or alterations in protein filament structure may be involved (Fleckenstein et al., 1991b). Regardless of the mechanism of this effect, it can be used to assess which muscles are reliably activated during a given exercise. This can help to optimize MRS studies so as to avoid errors inherent to the use of 'blindly' placed surface coils (Fig. 16.6) (Fleckenstein et al., 1991b).

Magnetic resonance spectroscopy

MRS has played an important role in improving the understanding of muscle metabolism. Assumptions about the biochemistry of muscle in vivo have been tested (and sometimes found to be incorrect), and new insights into the regulation of energetics and adaptation of muscle to disease have been achieved. It is often an overall pattern of abnormality detected by MRS rather than a single feature that distinguishes different myopathies. For example, a high Pi/PCr ratio is a common finding in mitochondrial myopathy but it is quite nonspecific, being seen in other

Table 16.1. Magnetic resonance spectroscopy data from a group of normal controls and patients with muscle disease

	Normal controls[a]	Mitochondrial myopathy	Phosphorylase deficiency	Becker muscular dystrophy
Age (years)	28.9 ± 8.4	22	47	53
Sex	15 men, 18 women	Male	Male	Male
Rest				
pH_i	7.02 ± 0.03	7.09	7.11	7.07
PCr/ATP	3.40 ± 0.25	2.98	4.24	3.00
Pi/ATP	0.37 ± 0.09	0.50	0.67	0.47
PCr/Pi	9.5 ± 2.1	6.0	6.4	6.4
PCr/(PCr + Pi)[b]	0.90 ± 0.02	0.86	0.86	0.86
PME/ATP	0.15 ± 0.10	0.18	0.0	0.12
PDE/ATP	0.13 ± 0.09	0.20	0.30	0.28
ADP (μmol/l)	13 ± 5	26	1	24
(1/phosphorylation potential) $\times 10^{6c}$	6.2 ± 2.4	16.3	0.6	14.2
Exercise (first min)				
pH_i	7.07 ± 0.02	7.11	7.15	7.07
PCr/(PCr + Pi)[b]	0.76 ± 0.07	0.73	0.77	0.67
ADP (μmol/l)	30 ± 12	48	26	47
Exercise (end)				
Time to exhaustion (min)	12.8 ± 2.8	9.9	5.5	8.8
pH_i	6.64 ± 0.14	6.85	7.19	6.80
PCr/(PCr + Pi)[b]	0.35 ± 0.13	0.30	0.22	0.35
ADP (mmol/l)	55 ± 21	108	243	78
Recovery				
Half-time PCr (s)	29 ± 10	55	85	20
Half-time Pi (s)	28 ± 14	30	74	21
Half-time ADP (s)	11 ± 5	19	26	6
PCr, initial rate (mmol/l per min)	33 ± 14	15	16	38
Maximum rate oxidative ATP synthesis (mmol/l per min)	52 ± 18	19	18	53

Notes:

PCr, phosphocreatine; Pi, inorganic phosphate; PME, phosphomonoesters; PDE, phosphodiesters.

[a] Data for normal controls are given as the mean ± 1 SD.

[b] PCr is expressed as the ratio PCr/(PCr + Pi) to correct for loss of signal owing to movement away from the MRS surface coil.

[c] The phosphorylation potential is given as its reciprocal in order to convert the values to a normal distribution.

disorders, including muscular dystrophy and muscle injury (McCully et al., 1988).

The basic metabolic picture presented by ^{31}P MRS can conveniently be divided into three parts: muscle at rest, the response to exercise, and recovery following exercise. The derived concentrations can be used to calculate the metabolically active ADP concentration and the phosphorylation potential, [ATP]/([ADP] × [Pi]), a measure of the energy available to the muscle fibre. Data from a group of normal, untrained subjects and three patients with

different metabolic muscle diseases are compared in Table 16.1. A diagram of the relevant biochemical pathways is shown in Fig 16.7.

In normal adult muscle at rest, metabolite concentrations show modest differences among individuals, similar to those found in biopsy samples, while pH_i is essentially invariant. In contrast, the response to exercise shows wide intersubject variability. It is important to minimize this as much as possible by optimizing and standardizing the MRS volume localization and exercise protocol. For example, standardization of the work performed according to muscle mass or maximum voluntary contraction force is needed if results are used for comparison with patient groups in whom there may be atrophy or other degenerative changes. Fig. 16.8*a* shows typical data from calf muscle exercise in a normal, untrained volunteer. The energy requirement for contraction leads to an immediate increase in the rate of ATP hydrolysis; however, even in the face of high energy demand, ATP is buffered against large changes in concentration by transfer of a high-energy phosphate group from PCr to ADP via the creatine kinase reaction (Eq. 16.1). On initiation of muscle contraction or at times when the work load or rate is increased, glycogen breakdown is rapidly activated to provide substrate for glycolysis, and any pyruvate that is not oxidized by the mitochondria is converted to lactic acid, thereby lowering pH_i (Fig. 16.7 and 16.8*b*) The extent of the change in pH_i is a balance between lactic acid accumulation, proton efflux and the pH-raising effect of PCr hydrolysis (Eq. 16.1). In fact, at the very beginning of exercise there is rapid PCr depletion before glycolysis is activated, so pH_i actually rises (Fig. 16.8*b*). As blood flow increases and fatty acids are mobilized to serve as substrates for mitochondrial metabolism, oxidative phosphorylation becomes increasingly able to provide ATP. The overall result of the changes in PCr and pH_i in exercise is to increase the concentrations of ADP and Pi (Fig. 16.8*a*), and this serves to stimulate mitochondrial ATP synthesis. Because the relative activities of the glycolytic and oxidative pathways depend on the intensity and duration of exercise (Kemp and Radda, 1994), the exercise regimen can be designed to accentuate a particular bioenergetic characteristic. The most extreme situation is ischaemia. If blood flow to the limb is occluded, ATP production is entirely via PCr and glycolysis; delivery of blood-borne glucose, washout of metabolites (including H^+) and oxidative phosphorylation are prevented until blood flow is restored (Taylor et al., 1983).

When muscle contraction ceases, the rate of ATP turnover is immediately and dramatically reduced. Even though glycolysis is no longer active, ATP synthesis through oxidative phosphorylation continues at a high rate, leading to the restoration of PCr to pre-exercise levels (Fig. 16.8*c*). The rate of PCr repletion, therefore, reflects the rate of mitochondrial ATP synthesis and is a sensitive index of mitochondrial activity (Argov et al., 1987d; Taylor et al., 1994). This recovery rate varies in relation to pH_i (Arnold et al., 1984b; Bendahan et al., 1990), so care must be taken in comparing results from studies in which pH_i at the end of exercise is substantially different (Iotti et al., 1993). Data from the recovery period can be used to derive other indices of mitochondrial activity (for example ADP recov-

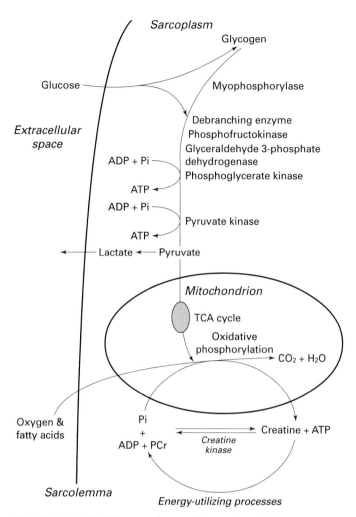

Fig. 16.7. A simplified diagram of some of the steps involved in energy production and utilization in skeletal muscle. For a more detailed description see Chapter 8. Defects in enzymatic steps indicated in this diagram may lead to changes in muscle bioenergetics detectable by ^{31}P MRS, as described in the text.

ery rate and the maximal rate of mitochondrial ATP synthesis (V_{max}) as shown in Table 16.1). All of these processes are independent of muscle mass, an important consideration in the investigation of any muscle-wasting disease. The return of metabolite concentrations toward pre-exercise values is rapid (Fig. 16.8*a,c*) and is independent of muscle cross-sectional area or volume. The initial time courses of PCr and Pi recovery are approximately exponential in the first minute or two, but recovery of pH_i is slower and follows a more complex time course. This is influenced mainly by two processes: proton efflux rate, which is dependent on the proton concentration, and the proton-producing effect of net PCr synthesis. During the initial

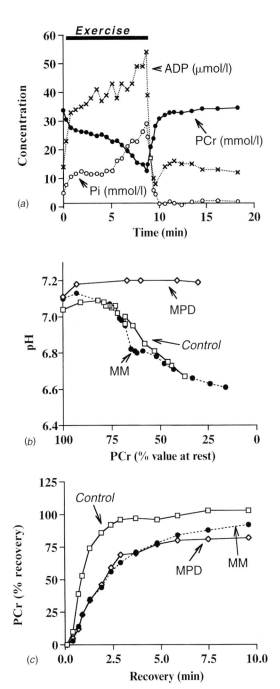

Fig. 16.8. MRS data (^{31}P) from calf muscle during exercise and recovery. (*a*) Data from a normal control showing the changes in phosphocreatine (PCr), inorganic phosphate (Pi) and ADP during 10 minutes of aerobic, dynamic exercise and in an 8 minute recovery period. (*b*) The relationship of intracellular pH and PCr during exercise in the normal control, a patient with mitochondrial myopathy (MM) and a patient with myophosphorylase deficiency (MPD). (*c*) Repletion of PCr after exercise in the normal control and the patients with MM and MPD.

stage of recovery, PCr repletion is rapid enough to cause a decrease in pH$_i$. An approximately linear recovery of pH$_i$ after this initial dip has been found for finger flexor muscle (Taylor et al., 1986), but in many studies the Pi must become tightly bound because it disappears from the spectra, making pH$_i$ impossible to measure for several minutes during recovery. The situation can also be complicated by different rates of recovery in different pools of Pi. The presence of different fibre types arguably accounts for the multiple Pi peaks sometimes seen in exercise and recovery (resulting from pools of P$_i$ in different pH environments) (Park et al., 1987; Vandenborne et al., 1991). However, heterogeneity of muscle activation within and between whole muscles may also contribute to the Pi peak splitting (Taylor et al., 1983; Fleckenstein et al., 1989a). The importance of anatomical determinants of physiological measures cannot be emphasized strongly enough. Macroscopic heterogeneity of muscle response may help to explain why attempts to use MRS to assess quantitatively the proportions of muscle fibre types have so far met with little success.

Control groups for MRS studies must be chosen carefully because there are many factors that influence muscle metabolism, including the muscle group investigated (Taylor et al., 1994), age of the subject (McCully et al., 1991; Taylor et al., 1997), degree of training (Kent-Braun et al., 1990; Guthrie et al., 1996) and systemic influences of disease. Some conditions known to affect the MRS findings are peripheral vascular disease (Hands et al., 1986, 1990; Zatina et al., 1986), respiratory insufficiency (Levy et al., 1997; Thompson et al., 1993), hypertension (Dudley et al., 1990), heart failure (Rajagopalan et al., 1988; Arnolda et al., 1990; Kemp et al., 1993b; Kao et al., 1995), denervation (Frostick et al., 1992, Zochodne et al., 1988), muscle injury (McCully et al., 1988) and malnutrition (Gupta et al., 1994). Certain drugs such as zidovudine can inhibit oxidative metabolism (Weissman et al., 1992; Sinnwell et al., 1995), while alcoholic myopathy affects glycogen metabolism (Bollaert et al., 1989).

Primary metabolic myopathies

Primary metabolic myopathies include inherited disorders of glycogen and glucose metabolism, lipid metabolism and defects affecting oxidative phosphorylation. In most forms of metabolic myopathies there is impairment of anaerobic and/or aerobic metabolism that can be assessed precisely by ^{31}P MRS. Selective muscle atrophy and fatty replacement of degenerated muscle fibres can be evaluated with high sensitivity by MRI.

Mitochondrial myopathies

Mitochondrial myopathies are a clinically heterogeneous group of disorders caused by biochemical defects affecting one or more of the many steps in the oxidation of substrates: substrate transport into mitochondria, tricarboxylic acid cycle, electron transport chain and oxidation/phosphorylation coupling (Chapter 29).

Imaging studies

There are few muscle imaging studies of patients with genetic defects of mitochondrial metabolism. One study of thigh muscles in 11 patients with mitochondrial myopathies disclosed that gross muscle structural deterioration, characterized by atrophy and a 'marbling' type of fatty replacement, was common, particularly in patients with ophthalmoplegia (Fleckenstein et al., 1996). In this subset of patients, selective deterioration of the sartorius and gracilis muscles was surprisingly common. This pattern is opposite to that seen in other types of myopathy (e.g. dystrophies, congenital myopathies and polymyositis).

Another interesting MRI feature of muscle abnormalities in these patients is a high incidence of fatty deterioration of muscle without associated oedema-like changes of deteriorating muscles, a feature reminiscent of muscular dystrophies and in contradistinction to most other muscle disorders including denervation, inflammation and myonecrosis. The paucity of oedematous changes was consistent with the minimal histopathological evidence of myonecrosis or inflammation and the minimal elevation in serum creatine kinase levels.

Spectral studies

Despite the diversity of the biochemical lesions involved, mitochondrial myopathies share a characteristic pattern of MRS-detectable abnormality, which reflects the common deficit of mitochondrial ATP synthesis. In comparison with other functional evaluations, testing for increased blood lactate in particular, ^{31}P MRS has demonstrated high sensitivity in the detection of abnormalities of oxidative metabolism. In the specialized centres where it is available, evaluation by MRS may precede muscle biopsy and genetic analysis in the diagnostic protocols of mitochondrial myopathy. Defects of respiratory chain enzymes are the most prevalent types of mitochondrial myopathy and the most frequently studied with MRS. Most reports have been on patients with chronic progressive external opthalmoplegia (Kearns–Sayre–Shy syndrome), MELAS (mitochondrial encephalomyopathy, lactic acidosis and stroke-like episodes), MERRF (mitochondrial encephalomyopathy with ragged-red fibres) and LHON (Leber's

hereditary optic neuropathy). Most patients show ^{31}P MRS abnormalities in resting muscle (Arnold et al., 1985; Argov et al., 1987d; Matthews et al., 1991; Taylor et al., 1994). Results from a single patient illustrating typical findings are shown in Figs. 16.8b,c and Table 16.1. The limited data on biochemical analyses of ATP concentration in mitochondrial myopathy suggest that it remains unaffected by the disease (Arnold et al., 1985; Taylor et al., 1994). The low PCr/ATP and increased Pi/ATP, therefore, imply that the absolute concentration of PCr is decreased and Pi is high. Some studies have shown an increase in Pi as the most prominent feature (Argov et al., 1987d; Matthews et al., 1991) and others a reduction in PCr concentration (Taylor et al., 1994; Lodi et al., 1997e). These differences do not seem to be related to the muscle group investigated (Taylor et al., 1994) or to the clinical or molecular phenotype. Abnormalities have also been detected in resting muscle in the absence of any muscle signs or symptoms in patients with LHON and symptom-free carriers of primary LHON mutations (Cortelli et al., 1991; Lodi et al., 1997e). There is no consistent finding with respect to pH_i at rest; it is most often in the normal range, but it may be high even in the presence of elevated plasma lactate. ADP concentration is found to be abnormally high in about two-thirds of patients. Not surprisingly, the phosphorylation potential is low in the majority of patients, and in some studies has been the most frequently detected abnormality.

The consequence of a deficit in mitochondrial ATP production during exercise is an increase in nonoxidative energy production (i.e. increased PCr consumption and glycolytic activity). Consequently, as illustrated in the example in Table 16.1 and Fig 16.8b, patients with mitochondrial myopathies tend to display a rapid rate of PCr depletion during exercise, consistent with their decreased exercise tolerance. Despite the increase in lactic acid synthesis in mitochondrial myopathy, pH_i during exercise may be prevented from falling excessively (Fig. 16.8b) because of an increased rate of proton efflux from muscle, as shown by a faster-than-normal pH_i recovery after exercise (Arnold et al., 1985; Taylor et al., 1994).

Enzyme activities measured in vitro do not always correspond to the results in vivo. Patients with LHON carrying a primary mtDNA point mutation at one of three nucleotide positions, 11 778, 14 484 or 3460, in genes coding for different subunits of complex I of the respiratory chain showed slow PCr recovery rate and low V_{max} for mitochondrial ATP synthesis (Cortelli et al., 1991; Barbiroli et al., 1995; Lodi et al., 1997e). In vitro, the specific activity of complex I was markedly decreased for 3460 and normal for 11 778 but in vivo, mitochondrial activity was lowest in subjects homoplasmic for 11 778, higher for 14 484 and just within the normal range for 3460 (V_{max}, 27, 53 and 65% of the normal mean, respectively) (Lodi et al., 1997e). The in vivo values for V_{max} in three subjects with the 3460 mutation correlated inversely with the percentage of mutated mtDNA, indicating that the level of wild-type mtDNA necessary for a complete functional complementation may be higher than suggested by the in vitro results (Carelli et al., 1997). The study of cybrids homoplasmic for the 3460 mutation showed that the nuclear background influences the expression of the biochemical defect (Cock et al., 1998) and this may help to explain the mild reduction in skeletal muscle oxidative ATP synthesis found in vivo.

Phosphorus-31 MRS of skeletal muscle has been widely used to evaluate objectively the response to specific treatments in different forms of mitochondrial myopathy. Classically, medical treatments have focused on improving mitochondrial metabolism by either bypassing the biochemical defect or enhancing electron transport chain activity. Administration of vitamins K_3 and C to a patient with complex III deficit resulted in clinical improvement in association with dramatic improvements of ^{31}P MRS indices (Eleff et al., 1984). Similarly, treatment with riboflavin and nicotinamide (niacinamide) of a patient with MELAS with complex I deficiency resulted in improved oxidative mitochondrial metabolism, and this paralleled the clinical response (Penn et al., 1992). Coenzyme Q_{10} administration was found to enhance oxidative metabolism in some patients but not in others (Bendahan et al., 1992b; Matthews et al., 1993; Barbiroli et al., 1997). Dichloroacetate, which stimulates the activity of pyruvate dehydrogenase, reduced blood levels of lactate but did not improve postexercise indices of mitochondrial ATP production (de Stefano et al., 1995). A similar effect on blood lactate was found in patients with mitochondrial myopathy undergoing moderate-intensity aerobic training, but in contrast with dichloroacetate administration, this was associated with a more than 60% improvement in ADP postexercise recovery rate (Taivassalo et al., 1998).

Disorders of carbohydrate metabolism

Deficits in carbohydrate metabolism can present either with exercise-induced symptoms such as painful cramps, contractures and rhabdomyolysis or with progressive weakness. Muscle fatty replacement is a typical feature of those glycogenoses in which the affected enzyme is not involved in energy generation, e.g. acid maltase and the glycogen branching enzymes. The fatty infiltration is possibly caused by muscle damage from excessive glycogen accumulation disrupting the normal myofibrillar organization. Progressive fatty deterioration may also be linked to rhabdomyolysis in glycogenolytic/glycolytic enzyme defects (myophosphorylase, debranching enzyme and phosphofructokinase deficiencies). MRI can be useful in observing these changes and in evaluating differences in exercise-induced changes in SI between normal subjects and patients with glycogenosis defects. A distinctive pattern of abnormality is observed by ^{31}P MRS in muscle deficient in glycogenolytic or glycolytic enzyme activity. There is a rapid depletion of energy reserves because of the diminished rate of ATP synthesis, and an abnormal pH_i response to exercise as a result of the decreased production of lactic acid (Fig. 16.8b and Table 16.1). This abnormal relationship between pH_i and PCr can form the basis of a sensitive alternative to the ischaemic lactate test that is often used as a diagnostic test for this kind of disorder. The investigator can monitor the PCr concentration to ensure that an adequate amount of work was performed, and the rate of change in pH_i is a measure of lactic acid synthesis.

Glycogenolytic disorders
Myophosphorylase deficiency (McArdle's disease)
Fatty changes of muscles may be present in myophosphorylase deficiency, although they occur less frequently and extensively than in other forms of glycogenosis, such as acid maltase deficiency. It has been suggested that the distribution of deteriorated muscles seen on lumbar imaging studies may help to differentiate between different forms of glycogenosis (Cinnamon et al., 1991). Of practical note, when oedematous foci are identified in imaging studies of patients with undiagnosed muscle conditions, these areas should be avoided during biopsy when myophosphorylase deficiency is suspected. In such patients, relatively normal appearing muscle is favoured as a site for biopsy because necrotic muscle may produce a small amount of fetal phosphorylase (Fleckenstein et al., 1989b). This contrasts with the situation in inflammatory myopathy, where oedematous muscle is favoured for biopsy. It is important for radiologists to be aware of this kind of issue as they are increasingly called upon to participate in muscle biopsies (Pitt et al., 1993; Schweitzer and Fort, 1995).

Compared with the MRI findings from exercising muscle in normal subjects, myophosphorylase-deficient patients exhibit a smaller increase in muscle volume, while T_1 and T_2 relaxation times fail to lengthen (Fleckenstein et al., 1991b). Similarly, after ischaemic handgrip, the SI of normal muscle but not of myophosphorylase-deficient muscle increases markedly on short tau-inversion recovery images. The contractures that these patients experience result in MRI-detectable changes which are fully reversible. Serial imaging reveals that these focal areas of oedematous change (Fig. 16.9) develop in the exercised

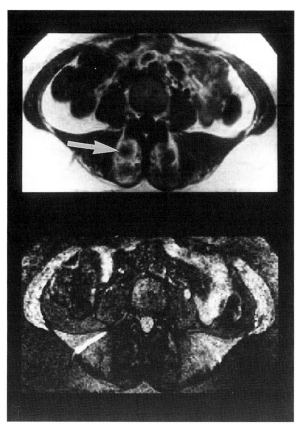

Fig. 16.9. Focal muscle lesions in generalized myopathy. The strikingly focal distribution of severe muscle deterioration in the glycogenoses is demonstrated in this patient with myophosphorylase deficiency (McArdle's disease). Note selective atrophy of the multifidus muscles in the lumbar paraspinal region (arrow).

muscles and are not detectable in the initial stages of contracture. They begin to develop within 24 hours and persist for at least several days (Fleckenstein et al., 1989b).

The first clinical MRS study was carried out in 1981 on a patient with myophosphorylase deficiency (Ross et al., 1981). The findings of rapid PCr depletion and a lack of muscle acidification, later confirmed by others (Argov et al., 1987b; Duboc et al., 1987), correlated with clinical aspects of this disorder. The characteristic cramp experienced by these patients was found to coincide with particularly high concentrations of ADP, a situation that develops as PCr concentration decreases but pH_i fails to fall. In the 'second wind' phenomenon, cramp diminishes and the ability to exercise is restored as delivery to the muscle of glucose, fatty acids and oxygen increases and pH_i and metabolite concentrations return toward normal (Radda et al., 1989). Exercise protocols must be designed carefully in

order to elicit these diagnostic features; short and intense exercise (Bendahan et al., 1992a; Siciliano et al., 1995) may prevent the 'second wind' phenomenon. Typical MRS findings are shown in Fig. 16.8 and Table 16.1.

Myophosphorylase-deficient muscle is unable to synthesize glucose 6-phosphate or other sugar phosphates of the glycolytic pathway (see Fig. 16.7), so there is no increase in the PME peak in the MRS spectrum during exercise (Duboc et al., 1987; Bendahan et al., 1992a; Siciliano et al., 1995). Infusion of glucose bypasses the block in glycogenolysis, thereby reducing net PCr depletion and generating pyruvate that can serve as mitochondrial substrate (Argov et al., 1987b). The slow recovery of PCr (Bendahan et al., 1992a; Siciliano et al., 1995) and ADP (de Stefano et al., 1996) after exercise in myophosphorylase deficiency are signs of inhibition of oxidative phosphorylation caused by lack of substrate, so recovery may not be delayed if the second wind has been reached. In spite of the evidence for reduced ATP synthesis by both glycolysis and oxidative phosphorylation, there is no simple correlation between symptoms and muscle ATP concentration. The high PCr/ATP ratio in resting muscle is consistent with a reduced ATP concentration but neither exercise, whether aerobic (Argov et al., 1987b) or ischaemic (Argov et al., 1987b; Siciliano et al., 1995), nor sustained muscular contracture has been found to lead to a further decrease in muscle ATP content.

Debranching enzyme deficiency

Debranching enzyme is essential for complete degradation of the tree-like structure of glycogen. In the experience of ourselves and others, the ^{31}P MRS findings in muscle of patients lacking debrancher activity are qualitatively similar to those in patients with myophosphorylase deficiency. Muscle glycogen can be broken down by myophosphorylase but only until the branch points are reached, explaining why a mild degree of acidification can be achieved in exercise (Duboc et al., 1987).

Glycolytic disorders
Phosphofructokinase deficiency
Phosphofructokinase is a key regulatory enzyme of glycolysis. In the absence of enzyme activity, glycolytic ATP production from both glycogen and glucose is prevented, so infusion of glucose does not reduce PCr depletion. The typical ^{31}P MRS features are a lack of pH_i decrease during either aerobic or ischaemic exercise and a striking increase in the PME peak as a result of accumulation of hexose phosphates (Chance et al., 1981; Edwards et al., 1982; Argov et al., 1987c; Duboc et al., 1987). As in myophosphorylase deficit, PCr/ATP at rest is increased, representing a

decrease in muscle ATP content of up to 30%, but in contrast with myophosphorylase deficiency, ATP concentration during either aerobic or ischaemic exercise has been found to fall dramatically by as much as half (Argov et al., 1987c; Grehl et al., 1998). Increased PCr consumption (Bertocci et al., 1993; Grehl et al., 1998) and slow PCr recovery (Duboc et al., 1987; Grehl et al., 1998) are commonly found. The Pi of the muscle cells, which is required for ATP synthesis, becomes effectively trapped in the sugar phosphate intermediate, contributing to ATP depletion and slow PCr recovery. The MRS findings are consistent with reduced oxidative activity, confirmed by a decreased maximal oxygen uptake (Lewis and Haller, 1989). Compatible with the site of the biochemical defect and the absence of the second wind phenomenon, intravenous glucose administration during exercise does not improve exercise kinetics (Argov et al., 1987c) but lactate infusion is able to bypass the enzymatic block and decrease the rate of PCr depletion (Bertocci et al., 1993).

Of the three patients with late-onset disease investigated by MRS, two showed a rapid depletion of PCr and a modest increase in PME, consistent with partial phosphofructokinase deficiency (in vitro activity in one of the subjects was 33% of normal) (Sivakumar et al., 1996). The third showed 4% of normal activity in vitro even though the only abnormality revealed by MRS was a mildly decreased acidification during exercise (Massa et al., 1996). The authors suggested that this discrepancy could be explained by enzyme instability rather than its absence, and this situation might be common in other patients with late-onset phosphofructokinase deficit (Vora et al., 1987).

Deficiencies of the distal glycolytic pathway
The ^{31}P MRS pattern of abnormality in phosphoglycerate kinase and phosphoglycerate mutase is similar to that in phosphofructokinase deficiency, being characterized by PME accumulation and reduced acidification during exercise. In the one patient with phosphoglycerate kinase deficiency investigated by ^{31}P MRS, there was a striking PME accumulation during exercise, but pH$_i$ revealed some degree of acidification (Duboc et al., 1987). This is probably a result of H$^+$ production by the synthesis of 1,3-diphosphoglycerate, which accumulates because of the enzymatic block, and this may help to differentiate phosphoglycerate kinase deficiency from deficit of phosphofructokinase. A deficit in oxidative metabolism was demonstrated in this patient by a very slow PCr recovery rate. Studies of two patients with residual phosphoglycerate mutase activities of 6% (Argov et al., 1987a) and 8% (Vita et al., 1994) of control values found that the degree of abnormality detected by MRS for a given residual enzyme

activity was proportional to the degree of glycolytic activation demanded by the exercise protocol. The patient with the lower residual activity showed a mildly reduced PCr recovery rate while the patient with the higher activity showed a small drop in pH$_i$ as the only abnormality during a mild aerobic exercise; a small PME accumulation was evident only during an intense aerobic exercise.

Other disorders of carbohydrate metabolism: acid maltase deficiency
Acid maltase is a lysosomal enzyme involved in the degradation of glycogen. The largest series of glycogenoses imaged to date described paraspinal muscle atrophy in the adult forms of acid maltase and myosphosphorylase deficiencies (Cinnamon et al., 1991). Fatty deterioration of the psoas and erector spinae muscles occurred in seven of nine patients with acid maltase deficiency. While erector spinae fatty deterioration was also common in myophosphorylase deficiency (6 of 10 patients), in none of those patients was there psoas atrophy (Fig. 16.9). The authors concluded that radiologists might suggest the type of myopathy present by the distribution of deteriorated muscles seen on lumbar imaging studies. However, this conclusion does not consider the many other diseases that may also preferentially involve the psoas and erector spinae, including muscular dystrophies, myositis and mitochondrial myopathies. Hence, paraspinal muscle atrophy, while important, is nonspecific in determining a specific myopathy.

In the authors' experience with adult patients with acid maltase deficiency, severe fatty deterioration of thigh muscles was identified in all nine patients assessed, correlating with advanced muscular weakness (unpublished observations). Muscles always involved included the vastus intermedius and the short head of the biceps femoris, with more variable and milder involvement of other muscles. In acid maltase deficiency, the muscle is replaced by fat and the overall configuration of the muscle is preserved without deformation of intermuscular fascia. This feature was described as the 'filling up process', a nonspecific feature most commonly seen in muscular dystrophies (Bulcke and Baert, 1982). Interestingly, this is in contrast to the appearance of other conditions, such as chronic polymyositis, in which muscle atrophy and increased adiposity are frequently associated with volume loss of the muscular compartment and resulting undulation of the intermuscular fasciae (see below).

Acid maltase does not contribute to energy production, and exercise-induced symptoms are not present in affected patients. MRS abnormalities have not been described.

Muscular dystrophies

The muscular dystrophies are heterogeneous with respect to both clinical presentation and underlying genetic defect. The structural alterations caused by fibre atrophy, necrosis and fatty replacement of muscle tissue are easily detectable by MRI. The physical changes revealed by MRI must ultimately derive from biochemical abnormalities that arise from the individual genetic defects, and some of these abnormalities can be detected by MRS. Not surprisingly, most of the MR studies of dystrophic muscle have been carried out on patients with Duchenne and Becker muscular dystrophies, in whom there is a deficit of the large subsarcolemmal protein dystrophin. Myotonic dystrophy is discussed separately.

Imaging studies

MRI of muscle in patients with Duchenne and Becker dystrophy reveal on a large scale the fatty degeneration and necrosis that can be seen under the microscope (Chapter 19). Such studies also clearly show that individual muscles and muscle groups are affected to different degrees even though all muscles are totally lacking in dystrophin. In the thigh, certain muscles such as gracilis and sartorius are peculiarly spared the atrophic process or are even hypertrophic (Fig. 16.10). Differential muscle involvement is also seen in the lower leg, in which soleus and tibialis anterior muscles are spared relative to gastrocnemius but are more affected than deep posterior muscles.

Standard, unquantified MRI scans showing focal fatty changes are typical of, but not specific to, muscular dystrophy. This type of study is limited not only in the specificity with which it can be used to diagnose dystrophy but also in its sensitivity (de Visser et al., 1996). However, in contrast to most other neuromuscular disorders, in Duchenne and Becker dystrophy the oedema-sensitive STIR pulse sequence frequently does not reveal a conspicuous oedema-like phase prior to the development of obvious fatty degeneration. This may explain why in the first few years of life, MRI findings in Duchenne dystrophy are often normal. A quantitative approach markedly improves the sensitivity of MRI to degeneration in dystrophies. In the relatively early stages of Duchenne dystrophy, T_1 relaxation times in muscle are elevated in the thighs and slightly decreased in the calves. With disease progression, T_1 values rapidly decrease as a result of replacement of muscle by fat. Although a significant correlation is found between MRI data and patients' functional status, age and disease duration, one MRI study showed that in half of patients there was progressive muscle degeneration at a subclinical level

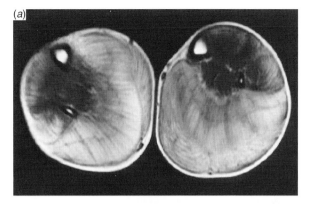

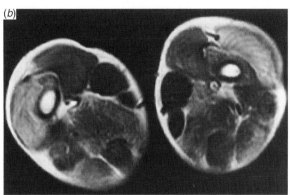

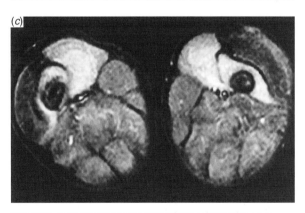

Fig. 16.10. Pseudohypertrophy in Duchenne dystrophy. (*a*) T_1-weighted image of the calves shows large girth with fatty replacement of much of the posterior compartments. (*b*) Note markedly symmetrical distribution of feathery fatty change in thigh muscles. Peculiar to this family of diseases is the focal sparing of adductors. (*c*) Short inversion time inversion recovery (STIR) has a high sensitivity to oedema and shows which volumes include substantial oedema-like change (high signal intensity). This finding is unusual for dystrophinopathies.

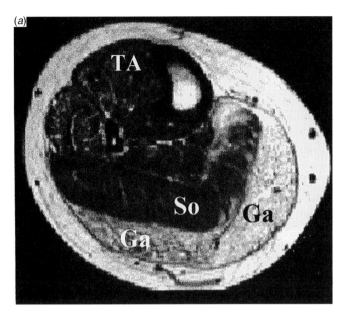 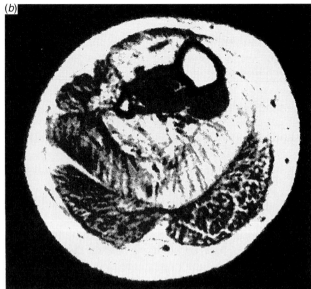

Fig. 16.11. T_1-weighted axial images at the level of the maximal calf circumference from (*a*) a patient with Becker muscular dystrophy and (*b*) a patient with sarcoglycan-deficient limb girdle muscular dystrophy. It should be noted that in (*a*) there is a marked increase in signal intensity as a result of fat replacement of degenerated fibres in the medial and lateral gastrocnemius (Ga) muscles while soleus (So) and tibialis anterior (TA) muscles are still relatively spared. In contrast, (*c*) shows a marked increase in signal intensity in So and TA, while Ga displays a much smaller increase.

(Lamminen et al., 1990). Female carriers of Duchenne dystrophy are also sometimes clinically affected and may show abnormalities on imaging studies similar to those found in mild cases of Becker dystrophy. Significantly higher T_1 values caused by degenerative muscular changes accompanied by interstitial oedema is found in proximal muscles of carriers compared with normal females. These 'manifesting carriers' may show asymmetric involvement of proximal muscles of the lower limbs (de Visser and Verbeeten, 1985).

Experience in imaging other muscular dystrophies such as limb girdle muscular dystrophy, Emery–Dreifuss muscular dystrophy, congenital muscular dystrophy, facioscapulohumeral muscular dystrophy, distal muscular dystrophies and oculopharyngeal muscular dystrophy is limited, but MR may be expected increasingly to reveal subtle differences as more quantitative methods are developed. Some of these disorders show patterns of abnormality that are of potential importance in diagnosis. A subgroup of the limb girdle dystrophies is known to be caused by deficits in the transmembrane sarcoglycan portion of the dystrophin complex. These patients have normal dystrophin expression but share many clinical features with Duchenne and Becker dystrophy. MRI reveals a pattern of muscle degeneration and fat replacement clearly distinguishable from dystrophin deficiency.

Gastrocnemius muscle is relatively less affected while soleus and tibialis anterior muscles are more severely involved (Fig. 16.11).

Spectral studies

Underlying the MRI-visible abnormalities in dystrophic muscle are the biochemical mechanisms that lead to these changes. Different types of dystrophy share many common clinical features even though they originate from different genetic defects, so it is not surprising that they also show common abnormalities on MRS. An increase in pH_i and changes in concentration ratios of PCr and Pi and ATP have been found in resting muscle in Becker dystrophy (Table 16.1), Duchenne dystrophy, carriers of Becker dystrophy/Duchenne dystrophy, as well as in those with oculopharyngeal dystrophy. These abnormalities generally become more pronounced with age and disease progression (Newman et al., 1982; Edwards et al., 1985; Younkin et al., 1987; Barbiroli et al., 1992; Kemp et al., 1993a). Typical results from a dystrophin deficient patient with Becker dystrophy are shown in Table 16.1.

Although the structure and localization of dystrophin are well defined, the functional role of this protein and the biochemical mechanisms leading to muscle necrosis are still unknown. There is still less known about the other components of the dystrophin complex: the transmembrane glycoproteins called sarcoglycans (also known as dystrophin-associated glycoproteins and the extracellular matrix protein merosin (also known as laminin). There are various hypotheses and much conflicting evidence from studies carried out in vitro about the possible role of defective cellular energetics in muscle fibre degeneration. Studies using ^{31}P MRS have been able to clarify some of these issues and raise others.

Early MRS investigations of Duchenne dystrophy revealed not only a high concentration of PDEs in skeletal muscle consistent with cell necrosis but also abnormally high pH_i. This is a feature of most dystrophies and is thought to arise from changes in the membrane-bound system that maintains the intracellular H^+ content of resting muscle, the Na^+/H^+ antiporter (Barnes et al., 1997). Investigations of dystrophin-deficient muscles at rest show that even in Becker dystrophy/Duchenne dystrophy carriers there are abnormalities in the concentrations of metabolites central to cellular energy processes (Barbiroli et al., 1992, 1993; Kemp et al., 1993a). Muscle fibres have a low phosphorylation potential and, therefore, less energy available from ATP hydrolysis. During exercise, a rapid depletion of energy reserves has been demonstrated in dystrophin deficiency (Barbiroli et al., 1992; Kemp et al., 1993a; Lodi et al., 1999), sarcoglycan deficiency (Lodi et al., 1997c) and oculopharyngeal dystrophy (Zochodne et al., 1992), consistent with low muscle mass and low phosphorylation potential. There are high ADP levels not only at rest but throughout exercise (Kemp et al., 1993a,b; Lodi et al., 1999). ADP is an important regulator of ATP synthesis, so maintaining a high concentration would help to increase ATP production as the progressively decreasing muscle mass struggles to cope with the relative increase in energy demand. There is evidence that the integrity of the cytoskeleton is necessary for the proper functioning of glycolysis and the tricarboxylic acid cycle (Letellier et al., 1993; Pagliaro, 1993), and this suggests a possible role for defective energy metabolism in muscle fibre degeneration. However, it is clear from quantitative analysis of MRS recovery data that in both dystrophin and sarcoglycan deficiencies there can be no marked decrease in mitochondrial ATP synthesis comparable with that seen in primary disorders of glycolysis and oxidative phosphorylation (Kemp et al., 1993a,b; Lodi et al., 1999). This would seem to rule out any major role for impaired energy production in the progressive fibre necrosis found in these patients but does not exclude the presence of more subtle abnormalities in energy production or utilization that could contribute to muscle dysfunction. In fact, MRS results provide evidence that there may be reduced glucose availability for dystrophin-deficient muscles during exercise (Lodi et al., 1999). It is glycolytically produced ATP that is thought to be used preferentially to provide energy for the ion pumps of the cell membrane, and in dystrophin deficiency there is a general imbalance of ionic homeostasis involving sodium, potassium and calcium ions. Whether or not this deficit in glycolytic ATP production owing to decreased glucose availability is severe enough to compromise ion transport has not been resolved. Delayed recovery of Pi after exercise has been reported in some studies of dystrophin deficiency and can be interpreted as an effect of altered ionic equilibrium (Barbiroli et al., 1992, 1993).

The general pattern of MRS-detectable abnormalities is similar for the various types of muscular dystrophy, but MRI and ^{31}P MRS have been used in combination to distinguish sarcoglycan-deficient limb girdle muscular dystrophy from dystrophin deficiency, even though the two disorders have a similar clinical presentation (Fig. 16.11) (Lodi et al., 1997c). In contrast to dystrophin-deficient muscle, in sarcoglycan deficiency, the pH_i correlated inversely and the phosphorus metabolite content correlated positively with the extent of fatty replacement. Such a finding is difficult to explain unless in sarcoglycan deficiency the muscle fibres that remain as the disease progresses are relatively unaffected compared with those which undergo fatty replacement.

Myotonic dystrophy

Myotonic dystrophy is the most common cause of myotonia. It is an inherited multisystem disorder associated with an unstable expansion of a CTG triplet repeat polymorphism (see Chapter 27). In addition to the myotonia, skeletal muscle exhibits weakness that may be out of proportion to the degree of wasting. On a cellular level, the sarcolemma is affected. There is abnormal sodium channel activity and altered intracellular concentrations of sodium, potassium and chloride ions.

Imaging studies

A relatively large quantitative study of many muscles offers a comprehensive summary of MRI-visible muscle changes (Reimers and Vogl, 1996). Common findings include atrophy of the tibialis anterior, triceps brachii, rectus femoris, vastus intermedius and sternocleidomastoid muscles. As in spinal muscular atrophy, the thickness of subcutaneous fat layers is associated with a decrease in muscle thickness. The sternocleidomastoid muscle becomes atrophic early in the disease and is progressively replaced with fat. This can be seen on routine MRI studies of the cervical spine; it may be asymmetrical. As the disease progresses, atrophy becomes obvious in the extensor muscles of the spine, initially in the thoracolumbar region, then in the tibialis anterior and the medial head of the gastrocnemius muscles. The lateral head of the gastrocnemius muscle and the soleus become involved later and to a lesser extent. As in other dystrophies, the sartorius and gracilis muscles often are only mildly abnormal. Both fatty and oedema-like changes of muscles are readily detected on MRI, particularly when a fat-suppression scheme, such as STIR, is used. As is apparent clinically, distal muscles are seen to be more severely damaged than proximal ones.

Spectral studies

In myotonic dystrophy, as in many other muscle diseases, the biochemical abnormalities detected by ^{31}P MRS increase in magnitude along with clinical severity. The MRS results provide evidence that some of the clinical weakness and fatigue experienced by patients may indeed be caused by defects in energy supply. The general findings are a decrease in phosphorylation potential, a higher ATP turnover than normal during exercise and a high free ADP concentration (Taylor et al., 1993; Barnes et al., 1997). Differences have been found between muscle groups, with calf muscles showing a pattern similar to dystrophin deficiency but forearm muscles maintaining a normal pH_i at rest regardless of clinical state. Recovery kinetics point to a small but significant reduction in mitochondrial function; ischaemic exercise in the forearm provides evidence of a relative reduction in the utilization of glycogen for ATP production. This may account for the reduced acidification seen during exercise in both limbs. The question remains as to how much of the abnormal bioenergetics results directly from the product of the affected gene, as the putative protein has a strong sequence homology to the serine-threonine group of protein kinases (Jansen et al., 1992; Mahadevan et al., 1993), and other members of this group are known to be involved in a wide variety of regulatory cell functions.

Ion channel disorders

The only ion channel disorder that has been thoroughly studied by ^{31}P MRS is malignant hyperthermia. This pharmacokinetic condition, in which a state of potentially life-threatening hypermetabolism and sustained muscle contraction is initiated by sensitivity to certain volatile anaesthetics and depolarizing muscle relaxants, has been widely investigated using ^{31}P MRS, both in humans and in the porcine animal model. Only the results from human studies are discussed here.

Malignant hyperthermia is genetically heterogeneous and may occur with or without association to other neuromuscular disorders. The underlying basis for the condition appears most commonly to be any one of a number of mutations in the gene for the ryanodine receptor on chromosome 19 (the calcium release channel RYR1 in the sarcoplasmic reticulum), although other genes may be involved in some families (see Chapter 30). An in vitro test in which muscle strips are exposed to caffeine and halothane is the standard method of determining which patients, considered to be at risk because of family history, are actually susceptible. However the abnormalities, which probably arise from abnormal calcium ion handling by the sarcoplasmic reticulum, cause changes in muscle bioenergetics that can be detected by ^{31}P MRS in vivo.

Subjects who are susceptible to malignant hyperthermia appear to have a high rate of ATP utilization, as shown by the rapid depletion of PCr in both aerobic and ischaemic exercise. The decrease in pH_i is also faster and more extensive than normal (Webster et al., 1990; Monsieurs et al., 1997; Bendahan et al., 1998b), suggesting that glycolytic activity is elevated in order to supply the increased demand for ATP. Differences in pH_i at the end of exercise may help to explain why slow PCr recovery has been found in some studies but not in others. There is no definitive explanation, however, for the finding in some (Olgin et al., 1991; Payen et al., 1993) but not all (Monsieurs et al., 1997; Bendahan et al., 1998b) laboratories of abnormal phosphorus metabolite concentrations in resting muscle. In vitro assays have established that the increase in PDE results from an increase in glycerophosphorylcholine, although the mechanism responsible remains unidentified (Payen et al., 1996).

The abnormal MRS profiles of the susceptible subjects have been compared with results from the in vitro contracture test and found to be diagnostically reliable both retrospectively and prospectively (Payen et al., 1993; Bendahan et al., 1998b). Sensitivity and specificity were greater than 90% in all studies and as high as 100% in some when several MRS parameters were combined. It may, however, be difficult to establish whether all genetic variations of the disease are detected equally reliably. Interstudy variations make clear the need for each laboratory to accumulate a substantial database on subjects with malignant hyperthermia and with susceptibility to malignant hyperthermia before using this method diagnostically.

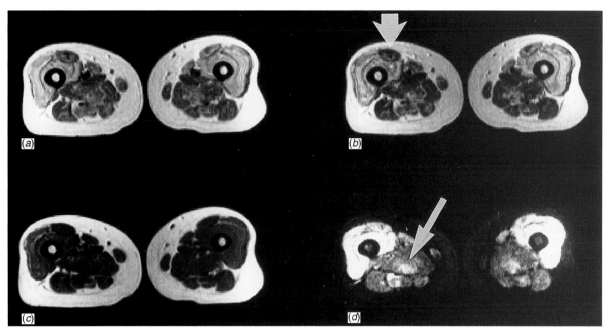

Fig. 16.12. In acute dermatomyositis there is oedema without fatty change. (*a*) Modestly T_2-weighted image shows slightly increased signal intensity in multiple thigh muscles. (*b*) With greater T_2 weighting, the contrast of abnormal muscles is greater. Note, for example, that each of the quadriceps muscles is abnormal, with the right rectus femoris less involved (arrowhead). (*c*) The signal intensity changes are caused by oedema and not fat, as is evident by the normality of signal intensity with T_1 weighting (500/30). (*d*) Oedematous change is most conspicuous using short inversion time inversion recovery (STIR) even in sites where it was difficult to identify without fat suppression (arrow). MRI support for improvement in this patient was provided by repeat MRI performed after 60 days of treatment with corticosteroids (not shown).

Myotonia congenita

Of the rarer myotonias, myotonia congenita is the most common. Patients frequently look athletic because muscles are hypertrophic. MRI can confirm muscle hypertrophy without associated SI changes.

Inflammatory myopathies

Idiopathic inflammatory myopathies

The idiopathic inflammatory myopathies comprise three main groups: polymyositis, dermatomyositis and inclusion body myositis. Although polymyositis and dermatomyositis share an autoimmune origin of the inflammatory process, they present distinctive mechanisms of disease and pathological characteristics. The pathogenic basis of inclusion body myositis remains uncertain. Each condition presents specific clinical features and ^{31}P MRS and MRI patterns.

Dermatomyositis and polymyositis

In acute polymyositis and DM, MRI shows oedema-like changes that are roughly symmetrical. This is characterized by a normal or nearly normal appearance on T_1-weighted images and focally or diffusely increased SI on T_2-weighted and/or STIR sequences (Fig. 16.12). Intravenous contrast does not provide more information than T_2-weighted images alone. Chronic PM, by comparison, is characterized by fatty replacement of many muscles, with or without concurrent oedematous changes (Fig. 16.13). Abnormalities tend to be symmetric and mostly proximal, although exceptions are well documented.

MRI-visible peculiarities of the subtypes of myositis have been sought in the hope of using MRI to refine the clinical diagnosis. While one group was unable to find any significant difference between polymyositis and DM, another found oedema-like abnormalities to be more common, and muscle atrophy less common, in the latter. Focal and diffuse patterns of MRI abnormalities occur with similar frequencies. Functional disability and disease activity correlate strongly with increased T_2-weighted and STIR SI (Reimers et al., 1994).

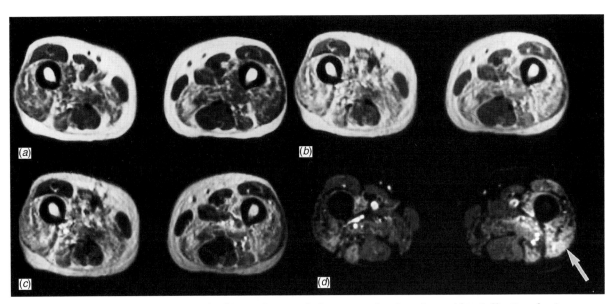

Fig. 16.13. Chronic polymyositis. (a) A T_1-weighted image shows patchy but symmetric volume loss and fatty infiltration of various muscles, with sparing of adductors. (b,c) Progressive T_2 weighting fails to show additional abnormality. (d) Short inversion time inversion recovery (STIR) shows to best advantage subvolumes of oedema that represent more 'active' disease (arrow).

As a practical matter, the value of MRI for clinical management of individual patients revolves around three issues. First, knowledge of the distribution of changes in a given patient can aid in individualizing invasive procedures such as electromyography and biopsy (Fig. 16.14 and 16.15). This is important because it is now confirmed that the number of biopsies with false-negative results is lower when the biopsy site is selected on the basis of MR images (Schweitzer and Fort, 1995). Second, the prognosis for the patient depends, in part, upon how much muscle is already replaced by fat, since that is an end-stage event that currently cannot be altered (Fig. 16.15). Third, muscle that is normal on MRI is at risk for subsequent deterioration (Fig. 16.16). Therefore, MRI findings at any point in time can provide a considerable amount of information as to the temporal position of a disease in a continuum from normal to oedematous to fatty mesenchymal change.

There is little information available from ^{31}P MRS of PM, but abnormalities in muscle bioenergetics in dermatomyositis have been reported (Park et al., 1994). The changes tend to correlate with the patients' symptoms and clinical findings. Quadriceps of amyopathic patients were normal at rest, but myopathic subjects had low PCr and ATP concentrations (Park et al., 1995); in patients with muscle weakness, PCr concentration was lower in the more severely affected (Park et al., 1990). Patients also show metabolic dysfunction during exercise, but in the amyopathic patients these differences were unmasked only at a high workload (Park et al., 1995). Slow recovery

from exercise has been reported in dermatomyositis (Park et al., 1990). All of the MRS findings are consistent with a deficit in oxidative metabolism. Reduced capillary density is present in dermatomyositis even in the absence of inflammation (Emslie-Smith and Engle, 1990). Consequently, an inadequate oxygen supply is the most likely cause of the oxidative deficit, although in amyopathic patients this becomes evident only when the oxygen requirement is high.

MRI and ^{31}P MRS show high sensitivity in DM: SI on T_2-weighted images may be increased even when serum creatine kinase is in the normal range and in some patients MRS changes precede the appearance of other abnormalities, including those detectable by MRI. The bioenergetic abnormalities may persist after resolution of inflammation, implying that damage to the capillaries precedes the inflammation (Park et al., 1994). SI normalizes after clinically successful treatment (Reimers et al., 1994), and in individual patients the ^{31}P MRS data reflect precisely the clinical response to therapy. On longitudinal follow-up, there was a good correlation between ^{31}P MRS data and severity of clinical features (Park et al., 1998a).

Sporadic inclusion body myositis

The clinical pattern of sporadic inclusion body myositis differs from polymyositis and dermatomyositis by the high frequency of weakness and atrophy affecting both proximal and distal muscle groups, a characteristic early involvement of the quadriceps and deep finger flexors, slow progression and unresponsiveness to steroid/immu-nosuppressant treatment (Dalakas, 1991; Griggs et al., 1995). Virtually all patients with sporadic inclusion body myositis show increased muscle SI on T_1-weighted imaging (Reimers et al., 1994; Sekul et al., 1997; Lodi et al., 1998). Consistent with the distribution of muscle weakness and atrophy, the highest degree of muscle lipomatosis (increased SI on T_1- and T_2-weighted imaging) is found in quadriceps and flexor digitorum profundus muscles (Reimers et al., 1994; Sekul et al., 1997). Oedema-like muscle abnormalities are uncommon, and SI on STIR is increased in less than 30% of patients (Sekul et al., 1997). MRI of forearm muscles shows a correlation between the degree of clinical involvement of the flexor digitorum profundus and T_1-weighted abnormality, although SI may be increased even in the absence of this muscle weakness (Sekul et al., 1997).

Reports of increased frequency in cytochrome oxidase-deficient fibres and ragged-red fibres in association with multiple deletions of mtDNA in skeletal muscle of patients with sporadic inclusion body myositis (Oldfors et al., 1993; Santorelli et al., 1996) raised the possibility that a defect of oxidative metabolism might play a role in the pathogenesis of this disorder and might be involved in the progressive skeletal muscle degeneration. This question has been addressed in two ^{31}P MRS studies (Argov et al., 1998; Lodi et al., 1998), both of which showed that the mitochondrial ATP production rate as measured from postexercise recovery data was normal. The conclusions were that the accumulation of mtDNA deletions and the presence of other mitochondrial abnormalities are a secondary process and do not contribute to the pathogenesis of the muscle weakness/atrophy. In contrast to the finding of normal oxidative metabolism, resting muscle in most patients with sporadic inclusion body myositis shows abnormalities in the concentrations of the phosphorus-containing metabolites and an increased pH_i. In our experience, the degree of MRS abnormality at rest in a particular muscle correlates positively with the degree of SI increase on the T_1-weighted image. This suggests that the MRS-detectable changes are nonspecific indices of muscle damage and disease progression in this disorder.

Sarcoid myositis

The nodular type of sarcoid myositis has a peculiar MRI appearance, characterized by a centre of low SI on T_1-weighted images, surrounded by a zone of oedema-like change. In the myopathic type of sarcoid myositis, MRI findings may be normal. Most frequently, fatty change dominates and oedema is less conspicuous.

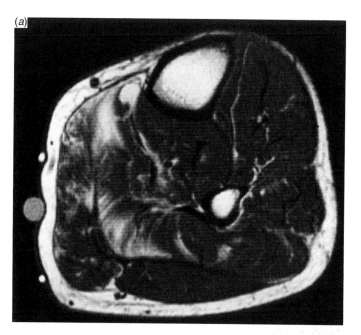

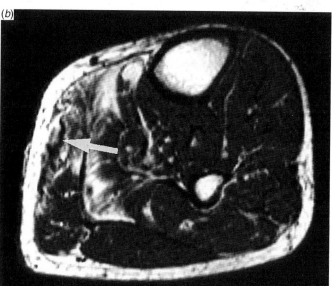

Fig. 16.14. Interventional MRI in muscle biopsy. (*a*) A T_1-weighted image of the leg in a patient with chronic leg pain and weakness long after lumbar discectomy shows moth-eaten foci of fatty change in medial gastrocnemius and soleus muscles. An external marker is used to mark the site of proposed biopsy. (*b*) Repeat imaging after biopsy shows where the needle tract was marked by undiluted intramuscular gadolinium-labelled diethylenetriamine pentaacetic acid (DTPA) (arrow).

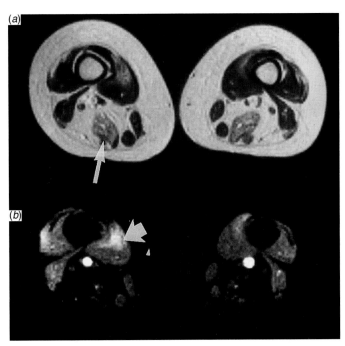

Fig. 16.15. Prognostication and biopsy selection in polymyositis. (*a*) A T$_2$-weighted image shows high signal intensity in muscle where there is fat or oedema (example, arrow). Fat will not return to normal while oedema may or may not. (*b*) Short inversion time inversion recovery (STIR) refines the assessment of mesenchymal changes of diseased muscle by distinguishing fat (suppressed signal) from oedema (high signal). Note that while the T$_2$W image in (*a*) does not distinguish fat from oedema, the STIR sequence does by virtue of the fact that fat is suppressed while oedema is highlighted (arrowhead). Hence, the posterior muscles (hamstrings) are markedly replaced by fat and are unlikely to improve but they also have no oedema and may not provide a useful biopsy result. The vastus medialis, by comparison harbours focal oedema which is at risk for subsequent deterioration to fat. Such a focus would be preferred when planning a biopsy.

Primary painful muscle syndromes

Two syndromes have been extensively investigated by ^{31}P-MRS: chronic fatigue and fibromyalgia. Controversies over pathogenesis in chronic fatigue are reflected in the contrasting results of MRS studies that followed the first case-report of a patient studied with this technique. The patient showed an excessive acidification in his forearm muscles during aerobic exercises, associated with normal mitochondrial oxidative metabolism (Arnold et al., 1984a). Excessive glycolytic activity was the explanation for this finding, which was supported by predominance of type II fibres on biopsy. Subsequent larger studies showed

that this is not a specific or consistent MRS pattern in these patients. In particular, most of the studies have shown that MRS abnormalities such as excessive acidification during exercise (Barnes et al., 1993) and reduced rate of mitochondrial ATP production (McCully et al., 1996; Lodi et al., 1997d) are present only in a small proportion of these patients. Taken together these findings point to chronic fatigue as a heterogeneous disorder. This has been confirmed studying patients with normal and increased lactate production in the subanaerobic threshold exercise test (Lane et al., 1998). In patients with chronic fatigue who had increased lactate production, pH$_i$ was significantly lower and mitochondrial ATP synthesis rate was slower than in controls or in patients with chronic fatigue and a normal test value. In addition, the proportion of type I fibres (which have the largest oxidative capacity) was lower in the group with increased lactate production than in the group with normal lactate production (Lane et al., 1998). These findings indicate that in a subpopulation of patients with the chronic fatigue syndrome there is a deficit of oxidative phosphorylation and a relative higher glycolytic capacity; consequently, for some patients there is a peripheral component to their fatigue.

Most of the MRS results on fibromyalgia would seem to rule out a role for a deficit of oxidative phosphorylation in the pathophysiology of this disorder (Simms et al., 1994; Vestergaard-Poulsen et al., 1995). Findings using ^{31}P MRS were negative even when the data were collected at tender sites (de Blecourt et al., 1991). Although in one study it was concluded that the greater changes in PCr/Pi relative to the work performed were the result of a deficit of oxidative phosphorylation (Park et al., 1998b), deconditioning and reduced muscle mass in the patient group could explain this result.

Summary

Muscle disorders commonly arise from biochemical defects that result in structural abnormalities. MRI and MRS offer specialized approaches to characterize these features further. This capability has also yielded specific tools to assist in the diagnosis and management of muscle disease. In addition, the techniques have allowed for the identification of pathophysiological clues not previously recognized by alternative techniques. Continued integration of these emerging technologies will impact positively on the clinical and scientific exploration of this family of diseases, with optimal treatment strategies being brought closer into focus as a result.

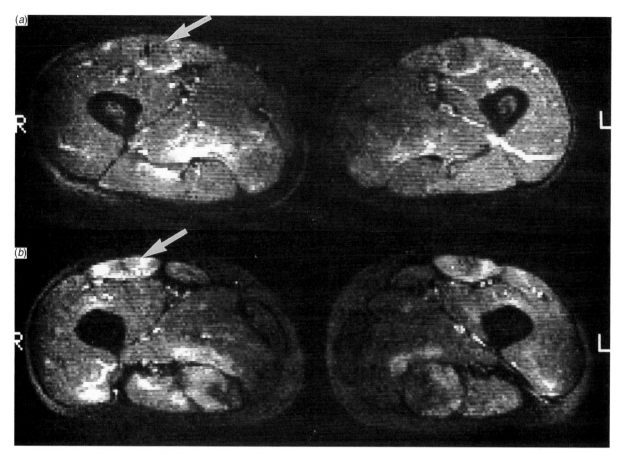

Fig. 16.16. MRI monitoring of the distribution of myopathy and response to treatment. (*a*) Short inversion time inversion recovery (STIR) image of mid-thighs during acute presentation shows patchy and approximately symmetrical oedema pattern. (*b*) Despite 4 weeks of aggressive treatment, there is progression of the volume of abnormality coinciding with the clinical course. Note that if biopsy were being considered, the right rectus femoris (arrows) would be a poor choice on the first occasion but an excellent choice on the second.

References

Andrew, E. R., Bydder, G., Griffiths, J., Iles, R. and Styles P. (1990). *Clinical Magnetic Resonance: Imaging and Spectroscopy*. Chichester: John Wiley.

Argov, Z., Bank, W. J., Boden, B., Ro, Y. I. and Chance, B. (1987a). Phosphorus magnetic resonance spectroscopy of partially blocked muscle glycolysis. An in vivo study of phosphoglycerate mutase deficiency. *Arch. Neurol.* 44, 614–617.

Argov, Z., Bank, W. J., Maris, J. and Chance, B. (1987b). Muscle energy metabolism in McArdle's syndrome by in vivo phosphorus magnetic resonance spectroscopy. *Neurology* 37, 1720–1724.

Argov, Z., Bank, W. J., Maris, J., Leigh, J. S., Jr and Chance, B. (1987c). Muscle energy metabolism in human phosphofructokinase deficiency as recorded by ^{31}P nuclear magnetic resonance spectroscopy. *Ann. Neurol.* 22, 46–51.

Argov, Z., Bank, W. J., Maris, J., Peterson, P. and Chance, B. (1987d). Bioenergetic heterogeneity of human mitochondrial myopathies: phosphorus magnetic resonance spectroscopy study. *Neurology* 37, 257–262.

Argov, Z., de Stefano, N. and Arnold, D. L. (1996). ADP recovery after a brief ischemic exercise in normal and diseased human muscle – a ^{31}P MRS study. *NMR Biomed.* 9, 165–172.

Argov, Z., Taivassalo, T., de Stefano, N., Genge, A., Karpati, G. and Arnold, D. L. (1998). Intracellular phosphates in inclusion body myositis – a ^{31}P magnetic resonance spectroscopy study. *Muscle Nerve* 21, 1523–1525.

Arnold, D. L., Bore, P. J., Radda, G. K., Styles, P. and Taylor, D. J. (1984a). Excessive intracellular acidosis of skeletal muscle on exercise in a patient with a post-viral exhaustion/fatigue syndrome. A ^{31}P nuclear magnetic resonance study. *Lancet*, i, 1367–1369.

Arnold, D. L., Matthews, P. M. and Radda, G. K. (1984b). Metabolic recovery after exercise and the assessment of mitochondrial function in vivo in human skeletal muscle by means of ^{31}P NMR. *Magn. Reson. Med.* 1, 307–315.

Arnold, D. L., Taylor, D. J. and Radda, G. K. (1985). Investigation of human mitochondrial myopathies by phosphorus magnetic resonance spectroscopy. *Ann. Neurol.* 18, 189–196.

Arnolda, L., Conway, M., Dolecki, M. et al. (1990). Skeletal muscle metabolism in heart failure: a ^{31}P nuclear magnetic resonance spectroscopy study of leg muscle. *Clin. Sci.* **79**, 583–589.

Avison, M. J., Rothman, D. L., Nadel, E. and Shulman, R. G. (1988). Detection of human muscle glycogen by natural abundance ^{13}C NMR. *Proc. Natl. Acad. Sci. USA* **85**, 1634–1636.

Barany, M., Venkatasubramanian, P. N., Mok, E. et al. (1989). Quantitative and qualitative fat analysis in human leg muscle of neuromuscular diseases by ^{1}H MR spectroscopy in vivo. *Magn. Reson. Med.* 10: 210–226.

Barbiroli, B., Funicello, R., Iotti, S., Montagna, P., Ferlini, A. and Zaniol, P. (1992). ^{31}P-NMR spectroscopy of skeletal muscle in Becker dystrophy and DMD/BMD carriers. Altered rate of phosphate transport. *J. Neurol. Sci.* **109**, 188–195.

Barbiroli, B., McCully, K. K., Iotti, S., Lodi, R., Zaniol, P. and Chance, B. (1993). Further impairment of muscle phosphate kinetics by lengthening exercise in DMD/BMD carriers. An in vivo ^{31}P-NMR spectroscopy study. *J. Neurol. Sci.* **119**, 65–73.

Barbiroli, B., Montagna, P., Cortelli, P. et al. (1995). Defective brain and muscle energy metabolism shown by in vivo ^{31}P magnetic resonance spectroscopy in nonaffected carriers of 11778 mtDNA mutation. *Ann. Neurol.* **45**, 1364–1369.

Barbiroli, B., Frassineti, C., Martinelli, P. et al. (1997). Coenzyme Q10 improves mitochondrial respiration in patients with mitochondrial cytopathies. An in vivo study on brain and skeletal muscle by phosphorous magnetic resonance spectroscopy. *Cell. Mol. Biol.* **43**, 741–749.

Barnes, P. R., Taylor, D. J., Kemp, G. J. and Radda, G. K. (1993). Skeletal muscle bioenergetics in the chronic fatigue syndrome. *J. Neurol. Neurosurg. Psychiatry* **56**, 679–683.

Barnes, P. R., Kemp, G. J., Taylor, D. J. and Radda, G. K. (1997). Skeletal muscle metabolism in myotonic dystrophy A ^{31}P magnetic resonance spectroscopy study. *Brain* **120**, 1699–1711.

Bendahan, D., Confort-Gouny, S., Kozak-Reiss, G. and Cozzone, P. J. (1990). Heterogeneity of metabolic response to muscular exercise in humans. New criteria of invariance defined by in vivo phosphorus-31 NMR spectroscopy. *FEBS Lett.* **272**, 155–158.

Bendahan, D., Confort-Gouny, S., Kozak-Ribbens, G. and Cozzone, P. J. (1992a). [31]P characterization of the metabolic anomalies associated with the lack of glycogen phosphorylase activity in human forearm muscle. *Biochem. Biophys. Res. Commun.* **185**, 16–21.

Bendahan, D., Desnuelle, C., Vanuxem, D. et al. (1992b). ^{31}P NMR spectroscopy and ergometer exercise test as evidence for muscle oxidative performance improvement with coenzyme Q in mitochondrial myopathies. *Neurology* **42**, 1203–1208.

Bendahan, D., Jammes, Y., Salvan, A. M. et al. (1996). Combined electromyography–[31]P-magnetic resonance spectroscopy study of human muscle fatigue during static contraction. *Muscle Nerve* **19**, 715–721.

Bendahan, D., Badier, M., Jammes, Y. et al. (1998a). Metabolic and myoelectrical effects of acute hypoxaemia during isometric contraction of forearm muscles in humans: a combined ^{31}P-magnetic resonance spectroscopy-surface electromyogram (MRS-SEMG) study. *Clin. Sci.* **94**, 279–286.

Bendahan, D., Kozak-Ribbens, G., Rodet, L., Confort-Gouny, S. and Cozzone, P. J. (1998b). [31]Phosphorus magnetic resonance spectroscopy characterization of muscular metabolic anomalies in patients with malignant hyperthermia: application to diagnosis. *Anesthesiology* **88**, 96–107.

Bertocci, L. A., Haller, R. G. and Lewis, S. F. (1993). Muscle metabolism during lactate infusion in human phosphofructokinase deficiency. *J. Appl. Physiol.* **74**, 1342–1347.

Boesch, C., Slotboom, J., Hoppeler, H. and Kreis, R. (1997). In vivo determination of intra-myocellular lipids in human muscle by means of localized [1]H-MR-spectroscopy. *Magn. Reson. Med.* **37**, 484–493.

Bollaert, P. E., Robin-Lherbier, B., Escanye, J. M. et al. (1989). Phosphorus nuclear magnetic resonance evidence of abnormal skeletal muscle metabolism in chronic alcoholics. *Neurology* **39**, 821–824.

Boska, M. (1991). Estimating the ATP cost of force production in the human gastrocnemius/soleus muscle group using ^{31}P MRS and ^{1}H MRI. *NMR Biomed.* **4**, 173–181.

Bottomley, P. A., Lee, Y. and Weiss, R. G. (1997). Total creatine in muscle: imaging and quantification with proton MR spectroscopy. *Radiology* **204**, 403–410.

Bulcke, J. A. L. and Baert, A. L. (1982). *Clinical and Radiological Aspects of Myopathies.* Berlin: Springer-Verlag.

Carelli, V., Ghelli, A., Ratta, M. et al. (1997). Leber's hereditary optic neuropathy: biochemical effect of 11778/ND4 and 3460/ND1 mutations and correlation with the mitochondrial genotype. *Neurology* **48**, 1623–1632.

Chance, B. and Bank, W. (1995). Genetic disease of mitochondrial function evaluated by NMR and NIR spectroscopy of skeletal tissue. *Biochim. Biophys. Acta,* **1271**, 7–14.

Chance, B., Eleff, S., Leigh J. A., Sokolov, D. and Sapega, A. (1981). Mitochondrial regulation of phosphocreatine/inorganic phosphate ratios in exercising human muscle: a gated ^{31}P NMR study. *Proc. Natl. Acad. Sci. USA* **78**, 6714–6718.

Chance, B., Leigh, J. S., Jr, Kent, J. and McCully, K. (1986). Metabolic control principles and ^{31}P NMR. *Fed. Proc.* **45**, 2915–2920.

Cinnamon, J., Slonim, A. E., Black, K. S., Gorey, M. T., Scuderi, D. M. and Hyman, R. A. (1991). Evaluation of the lumbar spine in patients with glycogen storage disease: CT demonstration of patterns of paraspinal muscle atrophy. *Am. J. Neuroradiol.* **12**, 1099–1103.

Cock, H., Tabrizi, S., Cooper, J. and Schapira, A. (1998). The influence of nuclear background on the biochemical expression of 3460 Leber's hereditary optic neuropathy. *Ann. Neurol.* **44**, 187–193.

Constantin-Teodosiu, D., Greenhaff, P. L., McIntyre, D. B., Round, J. M. and Jones, D. A. (1997). Anaerobic energy production in human skeletal muscle in intense contraction: a comparison of ^{31}P magnetic resonance spectroscopy and biochemical techniques. *Exp. Physiol.* **82**, 593–601.

Cortelli, P., Montagna, P., Avoni, P. et al. (1991). Leber's hereditary optic neuropathy: genetic, biochemical and phosphorus magnetic resonance spectroscopy study in an Italian family. *Neurology* **41**, 1211–1215.

Dalakas, M. C. (1991). Polymyositis, dermatomyositis and inclusion-body myositis. *N. Engl. J. Med.* **325**, 1487–1498.

de Blecourt, A. C., Wolf, R. F., van Rijswijk, M. H., Kamman, R. L., Knipping, A. A. and Mooyaart, E. L. (1991). In vivo ^{31}P magnetic resonance spectroscopy (MRS) of tender points in patients with primary fibromyalgia syndrome. *Rheumatol. Int.* **11**, 51–54.

de Stefano, N., Matthews, P. M., Ford, B., Genge, A., Karpati, G. and Arnold, D. L. (1995). Short-term dichloroacetate treatment improves indices of cerebral metabolism in patients with mitochondrial disorders. *Neurology* **45**, 1193–1198.

de Stefano, N., Argov, Z., Matthews, P. M., Karpati, G. and Arnold, D. L. (1996). Impairment of muscle mitochondrial oxidative metabolism in McArdles's disease. *Muscle Nerve* **19**, 764–769.

de Visser, M. and Verbeeten, B. (1985). Computed tomographic findings in manifesting carriers of Duchenne muscular dystrophy. *Clin. Genet.* **27**, 269–275.

de Visser, M., Schalke, B. and Reimers, C. (1996). Muscular dystrophies. In: *Muscle Imaging in Health and Disease*, eds. J. C. Fleckenstein, C. D. Reimers and J. V. Crues, pp. 218–236. New York: Springer Verlag.

Duboc, D., Jehenson, P., Tran-Dinh, S., Marsac, C., Syrota, A. and Fardeau, M. (1987). Phosphourus NMR spectroscopy study of muscular enzyme deficiencies involving glycogenolysis and glycolysis. *Neurology* **37**, 663–671.

Dudley, C. R., Taylor, D. J., Ng, L. L. et al. (1990). Evidence for abnormal Na^+/H^+ antiport activity detected by phosphorus nuclear magnetic resonance spectroscopy in exercising skeletal muscle of patients with essential hypertension. *Clin. Sci.* **79**, 491–497.

Dwyer, A. J., Frank, J. A., Sank, V. J., Reinig, J. W., Hickey, A. M. and Doppman, J. L. (1988). Short-T_1 inversion-recovery pulse sequence: analysis and initial experience in cancer imaging. *Radiology* **168**, 827–836.

Edwards, R. H. T., Dawson, M. J., Wilkie, D. R., Gordon, R. E. and Shaw, D. (1982). Clinical use of nuclear magnetic resonance in the investigation of myopathy. *Lancet* **i**, 725–731.

Edwards, R. H., Griffiths, R. D. and Cady, E. B. (1985). Topical magnetic resonance for the study of muscle metabolism in human myopathy. *Clin. Physiol.* **5**, 93–109.

Eleff, S., Kennaway, N., Buist, N. et al. (1984). ^{31}P NMR study of improvement in oxidative phosphorylation by vitamins K_3 and C in a patient with a defect in electron transport at complex III in skeletal muscle. *Proc. Natl. Acad. Sci. USA* **81**, 3529–3533.

Emslie-Smith, A. M. and Engel, A. G. (1990). Microvascular changes in early and advanced dermatomyositis: a quantitative study. *Ann. Neurol.* **27**, 343–356.

Fleckenstein, J. L., Canby, R. C., Parkey, R. W. and Peshock, R. M. (1988). Acute effects of exercise on MR imaging of skeletal muscle in normal volunteers. *Am. J. Roentgenol.* **151**, 231–237.

Fleckenstein, J. L., Bertocci, L. A., Nunnally, R. L., Parkey, R. W. and Peshock, R. M. (1989a). Exercise-enhanced MR imaging of variations in forearm muscle anatomy and use: importance in MR spectroscopy. *Am. J. Roentgenol.* **153**, 693–698.

Fleckenstein, J. L., Peshock, R. M., Lewis, S. F. and Haller, R. G. (1989b). Magnetic resonance imaging of muscle injury and atrophy in glycolytic myopathies. *Muscle Nerve* **12**, 849–855.

Fleckenstein, J. L., Archer, B. T., Barker, B. A., Vaughan, J. T., Parkey, R. W. and Peshock, R. M. (1991a). Fast short-tau inversion-recovery MR imaging. *Radiology* **179**, 499–504.

Fleckenstein, J. L., Haller, R. G., Lewis, S. F. et al. (1991b). Absence of exercise-induced MRI enhancement of skeletal muscle in McArdle's disease. *J. Appl. Physiol.* **71**, 961–969.

Fleckenstein, J. L., Weatherall, P. T., Bertocci, L. A. et al. (1991c). Locomotor system assessment by muscle magnetic resonance imaging. *Magn. Reson. Q.* **7**, 79–103.

Fleckenstein, J. L., Reimers, C. D. and Haller, R. G. (1996). Inherited defects of muscle energy metabolism. In: *Muscle Radiology*, eds. J. L. Fleckenstein, C. D. Reimers and R. G. Haller, pp. 253–267. New York: Springer Verlag.

Frostick, S. P., Taylor, D. J., Dolecki, M. J. and Radda, G. K. (1992). Human muscle cell denervation: the results of a 31-phosphorus magnetic resonance spectroscopy study. *J. Hand Surg.* **17**, 33–45.

Grehl, T., Muller, K., Vorgerd, M., Tegenthoff, M., Malin, J.-P. and Zange, J. (1998). Impaired aerobic glycolysis in muscle phosphofructokinase deficiency results in biphasic post-exercise phosphocreatine recovery in ^{31}P magnetic resonance spectroscopy. *Neuromusc. Disord.* **8**, 480–488.

Griggs, R. C., Askanas, V., DiMauro, S. et al. (1995). Inclusion body myositis and myopathies. *Ann. Neurol.* **38**: 705–713.

Gupta, R. K., Gupta, P., Yushok, W. D. and Rose, Z. B. (1983). On the noninvasive measurement of intracellular free magnesium by ^{31}P NMR spectroscopy. *Physiol. Chem. Physi. Med. NMR* **15**, 265–280.

Gupta, R. K., Mittal, R. D., Agarwal, K. N. and Agarwal, D. K. (1994). Muscular sufficiency, serum protein, enzymes and bioenergetic studies (31-phosphorus magnetic resonance spectroscopy) in chronic malnutrition. *Acta Paed.* **83**, 327–331.

Guthrie, B. M., Frostick, S. P., Goodman, J., Mikulis, D. J., Plyley, M. J. and Marshall, K. W. (1996). Endurance-trained and untrained skeletal muscle bioenergetics observed with magnetic resonance spectroscopy. *Can. J. Appl. Physiol.* **21**, 251–263.

Hands, L. J., Bore, P. J., Galloway, G., Morris, P. J. and Radda, G. K. (1986). Muscle metabolism in patients with peripheral vascular disease investigated by ^{31}P nuclear magnetic resonance spectroscopy. *Clin. Sci.* **71**, 283–290.

Hands, L. J., Sharif, M. H., Payne, G. S., Morris, P. J. and Radda, G. K. (1990). Muscle ischaemia in peripheral vascular disease studied by 31P-magnetic resonance spectroscopy. *Eur. J. Vasc. Surg.* **4**, 637–642.

Harris, R., Hultman, E. and Nordesjo, L.-O. (1974). Glycogen, glycolytic intermediates and high energy phosphates determined in biopsy samples of musculus quadriceps femoris of man at rest. Methods and variance of values. *Scand. J. Clin. Lab. Invest.* **33**, 109–120.

Iotti, S., Lodi, R., Frassineti, C., Zaniol, P. and Barbiroli, B. (1993). *In vivo* assessment of mitochondrial functionality in human gastrocnemius muscle by ^{31}P MRS. The role of pH in the evaluation of phosphocreatine and inorganic phosphate recoveries from exercise. *NMR Biomed,* **6**, 248–253.

Jansen, G., Mahadevan, M., Amemiya, C. et al. (1992). Characterization of the myotonic dystrophy region predicts multiple protein isoform-encoding mRNAs. *Nat. Genet.* **1**, 261–266.

Kao, W., Helpern, J. A., Goldstein, S., Gheorghiade, M. and Levine, B. (1995). Abnormalities of skeletal muscle metabolism during nerve stimulation determined by ^{31}P nuclear magnetic resonance spectroscopy in severe congestive heart failure. *Am. J. Cardiol.* **76**, 606–609.

Kemp, G. J. and Radda, G. K. (1994). Quantitative interpretation of bioenergetic data from ^{31}P and ^{1}H magnetic resonance spectroscopic studies of skeletal muscle: an analytical review. *Magn. Reson. Q.* **10**, 43–63.

Kemp, G. J., Taylor, D. J., Dunn, J. F., Frostick, S. P. and Radda, G. K. (1993a). Cellular energetics of dystrophic muscle. *J. Neurol. Sci.* **116**, 201–206.

Kemp, G. J., Taylor, D. J., Thompson, C. H. et al. (1993b). Quantitative analysis by ^{31}P magnetic resonance spectroscopy of abnormal mitochondrial oxidation in skeletal muscle during recovery from exercise. *NMR Biomed.* **6**, 302–310.

Kent-Braun, J. A., McCully, K. K. and Chance, B. (1990). Metabolic effects of training in humans: a ^{31}P-MRS study. *J. Appl. Physiol.* **69**, 1165–1170.

Lamminen, A. E., Tanttu, J. I., Sepponen, R. E., Suramo, I. J. and Pihko, H. (1990). Magnetic resonance of diseased skeletal muscle: combined T1 measurement and chemical shift imaging. *Brit. J. Radiol.* **63**, 591–596.

Lane, R. J., Barrett, M. C., Taylor, D. J., Kemp, G. J. and Lodi, R. (1998). Heterogeneity in chronic fatigue syndrome: evidence from magnetic resonance spectroscopy of muscle. *Neuromusc. Disord.* **8**, 204–209.

Letellier, T., Malgat, M. and Mazat, J. P. (1993). Control of oxidative phosphorylation in rat muscle mitochondria: implications for mitochondrial myopathies. *Biochim. Biophys. Acta,* **1141**, 58–64.

Levy, P., Wuyam, B., Pepin, J. L., Reutenauer, H. and Payen, J. F. (1997). Skeletal muscle abnormalities in chronic obstructive lung disease with respiratory insufficiency. Value of P31 magnetic resonance spectroscopy. *Rev. Mal. Resp.* **14**, 183–191.

Lewis, S. F. and Haller, R. G. (1989). Skeletal muscle disorders and associated factors that limit exercise performance. *Exercise Sport Sci. Rev.* **61**, 67–113.

Lodi, R., Kemp, G. J., Iotti, S., Radda, G. K. and Barbiroli, B. (1997a). Influence of cytosolic pH on in vivo assessment of human muscle mitochondrial respiration by phosphorus magnetic resonance spectroscopy. *Magma* **5**, 165–171.

Lodi, R., Montagna, P., Soriani, S. et al. (1997b). Deficit of brain and skeletal muscle bioenergetics and low brain magnesium in juvenile migraine: an in vivo ^{31}P magnetic resonance spectroscopy interictal study. *Ped. Res.* **42**, 866–871.

Lodi, R., Muntoni, F., Taylor, J. et al. (1997c). Correlative MR imaging and ^{31}P-MR spectroscopy study in sarcoglycan deficient limb girdle muscular dystrophy. *Neuromusc. Disord.* **7**, 505–511.

Lodi, R., Taylor, D. J. and Radda, G. K. (1997d). Chronic fatigue syndrome and skeletal muscle mitochondrial function. *Muscle Nerve* **20**, 765–766.

Lodi, R., Taylor, D. J., Tabrizi, S. J. et al. (1997e). In vivo skeletal muscle mitochondrial function in Leber's hereditary optic neuropathy assessed by ^{31}P magnetic resonance spectroscopy. *Ann. Neurol.* **42**, 573–579.

Lodi, R., Taylor, D. J., Tabrizi, S. J. et al. (1998). Normal in vivo skeletal muscle oxidative metabolism in sporadic inclusion body myositis assessed by ^{31}P-magnetic resonance spectroscopy. *Brain* **121**, 2119–2126.

Lodi, R., Kemp, G. J., Muntoni, F. et al. (1999). Reduced cytosolic acidification during exercise suggests defective glycolytic activity in skeletal muscle of patients with Becker muscular dystrophy. An *in vivo* [31]P magnetic resonance spectroscopy study. *Brain* **122**, 121–130.

Mahadevan, M. S., Amemiya, C., Jansen, G. et al. (1993). Structure and genomic sequence of the myotonic dystrophy (DM kinase) gene. *Hum. Mol. Genet.* **2**, 299–304.

Massa, R., Lodi, R., Barbiroli, B. et al. (1996). Partial block of glycolysis in late-onset phosphofructokinase deficiency myopathy. *Acta Neuropatholog.* **91**, 322–329.

Matthews, P. M., Allaire, C., Shoubridge, E. A., Karpati, G., Carpenter, S. and Arnold, D. L. (1991). In vivo muscle magnetic resonance spectroscopy in the clinical investigation of mitochondrial disease. *Neurology* **41**, 114–120.

Matthews, P. M., Ford, B., Dandurand, R. J. et al. (1993). Coenzyme Q10 with multiple vitamins is generally ineffective in treatment of mitochondrial disease. *Neurology* **43**, 884–890.

McCully, K. K., Kent, J. A. and Chance, B. (1988). Application of ^{31}P magnetic resonance spectroscopy to the study of athletic performance. *Sports Med.* **5**, 312–321.

McCully, K. K., Forciea, M. A., Hack, L. M. et al. (1991). Muscle metabolism in older subjects using ^{31}P magnetic resonance spectroscopy. *Can. J. Physiol. Pharmacol.* **69**, 576–580.

McCully, K. K., Iotti, S., Kendrick, K. et al. (1994). Simultaneous in vivo measurements of HbO_2 saturation and PCr kinetics after exercise in normal humans. *J. Appl. Physiol.* **77**, 5–10.

McCully, K. K., Natelson, B. H., Iotti, S., Sisto, S. and Leigh, J. S., Jr. (1996). Reduced oxidative muscle metabolism in chronic fatigue syndrome. *Muscle Nerve* **19**, 621–625.

Monsieurs, K., Heytens, L., Kloeck, C., Martin, J. J., Wuyts, F. and Bossaert, L. (1997). Slower recovery of muscle phosphocreatine in malignant hyperthermia-susceptible individuals assessed by ^{31}P-MR spectroscopy. *J. Neurol.* **244**, 651–656.

Morvan, D., Leroy-Willig, A., Jehenson, P., Cuenod, C. A. and Syrota, A. (1992). Temperature changes induced in human muscle by radio-frequency H-1 decoupling: measurement with an MR imaging diffusion technique. Work in progress. *Radiology* **185**, 871–874.

Newman, R. J., Bore, P. J., Chan, L. et al. (1982). Nuclear magnetic resonance studies of forearm muscle in Duchenne dystrophy. *Brit. J. Med.* **284**, 1072–1074.

Oldfors, A., Larsson, N. G., Lindberg, C. and Holme, E. (1993). Mitochondrial DNA deletions in inclusion body myositis. *Brain* **116**, 325–336.

Olgin, J., Rosenberg, H., Allen, G., Seestedt, R. and Chance, B. (1991). A blinded comparison of noninvasive, in vivo phosphorus nuclear magnetic resonance spectroscopy and the in vitro halothane/caffeine contracture test in the evaluation of malignant hyperthermia susceptibility. *Anesth. Analg.* **72**, 36–47.

Pagliaro, L. (1993). Glycolysis revisited. *News Physiol. Sci.* **8**, 219–223.

Pan, J. W., Hamm, J. R., Hetherington, H. P., Rothman, D. L. and Shulman, R. G. (1991a). Correlation of lactate and pH in human skeletal muscle after exercise by ^{1}H NMR. *Magn. Reson. Med.* **20**, 57–65.

Pan, J. W., Hetherington, H. P., Hamm, J. R. and Shulman, R. G. (1991b). Quantitation of metabolites by ^{1}H NMR. *Magn. Reson. Med.* **20**, 48–56.

Park, J. H., Brown, R. L., Park, C. R. et al. (1987). Functional pools of oxidative and glycolytic fibers in human muscle observed by ^{31}P magnetic resonance spectroscopy during exercise. *Proc. Natl. Acad. Sci. USA* **84**, 8976–8980.

Park, J. H., Vansant, J. P., Kumar, N. G. et al. (1990). Dermatomyositis: correlative MR imaging and P-31 MR spectroscopy for quantitative characterization of inflammatory disease. *Radiology* **177**, 473–479.

Park, J., Vital, T., Ryder, N. et al. (1994). Magnetic resonance imaging and P-31 magnetic resonance spectroscopy provide unique quantitative data useful in the longitudinal management of patients with dermatomyositis. *Arthritis Rheum.* **37**, 736–746.

Park, J. H., Olsen, N. J., King, L., Jr et al. (1995). Use of magnetic resonance imaging and P-31 magnetic resonance spectroscopy to detect and quantify muscle dysfunction in the amyopathic and myopathic variants of dermatomyositis. *Arthritis Rheum.* **38**, 68–77.

Park, J. H., Kari, S., King, L. E. and Olsen, N. J. (1998a). Analysis of ^{31}P MR spectroscopy data using artificial neural networks for longitudinal evaluation of muscle diseases: dermatomyositis. *NMR Biomed.* **11**, 245–256.

Park, J. H., Phothimat, P., Oates, C. T., Hernanz-Schulman, M. and Olsen, N. J. (1998b). Use of P-31 magnetic resonance spectroscopy to detect metabolic abnormalities in muscles of patients with fibromyalgia. *Arthritis Rheum.* **41**, 406–413.

Payen, J. F., Bosson, J. L., Bourdon, L. et al. (1993). Improved non-invasive diagnostic testing for malignant hyperthermia susceptibility from a combination of metabolites determined in vivo with ^{31}P-magnetic resonance spectroscopy. *Anesthesiology* **78**, 848–855.

Payen, J. F., Fouilhe, N., Sam-Lai, E. et al. (1996) In vitro ^{31}P-magnetic resonance spectroscopy of muscle extracts in malignant hyperthermia-susceptible patients. *Anesthesiology* **84**, 1077–1082.

Penn, A. M., Lee, J. W., Thuillier, P. et al. (1992). MELAS syndrome with mitochondrial tRNA(Leu)(UUR) mutation: correlation of clinical state, nerve conduction and muscle ^{31}P magnetic resonance spectroscopy during treatment with nicotinamide and riboflavin. *Neurology* **42**, 2147–2152.

Pitt, A. M., Fleckenstein, J. L., Greenlee, R. G., Jr, Burns, D. K., Bryan, W. W. and Haller, R. (1993). MRI-guided biopsy in inflammatory myopathy: initial results. *Magn. Res. Imaging* **11**, 1093–1099.

Porter, B. A., Hastrup, W., Richardson, M. L. et al. (1987). Classification and investigation of artifacts in magnetic resonance imaging. *Radiographics* **7**, 271–279.

Radda, G. K., Rajagopalan, B. and Taylor, D. J. (1989). Biochemistry in vivo: an appraisal of clinical magnetic resonance spectroscopy. *Magn. Reson. Q.* **5**, 122–151.

Rajagopalan B., Conway M. A., Massie B. and Radda G. K. (1988). Alterations of skeletal muscle metabolism in humans studied by phosphorus 31 magnetic resonance spectroscopy in congestive heart failure. *Am. J. Cardiol.* **62**, 53E–57E.

Reimers, C. D. and Vogl, T. J. (1996). Myotonic dystrophy. In: *Muscle Radiology*, eds. C. D. Reimers and T. J. Vogl, pp. 237–243. New York: Springer Verlag.

Reimers, C. D., Schedel, H., Fleckenstein, J. L. et al. (1994). Magnetic resonance imaging of skeletal muscles in idiopathic inflammatory myopathies of adults. *J. Neurol.* **241**, 306–314.

Roman, W. J., Fleckenstein, J., Stray-Gundersen, J., Alway, S. E., Peshock, R. and Gonyea, W. J. (1993). Adaptations in the elbow flexors of elderly males after heavy-resistance training. *J. Appl. Physiol.* **74**, 750–754.

Ross, B. D., Radda, G. K., Gadian, D. G., Rocker, G., Esiri, M. and Falconer-Smith, J. (1981). Examination of a case of suspected McArdle's syndrome by ^{31}P nuclear magnetic resonance. *N. Engl. J. Med.* **304**, 1338–1342.

Santorelli, F. M., Sciacco, M., Tanji, K. et al. (1996). Multiple mitochondrial DNA deletions in sporadic inclusion body myositis: a study of 56 patients. *Ann. Neurol.* **39**, 789–795.

Schweitzer, M. E. and Fort, J. (1995). Cost-effectiveness of MR imaging in evaluating polymyositis. *Am. J. Roentgenol.* **165**, 1469–1471.

Sekul, E. A., Chow, C. and Dalakas, M. C. (1997). Magnetic resonance imaging of the forearm as a diagnostic aid in patients with sporadic inclusion body myositis. *Neurology* **48**, 863–866.

Siciliano, G., Rossi, B., Martini, A. et al. (1995). Myophosphorylase deficiency affects muscle mitochondrial respiration as shown by ^{31}P-MR spectroscopy in a case with associated multifocal encephalopathy. *J. Neurol. Sci.* **128**, 84–91.

Simms, R., Roy, S., Hrovat, M. et al. (1994). Lack of association between fibromyalgia syndrome and abnormalities in muscle energy metabolism. *Arthritis Rheum.* **37**, 794–800.

Sinnwell, T. M., Sivakumar, K., Soueidan, K., Frank, J. A., McLaughlin, A. C. and Dalakas, M. C. (1995). Metabolic abnormalities in skeletal muscle of patients receiving zidovudine therapy observed by ^{31}P in vivo magnetic resonance spectroscopy. *J. Clin. Invest.* **95**, 126–131.

Sivakumar, K., Vasconcelos, O., Goldfarb, L. and Dalakas, M. C. (1996). Late-onset muscle weakness in partial phosphofructokinase deficiency: a unique myopathy with vacuoles, abnormal mitochondria and absence of the common exon 5/intron 5 junction point mutation. *Neurology* **46**, 1337–1342.

Taivassalo, T., de Stefano, N., Argov, Z. et al. (1998). Effects of aerobic training in patients with mitochondrial myopathies. *Neurology* **50**, 1055–1060.

Taylor, D. J., Bore, P. J., Styles, P., Gadian, D. G. and Radda, G. K. (1983). Bioenergetics of intact human muscle. A ^{31}P nuclear magnetic resonance study. *Mol. Biol. Med.* **1**, 77–94.

Taylor, D. J., Styles, P., Matthews, P. M. et al. (1986). Energetics of human muscle: exercise-induced ATP depletion. *Magn. Reson. Med.* **3**, 44–54.

Taylor, D. J., Kemp, G. J., Woods, C. G., Edwards, J. H. and Radda, G. K. (1993). Skeletal muscle bioenergetics in myotonic dystrophy. *J. Neurol. Sci.* **116**, 193–200.

Taylor, D. J., Kemp, G. J. and Radda, G. K. (1994). Bioenergetics of skeletal muscle in mitochondrial myopathy. *J. Neurol. Sci.* **127**, 198–206.

Taylor, D. J., Kemp, G. J., Thompson, C. H. and Radda, G. K. (1997). Ageing: effects on oxidative function of skeletal muscle in vivo. *Mol. Cell. Biochem.* **174**, 321–324.

Thompson, C. H., Davies, R. J., Kemp, G. J., Taylor, D. J., Radda, G. K. and Rajagopalan B. (1993). Skeletal muscle metabolism during exercise and recovery in patients with respiratory failure. *Thorax* **48**, 486–490.

Vandenborne, K., McCully, K., Kakihira, H. et al. (1991). Metabolic heterogeneity in human calf muscle during maximal exercise. *Proc. Natl. Acad. Sci. USA* **88**, 5714–5718.

Veech, R., Lawson, J., Cornell, N. and Krebs, H. (1979). Cytosolic phosphorylation potential. *J. Biol. Chem.* **254**, 6538–6547.

Vestergaard-Poulsen, P., Thomsen, C., Sinkjaer, T. and Henriksen, O. (1994). Simultaneous ^{31}P NMR spectroscopy and EMG in exercising and recovering human skeletal muscle: technical aspects. *Magn. Reson. Med.* **31**, 93–102.

Vestergaard-Poulsen, P., Thomsen, C., Norregaard, J., Bulow, P., Sinkjaer, T. and Henriksen, O. (1995). ^{31}P NMR spectroscopy and electromyography during exercise and recovery in patients with fibromyalgia. *J. Rheumatol.* **22**, 1544–1551.

Vita, G., Toscano, A., Bresolin, N. et al. (1994). Muscle phosphoglycerate mutase (PGAM) deficiency in the first Caucasian patient: biochemistry, muscle culture and ^{31}P-MR spectroscopy. *J. Neurol.* **241**, 289–294.

Vora, S., DiMauro, S., Spear, D., Harker, D. and Danon, M. (1987). Characterization of the enzymatic defect in late-onset muscle phosphofructokinase deficiency. New subtype of glycogen storage disease type VII. *J. Clin. Invest.* **80**, 1479–1485.

Ward, K. M., Rajan, S. S., Wysong, M., Radulovic, D. and Clauw, D. J. (1996). Phosphorus nuclear magnetic resonance spectroscopy: in vivo magnesium measurements in the skeletal muscle of normal subjects. *Magn. Reson. Med.* **36**, 475–480.

Webster, D. W., Thompson, R. T., Gravelle, D. R., Laschuk, M. J. and Driedger, A. A. (1990). Metabolic response to exercise in malignant hyperthermia-sensitive patients measured by ^{31}P magnetic resonance spectroscopy. *Magn. Reson. Med.* **15**, 81–89.

Weissman, J. D., Constantinitis, I., Hudgins, P. and Wallace, D. C. (1992). ^{31}P magnetic resonance spectroscopy suggests impaired mitochondrial function in AZT-treated HIV-infected patients. *Neurology* **42**, 619–623.

Younkin, D. P., Berman, P., Sladky, J., Chee, C., Bank, W. and Chance, B. (1987). ^{31}P NMR studies in Duchenne muscular dystrophy: age-related metabolic changes. *Neurology* **37**, 165–169.

Zatina, M. A., Berkowitz, H. D., Gross, G. M., Maris, J. M. and Chance, B. (1986). ^{31}P nuclear magnetic resonance spectroscopy: noninvasive biochemical analysis of the ischemic extremity. *J. Vasc. Surg.* **3**, 411–420.

Zochodne, D. W., Thompson, R. T., Driedger, A. A., Strong, M. J., Gravelle, D. and Bolton, C. F. (1988). Metabolic changes in human muscle denervation: topical ^{31}P NMR spectroscopy studies. *Magn. Reson. Med.* **7**, 373–383.

Zochodne, D. W., Koopman, W. J., Witt, N. J. et al. (1992). Forearm P-31 nuclear magnetic resonance spectroscopy studies in oculopharyngeal muscular dystrophy. *Can. J. Neurol. Sci.* **19**, 174–179.

Part III

Description of muscle disease

17

The examination and investigation of the patient with muscle disease

David Hilton-Jones and John T. Kissel

Introduction

The evaluation of the patient with suspected muscle disease traditionally followed a simple and reproducible pattern. Following the history and examination that suggested the presence of a myopathy, the patient underwent a few blood tests (often only a creatine kinase (CK) level), electrophysiological studies to confirm that the process involved muscle and then a muscle biopsy for histological and histochemical analysis. Although occasional patients might undergo more specialized evaluations, it was the rare patient who avoided a muscle biopsy. This was largely because there were few other practical methods to investigate muscle structure and function.

Since the last edition of this textbook appeared, the molecular genetics revolution has resulted in a wealth of new information on the pathogenesis of most myopathies. These advances, coupled with technological improvements in laboratory medicine, have broadened the scope of testing available to the neuromuscular clinician (Table 17.1), and resulted in a fundamental change in the traditional diagnostic approach. For example, a boy with suspected Duchenne dystrophy may now be evaluated through a serum CK assay and direct genetic analysis for an Xp21 mutation, before electrodiagnostic testing and muscle biopsy are even considered.

It is ironic, however, that this increase in the number and sophistication of diagnostic tests has, if anything, only increased the importance of the bedside history and examination in the diagnostic process. It is still only through a careful history and examination that the clinician can make the initial determination that a disorder is likely to be myopathic, rather than involving some other part of the nervous system. In addition, some muscle disorders (Table 17.2) have findings so characteristic that they can be diagnosed with relative certainty at the bedside. More frequently, the data gathered from the history and examination permit the generation of diagnostic hypotheses, which can then be assessed through appropriate diagnostic studies. Thus, the clinical features may suggest a form of muscular dystrophy, inflammatory myopathy or a metabolic disorder, a deduction of obvious crucial importance in planning the subsequent work-up. No amount of laboratory testing, including genetic testing, can compensate for an erroneous impression based on an incomplete, hastily performed history and examination. Equally as important is the fact that the process of history taking and performing the examination through the 'laying on of hands' represents the first and most important interaction between physician and patient. It is during this initial contact that the patient develops trust in the clinician and the rapport necessary for a successful therapeutic relationship is established. This chapter will, therefore, begin with a discussion of the neuromuscular history and examination as a prelude to discussing other aspects of the evaluation of patients with suspected muscle disease. The aim throughout is to provide practical advice that will be of benefit to the clinician at the bedside.

History

Although the basic elements of the history (presenting complaint, history of the present illness, past medical history, family history, social history, review of symptoms and drug history) are the same for neuromuscular complaints as for other medical problems, certain features are unique to the patient with suspected myopathy. One of the most notable differences is that some of the more common muscle symptoms, such as pain and fatigue, are not amenable to direct observation or quantification by the examiner, and they often occur in patients with no definable

Table 17.1. Diagnostic testing useful in patients with suspected muscle disease

Clinical history and examination
Computed quantitative muscle testing
Biochemical tests
    Blood and urine analyses (e.g. serum creatine kinase)
    Exercise tests (forearm exercise test, treadmill or bicycle
        ergometry)
    Enzyme assay
Neurophysiological studies
    Nerve conduction studies
    Electromyography: single fibre electromyography
    Repetitive stimulation studies
Muscle imaging
Muscle biopsy
    Routine histology and histochemistry
    Immunocytochemistry
    Specific enzyme assays
    Genetic tests
Molecular genetic testing
    Specific gene tests for disease (e.g. Xp21 deletion in Duchenne
        dystrophy)
    Genetic tests associated with disease (e.g. 4q5 deletion in
        facioscapulohumeral dystrophy)
    Linkage analysis

Table 17.2. Myopathies that can be diagnosed or strongly suspected after examination

Duchenne muscular dystrophy
Emery–Dreifuss syndrome
Facioscapulohumeral muscular dystrophy
Oculopharyngeal muscular dystrophy
Rigid spine syndrome
Myotonic dystrophy
Myotonia congenita
Dermatomyositis
Inclusion body myositis
Some endocrine myopathies (e.g. hypothyroid myopathy)
Some mitochondrial disorders (e.g. Kearns–Sayre syndrome)
Acid maltase deficiency (if there is diaphragmatic involvement)

muscle disease. Conversely, other symptoms, such as weakness, may develop so slowly that patients may not realise it and not complain of it during the history.

Presenting complaint

Skeletal muscle has a limited repertoire of responses to many insults; consequently, the chief complaint in most myopathic patients is usually limited to one or more of the following: weakness, muscle pain at rest or with exercise, muscle enlargement or atrophy, muscle 'overactivity' or delayed relaxation (e.g. cramps, myotonia), fatigue or (rarely) myoglobinuria. Such symptoms may point to a multisystem disorder of which myopathy is just a part, or a primary myopathy with secondary effects (e.g. renal failure caused by myoglobinuria).

Weakness

Weakness is by far the most common presenting symptom of patients with a definable muscle disease. Patients may use the term 'weakness' to refer to any of a number of symptoms, including fatigue, restricted movement owing to orthopaedic or mechanical problems, reduced exercise capacity, or occasionally even sensory disturbances. Conversely, patients frequently use words such as deadness, heaviness, aching or even numbness to describe what is actually muscle weakness. It is obviously crucial for the examiner to pin down precisely the nature of the presenting complaint, and what the patient means by 'weakness'. Questions detailing functional limitations induced by the weakness are usually required to make this determination.

Accurate delineation of the duration of weakness, rate of progression, distribution of involved muscles and whether the weakness is persistent or intermittent is also crucial. Making these determinations by history alone can be difficult, particularly in slowly progressive disorders that have their onset years or decades prior to the patient's initial presentation. Weakness may be relatively static, as in some congenital myopathies, progressive, as in most dystrophies, fluctuating, as in the myasthenic disorders, intermittent, as in the periodic paralyses and some myotonic disorders, or exercise related, as in many metabolic disorders.

The distribution of weakness is in many respects the most important aspect to be determined from the history and examination, as it provides important clues to the diagnosis. Although there are many exceptions to any rule concerning distribution of involved muscles, most patients with myopathy have one of three predominant patterns of weakness (Lane and Fuller, 1996). By far the most common pattern involves predominant involvement of the proximal and axial muscles (including neck muscles) compared with more distal groups. This pattern results in difficulty getting out of chairs or car seats, going up and down steps, arising from a squat or getting off the floor. Proximal arm weakness manifests historically as difficulty reaching to get things from shelves, or difficulty with self-care activities such as shaving, combing or setting hair, brushing teeth or even raising the arms enough to put on a shirt or sweater. Less commonly, disorders like myotonic dystrophy, distal myopathies and inclusion body myositis (IBM) can cause predominantly distal weakness, which results in leg complaints such as tripping over curbs and difficulty walking in fields or over uneven ground or thick carpeting. Patients may notice difficulty standing on their toes while reaching for objects or during exercise classes. Patient's may notice 'slapping' feet caused by foot drop, and patients may begin wearing high-topped shoes or boots to stabilize the ankle. Distal arm weakness produces difficulty opening car doors, turning keys, opening jars, wringing-out a cloth, picking up cartons of milk or similar objects while shopping, and buttoning-up clothes.

The third category of myopathic weakness is produced by muscle diseases that result in selective involvement of certain muscles and, therefore, do not result in a predominantly proximal or distal pattern. In many of these conditions, such as facioscapulohumeral (FSH) dystrophy, inclusion body myositis and some mitochondrial disorders, the involvement may also be asymmetric. In other cases, isolated groups of muscles, such as the facial and pharyngeal muscles in oculopharyngeal dystrophy and the ocular muscles in the mitochondrial disorders, may be predominantly affected. Symptoms relating to weakness in particular areas are discussed below.

Muscles innervated by cranial nerves

Patients may complain of ptosis because of the cosmetic appearance noticed while shaving or putting on make-up, or because it is severe enough to cover the pupil and obscure vision. With mild or chronic ptosis, the lid droop is often first noticed by an acquaintance. When the onset of ptosis is uncertain, the examiner should request old pictures of the patient, which frequently will reveal mild ptosis long before it was noticed by the patient. Constant ptosis occurs in myotonic dystrophy, mitochondrial cytopathies, oculopharyngeal dystrophy and several congenital muscle syndromes. Weakness of extraocular muscles may cause diplopia, although in mitochondrial disorders diplopia is uncommon despite restricted eye movements because of the chronicity of the symptoms (Petty et al., 1986). Diplopia rarely occurs in oculopharyngeal dystrophy and myotonic dystrophy. Variable ptosis and diplopia are pathognomonic of myasthenia gravis. Thyroid ophthalmopathy can produce ptosis, although it is more commonly causes lid retraction; diplopia may be constant or fluctuating in this disorder.

Facial weakness in muscle disease is usually bilateral and relatively symmetric; consequently, subtle facial weakness may be overlooked until it becomes severe. Frequently, patients are asymptomatic even with marked

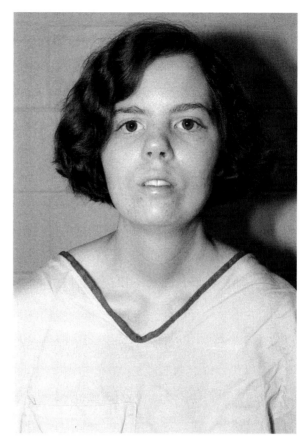

Fig. 17.1. Transverse smile in facioscapulohumeral muscular dystrophy.

objective weakness. Questioning may elicit a history of having a 'funny smile' (Fig. 17.1), or difficulty blowing-up balloons, whistling, drinking through a straw and clearing food caught between the lips and gums. Severe facial weakness may also cause dysarthria.

Limb muscles

Common complaints associated with limb weakness have already been discussed. Various myopathies produce isolated or restricted limb involvement that leads to specific complaints and symptoms. Preferential quadriceps weakness, for example, occurs in disorders such as inclusion body myositis and X-linked myopathy with excessive autophagy. Such patients complain of falls caused by their 'knees giving out', and difficulties going down stairs. Scapular stabilizer muscles, by definition, are affected early in FSH and scapuloperoneal syndromes. These patients often relate a history of prominent scapulae and 'sloped-shoulders' noticed by classmates during gym class or sporting events at school (Fig. 17.2). Some are criticized for their 'poor posture'. Others are noticed to have these

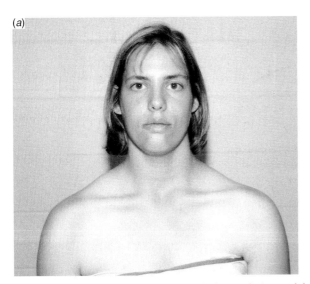

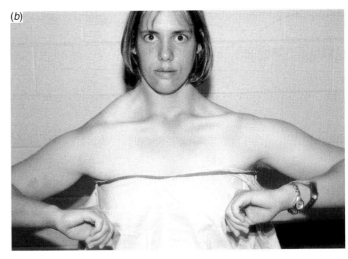

Fig. 17.2. Shoulder and pectoral findings in facioscapulohumeral muscular dystrophy.

features while trying on clothes or during a medical examination. Frequently, children or teenagers note difficulty doing activities involving the shoulders that are performed easily by peers, such as climbing trees or a rope, throwing a ball or swinging a golf club. Another example of selective muscle involvement is seen in inclusion body myositis, where wrist and finger flexor muscles can be preferentially affected (Sekul et al., 1997). These patients complain of difficulty lifting objects and doing fine manipulations, such as picking up coins, winding their wrist-watch, or doing crafts and hobbies.

Respiratory muscles

Mild respiratory muscle weakness is usually asymptomatic. The earliest symptoms of respiratory failure are typically caused not by hypoxia but rather by retention of carbon dioxide. This causes nightmares, frequent needs to be turned at night, early morning headache and excessive daytime sleepiness. With increased severity, patients complain of shortness of breath on exertion and orthopnoea. Respiratory insufficiency typically occurs in the later stages of disorders causing progressive weakness, such as Duchenne dystrophy (Emery, 1987). Certain disorders, however, such as acid maltase deficiency, myasthenia gravis (rarely), critical illness myopathy and carnitine palmitoyltransferase deficiency may present with respiratory failure (Trend et al., 1985; Howard et al., 1993; Zierz, 1994).

Pain

Muscle pain is the most common muscle complaint encountered by clinicians. In some population studies, up to 10% of individuals complained of diffuse muscle dis-

comfort. Muscle pain is a nonspecific symptom that can arise from a variety of general medical, rheumatological, orthopaedic, neurological and psychiatric conditions. Even intense muscle pain may be unrelated to primary muscle disease, originating instead from a disorder of peripheral nerves, anterior horn cells, or the central nervous system (CNS). In fact, evaluation of patients with muscle pain *alone* (i.e. without accompanying weakness) usually does not reveal a muscle disease in the usual sense (Mills and Edwards, 1983); many of these patients are diagnosed with fibromyalgia. Muscle pain is also often a major feature of the chronic fatigue syndrome, in which in the majority of patients there is no evidence of muscle pathology (Hilton-Jones, 1994; Kissel and Miller, 1999). Part of the difficulty in evaluating muscle pain relates to confusion in the patients' descriptions of their symptoms. Patients frequently use the word 'pain' to refer to a number of abnormal sensations, including aching, stiffness, numbness, burning, restlessness and swelling. Patients with cramping and contractures (see below) will also usually complain of muscle pain.

The most common muscle pain is a deep discomfort, often described as 'burning' or 'dull ache'. This pain can be either focal and localized to an individual muscle or group of muscles or widespread and generalized (Table 17.3). Muscle conditions that cause focal pain usually involve local trauma, an infiltrating process (such as tumour or sarcoidosis), vascular disorders (either arterial ischaemia or venous thrombophlebitis) or a local bacterial or parasitic infection. Diffuse myalgia is most common after viral infection but also occurs in polymyositis and dermatomyositis (but usually only when the onset is acute or subacute), toxic or infectious myopathies and a few rare

Table 17.3. *Muscle disorders causing localized or diffuse myalgia*

Myalgia	Disorders
Localized myalgia	Postexercise myalgia
	Focal pressure necrosis
	Trauma
	Focal infiltrating processes: tumour; sarcoidosis, focal myositis
	Localized infections (bacterial, parasitic)
	Vascular occlusion: arterial ischaemia (thrombotic or embolic), venous occlusion
	Referred 'muscle' pain from neuropathic, orthopaedic rheumatological causes
Generalized myalgia	Infectious myalgia (especially viral): diffuse parasitic or bacterial infections
	Inflammatory muscle disease (polymyositis, dermatomyositis)
	Eosinophilia-myalgia syndrome
	Toxic myopathies associated with drugs (e.g. lovastatin, chloroquine)
	Hypothyroidism
	Mitochondrial myopathies
	Myoadenylate deaminase deficiency (association with myalgia controversial)
	Rare myopathies: paraspinal vacuolar myopathies with myalgia, myalgia with tubular aggregates, X-linked myalgia and cramps (Becker dystrophy variant)
	Polymyalgia rheumatica
	Fibromyalgia

Table 17.4. *Muscle disorders associated with contractures*

Myopathies associated with glycolytic/glycogenolytic enzyme defects
    Phosphorylase deficiency (McArdle's disease)
    Phosphofructokinase deficiency
    Phosphoglycerate kinase deficiency
    Phosphoglycerate mutase deficiency
    Lactate dehydrogenase deficiency
    Debrancher enzyme deficiency
Paramyotonia congenita
Hypothyroid myopathy with myoedema
Rippling muscle syndrome
Brody's disease

endocrine myopathies. In most of these disorders, pain is accompanied by weakness, which can be mild to devastating. Diffuse myalgia without weakness is seen in polymyalgia rheumatica and fibromyalgia. It is also useful to distinguish between pain present at rest (most of the conditions listed in Table 17.3) and that which comes on only during exercise, which usually suggests one of the metabolic myopathies. Numerous drugs may also cause a painful myopathy (Argov and Mastaglia, 1994). The origin of muscle pain in most conditions is uncertain (for a review, see Chapter 34).

Contractures

The term contracture is used to refer to two different phenomena. In many chronic neuromuscular disorders, there is shortening of muscles and an inability to stretch the muscle passively to its proper length because of fibrosis. Such fixed contractures, which are in themselves painless, are rarely the presenting complaint in patients with muscle disease since they are usually a late feature of most diseases. In a few disorders, such as Emery–Dreifuss dystrophy (Fig. 17.3), Bethlem myopathy and the rigid spine syndrome, contractures may be an early and striking feature affecting both limbs and spine. The term contracture is also used to describe sustained, electrically silent, muscle contractions that produce hard nodules in the muscle and may persist for hours, in severe cases leading to myoglobinuria. Such contractures are painful, usually occur with exercise and are the hallmark of the glycolytic metabolic myopathies and a few other muscle disorders (Table 17.4). The pathogenesis of contractures in these conditions is poorly understood, although they probably result from a disturbance of high-energy metabolic pathways.

Cramps

Cramping is also accompanied by intense muscle pain and can produce a palpable mass in the muscle. Unlike contractures, cramps may occur at rest, are explosive in onset and short in duration and may be relieved by passive stretching of the muscle. Electromyographic (EMG) study of a cramp reveals high-frequency motor unit discharges similar to a maximal contraction (Layzer, 1994). Cramps, particularly those in the gastrocnemius muscle, occur in all normal individuals. Although the aetiology of cramps is uncertain, evidence suggests they are originate in the intramuscular motor nerve terminals (Auger, 1994). As such, widespread cramps usually indicate neurogenic disease (e.g. amyotrophic lateral sclerosis, peripheral neuropathy) or metabolic disorders that alter the nerve

(a)

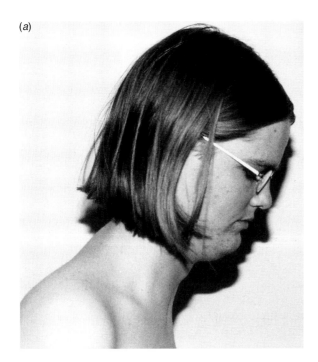

(b)

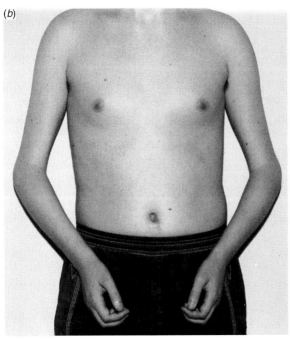

(c)

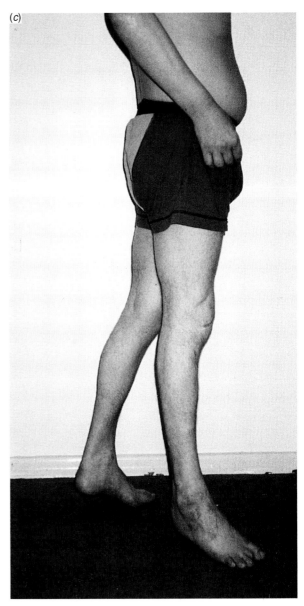

Fig. 17.3. Contractures in Emery–Dreifuss muscular dystrophy. Note limited neck flexion (a), inability to extend elbows fully (b) and Achilles tendon contractures (c), causing toe-walking.

microenvironment (e.g. hypothyroidism, dehydration and uraemia) (Table 17.5).

Stiffness and other muscle hyperactivity states

'Stiffness' is another word often used by patients to describe a number of different phenomena, some of which may be painful. Most commonly, the term is used to describe muscle that feels tight, is resistant to passive stretch and does not relax normally. Stiffness can arise from a wide range of neurological disorders affecting every part of the neuraxis, as well as medical conditions that cause metabolic derangements which disrupt muscle relaxation (Auger, 1994). Although stiffness and pain frequently overlap, many patients with excessive stiffness

Table 17.5. Conditions associated with cramps

Type of cramps	Conditions
Idiopathic (normal cramps)	Exertional and postexertional cramps
	Nocturnal leg cramps
Neurogenic cramps	Motor neuron disease
	Peripheral neuropathies
	Radiculopathies
Cramps owing to altered neuronal environment	Pregnancy
	Metabolic disorders: renal failure; hepatic failure, hypothyroidism, adrenal insufficiency
	Electrolyte disturbances/volume depletion

Table 17.6. Muscle disorders associated with muscle stiffness

Hypothyroidism
Myotonic disorders
Myotonic dystrophy
Myotonia congenita
Proximal myotonic myopathy
Hyperkalaemic periodic paralysis
Paramyotonia congenita
Brody's disease
Polymyalgia rheumatica
Fibromyalgia

related to central mechanisms (e.g. spasticity or rigidity) do not have significant pain. Table 17.6 lists the muscle disorders associated with prominent stiffness.

Myotonia is the most common muscle phenomenon that results in stiffness. It is caused by recurrent depolarization of the muscle membrane, characterized on electrophysiological studies by waxing and waning rhythmical discharges. Patients experience stiffness and slowed relaxation, most evident after voluntary contraction and percussion of the muscle. Myotonia is seen in four main conditions. In myotonic dystrophy, patients complain of difficulty releasing objects after a firm grasp, or of stiffness in the hands and forearms (Harper, 1989). Myotonia may also affect tongue movements and chewing, and some patients notice dysphagia because of myotonia in the upper oesophagus. Patients usually complain more of weakness than myotonia. Patients with myotonic dystrophy may be asymptomatic, even when myotonia is evident on examination. Proximal myotonic myopathy is characterized, as the name suggests, by predominantly proximal

weakness and myotonia. In these patients, the myotonia is frequently subclinical, and often detectable only with EMG, although patients frequently complain of stiffness and aching in affected muscles. In myotonia congenita, a chloride channelopathy, there is severe generalized myotonia, which is usually worse after rest and on initiation of movement (Hudson et al., 1995). A severe episode of myotonia may be followed by transient weakness of the affected muscles. Facial muscles can be involved, resulting in a blepharospasm-like appearance after forceful eye closure. In the sodium channelopathies (paramyotonia congenita and hyperkalaemic periodic paralysis), myotonia may be exacerbated by continued activity (paradoxical myotonia), whereas in the other conditions myotonia lessens with sustained action. It may also be markedly exacerbated by cold. The facial, forearm and hand muscles tend to be the most affected (Hudson et al., 1995).

Some rare muscle disorders can also be associated with muscle stiffness. Brody's syndrome is caused by a deficiency of sarcoplasmic reticulum calcium-ATPase, which causes exercised-induced stiffness and cramping, and slowed muscle relaxation (Hiel et al., 1996). Rippling muscle syndrome is sporadic or dominantly inherited. Patients complain of stiffness; on examination, stretching or percussion of muscle sets off waves of rippling (Ricker et al., 1989).

Two neurogenic disorders with prominent muscle overactivity are *neuromyotonia* and *stiff-person syndrome*. Neuromyotonia, characterized by stiffness, cramps, myokymia, increased sweating and occasionally sensory symptoms, may be associated with a variety of inherited and acquired disorders. Autoimmunity is involved in at least some acquired disease (Shillito et al., 1995; Hart and Newsom-Davis, 1996). In stiff-person syndrome, the axial and then limb muscles develop severe painful spasms and stiffness giving rise to spinal deformity and gait disturbance. Most cases are associated with antibodies to glutamic acid decarboxylase, an enzyme crucial in inhibitory GABAergic pathways (Kissel and Elble, 1998).

Fatigue

Fatigue refers to a sense of tiredness, lack of energy and a tendency to avoid physical (and often mental) activities because of exhaustion (Krupp and Pollina, 1996). Fatigue is a multifactorial phenomenon, depending upon the individual's emotional state, sleep habits, cardiopulmonary status, conditioning, and overall medical status (Layzer, 1994; Krupp and Pollina, 1996). Although some myopathies (most notably mitochondrial disorders, some metabolic myopathies and myotonic dystrophy), and neuromuscular junction disorders can be associated with significant fatigue, fatigue *in isolation* almost never indicates a

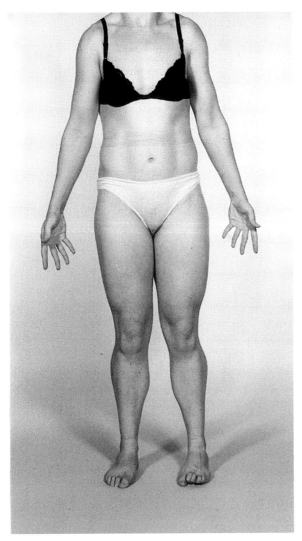

Fig. 17.4. Generalized muscle enlargement in myotonia congenita.

Table 17.7. Muscle disorders associated with muscle enlargement

Muscular dystrophies
   Duchenne/Becker
   Manifesting carriers of Duchenne
   Limb girdle dystrophies
Myotonia congenita
Neuromyotonia
Debrancher enzyme deficiency
Cysticercosis

Muscle wasting and enlargement

Patients with myopathic disorders rarely complain of muscle wasting as their *primary* complaint. Unlike neurogenic disease, where the degree of wasting often parallels weakness, wasting may be slight or absent in myopathies, even with severe weakness. Early wasting is often difficult for the patient (or examiner) to see, particularly if the patient is obese. In some diseases, wasting may be focal and affects only certain muscles. This can result in an unusual appearance that may bring the patient to medical attention; the marked gastrocnemius atrophy seen in some of the distal myopathies (e.g. Miyoshi myopathy) is an example. In other disorders, wasting is evident only as the disease progresses and weakness becomes severe.

Muscle enlargement, either focal or generalized, is seen in a number of disorders (Table 17.7). True hypertrophy, which involves enlargement of muscle fibres as a result of repetitive activity, is seen in some cases of myotonia congenita (Fig. 17.4) and neuromyotonia. In other instances, enlargement is better termed pseudo-hypertrophy and results from replacement of damaged muscle by fat and connective tissue. The pattern of muscle enlargement can help to suggest the diagnosis; the calf enlargement seen in boys with dystrophin-related dystrophies being the best example.

Myoglobinuria

Any disorder that disrupts muscle membranes may allow release of myoglobin into the blood (myoglobinaemia) and then excretion in urine (myoglobinuria) (Rowland and Penn, 1972; Penn, 1994). Patients typically notice discoloration of the urine ranging from light-brown to dark brown-black; they describe the urine as dark, smoky, rusty or like Coca-Cola or whisky. Such discoloration must be distinguished from other causes of pigmenturia, including drugs, haemolysis and porphyria (Hilton-Jones et al., 1995). Myoglobinuria, which may cause renal failure from

primary myopathy. However, many patients with muscle disease and weakness complain of fatigue and decreased endurance, since they must perform routine activities with less muscle (the so-called overuse syndrome).

In patients complaining of fatigue and decreased endurance, it is important to determine exactly why certain activities cannot be performed, particularly in relation to other complaints. Patients often use the term weakness when trying to describe fatigue. For example, many fatigued patients will complain of inability to perform some routine activity, such as going up a flight of stairs or walking one block, because of weakness when in reality they are simply too fatigued and exhausted and could accomplish the activity if strength alone were the issue.

Table 17.8. Causes of myoglobinuria

Prolonged, intensive exercise
Metabolic myopathies
    Glycogenoses (e.g. myophosphorylase deficiency)
    Lipid disorders (e.g. carnitine palmitoyltransferase deficiency)
    Malignant hyperthermia
Muscular dystrophies (e.g. Duchenne and Becker)
Dermatomyositis and polymyositis
Viral and bacterial infections
Ischaemia and trauma (e.g. crush or compression injuries,
    electric shock, arterial insufficiency)
Drugs and toxins: alcohol; bacterial toxins, carbon monoxide,
    snake venom, opiates, clofibrate
Neuroleptic malignant syndrome
Severe metabolic disturbances
Fever and heat stroke
Idiopathic causes

Table 17.9. Myopathies with cardiac involvement

Effects	Myopathies
Conduction system defects and arrhythmias	Myotonic dystrophy
	Emery–Dreifuss muscular dystrophy
	Mitochondrial cytopathies (especially Kearns–Sayre syndrome)
	Periodic paralysis (particularly Andersen's syndrome)
Cardiomyopathy	Duchenne and Becker muscular dystrophy
	Limb–girdle muscular dystrophy (rare)
	Emery–Dreifuss syndrome (late)
	Dermatomyositis
	Infantile acid maltase deficiency
	Disorders of lipid metabolism
	Debranching enzyme deficiency
	Mitochondrial cytopathies
	Some endocrine myopathies

acute tubular necrosis, is always paralleled by markedly increased serum CK. Some common causes of myoglobinuria are listed in Table 17.8.

Systemic symptoms

Patients with myopathic complaints frequently will have symptoms related to other organ systems that can be very helpful in suggesting the type of muscle disease present. Other patients may present with chief complaints unrelated to skeletal muscle per se. The review of systems is often neglected in the history. Although frequently tedious, an accurate review of systems allows for the early identification of symptoms that suggest a myopathy and yet may have been overlooked by the patient or that point towards a disease that involves systems other than muscle. Significant symptoms must be pursued by a review of old records or by discussions with the patient's primary care physician or other involved specialists. The following symptoms are discussed according to organ-system involvement.

Heart

Cardiac involvement in myopathies is common (Table 17.9) and may cause significant morbidity and mortality. It can assume many forms and involve either the contractile or conduction systems, producing symptoms of cardiac failure or arrhythmias, respectively. It can occasionally be difficult to distinguish respiratory symptoms caused by cardiac failure from those resulting from primary respiratory failure, and consultation with medical specialists is often indicated. It is crucial to identify cardiac involvement early since it may be amenable to therapy.

Liver

In both childhood and adult debranching enzyme deficiency, hepatomegaly may cause symptomatic protrusion of the abdomen. In branching enzyme deficiency, hepatomegaly is associated with ascites; without liver transplantation death ensues from hepatic failure. Neonatal and childhood liver involvement is common in disorders of carnitine metabolism and fatty acid β-oxidation and may be seen in the mitochondrial cytopathies.

Central nervous system

Mitochondrial cytopathies are frequently associated with CNS symptoms and signs. CNS involvement, including ocular symptoms, may even be the presenting feature of these disorders (Table 17.10). Some CNS involvement also occurs in dystrophinopathies, where the intelligence quotient (IQ) of patients averages lower than controls. This difference is often not apparent in individual patients and seldom helps in making a diagnosis. In contrast, the lower IQ and personality differences seen in myotonic dystrophy are usually more apparent; patients with congenital myotonic dystrophy are severely mentally handicapped. A lower than average IQ is also a feature of some congenital myopathies. An interesting example of CNS involvement

Table 17.10. Central nervous system and ocular involvement in respiratory chain (mitochondrial) disorders

Type of involvement	Symptoms
Intermittent or episodic involvement	Stroke-like episodes, headache, myoclonus, epilepsy
Persistent involvement	Deafness, ataxia, movement disorders, encephalopathy, dementia, dysphagia
Ocular findings	Pigmentary retinopathy, optic atrophy, progressive external ophthalmoplegia

Table 17.11. Conditions that may affect both skeletal muscle and peripheral nerve

Alcohol abuse
Amyloidosis (familial or acquired)
Chronic renal failure
Collagen vascular disorders
    Rheumatoid arthritis
    Systemic lupus erythematosus
    Systemic vasculitis
    Primary or secondary vasculitides
Drugs (e.g. vincristine, gold)
Endocrine disorders (e.g. acromegaly, hypothyroidism)
HIV infection
Malnutrition
Mitochondrial cytopathies
Sarcoidosis

with muscle disease occurs in congenital muscular dystrophy with laminin α_2-chain deficiency, where white matter hypomyelination is seen by magnetic resonance imaging (MRI), but patients rarely have intellectual impairment (Tsao et al., 1998; Tsao and Mendell, 1999).

Peripheral nervous system

As already discussed, patients often use words like deadness or numbness to describe true muscle weakness. Occasionally, patients may even say that touching the affected extremity does not 'feel' normal. There are, however, many disorders that may involve both muscle and peripheral nerve and, therefore, produce symptoms referable to both systems (Table 17.11). In these patients, it is important not to misinterpret the sensory complaints as indicating involvement of only the peripheral nervous system.

Table 17.12. Endocrinopathies causing myopathy

Hypothyroidism
Hyperthyroidism
Graves' ophthalmopathy
Cushing's syndrome
Addison's disease
Hyperparathyroidism
Hypoparathyroidism
Acromegaly
Hypopituitarism
Primary hyperaldosteronism
Phaeochromocytoma

Eyes

Ptosis and altered ocular motility are the most common ocular symptoms related to muscle disease (as discussed above). Other ocular problems, however, may also be associated with myopathies. Pigmentary retinopathy, optic atrophy or both may occur with mitochondrial disorders, but symptomatic visual impairment is unusual (Mullie et al., 1985). Eye involvement with severe visual failure may be seen in some congenital muscular dystrophies.

Endocrine system

Although most endocrinopathies can, if severe enough, produce a myopathy (Table 17.12), the almost universal availability of rapid biochemical screening for most hormones has rendered clinically significant endocrine myopathies very uncommon (Kissel and Mendell, 1992). It is still important, however, to question patients about symptoms that may be related to an underlying endocrinological disorder. Myasthenia gravis is associated with an increased incidence of thyroid dysfunction (and vice versa), which may exacerbate the myasthenia. Mitochondrial cytopathies have been linked with several endocrine disorders, including diabetes mellitus. A specific form of periodic paralysis is linked to hyperthyroidism.

Kidneys

Myoglobinuria as a cause of renal damage has already been discussed. Chronic renal failure from any cause, along with dialysis and subsequent renal tubular acidosis, can cause myopathy through several mechanisms (Kissel and Mendell, 1992).

Gastrointestinal system

Many neuromuscular disorders affect the gastrointestinal tract; conversely, a number of bowel disorders cause myopathy. The most common gastrointestinal-related symptom in myopathic patients is dysphagia, which usually relates to weakness of the pharyngeal muscles and upper third of the oesophagus. Dysphagia is particularly prominent in myotonic dystrophy, oculopharyngeal dystrophy, inclusion body myositis and myasthenia gravis. Gastric stasis and intestinal dysmotility causing bowel pseudo-obstruction, and constipation may result from involvement of smooth muscle, as in Duchenne dystrophy. More frequently, constipation can arise from simple immobility resulting from generalized weakness. In myotonic dystrophy, symptoms similar to irritable bowel syndrome, and fecal soiling in childhood, are common. In the rare MNGIE syndrome (mitochondrial myopathy, peripheral neuropathy, gastrointestinal disease and encephalopathy), nausea, vomiting and diarrhoea are caused by gut dysmotility (Hirano et al., 1994).

Skin

The muscle disease most commonly associated with skin involvement is dermatomyositis. The 'classic' heliotrope discoloration of the eyelids is much less frequent than erythema of the face and upper chest (sun-exposed areas) and of the hands, particularly over the knuckles. Raynaud's phenomenon can also occur in this disorder. Various types of skin rash can result from underlying vasculitis, which may also involve muscle. Such rashes occasionally bring patients to medical attention before weakness is symptomatic. Other rare cutaneous manifestations of myopathy include lipomatosis, a feature of some mitochondrial disorders, and jaundice, which is seen in approximately 25% of those with phosphofructokinase deficiency.

Past medical history

The past medical history should focus predominantly on four key areas. First and most importantly, the presence of any underlying illnesses associated with muscle involvement needs to be identified. These disorders include the various connective tissue disorders, endocrine disturbances, and renal or hepatic failure. Second, any disorder associated with peripheral neuropathy or other symptoms that may be confused with a myopathy must be identified (e.g. diabetes mellitus). Similarly, it is crucial to recognize prior surgery (such as cervical or lumbar laminectomies, thoracic outlet surgery, carpal tunnel release) that may affect the neurological history or examination and the patient's functional status. A third key area concerns anaesthetic exposure. Many myopathies cause subclinical respiratory muscle involvement that is asymptomatic until the patient is stressed with general anaesthesia. A history of being 'difficult to wake up' or needing prolonged

Table 17.13. Drugs associated with myopathy

	Drugs
Often associated with pain	Amiodarone, cimetidine, clofibrate, cyclosporin (cyclosporine), E-aminocaproic acid (EACA), emetine, gemfibrozil, gold, heroin, labetalol, lovastatin, nifedipine, D-penicillamine, procainamide, salbutamol, L-tryptophan, vincristine, zidovudine
Usually painless	Chloroquine, colchicine, corticosteroids, hypokalaemia-inducing drugs (e.g. diuretics), perhexiline

assisted ventilation after general anaesthesia can be important clues to the presence of an underlying muscle disorder. Such a history is often obtained from patients with myotonic dystrophy, who also may give a history of peri- or postoperative cardiac arrhythmias. Patients with subclinical myasthenia gravis also may present with acute deterioration following either anaesthetic agents or neuromuscular blockers. A history of malignant hyperthermia with general anaesthesia is also a 'red flag' for an occult myopathy. Although malignant hyperthermia frequently occurs in isolation or in association with central core disease, anaesthesia-induced hyperthermic reactions may also occur in patients with Duchenne or Becker muscular dystrophy.

A final important area in the history relates to past and current medication use and toxin exposure. The examiner must identify all legal or illicit medications the patient is taking, over-the-counter products as well as all nutritional or vitamin supplements and even homoeopathic remedies. The common pharmacological agents associated with myopathy are listed in Table 17.13.

Family history

The family history is of obvious importance in patients with suspected muscle disease, but obtaining an accurate family history can sometimes require a great deal of effort by the examiner. A common mistake is asking vague general questions concerning whether any family members have a similar disease as the patient, an approach that is often unproductive. Rather, it is essential to ask specifically about the health, functional status and associated medical conditions of each family member in the nuclear group (parents, siblings and children).

Questions addressed to specific issues, such as the need for canes or wheelchairs, functional limitations and postural or skeletal deformities are often more rewarding than questions about muscle diseases. Frequently, family members have been diagnosed with 'arthritis' or various orthopaedic disorders when a muscle disorder was actually present. The examiner also must address the fact that family members may be very reluctant to discuss the possibility of a genetic disorder and even try to deceive family members and physicians. In some families, particularly those with certain autosomal dominant disorders (e.g. FSH dystrophy), phenotypic variability may be such that even affected parents can be asymptomatic. This phenomenon is typical in conditions such as myotonic dystrophy, which show true genetic anticipation. If an inherited disorder is being considered and the parents are living, they should be examined even if asymptomatic.

Social history

Relatively few aspects of the social history are pertinent to the patient with suspected myopathy. Information about alcohol consumption and tobacco use is of obvious importance, although 'alcoholic myopathy' is an uncommon and controversial entity. Information on recreational drug exposure and sexual preference are important clues to possible muscle disease related to human immunodeficiency virus (HIV). Even initial denial of such risk factors should not be accepted without question in the appropriate clinical situation.

Physical examination

The examination of the patient with a suspected muscle disorder flows naturally from, and is directed by, information gleaned from the history. Given the associations between myopathies and general medical disorders, the examination cannot be confined to assessment of the muscles alone but rather must encompass a general examination. Systems suspected to be involved because of information obtained in the history of the present illness or review of systems must receive special attention. Examination of the cardiovascular and pulmonary systems is always indicated. The goal is to identify a systemic disorder that may be associated with myopathy.

A neurological examination to exclude possible central or peripheral nervous system disorders that might explain the patient's symptoms should be performed in all patients. A more detailed CNS examination is essential in patients suspected of having a mitochondrial cytopathy

(Table 17.10). The retinopathy in these disorders is mainly peripheral and, therefore, it may be necessary to dilate the pupils to detect it. Hearing loss may be mild and easily overlooked. Examination of the peripheral nervous system, including sensory examination, is also vital, not only to exclude neurogenic disorders from the differential diagnosis but also because a number of conditions can involve both nerves and muscle (Table 17.11). The following section will focus on the muscle examination but will not review basic techniques, which should be familiar to all clinicians.

Muscle examination

All too often, the muscle assessment is restricted to 'pushing and pulling' on muscles to assess strength, with little attention paid to other aspects of the examination. A complete skeletal muscle examination includes the classic components of inspection, palpation, and percussion.

Inspection and palpation

The muscle examination should always begin with an adequate inspection of the undressed and gowned patient. The muscles under inspection should be completely relaxed, so that patient efforts to support the limb do not result in subtle voluntary contractions that may be misinterpreted as fasciculations. Any wasting or hypertrophy and any involuntary movements (e.g. fasciculation, rippling, myokymia) should be noted, in addition to any skeletal abnormalities, such as pectus excavatum, kyphoscoliosis or scapular winging. Inspection is best performed by region, including the individual limbs and the entire back or trunk. Such an approach helps to identify patterns of muscle and orthopaedic findings that can be useful diagnostically, such as the shoulder and pectoral findings in FSH dystrophy (Fig. 17.2). Palpating the muscles is appropriate during this phase of the examination. Palpation may help to detect subtle atrophy not readily apparent on inspection. Rarely, a mass or nodule can be palpated, as with an abscess or diabetic muscle infarction. Palpation also permits assessment of muscle texture; for example, the doughy feel of the gastrocnemius in patients with Duchenne dystrophy or the fibrotic, ropey, feel of muscles replaced by connective tissue and fat in patients with various dystrophies can be appreciated.

Strength assessment

Strength assessment is clearly the most important aspect of the muscle examination. In general, groups of muscles having specific actions on a joint should be tested rather than individual muscles (Table 17.14). With rare exceptions,

Table 17.14. Muscles groups to be tested in all patients with muscle disease

Groups	Assessment
Cranial nerve innervated muscles	Eyelid elevation
	Extraocular muscle function
	Facial muscle strength
	Palate movement and speech
	Neck flexion/extension, and rotational strength
	Shoulder shrugging
	Tongue protrusion and strength
Limbs and trunk	Scapula stabilizers
	Shoulder abductors and adductors
	Elbow flexors and extensors
	Wrist flexors and extensors
	Finger flexors, extensors, and abductors
	Grip strength
	Hip flexors and extensors
	Knee flexors and extensors
	Ankle dorsiflexors and everters
	Ankle inverters and plantar flexors
	Trunk and abdominal muscles performing sit up
Respiratory muscles	Diaphragm movement on inspiration
	Seconds patient can count out on single inspiration

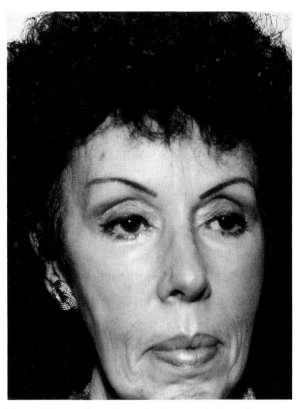

Fig. 17.5. Temporal muscle wasting in myotonic dystrophy.

it is important that a standard group of muscles be tested in every patient, with more specific testing performed as indicated by the presenting symptoms. For example, in patients with mainly proximal involvement, the examiner should assess other shoulder muscles, such as the supra- and infraspinatus, as well as other muscles around the hips, such as the hip abductors, adductors and internal and external rotators. If there is evidence of mainly distal weakness, other distal functions should be examined, such as the long finger flexors and extensors, intrinsic hand muscles, ankle eversion and inversion and the small muscles of the feet. Selective involvement of specific muscles in the same anatomical area is typical for many muscular dystrophies. In FSH dystrophy, for example, the biceps and triceps are significantly affected but the deltoids are relatively spared. No aspect of the muscle examination is more important in providing clues to the diagnosis than the pattern of muscle weakness. In this regard, it is convenient to consider separately muscles innervated by the cranial nerves, limb and trunk muscles, and the respiratory muscles, since different methods are involved in testing these areas.

Cranial nerve innervated muscle

Mild ptosis and ophthalmoplegia may be subtle and difficult to detect on examination. Patients with significant ptosis may tilt their head backwards, raise their eyebrows or wrinkle their foreheads in an attempt to look out from under ptotic lids (referred to as 'overactivity of frontalis'). When assessing ptosis and eye movement, it is crucial to check for fatigability in addition to weakness and restriction of movement. Wasting and atrophy of the temporalis muscle is characteristic of myotonic dystrophy (Fig. 17.5), although it may occur in other disorders. The masseters are best tested by having the patient clench their teeth and move the jaw from side to side while the masseter is palpated. The most common disorder resulting in masseter weakness is myasthenia gravis.

Mild symmetric facial weakness can also be difficult to detect. Although patients often have a somewhat blank, drooped, 'myopathic' expression, this may easily be overlooked on cursory examination, particularly if it is the examiner's first encounter with the patient. Asking the patient to smile broadly, show their teeth, wrinkle their forehead, blow a kiss and whistle may bring out the abnormalities. One sensitive test is to ask the patient to close their

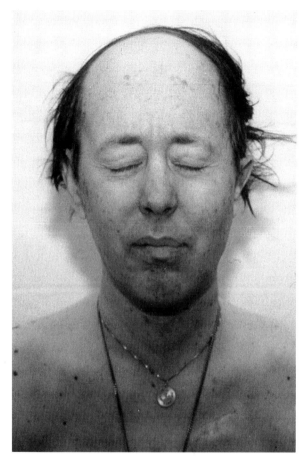

Fig. 17.6. Facial diplegia: failure to bury eyelashes with eye closure.

Table 17.15. Medical Research Council grading scale for muscle testing

Grade	Muscle response
0	No contraction
1	Flicker of contraction
2	Active movement, with gravity eliminated
3	Active movement against gravity
4−	Active movement against slight resistance
4	Active movement against moderate resistance
4+	Active movement against strong resistance
5	Normal power

and sideways against a tongue-blade is another way to assess tongue strength. Swallowing can be assessed by observing the patient eat and drink. The time taken to swallow a certain fluid volume, or the number of swallows taken, may be recorded as an objective measure of swallowing.

Many muscle disorders cause weakness of the neck flexors and extensors. These muscles can be tested in the supine and prone positions, respectively, so that their actions against gravity can be determined. Neck flexor weakness with relatively preserved extensor strength can be seen in many conditions and is common in disorders such as myotonic dystrophy, myasthenia gravis and the inflammatory myopathies. Preferential involvement of the neck extensors is much less common but may be seen in myasthenia gravis, poly- or dermatomyositis, myotonic dystrophy and the so-called dropped head syndrome (Suarez and Kelly, 1992).

Limb and trunk muscles

Table 17.14 lists muscle groups that should be tested in all patients presenting with a suspected muscle problem. The findings on this basic screening, as well as the patient's specific symptoms, will indicate if other limb muscles should be tested. Although the basic procedure of manual muscle testing is familiar to all clinicians, several aspects deserve comment. The first point when assessing strength is that it is crucial to have the patient in the appropriate position for testing each muscle, both to assess function against gravity and to provide the optimum opportunity to detect subtle weakness. Hip abductors, for example, should never be tested in the seated position; rather the patient should be placed on their side. Most clinicians employ the positions, methods and 5-point grading scale outlined in the *Aids to the Examination of the Peripheral Nervous System* by the Medical Research Council (1986) (Table 17.15). Although

eyes tightly: failure to bury the eyelashes completely indicates weakness (Fig. 17.6). Another method is to try to force the eyelids open with the thumbs, although this is often poorly tolerated. Pursing the lips can be helpful in patients with FSH dystrophy, where involvement is often asymmetric, particularly in the orbicularis oris muscle, resulting in an odd, twisted smile with dimpling at the corner of the mouth and a depressed and 'flat' appearance to the patient's face. When asked to whistle or blow a kiss, the lips frequently form a characteristic transverse or horizontal configuration (Fig. 17.1). Significant facial weakness also results in hollow sounding speech, and if the lips are affected, difficulty pronouncing consonants such as b, f, m and p.

Speech is an excellent method for assessing tongue and palate strength. Palatal weakness produces speech that is nasal and 'airy', with difficulty pronouncing sounds such as k and the hard g. In contrast, tongue weakness produces thick, slurred speech and difficulty with sounds such as d, l, n and t. Having the patient protrude the tongue and push forward there may be considerable inter- and intraobserver variability with this grading scale, clinical trials have shown that manual testing can be accurate and reproducible if performed by experienced evaluators (Tawil et al., 1994). Clinicians familiar with this scheme who use it routinely find it invaluable in documenting the status of their patients. Various computerized systems have been developed, most of which employ strain gauge tensiometers that record the maximal force a muscle can generate and then compare the values with those of age- and sex-matched controls (Munsat, 1989; Personius et al., 1994). These systems are widely used in clinical trials but are not available to most clinicians for routine clinical use.

A second major point concerning muscle testing is that accurate strength determinations cannot be made in patients who do not give a maximal effort or who are in significant pain. Frequently, joint pain results in a rapid collapse of the extremity during manual muscle testing that is misinterpreted as weakness. Patients with psychogenic or functional 'weakness' may also give-way suddenly when tested. These patients often adjust the resistance they offer to match the force applied by the examiner. Patients with genuine weakness rarely 'give-way' in this fashion; rather, they offer resistance that, although not normal, is uniform through the range of motion.

The final, and perhaps most important, point concerning manual muscle testing is that it represents only part of the strength assessment and should *never* be interpreted in isolation. Rather, the results of manual muscle testing must always be assessed in conjunction with simple bedside functional tests, which, although not truly quantitative, nevertheless give a clearer picture of the patient's abilities and how they are compromised by weakness. Such functional analyses are also informative in younger children, where detailed manual muscle testing is usually not feasible. Table 17.16 lists the most useful functional tests performed in the clinic. Many experienced clinicians feel that this type of functional testing is superior to manual muscle testing in determining whether a patient's weakness is improving or worsening and is less subject to interobserver variability (Brooke, 1986). A patient with mild lower limb weakness, for example, may be able to walk normally and get up from a chair without pushing with the arms but may not be able to rise from a squat. The subsequent ability to rise from a squat provides convincing evidence that improvement has occurred. Conversely, an inability to arise from a chair as well as rise from a squat would indicate that there has likely been deterioration.

Functional testing is also the best way to assess axial strength and muscle fatigability. Weakness of truncal muscles may be evident when the patient tries to sit up

Table 17.16. Bedside functional motor tests

Lying supine on examining table and lifting head
Lying supine on examining table and lifting lower limb straight up; measure heel–couch distance
Sitting up from lying
Standing up from 'standard' chair – with or without arm assist
Rising from a squat
Getting up from a cross-legged position on the floor
Time to walk a specific distance
Ability to run
Ability to stand, hop on either foot
Ability to walk on heels and toes
Ability to step up to standard 8 inch (20 cm) step, beginning with either foot
Ability to climb steps in 'child' or 'adult' fashion
Raising arms over the head, either with forward flexion or abduction

from lying. With greater weakness there may be spinal deformity in the form of scoliosis or kyphosis, a common finding in Duchenne dystrophy, many of the congenital and limb girdle dystrophies, and several congenital myopathies. Fatigue, a pronounced feature in myasthenia gravis and some metabolic myopathies, may be assessed by timing the number of seconds a patient can stand with outstretched arms, or by counting the number of squats the patient can perform before 'giving out'.

Respiratory muscles
Patient may have advanced respiratory muscle insufficiency before they develop symptoms of respiratory failure and signs at the bedside become obvious. It is imperative to assess respiratory function, particularly in patients with muscle disorders associated with diaphragmatic weakness, such as Duchenne dystrophy, acid maltase deficiency, myotonic dystrophy and some congenital myopathies. At the bedside, respiratory reserve can be estimated by having the patient take a deep breath and count slowly while exhaling. The availability of hand-held spirometers permits easy and more accurate testing of forced vital capacity (Hughes and Bihari, 1993). As respiratory weakness progresses, paradoxical movement of the abdominal wall may be observed. Normally, on inspiration, the upper abdomen moves outward as the diaphragm descends. If the diaphragm is weak it is drawn *up* on inspiration by negative intrathoracic pressure, and the abdominal wall moves inwards. The use of accessory muscles, including the sternocleidomastoid and other cervical muscles, may also be observed.

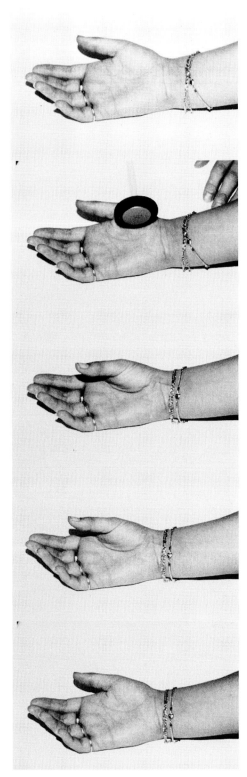

Fig. 17.7. Percussion myotonia in myotonic dystrophy. The thenar eminence is given a sharp tap with the tendon hammer – subsequent pictures taken at 2-second intervals.

(a)

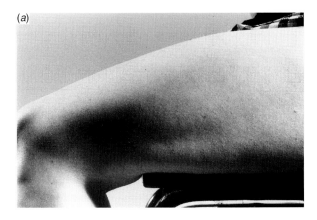

(b)

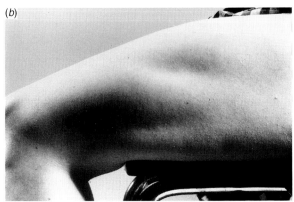

Fig. 17.8. Percussion myotonia in myotonia congenita. Following a sharp tap with a tendon hammer, there is a sustained localized depression that lasted about 5 seconds.

Percussion of muscle and abnormal relaxation phenomena

Although usually not a major part of the muscle examination, muscle percussion can elicit several reactions helpful in suggesting diagnoses. By far the most common of these phenomena is percussion myotonia, best elicited by sharply tapping the thenar eminence with a reflex hammer (Fig. 17.7). Percussion myotonia is most commonly seen in myotonic dystrophy but is more widespread and severe in myotonia congenita (Fig. 17.8). Patients with one of the sodium channelopathies or proximal myotonic myopathy may also have percussion myotonia. Most of these disorders also cause grip myotonia, demonstrated by asking the patient to grip the examiner's fingers tightly for several seconds and then release rapidly (Fig. 17.9). Muscle percussion can also elicit myo-oedema, or mounding-phenomenon, which manifests as a muscle ridge or lump that may persist for many seconds. This rare phenomenon is usually seen in the setting of myxoedema or severe malnutrition.

Reflex testing

As in all neurological disease, reflex testing is an important part of the examination of patients with suspected muscle disease. As a rule, tendon reflexes are normal in myopathies until late in the course, when wasting and weakness are advanced. There are, however, several important exceptions to this rule. In the Lambert–Eaton syndrome, absent tendon reflexes may reappear after sustained contraction of the appropriate muscle (i.e. reflex potentiation). In contrast, the reflexes in myasthenia gravis are often relatively brisk. Delayed or slowed relaxation of the reflexes is typical of hypothyroidism, although this can be difficult to detect in an individual patient unless the relaxation is quite abnormal. This is perhaps most often elicited in the ankle jerks but is sometimes better seen with the supinator reflex.

Muscle examination in children

Disorders beginning in early infancy and childhood cause particular problems for the clinician, since the patient cannot present their own history and the standard adult neurological examination is in many respects not appropriate or applicable (or even possible!) in infants or very young children. An excellent review of the approach to neuromuscular problems in childhood is Dubowitz's classic monograph (Dubowitz, 1995). Areas unique to the childhood assessment include details of the pregnancy, labour and delivery, and early motor and intellectual milestones.

Weakness in young children usually manifests initially as delayed motor milestones, although in some congenital myopathies the mother may notice reduced fetal movements during pregnancy. Perinatal features of note include hypotonia (floppy baby) and feeding and breathing difficulties. In older children, it is crucial, but often difficult, to determine the age of onset and whether the weakness is static, improving or progressive. Children with muscle diseases are frequently thought to be simply 'a little slow' or 'kind of clumsy' by their parents, siblings and paediatricians, and the seriousness of the problem may be overlooked until the weakness is advanced. It may take many years of observation before one can determine with any certainty the rate of progression of the disorder, an important feature in determining prognosis. The family may be able to comment on muscle atrophy or hypertrophy, and even in very young children it may be evident that exercise induces pain. The parents' description of the child's problems, watching the child play in the examining room, and performing functional tests as discussed above usually reveal more than a rigid, structured interview and formal examination.

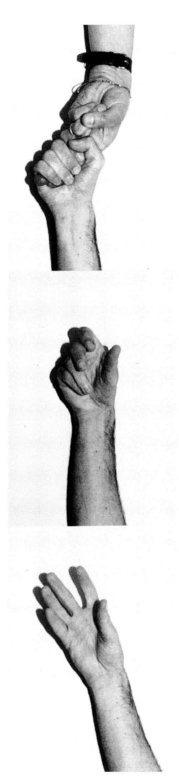

Fig. 17.9. Grip myotonia in myotonic dystrophy. The patient was asked to grip the examiner's fingers tightly for 3 seconds, and then to release and open their hand fully as quickly as possible. The following two pictures were taken at 3 second intervals.

Initial differential diagnosis

Based on findings gleaned from the history and examination, the clinician should be able to formulate a differential diagnosis that can be refined by subsequent laboratory investigations. A discussion of the differential diagnosis for each set of symptoms and signs that patients may manifest is beyond the scope of this chapter; much of this material is covered in subsequent chapters on specific disorders. Two fundamental issues, however, need to be addressed in all patients and deserve discussion here. The first issue concerns making the initial distinction between whether the patient is likely to have a primary muscle disorder, as opposed to a disease of the neuromuscular junction, anterior horn cells, peripheral nerves, CNS structures or even a non-neurological process. While this may seem straightforward, the distinction between these entities can often be difficult on clinical grounds alone. Features favouring a peripheral nerve disorder are sensory symptoms and signs; however, not all neuropathies (e.g. demyelinating polyneuropathies) cause demonstrable sensory involvement. Distal myopathies can simulate the Charcot–Marie–Tooth syndromes (in which sensory features can be slight or absent) as well as the distal spinal muscular atrophies. A possible additional source of confusion is that most myopathies causing severe disability and immobility may result in sensory symptoms because of secondary compressive neuropathies.

Once the determination is made that the disorder *is* likely to be myopathic, the second fundamental issue concerns identification of the specific myopathy present. Obviously, a family history of similar difficulties is strong evidence that the condition is inherited, but coincidental disorders in other family members may be unrelated and can be very misleading. Age of onset is often a powerful discriminator. Duchenne dystrophy, for example, does not present at age 15 years, and the primary periodic paralyses do not present in old age. In contrast, oculopharyngeal muscular dystrophy rarely presents in early adult life, but mitochondrial external ophthalmoplegia can present at any age. Rate of progression may also be informative. Many congenital disorders are nonprogressive or change only slowly with time. Inflammatory myopathies, but not dystrophies, may have a very acute onset with severe weakness developing within days. Metabolic disorders and channelopathies may cause slowly progressive weakness, over many decades, but with superimposed acute exacerbations. The pattern of weakness may also be highly informative. Dystrophies tend to 'pick out' certain muscles, whereas inflammatory myopathies are less selective. Cardiac involvement occurs in only certain myopathies,

and the mitochondrial cytopathies have many nonmyopathic features. By the end of the interview and examination, therefore, a relatively short list of possible diagnoses should be under consideration. This list can then be refined further through judicious testing, as discussed in the next section.

Approach to laboratory investigations

With few exceptions (e.g. typical myotonic dystrophy), all patients suspected of having a muscle disorder should have a serum CK determination. Although many patients should also undergo neurophysiological studies, these are not necessary in all patients, since other tests may be more specific (e.g. genetic testing in myotonic dystrophy). If these evaluations indicate a myopathy, and there is no evidence for a systemic disorder (e.g. endocrinopathy), then the patient's condition is likely to fall into one of the broad categories of myopathy listed in Table 17.17, which also lists the investigations most useful in reaching a diagnosis. It is important to remember that testing in the muscle diseases may serve different purposes depending on the type of test and the nature of the problem. Some tests, such as enzyme assays in metabolic disorders and DNA analyses in genetic disorders, provide a specific diagnosis. Other tests, such as the forearm exercise test, suggest the type of problem but not an exact diagnosis. Still other studies, such as electrocardiography, reveal abnormalities that are a consequence of the primary myopathy but provide few clues to the underlying disorder. Finally, there are investigations, such as magnetic resonance spectroscopy, which are currently mainly of research value.

In some muscular dystrophies (e.g. FSH dystrophy), the diagnosis can often be strongly suspected on the basis of clinical features and family history. Gene studies are becoming increasingly important and in many situations (myotonic dystrophy, FSH dystrophy, oculopharyngeal dystrophy and 70% of patients with Duchenne dystrophy) have made muscle biopsy unnecessary. This is an important concept, especially since routine histochemical and electron microscopy studies in the dystrophies are rarely unique or diagnostic anyway, an exception being the characteristic intranuclear inclusions seen in oculopharyngeal muscular dystrophy (Tomé et al., 1997). Immunochemistry and immunoblotting are major tools in the study of the dystrophin disorders, especially if there is no Xp21 mutation, and some limb girdle and congenital dystrophies. For inflammatory myopathies, muscle biopsy remains the *sine qua non* of diagnosis. Electromyography may be suggestive but is never diagnostic and serum CK

Table 17.17. Major categories of muscle disease and investigations useful in their diagnosis

Category	Investigations
Muscular dystrophies	Muscle biopsy for histology, histochemistry and immunocytochemistry
	Immunoblotting of muscle specimen for a specific defective protein
	DNA studies for gene defect
Congenital myopathies	Muscle biopsy for histology, histochemistry and immunocytochemistry
	DNA studies for gene defect
Inflammatory myopathies	Muscle biopsy for histology and histochemistry: immunocytochemistry for complement, mononuclear cell analysis, staining for amyloid deposits (i.e. for inclusion body myositis), electron microscopy
	Skin biopsy (in dermatomyositis)
Primary metabolic myopathies affecting carbohydrate metabolism	Forearm exercise test (assay lactate and ammonia)
	Muscle biopsy for histology and histochemical staining; enzyme assay on muscle tissue
	Leukocyte glycogen storage (acid maltase deficiency)
	Blood cells, fibroblasts, or leukocyte assay for enzyme defect
	DNA studies
Primary metabolic myopathies affecting lipid metabolism	Urinalysis
	Organic acid serum assay
	Acylcarnitine and carnitine assay
	Serum tandem mass spectrometry
	Prolonged fasting (assay free fatty acids, lactate, pyruvate, uric acid, ammonia, ketone bodies, glucose, creatine kinase)
	Aerobic exercise stress test
	Muscle biopsy for histology, histochemistry, lipid analysis: enzyme assay on muscle tissue
	Fibroblast assay
	Liver biopsy
	DNA studies
Mitochondrial cytopathies	Resting blood lactate and pyruvate
	Aerobic exercise (assay lactate, pyruvate, ammonia, glucose)
	Muscle biopsy for histology ('ragged-red' fibers), histochemistry: mitochondrial DNA studies
	Magnetic resonance spectroscopy
Channelopathies	Neurophysiological studies
	Serum potassium changes during attacks (for periodic paralysis)
	Provocation tests (for periodic paralysis)
	DNA studies

may be normal. Inflammatory changes within muscle may be patchy, however, and result in a noninformative biopsy. Routine histology may be diagnostic but electron microscopy (for filaments in inclusion body myositis) and immunocytochemistry (for complement membrane attack complex in dermatomyositis) may provide additional information.

The metabolic myopathies are rare but among the most complicated and difficult of the myopathies to investigate (Hilton-Jones et al., 1995). Exercise tests, if performed correctly by experienced personnel, may help to determine the site of metabolic dysfunction as a prelude to specific biochemical investigations or muscle biopsy (Haller and Bertocci, 1994; Lane and Fuller, 1996). Histochemical staining of biopsy material may sometimes demonstrate directly the enzyme deficiency or show accumulated products (e.g. glycogen, lipid) resulting from the blocked metabolic pathway. Enzyme assay may also be performed on a biopsy sample. For disorders where the genetic defect is known, DNA analysis can often be performed on a blood sample, but at a research level mRNA studies on muscle may be useful. An important exception is mitochondrial DNA deletion/duplication syndromes in which the genetic defect is best detected in muscle, not lymphocytes. For the channelopathies, electromyography is useful, particularly if myotonia is present. In the periodic paralyses, monitoring potassium levels during spontaneous attacks may be diagnostic and obviate the need for more risky provocative tests. Direct gene analysis is rapidly becoming the investigation of choice for these disorders.

Neurophysiology

It is frustrating but all too true that even after the most thorough assessment it may be impossible at the bedside to make even the fundamental determination of whether the patient has a myopathy or a disorder affecting some other part of the neuraxis. Neurophysiological studies are the most valuable method to make this distinction. Although many techniques are now available in clinical neurophysiology departments, those most pertinent to the assessment of possible muscle disorders include nerve conduction studies, electromyography, and studies of neuromuscular transmission. These are all discussed in more detail elsewhere, and only two points will be stressed here. The first is that although these techniques will *usually* clearly indicate whether the patient has a neurogenic or myopathic disorder, this is not invariably true. For example, there are some diseases that mainly produce a myopathy but that may also be associated with a subclinical neuropathy (e.g. mitochondrial disorders, myotonic dystrophy and inclusion body myositis). The second point is that the neurophysiological studies, like any test in medicine, cannot be interpreted in isolation but must always be analysed in light of the clinical findings and the results of other testing.

Biochemical studies

The biochemical tests available to evaluate patients with muscle disease range from the simple and inexpensive serum CK assay to complex and time-consuming exercise protocols and phosphorus magnetic resonance spectroscopy. Other biochemical studies are useful for diagnosing various endocrinological or metabolic disorders (such as thyroid disease) that may be associated with muscle disease. The CK is by far the most common, and useful, serum test obtained in the muscle clinic.

Creatine kinase assay

CK is an enzyme that catalyses the reversible reaction by which adenosine diphosphate (ADP) and phosphocreatine form adenosine triphosphate (ATP) and creatine, but knowledge of this reaction is not important in understanding the significance of the assay in clinical practice.

Elevation of the serum CK is a nonspecific marker of muscle damage and occurs in a wide variety of muscle diseases. Simply put, damaged muscle allows the enzyme to leak-out into the circulation. It is important to remember that CK elevation can occur in diseases not of muscle origin; conversely, many muscle diseases do not cause an increase in CK. For example, CK is often normal in the two common forms of adult muscular dystrophy, namely myotonic dystrophy and FSH dystrophy. It is also crucial to remember that CK levels vary among normal individuals on the basis of gender, race, age and physical activity. Black males, for example, may have CK values two or three times higher than standard laboratory grouped control values (Wong et al., 1983). Fractionating the CK isoforms is not helpful in assessing muscle disease.

The highest CK elevations are seen with rhabdomyolysis from any cause. In Duchenne and Becker dystrophies, the serum CK is markedly elevated in the early stages but declines later on as muscle mass is reduced. In the inflammatory myopathies, serum CK is usually, but not always, elevated, more so in dermatomyositis and polymyositis than in inclusion body myositis. Although it is tempting in these disorders to use the CK level to monitor progress, there is an imprecise relationship between serum CK and strength. For example, serum CK typically falls to normal within weeks of starting steroids but weakness may take much longer to improve. Serum CK elevation may also result from muscle injury that does not involve a muscle disease in the usual sense, such as muscle trauma (e.g. intramuscular injections, electric shock), sepsis, hypothermia, vigorous exercise, cardiac injury and severe dyskinesias. More common is the patient with elevated serum CK without obvious cause or weakness. Common causes of elevated CK in an otherwise asymptomatic individual are shown in Table 17.18. It is unusual to make a specific diagnosis in a patient with no weakness or pain and a *modest* elevation in CK (up to three to five times normal). Many of these patients have idiopathic, or hereditary, 'hyper-CK-aemia' and do not develop serious muscle disease, even on long-term follow-up.

Other serum and urine tests

Although other muscle enzymes and proteins can be assayed (e.g. myoglobin, aldolase, carbonic anhydrase III, aspartate transaminase (AST)), none offers an advantage over the CK test. A relatively common situation in this regard concerns patients found on routine blood testing to have an elevated AST level. Since AST is a marker of hepatic function, these patients are often suspected of having liver disease, even though other liver function tests are normal.

Table 17.18. Causes of elevated creatine kinase in patients without overt muscle disease

Intense physical exercise
Black race
Frequent trauma
Sustained alcohol use
Hypothyroidism
Female carriers of the Duchenne/Becker muscular dystrophy gene
Asymptomatic (or presymptomatic) McArdle's disease
Susceptibility to malignant hyperthermia
Drugs causing subclinical myopathy (e.g. lovastatins)
Hereditary persistent high creatine kinase ('hyper-CK-aemia')

Some patients undergo liver biopsy before a CK value is obtained and it is realized that the AST is of muscle origin. In mitochondrial disorders, serum (and spinal fluid) lactate may be elevated at rest, a finding that can be a useful screening test. In the rare disorders of lipid metabolism, blood and urine carnitine and acylcarnitine assays are helpful. Tandem mass spectrometry is a recently developed method to study disorders of fatty acid β-oxidation. Myoglobin levels may be elevated in patients with rhabdomyolysis, although a more obvious manifestation of this disorder is myoglobinuria, which causes a positive dipstick reaction that may be confused with the presence of blood.

Enzyme assays

In many metabolic myopathies, the diagnosis is secured only after enzyme assay on a muscle biopsy specimen frozen immediately in liquid nitrogen and stored at −70°C. In some disorders, assays can be performed on blood, urine, fibroblast cultures and liver biopsy specimens.

Exercise tests

Exercise tests are used chiefly in the investigation of metabolic myopathies but they may also be beneficial in some channelopathies. Forearm exercise testing can be performed at the bedside, while aerobic bicycle exercise is more complex and requires specialized equipment; both should be performed at neuromuscular referral centres by experienced staff. Phosphorus magnetic resonance spectroscopy has proven useful in the research setting but is available in few centres and is not yet practical for routine diagnosis. These tests are discussed in more detail elsewhere in this book and in other reviews (Hilton-Jones et al., 1995).

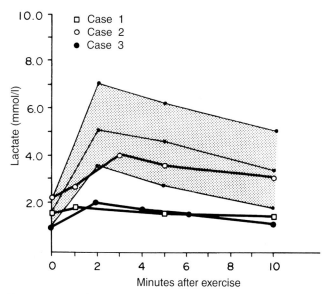

Fig. 17.10. Venous lactate response to 1-minute of forearm exercise in three patients with phosphoglycerate mutase deficiency. The shaded area represents the mean and range of normal control responses to the same exercise protocol. None of the patients shows even a twofold rise in lactate above baseline. (Reproduced with permission from Kissel, J. T., Beam, W., Bresolin, N. et al. (1985). Physiologic assessment of phosphoglycerate mutase deficiency: Incremental exercise tests. *Neurology* **35**, 828–833.)

Forearm exercise test

The forearm exercise test is a simple screen for defects of glycogenolysis and glycolysis. The test is not without risk, and compartment syndromes or rhabdomyolysis with secondary renal compromise can occur, especially if the test is done under ischaemic conditions (i.e. forearm ischaemic exercise test). Because of these concerns, and the fact that oxidative metabolism contributes little in early intense exercise, most muscle centres perform the test under non-ischaemic conditions. In this test, an intravenous line is placed in an antecubital vein and kept patent with heparin. After baseline blood samples are obtained, the patient exercises by squeezing a sphygmomanometer bulb to exhaustion (usually over 1–2 minutes). After exercise stops, further blood samples are taken at 1, 2, 3, 5, 10 and 15 minutes. Samples are assayed for lactate and ammonia, which requires pre-iced sample tubes and rapid processing. The normal response is a three- to fivefold increase over baseline for both lactate and ammonia (Fig. 17.10). In disorders of glycogenolysis and glycolysis, the lactate response curve is reduced (or absent) and the rise in ammonia excessive. Conversely, myoadenylate deaminase deficiency results in a normal lactate rise but little or no increase in ammonia. With submaximal effort, neither lactate nor ammonia increase (Coleman et al., 1986; Sinkeler et al., 1986).

Aerobic bicycle exercise test

The main clinical value of aerobic exercise testing is in the investigation of patients suspected of having disorders of oxidative metabolism, such as the mitochondrial disorders. In the test, the patient typically exercises for 15 minutes, and lactate and pyruvate are measured during exercise and recovery. Many protocols are used; one of the most satisfactory being the subanaerobic threshold exercise test (Nashef and Lane, 1989; Lane and Fuller, 1996). A defect in the Krebs' cycle or respiratory chain results in the pyruvate formed during glycolysis being reduced to lactate. In disorders of oxidative metabolism, there is an abnormal increase in serum lactate and also an abnormal lactate/pyruvate ratio.

Phosphorus magnetic resonance spectroscopy

Although phosphorus magnetic resonance spectroscopy is available routinely in relatively few muscle centres, it has already contributed significantly to the understanding of a number of disorders, principally the metabolic myopathies (Hilton-Jones et al., 1995). This method measures changes in parameters reflecting cellular responses to demands such as exercise (see Chapter 16).

Muscle imaging

Although muscle imaging can prove invaluable in selected patients, such as those with diabetic thigh muscle infarction (Fig. 17.11), it is a rare patient in whom imaging is an indispensable part of the diagnostic process. The standard imaging modalities, ultrasound, computed tomography (CT) scanning and MRI, can all be used and each provides somewhat different information. Imaging may demonstrate early and selective muscle involvement not evident to even the most experienced clinical eye (Swash et al., 1995). For example, forearm flexor muscle involvement may be detected by MRI scanning in patients with inclusion body myositis prior to the onset of the characteristic finger flexor weakness (Sekul et al., 1997). Imaging may also be used to evaluate the severity of the disease process in a given area, assess disease progression or regression demonstrate fatty replacement in degenerating muscles or help to localize inflammatory deposits in disorders such as sarcoidosis.

Ultrasound

Ultrasound has distinct advantages over other modalities in that the equipment is portable and the study can be per-

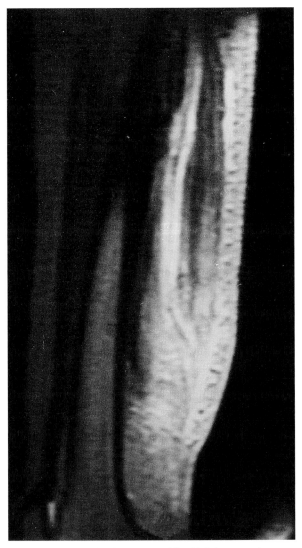

Fig. 17.11. A T_2-weighted MRI scan of the thigh from a patient with diabetic thigh muscle infarction. There is diffuse high signal in the posterior muscles, including the biceps femoris, semimembranosus and semitendinosus muscles. The bone and quadriceps muscles (on the left of the figure) appear normal. (From Barohn, R. J. and Kissel, J. T. Case of the month: painful thigh mass in a young woman: diabetic muscle infarction. *Muscle Nerve* 15, 850–855, copyright ©1992 John Wiley. Reprinted by permission of John Wiley & Sons Inc.)

formed by the clinician. Muscle bulk can be easily measured with this technique, and various pathological processes alter muscle echogenic properties. It is most useful in studying dystrophies and, to a lesser extent, inflammatory myopathies. Ultrasound has proven particularly helpful in paedriatic patients in selecting an appropriate muscle for biopsy (Dubowitz, 1995).

Computed tomographic scanning

Muscle bulk is readily measured by CT scanning, and densities within muscle can be determined and measured. Like ultrasound, CT can identify focal abnormalities such as cysts and tumours. Radiation concerns have led to CT scanning being supplanted by MRI.

Magnetic resonance imaging

Given its safety and sensitivity, MRI has rapidly become the method of choice for investigating muscle disorders, although it currently has limited availability in many parts of the world. A number of reports have documented its use in the clinical setting (Reimers et al., 1994; Sekul et al., 1997), confirming this modality's value in demonstrating selective muscle involvement (Fig. 17.11).

Muscle biopsy

Despite advances in genetics and molecular biology, muscle biopsy remains an important diagnostic tool in evaluating many types of muscle disorder. The material obtained through biopsy can be studied through histological, histochemical, immunocytochemical, biochemical, electron microscopic or genetic techniques; these methodologies, along with interpretive aspects related to muscle biopsies, are reviewed in Chapters 13–16. Like neurophysiological studies, biopsy results must always be interpreted in the light of the clinical presentation and other laboratory studies. It is also important to remember that pathological changes may be very focal, both between muscles and within a given muscle. This is particularly common in the inflammatory myopathies, where an initial biopsy may show no abnormality while a second specimen from an adjacent area shows striking pathology. It is often helpful in such cases to sample multiple levels through the specimen. Biopsy appearances in specific disorders are considered throughout this volume, and there are also several excellent monographs on muscle biopsy (Carpenter and Karpati, 1984; Dubowitz, 1985).

Molecular genetic diagnosis

The impact of molecular genetics on the understanding of the hereditary muscle disorders cannot be overstated. Since the mid-1980s, the field has advanced so rapidly that genetic testing has become a routine part of the evaluation of many muscle diseases, and it is crucial for all clinicians to have at least some understanding of the main methodologies involved. These are reviewed in Chapter 4 and will not be discussed here, except in terms of their impact on diagnosis. The single most important technique has been that of positional cloning (also called reverse genetics), which allows the defective gene responsible for a disease to be isolated so that the protein product of the gene can be identified. This is accomplished by studying large informative families with a clearly defined disorder using polymorphic markers to identify the approximate chromosomal location of the gene. The exact position of the gene is then determined using finer mapping techniques. Expressed transcripts of candidate genes from the area are assessed until the responsible gene is identified. The protein product can then be deduced from the nucleotide sequence. Another approach is to study candidate genes likely to be responsible for a given disorder, based on specific pathophysiological or biochemical features of that disease. This technique will become increasingly important in the future as the Human Genome Project results in identification of the entire human genome.

Several different types of mutation have been identified in muscle disorders, as summarized in Table 17.19. The disorders for which commercial tests were available at the time this chapter was written are also indicated. The identification of the gene defect responsible for a given disease may have immediate clinical import from a number of perspectives. Most obviously, such an identification is likely to be a major prerequisite to the development of effective therapy, whether by gene therapy or by some pharmacological or biochemical means (see Chapters 35 and 36). There are also immediate practical benefits to the patient and their family of having a specific genetic marker:

- provides precise diagnosis and information about disease pathogenesis
- usually limits need for additonal testing
- often permits carrier detection
- allows identification of presymptomatic or at-risk individuals
- in some instances, may permit prenatal diagnosis and accurate genetic counselling
- provides diagnostic homogeneity for patients participating in clinical trials
- may eventually be useful in identifying patients for gene therapy trials
- occasionally, may *suggest* phenotypic expression and severity of disease (but should never replace clinical determinations of disease severity or be used only rarely to provide detailed prognostic information to patient or family).

Most of these benefits are self-evident and are considered further in Chapter 35 and in the discussions of each disorder.

Table 17.19. Mutations in some muscle disorders

Mutation	Disorder
Genomic DNA	
Large deletions	Duchenne/Becker muscular dystrophy (~60% of patients)[a]
Duplication	Some patients with Duchenne/Becker dystrophy (~5% of patients)[a]
Point mutations	Some patients with Duchenne/Becker dystrophy (~5%), sarcoglycanopathies, limb girdle dystrophy type 2A (calpain-deficient), congenital muscular dystrophy (merosin deficient), many metabolic disorders, channelopathies, myotonia congenita, Emery–Dreifuss X-linked muscular dystrophy[a], congenital myasthenic syndromes
Trinucleotide repeat expansion	Myotonic dystrophy[a], oculopharyngeal dystrophy
Deletion of repeat units	Facioscapulohumeral muscular dystrophy[a]
Mitochondrial DNA	
Deletion	Kearns–Sayre syndrome (single deletion)[a], autosomal dominant progressive external ophthalmoplegia (multiple deletions)[a]
Point mutations	Other mitochondrial syndromes (e.g. myoclonus epilepsy with ragged-red fibres (MERRF), mitochondrial encephalomyopathy – lactic acidosis – stroke-like symptoms (MELAS)[a]

Notes:

[a] Genetic assay commercially available.

References

Argov, Z. and Mastaglia, F. L. (1994). Drug-induced neuromuscular disorders in man. In: *Disorders of Voluntary Muscle*, 6th edn, eds. J. Walton, G. Karpati and D. Hilton-Jones, pp. 989–1029. Edinburgh: Churchill Livingstone.

Auger, R. G. (1994). Diseases associated with excess motor unit activity. *Muscle Nerve* **17**, 1250–1263.

Brooke, M. H. (1986). *A Clinician's View of Neuromuscular Disease*, 2nd edn. Baltimore, MD: Williams & Wilkins.

Carpenter, S. and Karpati, G. (1984). *Pathology of Skeletal Muscle*. New York: Churchill Livingstone.

Coleman, R. A., Stajich, J. M., Pact, V. W. and Pericak-Vance, M. A. (1986). The ischemic exercise test in normal adults and in patients with weakness and cramps. *Muscle Nerve* **9**, 216–221

Dubowitz, V. (1985). *Muscle Biopsy. A Practical Approach*, 2nd edn. London: Baillière Tindall.

Dubowitz, V. (1995). *Muscle Disorders in Childhood*, 2nd edn. London: Saunders.

Emery, A. E. H. (1987). *Duchenne Muscular Dystrophy*. Oxford: Oxford University Press.

Eneas, J. F., Schoenfeld, P. Y. and Humphries, M. H. (1979). The effect of infusion of mannitol–sodium bicarbonate on the clinical course of myoglobinuria. *Arch. Int. Med.* **139**, 801–810.

Haller, R. G. and Bertocci, L. A. (1994). Exercise evaluation of metabolic myopathies. In: *Myology*, eds. A. G. Engel and C. Franzini-Armstrong, pp. 807–821. New York: McGraw-Hill.

Harper, P. S. (1989*). Myotonic dystrophy*, 2nd edn. London: Saunders.

Hart, I. K. and Newsom-Davis, J. (1996). Neuromyotonia. In: *Handbook of Muscle Disease*, ed. R. J. M. Lane, pp. 355–364. New York: Marcel Dekker.

Hiel, J. A. P., Jongen, P. J. H., Poels, P. J. E. et al. (1996). Sarcoplasmic reticulum Ca^{2+}-adenosine triphosphate deficiency (Brody's disease). In: *Handbook of Muscle Disease*, ed. R. J. M. Lane, pp. 473–478. New York: Marcel Dekker.

Hilton-Jones, D. (1994). The clinical features of some miscellaneous neuromuscular disorders. In: *Disorders of Voluntary Muscle*, 6th edn, eds. J. Walton, G. Karpati and D. Hilton-Jones. Edinburgh: Churchill Livingstone.

Hilton-Jones, D., Squier, M., Taylor, D. and Matthews, P. (1995). *Metabolic Myopathies*. London: Saunders.

Hirano, M., Silvestri, G., Blake, D. M. et al. (1994). Mitochondrial neurogastrointestinal encephalomyopathy (MNGIE): clinical, biochemical and genetic features of an autosomal recessive mitochondrial disorder. *Neurology* **44**, 721–727.

Howard, R. S., Wiles, C. M., Hirsch, N. P. and Spencer, G. T. (1993). Respiratory involvement in primary muscle disorders: assessment and management. *Q. J. Med.* **86**, 175–189.

Hudson, A. J., Ebers, G. C. and Bulman, D. E. (1995). The skeletal muscle sodium and chloride channel diseases. *Brain* **118**, 547–563.

Hughes, R. A. C. and Bihari, D. (1993). Acute neuromuscular respiratory paralysis. *J. Neurol. Neurosurg. Psychiatry* **56**, 334–343.

Kissel, J. T. and Elble, R. (1998). Stiff-person syndrome. Stiff opposition to a simple explanation. *Neurology* **51**, 11–14.

Kissel, J. T. and Mendell, J. R. (1992). Endocrine myopathies. In: *Handbook of Clinical Neurology*, Vol. 19, *Myopathies*, eds. L. P. Rowland and S. DiMauro, pp. 527–551. New York: Elsevier Science.

Kissel, J. T. and Miller, R. (1999). Muscle pain and fatigue. In: *Muscle Diseases*, eds. A. H. V. Schapira and R. C. Griggs, pp. 33-58. Woburn: Butterworth-Heinemann.

Krupp, L. B. and Pollina, D. A. (1996). Mechanisms and management of fatigue in progressive neurological disorders. *Curr. Opin. Neurol.* **9**, 456–460.

Lane, R. J. M. and Fuller, G. N.. (1996). Clinical presentation. Symptoms and signs of muscle disease and their interpretation. In: *Handbook of Muscle Disease*, ed. R. J. M. Lane, pp. 1–17. New York: Marcel Dekker.

Layzer, R. B. (1994). Muscle pain, cramps and fatigue. In: *Myology*, 2nd edn, eds. A. G. Engel and C. Franzini-Armstrong, pp. 1754–1768. New York: McGraw-Hill.

Medical Research Council (1986). *Aids to the Examination of the Peripheral Nervous System*. London: Ballière Tindall.

Mills, K. R. and Edwards, R. H. T. (1983). Investigative strategies for muscle pain. *J. Neurolog. Sci.* **58**, 73–88.

Morita, H., Kondo, K., Hoshino, K., Maruyama, K. and Yanagisawa, N. (1990). Rigid spine syndrome with respiratory failure. *J. Neurol. Neurosurg. Psychiatry* **53**, 782–784.

Mullie, M. A., Harding, A. E., Petty, R. K. H., Ikeda, H., Morgan-Hughes, J. A. and Sanders, M. D. (1985). The retinal manifestations of mitochondrial myopathy. *Arch. Ophthalmol.* **103**, 1825–1830.

Munsat, T. L. (1989). *Quantification of Neurologic Deficit*. Stoneham: Butterworth.

Nashef, L. and Lane, R. J. M. (1989). Screening for mitochondrial cytopathies: the sub-anaerobic threshold exercise test (SATET). *J. Neurol. Neurosurg. Psychiatry* **52**, 1090–1094.

Penn, A. S. (1994). Myoglobinuria. In: *Myology*, 2nd edn, eds. A. G. Engel and C. Franzini-Armstrong, pp. 1577–1586. New York: McGraw-Hill.

Personius, K. E., Pandya, S., King, W. M., Tawil, R. and McDermott, M. P. (1994). Facioscapulohumeral dystrophy natural history study: standardization of testing procedures and reliability measurements. The FSHDY Group. *Phys. Ther.* **74**, 253–263.

Petty, R. K. H., Harding, A. E. and Morgan-Hughes, J. A. (1986). The clinical features of mitochondrial myopathy. *Brain* **109**, 915–938.

Reimers, C. D., Schedel, H., Fleckenstein, J. L. et al. (1994). Magnetic resonance imaging of skeletal muscles in idiopathic inflammatory myopathies of adults. *J. Neurol.* **241**, 306–314.

Ricker, K., Moxley, R. T. and Rohkamm, R. (1989). Rippling muscle disease. *Arch. Neurol.* **46**, 405–408.

Rowland, L. P. and Penn, A. S. (1972). Myoglobinuria. *Med. Clin. North Am.* **56**, 1233–1256.

Sekul, E .A., Chow, C. and Dalakas, M. C. (1997). Magnetic resonance imaging of the forearm as a diagnostic aid in patients with sporadic inclusion body myositis. *Neurology* **48**, 863–866.

Shillito, P., Molenaar, P. C., Vincent, A. et al. (1995). Acquired neuromyotonia: evidence for autoantibodies directed against K^+ channels of peripheral nerves. *Ann. Neurol.* **38**, 714–722.

Sinkeler, S. P., Wevers, R. A., Joosten, E. M. et al. (1986). Improvement of screening in exertional myalgia with a standardized ischemic forearm test. *Muscle Nerve* **9**, 731–737.

Suarez, G. A. and Kelly, J. J. (1992). The dropped head syndrome. *Neurology* **42**, 1625–1627.

Swash, M., Brown, M. M. and Thakkar, C. (1995). CT muscle imaging and the clinical assessment of neuromuscular disease. *Muscle Nerve* **18**, 708–714.

Tawil, R., McDermott, M. P., Mendell J. R. and the FSH-DY Group (1994). FSHD: design of natural history and results of baseline testing. *Neurology* **44**, 442–446.

Tomé, F. M. S., Chateau, D., Helbling-Leclerc, A. and Fardeau, M. (1997). Morphological changes in muscle fibres in oculopharyngeal muscular dystrophy. *Neuromusc. Disord.* **7**(Suppl. 1), S63–S69.

Trend, P. S. J., Wiles, C. M., Spencer, G. T., Morgan-Hughes, J. A., Lake, B. D. and Patrick, A. D. (1985). Acid maltase deficiency in adults. *Brain* **108**, 845–860.

Tsao, C.-Y. and Mendell, J. R. (1999). The childhood muscular dystrophies: making order out of chaos. *Semin. Neurol.* **19**, 9–23.

Tsao, C. Y., Mendell, J. R., Rusin, J. and Luquette, M. (1998). Congenital muscular dystrophy with complete lamin-alpha-2 deficiency, cortical dysplasia and cerebral white-matter changes in children. *J. Child Neurol.* **13**, 253–256.

Wong, E. T., Cobb, C. and Umahara, M. K. (1983). Heterogeneity of serum CK activity among racial and gender groups of the population. *Am. J. Clin. Pathol.* **79**, 582–586.

Zierz, S. (1994). Carnitine palmitoyltransferase deficiency. In: *Myology*, eds. A. G. Engel and C. Franzini-Armstrong, pp. 1577–1586. New York: McGraw-Hill.

18

The classification of muscle diseases

Michael H. Brooke

Order is Heaven's first law.
An essay on Man: ALEXANDER POPE

Introduction

It is a mundane observation that humans create chaos out of order. From the history of this world to the appearance of my desk top there is evidence that humans have a natural tendency to litter, waste and upset things. Perhaps in compensation for this, humans have also developed a contrary tendency to try to create form where none exists. To see shapes in clouds, snow on the television screen or figures in the embers; these are all of course illusions, but continue to entertain us.

At an intellectual level, humans have a similar need to give form to the environment. This is best accomplished by inventing classifications. These are often useful. Dewey, Linnaeus, Bentham and Hooker, the supermarket: all are responsible for classifications that allow us to find our way through a labyrinth of things which are otherwise unrelated.

This brings us to the classification of muscle diseases. For more than a century, muscle diseases have been categorized by their clinical appearance. Often this was by their original patrons, beginning with the best known and easiest to recognize, Duchenne dystrophy, followed by Erb, Landouzy, Dejerine, Steinert and the other luminaries. Sometimes the classification was by age, in which case it began with Duchenne dystrophy, followed by limb girdle, facioscapulohumeral and myotonic. As classifications go, these were useful enough to be able to persuade patients that they had, at least, a recognizable disease, but anyone with more than two weeks' experience in the average muscle clinic began to realize that there were many, perhaps the majority, of patients who refused to be neatly pigeon-holed into this system.

The discoveries of the period since the mid-1980s have demolished all sense of order in the old classification. Patients with identical histories and findings have totally different genetic abnormalities. Patients with the same molecular defect appear radically different. It is enough to make the great clinicians turn in their grave and the diagnosticians slink back to their lairs. Chaos reigns. But out of the fog, as always, a new figure can be glimpsed emerging. A figure, not yet fully limned, which holds out to us a new classification. Will it improve upon the old? Time will tell.

Until 1984 the causes of muscular dystrophy were a subject of happy speculation. The early pioneering studies narrowed the cause of Duchenne dystrophy to an abnormality in dystrophin consequent upon an alteration in the gene on the short arm of the X chromosome. There then followed a cascade of discoveries identifying various genetic abnormalities. This had several effects, some desirable.

Patients were often detoured from the muscle clinic and sent for DNA studies before the examining physician had a chance to ply his trade, akin to the neurologist who prefers to view the magnetic resonance image before checking the reflexes. In fairness, this is not unique: chest physicians used to murmur learnedly about whispering pectoriloquy and would percuss out the lesion with a good deal more confidence once they had seen the chest radiograph. More of a mixed blessing was the disappearance into the genetic laboratory of every aspiring fellow, together with much of the funding, leaving biochemists and physiologists to bemoan their fate.

At the start of the 1990s, I would have confidently predicted that the next long-lasting classification of muscle disease would be based on genetic abnormalities. This is no longer tenable and it is now apparent that any future classification will have to be based on the molecular abnormalities themselves. This should, in fact, have been self-evident. Except for the muscle diseases that are caused by remote factors such as vascular insufficiency or immunological attack, the root cause has to be an abnormality in

Table 18.1. Proposed system for classifying muscle disease

Group	Associated with
Structural/linking proteins	Nucleus: membrane or other
	Mitochondria
	Contractile apparatus
	Sarcolemmal membrane
	Other
Contractile proteins	
Ion channel proteins	
Associated with enzyme activity	Energy-related processes: glycolysis, lipid oxidation, mitochondrial enzymes, adenylate deaminase
	Non-energy-related processes: proteases, protein kinases, phosphatases
Other proteins	Nucleus
	Mitochondria
	Contractile apparatus
	Membranes
	Other
Protein storage	
Secondary diseases	Inflammation and autoimmunity
	Immunological disease
	Infectious disease
	Systemic disease
	Toxins

the component mechanisms of the muscle 'machine'. These are all proteins, each of which may be governed by one or several genes. We should turn our attention to these proteins and assemble them into some order. The muscle machinery is crafted by the nucleus and other subcellular components. Some of the proteins thus formed are directly involved in the contractile mechanism, the thick and thin filaments. Others participate as structural proteins forming a framework or linking other proteins to each other. Many of these proteins are associated with the sarcolemmal membrane. There are proteins that participate in energy metabolism to fuel the cell as well as the proteins that make up the structure of the mitochondria. If we arrange the known diseases according to this schema, there will still be plenty of room to assimilate those diseases that are, as yet, undefined and that will be found in later years to be caused by one or other new protein abnormality.

The system of classification proposed is outlined in Table 18.1.

Most of the known diseases are linked with abnormalities in structural proteins. This may simply reflect that these are easier to find than others or may be an indication that survival is only possible when the abnormality is of supporting structures and that a mutation affecting more fundamental properties would be lethal.

The proposed classification looks nothing like the older classifications. Table 18.2 compares old terms with the new protein defect terminology. It may bear little resemblance to classifications to come. That is a danger inherent in trying to establish a permanent foundation during a time of transition. Perhaps the clarion message of this chapter should be that all is changing, nothing is fixed. We are between two eras. This is an interesting, if not enviable position. It might be well to remember the old ritual cry that went up at the death of a ruler that recognized the transfer of the monarchy: 'The King is dead! Long live the King!'. The ideas that many of us grew to treasure and that became so familiar are dead. Those of the future, although uncertain, are likely to take us into hitherto undreamed of areas. Long live the King!

Structural/linking proteins

Associated with the nucleus

Nuclear membrane

Emerin

Emerin is a membrane-spanning 34 kDa serine-rich protein that is a component of the nuclear lamina associated with the nuclear envelope. It is one member of a family of lamina-associated proteins which includes LAP1,

Table 18.2. *Correlation of the older terminology for muscle diseases with the underlying molecular defects, where known*

Older terminology	'New' terminology
Emery–Dreifuss dystrophy	Emerin deficiency, lamin A deficiency
Nemaline myopathy	Nebulin deficiency, α-tropomyosin deficiency
Duchenne/Becker dystrophies	Dystrophin deficiency
'Limb Girdle' dystrophies	Deficiencies of α-, β-, γ- and δ-sarcoglycan, laminin α_2- and β_1-chains, dysferlin, caveolin, calpain 3
Epidermolysis bullosa muscular dystrophy	Plectin deficiency
Bethlem myopathy	Collagen VI deficiency
Fukuyama dystrophy	Fukutin deficiency
Hypokalaemic periodic paralysis (autosomal dominant)	Calcium channel
Hyperkalaemic periodic paralysis (autosomal dominant)	Sodium channel
Paramyotonia congenita	Sodium channel
Myotonia congenita	Chloride channel
Malignant hyperthermia	Ryanodine receptor
Central core disease	Ryanodine receptor
Congenital muscular dystrophy	Deficiencies of laminin α_2-chain and γ-sarcoglycan
Myoshi myopathy	Dysferlin deficiency
Myotonic dystrophy	Myotonin protein kinase deficiency
Myotubular myopathy	Myotubularin deficiency
Oculopharyngeal dystrophy	Poly-A-binding protein

LAP2 and lamin B receptor. It is found in almost all tissues on the inner nuclear membrane. The gene for emerin has been mapped to chromosome X (q28).

In addition to domains that target the membrane, emerin has been reported to interact with A and B type lamins and actin in the nucleus. The hydrophobic C-terminal region appears to be the important domain in targeting emerin to the membrane. The N-terminal region is directed to the nucleoplasm. One postulated function of emerin is to stabilize the nuclear membrane and provide structural support in an environment in which the nucleus is subject to mechanical stress. This might explain the effect of a deficiency on muscle, heart and joints: all of which are actively moving organs (Ellis et al., 1999; Fairley et al., 1999; Ognibene et al., 1999; Ostlund; et al., 1999; Tsuchiya et al., 1999)

Absence or abnormalities of a protein that weaken the interaction of the neuroplasm with the nuclear envelope may be associated with a characteristic clinical picture with cardiac abnormalities, conduction defects, joint contractures and slowly progressive weakness in a scapuloperoneal distribution (see Chapter 23). This is known as Emery–Dreifuss dystrophy and, as expected, is inherited as an X-linked recessive.

Lamin A

Lamin A is a member of another family of nuclear laminar proteins. It is coded by a gene on chromosome 1q11–23.

The same gene codes lamin C, which is produced by alternate splicing. Lamin A, B_1, B_2 and C co-localize with emerin, but B_1 is absent in skeletal muscle and heart. Perhaps the absence of a protein that could potentially compensate for the absence of lamin A/C or emerin is another reason why there is selective involvement of these tissues. Abnormalities in the gene for lamin A are associated with an autosomal dominant illness that is clinically identical to emerin deficiency. (Manilal et al., 1999; Taylor et al., 1998; Manilal et al., 1998; Bonne et al., 1999).

Other

None is known as yet.

Associated with the mitochondria

Most of the muscle mitochondrial diseases, and they are legion, result from perturbations in enzyme activity rather than from structural abnormalities. The large-scale deletion seen in Kearns–Sayre syndrome causes structural alterations in the mitochondria as well as enzymatic abnormalities.

Associated with the contractile apparatus

The basic structure of the myofibril is the familiar array of thick and thin filaments with actin and myosin as the main constituents. It is probable that a serious mutation in either of these proteins would be lethal. Troponin and tropomyosin are other familiar proteins involved in the process of contraction. The other structural proteins are less well known and, athough the integrity of the sarcomere is a major part of their function, they may also have a more active role. For the purpose of this classification they will be termed structural proteins.

Titin

Titin is a giant protein of 3 MDa. It extends from the Z line to the M line and maintains the integrity of the sarcomere. It is the third most abundant protein in muscle and is encoded by a gene on chromosome 2q24. It is thought to contribute to the passive elastic force in muscle. It also provides the blueprint for sarcomere assembly and positions myosin filaments by linking them to the Z line. It binds to and promotes the polymerization of actin. It associates with alpha actinin and stabilizes actomyosin.

At the time of writing, no diseases have been associated with titin abnormalities (Eilertsen et al., 1997; Granzier et al., 1997; Pelin et al., 1997; Astier et al., 1998; Fougerousse et al., 1998; Gilbert et al., 1998; Linke et al., 1998; Littlefield and Fowler, 1998; Means, 1998; Stromer, 1998; Tatsumi et al., 1998; Trombitas et al., 1998; Gregorio et al., 1999; Soeno et al., 1999)

Nebulin

Nebulin is another of the large proteins (800 kDa). Its C-terminal region integrates into the Z disc and the N-terminal region projects into the I band. It may provide a molecular template to regulate the length of the actin filament. The genetic defect in autosomal recessive nemaline myopathy, one of the congenital myopathies often associated with respiratory difficulties, has been localized to chromosome 2q21–q22, the locus of the nebulin gene but outside the locus for titin (Pelin et al., 1997; Littlefield and Fowler, 1998; Stromer, 1998; Tatsumi et al., 1998).

Alpha-tropomyosin

Nemaline myopathy has also been inherited in autosomal dominant form, and an abnormality of the gene for tropomyosin has been found in an affected family (Goebel, 1996, 1998; Wallgren-Pettersson and Laing, 1996; North et al., 1997; Thomas, 1997; Pelin et al., 1999)

Associated with the sarcolemmal membrane

There are a number of structural proteins that form a chain linking the contractile apparatus with the extracellular matrix. They confer stability to membranes that are subject to the considerable mechanical stress of contraction. The first described and best known is dystrophin, but a number of others are of importance. Absence of all or any of these proteins may cause a progressive weakness marked by very high serum creatine kinase levels, muscle pains and a good deal of clinical heterogeneity in terms of the severity of the illness.

Dystrophin

Dystrophin is a large protein (427 kDa) that is coded by a gene on the short arm of the X chromosome. Dystrophin is related to spectrin and other structural proteins and consists of two ends separated by a long, flexible, rodlike region. The N-terminus binds to the actin molecule, and the C-terminus, which is rich in cysteine, links dystrophin to a complex of glycoproteins in the sarcolemma. This dystrophin–glycoprotein complex is vital for normal muscle function. There are also two shortened forms of dystrophin, Dp140 and Dp71, which may play a role in other tissues such as brain, although this role has not yet been defined.

Dystrophin deficiency causes the well-known clinical entity Duchenne muscular dystrophy, or pseudohypertrophic muscular dystrophy. There is some correlation between the cognitive problems in Duchenne dystrophy and the quantity of Dp140 and Dp71. Becker dystrophy, the milder form, is often associated with a reduced amount of an abnormal dystrophin rather than its complete absence. There are however, some striking exceptions to the correlation between genotype and phenotype (Culligan et al., 1998; Roberts and Bobrow, 1998).

Utrophin

Utrophin is coded by an autosomal gene and is a striking homologue of dystrophin. In normal muscle this 395 kDa protein is concentrated at the neuromuscular and myotendinous junctions, and only in the case of some of the muscular dystrophies does its territory spread to include other regions of the sarcolemmal membrane. As for dystrophin, there are isoforms (Up71 and Up140) which are present in skeletal muscle. At the present time, there is no disease linked to utrophin deficiency (Culligan et al., 1998; Teijeira et al., 1998; Gramolini et al., 1999; Infante and Huszagh, 1999; Wilson et al., 1999).

The glycoprotein complex

Dystrophin is attached to a complex of glycoproteins. These are often described as the dystrophin-related proteins. One is a 156 kDa transmembrane protein, β-dystroglycan, which is connected to α-dystroglycan, itself attached to laminin. This forms the essential link between the contractile protein actin and the extracellular matrix.

The normal function of this link also depends upon the presence of other members of the complex, the sarcoglycans. There are four or possibly five sarcoglycans, sarcoglycans, α, β, γ and δ and these are associated with each other as a complex that is inserted into the membrane. This complex assembly is dependent on the simultaneous synthesis of all four sarcoglycans. This probably accounts for the fact that if any one is abnormal, the others are not likely to find their place in the sarcolemma.

Recent additions to the group are the syntrophins, sarcospan and dystrobrevin. Sarcospan is a unique 25 kDa member of the group. It localizes and co-purifies with dystrophin and spans the sarcolemmal membrane. Syntrophins are a family of proteins (α_1, β_1 and β_2) that are part of the sarcoglycan complex. They are involved in nitric oxide synthase activity and may confer some signalling potential on the complex. Dystrobrevin was initially identified as a synaptic protein in the electric organ of the electric eel. It is a protein that is phosphorylated by tyrosine kinase. There are two forms, α and β. Beta-dystrobrevin is present in many tissues. Alpha-dystrobrevin is found largely in muscle and brain and complexes with dystrophin (enriched at the neuromuscular junction), utrophin and Dp71. This form is tightly associated with the membrane and with syntrophin. It may render the glycoprotein complex sensitive to phosphorylation (Culligan et al., 1998; Holt and Campbell, 1998; Peters et al., 1998; Araishi et al., 1999; Crosbie et al., 1999; Fuhrer et al., 1999; Lumeng et al., 1999; Montanaro et al., 1999; Vainzof et al., 1999; Wakayama et al., 1999)

Abnormalities in the dystroglycans, dystrobrevins, syntrophins and sarcospan are likely but are yet to be discovered.

Deficiencies in the sarcoglycans may explain our historical confusion in regard to limb girdle dystrophies (Bushby, 1999). Some of these are inherited as autosomal dominants (type 1 or LGMD1) others as autosomal recessive (LGMD2). In the category that follows, the relevant limb girdle dystrophy is indicated.

Alpha-sarcoglycan deficiency (LGMD2D)
Alpha-sarcoglycan is coded by a gene on chromosome 17q12–21. It is inherited as an autosomal recessive. Manifesting with varying degrees of severity, the clinical picture may resemble dystrophin deficiency with features common to the whole group of high serum creatine kinase levels, weakness and some muscle pains.

Beta-sarcoglycan deficiency (LGMD2E)
Beta-sarcoglycan is coded on chromosome 4q12 and is also inherited as an autosomal recessive. Originally described in the Amish population southern Indiana, it has now been seen in other areas.

Gamma-sarcoglycan deficiency (LGMD2C)
The gene for γ-sarcoglycan is on chromosome 13q12. Gamma-sarcoglycan deficiency is another autosomal recessive disorder and causes a severe congenital autosomal recessive muscular dystrophy that was described several years ago.

Delta-sarcoglycan deficiency (LGMD2F)
LGMD2F is an autosomal recessive disease caused by an abnormality in δ-sarcoglycan with the affected gene on chromosome 5q33–34.

Laminin
Laminin-2 is a constituent of the basal lamina that links to dystroglycan and that provides structural support in the extracellular matrix. It comprises three dissimilar chains: α2, formerly known as merosin, β1 and γ1. The N-termini separate to form a cross-like structure, and the other end of the molecule attaches to the dystroglycan complex.

Deficiency of the α2-chain
The α2-chain is coded on chromosome 6q2 and the defect causes another autosomal recessive disease. The deficiency was originally described as causing a severe congenital dystrophy, but there is a good deal of heterogeneity in the clinical picture. An unusual feature is the presence of white matter changes seen by magnetic resonance imaging in many of the patients.

Deficiency of the β1-chain
When any of the membrane-associated glycoproteins are missing, it is possible, even probable, that others will be absent as a secondary phenomenon. Isolated deficiency of laminin β1-chain has been described in a clinical entity similar to limb girdle dystrophy (Li et al., 1997). Confirmatory reports will be needed.

Integrins
Integrins are important structural molecules joining fibres and providing structural strength. The α_7-subunit, which is involved in differentiation and myogenesis, is expressed mainly in skeletal and cardiac muscle. In adult muscle, the α_{7A}- and α_{7B}-subunits are mainly found at myotendinous junctions, but they also occur in the neuromuscular junctions and along the sarcolemmal membrane. Integrin $\alpha_7 \beta_1$ is a specific receptor for laminin-1 and provides a linkage between fibre and extracellular matrix that is independent

of the dystrophin–glycoprotein complex (Mayer et al., 1997; Wei et al., 1999).

Integrin α_7 deficiency has been described associated with a congenital myopathy. The responsible gene is on chromosome 12q13 and the disorder is inherited as an autosomal recessive.

Caveolin 3

Caveolae or little caves are small invaginations in the plasma membrane that are present in most types of cell. One family of proteins in this structure are the caveolins. These are integrated into the structural framework of the caveolae and also play a part in signal transduction and cellular transport, particularly cholesterol transport. Caveolin 3 is specific to muscle. Caveolins form a scaffold onto which many signalling molecules can assemble. In muscle, caveolin 3 is found in the region of the T-tubules in the plasma membrane (Crosbie et al., 1998; Gossrau, 1998; McNally et al., 1998; Minetti et al., 1998; Schlegel et al., 1998, 1999; Galbiati et al., 1999; Ralston and Ploug, 1999).

Caveolin deficiency has been described in association with a form of limb girdle dystrophy (LGMD1C) that is dominantly inherited.

Dysferlin

Dysferlin is an unique protein associated with the sarcolemmal membrane and coded by a gene on chromosome 2p12–14. This gene shows no homology to any known mammalian gene but does have a relative in the *Caenorhabditis elegans* spermatogenesis factor fer-1, hence the name dysferlin. It may turn out to be a structural protein and is listed here because of its membrane association, but it may be better placed in the 'other structural proteins'. Two clinical pictures are associated with a seemingly identical abnormality of the protein: Miyoshi myopathy is a predominantly distal muscle wasting and LGMD2B is a proximal weakness. Both are inherited as autosomal recessive disorders. The different phenotypes may be associated with some modifier gene or factor (Bashir et al., 1998; Anderson et al., 1999).

Other structural proteins

Plectin

Plectin is a widely distributed protein that is a cytoskeletal linker and provides a scaffold for the cell. It maintains the integrity of mechanically stressed cells and is present in heart, skin and muscle. It interacts with other proteins including actin. In muscle it is associated with the Z disc which it links with intermediate filaments (Schroder et al., 1997; Andra et al., 1998; Gregory and Brown, 1998; Wiche, 1998).

A defect in plectin is responsible for the disease epidermolysis bullosa muscular dystrophy. This is inherited as an autosomal recessive and is caused by an abnormality in the plectin gene. Skin blistering and scarring occur in early childhood and are followed by later proximal weakness.

Collagen VI

Collagen exists in several different forms. Microfibrillar collagen VI is a major factor in cell-matrix adhesion in muscle. It links strongly with the collagen in the basement membrane. The various subunit chains, $\alpha 1$, $\alpha 2$ and $\alpha 3$, form dimers and tetramers during the assembly and secretion process. The $\alpha 1$- and $\alpha 2$-subunits are coded on chromosome 21q22.3 and the $\alpha 3$-subunit is coded on chromosome 2q37. Mutation in these genes is responsible for an autosomal dominant childhood muscle weakness associated with contractures (Bethlem myopathy). The mutant collagen is incapable of proper assembly into the normal structure (Bonaldo et al., 1998; Jobsis et al., 1999; Lamande et al., 1999; Pepe et al., 1999).

Fukutin

Fukutin is a secreted protein that is probably found in the extracellular matrix. At present, it is thought not to be associated with the membrane although it may interact with membrane proteins and reinforce the stability of the membrane. The gene for fukutin is on chromosome 9 and is different from any gene of known function. In patients with an autosomal recessive severe muscular dystrophy with neurological abnormalities, there is a segment inserted into the untranslated $3'$ region of the gene. This dystrophy is known as Fukuyama disease, hence the name of the protein (Kobayashi et al., 1998).

Contractile proteins

Primary disorders of actin and myosin have not yet been characterized even in those diseases such as the fulminant myopathy seen in the intensive care environment (critical illness myopathy), which seem to show lysis of the filaments. Perhaps a mutation in the contractile apparatus would be a disturbance so fundamental that it would not be compatible with life.

Proteins of the ion channels

The various channels that control the flow of electrolytes into and out of the muscle are of fundamental importance. They are of several types. Disorders resulting from malfunctioning ion channels are known as channelopathies.

The calcium channel

The calcium channel is made of five subunits, α_1, which is the most important and forms the ion pore across the membrane, α_2, β, γ and δ. The type of α_1-subunit determines the sensitivity of the calcium channel. In muscle, this is sensitive to dihydropyridine (an L-type channel). The subunit is formed from four similar transmembrane regions or domains, I–IV, each made of six membrane-spanning proteins, S1–S6, all linked in series by loops that extend into the cytoplasm or extracellularly. S4 is highly charged, by virtue of the richness of positively charged amino acids, and may confer voltage sensitivity to the channel.

Mutations in the gene on chromosome 1q31–32, are associated with the autosomal dominant hypokalaemic periodic paralysis.

The ryanodine receptor

In muscle, the calcium channels are linked to the ryanodine receptor calcium release channel, which controls the flux of calcium from the sarcoplasmic reticulum into the cytoplasm. The ryanodine receptor exists in several forms, RYR1 and RYR3 being important in muscle. It is located in the triadic junctions and provides a means of calcium release and mobilization in excitation contraction–coupling. Ryanodine receptors are made of four identical subunits, each of which is about 550 kDa.

The gene for the ryanodine receptor is located on chromosome 19q13.1. Mutations result in central core disease, a congenital myopathy, and malignant hyperthermia, a potentially devastating and fatal condition.

The sodium channel

The sodium channel is very similar in its make-up to the calcium channel. The α-subunit, a 260 kDa protein, confers the channel activity with four domains made of six membrane-spanning proteins connected in similar fashion. Again the S4 segment is highly charged, which might make it suitable for responding to voltage changes.

Mutations of chromosome 17q31 alter channel activity and give rise to autosomal dominant hyperkalaemic (potassium-sensitive) periodic paralysis. Paramyotonia congenita and an unusual myotonic condition are also associated with sodium channel abnormalities.

The chloride channel

The chloride channel has a different structure to that of the sodium and calcium channels, being a homotetramer in which each unit contains about 1000 amino acid residues.

Autosomal dominant and autosomal recessive forms of myotonia congenita are seen with abnormalities in the gene for the chloride channel on chromosome 7q35.

Proteins associated with enzyme activity

Energy-related processes

The energy-related enzymes may be broadly classed as glycolytic, lipid metabolizing, mitochondrial and other ATP support systems. The glycolytic defects predictably cause fatigue weakness and pain early in exercise. Disorders of lipid or fatty acid metabolism are only symptomatic later in exercise when fatty acids are mobilized. Mitochondrial disorders may cause symptoms of heavy exercise at a low work load

Enzymes of glycolysis known to cause muscle diseases when defective include: muscle phosphorylase, phosphorylase kinase, phosphofructokinase, phosphoglycerate kinase, phosphoglycerate mutase and lactic dehydrogenase (see Chapter 28).

Muscle disease is also caused by defects in lipid metabolism, including carnitine palmityltransferase deficiency and defects affecting β-oxidation.

There are a number of mitochondrial enzyme defects that have been identified in muscle diseases including those involved in complexes I and III and cytochrome oxidase. Mitochondrial defects are myriad and often cause neurological problems rather than muscular symptoms. The listing of these is out of the scope of this chapter.

Adenylate deaminase deficiency

Deficiency of adenylate deaminase is a common autosomal recessive disease. The association of this with a muscle disease is controversial. Although this enzyme provides ATP to the cell, muscle performance is not impeded by its absence.

Non-energy-related processes

Calcium-activated neutral protease 3 (calpain 3)

Calpain 3 is a cytosolic protease. Proteases are ubiquitous and the muscle-specific enzyme is the p94 homologue. Being a protease, it plays a part in the disassembly of sarcomeric proteins, but it may also have a regulatory role in modulation of transcription factors. Loss of the function of this enzyme leads to activation of other proteases. Interestingly it also interacts with titin.

The gene for this enzyme is on chromosome 15q15.1–21.1 and a deficiency of calpain 3 is the cause of a form of muscular dystrophy first identified in the Isle Reunion, later in the Amish of northern Indiana and still later worldwide. The illness has been categorized as limb girdle dystrophy type 2A. This is another of the dystrophies with marked elevation of serum creatine kinase (Huang and Forsberg, 1998; Kinbara et al., 1998; Baghdiguian et al., 1999; Herasse et al., 1999; Richard et al., 1999).

Myotonin protein kinase

Myotonic dystrophy is a disease that is difficult to classify. Clinically, it should involve an abnormality in the membrane. The genetic abnormality is a CTG repeat in the 3′ untranslated region of a gene located on chromosome 19q13.3. The function of the gene product is not precisely known, although from the projected structure it is thought to be a serine protein kinase.

Myotubularin

Myotubularin is a protein of a family that is conserved in many species. It is a phosphatase with dual specificity, acting on tyrosine and serine. It probably acts with components of the regulatory machinery and signalling pathways involved in growth and differentiation (Cui et al., 1998; Laporte et al., 1998).

Myotubularin is coded in part by a gene on chromosome Xq28 and abnormalities in myotubularin are associated with the X-linked illness myotubular myopathy.

Other proteins

Although other proteins associated with the nucleus, mitochondria, contractile apparatus and membrane could be defective in muscle disease, only one protein, associated with the nucleus, has been identified to date.

Associated with the nucleus

PolyA-binding protein

Oculopharyngeal dystrophy is an autosomal dominant disease with preferential involvement of eye and pharyngeal muscles in the older person. It has been associated with abnormalities in a gene on chromosome 14q11–13. This gene encodes a protein that is a polyA-binding protein. It is localized to the nucleus and is involved in the process of polyadenylation of messenger RNA among other things (Brais et al., 1998; Mezei et al., 1999).

Abnormal protein storage

Desmin

Desmin is a protein of the intermediate filament family (type III). It accumulates in a number of myopathies; in particular there is one that affects the muscle, heart and intestine and may cause mental retardation.

A French family with such a myopathy demonstrated an abnormality in a gene on chromosome 11q21–23, which codes for a small heat shock protein with molecular chaperone activity known as α_B-crystallin. Transfection of this gene in muscle cell culture resulted in accumulations of desmin (Vicart et al., 1998; Caron et al., 1999; Fidzianska et al., 1999).

'Amyloid' type proteins

In the disorder known as inclusion body disease there is an accumulation of abnormal proteins including amyloid, β-amyloid precursor protein, ubiquitin and tau protein. There are two forms of inclusion body disease: the common sporadic disease is associated with inflammatory changes (sporadic inclusion body myositis); the familial form has been linked to chromosome 9 and is a quadriceps-sparing myopathy without inflammatory cells.

Secondary diseases

Inflammatory and autoimmune myopathies

There are a number of inflammatory and autoimmune disorders giving rise to muscle disease: polymyositis, dermatomyositis, polymyalgia rheumatica, myositis associated with various infections (acquired immunodeficiency syndrome, *Staphylococcus aureus* abscess, viral myositis, cystocercosis, trichinosis, toxoplasmosis, etc.), sarcoidosis and eosinophilic myositis.

Associated with external toxins

Myopathies can also result from external toxins, particularly cholesterol-lowering agents, myotoxins (venom, nofensin, chloroquine) and from myoglobinuria associated with various drugs.

Remote effects of systemic disease

Cachexia, disuse and muscle-wasting conditions following solid organ transplantation and immunosuppression can all result in muscle dysfunction. Myopathies can also be associated with endocrine abnormalities: thyroid, adrenal, pituitary.

Table 18.3. Conditions for which a gene but not a gene product is identified

Chromosome	Locus	Disorder
1	q11–21	Autosomal dominant limb girdle dystrophy type 1B
2	p12–14	Autosomal recessive distal myopathy
4	q35	Facioscapulohumeral dystrophy
5	q22–34	Autosomal dominant limb girdle dystrophy type 1A
9	p1–q1	?Distal myopathy with rimmed vacuoles
	q31–34.1	Autosomal recessive limb girdle dystrophy type 2H
17	q11–12	Autosomal recessive limb girdle dystrophy type 2G

Conditions for which only the gene has been identified

There are a number of conditions that have been associated with a genetic abnormality without identification of the protein product. It is only a matter of time before this is achieved. The entity will then move into one of the above categories. In the meantime, these conditions are listed by the chromosome involved (Table 18.3).

Whatever is; is

All nature is but art unknown to thee
All chance, direction which thou canst not see;
All discord, harmony not understood;
All partial evil, universal good;
And, spite of pride, in erring reason's spite,
One truth is clear, Whatever is, is right.

An essay on Man. Alexander Pope

There are still those entities that, either by clinical art or laboratory science, have been recognized, for which no clue has yet fallen as to their fundamental nature. They are simply listed here and will hopefully be moved as progress is made.

    proximal myotonic myopathy
    Walker Warburg disease
    Muscle–eye–brain disease
    Aches, cramps, pains and fatigue disease
    Fibromyalgia?
    Exercise intolerance
    Chronic fatigue syndrome?

It would be meet to close this section with some deep insights into the nature of neuromuscular diseases. My successors in future years will undoubtedly be able to do so. For me to attempt this would be ludicrous; the blind man giving order to the rainbow. It is yet perhaps worth remembering that the retina and cortex of the sighted are simply interpreting electromagnetic radiations and converting them into an unverifiable illusion of grace and beauty. 'One truth is clear, Whatever is; is right.'

References

Anderson, L. V., Davison, K., Moss, J. A. et al. (1999). Dysferlin is a plasma membrane protein and is expressed early in human development. *Hum. Mol. Genet.* **8**, 855–861.

Andra, K., Nikolic, B., Stocher, M., Drenckhahn, D. and Wiche, G. (1998). Not just scaffolding: plectin regulates actin dynamics in cultured cells. *Genes Dev.* **12**, 3442–3451.

Araishi, K., Sasaoka, T., Imamura, M. et al. (1999). Loss of the sarcoglycan complex and sarcospan leads to muscular dystrophy in beta-sarcoglycan-deficient mice. *Hum. Mol. Genet.* **8**, 1589–1598.

Astier, C., Raynaud, F., Lebart, M. C., Roustan, C. and Benyamin, Y. (1998). Binding of a native titin fragment to actin is regulated by PIP2. *FEBS Lett.* **429**, 95–98.

Baghdiguian, S., Martin, M., Richard, I., Pons, F., Astier, C. and Bourg, N. (1999). Calpain 3 deficiency is associated with myonuclear apoptosis and profound perturbation of the IkappaB alpha/NF-kappaB pathway in limb-girdle muscular dystrophy type 2A. *Nat. Med.* **5**, 503–511.

Bashir, R., Britton, S., Strachan, T. et al. (1998). A gene related to *Caenorhabditis elegans* spermatogenesis factor fer-1 is mutated in limb-girdle muscular dystrophy type 2B. *Nat. Genet.* **20**, 37–42.

Bonaldo, P., Braghetta, P., Zanetti, M., Piccolo, S., Volpin, D. and Bressan, G. M. (1998). Collagen VI deficiency induces early onset myopathy in the mouse: an animal model for Bethlem myopathy. *Hum. Mol. Genet..* **7**, 2135–2140.

Bonne, G., Di Barletta, M. R., Varnous, S. et al. (1999). Mutations in the gene encoding lamin A/C cause autosomal dominant Emery–Dreifuss muscular dystrophy. *Nat. Genet.* **21**, 285–288.

Brais, B., Bouchard, J. P., Xie, Y. G. et al. (1998). Short GCG expansions in the *PABP2* gene cause oculopharyngeal muscular dystrophy. *Nat. Genet.* **18**, 164–167.

Bushby, K. M. (1999). Making sense of the limb-girdle muscular dystrophies. *Brain* **122**, 1403–1420.

Caron, A., Gohel, C., Mollaret, K., Morello, R. and Chapon, F. (1999). Study of some components of the cytoskeleton in muscular disorders with nonspecific cytoplasmic bodies. *Acta Neuropathol.* **97**, 267–274.

Crosbie, R. H., Yamada, H., Venzke, D. P., Lisanti, M. P. and Campbell, K. P. (1998). Caveolin-3 is not an integral component of the dystrophin glycoprotein complex. *FEBS Lett.* **427**, 279–282.

Crosbie, R. H., Lebakken, C. S., Holt, K. H. et al. (1999). Membrane targeting and stabilization of sarcospan is mediated by the sarcoglycan subcomplex. *J. Cell Biol.* **145**, 153–165.

Cui, X., De Vivo, I., Slany, R., Miyamoto, A., Firestein, R. and Cleary, M. L. (1998). Association of SET domain and myotubularin-related proteins modulates growth control. *Nat. Genet.* **18**, 331–337.

Culligan, K. G., Mackey, A. J., Finn, D. M., Maguire, P. B. and Ohlendieck, K. (1998). Role of dystrophin isoforms and associated proteins in muscular dystrophy (review). *Int. J. Mol. Med.* **2**, 639–648.

Eilertsen, K. J., Kazmierski, S. T. and Keller, T. C. III (1997). Interaction of alpha-actinin with cellular titin. *Eur. J. Cell. Biol.* **74**, 361–364.

Ellis, J. A., Yates, J. R., Kendrick-Jones, J. and Brown, C. A. (1999). Changes at P183 of emerin weaken its protein–protein interactions resulting in X-linked Emery–Dreifuss muscular dystrophy. *Hum. Genet.* **104**, 262–268.

Fairley, E. A., Kendrick-Jones, J. and Ellis, J. A. (1999). The Emery–Dreifuss muscular dystrophy phenotype arises from aberrant targeting and binding of emerin at the inner nuclear membrane. *J. Cell. Sci.* **112**, 2571–2582.

Fidzianska, A., Drac, H. and Kaminska, A. M. (1999). Familial inclusion body myopathy with desmin storage. *Acta Neuropathol.* **97**, 509–514.

Fougerousse, F., Durand, M., Suel, L. et al. (1998). Expression of genes (*CAPN3*, *SGCA*, *SGCB* and *TTN*) involved in progressive muscular dystrophies during early human development. *Genomics* **48**, 145–156.

Fuhrer, C., Gautam, M., Sugiyama, J. E. and Hall, Z. W. (1999). Roles of rapsyn and agrin in interaction of postsynaptic proteins with acetylcholine receptors. *J. Neurosci.* **19**, 6405–6416.

Galbiati, F., Volonte, D., Minetti, C., Chu, J. B. and Lisanti, M. P. (1999). Phenotypic behavior of caveolin-3 mutations that cause autosomal dominant limb girdle muscular dystrophy (LGMD-1C). Retention of LGMD-1C caveolin-3 mutants within the Golgi complex. *J. Biol. Chem.* **274**, 25632–25641.

Gilbert, R., Cohen, J. A., Pardo, S., Basu, A. and Fischman, D. A. (1998). Identification of the A-band localization domain of myosin binding proteins C and H (MyBP-C, MyBP-H) in skeletal muscle. *J. Cell Sci.* **112**, 69–79.

Goebel, H. H. (1996). Congenital myopathies. *Semin. Pediatr. Neurol.* **3**, 152–161.

Goebel, H. H. (1998). Congenital myopathies with inclusion bodies: a brief review. *Neuromusc. Disord.* **8**, 162–168.

Gossrau, R. (1998). Caveolin-3 and nitric oxide synthase I in healthy and diseased skeletal muscle. *Acta Histochem.* **100**, 99–112.

Gramolini, A. O., Angus, L. M., Schaeffer, L. et al. (1999). Induction of utrophin gene expression by heregulin in skeletal muscle cells: role of the N-box motif and GA binding protein. *Proc. Natl. Acad. Sci. USA* **96**, 3223–3227.

Granzier, H., Kellermayer, M., Helmes, M. and Trombitas, K. (1997). Titin elasticity and mechanism of passive force development in rat cardiac myocytes probed by thin-filament extraction. *Biophys. J.* **73**, 2043–2053.

Gregorio, C. C., Granzier, H., Sorimachi, H. and Labeit, S. (1999). Muscle assembly: a titanic achievement? *Curr. Opin. Cell. Biol.* **11**, 18–25.

Gregory, S. L. and Brown, N. H. (1998). *Kakapo*, a gene required for adhesion between and within cell layers in *Drosophila*, encodes a large cytoskeletal linker protein related to plectin and dystrophin. *J. Cell. Biol.* **143**, 1271–1282.

Herasse, M., Ono, Y., Fougerousse, F. et al. (1999). Expression and functional characteristics of calpain 3 isoforms generated through tissue-specific transcriptional and posttranscriptional events. *Mol. Cell Biol.* **19**, 4047–4055.

Holt, K. H. and Campbell, K. P. (1998). Assembly of the sarcoglycan complex. Insights for muscular dystrophy. *J. Biol. Chem.* **273**, 34667–34670.

Huang, J. and Forsberg, N. E. (1998) Role of calpain in skeletal-muscle protein degradation. *Proc. Natl. Acad. Sci. USA* **95**, 12100–12105.

Infante, J. P. and Huszagh, V. A. (1999). Mechanisms of resistance to pathogenesis in muscular dystrophies. *Mol. Cell. Biochem.* **195**, 155–167.

Jobsis, G. J., Boers, J. M., Barth, P. G. and de Visser, M. (1999). Bethlem myopathy: a slowly progressive congenital muscular dystrophy with contractures. *Brain* **122**, 649–655.

Kinbara, K., Sorimachi, H., Ishiura, S. and Suzuki, K. (1998). Skeletal muscle-specific calpain, p49: structure and physiological function. *Biochem. Pharmacol.* **56**, 415–420.

Kobayashi, K., Nakahori, Y., Miyake, M. et al. (1998). An ancient retrotransposal insertion causes Fukuyama-type congenital muscular dystrophy. *Nature* **394**, 388–392.

Lamande, S. R., Shields, K. A., Kornberg, A. J., Shield, L. K. and Bateman, J. F. (1999). Bethlem myopathy and engineered collagen VI triple helical deletions prevent intracellular multimer assembly and protein secretion. *J. Biol. Chem.* **274**, 21817–21822.

Laporte, J., Blondeau, F., Buj-Bello, A. et al. (1998). Characterization of the myotubularin dual specificity phosphatase gene family from yeast to human. *Hum. Mol. Genet.* **7**, 1703–1712.

Li, M., Dickson, D. W. and Spiro, A. J. (1997). Abnormal expression of laminin beta 1 chain in skeletal muscle of adult-onset limb-girdle muscular dystrophy. *Arch. Neurol.* **54**, 1457–1461.

Linke, W. A., Stockmeier, M. R., Ivemeyer, M., Hosser, H. and Mundel, P. (1998). Characterizing titin's I-band Ig domain region as an entropic spring. *J. Cell. Sci.* **111**, 1567.

Littlefield, R. and Fowler, V. M. (1998). Defining actin filament length in striated muscle: rulers and caps or dynamic stability? *Annu. Rev. Cell. Dev. Biol.* **14**, 487–525

Lumeng, C., Phelps, S., Crawford, G. E., Walden, P. D., Barald, K. and Chamberlain, J. S. (1999). Interactions between beta 2-syntrophin and a family of microtubule-associated serine/threonine kinases. *Nat. Neurosci.* **2**, 611–617.

Manilal, S., Nguyen, T. M. and Morris, G. E. (1998). Colocalization of emerin and lamins in interphase nuclei and changes during mitosis. *Biochem. Biophys. Res. Commun.* **249**, 643–647.

Manilal, S., Sewry, C. A., Pereboev, A. et al. (1999). Distribution of emerin and lamins in the heart and implications for Emery–Dreifuss muscular dystrophy. *Hum. Mol. Genet.* **8**, 353–359.

Mayer, U., Saher, G., Fassler, R. et al. (1997). Absence of integrin alpha 7 causes a novel form of muscular dystrophy. *Nat. Genet.* **17**, 318–323.

McNally, E. M., de Sa Moreira, E., Duggan, D. J. et al. (1998). Caveolin-3 in muscular dystrophy. *Hum. Mol. Genet.* **7**, 871–877.

Means, A. R. (1998). The clash in titin [news; comment]. *Nature* **395**, 846–847.

Mezei, M. M., Mankodi, A., Brais, B. et al., (1999). Minimal expansion of the GCG repeat in the PABP2 gene does not predispose to sporadic inclusion body myositis. *Neurology* **52**, 669–670.

Minetti, C., Sotgia, F., Bruno, C. et al. (1998). Mutations in the caveolin-3 gene cause autosomal dominant limb-girdle muscular dystrophy. *Nat. Genet.* **18**, 365–368.

Montanaro, F., Lindenbaum, M. and Carbonetto, S. (1999). Alpha-dystroglycan is a laminin receptor involved in extracellular matrix assembly on myotubes and muscle cell viability. *J. Cell. Biol.* **145**, 1325–1340

North, K. N., Laing, N. G. and Wallgren-Pettersson, C. (1997). Nemaline myopathy: current concepts. The ENMC International Consortium on Nemaline Myopathy. *J. Med. Genet.* **34**, 705–713.

Ognibene, A., Sabatelli, P., Petrini, S. et al. (1999). Nuclear changes in a case of X-linked Emery–Dreifuss muscular dystrophy. *Muscle Nerve* **22**, 864–869.

Ostlund, C., Ellenberg, J., Hallberg, E., Lippincott-Schwartz, J. and Worman, H. J. (1999). Intracellular trafficking of emerin, the Emery–Dreifuss muscular dystrophy protein. *J. Cell. Sci.* **122**, 1709–1719.

Pelin, K., Ridanpaa, M., Donner, K. et al. (1997). Refined localisation of the genes for nebulin and titin on chromosome 2q allows the assignment of nebulin as a candidate gene for autosomal recessive nemaline myopathy. *Eur. J. Hum. Genet.* **5**, 229–234.

Pelin, K., Hilpela, P., Donner, K. et al. (1999). Mutations in the nebulin gene associated with autosomal recessive nemaline myopathy. *Proc. Natl. Acad. Sci. USA* **96**, 2305–2310

Pepe, G., Bertini, E., Giusti, B. et al. (1999). A novel de novo mutation in the triple helix of the *COL6A3* gene in a two-generation Italian family affected by Bethlem myopathy. A diagnostic approach in the mutations' screening of type VI collagen. *Neuromusc. Disord.* **9**, 264–271.

Peters, M. F., Sadoulet-Puccio, H. M., Grady, M. R. et al. (1998). Differential membrane localization and intermolecular associations of alpha-dystrobrevin isoforms in skeletal muscle. *J. Cell. Biol.* **142**, 1269–1278.

Ralston, E. and Ploug, T. (1999). Caveolin-3 is associated with the T-tubules of mature skeletal muscle fibers. *Exp. Cell Res.* **246**, 510–515.

Richard, I., Roudaut, C., Saenz, A. et al. (1999). Calpainopathy – a survey of mutations and polymorphisms. *Am. J. Hum. Genet.* **64**, 1524–1540.

Roberts, R. G. and Bobrow, M. (1998). Dystrophins in vertebrates and invertebrates. *Hum. Mol. Genet.* **7**, 589–595.

Schlegel, A., Volonte, D., Engelman, J. A. et al. (1998). Crowded little caves: structure and function of caveolae. *Cell Signal.* **10**, 457–463.

Schlegel, A., Schwab, R. B., Scherer, P. E. and Lisanti, M. P. (1999). A role for the caveolin scaffolding domain in mediating the membrane attachment of caveolin-1. The caveolin scaffolding domain is both necessary and sufficient for membrane binding in vitro *J. Biol. Chem.* **274**, 22660–22667.

Schroder, R., Mundegar, R. R., Treusch, M. et al. (1997). Altered distribution of plectin/HD1 in dystrophinopathies. *Eur. J. Cell. Biol.* **74**, 165–171.

Soeno, Y., Yajima, H., Kawamura, Y., Kimura, S., Maruyama, K. and Obinata, T. (1999). Organization of connectin/titin filaments in sarcomeres of differentiating chicken skeletal muscle cells. [In process citation] *Mol. Cell. Biochem.* **190**, 125–131

Stromer, M. H. (1998). The cytoskeleton in skeletal, cardiac and smooth muscle cells. *Histol. Histopathol.* **13**, 283–291.

Tatsumi, R., Hattori, A. and Takahashi, K. (1998). Deterioration of connectin/titin and nebulin filaments by an excess of protease inhibitors. *Biosci. Biotechnol. Biochem.* **62**, 927–934.

Taylor, J., Sewry, C. A., Dubowitz, V. and Muntoni, F. (1998). Early onset, autosomal recessive muscular dystrophy with Emery–Dreifuss phenotype and normal emerin expression. *Neurology* **51**, 1116–1120.

Teijeira, S., Teijeiro, A., Fernandez, R. and Navarro, C. (1998). Subsarcolemmal expression of utrophin in neuromuscular disorders: an immunohistochemical study of 80 cases. *Acta Neuropathol.* **96**, 481–486.

Thomas, C. (1997). Nemaline rod and central core disease: a coexisting Z-band myopathy. *Muscle Nerve* **20**, 893–896.

Trombitas, K., Greaser, M., Labeit, S. et al. (1998). Titin extensibility in situ: entropic elasticity of permanently folded and permanently unfolded molecular segments. *J. Cell. Biol.* **140**, 853–859

Tsuchiya, Y., Hase, A., Ogawa, M., Yorifuji, H. and Arahata, K. (1999). Distinct regions specify the nuclear membrane targeting of emerin, the responsible protein for Emery–Dreifuss muscular dystrophy. *Eur. J. Biochem.* **259**, 859–865.

Vainzof, M., Passos-Bueno, M. R., Pavanello, R. C., Marie, S. K., Oliveira, A. S. and Zatz, M. (1999). Sarcoglycanopathies are responsible for 68% of severe autosomal recessive limb-girdle muscular dystrophy in the Brazilian population. [See comments] *J. Neurol. Sci.* **156**, 44–49.

Vicart, P., Caron, A., Guicheney, P., Li, Z., Prevost, M. C. and Faure, A. (1998). A missense mutation in the alphaB-crystallin chaperone gene causes a desmin-related myopathy. *Nat. Genet.* **20**, 92–95.

Wakayama, Y., Inoue, M., Kojima, H., Murahashi, M., Shibuya, S. and Jimi, T. (1999). Ultrastructural localization of alpha-, beta- and gamma-sarcoglycan and their mutual relation and their relation to dystrophin, beta-dystroglycan and beta-spectrin in normal skeletal myofibre. *Acta Neuropathol.* **97**, 288–296.

Wallgren-Pettersson, C. and Laing, N. (1996). Workshop report: the 40th ENMC sponsored international workshop: nemaline myopathy. *Neuromusc. Disord.* **6**, 389–391.

Wei, Y., Yang, X., Liu, Q., Wilkins, J. A. and Chapman, H. A. (1999). A role for caveolin and the urokinase receptor in integrin-mediated adhesion and signaling. *J. Cell Biol.* **144**, 1285–1294.

Wiche, G. (1998). Role of plectin in cytoskeleton organization and dynamics. [In process citation] *J. Cell Sci.* **111**, 2477–2486

Wilson, J., Putt, W., Jimenez, C. and Edwards, Y. H. (1999). Up71 and Up140, two novel transcripts of utrophin that are homologues of short forms of dystrophin. *Hum. Mol. Genet.* **8**, 1271–1278.

19

Dystrophinopathies

Eric P. Hoffman

Introduction

The dystrophinopathies are the most common form of muscle disease. Clinical presentations generally involve proximal muscle weakness and highly elevated serum creatine kinase levels. Dystrophinopathies are most often progressive disorders, although there are many variants that show variable presentations and progressions.

The dystrophin gene resides on the X chromosome and, consequently, most patients are boys or men. However, approximately 10% of female dystrophy patients can be shown to be manifesting carriers of a primary dystrophinopathy. Complete or near-complete dystrophin deficiency causes Duchenne muscular dystrophy, the most common subtype of muscular dystrophy. Patients present in early childhood and are typically wheelchair-bound by age 11 years. Patients succumb to respiratory or cardiac failure in their teens, unless ventilated. Patients with milder phenotypes have partial deficiencies of dystrophin, typically caused by deletion mutations of the dystrophin gene that are still compatible with translation of a semifunctional protein. Animal models of dystrophin deficiency have been identified (dogs, cats and mice), which have provided a wealth of information on dystrophin biochemistry and the pathophysiology of dystrophin deficiency.

The dystrophin gene is by far the largest gene identified to date, a feature that seems to result in a very high spontaneous mutation rate (1 in 10000 eggs or sperm). The gene is about 2.5 million base pairs, with about 80 exons. The encoded protein is a 427 kDa component of the membrane cytoskeleton of muscle fibres, smooth muscle and neurons. However, there are many additional protein isoforms produced by the gene, most of which have undefined functions in various tissues.

The primary function of 'full-length' muscle dystrophin is to reinforce the myofibre plasma membrane against contraction-induced injury. As such, lengthening contractions and other types of membrane stress are particularly damaging to dystrophin-deficient muscle. The membrane fragility is exacerbated by a series of additional cellular and tissue changes, including inability to regulate local vascular perfusion during exercise as a result of loss of the neuronal isoform of nitric oxide synthetase (nNOS) in myofibres, difficulty in maintaining calcium homeostasis and difficulty in repairing membrane damage from proteases and other physiological and cellular insults to the myofibre.

Treatment of dystrophinopathic patients is generally palliative, although some patients respond well to corticosteroids (prednisone, deflazacort). Considerable recent effort is being placed on experimental therapeutics. These approaches include viral-mediated delivery of the dystrophin gene (adenovirus, adeno-associated virus (AAV)), upregulation of a related protein (utrophin), altering the progressive pathophysiology of the disorder via drug screening and attempts to over-ride certain types of gene mutation in patient muscle.

Historical perspectives

I can well appreciate the difficulty of weaning the mind from the belief that, as all other forms of paralysis are dependent on affections of the nervous system, this must be so too. It is part of our education to learn that the muscular system would be a mass of inert matter, were it not animated by nervous tissue; that by virtue of the association of nervous fibres the latter are endowed with their sensibility and contractility; and I admit that the disturbance of nervous centres may favour the development of granular degeneration in individuals predisposed to it; but my observations have led me to the belief that this same degeneration may and does exist independent of nervous lesion.

> Meryon (1864, p. 210), in response to the suggestion of Duchenne de Bologne that 'granular degeneration of the voluntary muscles' (muscular dystrophy) was a neurogenic disorder.

Worldwide, muscular dystrophy is the most common childhood-lethal inherited disorder of humans. Other well-known paedriatic conditions, such as cystic fibrosis or Tay–Sachs disease, may show a higher incidence than muscular dystrophy in certain ethnic populations (Caucasians or Ashkenazum) but are not as common worldwide. The high incidence of muscular dystrophy in children results from one specific X-linked condition known as 'Duchenne muscular dystrophy', and initial discussions of historical perspectives here will focus on this subtype. For a very thorough, and well-written scholarly record of clinical and scientific discoveries leading to our current state of understanding of this disorder, the reader is referred to Emery and Emery (1995).

The disease which we know as 'Duchenne muscular dystrophy' shows certain enigmatic clinical features, which can be found described in written case reports as early as 1836 (Conte and Gioja, reprinted 1986). In this paper, Conte and Gioja describe two Napolitan brothers who showed proximal weakness beginning around age 8 years. The boys showed increasing clinical severity with age, with progressive tendon flexion contractions of the hips and knees. The calf and deltoid muscles showed marked enlargement, but this hypertrophy of muscle was abnormal in having a wooden, nonpliable texture upon palpation. Nerve sensation and cognitive function appeared intact. Both died in their late teens, one with signs of cardiac hypertrophy. These authors lumped their description of these patients in with many others from their 'Ospedale degl' Incurabili' in Naples, most of whom probably had sequelae of tuberculosis. Without the aid of histopathology, retrospective diagnosis of these patients as having Duchenne muscular dystrophy is speculative. Moreover, no additional patients with similar symptoms were reported. However, the hallmark clinical features of Duchenne muscular dystrophy seemed to be present: early childhood presentation of proximal muscle weakness in male relatives, progressive weakness and wasting, prominent flexion contractures and marked enlargement of the calves and certain other muscles (tongue, deltoid) (Emery and Emery, 1995).

Ten years later, case reports on a pair of affected brothers were published independently by British physicians Richard Partridge (1847, 1848) and William J. Little (1853). Dr Little was quite obviously impressed with the symptoms of these brothers (age 12 years, and 14 years), as he describes in the preface to a series of medical school lectures on various skeletal deformities (Little, 1853, p. 14): 'I append two of the most remarkable cases of abnormal increase in bulk of muscle, combined with contraction and adipose degeneration, with which I have been favoured.' In these reports, the natural history of the patients was described in more detail. Both reported normal birth, but the age at which walking was achieved was considerably later than normal. The gait of one brother was described as remarkable, with the upper body inclined backwards (lordosis) and toe-walking (contractures of the Achilles tendons). Both lost ambulation around age 11 years, with ensuing scoliosis and severe limb contractures. One boy died from pneumonia at around age 14 years. A postmortem of this patient showed enlargement of the gastrocnemius and soleus muscles; however, the tissue was noted as being largely replaced with fat. The tibial muscles were noted to show better preservation of myofibres. Of particular interest was the clear description of Achilles tendon contractures and shoulder girdle weakness (Little, 1853, p. 14): 'Contraction "behind the heels" appeared to commence at age of six, and has gradually increased to the present period [age 14 years]. The shoulders appeared loose, and upper arm very small, "so that a stranger would fear to grasp him by the arms".'

Edward Meryon (1807–80) was the first physician to describe a series of boys from different families, the first to insist that this was a disorder of muscle (and not nerve) and the first to point out the maternal nature of the inheritance pattern (Meryon, 1851, 1852, 1864). He noted that the boys all showed similar clinical symptoms, thus comprising a diagnostic entity of 'granular degeneration of voluntary muscle' leading to progressive muscle weakness (Meryon, 1851, 1852). Nine boys from three unrelated families were studied, with two of the families (six affected boys) showing early childhood onset of proximal muscle weakness, difficulty with running or jumping and problems with climbing stairs. Patients became wheelchair-bound around 11 years of age, and died in their teens. The remaining family with three affected patients showed a later onset and slower progression of the disease; this was likely the condition later to be dubbed Becker muscular dystrophy. Meryon published detailed pathological and microscopic studies emphasizing the normal appearance of the spinal cord and nerves, and he recruited the opinions of other noted histologists of the time who arrived at the same conclusion (Meryon, 1852; Emery and Emery, 1995).

Meryon continued to pursue his interest in cases of granular degeneration of muscle. In his book on forms of paralysis in 1864, he noted the familial nature of the disease and commented on the inheritance pattern (Meryon, 1864, pp. 200–215). He reported seven families with 14 affected males, including a sibship where three sisters each had sons with the disease, and a second family where a father had sons with the disorder with one wife, and not a second, '. . . thus exempting him from suspicion of personal trait'.

He also published an excerpt from a letter of a father who had nine affected sons, with none of his daughters affected (Meryon, 1864, p. 213). Meryon pointed out that the disease could be hereditary and, if so, was through maternal lineages. Definitions of 'heredity', as applied to familial traits, were not yet well codified at this time; the seminal genetic studies of Galton and Mendel were published later in the 1860s. The precise pattern of familial transmission of X-linked recessive traits had been established for haemophilia 60 years earlier, but the conformity of inheritance patterns for haemophilia and muscular dystrophy were not noted until the writings of Gowers (1879).

Given the clear contribution of Edward Meryon to the description of X-linked recessive muscular dystrophy, one might question why the disorder is currently referred to as Duchenne muscular dystrophy instead of 'Meryon's disease'. Emery and Emery (1995) point out that it may simply be a matter of volume of material published, and subsequent promotion of the findings to the medical public. Meryon's primary contribution was a 12 page article in 1852. Sixteen years later, the renowned Duchenne de Boulogne published five extensive articles on the disorder in a single year, totalling 124 pages of text (Duchenne, 1868). Another factor seems to have been the misinterpretation of Meryon's findings by Duchenne (Emery and Emery, 1995). Specifically, Duchenne claimed that Meryon had studied a muscular atrophy secondary to nerve dysfunction, rather than a muscular dystrophy (Duchenne, 1868). Meryon emphatically denied this assertion (Meryon, 1864), although the reluctance of physicians to acknowledge the existence of primary muscle disorders seems to have contributed to the greater visibility of Duchenne's contribution to the description of the disorder.

To underscore the sensitive issue of whether this was a disorder of muscle (Meryon) and not of nerve (Duchenne) is the following quote from Meryon (1864, p. 204). It may also be pertinent to point out that Meryon aptly describes the progressive nature of the histopathology, and in other writings refers to the 'breakdown of the sarcolemma' as a distinctive feature of the histopathology. Both these features become key aspects of the molecular pathophysiology to be discovered much more recently.

I have not observed the great abundance of fat globules which he [Duchenne] speaks of, except where every vestige of striated muscular fibres has disappeared; and there the vital power which belongs to the higher products of animal organization is so far weakened as to allow those tissues to yield to the physical and chemical influences that surround them, and to degenerate into fat.

While Duchenne de Bologne (1806–75) was slightly off the mark in his assertion that this was a disorder of nerve,

with secondary muscle involvement, he nevertheless published an impressive series of articles on the clinical features and histopathology (Duchenne, 1868). He also published compelling artwork, which clearly illustrates the typical patient habitus at presentation (Figs. 19.1 and 19.2). Duchenne first became interested in neurology through his chance observations on the effect of electricity on muscles and nerves of his patients (Duchenne, 1855). He interacted extensively with Jean-Martin Charcot in Hôpital de la Salpetriere in Paris, where Duchenne taught Charcot about electrical stimulation and photography, while Charcot taught Duchenne histopathology and anatomy (Emery and Emery, 1995) – and where a contributor to this volume (M. Fardeau) works today. It was in 1861 that Duchenne first published a case report of a 9-year-old boy with classic symptoms of the disease that would bear his name: delayed motor milestones, calf hypertrophy, lordosis, difficulty with ambulation and inability to stand from a sitting position without the use of hands. The presence of cognitive deficits in this boy caused Duchenne to question whether the disease had a central nervous system (CNS) component. No histopathology was reported in this initial case.

Duchenne continued his interest in this disorder, reviewing reports of 15 cases in Germany, in nine papers published between 1862 and 1867 (Emery and Emery, 1995), in addition to 12 new cases of his own. He mentions Meryon's publication of 1852 but dismisses his case as a type of congenital spinal muscular atrophy (Duchenne, 1868). It should be noted that the British, German and French series of patient reports included rare girls with a similar disorder. In these cases, it is likely that some represented autosomal recessive pedigrees (SCARMD) and others manifesting carriers of Duchenne dystrophy (see below). Duchenne dubbed the disorder pseudohypertrophic muscular paralysis (paralysie musculaire pseudohypertrophique) and paralytic sclerosis of muscle (paralysie myo-sclerosique) (Duchenne, 1868).

Perhaps the most significant and novel contribution to the descriptions of muscular dystrophy by Duchenne was the systematic study of punch muscle biopsies of living patients. He designed and used a needle biopsy apparatus and conducted longitudinal studies of muscle histology in different muscle groups. He noted the early, aggressive proliferation of connective tissue in muscle (fibrosis), which then resolved into fatty infiltration in later stages of the disease. As described below, the fibrotic proliferation in Duchenne dystrophy appears to be a critical component in the progressive pathophysiology of the disease. Duchenne did *not* report many other important features of the disease, which were astutely recognized by Meryon many

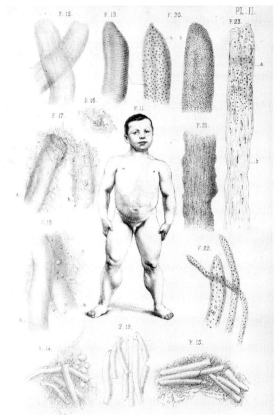

Fig. 19.1. Duchenne's original artwork. (Plate I from Duchenne, 1879, p. 179.)

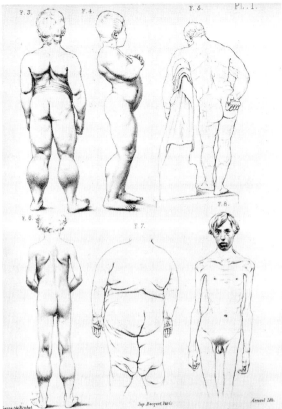

Fig. 19.2. Duchenne's original artwork. (Plate II from Duchenne, 1879, p. 188.)

years earlier: specifically, the heritable nature of the condition, the normal anatomy and histopathology of the spinal cord and the suggestion that the myofibre membrane (sarcolemma) appeared abnormal.

The British physician William Gowers (1845–1915) subsequently published extensively on 'psuedo-hypertrophic muscular paralysis', including a summary of 220 cases of which 24 were seen by him personally (Gowers, 1879). Like Duchenne, Gowers made substantial contributions to a number of aspects of medicine, and the eloquence of Gowers' writings have long been recognized. He expanded upon the earlier clinical descriptions and emphasized the maternal inheritance. His name is strongly associated with the 'Gowers' manoeuvre' or 'sign', which he himself describes as follows (Gowers, 1879, p. 36):

In getting up they first put the hands on the ground, then stretch out the legs behind them far apart, and, the chief weight of the trunk resting on the hands, by keeping the toes on the ground and pushing the body backwards, they manage to get the knees extended, so that the trunk is supported by the hands and feet, all placed as widely apart as possible. Next the hands are moved alternately along the ground backwards, so as to bring a larger portion of the weight of the trunk over the legs. Then one hand is placed upon the knee, and a push with this and with the other hand on the ground is sufficient to enable the extensors of the hip to bring the trunk into the upright posture.

It is important to point out the variable early descriptions of Duchenne dystrophy as 'hypertrophic muscular dystrophy' or 'pseudo-hypertrophic muscular dystrophy'. It was clearly noted by Conte, Meryon and Duchenne that certain muscle groups showed impressive bulk, particularly the calves (Figs. 19.1 and 19.2). This hypertrophy was clinically enigmatic, as patients were clearly losing strength despite the abnormally large size of some muscles. The first histological studies of patient muscle by Meryon used postmortem material, where he observed that many end-stage muscles were replaced by fat, while others contained higher numbers of myofibres. The variable presence of gross muscle hypertrophy, fatty replacement of muscles in older patients and marked muscle weakness caused early authors to vacillate between 'hypertrophy' and 'pseudo-hypertrophy' in their writings. Both Duchenne and his son published descriptions of the disease as paralysie hypertrophique de l'Enfance, clearly pointing out the nosological importance of the finding of hypertrophied muscles. Duchenne's later more systematic studies of muscle biopsies from patients of different ages showed that the fatty infiltration seen by Meryon was a later event in the disease, whereas proliferation of connective tissue occurred earlier (fibrosis). He concluded that the connective tissue proliferation was responsible for the hypertrophy, and hence began using the term pseudo-hypertrophique. This term then became embedded in the literature, with Duchenne muscular dystrophy being synonymous with pseudo-hypertrophic muscular dystrophy in young boys.

More recent studies of younger patients, and the systematic histological and clinical studies of cat, dog and mouse models of Duchenne dystrophy, have altered our perception regarding the nature of the increased bulk. Evidence is accumulating that the disease shows true hypertrophy of muscle and muscle fibres early in the disease process. This hypertrophy later changes to pseudo-hypertrophy as the muscle is gradually replaced first by fibrotic tissue and then by fat (Hoffman and Gorospe, 1991). Therefore, the term pseudo-hypertrophic muscular dystrophy does not accurately reflect the entire disease process and is an inappropriate description of the disease given current knowledge.

Major strides were made in differential diagnosis and categorization of the different types of muscular dystrophy in the period 1950–80. It was noted early on that affected brother–sister pairs could be found, albeit at a low frequency relative to typical Duchenne dystrophy in males. Also, milder phenotypes were evident, some of which showed X-linked inheritance patterns, and some of which did not. Critical in this phase of muscular dystrophy research was the emerging ability to conduct large-scale, nationwide studies of patients and their families, and the emerging fields of genetics and statistics. Discussions of other important types of muscular dystrophy can be found

elsewhere in this book. However, particularly important to mention here are those who made major contributions to the nosology of the X-linked muscular dystrophies. John Walton, the founding editor of Disorders of Voluntary Muscle, was hired as a young physician to survey all muscular dystrophy cases in England, specifically to address the question of why some cases seemed to show clinical improvement (Emery and Emery, 1995). His mentor, Frederick Nattrass, soon showed that these patients had autoimmune disease (Walton and Nattrass, 1954). However, Walton went on to publish a classification of the types of muscle disease in England, with interviews of family members and systematic electromyographic (EMG) and biopsy studies (Walton and Nattrass, 1954). Walton went on to lead the Newcastle group of muscular dystrophy laboratories, which have made important contributions to muscular dystrophy research, including epidemiological, microscopic and biochemical studies.

There were two additional, relatively common, X-linked muscular dystrophies that began to be viewed as distinct from that of Duchenne muscular dystrophy. Peter Emil Becker (b. 1908) examined an extended German X-linked muscular dystrophy pedigree where the age of onset was generally in the second decade (Becker and Kiener, 1955). While milder forms of muscular dystrophy in males had been observed since the time of Meryon, Becker was the first to point out that this disease 'bred true' within affected families and was, therefore, clinically distinct from Duchenne muscular dystrophy. He subsequently published observations on an additional two pedigrees (Becker, 1962), showing that the calf hypertrophy and proximal muscle weakness were strikingly similar to Duchenne dystrophy, although the age of onset was later, and progression slower. This disorder is now known to be allelic to Duchenne dystrophy.

The second type of X-linked dystrophy was initially described in a Virginia family by neurologist Fritz Dreifuss (Dreifuss and Hogan, 1961). This family showed clear X-linked recessive inheritance but had early-onset contractures, lack of hypertrophy of the calves and a slow and relatively benign clinical course. A few years later, Alan Emery restudied the family, and documented clinical and cardiac features quite distinct from Duchenne dystrophy, namely, weakness distributed more distally in the lower limbs (humeroperoneal), early contractures that seemed to precede significant muscle weakness, and cardiac conduction defects (Emery and Dreifuss 1966). This disorder, now known as Emery–Dreifuss, muscular dystrophy, is nonallelic to Duchenne and Becker muscular dystrophies, with the gene location in Xq28.

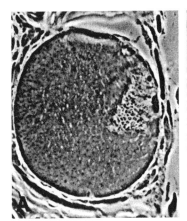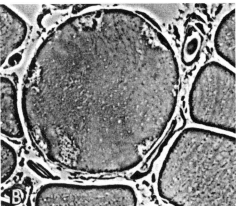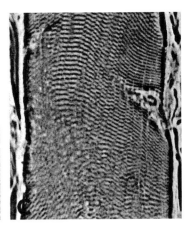

Fig. 19.3. Delta lesions in isolated myofibres as seen in epon-embedded muscle biopsies from patients with Duchenne muscular dystrophy. Phase micrographs, from three muscle fibres are shown; the longitudinal section at the right shows hypercontracted sarcomeres directly adjacent the lesion. (Taken from Mokri and Engel (1975) with permission.)

Premolecular histological and biochemical studies of Duchenne dystrophy

The paper of Mokri and Engel (1975) is credited as a milestone in the evolution of the fragile plasma membrane model, and was recently cited as a 'Landmark Article' by the American Academy of Neurology. The authors stated:

The present study directly implicates the plasma membrane in muscle fiber degeneration in Duchenne muscular dystrophy. The membrane abnormality is an early one, and it may be a basic one. Nonetheless, it would be shortsighted to overlook the possibility that this particular lesion could not be conditioned by or be secondary to a biochemical lesion elsewhere in the muscle fiber. Further, it is also conceivable that a pathogenetic factor not residing in the muscle fiber could cause or abet the membrane defects. On the other hand, if the cause of the structural defects resided in the membrane itself (as it very well might), it could be caused by an abnormal lipid component or by a defective structural protein in the membrane. Further studies directed at the molecular architecture of the muscle fiber plasma membrane will clarify these questions.

The continued development of light microscopy, and the evolution of both electron microscopy and biochemistry, resulted in a flurry of publications that proposed a model for the pathogenesis of Duchenne muscular dystrophy. Perhaps the first important early advance was in blood chemistry; it became apparent that all patients with Duchenne muscular dystrophy showed striking elevations of first aldolase (Schapira et al., 1953), and then serum creatine kinase (Ebashi et al., 1959). Serum creatine kinase levels were found to be quite high at birth in Duchenne patients, and subsequent studies showed that about 70% of female carriers showed serum creatine kinase levels above the upper limit of normal (Emery, 1967). The release

of muscle enzymes from myofibres affected by Duchenne dystrophy appeared to be quite high relative to other muscle diseases. Indeed, the muscle concentrations of creatine kinase were reduced in patients with Duchenne dystrophy, suggesting a large-scale efflux from fibres (Dreyfus et al., 1954; Rowland, 1964).

Histopathological studies, both at the light and electron microscopic levels, found considerable evidence for a faulty plasma membrane. A consistent finding of the early histopathological studies were prominent eosinophilic 'hypercontracted' or 'hyaline' fibres in patient muscle. Hypercontracted fibres were originally felt to represent the initial stages of myofibre necrosis ('prenecrotic'); however, they were observed very early in the disease process (fetal and neonatal muscle) at points where necrosis was not a conspicuous feature (Hudgson et al., 1967). Mokri and Engel (1975) used both light and electron microscopy to visualize directly breaks of the plasma membrane of otherwise healthy myofibres in muscle biopsies from patients with Duchenne dystrophy (delta lesions) (Fig. 19.3). A series of papers studying both symptomatic and presymptomatic cases of Duchenne dystrophy, using a variety of markers of cell damage, obtained data consistent with the 'leaky membrane theory' (Emery, 1977, 1993; Bodensteiner and Engel, 1978; Bradley and Fulthorpe, 1978; Carpenter and Karpati, 1979; Guibaud et al., 1981; Bertorini et al., 1982, 1984; Wakayama et al., 1983; Cornelio and Dones, 1984). By 1980, the leaky membrane was a prominent model for the pathophysiology of Duchenne dystrophy (Rowland, 1980).

The early writings of Meryon (1852, p. 76) mentioned that the plasma membrane seemed a possible site of the problem in Duchenne dystrophy: '. . . whilst the sarcolemma or tunic of the elementary fibre was broken down and destroyed'. The finding of physical breaks in the plasma membrane by Mokri and Engel (1975) was likewise visionary and absolutely accurate. It is important to point out that the leaky membrane hypothesis was only one model of many that were circulated at the time, and there were valid criticisms of this model. For example, it was well established that many different types of insult to muscle tissue could induce calcium influx, creatine kinase efflux and myofibre necrosis, including vigorous exercise (Fowler et al., 1968), and ischaemia (Hearse, 1979). There was, therefore, considerable debate as to whether or not the membrane damage was primary, or whether it was secondary to some other problem. Indeed, some features of the histopathology did not agree with a primary membrane problem (Engel, 1977). For example, myofibre necrosis often occurs in groups of adjacent fibres (grouped necrosis). If a myofibre has a problem maintaining its own plasma membrane, why should neighbouring fibres undergo necrosis at the same time? This feature of the histopathology evoked the 'vascular hypothesis' (Hathaway et al., 1970; Mendell et al., 1971, 1972), which, as we will show below, is strongly bolstered by new insights regarding nitric oxide control of blood flow in Duchenne muscle. Likewise, a model of a primary role for connective tissue proliferation in the disease pathogenesis was proposed in 1959 (Bourne and Golarz, 1959; Duance et al., 1980). Current understanding of the disease is that connective tissue proliferation is, in fact, the pathological process that limits the life of Duchenne patients.

To conclude the description of the premolecular era of Duchenne dystrophy research, many reviews of the literature to date imply that the postgene findings validate *only* the leaky membrane theory. As we learn more and more about the pathophysiological processes caused by dystrophin deficiency, it is clear that many of the previously proposed pathogenesis models explain different and important direct consequences of the primary biochemical defect.

Identification of the dystrophin gene and protein

The X-linked recessive inheritance pattern of Duchenne muscular dystrophy strongly implied loss of function of some biochemical component of muscle tissue; a single protein was likely missing, and the key to the pathogenesis was the identification of this protein. There were clearly many histological changes in a patient's muscle, and one could assume that there were many consequent secondary biochemical changes. It, therefore, became critical to dis-

tinguish the primary biochemical defect from all the secondary changes in protein expression. This is not a trivial task, and efforts to do this had not proved successful. An alternative approach was needed, and the emergence of analysis methods in human molecular genetics in the 1980s set the stage for the application of these techniques to Duchenne dystrophy.

Duchenne muscular dystrophy is considered the first successful use of molecular genetics to identify a causative gene and protein in a human inherited disorder, where little or nothing was known of the biochemical defect prior to the application of genetics. There are a number of features of Duchenne dystrophy that facilitated the gene search. First, the high mutation rate meant that many cases represented new mutations and that most patients probably had independent (possibly different) mutations of the gene. Second, the disease was X-linked, and patients were hemizygous, with only a single mutant gene to study. Third, extensive X-linked pedigrees existed for genetic linkage analyses. Fourth, there was an international collaborative effort in place for sharing reagents, which was promoted and fostered by nonprofit foundations (particularly the muscular dystrophy associations of USA, UK and Canada).

The critical initial step in the identification of the Duchenne dystrophy gene was the identification of female manifesting carriers, who had severe symptoms of muscular dystrophy resembling Duchenne dystrophy in males and who consistently showed X:autosome translocations (Greenstein et al., 1977; Zatz et al., 1981; Verellen-Dumoulin et al., 1984). The specific autosome involved in each translocation was different but the X chromosome breakpoint was always the same, namely the short arm of the X chromosome (Xp21). These girls were thought to be heterozygous carriers for Duchenne dystrophy but showed symptoms because of the preferential inactivation of the nontranslocated (normal) X chromosome. The reasons for the preferential inactivation of the normal X chromosome is fairly well established; X inactivation occurs at around the 100-cell stage of embryogenesis, at which point each cell makes an independent decision as to which X chromosome to inactivate (maternal or paternal). In the females with a X:autosome translocation, the cells that inactivate the translocated (abnormal) X will also inactivate a section of the autosome translocated to it, leading to partial monosomy for that autosome. In addition, the Xp-ter section of the abnormal X, which is translocated to an autosome, is *not* inactivated, leading to inappropriate double dosage of Xp-ter. The cells with the *abnormal* X *inactive* die (or show growth disadvantage) because of dosage problems, leaving only the cells with the *abnormal* X *active* viable in the embryo. Hence, the girls resulting from these embryos have all, or nearly all, cells with the *translocated abnormal X active*, which has the Duchenne muscular dystrophy gene cut in half by the translocation and, therefore, cannot make any of the protein product (loss-of-function) despite being a heterozygote.

Genetic linkage studies using polymorphic markers around Xp21 confirmed the localization of the Duchenne muscular dystrophy gene by the early 1980s (Murray et al., 1982; Davies et al., 1983). In fact, these early studies were the first to show genetic linkage between an anonymous restriction fragment length polymorphism (RFLP) probe and a human disease with no known biochemical defect. Soon thereafter, genetic linkage between the same genetic markers and Becker muscular dystrophy families was shown, indicating that Duchenne and Becker dystrophies were in fact allelic (caused by different mutations in the same gene) (Kingston et al., 1984).

Two approaches were then used by different laboratories to identify the specific gene sequences responsible for the disease. One, used by the laboratory of Ronald Worton, was to employ the DNA of an X:autosome translocation-bearing female Duchenne patient. The translocation in this patient was between Xp21 and chromosome 21, in the ribosomal gene cluster. The goal was to cross the translocation breakpoint, using the already cloned ribosomal genes to 'walk' into the region of Xp21 containing the dystrophin gene. As the dystrophin gene was presumably cut in half in this girl, the part of the X chromosome at the translocation breakpoint should be a part of the Duchenne muscular dystrophy gene (Worton et al., 1984). This group went on to identify X chromosome sequences flanking the breakpoint (Ray et al., 1985) and found that these sequences were deleted in some males with Duchenne muscular dystrophy, suggesting that they had in fact landed in the Duchenne dystrophy gene. This group was unable to find any exons (coding sequence) of a gene in the area sufficiently quickly, and the Duchenne gene was first identified by Louis Kunkel and co-workers (1985), as described below. In retrospect, this was because there were very few exon sequences in the area of the gene that Worton's group had cloned, whereas exon sequences were more common in the region identified by Kunkel.

The experimental rationale that was employed in the identification of the Duchenne dystrophy gene, and ultimately its protein product, is shown schematically in Fig. 19.4. The initial step was the identification of a patient, called BB, who was not only afflicted with Duchenne dystrophy but also with chronic granulomatous disease, X-linked retinitis pigmentosa and the McLeod red blood cell phenotype (Francke et al., 1985). Because all of these disorders were thought to reside on the X chromosome, it

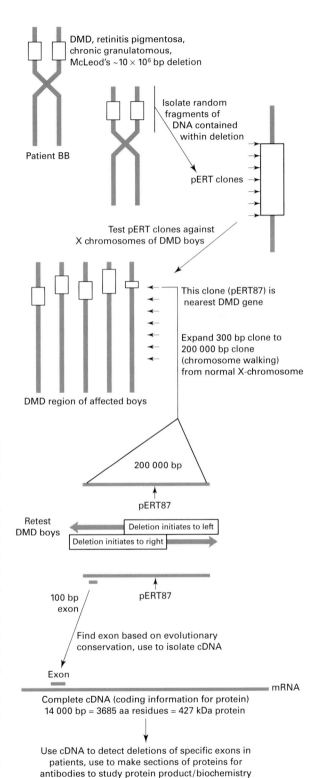

Fig. 19.4. Schematic of the experimental protocol used for identification of the Duchenne muscular dystrophy gene. (Taken from Hoffman (1989) with permission.)

seemed likely that this particular patient would exhibit a deletion mutation encompassing all of these genes. Indeed, using cytological methods, a relatively small region of this patient's X chromosome was found to be deleted (Francke et al., 1985). It was then reasoned that if random fragments (clones) of genomic DNA could be isolated that were contained within this deletion (and thus absent in the DNA of this patient), each of these fragments could be a candidate for being near one of the normal genes responsible for preventing these disorders. Using a competitive hybridization strategy, a number of such clones were obtained (Fig. 19.4) (Kunkel et al., 1985).

Of the nearly 1000 cloned sequences studied, only eight were unique copy sequence and missing from patient BB (i.e. within the approximately 10 million base pair deletion containing the Duchenne dystrophy gene). To determine which of these eight clones was probably nearest the Duchenne gene, a series of other boys with Duchenne dystrophy, and no other genetic disorder, were tested for the presence or absence of each. In a large collaborative study, it was found that one of the clones, pERT87, was missing (deleted) from 5–8% of males with either Duchenne or Becker muscular dystrophy (Fig. 19.4) (Kunkel et al., 1985, Monaco et al., 1986a). This analysis strongly suggested that the pERT87 clone was in or near the Duchenne muscular dystrophy gene. A 200 kb chromosome walk was initiated from the pERT87 clone, and it was soon found that deletions were present throughout the cloned region, indicating that the cloned area was in fact in the centre of the Duchenne dystrophy gene (Monaco et al., 1987). Unique sequences within the cloned area were then used to probe Southern blots of genomic DNA isolated from various species of animals to see if any could detect an evolutionarily conserved exon. One such conserved sequence was identified, and it showed hybridization to a very large 14 kb mRNA in Northern blots from fetal skeletal muscle (Monaco et al., 1986b). This exon was used to probe a cDNA library from human fetal muscle, and the first 1000 bp fragment of the Duchenne dystrophy gene RNA was identified and sequenced (Monaco et al., 1986b). Large insert cDNA libraries were then produced from mouse muscle with sequence data published for the first 25% of the RNA for both human and mouse (Hoffman et al., 1987a). This analysis showed that the gene was very highly conserved between these two species.

The full-length 14 kb cDNA of the Duchenne dystrophy gene was then cloned from human fetal skeletal muscle (Fig. 19.5) (Koenig et al., 1987). The cDNA was shown to recognize over 70 exons distributed over 2 million bases of genomic DNA (Fig. 19.5) (Koenig et al., 1987). Approximately 65% of patients with Duchenne and Becker

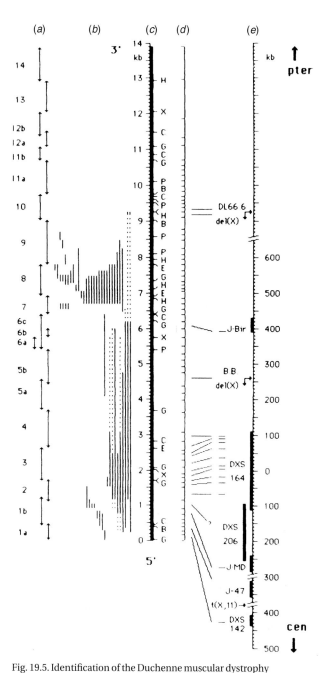

Fig. 19.5. Identification of the Duchenne muscular dystrophy mRNA (cDNA) and alignment of the cDNA with the genomic locus, and location of patient deletion mutations. (a) cDNA clones identified; (b) deletion mutations observed in 53 patients with Duchenne dystrophy; (c) complete cDNA (14 kb) with restriction enzyme map; (d) schematic of the 79 exons making up the muscle dystrophin mRNA; (e) schematic of the genomic locus of the gene, showing the chromosomal walk done by Kunkel's group (DXS164) and that done by Worton's group (DXS206). The deletion breakpoint of patient BB is also shown (BB del(X)). Orientation relative to the X chromosome centromere (cen) and telomere (pter) are also shown. (Taken from Koenig et al. (1987) with permission.)

dystrophy were found to have deletion mutations of one or more exons of the enormous gene (Koenig et al., 1987). Deletion hotspots were found around exons 45–50, and also in the 5′ end of the gene (Fig. 19.5).

It was quickly clear from the deletion mutation analysis of patients that clinical severity could not be predicted based on the extent of the deletion mutation, or on the region of the gene deleted (Koenig et al., 1987). Anthony Monaco studied some deletions carefully and developed the reading frame hypothesis (Fig. 19.6) (Monaco et al., 1988). He found that the critical issue that determines clinical severity was whether or not the exons that remained in the patient's gene could be spliced together into a 'functional' mRNA (Monaco et al., 1988). Specifically, if the exons flanking the deletion mutation happened to share the same reading frame of the triplet codon translational sequence, then protein translation could continue unabated through the new junction of exons (Fig. 19.6), and this would result in the production of the protein product through the end of the gene. This protein product would be missing amino acids corresponding to the deleted exons, but it would retain some biochemical function and result in a milder Becker muscular dystrophy phenotype in the patient. In those cases where flanking exons did *not* share the same reading frame, a translational frameshift would occur, and no functional protein would be produced. This hypothesis was later validated for the large majority of patients.

The sequence of the complete cDNA (mRNA) was then determined, and the sequence decoded into an amino acid sequence of 3600 residues (Koenig et al., 1988). The protein was found to have a long rod shape, with homology to previously characterized cytoskeletal proteins spectrin and α-actinin (Koenig et al., 1988). Four distinct domains were identified from the sequence, including an N-terminal actin-finding domain, a large coiled-coil central rod domain, and two C-terminal domains, one rich in cysteine residues and a second larger globular domain. The molecular mass was calculated at 427 kDa by computer programs.

To identify the protein product of the gene, sections of the cDNA were cloned into bacterial expression vectors, and peptide fragments of 500 and 250 amino acid residues produced. Antibodies raised against these fusion proteins detected the expected 427 kDa protein, which was then named dystrophin (Hoffman et al., 1987b). The dystrophin protein was found to be absent in muscle from patients with Duchenne dystrophy and of abnormal size and amount in those with Becker muscular dystrophy (consistent with the reading frame hypothesis) (Fig. 19.7) (Arahata et al., 1988; Bonilla et al., 1988; Hoffman et al., 1988a). The

protein was found to be a membrane-bound component of skeletal muscle, heart, smooth muscle (vascular and visceral) and neurons (Arahata et al., 1988; Bonilla et al., 1988; Hoffman et al., 1988b). The protein was absent from the *mdx* mouse, suggesting that it was a homologous animal model for Duchenne muscular dystrophy (Fig. 19.8) (Hoffman et al., 1987b, 1988b).

A literature search of dystrophin now retrieves over 2500 journal publications. The rate of publication has been at approximately 250 publications per year in the 1990s. The dystrophin gene remains the largest and most complex gene yet identified. The dystrophin protein provided a starting point for investigations of the structure and function of the membrane cytoskeleton of the muscle fibre. These latter studies have had a major impact on our understanding of many muscle disorders, and a number of important infectious diseases as well. Finally, the dystrophin gene and protein paved the way for the extensive use of 'molecular diagnostics' in neurology.

The animal models of Duchenne muscular dystrophy

Discussions of the recent findings concerning the biochemistry of dystrophin, and the pathophysiology of its deficiency, require frequent citation of results obtained in the animal models. Spontaneous mutations of the dystrophin gene have been identified in many dogs, cats and mice. These biochemically and genetically identical animal models for the human disease have been instrumental in research into dystrophin function and dysfunction.

The dystrophin protein is highly homologous between species, with >93% identity in amino acid sequence between human, mouse, chicken, fish and frogs through the more conserved C-terminal 20% of the protein (Fig. 19.9). The large size of the gene also seems conserved, at least through placental mammals. These features, coupled with the specificity of muscle dystrophin deficiency for mutations in the dystrophin gene, and the fact that X-linked genes in humans are X-linked throughout all placental mammals, greatly facilitated the identification of homologous animal models for Duchenne dystrophy.

The first animal model to be identified was the *mdx* mouse. This mouse mutation occurred spontaneously on a C57Bl10 background and was fortuitously identified during a screen for red blood cell defects in a C57Bl10 colony (Bulfield et al., 1984). Serum creatine kinase levels were highly elevated, and this trait was inherited in an X-linked recessive pattern. Dystrophin deficiency in the

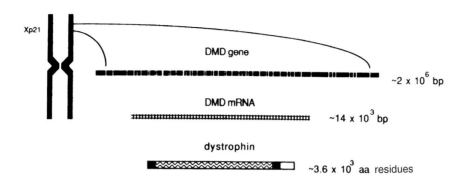

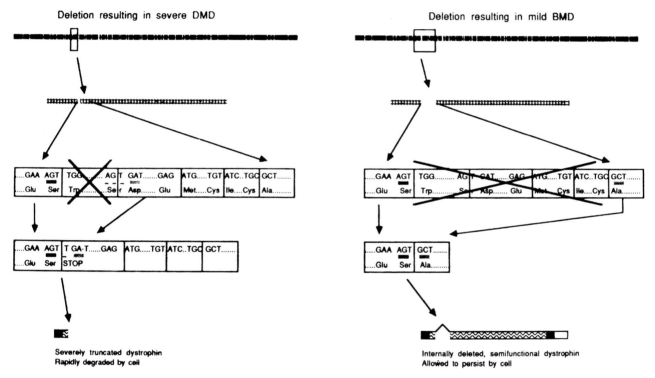

Fig. 19.6. The reading frame hypothesis. A schematic diagram of the dystrophin gene, mRNA and protein. In the lower panels, two different deletion mutations are shown, one leading to severe Duchenne dystrophy (DMD, left), and one leading to milder Becker dystrophy (right). The Becker dystrophy deletion is larger in size (4 exons) than the DMD example given (1 exon). The reason that the larger deletion leads to a clinically milder phenotype in Becker dystrophy is that the translational reading frame of the remaining exons is shared, leading to translation continuing through the newly spliced exons, and an internally deleted dystrophin protein (right). The muscle in the patient with Duchenne dystrophy is unable to maintain the correct reading frame in the newly spliced exons, leading to a translational reading frame shirt and an early stop codon. This leads to grossly truncated dystrophin, which is usually rapidly degraded by the myofibre. (Taken from Hoffman and Kunkel (1989) with permission.)

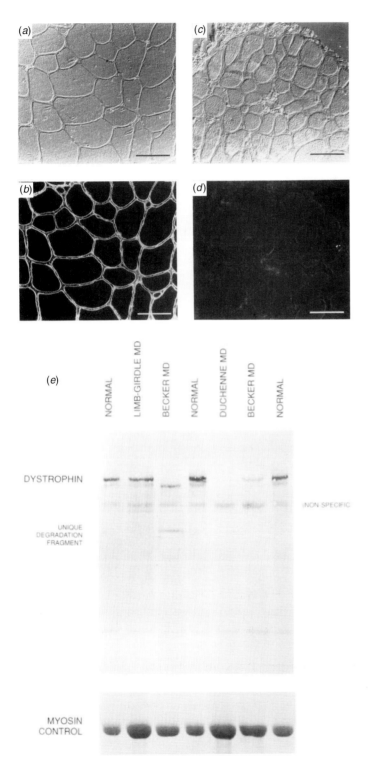

Fig. 19.7. Dystrophin abnormalities in muscle biopsies from patients with Duchenne and Becker muscular dystrophy. (*a–d*) Immunofluorescence analysis of muscle biopsies from a normal individual (*a,b*) and a patient with Duchenne muscular dystrophy (*c,d*). (*a,c*) Paired nomarski optics. (*b,d*) Immunofluorescence using anti-dystrophin antibodies. Dystrophin is seen as a plasma membrane protein in the normal biopsy (*b*) but is absent in Duchenne dystrophy muscle (*d*). (*e*) In an immunoblot analysis, dystrophin is seen as a large, 427 kDa protein in muscle from normal individuals and patients with nondystrophinopathies (limb girdle muscular dystrophy (limb-girdle MD)). The patient with Duchenne dystrophy (Duchenne MD) shows no detectable dystrophin, while the two patients with Becker muscular dystrophy (Becker MD) have dystrophin of abnormal molecular weight and/or abnormal quantity. (*a–d* from Hoffman and Gorospe (1991) with permission; *e* from Miller and Hoffman (1994) with permission.)

mdx muscle was documented, proving the *mdx* mouse shared the same biochemical defect with patients with Duchenne (Fig. 19.8) (Hoffman et al., 1987b). A stop codon mutation in exon 23 was subsequently identified (Sicinski et al., 1989). A series of new alleles of the *mdx* strain were induced by mutagenesis; all showed a phenotype consistent with the original *mdx* allele, and all mutations are known (Im et al., 1996).

A sporadically occurring mutation in Golden Retriever dogs was found that caused muscular dystrophy and was again inherited in an X-linked recessive pattern. The dogs were first identified in upstate New York by de Lahunta (1983) and then characterized in North Carolina by Kornegay et al. (1988), and at Cornell University by Cooper et al. (1988). The dogs show dystrophin deficiency in muscle that was inherited as an X-linked trait (Cooper et al., 1988), with the causative mutation being a splicing mutation in exon 8 (Sharp et al., 1992). Independent alleles have been identified in a series of dog breeds, including Rottweilers, Wire-hair Fox Terriers, Shelties and German Short-haired Pointers (Gorospe et al., 1997; Schatzberg et al. 1999). The Golden Retriever shows two alternatively spliced transcripts that exclude the exon 8 mutation and thus produce a low level of dystrophin, which may contribute to clinical variability between individual dogs (Schatzberg et al., 1998). At least two independent isolates of dystrophinopathy in domestic cats have been identified (Carpenter et al., 1989; Gaschen et al., 1992), and the mutation has been identified in one of these lines (Winand et al., 1994).

The animal models of Duchenne dystrophy have evoked considerable angst in the scientific community, with many questioning the 'appropriateness' of these models. This angst arose because the clinical symptoms of each animal

Fig. 19.8. Dystrophin deficiency in muscle membrane preparations and total brain protein extracts from normal (B6) and *mdx* mice. The dystrophin protein is seen as a 427 kDa protein in microsomes from muscle from normal (B6) mice but is absent from *mdx* mice. Low levels of dystrophin are seen in total protein homogenates from normal mouse brain (arrow), which are similarly lacking from *mdx* brain. (Taken from Hoffman et al. (1988b) with permission.)

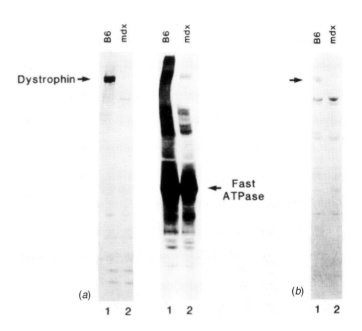

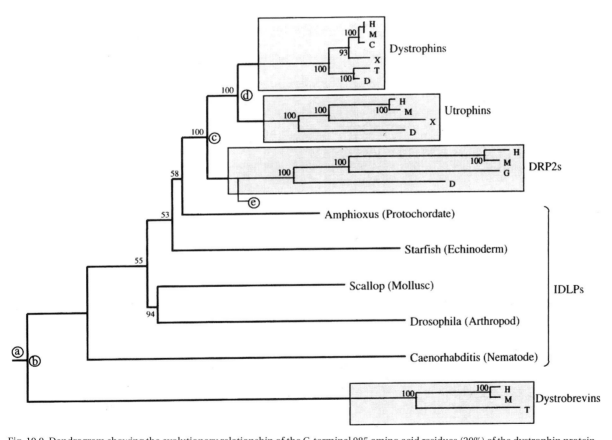

Fig. 19.9. Dendrogram showing the evolutionary relationship of the C-terminal 985 amino acid residues (20%) of the dystrophin protein to other related vertebrate (utrophin, DRP2, dystrobrevin) proteins and invertebrate dystrophin-like proteins (IDLPs). Numbers noted at each branch point indicate the percentage of 1000 bootstrap trials that supported that cluster. DRP, dystrophin-related protein. (Taken from Roberts and Bobrow (1998) with permission.)

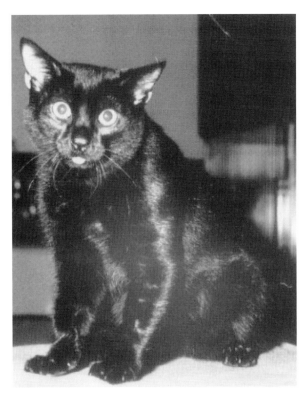

Fig. 19.10. Generalized muscle hypertrophy in a dystrophin-deficient cat. This cat is shown at 5 months of age. There is generalized muscle hypertrophy and a tendency to keep the tip of the tongue protruding out of the mouth because of lingual hypertrophy. (Taken from Gaschen et al. (1992) with permission.)

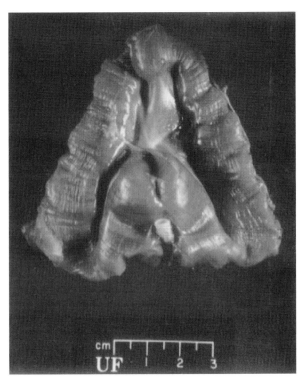

Fig. 19.11. Diaphragmatic hypertrophy in dystrophin-deficient cats. Diaphragmatic hypertrophy led to oesophogeal constriction in this cat, leading to its demise. (Taken from Gaschen et al. (1992) with permission.)

model differ from the human disease, and from each other. Dystrophin-deficient cats show marked muscular hypertrophy (Fig. 19.10), which becomes so severe as to cause the cats to succumb from dehydration (lingual hypertrophy) or starvation (diaphragmatic hypertrophy) (Fig. 19.11) (Cooper et al., 1988; Gaschen et al., 1992, 1998). The cats show considerable stiffness and have cardiac involvement but are not very weak. Dystrophin-deficient dogs show a rapidly progressive course of muscle weakness, wasting and contractures; onset is around 3 months of age, with death occurring anywhere from the neonatal period to adulthood. Significant disability is frequently observed by age 6 months (Cooper et al., 1988; Kornegay et al., 1988). Dystrophin-deficient mice show marked muscular hypertrophy (Hoffman and Gorospe, 1991) and are often stronger than age-matched control mice. However, if the strength is normalized for cross-sectional area of the muscle, then they are weaker than controls. Mice do eventually show some progressive disease and weakness near the end of their normal lifespan (Lefaucheur et al., 1995; Pastoret and Sebille, 1995; Pagel and Partridge, 1999).

Are the animals 'good' models for Duchenne muscular dystrophy? They all have loss-of-function mutations in the same highly conserved dystrophin gene, so they are certainly analogous at the gene level. They all lack the highly conserved dystrophin protein in muscle tissue, so they are biochemically homologous. Muscle tissue itself is exceedingly highly conserved through evolution, and, in fact, all the animal models share many of the histological features of the human disease, including fibre size variation and degeneration/regeneration of fibres (Figs. 19.12 (cat), 19.13 (mouse), 19.14 (human)). All show cardiac involvement, preferentially affecting the basolateral free wall of the left ventrical (Gaschen et al., 1999). All have striking elevations of serum creatine kinase. Consequently, the animals are excellent models for the genetics, biochemistry and early histology of Duchenne dystrophy.

The clinical differences find their origin in the *progressive* aspects of the disease, particularly with regards to connective tissue proliferation in muscle and failure of regeneration over time. All dystrophin-deficient species show marked muscular hypertrophy at a young age, but in dogs and humans the hypertrophy changes to loss of

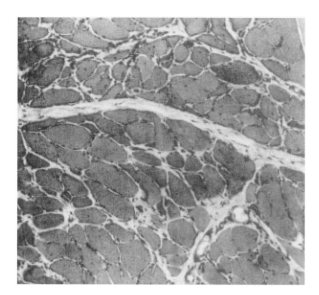

Fig. 19.12. Histopathology of dystrophin-deficient cats. The histology is consistent with early-stage Duchenne muscular dystrophy in humans. Fibre size variation and focal endomysial fibrosis is seen. (Taken from Gaschen et al. (1992) with permission.)

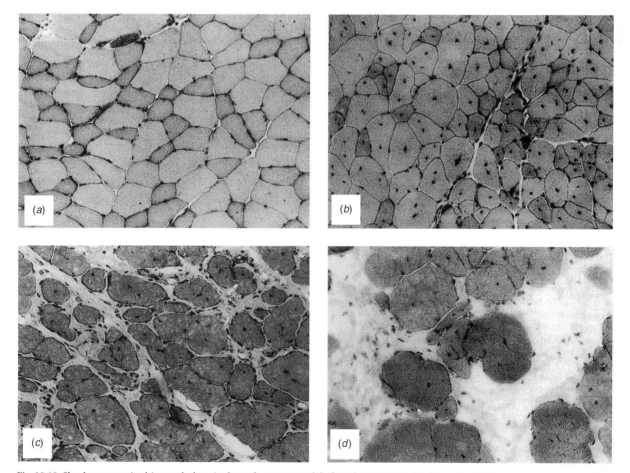

Fig. 19.13. Slowly progressive histopathology in the *mdx* mouse model of Duchenne muscular dystrophy. (*a*) Normal mouse muscle. (*b*) A 1-year-old mouse showing variable histopathology with mild centronucleated pathology. (*c*) More severe dystrophic pathology from a different region of the same muscle as in (*b*). (*d*) At older ages (1.5 years), some muscles can show significant fibrofatty infiltration with loss of muscle fibres. (Taken from Hoffman and Kunkel (1989) with permission.)

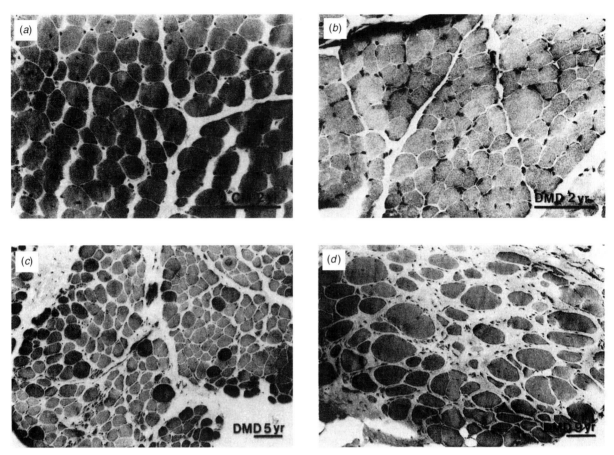

Fig. 19.14. Progressive histopathology of Duchenne muscular dystrophy (dystrophin-deficient boys). (*a*) Muscle from a 2-year-old boy with congenital myopathy is shown for comparison. The histopathology of Duchenne muscular dystrophy shows a marked progression from milder picture to a more severely dystrophic picture as patients age: (*b*) 2 year old; (*c*) 5 year old; (*d*) 9 year old child. (Taken from Hoffman and Gorospe (1991) with permission.)

muscle (wasting) and loss of strength. In this context, it is important to refer to the early drawings of Duchenne (Figs. 19.1 and 19.2), and the early writings of both Meryon and Duchenne, which point out the extreme hypertrophy present in patient muscle. Even more extreme examples of hypertrophy can be found in human patients with Duchenne dystrophy (Fig. 19.15) however, this is variable, apparently depending to some extent on extragenic or multigenic factors.

There is an emerging consensus that the dystrophin-deficient mice, dogs and cats are indeed outstanding models for Duchenne muscular dystrophy. The fact that they show differences in clinical phenotype is particularly valuable, as they provide insight into the *secondary* consequences of *primary* dystrophinopathy.

Dystrophin structure and function

Biochemistry of dystrophin

Many different isoforms of dystrophin have been identified, which arise from alternative splicing of the dystrophin gene and from use of alternative promoters within the gene (Fig. 19.16). Full-length or 'muscle dystrophin' generally refers to the product of the muscle promoter (MD in Fig. 19.16), which includes all exons, with alternatively spliced isoforms at the C-terminus. This isoform is present at high levels in skeletal muscle, cardiac muscle and smooth muscle. Critically, deficiency of this isoform is clearly responsible for the large majority of clinical symptoms in patients with Duchenne dystrophy and in all the animal models.

Myogenic cells require about 16 hours to transcribe one mRNA molecule, and it has been calculated that only

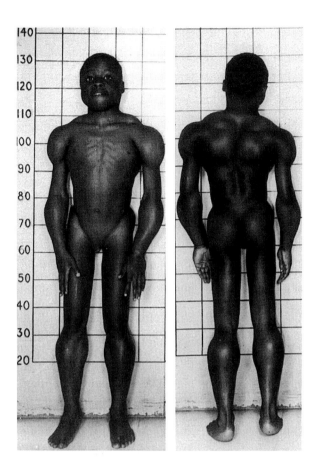

Fig. 19.15. Marked muscle hypertrophy in a patient with Duchenne muscular dystrophy. Shown is an extreme example of muscles showing marked hypertrophy (calves, forearms, deltoids, masseters), with other groups showing wasting (biceps, quadriceps). (Taken from Bundy (1972) with permission.)

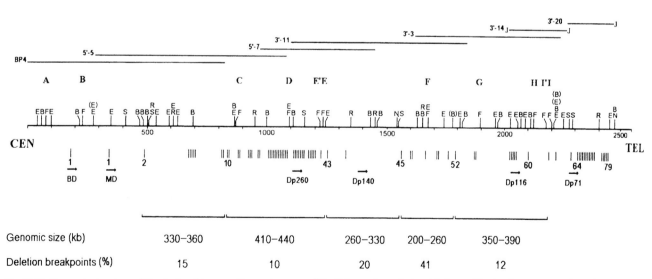

Fig. 19.16. Genomic structure of the dystrophin gene. Shown is a map of the 2.5 megabase dystrophin locus. The top lines represent yeast artificial chromosomes (YACs) used to localize exons. The A–I letters underneath the YACs represent rare-cutting *SfiI* sites. A representation of the genomic locus is next, with size (in kilobase pairs; 1–2500 kb), and a restriction map. Beneath this is an indication of the location of each exon (1–79), followed by a representation of each of the promoters of the gene (BD, brain dystrophin; MD, muscle dystrophin; Dp260, Dp140, Dp116 and Dp71 are the different isoforms characterized to date). (Taken from Nobile et al. (1997) with permission.)

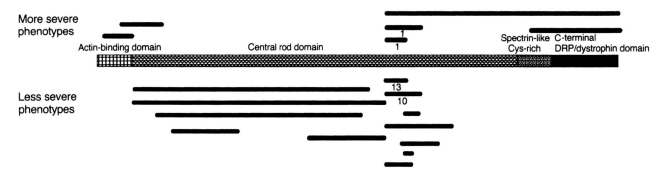

Fig. 19.17. Schematic diagram of dystrophin domains, and clinical severity in patients with Becker muscular dystrophy. The cysteine-rich and N-terminal actin-binding domains appear particularly critical for dystrophin function in muscle. (Taken from Hoffman (1993) with permission.)

about half of the initiated transcripts are successfully completed by the transcriptional machinery (Tennyson et al., 1995). There are approximately five to ten copies of dystrophin mRNA per nucleus, and the half-life of the mRNA in myogenic cell cultures is about 15 hours (Tennyson et al., 1996). The difficulty that cells have in making the dystrophin mRNA and protein leads to a low quantity of dystrophin mRNA and protein in mature muscle (approximately 0.03% of muscle transcripts and protein; Hoffman et al., 1987b). By comparison, the dystrophin protein appears to be very long lived: as long as 6 months in inducible transgenic mice (Ahmad et al., 2000).

Considerable data have accumulated regarding the relative importance of the four dystrophin domains from both human patients and transgenic mice (Fig. 19.17). Genotype/phenotype correlations established that the penultimate cysteine-rich domain and the beginning of the C-terminal globular domain are absolutely critical for dystrophin function (Beggs et al., 1991; Rafael et al., 1996; Corrado et al., 1996). The N-terminal actin-binding domain is likewise very important, with patients or mice deleted for this region showing a severe Becker phenotype, although not as severe as complete dystrophin deficiency (Duchenne dystrophy). The large central rod domain is considerably less important, with boys or mice deleted for much of this domain still showing a relatively mild phenotype. Similarly, the C-terminal domain appears relatively unimportant, despite the many alternatively spliced isoforms in this domain. Importantly, mouse knock-outs of the Dp71 isoform of dystrophin, which is expressed at a high level in many tissues, show no discernible phenotype, agreeing with the human studies (Lumeng et al., 1999a; Sarig et al., 1999).

Full-length muscle and brain dystrophin shows considerable homology to proteins that form anti-parallel dimers; however, the sequence of the rod domain has diverged to the point where it probably does not dimerize in the same manner as its distant relatives (spectrin, α-actinin) (Thomas et al., 1997). Studies have been contradictory with regards to the monomeric or dimeric structure of dystrophin, with most biochemical studies suggesting that it is a monomer, while electron microscopy has suggested that it may be a dimer (Watkins et al., 1988; Chan and Kunkel, 1997; Kahana et al., 1997; Winder et al., 1995; Rybakova and Ervasti, 1997). It is possible that it may be a conditional dimer, where dimerization is facilitated by actin binding along the rod domain (Fig. 19.18) (Rybakova and Ervasti, 1997). The dystrophin rod domain is able to associate directly with lipid bilayers containing phosphatidylserine, where it induces a large increase in the surface shear viscosity of the membrane (DeWolf et al., 1997). Importantly, the ability of the dystrophin rod domain to increase the viscosity of the membrane is dependent on the native state of the protein; denatured dystrophin is unable to strengthen the membrane (DeWolf et al., 1997).

Function of dystrophin in the membrane cytoskeleton

An impressive amount has been learned in the late 1990s concerning the structure and function of dystrophin, particularly with regards to the other proteins to which it binds at the plasma membrane (so-called dystrophin-associated proteins).

Actin

Dystrophin binds actin filaments at many positions along the molecule, with the highest affinity at the N-terminus (Rybakova and Ervasti, 1997; Howard et al., 1998, 1999). Dystrophin binds both myofibrillar actin and nonmuscle actins with similar affinity; this provides a functional link to the intracellular cytoskeleton and/or myofibrils (Renley et al., 1998). This actin-binding function of dystrophin is undoubtedly critical for its function; however, the multiple binding sites suggest that deletion of one actin-binding domain can be functionally rescued to some extent by the other actin-binding domains along the molecule.

Dystroglycan

The second critical protein–protein association is between dystrophin and the transmembrane β-dystroglycan (Fig. 19.18). Beta-dystroglycan, and the larger extracellular α-dystroglycan, are proteolytic products of the same larger precursor (Ervasti and Campbell, 1993). The dystroglycans provide a link between dystrophin and the extracellular basal lamina, via laminin (Campbell, 1995). The binding site between dystrophin and β-dystroglycan has been well studied and appears to be a Pro–Pro–X–Tyr motif on the C-terminal region of β-dystroglycan, and the cysteine-rich domain of dystrophin (Fig. 19.19) (Rentschler et al., 1999). Dystroglycan is not muscle specific and is expressed in a wide variety of tissues throughout development. Dystroglycan is used by many cells for correct orientation and interaction with the basal lamina, and mouse knockouts of dystroglycan show early embryonic lethality (Williamson et al., 1997; Henry and Campbell, 1998). Dystroglycan has also been found to be the attachment site for a number of infectious pathogens in nonmuscle tissues, including lymphocytic choriomeningitis virus, *Mycobacterium leprae* and Lassa fever virus (Cao et al., 1998; Rambukkana et al., 1998). In muscle, coxsackievirus B3 seems to cleave dystrophin soon after entry, and this cleavage may contribute to infectious dilated cardiomyopathy seen in coxsackievirus infection (Badorff et al., 1999).

Other dystrophin-associated proteins

The primary protein associations involved in the dystrophin-based transmembrane cytoskeletal network are actin, dystrophin, dystroglycans and laminin (Fig. 19.18). The sarcoglycans are also critical dystrophin-associated proteins. The sarcoglycan complex is a series of four related proteins, each of which shows a single transmembrane domain, with the majority of protein occurring at the external face of the plasma membrane. These four proteins do not directly interact with dystrophin; however, they appear to be responsible for stabilizing the dystrophin–dystroglycan–laminin network (Fig. 19.18) (Henry and Campbell, 1998; Lumeng et al., 1999b). Consistent with this, cells that produce the dystrophin–dystroglycan–laminin network but do not synthesize the sarcoglycans seem to show weaker interactions between

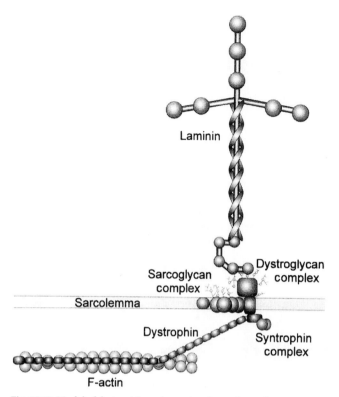

Fig. 19.18. Model of dystrophin and associated proteins at the plasma membrane cytoskeleton. Dystrophin is shown with the C-terminal domains bound to the transmembrane dystroglycan complex and cytoplasmic syntrophin complex. The rod domain and N-terminal domains bind filamentous actin. (Taken from Rybakova and Ervasti (1997) with permission.)

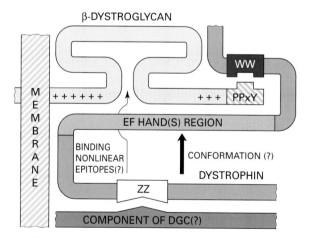

Fig. 19.19. The interaction between dystrophin and β-dystroglycan showing the sites of interactions, and specific subdomains, of dystrophin and β-dystroglycan. This association is critical for the function of dystrophin in stabilization of the plasma membrane and the linkage of the myofibre to the extracellular matrix. (Taken from Rentschler et al. (1999) with permission.)

dystrophin and dystroglycan (Li et al., 1998; Saito et al., 1999). The four sarcoglycans form a heterotetramer and are linked with intermolecular disulphide bonds (Chan et al., 1998). Mutations in any one of the four sarcoglycan genes results in a muscular dystrophy clinically similar to a dystrophinopathy (Duggan et al., 1997). (See Chapter 20). In dystrophin-deficient muscle, the sarcoglycans, and all the dystrophin-associated proteins, show dramatic secondary reductions. There are animal models of the sarcoglycanopathies that share many histological and clinical features with the dystrophin-deficient *mdx* mouse, although there is variability in heart involvement and clinical severity (Sakamoto et al., 1997; Duclos et al., 1998; Hack et al., 1998).

There are a number of additional dystrophin-associated proteins; however, most research to date suggests that these are not as important for the structural integrity of the membrane as the sarcoglycan-stabilized dystrophin–dystroglycan–laminin network. Instead, these additional proteins (syntrophins, NOS, dystrobrevins) are responsible for localizing other proteins to the dystrophin-based membrane cytoskeleton. Alpha-syntrophin is a cytoplasmic protein composed entirely of protein–protein interaction motifs, including PDZ and pleckstrin homology domains (Kachinsky et al., 1999; Kameya et al., 1999). Mouse knockout strains for α-syntrophin show unaltered phenotype and normal muscle histology, although the neuromuscular junction exhibits some structural changes (Adams et al., 2000). The PDZ domain is responsible for binding and localizing sodium channels and NOS. The involvement of NOS in Duchenne dystrophy has received considerable attention because it produces nitric oxide, which is implicated in modulating a variety of important cell functions. Loss of dystrophin at the membrane leads to secondary loss of syntrophin, which in turn leads to loss of NOS localization at the membrane cytoskeleton. The involvement of NOS in the pathophysiology of dystrophin deficiency is described below.

Two final, less-well characterized, dystrophin-associated proteins are sarcospan and the dystrobrevins. Sarcospan is a small plasma membrane protein, with four transmembrane domains, which is most highly concentrated at the neuromuscular and myotendinous junctions (Crosbie et al., 1997, 1999). Like the sarcoglycans, sarcospan appears to stabilize the dystrophin–dystroglycan–laminin membrane network, perhaps through stabilization of the extracellular α-dystroglycan to the assembled complex (Crosbie et al., 1999). Dystrobrevin is a class of related molecules produced by alternative splicing that share homology to the C-terminus of dystrophin (Peters et al., 1997, 1998; Roberts and Bobrow, 1998) (Fig. 19.9)). Dystrobrevins bind syntrophin and co-purify with the dystrophin-associated proteins (Kachinsky et al., 1999). Mouse knock-outs for α-dystrobrevin show a subclinical myopathy and cardiomyopathy, with retention of the dystrophin-based cytoskeleton but loss of NOS at the membrane (Grady et al., 1999).

Other membrane cytoskeleton networks

It appears that there are two means by which myofibres maintain their contact with the extracellular environment (basal lamina); one is the dystrophin–dystroglycan–laminin link (Fig. 19.18) and the second a vinculin–integrin–laminin link (not shown). These are somewhat redundant systems, as mutations of either link leads to muscle disease, yet myofibres do remain viable to some extent. Consistent with this partial redundancy, laminin polymerization into a cell-associated polygonal network is promoted by *either* α-dystroglycan or $\alpha_7\beta_1$-integrin; the resulting laminin network results in the redistribution of both the transmembrane proteins (α-dystroglycan, integrin) and the underlying membrane cytoskeleton (dystrophin, vinculin) into reciprocal networks (Colognato et al., 1999). Disruptions of either membrane link can lead to myogenic cell death, possibly via apoptosis (Vachon et al., 1996, 1997; Angoli et al., 1997; Montanaro et al., 1998; Brown et al., 1999). Interestingly, these two networks can coincide in localization, with enrichment at the costameres (binding sites for myofibrils to the plasma membrane) (Fig. 19.20). Recent studies suggest that there may be some protein connections between the two networks, possibly through α-actinin and/or actin filaments (Hance et al., 1999). Also consistent with the reciprocal nature of these two networks is the observation that $\alpha_7\beta_1$-integrin is upregulated in Duchenne dystrophy muscle, as an apparent effort to compensate for loss of the dystrophin–dystroglycan–laminin network (Hodges et al., 1997).

It is clear that the vinculin–integrin–laminin network exists almost exclusively at costameres and myotendinous junctions, while the dystrophin–dystroglycan–laminin network exists throughout the plasma membrane, although it is *enriched* at the costameres (both skeletal muscle and heart) and myotendinous junctions (Minetti et al., 1992; Kostin et al., 1998; Vohra et al., 1998). Laminin, in turn, binds to the other components of the basal lamina and extracellular matrix, including perlecan, fibulins and nidogens (Andac et al., 1999; Talts et al., 1999). Consistent with findings in other tissues, the integrin–laminin association is particularly important for development and regeneration of muscle. Inherited disorders of α_7-integrin

(Hayashi et al., 1998) and the laminin α2-chain (Pegoraro et al., 1998) result in muscle disorders that show features of both congenital myopathy (developmental problem) and congenital muscular dystrophy (degeneration/regeneration). The specific isoforms of the laminins and integrins involved in muscle disease are covered in other chapters of this volume.

There is a third protein network that can be considered conditionally redundant, namely the utrophin–dystroglycan–laminin network. Utrophin was first identified by immunoblots, which showed a protein of the same molecular weight as dystrophin cross-reacting with some anti-dystrophin antibodies (Hoffman et al., 1989a), and, independently, by sequence analysis of cross-hybridizing cDNA clones from the C-terminal domains of dystrophin (Love et al., 1989). Utrophin shares considerable homology with dystrophin throughout most of its amino acid sequence, and it was hypothesized that utrophin might be able to compensate functionally for dystrophin (Love et al., 1989). Utrophin is relatively highly expressed in many cells of the body and was named for this 'ubiquitous' expression pattern. In muscle, expression of utrophin is relatively high in fetal muscle then declines after birth. In dystrophin-deficient mice, utrophin levels persist in muscle, while in humans with Duchenne dystrophy utrophin declines after birth then rises again (Taylor et al., 1997; Gramolini et al., 1999a).

Utrophin itself is not critical for life: mouse knock-outs for utrophin show no evident phenotype and no muscle pathology (Grady et al., 1997a; Deconinck et al., 1997a; Rafael et al., 1999). However, utrophin is conditionally essential in the context of dystrophin deficiency, as it can substitute for dystrophin in the dystrophin–dystroglycan–laminin network. The ability of utrophin to compensate for dystrophin deficiency has been unambiguously proven using transgenic mice; mice lacking *both* dystrophin and utrophin show a very severe clinical phenotype, dying at an early age with a severe dystrophic process in their muscle (Deconinck et al., 1997b; Grady et al., 1997b). In agreement with the ability of utrophin to rescue muscles functionally in patients with Duchenne dystrophy, the amount of utrophin upregulation in extraocular muscles correlates with the severity of the clinical involvement (Porter et al., 1998). Utrophin upregulation as a potential route for therapy of Duchenne dystrophy will be further described below. However, it is important to recognize utrophin as a 'conditionally redundant' system: dystroglycan preferentially associates with dystrophin in the myofibre; in the absence of dystrophin it will associate with utrophin where the same function is accomplished.

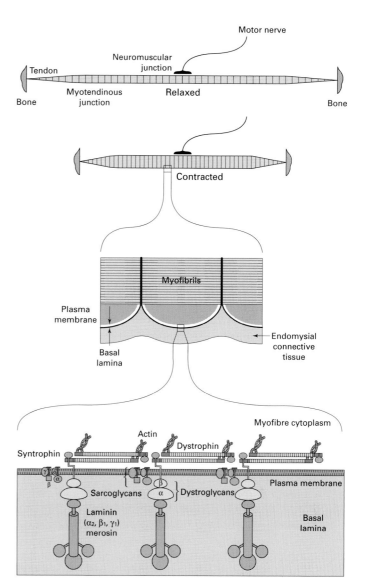

Fig. 19.20. Membrane stability during myofibre contraction and the requirement for the dystrophin-based membrane cytoskeleton. Shown is a syncytial muscle fibre, extending from bone attachment site at each end. After activation, the fibre contracts, with redistribution of the myofibre cytoplasm. Costameres at the level of the Z line keep the sarcolemmal membrane attached to the underlying myofibrils (centre panel); this area has enrichment of the dystrophin–dystroglycan–laminin network and is also the sole location of the vinculin–integrin–laminin network (not shown). Throughout the plasma membrane, dystrophin interacts with a series of associated proteins to enable attachment to both actin filaments and the extracellular basal lamina (dystrophin–dystroglycan–laminin network) (bottom panel). (Taken from Hoffman (1997) with permission.)

Dystrophin in invertebrates

Considerable research has been conducted on the evolutionary conservation of dystrophin-like genes and the consequences of their deficiency in distantly related species. In *Caenorhabditis elegans*, a gene showing high homology to the C-terminus of dystrophin has been dubbed *dys-1* (Fig. 19.9). Mutation of *dys-1* leads to hyperactivity and hypercontracted muscle in worms, and replacement of *dys-1* with human dystrophin sequences partially rescues this phenotype (Bessou et al., 1998). The Dys-1 protein in worms seems to be involved in cholinergic transmission and may be more similar in function to utrophin than dystrophin (Bessou et al., 1998). In fruit flies (*Drosophila*), a gene related to dystrophin dubbed *kakapo* is required for integrin-mediated attachment of muscle and other cell types to the epithelium (Gregory and Brown, 1998; Strumpf and Volk, 1998). *Kakapo* is expressed in tedons and is responsible for localization of a neuregulin-like factor (Vein). These dystrophin-related proteins in flies and worms follow the general theme of critical involvement in muscle cell anchorage in the extracellular matrix, although the specific interacting proteins seems to diverge with evolution.

Pathophysiology of dystrophin deficiency

The finding of full-length dystrophin in different cell types (skeletal muscle, heart, neurons, vascular and visceral smooth muscle) opened the possibility that the pathophysiology of Duchenne dystrophy might not be limited to muscle alone, and that Duchenne dystrophy could be a multisystemic disorder (Hoffman and Kunkel, 1989). Moreover, the marked clinical differences between the different dystrophin-deficient animal models and the human disease suggested that there were many aspects of the progressive pathophysiology that were secondary, for example induced by chronic muscle injury, and not directly caused by lack of dystrophin (Hoffman et al., 1987b; Hoffman and Gorospe, 1991). Here, the literature concerning dystrophin physiology and pathophysiology is discussed, drawing upon many recent insights gained through the study of dystrophin-deficient animals (particularly the *mdx* mouse).

Dystrophin and dystrophin deficiency in myofibres

The loss of dystrophin leads to some immediate consequences for the myofibre, which include a change in membrane shear viscosity as a result of loss of the direct stabilizing effect of the rod domain on membranes (DeWolf et al., 1997) and the loss of attachments to the intracellular membrane cytoskeleton owing to loss of actin filament binding at multiple sites along dystrophin (Figs. 19.18 and 19.20; Table 19.1) (Rybakova and Ervasti, 1997). This membrane instability likely predisposes the myofibre to stress-induced injury; however, these changes alone are relatively unlikely to cause substantial pathology.

The loss of dystrophin leads to secondary protein deficiencies, which have additional cumulative effects on cell damage and viability (Table 19.1). It is likely that the loss of the sarcoglycans ensues as the next step, which in turn destabilizes the dystroglycan–laminin interactions. Evidence for this temporal change is that mutations in any one of the sarcoglycans results in secondary deficiency of all sarcoglycans, and also of dystroglycan, while dystrophin is relatively well preserved. The destabilization of the dystroglycan–laminin binding leads to secondary loss of the dystroglycans, and consequent loss of a major attachment of the myofibre to the extracellular matrix. This, in turn, causes difficulty in maintaining synchronized contraction of the fibre per unit length, which adds further stress to the plasma membrane during activity. The additional membrane stress leads to greater damage, and more unrestained flow of material across the membrane. The vinculin–integrin–laminin network seems secondarily disrupted intracellularly, although spectrin and integrin attempt to compensate and the integrin–laminin link of the myofibre to the extracellular matrix appears intact (Minetti et al., 1998; Williams et al., 1999).

The consequence of the increased membrane instability is a particular sensitivity to membrane stress, such as with eccentric (lengthening) contractions of muscle. This increased membrane instability is initially interpreted as a cue for myofibre hypertrophy, which itself can exacerbate stress on the membrane and increase membrane damage. The loss of a major link to the extracellular matrix appears to be a cue for apoptosis of some myonuclei, which can decrease local protein synthesis at regions of a myofibre, again exacerbating membrane stability (Table 19.1). The end result of all the above processes is contraction-induced myofibre necrosis owing to an inability to compensate for unregulated calcium influx.

Additional secondary consequences of dystrophin deficiency have been recently documented, and all of these, while less important with regards to the primary function of the cell, may exacerbate myofibre dysfunction and hasten necrosis (Table 19.1; Fig. 19.21). First, the membrane instability leads to transient breaks in the plasma membrane, which allow unregulated calcium influx. Mitochondria attempt to buffer this abnormal calcium

Table 19.1. Consequences of dystrophin deficiency

Area affected	Importance	Consequences
Skeletal muscle and heart: membrane instability	Acutely important	Decrease in plasma membrane surface shear viscosity (rod domain)
		Loss of cell cytoskeleton connection to membrane by actin filaments
		Secondary loss of sarcoglycans, destabilization of α/β-dystroglycan association with laminin
		Secondary loss of α/β-dystroglycan
		Secondary loss of myfibre anchorage to extracellular matrix via laminin (basal lamina)
		Secondary loss of vinculin links to the integrin–laminin network
		Sensitivity to eccentric exercise, myofibre leakage of creatine kinase, other soluble proteins
		Misuses signals for myofibre hypertrophy, exacerbation of membrane injury
		Increased sensitivity of myofibres to proteases; increased mast cell degranulation; exacerbation of membrane damage
		Apoptosis of some nuclei
		Contraction-induced myofibre membrane damage and occasional necrosis
Skeletal muscle: vascularization and metabolic abnormalities	Chronically important	Abnormal calcium regulation, including overload of mitochondria; metabolic dysfunction, exacerbation of calcium homeostasis, apoptosis
		Secondary deficiencies of syntrophin/neuronal nitric oxide synthetase (nNOS): loss of localization of nNOS in the myofibre; inability to modulate α-adrenergic vasoconstriction during exercise; localized functional ischaemia during exercise; exacerbation of calcium homeostasis, apoptosis; grouped necrosis
Skeletal muscle: secondary biochemical deficiencies	Uncertain	Secondary deficiencies of dystrobrevin, sarcospan
		Secondary loss of aquaporin, increased sensitivity to osmotic stress
Visceral smooth muscle	Chronic	Loss of coordinated colonic peristaltic waves owing to nNOS mislocalization
Brain, neurons	Uncertain	Increased potentiation of NMDA (N-methyl-D-aspartate) receptor in hippocampal CA1 slices but no clinical abnormality of long-term potentiation
		Reduced cortical excitability observed by transcranial stimulation and electromyography
Vascular smooth muscle	Uncertain	nNOS mislocalization, vascular disturbance

load, while the strong calcium trafficking machinery of the sarcoplasmic reticulum works to sequester cytoplasmic calcium. However, it is well documented that the mitochondria in Duchenne and *mdx* muscle becomes overloaded with calcium, with subsequent dysfunction of mitochondria, and metabolic dysfunction of the myofibre. Also involved is the loss of NOS localization, with subsequent abnormalities in local control of vascular perfusion of myofibres. Transient ischaemia will only add to the increased calcium influx and exacerbate the calcium trafficking difficulties of the myofibre. Aquaporin, the membrane water channel, also seems mislocalized or disrupted in dystrophin-deficient fibres, and this may result in changes of osmolality and increased sensitivity to osmotic stress (Liu et al., 1999).

The data accumulating for this model are considerable (Table 19.1; Fig. 19.21). With regards to calcium traffic abnormalities, important studies have been done in cul-

tured *mdx* myotubes, both innervated and noninnervated. Under normal physiological ion conditions, calcium handling was similar in *mdx* and normal myotubes (Imbert et al., 1996; Leijendekker et al., 1996). However, when the extracellular calcium level was raised, or osmolality decreased, the *mdx* myotubes begin to show abnormal influx of calcium, of which only part could be blocked by a calcium channel blocker (gadolinium) (Leijendekker et al., 1996). Dystrophin-deficient myotubes and myoblasts seem very sensitive to apoptosis-inducing agents such as treatment with free radicals, suggesting that they are already near the threshold for apoptosis (Disatnik et al., 1998; Rando et al., 1998; Sandri et al., 1998a). Exercise of *mdx* mice induces an inappropriate increase in ubiquitination, and decrease in Bcl-2 expression, leading to apoptotic nuclei (Sandri et al., 1997). This increased sensitivity to cell-damaging agents is not directly related to misregulation of NOS, as there is no evidence of nitrotyrosine

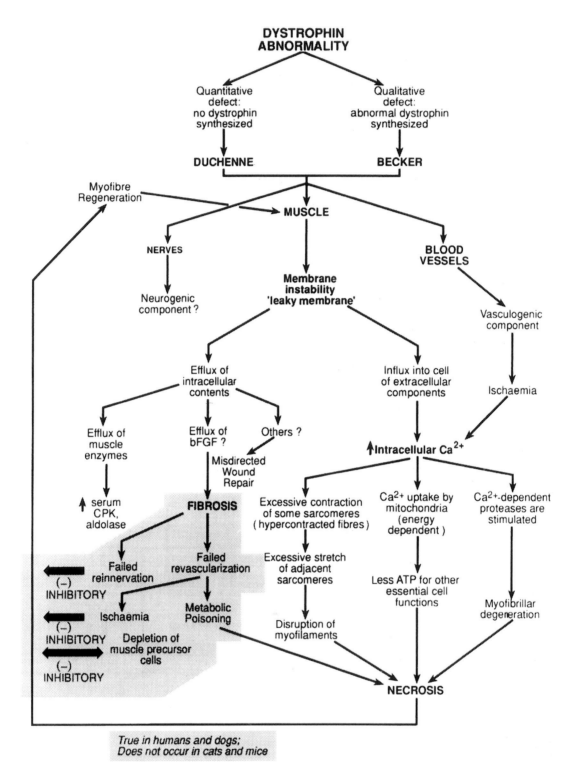

Fig. 19.21. Pathophysiology of dystrophin deficiency in humans and animals. Shown is a modification of a schematic diagram of Rowland (1980), as published in Hoffman and Gorospe (1991). This model has gained considerable validity with the finding of vascular perfusion defects secondary to nitric oxide synthetase (NOS) mislocalization, mitochondrial dysfunction owing to calcium overload, and the differences between the phenotypes of the animals models of dystrophin deficiency (see text). bFGF, basic fibroblast growth factor; CPK, creatine phosphokinase. (Taken from Hoffman and Gorospe (1991) with permission.)

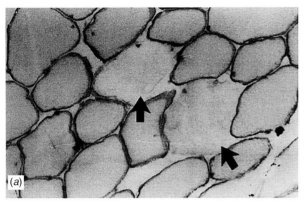 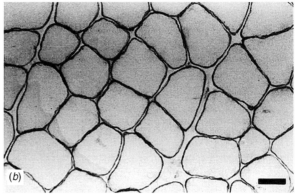

Fig. 19.22. Dystrophin remodelling is an early event in strenuous exercise of normal muscle. (*a*) Normal rats that had been exposed to 130 minutes of intermittent downhill running (eccentric contractions) showed an immediate loss of dystrophin in a subset of myofibres in the quadriceps femoris. (*b*) Interestingly, female rats showed considerably less damage to muscle after the same exercise, as shown by either dystrophin immunostaining (*b*) or by β-glucuronidase levels taken 48 hours after exercise. (Taken from Komulainen et al. (1999) with permission.)

formation in *mdx* muscle (Rando et al., 1998), and mice that are knock-out for both dystrophin and NOS show no worsening of phenotype or histopathology (Chao et al., 1998; Crosbie et al., 1998).

The role of exercise in exacerbation of the membrane instability, and the deleterious consequences of this instability, is becoming increasingly clear. Patients with Duchenne muscular dystrophy who show developmental arrest of muscle and muscle activity show far less necrosis and other 'dystrophic' features (Kimura et al., 1998). If sedentary *mdx* mice are exposed to exercise, then the number of apoptotic nuclei increases to 4% of all nuclei within 2 days by a variety of apoptosis assays (Podhorska-Okolow et al., 1998). Patients have been more difficult to study for apoptosis, though both apoptotic nuclei and anti-apoptotic proteins show increased expression in biopsies from patients with Duchenne dystrophy (Sandri et al., 1998b). It is important to note that apoptosis is probably only one route to myofibre damage, and that contraction-induced injury is still likely the primary end-point for a myofibre (Table 19.1; Fig. 19.21). A recent elegant study showed that elimination of apoptosis from dystrophin-deficient muscle by production of a double knock-out mouse (dystrophin and perforin deficient) resulted in a complete lack of apoptosis in *mdx* muscle (Spencer et al., 1997). However, these apoptosis-deficient *mdx* mice showed the same amount of myofibre necrosis as did apoptosis-competent mice, suggesting that contraction-induced injury may be the major mediator of cell death in the dystrophinopathies (Spencer et al., 1997).

Reinforcing the notion of miscued muscle hypertrophy through membrane damage are data accumulating in normal skeletal muscle exposed to hypertrophy-inducing eccentric contraction. Two recent studies have shown that loss of dystrophin is an immediate consequence of lengthening (eccentric) contractions in myofibres, after either downhill exercise or 240 forced lengthening contractions (Komulainen et al., 1998, 1999). Muscle was studied at 0 and 6 hours and two, four and seven days after the exercise, and myofibre damage was assayed by both β-glucuronidase activity and immunostaining changes of the membrane cytoskeleton. A percentage of normal muscle fibres showed swelling immediately after exercise (time 0), and these same fibres showed loss of dystrophin at the plasma membrane (Fig. 19.22) (Komulainen et al., 1998, 1999). As lengthening contractions are known to be a strong hypertrophic stimulus for muscle, these data suggest that dystrophin degradation is a very early event in the signal for muscle hypertrophy. Interestingly, female rats showed much less myofibre damage from downhill running and are also known to show less hypertrophic response to eccentric exercise (Komulainen et al., 1998).

A critical recent finding is that dystrophin-based localization of nNOS is necessary for local regulation of blood flow in muscle during exercise (Thomas et al., 1998). The evidence provided in this paper is quite compelling and makes it highly likely that dystrophin-deficient muscle experiences transient ischaemia during exercise (Table 19.1). The authors studied skeletal muscle at rest and during exercise in normal mice, *mdx* mice and nNOS knock-out mice. They found that vascularization and response to modulation of NOS was normal at rest, and there were normal levels of endothelial NOS (eNOS), suggesting that the eNOS responses of endothelium were intact. During exercise, there was a clear inhibition of sympathetic vasoconstriction in normal mice that was lacking in both dystrophin-deficient and nNOS-deficient mice. The authors could show that this inability to attenuate α-adrenergic vasoconstriction resulted from the loss of nNOS activity in muscle fibres (Thomas et al., 1998). This defect in local vascularization of muscle during exercise almost certainly causes transient functional ischaemia, with attending exercise intolerance (as is seen in both *mdx* mice and patients with Duchenne dystrophy). Importantly, myofibrillar nNOS modulation of blood flow appears more important for fast-twitch glycolytic fibres, than it does for slow-twitch oxidative fibres; this may explain some of the preferential loss of fast-twitch fibres in Duchenne muscle, which has been recognized for many years.

Given the growing evidence for exercise/contraction-induced injury in dystrophin-deficient muscle, one might jump to the conclusion that exercise is deleterious for humans (or animals) with dystrophin deficiency. This may be true for *damaging* types of exercise (e.g. eccentric contractions), but it may not be for low-intensity, low-load types of exercise. Indeed, recent studies suggest that low-intensity (noneccentric) exercise may be more beneficial to dystrophin-deficient muscle than it is harmful. For example, swimming exercise of both young and old *mdx* mice resulted in a 25% increase in normalized tetanic tensions for the extensor digitorum longus and a 45% increase for soleus (Hayes and Williams, 1998; Wineinger et al., 1998). This increase in strength was in spite of the severely dystrophic phenotype of the aged *mdx* mice.

Finally, there is growing evidence for calcium overload and subsequent dysfunction of mitochondria in dystrophin-deficient muscle. Mitochondrial oxidative phosphorylation in *mdx* mouse muscle was approximately half of that in age-matched controls, presumably as a result of calcium overload of the mitochondria (Kuznetsov et al., 1998). Oxidative damage was also evident (Haycock et al., 1996). Downregulation of mitochondrial function is indicated by a twofold reduction in mRNA expression for many nuclear-encoded mitochondrial proteins in patients with Duchenne dystrophy (Chen et al., 2000). Nuclear magnetic resonance studies with phosphorus-31 have shown that glycolytic lactate production is compromised in Becker muscular dystrophy, resulting in reduced glucose availability after exercise (Lodi et al., 1999).

One of the more intriguing aspects of the histopathology of all the dystrophin-deficient (and sarcoglycan-deficient) species is the sudden onset of grouped necrosis in mice at around three weeks of age. In humans, dogs and cats, myofibrillar necrosis is seen much earlier in life, and while

there are small groups of necrotic fibres, the histopathology does not include the large-scale sudden onset of dozens to hundreds of myofibres synchronously undergoing necrosis, as is seen in the dystrophin-deficient mice, and sarcoglycan-deficient mice and hamsters. Some studies have shown that mast cell degranulation can induce grouped necrosis (Gorospe et al., 1994a,b, 1996), and this will be discussed further. However, 'bystander effect' for grouped necrosis does not explain the remarkable postnatal onset at 3 weeks. A recent study found that this timing of necrosis coincides with postnatal maturation of the thyroid endocrine system, with serum thyroxine and triiodothyronine concentrations rising immediately prior to the onset of necrosis (McArdle et al., 1998). In keeping with a role of thyroid hormone in the succeptibility of rodent myofibres to dystrophin deficiency, induction of hypothyroidism with propylthiouracil resulted in a delayed onset of necrosis (McArdle et al., 1998). Mice at three weeks of age show an increase in physical activity (this is around the time of weaning), and inhibition of muscle movement at this time delays the onset of necrosis (Mokhtarian et al., 1995, 1999).

In conclusion, there is increasing evidence that muscle activity induces myofibre damage, which is exacerbated by a number of other cellular and tissue factors, eventually leading to necrosis in a subset of cells (Table 19.1; Figs. 19.20 and 19.21). However, the dystrophin-deficient muscle still responds positively to exercise, increasing in strength and bulk. The normal role of dystrophin appears to be to regulate stability of the plasma membrane, and part of this role seems to be to mediate early signals for muscle adaptation to excessive exercise (hypertrophic response to eccentric activity) and to increase local blood flow during exercise through localization of nNOS.

Dystrophin and dystrophin deficiency in smooth muscle

Patients with Duchenne dystrophy can show pseudo-obstruction of the gastrointestinal tract. Vascular involvement in the pathology of Duchenne dystrophy muscle has also long been hypothesized. The finding of full-length dystrophin expression in both visceral and vascular smooth muscle opened the possibility that the gastrointestinal and vascular differences seen in Duchenne dystrophy could be *primary* consequences of dystrophin deficiency, rather than secondary, downstream events.

Recent studies have made it clear that dystrophin deficiency has a primary effect on peristalsis of the colon (Mancinelli et al., 1995; Azzena and Mancinelli, 1999). These authors have documented abnormalities in the peristaltic reflex of *mdx* colon and then went on to show that this reflex could be modulated by using antagonists or agonists of nitric oxide; addition of ʟ-arginine restored 90% of the peristaltic waves of the *mdx* colon (Azzena and Mancinelli, 1999).

These studies, together with the studies of Thomas et al. (1998) showing that lack of myofibrillar dystrophin leads to loss of NOS-induced modulation of the α-adrenergic response for vascularization, suggests that dystrophin is important for regulation of NOS activities in multiple organ systems. This also suggests that dystrophin deficiency may have a direct effect on vascular smooth muscle in arteries and arterioles through similar NOS-based mechanisms, although there is no experimental evidence for this to date.

It is important to reiterate the fact that *mdx* mice with the gene for nNOS also knocked-out showed no difference in overt clinical phenotype compared with *mdx* mice with an intact nNOS gene (Chao et al., 1998; Crosbie et al., 1998). While this might sound counterintuitive when arguing for a central role of nNOS in the pathophysiology of dystrophin deficiency, this is, in fact, expected: nNOS is already 'dysfunctional' in *mdx* mice owing to mislocalization, hence the loss of the gene for nNOS might not be expected to exacerbate cellular dysfunction further.

Dystrophin and dystrophin deficiency in neurons and retina

It has been well established that full-length dystrophin and/or specific smaller dystrophin isoforms appear in the subsynaptic densities of some neurons, including the synapse of the rods at the bipolar cells of the retina (Ueda et al., 1997; Fitzgerald et al., 1999; Pillers et al., 1999). Perhaps the best-characterized neuronal defect is that of the retinal rod cells. The Dp260 and Dp71 isoforms of dystrophin (see Fig. 19.16) are expressed in rod spherules (submembranous dense regions facing bipolar cell processes), and the lack of expression of these dystrophin isoforms results in specific electroretinographic (ERG) abnormalities (reduction in B/A wave amplitude ratio) (Ueda et al., 1997; Pascual et al., 1998; Blank et al., 1999; Fitzgerald et al., 1999; Pillers et al., 1999).

Abnormalities in other neuronal cells have been less conclusive to date. In a hippocampal slice preparation from *mdx* mice, CA1 pyramidal neurons have been shown to display a hypoxia-induced loss of synaptic transmission (Mehler et al., 1992). As approximately one-third of patients with Duchenne dystrophy show nonprogressive mental retardation, it is possible that transient ischaemia during development or at birth could induce irreversible

brain damage leading to the observed mental retardation. This ischaemia could be exacerbated by the vascular smooth muscle defect in perfusion, discussed above. Consistent with a vascular aetiology of the mental retardation in Duchenne dystrophy, dystrophin isoforms have been localized on the pericapillary endfeet of astrocytes at the blood–brain barrier in both hippocampus and cerebral cortex (Chen et al., 1999a; Jancsik and Hajos, 1999).

Complicating the interpretation of cellular abnormalities of specific cell types in brain is the plethora of dystrophin isoforms in the brain (Moizard et al., 1998), and the many different cell types expressing certain isoforms. For example, in the mouse superior cervical ganglion, dystrophin isoforms of different types are expressed in the ganglionic neurons, satellite cells and Schwann cells and they are associated with a variety of cytoplasmic organelles and specialized membrane structures (de Stefano et al., 1997).

Functional studies of brain in *mdx* mouse or patients with Duchenne muscular dystrophy are few, and results somewhat contradictory. In looking at brain slices of *mdx* hippocampal CA1 area, normal synaptic responses were observed, but there was a greater potentiation of glutamatergic transmission after conditioning pulses (Vaillend et al., 1999). However, *mdx* mice seem to act normally for both spatial learning and hippocampal long-term potentiation (Sesay et al., 1996). Transcranial stimulation in patients with Duchenne dystrophy, with detection of cortical excitability by EMG, showed that the required threshold for stimulation was higher than normal, suggesting reduced cortical excitability (Di Lazzaro et al., 1998).

Dystrophin and dystrophin deficiency in the heart

All dystrophin-deficient organisms show significant cardiac involvement, and this is likely a combined consequence of dystrophin deficiency in cardiocytes and in vascular smooth muscle (Hoffman et al., 1987b; Hoffman and Gorospe 1991). Given the concentric nature of heart contractions, it is probably safe to assume that the heart does not show sheer-force-induced membrane instability as frequently as is seen in actively contracting skeletal myofibres. However, heart tissue is unable to regenerate; consequently, any destruction of cardiocytes is irreversible. Importantly, the basolateral free wall of the left ventricle is the region most highly affected, and this same region is most susceptible to damage from global ischaemia. The preferential involvement of this region of the heart may imply that the NOS-mediated vascular abnormalities seen in skeletal muscle and in visceral smooth muscle may affect the heart vasculature as well. A recent study has shown that breeding of a mouse lacking both dystrophin and a muscle transcriptional factor (MyoD) results in quite severe cardiac disease (Megeney et al., 1999). The molecular basis for this is not clear, as MyoD is thought to be most important for muscle regeneration, and cardiac tissue does not regenerate.

The progressive aspects of dystrophinopathies: secondary histological changes leading to wasting and weakness

The gradual failure of regeneration in the skeletal muscle of humans and dogs appears to be the cause of muscle wasting, weakness and early death (Fig. 19.21). Although age-dependent wasting is not as obvious in dystrophin-deficient mice and cats, *mdx* mice do, in fact, show relatively late-onset muscle weakness, and a decreased lifespan, and the muscle weakness is exacerbated by muscle overload (Dick and Vrbova, 1993; Lefaucheur et al., 1995; Pastoret and Sebille, 1995; Morgan et al., 1996; Pagel and Partridge, 1999). Similarly, in the dystrophin-deficient cat, muscle hypertrophy slowly gives way to loss of muscle tissue, although, as in the mouse, this takes much longer in the relative lifespan than in humans or dogs (F. Gaschen, personal communication).

Part of the progressive muscle wasting may also be the result of a deteriorating symbiotic relationship between muscle tissue and the rest of the organism. For example, glutamine is recognized as a 'conditionally essential' amino acid, where circulating levels must reach a certain critical threshold in certain infection or disease states, otherwise general metabolic failure can ensue. As muscle is the major source of circulating glutamine, patients with severely wasted muscular dystrophy may be unable to supply sufficient glutamine from their muscles, thereby exacerbating other infections, leading to sepsis and death (Hankard, 1998; Hankard et al., 1998). Moreover, when muscle tissue is severely compromised by dystrophin deficiency, it probably becomes more sensitive to systemic stress. For example, decreasing the food intake of *mdx* mice (fasting) has been shown to lead to an increase in necrosis and hypothermia, which was not seen in controls (Helliwell et al., 1996).

Another suggestive example of interaction between compromised myofibres and the host tissue milieu is with regard to mast cells. Tissue mast cells are at a very low concentration in normal muscle and are generally localized adjacent to major blood vessels (Gorospe et al., 1994a,b, 1996). However, in dystrophin-deficient muscle, there is a striking proliferation of mast cells that are in various states of degranulation. Purified mast cell granules, when injected into dystrophin-deficient muscle, cause wide-spread (complete) necrosis, while no damage is seen in normal muscle (Gorospe et al., 1994b). These findings imply that mast cells are attracted to the dysfunctional dystrophin-deficient muscle, where they degranulate, and the released proteases and immune mediators exacerbate the membrane defect of the myofibres. Consistent with this model, injection of saline into normal muscle caused a rapid invasion of the muscle by mast cells (Gorospe et al., 1996). Moreover, the ingress of mast cells in normal skeletal muscle was found to be rapidly induced by myofibre membrane damage (notexin injection), where mast cell counts increased from 3 to 118 cells/mm^2 (Lefaucheur et al., 1996). Ischaemia did not induce the same rapid influx of mast cells (Lefaucheur et al., 1996).

The progressive nature of the pathophysiology of Duchenne muscular dystrophy makes it a complicated disorder. However, identification of the many different cascades in the diseased muscle provides a large number of points at which the disease could be slowed or halted. Vasodilators may compensate for the NOS deficiency, mast cell stabilizers may prevent grouped necrosis, and muscle performance enhancers may improve the mitochondrial function. Therapeutic approaches are discussed below.

Complete dystrophin-deficiency: Duchenne muscular dystrophy

Patients with Duchenne muscular dystrophy typically have less than 3% of normal dystrophin levels in their muscle (Hoffman et al., 1988a; Nicholson et al., 1989). A recent survey of all publications reporting dystrophin findings in patient muscle biopsies showed 323 biopsies studied to date, with 320 showing marked dystrophin deficiency (99%) (Tables 19.2 and 19.3) (Hoffman, 1993). There are a few notable exceptions. Goldberg et al. (1998) reported an extensive X-linked Polish pedigree with Duchenne-like symptoms, but normal dystrophin and normal dystrophin-associated protein findings by both immunoblot and immunofluorescence assays. This family showed statistically significant genetic linkage to the dystrophin gene, and a single amino acid change was subsequently identified (D3335H) in the critical C-terminal dystroglycan-binding domain (Goldberg et al., 1998). This type of 'normal dystrophin' Duchenne dystrophy raises concerns with regards to molecular diagnosis; patients such as those in this family would likely be given a diagnosis of limb girdle muscular dystrophy in the absence of an X-linked family history.

The types of mutation found in patients with Duchenne muscular dystrophy have been extensively studied (Table

Table 19.2. DNA findings in Duchenne and Becker dystrophies

	Total studied	Deletion	Duplication	Point mutation(?)
Duchenne muscular dystrophy				
Hoffman (1993)	687	375 (55%)	13 (2%)	299 (43%)
Zatz et al. (1998)	615	385 (62%)	–	232 (38%)
Total	1302	58%	1%	40%
Becker muscular dystrophy				
Hoffman (1993)	158	107 (68%)	7 (4%)	44 (28%)

Table 19.3. Protein findings in Duchenne and Becker dystrophies

	Total studied	No. affected (%)
Duchenne muscular dystrophy: dystrophin deficient	323	320 (99%)
Becker muscular dystrophy: abnormal dystrophin	236	227 (96%)
Female Duchenne carriers: familial mosaic	58	52 (90%)

19.2). A compilation of published reports shows 58% of patients to have deletion mutations of one or more exons, and 40% to have nondetectable mutations (Hoffman, 1993; Zatz et al., 1998). Duplication mutations are technically problematic to identify, and the 2% cited is almost certainly an underascertainment (Hoffman, 1993); more focused studies have found about 10% of patients to have duplication mutations (Hu et al., 1990). If the deletion breakpoints can be identified, then the reading frame can be used to predict whether a presymptomatic patient is 'out-of-frame' and, therefore, has Duchenne muscular dystrophy. However, deletions in the 5′ end of the gene often do not follow the reading frame rule, so care must be taken in interpreting reading frame.

The clinical course of Duchenne muscular dystrophy has not changed considerably since the original descriptions in the 1850s. Indeed, a survey of British patients ascertained in 1934–83 did not show much difference in average age of death compared with the series by Gowers in 1879 (Emery and Emery, 1995, p. 97). Ventilatory support of patients can considerably prolong life, and some countries with nationalized health care boast an impressive lifespan of Duchenne patients, and equally impressive quality-of-life ratings (Danish Muscular Dystrophy

Association; http://www.muskelsvindfonden.dk). About 30% of patients with Duchenne dystrophy show nocturnal hypoxaemia, and most show ventricular cardiac defects (Melacini et al., 1996; Saito et al., 1996). Cardiac involvement is very common, though only a relatively small fraction of Duchenne patients succumb to overt heart failure. More typically, patients succumb to respiratory failure.

Tendon lengthenings of the Achilles tendon can prolong ambulation, and scoliosis surgery is often considered for increased comfort in wheelchair-bound patients (Nordeen et al., 1999). There is considerably more blood loss during scoliosis surgery compared with that in other neuromuscular disorders, and this is thought to be a consequence of the poor vasoconstrictive response (possibly caused by dystrophin deficiency in vascular smooth muscle) (Noordeen et al., 1999). An alternative to spinal fusions are plaster casts; experience with 28 patients with such orthoses has recently been published (Heller et al., 1997).

For more detailed descriptions of patient diagnosis and care, the reader is referred to excellent volumes by Brooke (1992) and Emery (1993).

Partial dystrophin deficiency: Becker muscular dystrophy and X-linked dilated cardiomyopathy

Partial dystrophin deficiency in males causes a wide range of clinical presentations and progressions, from asymptomatic high serum levels of creatine kinase, to weakness limited to certain muscles, dilated cardiomyopathy and disorders just slightly milder than Duchenne dystrophy. About 50% of patients with isolated, later-onset muscular dystrophy show abnormalities of dystrophin, by immunoblot, DNA studies or both. The remaining 50% have some form of autosomal recessive muscular dystrophy, such as a primary sarcoglycanopathy or calpain III disorder (see Hoffman, 1999 and Chapter 20).

Patients with Becker muscular dystrophy have a higher incidence of deletion mutations (68%) than do those with Duchenne muscular dystrophy (Table 19.2). Deletion of as much as 50% of the dystrophin gene can still be compatible with a relatively mild clinical phenotype; a patient with a deletion of exons 17–51 (68% of the rod domain) still shows normal localization of the dystrophin-associated proteins and a mild phenotype (Mirabella et al., 1998). Patients with milder phenotypes almost invariably have mutations of the central rod domain, as mutation of the N-terminal actin-binding domain, or C-terminal dystroglycan-binding site is correlated with a poor prognosis (Angelini et al., 1996). Cramps and myalgia are common presenting symptoms of mild dystrophinopathy, as is myoglobin-urea/rhabdomyolysis (Hoffman et al., 1989b; Angelini et al., 1996; Doriguzzi et al., 1997). The majority of patients with mild dystrophinopathy show cardiac involvement, with 25% showing left ventricle dilatation, 29% showing decreased ejection fraction and 66% showing mitral regurgitation (Angelini et al., 1996; Saito et al., 1996).

Patients with Duchenne muscular dystrophy may show cardiac failure late in the disease process but do not present with cardiac problems. In contrast, patients with Becker muscular dystrophy can often present with cardiac failure. The 'greater involvement' of the heart in Becker dystrophy is most often a consequence of the greater demands placed on the dystrophin-deficient heart by the more active skeletal muscles of a Becker patient. However, a few specific dystrophin gene mutations have been found that preferentially affect cardiac dystrophin, and *not* skeletal muscle dystrophin (Muntoni et al., 1997; Ferlini et al., 1998, 1999). The increasing attention paid to patients with dilated cardiomyopathy with an underlying primary dystrophinopathy has led to the term XLDC (X-linked dilated cardiomyopathy) to describe these patients with abnormal dystrophin. Most of these patients have biochemical and/or histological evidence of skeletal muscle disease, although the muscle disease is often preclinical or asymptomatic. A recent Italian study of 60 patients with dilated cardiomyopathy found that about 10% was probably caused by a primary dystrophinopathy (Mestroni et al., 1999).

Mosaicism for dystrophin: symptomatic and nonsymptomatic female carriers

The X-linked recessive inheritance pattern of the dystrophinopathies dictates that the majority of patients are male. However, Meryon noticed that female relatives of patients with Duchenne dystrophy could show large calves, and rare female family members could show overt muscle weakness (Meryon, 1864). Female heterozygous carriers of a dystrophinopathy who exhibit clinical symptoms are often called manifesting carriers.

The advent of molecular diagnostics has increased the identification of manifesting carriers. Approximately 10% of isolated female patients with muscular dystrophy, high serum creatine kinase and proximal muscle weakness can be shown to be manifesting carriers (Arikawa et al., 1991; Hoffman et al., 1992). These girls and women are 'mosaics' for dystrophin expression in muscle, with a certain percentage of myonuclei capable of making dystrophin and a certain percentage dystrophin negative (explained below) (Fig. 19.23). This mosaicism for dystrophin in female carriers has permitted a series of human and mouse studies addressing the ability of the dystrophin protein to diffuse within muscle, and the critical amount of dystrophin that is needed for functional rescue of muscle (Watkins et al., 1989; Pegoraro et al., 1995). These studies have found that dystrophin can diffuse only a limited distance from the site of production. While this limits the amount of dystrophin that can be contributed to a syncytial myofibre by a single nucleus, the persistent selection against dystrophin-negative myofibres, with the possibility of regeneration by dystrophin-positive myoblasts, leads to a great increase in the dystrophin content of muscle as a function of time (Pegoraro et al., 1995). The genetic basis for dystrophin deficiency in manifesting carriers is very well established; these patients all show skewed X inactivation, with the majority of myofibre nuclei preferentially using the X chromosome with the mutant dystrophin gene (Pegoraro et al., 1994, 1995). However, the 'skewing' of X inactivation must occur by some process independent of the dystrophinopathy. Recent studies have shed light on this enigma; most manifesting carriers appear to harbour a dystrophin mutation on one X chromosome and an X-linked lethal mutation on the other X chromosome (Pegoraro et al., 1994, 1997; Lanasa and Hoffman, 1999; Lanasa et al., 1999). During embryonic life, those cells with the active X chromosome harbouring the lethal gene are largely lost, leaving most cells with the X chromosome harbouring the mutant dystrophin gene as the active one. This is much the same mechanism that is presumed to take place in girls showing X:autosome translocations, where chromosomal dosage abnormalities effectively eliminate cells with the normal nontranslocated X (normal dystrophin gene) active. The X-linked lethal gene loci that appear to be responsible for many manifesting carriers have recently been shown to be a significant cause of recurrent pregnancy loss in the general population (Lanasa et al., 1999).

Given a positive family history for Duchenne muscular dystrophy in males, the finding of elevated serum creatine

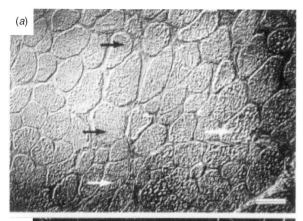

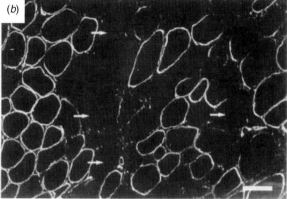

Fig. 19.23. Mosaic expression of dystrophin in an isolated female manifesting carrier of Duchenne muscular dystrophy. Paired Nomarski optics (*a*) and dystrophin immunofluorescence (*b*) of a muscle biopsy from a 28-year-old woman who was found to have chronically elevated serum creatine kinase levels, with no clinically detectable weakness. Arrows indicate specific dystrophin-negative fibres in the paired panels. (Taken from Miller and Hoffman (1994), with permission.)

because some regions of muscle tissue, or entire limbs, can receive a higher proportion of dystrophin-negative myonuclei. This can complicate the interpretation of muscle biopsy results. A recent case report is instructive in this regard. A 60-year-old nun with a history of a recent onset of cramps and proximal muscle weakness, and no family history for Duchenne dystrophy, was found to have 7% dystrophin-negative muscle fibres in one biopsy, and 60% negative fibres in a second (Doriguzzi et al., 1999). Her X-inactivation studies showed the abnormal X to be active in 90% of blood cells. As her muscle presumably began with 90% dystrophin-negative myonuclei, this case also demonstrates the selection for dystrophin-positive myonuclei that occurs over extended time in a patient's muscle.

It is important to make a distinction between *isolated* female manifesting carriers and *familial* manifesting carriers, the latter showing Duchenne muscular dystrophy in male family members. Correlations between serum creatine kinase, muscle weakness and blood X-inactivation patterns show relatively good concordance in isolated cases, but not familial cases (Pegoraro et al., 1995). The reasons underlying this distinction are not completely understood, although ascertainment bias may be a significant variable. It is important to rule out a manifesting carrier diagnosis in all isolated cases of muscular dystrophy in a female, as the incidence of these patients approaches the incidence of any other single cause (calpain 3 deficiency, sarcoglycanopathies, etc.). Testing for a manifesting carrier diagnosis is best done by immunostaining studies of open muscle biopsies, although X inactivation assays can be considered as well.

Cardiac involvement can be seen in female carriers who show no overt clinical weakness. In discussing heart involvement, it is important to note that cardiac muscle should not show an increase in dystrophin content of the tissue over time, as is seen in skeletal muscle. This is because cardiac muscle does not show the same syncytial structure as skeletal muscle, and cardiac muscle is unable to regenerate after damage. Therefore, all female carrier hearts are truly mosaic, with little or no change in the mosaicism state over time. Also, the heart is derived from comparatively fewer progenitor cells, and earlier in development, relative to skeletal muscle. This can lead to a type of 'sampling error', where a female carrier's heart may have the misfortune of being derived from predominantly dystrophin-negative cardiocytes, despite a 50:50 ratio in the remainder of her body. One recent publication reported the extent of heart and skeletal muscle involvement in 129 female carriers of Duchenne and Becker dystrophy (Hoogerwaard et al., 1999). The authors found that about 17% of carriers show some clinically detectable weakness,

kinase levels in a female is a strong indication that she is a carrier of Duchenne muscular dystrophy. It has recently become clear that the finding of chronically elevated serum creatine kinase levels, in the *absence* of a family history can also indicate carrier status (Hoffman et al., 1992; Doriguzzi et al., 1997). In one recent survey of patients seen in Torino, Italy, five out of nine females seen for asymptomatic elevations of serum creatine kinase were found to be female carriers of Duchenne dystrophy by muscle biopsy, while none of 34 males studied for elevated creatine kinase levels showed a dystrophinopathy (Doriguzzi et al., 1997).

The clinical presentations of manifesting carriers of Duchenne dystrophy are as varied as they are in Becker muscular dystrophy. A major difference with manifesting carriers is that weakness can often be *asymmetric*. This is and 8% showed evidence of a dilated cardiomyopathy. Cardiac imaging studies were more sensitive in detecting heart abnormalities, with an additional 15% showing sub-clinical ventricular dilatation in the study of Hoogerwaard et al. (1999) and 84% in that of Politano et al. (1996). Female carriers also show a higher incidence of breech position of pregnancies, presumably because of dystrophin mosaicism in uterine smooth muscle (Geifman-Holtzman et al., 1997). Cardiac transplantation in a female manifesting carrier has been reported (Melacini et al., 1998).

Molecular diagnosis and genetic counselling

The dystrophinopathies can be challenging for most of the medical subspecialties involved in diagnosis and genetic counselling. The neurologist (and cardiologist) needs to recognize the wide variation in clinical presentations and progressions that can occur as a result of dystrophin abnormalities. The pathologist often faces the difficulty in interpreting results for female carriers for dystrophin deficiency (mosaicism on muscle biopsy), and the specificity of changes in immunostaining patterns for dystrophin and associated proteins. The medical geneticist and genetic counsellor must struggle with the high mutation rate of the gene, and many potential female carriers with 'ambiguous' carrier risks. The molecular diagnostician must deal with the ability to detect only deletion mutations with relative ease (60% of patients), the daunting task of finding point mutations in a 2.5 million base pair gene and a high recombination rate when doing genetic linkage studies.

For consideration of a primary dystrophinopathy, the only prerequisite is a high serum creatine kinase level, with or without proximal muscle weakness (Fig. 19.24). Associated clinical findings may be mental impairment (30% in Duchenne dystrophy, less in Becker dystrophy or female manifesting carriers) and cardiac involvement (hypertrophic or dilated cardiomyopathy). An X-linked family history may, or may not, be present. The literature quotes 33% of Duchenne dystrophy cases as 'isolated, new mutations'; however, the advent of genetic counselling in more developed countries has led to the rapid decline in familial cases and a consequent increase in the proportion of isolated cases.

Serum creatine kinase levels are usually consistently elevated, although there have been a few isolated reports of patients with transiently normal, or near normal, serum levels (Ferlini et al., 1999). If there is a positive X-linked family history for Duchenne or Becker muscular dystrophy in males, then diagnosis and prognosis of a new male family member may be based on that of the older male relatives (Fig. 19.24). Female family members can often also be provided a carrier status simply based on serum creatine kinase measurements; the finding of a significantly elevated creatine kinase level strongly suggests that the girl or woman is a carrier, but normal creatine kinase does *not* rule out a carrier diagnosis.

If the patient is a male, with or without clinically evident weakness, then a dystrophin gene deletion test can be done; the identification of a deletion is diagnostic of a primary dystrophinopathy. About 40% of patients with a dystrophinopathy do not have deletion mutations, so protein testing of a muscle biopsy is generally necessary in isolated, deletion-negative cases (Table 19.3; Fig. 19.24). There are two methods for testing for deletions of one or more of the 80 exons of the dystrophin gene: multiplex polymerase chain reaction (PCR) (Chamberlain et al., 1988; Beggs et al., 1990; Anderson and Davis, 1999), or Southern blot (Koenig et al., 1987). Multiplex PCR is considerably faster and less expensive, although approximately 2% of deletions are missed using this assay. Also, different laboratories have varying success rates with detection of duplication mutations or female carriers of deletion mutations by this method. Those patients having a positive deletion test can sometimes be given a prognosis based on the reading frame of the remaining exons; an in-frame deletion suggests a milder phenotype (Becker muscular dystrophy), while an out-of-frame deletion suggests a Duchenne muscular dystrophy diagnosis (Monaco et al., 1988; Koenig et al., 1989). However, about 10% of deletion mutations do *not* follow the 'reading frame rule', and these deletions are most typically located at the beginning of the gene, where use of alternative AUG protein initiation codons is possible.

Dystrophin protein testing is done to identify *isolated* female carriers of Duchenne dystrophy and to diagnose males with no deletion mutation. Protein testing can also give a more accurate prognosis than DNA testing, and muscle biopsy should be considered in isolated male patients with deletion mutations for this reason (Fig. 19.24). In general, patients with Duchenne muscular dystrophy have less than 3% of normal dystrophin levels by immuno-blotting; patients with severe Becker muscular dystrophy (wheelchair-bound at 14–20 years of age) have 3–15% of normal levels, and patients with milder Becker dystrophy (wheelchair-bound >20 years of age) have 15% or more of normal levels. Substantial clinical variability is seen between patients with the same deletion mutations and similar amounts of dystrophin (Beggs et al., 1991). Any attempts at prognosis should be provided with this in mind.

For genetic counselling of the patients and their families, deletion mutations can be identified in potential female

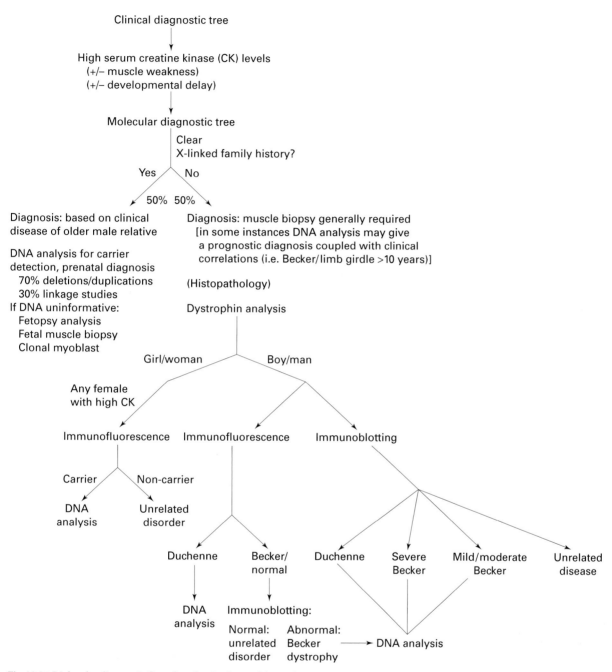

Fig. 19.24. Molecular diagnostic flow chart for the dystrophinopathies.

carriers or presymptomatic male patients, or genetic linkage studies can be done if no deletion mutation is found (Miller and Hoffman, 1994). Genetic linkage assays for the dystrophin gene are well developed, but results are often 'ambiguous' given the nature of the genetics of dystrophinopathies. There are many intragenic, highly polymorphic loci that can be used for linkage studies in families, and different loci are used by different groups. It is important that multiple markers distributed throughout the gene be tested, as there is approximately 9% recombination across the dystrophin gene. In nondeletion cases, a female relative is typically assigned a 'risk', which is only rarely absolute (0% or 100%). These risks take into account the family history, high mutation rate of the dystrophin gene, chance of recombination between informative markers and laboratory data (serum creatine kinase). These risks are calculated using Bayesian statistics and can be quite complicated; they are, therefore, best left for the medical geneticist or genetic counsellor.

Some additional tests can be employed where routine molecular diagnosis has led to an ambiguous risk assigned to the fetus or female carrier. Fetal muscle biopsy of male fetuses, with dystrophin testing of the biopsy, has been used in about 20–25 fetuses carrying an 'ambiguous' risk that was unacceptable to the family (Evans et al., 1994; Heckel et al., 1999; E. P. Hoffman, personal observations). In our experience with fetal muscle biopsies, we have found that some families consider 1% risk of Duchenne dystrophy to a fetus as 'unacceptably high' and have opted for fetal muscle biopsy, despite counselling where it is pointed out that the procedure has a 5–10% morbidity risk to the fetus. Other families continue pregnancies with 100% risk of Duchenne dystrophy to the fetus after molecular diagnosis. Again, the involvement of genetic counsellors and medical geneticists in the process of genetic counselling is critical, as the concept of 'relative risk' is a difficult one for most families to grapple with, and religious and moral value systems modify what are considered 'acceptable risks' to a very great degree. Some new methods to detect female carriers may prove important, such as electroretinograms (Fitzgerald et al., 1999) and dystrophin testing of endomyocardial biopsies or skin biopsies (Marbini et al., 1995).

A major impediment to unambiguous molecular diagnosis of families with nondeletion Duchenne and Becker muscular dystrophy is the unavailability of rapid and sensitive methods for detection of nondeletion mutations (point mutations). Some studies have been published on detecting point mutations in cohorts of patients (Prior et al., 1995; Tuffery et al., 1998; Dubourg et al., 1999); however, these are highly labour intensive, and expensive, and sensitivity is not 100% even after considerable effort. An excellent database of different types of mutation identified to date in Duchenne/Becker muscular dystrophy is available on the web, sponsored by University of Leiden, Holland.

The genetic counselling of isolated female manifesting carriers is considerably more complicated. New mutations can be derived from the maternal or paternal germline, and phase of polymorphic markers with abnormal dystrophin genes must often be done through correlation with X-inactivation studies (Hoffman et al., 1996). In addition, families of isolated female manifesting carriers may be at high risk for X-linked lethal gene mutations and recurrent pregnancy loss (Pegoraro et al., 1997; Lanasa and Hoffman, 1999; Lanasa et al., 1999).

Current and future therapeutics

Meryon commented 136 years ago (Meryon, 1864, p. 214):

And in spite of exercise regulated by the most careful and constant supervision; of food prescribed by the last word of physiology as the most appropriate; of climate varying from alpine heights to the sea level, and from the shores of the Mediterranean to those of the German Ocean; of electricity in all its forms; of almost every nervine tonic contained in the pharmacopaeia; and of every conceivable hygienic appliance; the disease has pursued a progressive course such as I have described.

Meryon's comment can be viewed as equally poignant today, and it epitomizes the frustration of neurologists and despair of parents as potential treatment after potential treatment is heralded from the newspaper or experienced first hand. Injections of myoblasts into muscle, transplantation of bone marrow-derived cells, Chinese alternative medicine, aggressive tendon resections and lengthenings, growth hormones, gene therapy, utrophin upregulation, mutation correction procedures and antibiotics, all hold promise but none has yet been shown substantially to halt the progression of Duchenne dystrophy. There are, however, many potential and promising paths being pursued simultaneously, and most are optimistic that it will not be long before the progression of Duchenne is substantially slowed or stopped.

There are five routes that are being actively investigated, each with mutiple subroutes: (i) cell transplantation (myoblast delivery); (ii) pharmacological interventions which target aspects of the pathophysiology; (iii) efforts to deliver the dystrophin gene to muscle; (iv) efforts to enable muscle to ignore the mutation in the patient's dystrophin gene; (v) upregulation of utrophin so that it can functionally replace dystrophin. Each of these is discussed separately here.

Cell transplantation (myoblast delivery)

Intact muscle tissue is difficult to transplant, as the loss of nerve and vascular supply leads to degeneration of the myofibres. An alternative is cell transplantation, using muscle precursor cells (satellite cells, myoblasts) from a normal donor and injection of these into dystrophin-deficient muscle. The first demonstration of this technique in *mdx* mice was in 1989; the authors showed that 3 of 70 immunocompromised *mdx* mice injected with myoblasts into the extensor digitorum longus muscle showed therapeutic levels of dystrophin protein from donor myoblasts (Partridge et al., 1989). While these authors cautioned against beginning human trials because of the very low efficiency of the technique, a number of human clinical trials were begun in patients with Duchenne and

Becker dystrophy. These trials consistently showed little or no dystrophin expression in injected muscle, using a variety of patient ages, number of injected myoblasts and immunosuppression protocols (Mendell et al., 1995; Miller et al., 1997; Neumeyer et al., 1998). While a single nonacademic laboratory in Tennessee (CTRF) has claimed success in achieving patient strength with myoblast injections; published reports from this laboratory are not convincing, with inadequate controls or quantification of dystrophin (Law et al., 1993). Muscle biopsies from one of the patients treated by CTRF was tested by independent groups, and no evidence of dystrophin production from donor cells was seen (Partridge et al., 1998). The US Food and Drug Administration (FDA) has recently published letters soundly criticizing the CTRF clinical trials: specifically, 'on the basis of the above listed violations, FDA asserts that you have repeatedly or deliberately failed to comply with the cited regulations and it proposes that you be disqualified as a clinical investigator' (http://www.fda.gov/foi/nidpoe/n98.pdf).

Over the last few years, the variables limiting the success of myoblast transfer have been studied in some detail. Myoblasts appear quite immunogenic, and dystrophin delivered by transplanted cells can serve as a neoantigen (Ohtsuka et al., 1998). Less than 10% of injected cells survive, and many of those appear unable to produce dystrophin despite presence in host myofibres (Gussoni et al., 1997). Myoblasts are unable to migrate very far from the injection site. The fibrosis present in most patient muscle was also thought to inhibit the migration, although recent studies using aged *mdx* mice found no significant reduction of myoblast 'take' in more fibrotic muscle (Morgan et al., 1996; Brussee et al., 1999).

Efforts have been targeted towards overcoming each of these barriers, with some success. Purification protocols for myogenic precursor cells have been improved, yielding subpopulations of cells that seem able to generate more muscle (muscle stem cells) (Qu et al., 1998; Irintchev et al., 1998). Alternative sources of myogenic cells have been sought, including bone marrow-derived cells (Bittner et al., 1999). However, the efficiency of these cells for generating muscle seems orders of magnitude less than muscle-derived cell populations, making the results more significant for developmental biologists (Partridge, 1998). To overcome immune barriers, *ex vivo* protocols have been attempted, where dystrophin genes are delivered to host myoblasts by some method, then the myoblasts are introduced back into the host (Floyd et al., 1998; Kinoshita et al., 1998). To improve the efficiency of delivery of myoblasts above that seen with intramuscular injection, a recent study used delivery by extracorporeal circulation, under high-pressure conditions, after induction of muscle regeneration (bupivacaine) and partial breakdown of basal lamina barriers (hyaluronidase) (Torrente et al., 1999). Even after these relatively heroic efforts, only a maximum of 4% of myofibres were successfully fused with donor myoblasts.

The most impressive results to date have been using an irradiated and immunosuppressed *mdx* model, with injection of purified primary myogenic cells. In this model, the *mdx* fibres gradually undergo necrosis as a result of dystrophin deficiency and can only be replaced by injected normal myoblasts as the endogenous myoblasts have been destroyed by radiation. Under this context, the large majority of the muscle can be converted to dystrophin-positive tissue, although the muscles are generally smaller than those originally present in the mouse (Morgan et al., 1990, 1996).

Myoblast transplantation will continue to be a promising path of research. However, cell procurement, systemic delivery and immunosuppression all remain significant significant hurdles to this approach, as they do for all dystrophin-based therapeutic lines of research.

Pharmacological interventions that target aspects of the pathophysiology

Prednisone and the related corticosteroid deflazacort have been shown to increase strength in patients and slow the progression of the disease to some extent (Angelini et al., 1994). The mechanism of action of steroids in muscular dystrophy is probably complex. They do not seem to work solely by immune suppression, as other more effective immune suppressants, such as intravenous immunoglobulin or cyclosporin, do not seem to show therapeutic benefit. Prednisone does not seem to mitigate contraction-induced injury in *mdx* diaphragm (Yang et al., 1998). A recent report using genome-wide expression profiling in biopsies from patients with Duchenne dystrophy suggested that corticosteroids may target activated dendritic cells (Chen et al., 2000).

Other targeted therapeutics are just beginning, but some are promising, such as the complementation of depleted systemic glutamine stores (Hankard, 1998; Hankard et al., 1998). Loss of chloride channel conductance in *mdx* mice by breeding to a knock-out of *ClC-1* leads to a decrease in severity, suggesting that alteration of salt balance in muscle may have a beneficial effect (Heimann et al., 1998; Kramer et al., 1998). Iron deprivation in *mdx* mice reduces necrosis, presumably through a reduction in stress enzymes (such as hsp70) (Bornman et al., 1998). Many other points in the pathophysiology of Duchenne dystrophy can be pinpointed and modulated via pharmacological intervention, including lack of nNOS activity and vascular disturbances, mitochondrial dysfunction, membrane stability, mast cell proliferation and degranulation, protease activity, connective tissue proliferation and others.

One of the more promising avenues is the large-scale screening of drugs using the *mdx* mouse model. The development of drug screening was slowed because of the relative lack of overt weakness in the mouse. However, some exercise models for inducing weakness in *mdx* mice have been published, and the first large-scale drug screen has been reported (Hudecki et al., 1993; Granchelli et al., 2000). From this study, a number of drugs were identified that improved the strength of *mdx* mice to an equal or greater degree than prednisone. These were glutamine (muscle-derived conditionally essential amino acid), creatinine (energy metabolism), oxpentifyline (pentoxifyline) (peripheral vascular agent), oxatamide (mast cell stabilizer) and insulin-like growth factor 1 (muscle growth factor). It can be difficult to predict the outcome of the effect on human patients using mouse model data; however, the beneficial effect of each of these drugs can be rationalized based on current understanding of the pathophysiological cascades consequent to dystrophin deficiency.

Efforts to deliver the dystrophin gene to muscle

There have been four different viral systems used to deliver the dystrophin gene (retrovirus, adenovirus, adeno-associated virus (AAV), herpesvirus), and two nonviral delivery systems (liposomes, direct DNA injection). Each of the delivery systems has advantages and disadvantages. Two have received the greatest recent attention because of very promising results: third-generation adenovirus (so-called 'gutted' adenovirus) and AAV.

Adenovirus has been extensively used as a delivery vehicle for gene therapy. First-generation adenoviral vectors are replication-defective as a result of deletion of critical viral genes needed for completion of the lifecycle and are able to package about 8 kb of foreign DNA. These vectors have been used to deliver truncated forms of the dystrophin gene (Becker constructs) and have resulted in substantial dystrophin expression after intramuscular injection in neonatal rodents (Guibinga et al., 1998; Yang et al., 1998; Yuasa et al., 1998) and dogs (Howell et al., 1998a,b). There have been a number of limitations with regards to use of first-generation adenoviral vectors in muscle tissue. First, they are unable to contain the full-length dystrophin gene because of size limitations.

Second, adenovirus infects neonatal muscle well but only very poorly transduces adult skeletal muscle fibres (Huard et al., 1996; Feero et al., 1997a). Third, first-generation adenovirus is highly immunogenic, presumably as a result of infection of dendritic cells in muscle and expression of viral antigens encoded by the many intact viral genes in the vector (Jooss et al., 1998). Fourth, adenovirus has been shown to be somewhat toxic to myofibres when large amounts of virus are injected (Yang et al., 1998). Methods have been devised to overcome some of these hurdles, such as the injection of a myotoxic agent into muscle prior to adenovirus injection to stimulate regeneration of muscle, and better infection of the immature cells by adenovirus. Immunosuppressive agents, such as cyclosporin (Howell et al., 1998b), tacrolimus (FK506) (Yang et al., 1998), and blocking of CD28 pathway (CTLA4Ig) (Guibinga et al., 1998) have been highly successful in mitigating the immune recognition and elimination of transduced fibres. With regards to infection of neonatal fibres being more effective than that of adult muscle fibres, promising results have been obtained using 'altered tropism' virus (Bouri et al., 1999). In this approach, the protein coat of the virion was modified to change the affinity and specificity for the cell-surface receptor of the virus through the addition of a series of lysine residues. This 'modified tropism' virus was found to infect adult myofibres fourfold more efficiently than the non-modified adenovirus (Bouri et al., 1999).

A new type of adenovirus that overcomes some of the above hurdles is third-generation, or 'gutted' adenovirus. This recombinant virus is able to package approximately 30 kb of exogenous DNA (Clemens et al., 1996). This large carrying capacity is produced by the elimination of viral coding sequences from the vector and the use of an attenuated helper virus for packaging of the recombinant vector. Using this virus in neonatal rodent muscle has shown high levels of dystrophin expression, with very little immune response against transfected fibres (Fig. 19.25, colour plate) (Clemens et al., 1996; Kochanek et al., 1996; Kumar-Singh and Chamberlain, 1996; Chen et al., 1997, 1999b). Importantly, the persistence of expression of this third-generation adenovirus is considerably longer than that of the first generation, presumably because of decreased adenoviral gene antigen presentation. If the host is tolerized against the transgene, then expression is persistent through at least 84 days (Chen et al., 1999b). The third-generation virus goes far in both reducing immunogenicity (though not eliminating it as a problem) and providing expanded packaging capacity capable of holding the full-length dystrophin cDNA. Adult myofibres are still only very poorly infected by both the first- and third-generation adenovirus, although altered tropism approaches may successfully navigate this hurdle. The major limitations to use of adenoviruses remain their toxicity and poor persistence. The adenovirus genome is maintained as extrachromosomal material, and expression is gradually lost over time (Chen et al., 1999b).

The most promising viral gene delivery vehicle for muscle is that using AAV (Fisher et al., 1997; Monahan et al., 1998; Xiao et al., 1998). AAV is a small picornavirus for which 80% of humans are seropositive and where muscle appears to be the natural tissue target for the virus (Tezak et al., 2000). The natural lifecycle of this virus seems ideal for gene therapy applications in muscle. It is nonpathogenic and nonimmunogenic, and in fact it may confer protection against autoimmunity (Tezak et al., 2000). It integrates stably into the host chromosomes and shows persistent, perhaps indefinite, expression of transgenes in muscle (Xiao et al., 1996). It infects adult skeletal muscle fibres very efficiently, where it can traverse the basal lamina and other connective tissue boundaries. The use of AAV is still in the early stages of development; however, it has been highly successful in delivering the gene for δ-sarcoglycan in the dystrophic hamster model of muscular dystrophy (Fig. 19.26) (Greelish et al., 1999; Li et al., 1999; Xiao et al., 2000). The major hurdle facing the use of AAV in Duchenne muscular dystrophy is the small capacity for exogenous DNA. AAV can only fit about 5 kb of foreign DNA, which makes it impossible to place the full-length dystrophin gene into the vector. A highly truncated form of the dystrophin gene has been successfully delivered to *mdx* mouse muscle using AAV, and the transduced muscle showed histological correction (Wang et al., 2000).

Two additional viruses that have been used are retrovirus and herpesvirus. Retrovirus has a relatively limited packaging capacity but is able to accept Becker-like truncated dystrophin constructs (Dunckley et al., 1993). Advantages of retrovirus are that it integrates stably into chromosomes and has been documented to be nonpathogenic. Disadvantages are difficulty in growing large quantities and the fact that the virus infects only actively dividing cells. As myofibres are postmitotic, retrovirus can only be used to infect regenerating muscle. A promising report in which retroviral producer cell lines were injected into muscle as a long-term source of therapeutic Becker-like constructs has recently been published (Fassati et al., 1997). Herpesvirus is a large virus, with considerable packaging capacity for exogenous DNA. This virus is complex and is still being refined for gene therapy applications. A single report has been published using herpesvirus to deliver the dystrophin gene, although the efficiency was not high, and stability questionable (Akkaraju et al., 1999).

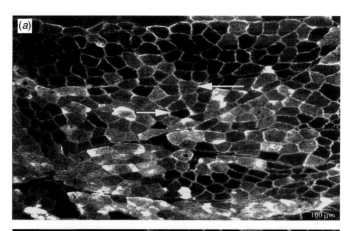

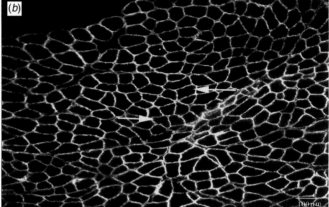

Fig. 19.26. Biochemical and histological rescue of a hamster model of musclar dystrophy using adeno-associated virus (AAV). The gastrocnemius muscle from a Biol4.6 hamster shows complete δ-sarcoglycan deficiency in its muscle as the result of a mutation in the gene for δ-sarcoglycan gene mutation. (*a*) A single injection of AAV virus carrying the human δ-sarcoglycan genes results in a high level of expression of human δ-sarcoglycan in the large majority of muscle fibres. Some fibres show both the expected membrane immunostaining (lower arrow), and inappropriate cytoplasmic localization (top arrow). (*b*) All dystrophic hamster muscle shows secondary loss of the other three sarcoglycan proteins (α-, β- and γ-sarcoglycan). The same region of muscle that is shown in (*a*) was also immunostained for α-sarcoglycan. This protein is restored in all fibres, and it shows the expected membrane localization. The appropriate membrane localization of α-sarcoglycan (*b*) is present in myofibres that show inappropriate cytoplasmic expression of δ-sarcoglycan (see arrows). (Taken from Li et al. (1999) with permission.)

Two nonviral delivery methods are being actively pursued. The first is intramuscular injection of purified plasmid DNA containing the dystrophin gene (Acsadi et al., 1991). The efficiency of this approach has been lower than that seen with viral vectors, and there is immunity induced against the transgene in the naive host. A recent report showed 17% of myofibres in the *mdx* diaphragm transduced after direct plasmid injection of a Becker-like construct (Decrouy et al., 1997). Another method used to improve stability and efficiency of expression is to use Epstein–Barr virus origin of replication encorporated into the plasmid construct (Tsukamoto et al., 1999). The second nonviral approach is to use liposomes, which can be formulated to approach viruses in size, although efficiency of transduction is typically much lower than seen with viral vectors. Efforts with liposomes in muscle disease have included identification of targeting ligands for systemic delivery (Feero et al., 1997b), and delivery of a Becker-like construct to dystrophic dog muscle using lipofectin (Howell et al., 1998a,b).

In summary, the viral gene delivery approaches using either gutted adenovirus or AAV vectors have shown biochemical, histological and functional rescue of relatively large areas of muscle in rodent muscular dystrophy models. Human clinical trials in limited muscle groups should be starting in the near future to test these two vectors. Major barriers facing all gene delivery efforts include large-scale growth of adequate virus to infect patient muscle, and development of some alternative to intramuscular injection. A single promising report describes systemic delivery to rodent limbs using high-pressure intra-arterial delivery with vascular permeabilizing agents (Greelish et al., 1999).

Efforts to enable muscle to ignore the mutation in the patient's dystrophin gene

A theoretically attractive, albeit technically difficult approach to therapy, would be to simply 'fix' the dystrophin gene mutation in each patient with Duchenne or Becker dystrophy. In many respects, patients have already shown us that this is possible. First, patients with Becker muscular dystrophy, with their in-frame deletions, have a partially repaired gene. Second, 'somatic reversion' events have been well-documented to occur, where dystrophin-positive fibres can be clearly seen in half of biopsies from patients with Duchenne muscular dystrophy and in all *mdx* muscle. These 'revertant' fibres result from second-site mutations, which give rise to an in-frame Becker-type deletion (Hoffman et al., 1990; Winder et al., 1995, 1996; Wilton et al., 1997).

The *mdx* mouse has been a critical tool in the efforts to develop gene correction methodologies. One approach is to use antisense oligoribonucleotides that are able to hybridize to the mutant *mdx* dystrophin mRNA. The oligoribonucleotides are constructed in such a manner that they force the RNA splicing machinery of the cell to skip over the exon containing the *mdx* mutation (exon 23). Some of the resulting RNAs contain in-frame deletions and make 'Becker-like' dystrophin in cultured *mdx* myogenic cells (Dunckley et al., 1998; Wilton et al., 1999). No reports of in vivo use of this method have yet been reported, and delivery of the oligoribonucleotide to skeletal muscle in vivo will be challenging.

Another approach is to use drugs that cause translational machinery to misread the premature stop codon in the *mdx* dystrophin gene. Gentamicin is a relatively commonly used antibiotic that causes bacteria to misread translational stop codons, thereby forcing them to produce many abnormal proteins, which are lethal to them. A recent promising report showed that use of gentamicin in *mdx* mice resulted in read-through of the *mdx* premature stop codon, with normal size dystrophin then produced in muscle in vivo (Barton-Davis et al., 1999). Gentamicin has considerable toxicity associated with chronic or high-level use; it remains to be determined if dystrophin production can be affected by this drug, without severe detrimental effects to all other proteins and tissues in a patient.

Upregulation of utrophin

As discussed above, it has become very clear that utrophin can functionally substitute for dystrophin (Tinsley et al., 1996; Deconinck et al., 1997c; Rafael et al., 1998). A corollary to this finding is that any methods that can produce higher levels of utrophin in dystrophin-deficient skeletal muscle should have a therapeutic effect. Two methods have been pursued to increase utrophin production in muscle; identification of drugs able to enhance production from the patient's endogenous utrophin gene (upregulation approach), or delivery of an overexpressing utrophin gene using viral vectors (gene therapy approach) (Tinsley et al., 1998). Based on the higher expression of utrophin at the neuromuscular junction in normal muscle, two drugs, agrin and heregulin, able to induce expression of proteins of this area have proven successful in inducing higher levels of utrophin throughout cultured myogenic cells (Gramolini et al., 1998, 1999b; Khurana et al., 1999). Neither compound has yet been tested in vivo, and delivery of these proteins systemically will be challenging. The second approach, using viral vectors, has been successfully accomplished using a truncated version of the utrophin gene in first-generation adenoviral vectors (Gilbert et al., 1999). Intramuscular injection into the tibialis anterior of mice aged three to five days led to about one-third of fibres being transduced. This truncated protein was able to restore the dystrophin-associated proteins and functionally rescue muscle (Gilbert et al., 1999). This approach is subject to the same hurdles and limitations of viral gene delivery systems. The advantage of using utrophin instead of dystrophin would be reduced immunological sequelae, as utrophin should not be a neoantigen to patients with Duchenne muscular dystrophy.

References

Acsadi, G., Dickson, G., Love, D. R. et al. (19910. Human dystrophin expression in *mdx* mice after intramuscular injection of DNA constructs. *Nature* **352**, 815–818.

Adams, M. E., Kramarcy, N., Krall, S. P. et al. (2000). Absence of α-syntrophin leads to structurally aberrant neuromuscular synapses deficient in utrophin. *J. Cell Biol.* **150**, 1385–1398.

Ahmad, A., Brinson, M., Hodges, B. L. et al. (2000). *mdx* mice inducibly expressing dystrophin provide insights into the potential of gene therapy for Duchenne muscular dystrophy. *Hum. Mol. Genet.* **9**, 2507–2515.

Akkaraju, G. R., Huard, J., Hoffman, E. P. et al. (1999). Herpes simplex virus vector-mediated dystrophin gene transfer and expression in mdx mouse skeletal muscle. *J. Gene Med.* **1**, 280–289.

Andac, Z., Sasaki, T., Mann, K. et al. (1999). Analysis of heparin, alpha-dystroglycan and sulfatide binding to the G domain of the laminin alpha1 chain by site-directed mutagenesis. *J. Mol. Biol.* **287**, 253–264.

Anderson, L. V. and Davison, K. (1999). Multiplex Western blotting system for the analysis of muscular dystrophy proteins. *Am. J. Pathol.* **154**, 1017–1022.

Angelini, C., Pegoraro, E., Turella, E. et al. (1994). Deflazacort in Duchenne dystrophy: study of long-term effect. *Muscle Nerve* **17**, 386–391.

Angelini, C., Fanin, M., Freda, M. P. et al. (1996). Prognostic factors in mild dystrophinopathies. *J. Neurol. Sci.* **142**, 70–78.

Angoli, D., Corona, P., Baresi, R. et al. (1997). Laminin-alpha2 but not -alpha1-mediated adhesion of human (Duchenne) and murine (*mdx*) dystrophic myotubes is seriously defective. *FEBS Lett.* **408**, 341–344.

Arahata, K., Ishiura, S., Ishiguro, T. et al. (1988). Immunostaining of skeletal and cardiac muscle surface membrane with antibody against Duchenne muscular dystrophy peptide. *Nature* **333**, 861–863.

Arikawa, E., Hoffman, E. P., Kairdo, M. et al. (1991). The frequency of patients having dystrophin abnormalities in a limb-girdle patient population. *Neurology* **41**, 1491–1496.

Azzena, G. B. and Mancinelli, R. (1999). Nitric oxide regenerates the normal colonic peristaltic activity in *mdx* dystrophic mouse. *Neurosci. Lett.* **261**, 9–12.

Badorff, C., Lee, G. H., Lamphear, B. J. et al. (1999). Enteroviral protease 2A cleaves dystrophin: evidence of cytoskeletal disruption in an acquired cardiomyopathy. *Nat. Med.* **5**, 320–326.

Barton-Davis, E. R., Cordier, L., Shoturma, D. I. et al. (1999). Aminoglycoside antibiotics restore dystrophin function to skeletal muscles of *mdx* mice. *J. Clin. Invest.* **104**, 375–381.

Becker, P. E. (1962). Two new families of benign sex-linked recessive muscular dystrophy. *Rev. Can. Biol.* **21**, 551–566.

Becker, P. E. and Kiener, F. (1955). Eine neue X-chromosomale Muskeldystrophie. *Arch. Psychiatr. Z. Neurol.*, **193**, 427–488.

Beggs, A. H., Koenig, M., Boyce, F. M. et al. (1990). Detection of 98% of DMD/BMD gene deletions by polymerase chain reaction. *Hum. Genet.* **86**, 45–48.

Beggs, A. H., Hoffman, E. P., Snyder, J. R. et al. (1991). Exploring the molecular basis for variability among patients with Becker muscular dystrophy: dystrophin gene and protein studies. *Am. J. Hum. Genet.* **49**, 54–67.

Bertorini, T. E., Bhattacharya, S. K., Palmieri, G. M. A. et al. (1982). Muscle calcium and magnesium content in Duchenne muscular dystrophy. *Neurology* **32**, 1088–1092.

Bertorini, T. E., Cornelio, F., Bhattacharya, S. K. et al. (1984). Calcium and magnesium content in fetuses at risk and prenecrotic Duchenne muscular dystrophy. *Neurology* **34**, 1436–1440.

Bessou, C., Giugia, J. B., Franks, C. J. et al. (1998). Mutations in the *Caenorhabditis elegans* dystrophin-like gene dys-1 lead to hyperactivity and suggest a link with cholinergic transmission. *Neurogenetics* **2**, 61–72.

Bittner, R. E., Schofer, C., Weipoltshammer, K. et al. (1999). Recruitment of bone-marrow-derived cells by skeletal and cardiac muscle in adult dystrophic *mdx* mice. *Anat. Embryol.* **199**, 391–396.

Blank, M., Koulen, P., Blake, D. J. and Kroger, S. (1999). Dystrophin and beta-dystroglycan in photoreceptor terminals from normal and *mdx*3Cv mouse retinae. *Eur. J. Neurosci.* **11**, 2121–2133.

Bodensteiner, J. B. and Engel, A. G. (1978). Intracellular calcium accumulation in Duchenne dystrophy and other myopathies: a study of 567000 muscle fibers in 114 biopsies. *Neurology* **28**, 439–446.

Bonilla, E., Samitt, C. E., Miranda, A. F. et al. (1998). Duchenne muscular dystrophy: deficiency of dystrophin at the muscle cell surface. *Cell* **54**, 447–452.

Bornman, L., Rossouw, H., Gericke, G. S. et al. (1998). Effects of iron deprivation on the pathology and stress protein expression in murine X-linked muscular dystrophy. *Biochem. Pharmacol.* **56**, 751–757.

Bouri, K., Feero, W. G., Myerburg, M. M. et al. (1999). Polylysine modification of adenoviral fiber protein enhances muscle cell transduction. *Hum. Gene Ther.* **10**, 1633–1640.

Bourne, G. H. and Golarz, M. N. (1959). Human muscular dystrophy as an aberration of the connective tissue. *Nature* **183**, 1741–1743.

Bradley, W. G. and Fulthorpe, J. J. (1978). Studies of sarcolemmal integrity in myopathic muscle. *Neurology* **28**, 670–677.

Brooke, M. H. (1992). *A Clinician's View of Neuromuscular Diseases*, 2nd edn. Baltimore, MD: Williams & Wilkins.

Brown, S. C., Fassati, A., Popplewell, L. et al. (1999). Dystrophic phenotype induced in vitro by antibody blockade of muscle alpha-dystroglycan-laminin interaction. *J. Cell Sci.* **112**, 209–216.

Brussee, V., Tardif, F., Roy, B. et al. (1999). Successful myoblast transplantation in fibrotic muscles: no increased impairment by the connective tissue. *Transplantation* **67**, 1618–1622.

Bulfield, G., Siller, W. G., Wight, P. A. et al. (1984). X chromosome-linked muscular dystrophy (*mdx*) in the mouse. *Proc. Natl. Acad. Sci. USA* **81**, 1189–1192.

Bundy, S. E. (1972). Extreme muscle hypertrophy in Duchenne muscular dystrophy. In: *Fifth Conference on the Clinical Delineation of Birth Defects*, ed. D. Bergsma, Vol. 10, p. 341.

Campbell, K. P. (1995). Three muscular dystrophies: loss of cytoskeleton–extracellular matrix linkage. *Cell* **80**, 675–679.

Cao, W., Henry, M. D., Borrow, P. et al. (1998). Identification of alpha-dystroglycan as a receptor for lymphocytic choriomeningitis virus and Lassa fever virus. *Science* **282**, 2079–2081.

Carpenter, S. and Karpati, G. (1979). Duchenne muscular dystrophy: plasma membrane loss initiates muscle cell necrosis unless it is repaired. *Brain* **102**, 147–161.

Carpenter, J. L., Hoffman, E. P., Romanul, F. C. A. et al. (1989). Feline muscular dystrophy with dystrophin deficiency. *Am. J. Pathol.* **135**, 909–919.

Chamberlain, J. S., Gibbs, R. A., Ranier, J. E. et al. (1988). Deletion screening of the Duchenne muscular dystrophy locus via multiplex DNA amplification. *Nucl. Acids Res.* **16**, 11141–11156.

Chan, Y. and Kunkel, L. M. (1997). In vitro expressed dystrophin fragments do not associate with each other. *FEBS Lett.* **410**, 153–159.

Chan, Y. M., Bonnemann, C. G., Lidov, H. G. W. et al. (1998). Molecular organization of sarcoglycan complex in mouse myotubes in culture. *J. Cell Biol.* **143**, 2033–2044.

Chao, D. S., Silvagno, F. and Bredt, D. S. (1998). Muscular dystrophy in *mdx* mice despite lack of neuronal nitric oxide synthase. *J. Neurochem.* **71**, 784–789.

Chen, H. H., Mack, L. M., Kelly, R., Ontell, M. et al. (1997). Persistence in muscle of an adenoviral vector that lacks all viral genes. *Proc. Natl. Acad. Sci. USA* **94**, 1645–1650.

Chen, D. H., Takeshima, Y., Ishikawa, Y. et al. (1999a). A novel deletion of the dystrophin S-promoter region cosegregating with mental retardation. *Neurology* **52**, 638–640.

Chen, H. H., Mack, L. M., Choi, S. Y. et al. (1999b). DNA from both high-capacity and first-generation adenoviral vectors remains intact in skeletal muscle. *Hum. Gene Ther.* **10**, 365–373.

Chen, Y.-W., Zhao, P., Borup, R. and Hoffman, E. P. (2000). Expression profiling in the muscular dystrophies: identification of novel aspects of molecular pathophysiology. *J. Cell Biol.* **151**, 1321–1336.

Clemens, P. R., Kochanek, S., Sunada, Y. et al. (1996). In vivo muscle gene transfer of full-length dystrophin with an adenoviral vector that lacks all viral genes. *Gene Therapy* **3**, 965–972.

Colognato, H., Winkelmann, D. A. and Yurchenco, P. D. (1999). Laminin polymerization induces a receptor-cytoskeleton network. *J. Cell Biol.* **145**, 619–631.

Conte, G. and Gioja, L. (reprinted 1986). Scrofola del sistema muscolare. [Annali Clinici dell' Ospedale degl'Incurabili di Napoli (1836) **2**, 66–79.] *Cardiomyology* 5.

Cooper, B. J., Winand, N. J., Stedman, H. et al. (1988). The homologue of the Duchenne locus is defective in X-linked muscular dystrophy of dogs. *Nature* **334**, 154–156.

Cornelio, F. and Dones, I. (1984). Muscle fibre degeneration and necrosis in muscular dystrophy and other muscle diseases: cytochemical and immunoctyochemical data. *Ann. Neurol.* **16**, 694–701.

Corrado, K., Rafael, J. A., Mills, P. L. et al. (1996). Transgenic *mdx* mice expressing dystrophin with a deletion in the actin-binding domain display a 'mild Becker' phenotype. *J. Cell Biol.* **134**, 873–874.

Crosbie, R. H., Heighway, J., Venzke, D. P. et al. (1997). Sarcospan, the 25-kDa transmembrane component of the dystrophin–glycoprotein complex. *J. Biol. Chem.* **272**, 31221–31224.

Crosbie, R. H., Straub, V., Yun, H. Y. et al. (1998). *mdx* muscle pathology is independent of nNOS perturbation. *Hum. Mol. Genetics* **7**, 823–829.

Crosbie, R. H., Lebakken, C. S., Holt, K. H. et al. (1999). Membrane targeting and stabilization of sarcospan is mediated by the sarcoglycan subcomplex. *J. Cell Biol.* **145**, 153–165.

Davies, K. E., Pearson, P .L., Harper, P. S. et al. (1983). Linkage analysis of two cloned DNA sequences flanking the Duchenne muscular dystrophy locus on the short arm of the human X chromosome. *Nucl. Acids Res.* **11**, 2303–2312.

Deconinck, A. E., Potter, A. C., Tinsley, J. M. et al. (1997a). Postsynaptic abnormalities at the neuromuscular junctions of utrophin-deficient mice. *J. Cell Biol.* **136**, 883–894.

Deconinck, A. E., Rafael, J. A., Skinner, J. A. et al. (1997b). Utrophin-dystrophin-deficient mice as a model for Duchenne muscular dystrophy. *Cell* **90**, 717–727.

Deconinck, N., Tinsley, J., de Backer, F. et al. (1997c). Expression of truncated utrophin leads to major functional improvements in dystrophin-deficient muscles of mice. *Nat. Med.* **3**, 1216–1221.

Decrouy, A., Renaud, J. M., Davis, H. L. et al. (1997). Mini-dystrophin gene transfer in *mdx*4cv diaphragm muscle fibers increases sarcolemmal stability. *Gene Ther.* **4**, 401–408.

de Lahunta, A. (1983). *Veterinary Neuroanatomy and Clinical Neurology*. Philadelphia, PA: Saunders.

de Stefano, M. E., Zaccaria, M. L., Cavaldesi, M. et al. (1997). Dystrophin and its isoforms in a sympathetic ganglion of normal and dystrophic *mdx* mice: immunolocalization by electron microscopy and biochemical characterization. *Neuroscience* **80**, 613–624.

DeWolf, C., McCauley, P., Sikorski, A. F. et al. (1997). Interaction of dystrophin fragments with model membranes. *Biophys. J.* **72**, 2599–25604.

Dick, J. and Vrbova, G. (1993). Progressive deterioration of muscles in *mdx* mice induced by overload. *Clin. Sci.* **84**, 145–150

Di Lazzaro, V., Restuccia, D., Servidei, S. et al. (1998). Functional involvement of cerebral cortex in Duchenne muscular dystrophy. *Muscle Nerve* **21**, 662–664.

Disatnik, M. H., Dhawan, J., Yu, Y. et al. (1998). Evidence of oxidative stress in *mdx* mouse muscle: studies of the pre-necrotic state. *J. Neurol. Sci.* **161**, 77–84.

Doriguzzi, C., Palmucci, L., Mongini, T. et al. (1997). Systematic use of dystrophin testing in muscle biopsies: results in 201 cases. *Eur. J. Clin. Invest.* **27**, 352–358.

Doriguzzi, C., Palmucci, L., Mongini, T. et al. (1999). Variable histological expression of dystrophinopathy in two females: *Acta Neuropathol.* **97**, 657–660.

Dreifuss, F. E. and Hogan, G. R. (1961). Survival in X-chromosomal muscular dystrophy. *Neurology* **11**, 734–737.

Dreyfus, J. C., Schapira, G. and Schapira, F. (1954). Biochemical study of muscle in progressive muscular dystrophy. *J. Clin. Invest.* **33**, 794–797.

Duance, V. C., Stephens, H. R., Dunn, M. et al. (1980). A role for collagen in the pathogenesis of muscular dystrophy? *Nature* **284**, 470–472.

Dubourg, C., Odent, S., Fergelot, P. et al. (1999). Identification of three novel mutations in the dystrophin gene detected by the heteroduplex/SSCA screening procedure. *Hum. Mutat.* **13**, 173.

Duchenne, G. B. A. (1855). *De l'Electrisation Localisee et de son Application a la Physiologie, a la Pathologie et a la Therapeutique.* Paris: J.-B. Baillière et Fils.

Duchenne, G. B. A. (1868). Recherches sur la paralysie musculaire pseudo-hypertrophique ou paralysie myo-sclerosique. *Arch. Gen. Med.* **11**, 5–25, 179–209, 305–321, 421–443, 552–588.

Duclos, F., Straub, V., Moore, S. A. et al. (1998). Progressive muscular dystrophy in alpha-sarcoglycan-deficient mice. *J. Cell Biol.* **142**, 1461–1471.

Duggan, D. J., Gorospe, J. R., Fanin, M. et al. (1997). Mutations in the sarcoglycan genes in patients with myopathy. *N. Eng. J. Med.* **336**, 618–624.

Dunckley, M. G., Wells, D. J., Walsh F. S. and Dickson, G. (1993). Direct retroviral-mediated transfer of a dystrophin minigene into *mdx* mouse muscle in vivo. *Hum. Mol. Genet.* **2**, 717–723.

Dunckley, M. G., Manoharan, M., Villiet, P. et al. (1998). Modification of splicing in the dystrophin gene in cultured Mdx muscle cells by antisense oligoribonucleotides. *Hum. Mol. Genet.* **7**, 1083–1090.

Ebashi, S., Toyokura, Y., Momoi, H. et al. (1959). High creatine phosphokinase activity of sera of progressive muscular dystrophy. *J. Biochem.* **46**, 103–104.

Emery, A. E. H. (1967). The use of serum creatine kinase for detecting carriers of Duchenne muscular dystrophy. In: *Exploratory Concepts in Muscular Dystrophy and Related Disorders,* ed. A. T. Milhorat, pp. 90–97. Amsterdam: Excerpta Medica.

Emery, A. E. H. (1977). Muscle histology and creatine kinase levels in fetuses in DMD. *Nature* **266**, 472–473.

Emery, A. E. H. (1993). Duchenne muscular dystrophy. In: *Oxford Monographs on Medical Genetics,* Vol. 24. Oxford: Oxford University Press.

Emery, A. E. H. and Dreifuss, F .E. (1966). Unusual type of benign X-linked muscular dystrophy. *J. Neurol. Neurosurg. Psychiatry* **29**, 338–342.

Emery, A. E. H. and Emery, M. L. H. (1995). *The History of a Genetic Disease: Duchenne Muscular Dystrophy or Meryon's Disease.* London: Royal Society of Medicine Press.

Engel, W. K. (1977). Integrative histochemical approach to the defect of Duchenne muscular dystrophy. In: *A Pathogenesis of Human Muscular Dystrophies,* ed. L. P. Rowland, pp. 277–309. Amsterdam: Excerpta Medica.

Ervasti, J. M. and Campbell, K. P. (1993). A role for the dystrophin–glycoprotein complex as a transmembrane linker between laminin and actin. *J. Cell Biol.* **122**, 809–823.

Evans, M. I., Hoffman, E. P., Cadrin, C. et al. (1994). Fetal muscle biopsy: collaborative experience with varied indications. *Obstetr. Gynecol.* **84**, 913–917.

Fassati, A., Wells, D. J., Serpente, P. A. et al. (1997). Genetic correction of dystrophin deficiency and skeletal muscle remodeling in adult *mdx* mouse via transplantation of retroviral producer Cells. *J. Clin. Invest.* **100**, 620–628.

Feero, W. G., Rosenblatt, J. D., Huard, J. et al. (1997a). Single fibres as a model system for viral gene delivery to skeletal muscle: Insights on maturation-dependent loss of fibre infectivity for adenovirus and herpes simplex type I viral vectors. *Hum. Gene Ther.* **8**, 371–380.

Feero, W. G., Li, S., Rosenblatt, J. D. et al. (1997b). Selection and use of ligands for receptor-mediated gene delivery to myogenic cells. *Gene Ther.* **4**, 664–674

Ferlini, A., Galie, N., Merlini, L. et al. (1998). A novel Alu-like element rearranged in the dystrophin gene causes a splicing mutation in a family with X-linked dilated cardiomyopathy. *Am. J. Hum. Genet.* **63**, 436–446.

Ferlini, A., Sewry, C., Melis, M. A. et al. (1999). X-linked dilated cardiomyopathy and the dystrophin gene. *Neuromusc. Disord.* **9**, 339–346.

Fisher, K. J., Jooss, K., Alston, J. et al. (1997). Recombinant adeno-associated virus for muscle directed gene therapy. *Nat. Med.* **3**, 306–312.

Fitzgerald, K. M., Cibis, G. W., Gettel, A. H. et al. (1999). ERG phenotype of a dystrophin mutation in heterozygous female carriers of Duchenne muscular dystrophy. *J. Med. Genet.* **36**, 316–22

Floyd, S. S. Jr, Clemens, P. R., Ontell, M. R. et al. (1998). Ex vivo gene transfer using adenovirus-mediated full-length dystrophin delivery to dystrophic muscles. *Gene Ther.* **5**, 19–30.

Fowler, W. M., Gardner, G. W., Kazerunian, H. H. et al. (1968). The effect of exercise on serum enzymes. *Arch. Phys. Med. Rehab.* **49**, 554–565.

Francke, U., Ochs, H. D., de Martinville, B. et al. (1985). Minor Xp21 chromosome deletion in a male associated with expression of Duchenne muscular dystrophy, chronic granulomatous disease, retinitis pigmentosa, and McLeod syndrome. *Am. J. Hum. Genet.* **37**, 250–267.

Gaschen, F., Hoffman, E. P., Gorospe, J. R. et al. (1992). Dystrophin deficiency causes lethal muscle hypertrophy in cats. *J. Neurol. Sci.* **110**, 149–159.

Gaschen, F., Gaschen, L., Seiler, G. et al. (1998). Lethal peracute rhabdomyolysis associated with stress and general anesthesia in three dystrophin-deficient cats. *Vet. Pathol.* **35**, 117–123.

Gaschen, L., Lang, J., Lin, S. et al. (1999). Cardiomyopathy in dystrophin-deficient hypertrophic feline muscular dystrophy. *J. Vet. Inter. Med.* **13**, 346–356.

Geifman-Holtzman, O., Bernstein, I. M., Capeless, E. L. et al. (1997). Increase in fetal breech presentation in female carriers of Duchenne muscular dystrophy. *Am. J. Med. Genet.* **73**, 276–278.

Gilbert, R., Nalbantoglu, J., Petrof, B. J. et al. (1999). Adenovirus-mediated utrophin gene transfer mitigates the dystrophic phenotype of *mdx* mouse muscles. *Hum. Gene Ther.* **10**, 1299–1310.

Goldberg, L. R., Hausmanowa-Petrusewicz, I., Fidzianska, A. et al. (1998). A dystrophin missense mutation showing persistence of dystrophin and dystrophin-associated proteins yet a severe phenotype. *Ann. Neurol.* **44**, 971–976.

Gorospe, J. R. M., Tharp, M. D., Hinckley, J. et al. (1994a). A role for mast cells in the progression of Duchenne muscular dystrophy? Correlations in dystrophin-deficient humans, dogs, and mice. *J. Neurol. Sci.* **122**, 44–56.

Gorospe, J. R. M., Tharp, M. D., Demitsu, T. et al. (1994b). Dystrophin-deficient myofibers are vulnerable to mast cell granule-induced necrosis. *Neuromusc. Disord.* **4**, 325–334.

Gorospe, J. R. M., Nishikawa, B. K. and Hoffman, E. P. (1996). Recruitment of mast cells to muscle after mild damage. *J. Neurol. Sci.* **135**, 10–17.

Gorospe, J. R. M., Nishikawa, B. K. and Hoffman, E. P. (1997). Pathophysiology of dystrophin deficiency: a clinical and biological enigma. In: *Dystrophin: Gene, Protein, and Cell*, eds. J. A. Lucy and S. C. Brown, pp. 201–232. Cambridge, UK: Cambridge University Press.

Gossrau, R. (1998). Nitric oxide synthase I (NOS I) is a costameric enzyme in rat skeletal muscle. *Acta Histochem.* **100**, 451–462

Gowers, W. R. (1879). Pseudo-hypertrophic muscular paralysis. In: *A Clinical Lecture*. London: J. and A. Churchill.

Grady, R. M., Merlie, J. P. and Sanes, J. R. (1997a). Subtle neuromuscular defects in utrophin-deficient mice. *J. Cell Biol.* **136**, 871–882.

Grady, R. M., Teng, H., Nichol, M. C. et al. (1997b). Skeletal and cardiac myopathies in mice lacking utrophin and dystrophin: a model for Duchenne muscular dystrophy. *Cell* **90**, 729–738.

Grady, R. M., Grange, R. W., Lau, K. S. et al. (1999). Role for α-dystrobrevin in the pathogenesis of dystrophin-dependent muscular dystrophies. *Nat. Cell Biol.* **1**, 215–220.

Gramolini, A. O., Burton, E. A., Tinsley, J. M. et al. (1998). Muscle and neural isoforms of agrin increase utrophin expression in cultured myotubes via a transcriptional regulatory mechanism. *J. Biol. Chem.* **273**, 736–743.

Gramolini, A. O.,. Karpati, G. and Jasmin, B. J. (1999a). Discordant expression of utrophin and its transcript in human and mouse skeletal muscles. *J. Neuropathol. Exp. Neurol.* **58**, 235–244.

Gramolini, A. O., Angus, L. M., Schaeffer, L. et al. (1999b). Induction of utrophin gene expression by heregulin in skeletal muscle cells: role of the N-box motif and GA binding protein. *Proc. Natl. Acad. Sc. USA* **96**, 3223–3227

Granchelli, J. A., Pollina, C. and Hudecki, M. S. (2000). Pre-clinical screening of drugs using the *mdx* mouse. *Neuromusc. Disord.* **10**, 235–239.

Greelish, J. P., Su, L.T., Lankford, E. B. et al. (1999). Stable restoration of the sarcoglycan complex in dystrophic muscle perfused with histamine and a recombinant adeno-associated viral vector. *Nat. Med.* **5**, 439–443.

Greenstein, R. M., Reardon, M. P. and Chan, T. S. (1977). A X-autosome translocation in a girl with Duchenne muscular dystrophy, evidence for DMD gene localisation. *Ped. Res.* **11**, 475A.

Gregory, S. L. and Brown, N. H. (1998). *kakapo*, a gene required for adhesion between and within cell layers in *Drosophila*, encodes a large cytoskeletal linker protein related to plectin and dystrophin. *J. Cell Biol.* **143**, 1271–1282.

Guibaud, P., Carrier, H. N., Planchu, H. et al. (1981). Manifestations musculaires precoces, cliniques et histopathologiques, chez 14 garcons presentant dans la premiere annee une activite serque elevee de creatine phosphokinase. *J. Genet. Hum.* **29**, 71–84.

Guibinga, G. H., Lochmuller, H., Massie, B. et al. (1998). Combinatorial blockade of calcineurin and CD28 signalling facilitates primary and secondary therapeutic gene transfer by adenovirus vectors in dystrophic (*mdx*) mouse muscles. *J. Virol.* **72**, 4601–4609.

Gussoni, E., Blau, H. M. and Kunkel, L. M. (1997). The fate of individual myoblasts after transplantation into muscles of DMD patients. *Nat. Med.* **3**, 970–977.

Hack, A. A., Ly, C. T,. Jiang, F. et al. (1998). Gamma-sarcoglycan deficiency leads to muscle membrane defects and apoptosis independent of dystrophin. *J. Cell Biol.* **142**, 1279–1287.

Hance, J. E., Fu, S. Y., Watkins, S. C. et al. (1999). alpha-actinin-2 is a new component of the dystrophin–glycoprotein complex. *Arch. Biochem.Biophys.* **365**, 216–222.

Hankard, R. G. (1998). Duchenne muscular dystrophy: a model for studying the contribution of muscle to energy and protein metabolism. *Reprod. Nutr. Dev.* **38**, 181–186.

Hankard, R. G., Hammond, D., Haymond, M. W. and Darmann, D. (1998). Oral glutamine slows down whole body protein breakdown in Duchenne muscular dystrophy. *Ped. Res.* **43**, 222–226.

Hathaway, P. W., Engel, W. K. and Zellweger, H. (1970). Experimental myopathy after microarterial embolization. *Arch. Neurol.* **22**, 365–378.

Hayashi, Y. K., Chou, F. L., Engvall, E. et al. (1998). Primary deficiency of integrin alpha7 as a cause of congenital myopathy. *Nat. Genet.* **19**, 94–97.

Haycock, J. W., MacNeil, S., Jones, P. et al. (1996). Oxidative damage to muscle protein in Duchenne muscular dystrophy. *Neuroreport* **8**, 357–361.

Hayes, A. and Williams, D. A. (1998). Contractile function and low-intensity exercise effects of old dystrophic (*mdx*) mice. *Am. J. Physiol.* **274**, C1138–C1144.

Hearse, D. J. (1979). Cellular damage during myocardial ischaemia: metabolic changes leading to enzyme leakage. In: *Enzymes in Cardiology; Diagnosis and Research*, eds. D. J. Hearse and J. de Leiris, pp. 1–20. Chichester: Wiley.

Heckel, S., Favre, R., Flori, J. et al. (1999). In utero fetal muscle biopsy: a precious aid for the prenatal diagnosis of Duchenne muscular dystrophy. *Fetal Diagn. Ther.* **14**, 127–132.

Heimann, P., Augustin, M., Wieneke, S. et al. (1998). Mutual interference of myotonia and muscular dystrophy in the mouse: a study on *adr-mdx* double mutants. *Neuromusc. Disord.* **8**, 551–560.

Heller, K. D., Forst, R., Forst, J. et al. (1997). Scoliosis in Duchenne muscular dystrophy: aspects of orthotic treatment. *Prosthet. Orthot. Int.* **21**, 202–209.

Helliwell, T. R., MacLennan, P. A., McArdle, A. et al. (1996). Fasting increases the extent of muscle necrosis in the *mdx* mouse. *Clin. Sci.* **90**, 467–472.

Henry, M. D. and Campbell, K .P. (1998). A role for dystroglycan in basement membrane assembly. *Cell* **95**, 859–870.

Hodges, B. L., Hayashi, Y. K., Nonaka, I. et al. (1997). Altered expression of the alpha7beta1 integrin in human and murine muscular dystrophies. *J. Cell Sci.* **110**, 2873–2881.

Hoffman, E. P. (1989). Human molecular genetics and the elucidation of the primary biochemical defect in Duchenne muscular dystrophy. *Cell Motil. Cytoskel.* **14**, 163–168.

Hoffman, E. P. (1993). Genotype/phenotype correlations in Duchenne/Becker dystrophy. In: *Molecular and Cell Biology of Muscular Dystrophy*, ed. T. Partridge, pp. 12–36. London: Chapman & Hall.

Hoffman, E. P. (1997). Muscular dystrophies. In: *Encyclopedia of Human Biology*, 2nd edn, ed. R. Dulbecco, pp. 901–906. San Diego, CA: Academic Press.

Hoffman, E. P. (1999). Counting dystrophies in the post-molecular census. *J. Neurol. Sci.* **164**, 44–49.

Hoffman, E. P. and Gorospe, R. J. M. (1991). The animal models of Duchenne muscular dystrophy: windows on the pathophysiological consequences of dystrophin deficiency. In: *Current Topics in Membranes*, Vol. 38, pp. 113–151. New York: Academic Press.

Hoffman, E. P. and Kunkel, L. M. (1989). Dystrophin abnormalities in Duchenne/Becker muscular dystrophy. *Neuron* **2**, 1019–1029.

Hoffman, E. P., Monaco, A. P., Feener, C. C. et al. (1987a). Conservation of the Duchenne muscular dystrophy gene in mice and humans. *Science* **238**, 347–350.

Hoffman, E. P., Brown, R. H. and Kunkel, L. M. (1987b). Dystrophin: the protein product of the Duchenne muscular dystrophy locus. *Cell* **51**, 919–928.

Hoffman, E. P., Fischbeck, K. H., Brown, R. H. et al. (1988a). Characterization of dystrophin in muscle biopsy specimens from patients with Duchenne's or Becker's muscular dystrophy. *N. Eng. J. Med.* **318**, 1363–1368.

Hoffman, E. P., Hudecki, M. S., Rosenberg, P. A. et al. (1988b). Cell and fiber-type distribution of dystrophin. *Neuron* **1**, 411–420.

Hoffman, E. P., Beggs, A. H., Koenig, M. et al. (1989a). Cross-reactive protein in Duchenne muscle. *Lancet* **ii**, 1211–1212.

Hoffman, E. P., Kunkel, L. M., Angelini, C. et al. (1989b). Improved diagnosis of Becker muscular dystrophy by dystrophin testing. *Neurology* **39**, 1011–1017.

Hoffman, E. P., Morgan, J. E., Watkins, S. C. et al. (1990). Somatic reversion/suppression of the mouse *mdx* phenotype in vivo. *J. Neurol. Sci.* **99**, 9–25.

Hoffman, E. P., Arahata, K., Minetti, C. et al. (1992). Dystrophinopathy in isolated cases of myopathy in females. *Neurology* **42**, 967–975.

Hoffman, E. P., Pegoraro, E., Scacheri, P. et al. (1996). Genetic counseling of isolated carriers of Duchenne muscular dystrophy. *Am. J. Med. Genet.* **63**, 573–580.

Hoogerwaard, E. M., Bakker, E., Ippel, P. F. et al. (1999). Signs and symptoms of Duchenne muscular dystrophy and Becker muscular dystrophy among carriers in the Netherlands: a cohort study. *Lancet* **353**, 2116–2119.

Howard, P. L., Klamut, H. J. and Ray, P. N. (1998). Identification of a novel actin binding site within the Dp71 dystrophin isoform *FEBS Lett.* **441**, 337–341.

Howard, P. L., Dally, G. Y., Ditta, S. D. et al. (1999). Dystrophin isoforms DP71 and DP427 have distinct roles in myogenic cells. *Muscle Nerve* **22**, 16–27.

Howell, J. M., Fletcher, S., O'Hara, A. et al. (1998a). Direct dystrophin and reporter gene transfer into dog muscle in vivo. *Muscle Nerve* **21**, 159–165.

Howell, J. M., Lochmuller, H., O'Hara, A. et al. (1998b). High-level dystrophin expression after adenovirus-mediated dystrophin minigene transfer to skeletal muscle of dystrophic dogs: prolongation of expression with immunosuppression. *Hum. Gene Ther.* **9**, 629–634.

Hu, X., Ray, P. N., Murphy, E. G. et al. (1990). Duplicational mutation at the Duchenne muscular dystrophy locus: its frequency, distribution, origin, and phenotype/genotype correlation. *Am. J. Hum. Genet.* **46**, 682–695.

Huard, J., Feero, W. G., Watkins, S. C. et al. (1996). The basal lamina is a physical barrier to viral mediated gene delivery to mature muscle fibres. *J. Virol.* **70**, 8117–8123.

Hudecki, M. S., Pollina, C. M., Granchelli, J. A. et al. (1993). Strength and endurance in thetherapeutic evaluation of prenisolone-treated *mdx* mice. *Res. Comm. Chem. Pathol. Pharmacol.* **79**, 45–60.

Hudgson, P., Pearce, G. W. and Walton, J. N. (1967). Pre-clinical muscular dystrophy: Histopathological changes observed on muscle biopsy. *Brain* **90**, 565–576.

Im, W. B., Phelps, S. F., Copen, E. H. et al. (1996). Differential expression of dystrophin isoforms in strains of *mdx* mice with different mutations. *Hum. Mol. Genet.* **5**, 1149–1153.

Imbert, N., Vandebrouck, C., Constantin, B. et al. (1996). Hypoosmotic shocks induce elevation of resting calcium level in Duchenne muscular dystrophy myotubes contracting in vitro. *Neuromusc. Disord.* **6**, 51–60.

Irintchev, A., Rosenblatt, J. D., Cullen, M. J., Zweyer, M. et al. (1998). Ectopic skeletal muscles derived from myoblasts implanted under the skin. *J. Cell Sci.* **111**, 3287–3297.

Jancsik, V. and Hajos, F. (1999). The demonstration of immunoreactive dystrophin and its developmental expression in perivascular astrocytes. *Brain Res.* **831**, 200–205.

Jooss, K., Yang, Y., Fisher, K. J. et al. (1998). Transduction of dendritic cells by DNA viral vectors directs the immune response to transgene products in muscle fibers. *J. Virol.* **72**, 4212–4223.

Kachinsky, A. M., Froehner, S. C. and Milgram, S. L. (1999). A PDZ-containing scaffold related to the dystrophin complex at the basolateral membrane of epithelial Cells. *J. Cell Biol.* **145**, 391–402.

Kahana, E., Flood, G. and Gratzer, W. B. (1997). Physical properties of dystrophin rod domain. *Cell Motil. Cytoskel.* **36**, 246–252

Kameya, S., Miyagoe, Y., Nonaka, I. et al. (1999). Alpha1-syntrophin gene disruption results in the absence of neuronal-type nitric-oxide synthase at the sarcolemma but does not induce muscle degeneration. *J. Biol. Chem.* **274**, 2193–2200.

Khurana, T. S., Rosmarin, A. G., Shang, J. et al. (1999). Activation of utrophin promoter by heregulin via the ets-related transcription factor complex GA-binding protein alpha/beta. *Mol. Biol. Cell* **10**, 2075–2086.

Kimura, S., Sugino, S., Ohtani, Y. et al. (1998). Muscle fibre immaturity and inactivity reduce myonecrosis in Duchenne muscular dystrophy. *Ann. Neurol.* **44**, 967–971.

Kingston, H. M., Sarfarazi, M., Thomas, N. S. T. et al. (1984). Localisation of the Becker muscular dystrophy gene on the short arm of the X chromosome by linkage to cloned DNA sequences. *Hum. Genet.* **67**, 6–17.

Kinoshita, I., Vilquin, J. T., Asselin, I. et al. (1998). Transplantation of myoblasts from a transgenic mouse overexpressing dystrophin prduced only a relatively small increase of dystrophin-positive membrane. *Muscle Nerve* **21**, 91–103.

Kochanek, S., Clemens, P. R., Mitani, K. et al. (1996). A new adenoviral vector: replacement of all viral coding sequences with 28 kb of DNA independently expressing both full-length dystrophin and beta-galactosidase. *Proc. Natl. Acad. Sci. USA* **93**, 5731–5736.

Koenig, M., Hoffman, E. P., Bertelson, C. J. et al. (1987). Complete cloning of the Duchenne muscular dystrophy (DMD) cDNA and preliminary genomic organization of the DMD gene in normal and affected individuals. *Cell* **51**, 509–517.

Koenig, M., Monaco, A. P. and Kunkel, L. M. (1988). The complete sequence of dystrophin predicts a rod-shaped cytoskeletal protein. *Cell* **53**, 219–228.

Koenig, M., Beggs, A. H., Moyer, M. et al. (1989). The molecular basis for Duchenne versus Becker muscular dystrophy: correlation of severity with type of deletion. *Am. J. Hum. Genet.* **45**, 498–506.

Komulainen, J., Takala, T. E., Kuipers, H. et al. (1998). The disruption of myofibre structures in rat skeletal muscle after forced lengthening contractions. *Pflugers Arch.* **436**, 735–741.

Komulainen, J., Koskinen, S. O., Kalliokoski, R. et al. (1999). Gender differences in skeletal muscle fibre damage after eccentrically biased downhill running in rats. *Acta Physiol. Scand.* **165**, 57–63.

Kornegay, J. N., Tuler, S. M., Miller, D. M. et al. (1988). Muscular dystrophy in a litter of golden retriever dogs. *Muscle Nerve* **11**, 1056–1064.

Kostin, S., Scholz, D., Shimada, T. et al. (1998). The internal and external protein scaffold of the T-tubular system in cardiomyocytes. *Cell Tissue Res.* **294**, 449–460.

Kramer, R., Lochmuller, H., Abicht, A. et al. (1998). Myotonic ADR-MDX mutant mice show less severe muscular dystrophy than MDX mice. *Neuromusc. Disord.* **8**, 542–550.

Kumar-Singh, R. and Chamberlain, J. S. (1996). Encapsidated adenovirus minichromosomes allow delivery and expression of a 14 kb dystrophin cDNA to muscle cells. *Hum. Mol. Genet.* **5**, 913–921.

Kunkel, L. M., Monaco, A. P., Middlesworth, W. et al. (1985). Specific cloning of DNA fragments absent from the DNA of a male patient with an X chromosome deletion. *Proc. Natl. Acad. Sci. USA* **82**, 4778–4782.

Kuznetsov, A. V., Winkler, K., Wiedemann, F. R. et al. (1998). Impaired mitochondrial oxidative phosphorylation in skeletal muscle of the dystrophin-deficient *mdx* mouse. *Mol. Cell Biochem.* **183**, 87–96

Lanasa, M. C. and Hoffman, E. P. (1999). The X chromosome and recurrent spontaneous abortion: the significance of transmanifesting carriers. *Am. J. Hum. Genet.* **64**, 934–938.

Lanasa, M. C., Hogge, W. A., Kubik, C. et al. (1999). Highly skewed X-chromosome inactivation is associated with idiopathic recurrent spontaneous abortion. *Am. J. Hum. Genet.* **65**, 252–254.

Law, P. K., Goodwin, T. G., Fang, Q. et al. (1993). Cell transplantation as an experimental treatment for Duchenne muscular dystrophy. *Cell Transplant.* **2**, 485–505.

Lefaucheur, J. P., Pastoret, C. and Sebille, A., (1995). Phenotype of dystrophinopathy in old *mdx* mice. *Anat. Rec.* **242**, 70–76.

Lefaucheur, J. P., Gjata, B. and Sebille, A., (1996). Factors inducing mast cell accumulation in skeletal muscle. *Neuropathol. Appl. Neurobiol.* **22**, 248–255.

Leijendekker, W. J., Passaquin, A. C., Metzinger, L. et al. (1996). Regulation of cytosolic calcium in skeletal muscle cells of the *mdx* mouse under conditions of stress. *Br. J. Pharmacol.* **118**, 611–616.

Li, M., Dickson, D. W. and Spiro, A. J. (1998). Sarcolemmal defect and subsarcolemmal lesion in a patient with gamma-sarcoglycan deficiency. *Neurology* **50**, 807–809.

Li, J., Dressman, D., Tsao, Y. P., Yoyo-oka, T., Hoffman, E. P. and Xiao, X. (1999). rAAV vector-mediated sarcoglycan gene transfer in a hamster model for limb–girdle muscular dystrophy. *Gene Ther.* **6**, 74–82.

Little, W. J. (1853). *On the Nature and Treatment of the Deformities of the Human Frame: being a Course of Lectures delivered at the Royal Orthopaedic Hospital in 1843.* London: Longman, Brown, Green and Longman.

Liu, J. W., Wakayama, Y., Inoue, M. et al. (1999). Immunocytochemical studies of aquaporin 4 in the skeletal muscle of *mdx* mouse *J. Neurol. Sci.* **164**, 24–28.

Lodi, R., Kemp, G. J., Muntoni, F. et al. (1999). Reduced cytosolic acidification during exercise suggests defective glycolytic activity in skeletal muscle of patients with Becker muscular dystrophy. An in vivo 31P magnetic resonance spectroscopy study. *Brain* **122**, 121–130.

Love, D. R., Hill, D. F., Dickson, G. et al. (1989). An autosomal transcript in skeletal muscle with homology to dystrophin. *Nature* **339**, 55–58.

Lumeng, C. N., Hauser, M., Brown, V. et al. (1999a). Expression of the 71 kDa dystrophin isoform (Dp71) evaluated by gene targeting. *Brain Res.* **830**, 174–178.

Lumeng, C. N., Phelps, S. F., Rafael, J. A. et al. (1999b) Characterization of dystrophin and utrophin diversity in the mouse. *Hum. Mol. Genet.* **8**, 593–599.

Mancinelli, R., Tonali, P., Servidei, S. et al. (1995). Analysis of peristaltic reflex in young dystrophic mouse. *Neurosci. Lett.* **192**, 57–60.

Marbini, A., Marcello, N., Bellanova, M. F. et al. (1995). Dystrophin expression in skin biopsy immunohistochemical. Localisation of striated muscle type dystrophin. *J. Neurol. Sci.* **129**, 29–33.

McArdle, A., Helliwell, T. R., Beckett, G. J. et al. (1998). Effect of propylthiouracil-induced hypothyroidism on the onset of skeletal muscle necrosis in dystrophin-deficient *mdx* mice. *Clin. Sci.*, **95**, 83–89.

Megeney, L. A., Kablar, B., Perry, R. L. et al. (1999). Severe cardiomyopathy in mice lacking dystrophin and MyoD. *Proc. Natl. Acad. Sci. USA* **96**, 220–225.

Mehler, M. F., Hass, K. Z., Kessler, J. A. et al. (1992). Enhanced sensitivity of hippocampal pyramidal neurons from *mdx* mice to hypoxia-induced loss of synaptic transmission. *Proc. Natl. Acad. Sci. USA* **89**, 2461–2465.

Melacini, P., Vianello, A., Villanova, C. et al. (1996). Cardiac and respiratory involvement in advanced stage Duchenne muscular dystrophy. *Neuromusc. Disord.* **6**, 367–376.

Melacini, P., Fanin, M., Angelini, A. et al. (1998). Cardiac transplantation in a Duchenne muscular dystrophy carrier. *Neuromusc. Disord.* **8**, 585–590.

Mendell, J. R., Engel, W. K. and Derrer, E. C. (1971). Duchenne muscular dystrophy: functional ischemia reproduces its characteristic lesions. *Science* **172**, 1143–1145.

Mendell, J. R., Engel, W. K. and Derrer, E. C. (1972). Increased plasma enzyme concentrations in rats, with functional ischaemia of muscle provide a possible model of Duchenne muscular dystrophy. *Nature* **239**, 522–524.

Mendell, J. R., Kissel, J. T., Amato, A. A. et al. (1995). Myoblast transfer in the treatment of Duchenne's muscular dystrophy. *N. Eng. J. Med.* **333**, 832–838.

Meryon, E. (1851). On fatty degeneration of the voluntary muscles. *Lancet* **ii**, 588–589.

Meryon, E. (1852). On granular and fatty degeneration of the voluntary muscles. *Med. Chirurg. Trans.* **35**, 73–84.

Meryon, E. (1864). *Practical and Pathological Researches on the Various Forms of Paralysis.* London: John Churchill and Sons.

Mestroni, L., Rocco, C., Gregori, D. et al. (1999). Familial dilated cardiomyopathy: evidence for genetic and phenotypic heterogeneity. Heart Muscle Disease Study Group. *J. Am. Coll. Cardiol.* **34**, 181–190.

Miller, R. G. and Hoffman, E. P. (1994). Molecular diagnosis and modern management of Duchenne muscular dystrophy. *Neurol. Clin.* **12**, 699–725.

Miller, R. G., Sharma, K. R., Pavlath, G. K. et al. (1997). Myoblast implantation in Duchenne muscular dystrophy: the San Francisco study. *Muscle Nerve* **20**, 469–478.

Minetti, C., Tanji, K. and Bonilla, E. (1992). Immunologic study of vinculin in Duchenne muscular dystrophy. *Neurology* **42**, 1751–1754.

Minetti, C., Cordone, G., Beltrame, F. et al. (1998). Disorganization of dystrophin costameric lattice in Becker muscular dystrophy. *Muscle Nerve* **21**, 211–216.

Mirabella, M., Galluzzi, G., Manfredi, G. et al. (1998). Giant dystrophin deletion associated with congenital cataract and mild muscular dystrophy. *Neurology* **51**, 592–595.

Moizard, M. P., Billard, C., Toutain, A. et al. (1998). Are Dp71 and Dp140 brain dystrophin isoforms related to cognitive impairment in Duchenne muscular dystrophy? *Am. J. Med. Genet.* **80**, 32–41.

Mokhtarian, A., Lefaucheur, J. P., Even, P. C. et al. (1995). Effects of treadmill exercise and high-fat feeding on muscle degeneration in *mdx* mice at the time of weaning. *Clin. Sci.* **89**, 447–452.

Mokhtarian, A., Lefaucheur, J. P., Even, P. C. et al. (1999). Hindlimb immobilization applied to 21-day-old *mdx* mice prevents the occurrence of muscle degeneration. *J. Appl. Physiol.* **86**, 924–931.

Mokri, B. and Engel, A. G. (1975). Duchenne dystrophy: electron microscopic findings pointing to a basic or early abnormality in the plasma membrane of the muscle fibre. *Neurology* **25**, 1111–1120.

Monaco, A. P., Bertelson, C., Middlesworth, W. et al. (1986a). Detection of deletions spanning the Duchenne muscular dystrophy locus using a tightly linked DNA segment. *Nature* **316**, 842–845.

Monaco, A. P., Neve, R. L., Colletti-Feener, C. et al. (1986b). Isolation of candidate cDNAs for portions of the Duchenne muscular dystrophy gene. *Nature* **323**, 646–650.

Monaco, A. P., Bertelson, C. J., Colleti-Feener, C. et al. (1987). Localization and cloning of Xp21 deletion breakpoints involved in muscular dystrophy. *Hum. Genet.* **75**, 221–227.

Monaco, A. P., Bertelson, C. J., Liechti-Gallati, S. et al. (1988). An explanation for the phenotypic differences between patients bearing partial deletions of the DMD locus. *Genomics* **2**, 90–95.

Monahan, P. E., Samulski, R. J., Tazelaar, J. et al. (1998). Direct intramuscular injection with recombinant AAV vectors results in sustained expression in a dog model of hemophilia. *Gene Ther.* **5**, 40–49.

Montanaro, F., Lindenbaum, M. and Carbonetto, S. (1998). Alpha-dystroglycan is a laminin receptor involved in extracellular matrix assembly on myotubes and muscle cell viability. *J. Cell Biol.* **145**, 1325–1340.

Morgan, J. E., Hoffman, E. P. and Partridge, T. A. (1990). Normal myogenic cells from newborn mice restore normal histology to degenerating muscles the *mdx* mouse. *J. Cell Biol.* **111**, 2437–2449.

Morgan, J. E., Fletcher, R. M. and Partridge, T. A. (1996). Yields of muscle from myogenic cells implanted into young and old *mdx* hosts. *Muscle Nerve* **19**, 132–139.

Muntoni, F., Di Lenarda, A., Porcu, M. et al. (1997). Dystrophin gene abnormalities in two patients with idiopathic dilated cardiomyopathy. *Heart* **78**, 608–612.

Murray, J. M., Davies, K. E., Harper, P. S. et al. (1982). Linkage relationship of a cloned DNA sequence on the short arm of the X chromosome to Duchenne muscular dystrophy. *Nature* **300**, 69–71.

Neumeyer, A. M., Cros, D., McKenna-Yasek, D. et al. (1998). Pilot study of myoblast transfer in the treatment of Becker muscular dystrophy. *Neurology* **51**, 589–592.

Nicholson, L. V. B., Davison, K., Johnson, M. A. et al. (1989). Dystrophin in skeletal muscle. II. Immunoreactivity in patients with Xp21 muscular dystrophy. *J. Neurol. Sci.* **94**, 137–146.

Nobile, C., Marchi, J., Nigro, V. et al. (1997). Exon–intron organization of the human dystrophin gene. *Genomics* **45**, 421–424.

Noordeen, M. H., Haddad, F. S., Muntoni, F. et al. (1999). Blood loss in Duchenne muscular dystrophy: vascular smooth muscle dysfunction? *J. Ped. Orthoped.* **8**, 212–215.

Ohtsuka, Y., Udaka, K., Yamashiro, Y. et al. (1998). Dystrophin acts as a transplantation rejection antigen in dystrophin-deficient mice: implication for gene therapy. *J. Immunol.* **160**, 4635–4640.

Pagel, C. N. and Partridge, T. A. (1999). Covert persistence of *mdx* mouse myopathy is revealed by acute and chronic effects of irradiation. *J. Neurol. Sci.* **164**, 103–116.

Partridge, R. (1847). Fatty degeneration of muscle. *Lond. Med. Gaz.* (New Series) **5**, 944.

Partridge, R. (1848). Fatty degeneration of voluntary muscle. *Trans. Pathol. Soc. Lond.* **35**, 73–84.

Partridge, T. (1998). The 'fantastic voyage' of muscle progenitor cells. [News] *Nat. Med.* **4**, 554–555

Partridge, T. A., Morgan, J. E., Coulton, G. R. et al. (1989). Conversion of *mdx* myofibres from dystrophin-negative to dystrophin-positive by injection of normal myoblasts. *Nature* **33**, 176–179.

Pascual Pascual, S. I., Molano, J. and Pascual-Castroviejo, I. (1998). Electroretinogram in Duchenne/Becker muscular dystrophy. *Ped. Neurol.* **18**, 315–320.

Pastoret, C. and Sebille, A. (1995). *mdx* mice show progressive weakness and muscle deterioration with age. *J. Neurol. Sci.* **129**, 97–105.

Pegoraro, E., Schimke R. N., Arahata, K. et al. (1994). Dystrophinopathy in females: paternal inheritance and genetic counseling. *Am. J. Hum. Genet.* **54**, 989–1003.

Pegoraro, E., Schimke, R. N., Garcia, C. et al. (1995). Genetic and biochemical normalization in female carriers of Duchenne muscular dystrophy: evidence for failure of dystrophin production in dystrophin competent myonuclei. *Neurology* **45**, 677–690.

Pegoraro, E., Whitaker, J., Mowery-Rushton, P. et al. (1997). Familial skewed X-inactivation: a molecular trait associated with high spontaneous abortion rate maps to Xq28. *Am. J. Hum. Genet.* **61**, 160–170.

Pegoraro, E., Marks, H., Garcia, C. A. et al. (1998). Genotype/phenotype correlations in 22 merosin-deficient congenital muscular dystrophy patients. *Neurology* **51**, 101–110.

Peters, M. F., O'Brien, K. F., Sadoulet-Puccio, H. M. et al. (1997). Beta-dystrobrevin, a new member of the dystrophin family. Identification, cloning, and protein associations. *J. Biol. Chem.* **272**, 31561–31569.

Peters, M. F., Sadoulet-Puccio, H. M., Grady, M. R. et al. (1998). Differential membrane localization and intermolecular associations of alpha-dystrobrevin isoforms in skeletal muscle. *J. Cell Biol.* **142**, 1269–1278.

Pillers, D. A., Weleber, R. G., Green, D. G. et al. (1999). Effects of dystrophin isoforms on signal transduction through neural retina: genotype-phenotype analysis of Duchenne muscular dystrophy mouse mutants. *Mol. Genet. Metab.* **66**, 100–110.

Podhorska-Okolow, M., Sandri, M., Zampieri, S. et al. (1998). Apoptosis of myofibres and satellite cells: exercise-induced damage in skeletal muscle of the mouse. *Neuropathol. Appl. Neurobiol.* **24**, 518–531.

Politano, L., Nigro, V., Nigro, G. et al. (1996). Development of cardiomyopathy in female carriers of Duchenne and Becker muscular dystrophies. *J. Am. Med. Assoc.* **275**, 1335–1338.

Porter, J. D., Rafael, J. A., Ragusa, R. J. et al. (1998). The sparing of extraocular muscle in dystrophinopathy is lost in mice lacking utrophin and dystrophin. *J. Cell Sci.* **111**, 1801–1811.

Prior, T. W., Bartolo, C., Pearl, D. K. et al. (1995). Spectrum of small mutations in the dystrophin coding region. *Am. J. Hum. Genet.* **57**, 22–33.

Qu, Z., Balkir, L., van Deutekom, J. C. et al. (1998). Development of approaches to improve cell survival in myoblast transfer therapy. *J. Cell Biol.* **142**, 1257–1267.

Rafael, J. A., Cox, G. A., Corrado, K. et al. (1996). Forced expression of dystrophin deletion constructs reveals structure–function correlations. *J. Cell Biol.* **134**, 93–102.

Rafael, J. A., Tinsley, J. M., Potter, A. C. et al. (1998). Skeletal muscle-specific expression of a utrophin transgene rescues utrophin–dystrophin deficient mice. *Nat. Genet.* **19**, 79–82.

Rafael, J. A., Trickett, J. I., Potter, A. C. et al. (1999). Dystrophin and utrophin do not play crucial roles in nonmuscle tissues in mice. *Muscle Nerve* **22**, 517–519.

Rambukkana, A., Yamada, H., Zanazzi, G. et al. (1998). Role of alpha-dystroglycan as a Schwann cell receptor for *Mycobacterium leprae. Science* **282**, 2076–2079.

Rando, T. A., Disatnik, M. H., Yu, Y. et al. (1998). Muscle cells from *mdx* mice have an increased susceptibility to oxidative stress. *Neuromusc. Disord.* **8**, 14–21.

Ray, P. N., Belfall, B., Duf, C. et al. (1985). Cloning of the breakpoint of an X:21 translocation associated with Duchenne muscular dystrophy. *Nature* **318**, 672–675.

Renley, B. A., Rybakova, I. N., Amann, K .J. et al. (1998). Dystrophin binding to nonmuscle actin. *Cell Motil. Cytoskel.* **41**, 264–270

Rentschler, S., Linn, H., Deininger, K. et al. (1999). The WW domain of dystrophin requires EF-hands region to interact with beta-dystroglycan. *Biol. Chem.* **380**, 431–442.

Roberts, R. G. and Bobrow, M. (1998). Dystrophins in vertebrates and invertebrates. *Hum. Mol. Genet.* **7**, 589–595.

Rowland, L. P. (1980). Biochemistry of muscle membranes in Duchenne muscular dystrophy. *Muscle Nerve* **3**, 3–20.

Rowland L. P. (1964). Muscular dystrophies and related diseases: metabolic aspects. *Manitoba Med. Rev.* **44**, 540–545.

Rybakova, I. N. and Ervasti, J. M. (1997). Dystrophin–glycoprotein complex is monomeric and stabilizes actin filaments in vitro through a lateral association. *J. Biol. Chem.* **272**, 28771–28778.

Saito, F., Masaki, T., Kamakura, K. et al. (1999). Characterization of the transmembrane molecular architecture of the dystroglycan complex in Schwann cells. *J. Biol. Chem.* **274**, 8240–8246.

Saito, M., Kawai, H., Akaike, M. et al. (1996). Cardiac dysfunction with Becker muscular dystrophy. *Am. Heart J.* **132**, 642–647.

Sakamoto, A., Ono, K., Abe, M. et al. (1997). Both hypertrophic and dilated cardiomyopathies are caused by mutation of the same gene, delta-sarcoglycan, in hamster: an animal model of disrupted dystrophin-associated glycoprotein complex. *Proc. Natl. Acad. Sci. USA* **94**, 13873–13878.

Sandri, M., Podhorska-Okolow, M., Geromel, V. et al. (1997). Exercise induces myonuclear ubiquitination and apoptosis in dystrophin-deficient muscle of mice. *J. Neuropathol. Exp. Neurol.* **56**, 45–57.

Sandri, M., Massimino, M. L., Cantini, M. et al. (1998a). Dystrophin deficient myotubes undergo apoptosis in mouse primary muscle cell culture after DNA damage. *Neurosci. Lett.* **252**, 123–126.

Sandri, M., Minetti, C., Pedemonte, M. et al. (1998b). Apoptotic myonuclei in human Duchenne muscular dystrophy. *Lab. Invest.* **78**, 1005–1016.

Sarig, R., Mezger-Lallemand, V., Gitelman, I. et al. (1999). Targeted inactivation of Dp71, the major non-muscle product of the DMD gene: differential activity of the Dp71 promoter during development. *Hum. Mol. Genet.* **8**, 1–10.

Schapira, G., Dreyfus, J. C. and Schapira, F. (1953). L'elevation du taux de l'adlolase serique, test biochimique des myopathies. *Semain. Hopit.* **29**, 1917–1920.

Schatzberg, S. J., Anderson, L. V., Wilton, S. D. et al. (1998). Alternative dystrophin gene transcripts in golden retriever muscular dystrophy. *Mol. Cell Biochem.* **183**, 87–96.

Schatzberg, S. J., Olby, N. J., Breen, M. et al. (1999). Molecular analysis of a spontaneous dystrophin 'knockout' dog. *Neuromusc. Disord.* **9**, 289–295.

Sesay, A. K., Errington, M. L., Levita, L. et al. (1996). Spatial learning and hippocampal long-term potentiation are not impaired in *mdx* mice. *Neurosci. Lett.* **211**, 207–210.

Sharp, N. J., Kornegay, J. N., van Camp, S. D. et al. (1992). An error in dystrophin mRNA processing in golden retriever muscular dystrophy, an animal homologue of Duchenne muscular dystrophy. *Genomics* **13**, 115–121.

Sicinski, P., Geng, Y., Ryder-Cook, A. S. et al. (1989). The molecular basis of muscular dystrophy in the *mdx* mouse: a point mutation. *Science* **244**, 1578–1580.

Spencer, M. J., Walsh, C. M., Dorshkind, K. A. et al. (1997). Myonuclear apoptosis in dystrophic *mdx* muscle occurs by perforin-mediated cytotoxicity. *J. Clin. Invest.* **99**, 2745–2751.

Strumpf, D. and Volk, T. (1998). A novel cytoskeletal-associated protein is essential for the restricted localization of the neuregulin-like factor, vein, at the muscle–tendon junction site. *J. Cell Biol.* **143**, 1259–1270.

Talts, J. F., Andac, Z., Gohring, W. et al (1999). Binding of the G domains of laminin alpha1 and alpha2 chains and perlecan to heparin, sulfatides, alpha-dystroglycan and several extracellular matrix proteins. *EMBO J.* **18**, 863–870.

Taylor, J., Muntoni, F., Dubowitz, V. et al. (1997). The abnormal expression of utrophin in Duchenne and Becker muscular dys-

trophy is age related. *Neuropathol. Appl. Neurobiol.* **23**, 399–405.

Tennyson, C. N., Klamut, H. J. and Worton, R. G. (1995). The human dystrophin gene requires 16 hours to be transcribed and is co-transcriptionally spliced. *Nat. Genet.* **9**, 184–190

Tennyson, C. N., Shi, Q. and Worton, R. G. (1996). Stability of the human dystrophin transcript in muscle. *Nucl. Acids Res.* **24**, 3059–3064.

Tezak, Z., Kanneboyina, N., Plotz, P. and Hoffman, E. P. (2000). Adeno-associated virus (AAV) in normal and myositis human skeletal muscle. *Neurology*, **55**, 1913–1917.

Thomas, G. D., Sander, M., Lau, K. S. et al. (1998). Impaired metabolic modulation of alpha-adrenergic vasoconstriction in dystrophin-deficient skeletal muscle. *Proc. Natl. Acad. Sci. USA* **95**, 15090–15095.

Thomas, G. H., Newbern, E. C., Korte, C. C. et al. (1997). Intragenic duplication and divergence in the spectrin superfamily of proteins. *Mol. Biol. Evol.* **14**, 1285–1295.

Tinsley, J. M., Potter, A. C., Phelps, S. R. et al. (1996). Amelioration of the dystrophic phenotype of *mdx* mice using a truncated utrophin transgene. *Nature* **384**, 349–353.

Tinsley, J. M., Deconinck, N., Fisher. R. et al. (1998). Expression of full-length utrophin prevents muscular dystrophy in *mdx* mice. *Nat. Med.* **4**, 1441–1444.

Torrente, Y., D'Angelo, M. G., Del Bo, R. et al. (1999). Extracorporeal circulation as a new experimental pathway for myoblast implantation in *mdx* mice. *Cell Transplant.* **8**, 247–258.

Tsukamoto, H., Wells, D., Brown, S. et al. (1999). Enhanced expression of recombinant dystrophin following intramuscular injection of Epstein–Barr virus (EBV)-based mini-chromosome vectors in *mdx* mice. *Gene Ther.* **6**, 1331–1335.

Tuffery, S., Chambert, S., Bareil, C. et al. (1998). Mutation analysis of the dystrophin gene in Southern French DMD or BMD families: from Southern blot to protein truncation test. *Hum. Genet.* **102**, 334–342.

Ueda, H., Baba, T., Terada, N. et al. (1997). Dystrophin in rod spherules; submembranous dense regions facing bipolar cell processes. *Histochem. Cell Biol.* **108**, 243–248.

Vachon, P. H., Loechel, F., Xu, H. et al. (1996). *J. Cell Biol.* **134**, 1483–1497.

Vachon, P. H., Xu, H., Liu, L. et al. (1997). Integrins (alpha7beta1) in muscle function and survival. Disrupted expression in merosin-deficient congenital muscular dystrophy. *J. Clin. Invest.* **100**, 1870–1881.

Vaillend, C., Ungerer, A. and Billard, J. M. (1999). Facilitated NMDA receptor-mediated synaptic plasticity in the hippocampal CA1 area of dystrophin-deficient mice. *Synapse* **33**, 59–70.

Verellen-Dumoulin, D., Freund, M., de Meyer, R. et al. (1984). Expression of an X-linked muscular dystrophy in a female due to translocation involving Xp21 and non-random X-inactivation. *Hum. Genet.* **67**, 115–119.

Vohra, M. S., Komiyama, M., Hayakawa, K. et al. (1998). Subcellular localization of dystrophin and vinculin in cardiac muscle fibers and fibers of the conduction system of the chicken ventricle. *Cell Tiss. Res.* **294**, 137–143.

Wakayama, Y., Bonilla, E. and Schotland, D. L. (1983). Muscle plasma membrane abnormalities in infants with Duchenne muscular dystrophy. *Neurology* **33**, 1368–1370.

Walton, J. N. and Nattrass, F. J. (1954). On the classification, natural history and treatment of the myopathies. *Brain* **3**, 219–261.

Wang, B., Li, J. and Xiao, X. (2000). Adeno-associated virus vector carrying human minidystrophin genes effectively ameliorates muscular dystrophy in the *mdx* mouse model. *Proc. Natl. Acad. Sci. USA* **97**, 13714–13719.

Watkins, S. C., Hoffman, E. P., Slayter, H. S. and Kunkel, L. M. (1988). Immunoelectron microscopic localization of dystrophin in myofibres. *Nature* **333**, 863–866.

Watkins, S. C., Hoffman, E. P., Slayter, H. S. et al. (1989). Dystrophin distribution in heterozygote MDX mice. *Muscle Nerve* **12**, 861–868.

Williams, M. W. and Bloch, R. J. (1999). Extensive but coordinated reorganization of the membrane skeleton in myofibers of dystrophic (*mdx*) mice. *J. Cell Biol.* **144**, 1259–1270.

Williamson, R. A., Henry, M. D., Daniels, K. J. et al. (1997). Dystroglycan is essential for early embryonic development: disruption of Reichert's membrane in Dag1-null mice. *Hum. Mol. Genet.* **6**, 831–841.

Wilton, S. D., Dye, D. E., Blechynden, L. M. et al. (1997). Revertant fibres: a possible genetic therapy for Duchenne muscular dystrophy? *Neuromusc. Disord.* **7**, 329–335.

Wilton, S. D., Lloyd, F., Carville, K. et al. (1999). Specific removal of the nonsense mutation from the *mdx* dystrophin mRNA using antisense oligonucleotides. *Neuromusc. Disord.* **9**, 330–338.

Winand, N. J., Edwards, M., Pradhan, D. et al. (1994). Deletion of the dystrophin muscle promoter in feline muscular dystrophy. *Neuromusc. Disord.* **4**, 433–445.

Winder, S. J., Gibson, T. J. and Kendrick-Jones, J. (1995). Dystrophin and utrophin: the missing links! *FEBS Lett.* **369**, 27–33.

Wineinger, M. A., Abresch, R. T., Walsh, S. A. et al. (1998). Effects of aging and voluntary exercise on the function of dystrophic muscle from *mdx* mice. *Am. J. Phys. Med.Rehab.* **77**, 20–27.

Winnard, A. V., Mendell, J. R., Prior, T. W., Florence, T. and Burghes A. H. (1995). Frameshift deletions of exons 3–7 and revertant fibres in Duchenne muscular dystrophy: mechanisms of dystrophin production. *Am. J. Hum. Genet.* **56**, 158–166.

Worton, R. G., Duff, C., Sylvester, J. E., Schmickel, R. D. and Willard, H. F. (1984). Duchenne muscular dystrophy involving translocation of the dmd gene next to ribosomal RNA genes. *Science* **224**, 1447–1449.

Xiao, X., Li, J. and Samulski, R. J. (1996). Efficient long-term gene transfer into muscle tissue of immunocompetent mice by adeno-associated virus vector. *J. Virol.* **70**, 8098–8108.

Xiao, X., Li, J. and Samulski, R. J. (1998). Production of high-titer recombinant adeno-associated virus vectors in the absence of helper adenovirus. *J. Virol.* **72**, 2224–2232.

Xiao, X., Li, J., Tsao, Y. P., Dressman, D., Hoffman, E. P. and Watchko, J. F. (2000). Full functional rescue of a complete muscle (TA) in dystrophic hamsters by AAV vector directed gene therapy. *J. Virol.* **74**, 1436–1442.

Yang, L., Lochmuller, H., Luo, J. et al. (1998). Adenovirus-mediated dystrophin minigene transfer improves muscle strength in adult dystrophic (*mdx*) mice. *Gene Ther.* **5**, 369–379.

Yuasa, K., Miyagoe, Y., Yamamoto, K., Nabeshima, Y., Dickson, G. and Takeda, S. (1998). Effective restoration of dystrophin-associated proteins in vivo by adenovirus-mediated transfer of truncated dystrophin cDNAs. *FEBS Lett.* **425**, 329–336.

Zatz, M., Vianna-Morgante, A. M., Campos, P. et al. (1981). Translocation (X;6) in a female with Duchenne muscular dystrophy, implications for the localisation of the DMD locus. *J. Med. Genet.* **18**, 442–447.

Zatz, M., Sumita, D., Campiotto, S. et al. (1998). Paternal inheritance or different mutations in maternally related patients occur in about 3% of Duchenne familial cases. *Am. J. Med. Genet.* **78**, 361–365.

20

Limb girdle muscular dystrophies

Jean-Claude Kaplan, Jacques S. Beckmann
and Michel Fardeau

Introduction

The limb girdle muscular dystrophies (LGMDs) are a clinically and genetically heterogeneous group of muscle dystrophies with either autosomal dominant or autosomal recessive mode of inheritance. The two common minimal denominators in this group of diseases are: (i) clinical manifestations characterized by weakness and wasting predominating in muscles of the pelvic and shoulder girdle, with occasional involvement of myocardium; and (ii) a histopathological pattern of necrosis/regeneration of muscle fibres. Time of onset and progression course are variable, both within groups and within families, with a broad spectrum of severity ranging from Duchenne-like to late-onset minor disability or only muscle fatigue. This heterogeneity for a long time confused the issue, and even the concept of LGMD was challenged.

To date, eight distinct loci for recessively inherited diseases (type 2) have been individualized (LGMD2A–H), with six genes already identified. These code for (i) five structural sarcolemmal proteins, comprising the four members of the sarcoglycan (SG) dystrophin-associated subcomplex (α-, β-, γ- and δ-SG) and dysferlin, (ii) and one nucleo-cytoplasmic proteolytic enzyme (calpain 3). While this chapter was in press, the gene for LGMD2G was identified. It codes for telethonin, a sarcomeric protein (Moreira et al., 2000). Five distinct loci leading to an autosomal dominant disease (type 1) have also been individualized (LGMD1A–E), with the *LGMD1C* locus known to code for the sarcolemmal caveolin 3 protein and the *LGMD1B* locus for the nuclear protein lamin A/C.

A number of salient features can be emphasized. A variable degree of allelic heterogeneity is exhibited by each of the genes identified. Many mutations cause a deficit of the protein (primary defect). Furthermore, a primary defect in one protein may lead to a secondary deficit in other proteins, pointing to shared pathophysiological pathways and raising some diagnostic difficulties.

Strict genotype-to-phenotype, and allele/phenotype correlations are not yet delineated. This precludes for the moment any integrated clinicogenetic nosology, and poses difficult diagnostic problems. The clinical diagnosis must be achieved by molecular analysis, mainly guided by (i) a normal or subnormal level of dystrophin, (ii) a decrease in any of the LGMD proteins known to date, (iii) and/or when possible genetic analysis of informative families.

Knowledge of the pathophysiology of the LGMDs is still in its infancy. At least six identified gene defects involve membrane proteins, pointing to sarcolemmal 'structuropathy'. In this category, the four sarcoglycanopathies are presumed to disrupt the mechanical dystrophin-mediated link between the cytoskeleton apparatus and the extracellular matrix. Calpain 3 stands apart since it is a proteolytic enzyme and its pathophysiology is not known. Animal models for these deficits are currently being constructed and analysed.

The general epidemiology of the LGMDs and the relative contribution of each locus in outbred populations are not firmly established as yet. Particular alleles, in the genes for γ-SG, calpain 3 and dysferlin, prevail in specific populations as a result of founder effects. In addition, it seems that in European populations the two most frequent loci involved give rise to LGMD2A (calpain 3 deficiency) and LGMD2D (α-SG deficiency).

The pending problems are (i) the identification of the remaining unsolved LGMD genes; (ii) the improvement in molecular diagnostics; (iii) the understanding of the pathophysiology and muscle selectivity of dystrophy; (iv) the discovery of possible modifier genes responsible for intrafamilial phenotypic heterogeneity; and (v) treatment (gene-based) and management development.

History

The term of limb girdle muscular dystrophy appeared in the early 1950s (Levison, 1951; Stevenson, 1953), and gained a worldwide acceptance after the classification by Walton and Nattrass of muscle diseases taking into consideration their mode of inheritance (Walton and Nattrass, 1954). Cardinal features of this type of muscular dystrophy are: (i) onset in the first decades; (ii) symptoms of muscular weakness in shoulder and/or pelvic girdle; (iii) relatively slow course, leading nevertheless to severe disablement and often premature death; and (iv) autosomal recessive mode of inheritance. In this classification, LGMD was clearly separated from the sex-linked Duchenne muscular dystrophy (DMD) and from the autosomal dominant facioscapulohumeral (FSH) dystrophy. Walton and Nattrass considered that most of the cases of LGMD would have been identified previously as the 'juvenile' form of progressive muscular dystrophy described 70 years earlier by Erb (1884).

In fact, the predominance of weakness and atrophy in limb girdle muscles in a number of hereditary and acquired muscular disorders led to frequent misdiagnosis, as revealed by muscle biopsies, and the concept of LGMD was soon challenged and severely criticized. The relevance of this term to designate an autonomous entity was even denied (Brooke, 1977). In the previous edition of this book (6th edition, 1994), D. Gardner-Medwin and J. Walton themselves wrote: 'in abandoning this term [limb girdle muscular dystrophy] as a definitive diagnosis and in attempting to list and describe the several entities which it disguises, we recognize that research in this long neglected group of muscular dystrophies is still in an early and transitional stage, that some of the entities we list are tentative and that before the next edition of this book this situation will have changed.'

Genetics of limb girdle dystrophies

The discovery of dystrophin as the defective protein in Duchenne and Becker dystrophy (BMD) opened the way to the elucidation of the other dystrophies. It showed the power of the 'reverse genetics' strategy (today's positional cloning) and provided a lead to uncover likely candidates among the proteins directly or indirectly associated with dystrophin (the dystrophin connection).

Another decisive element in this progress was the identification of a number of genetic niches with high preponderance of patients presenting an autosomal recessively inherited dystrophy that fitted well with the criteria defined by Walton and Nattrass (1954). Such patients were reported in inbred communities such as the Amish (Jackson and Carey, 1961; Jackson and Strehler, 1968) and Mennonite communities (Shokeir and Kobrinsky, 1976; Shokeir and Rozdilsky, 1985), in Tunisian families (Ben Hamida and Fardeau, 1980; Ben Hamida et al., 1983), in a group of Reunion Island families and in other large consanguineous pedigrees (Azibi et al., 1991; Passos-Bueno et al., 1991).

From the early 1990s, linkage analysis was applied to dissect the genetic basis of the progressive muscular dystrophies for which dystrophin deficiency had been excluded. The study of large families (both genetically and clinically homogeneous as well as genetically informative), sorted according to their dominant or recessive inheritance mode, resulted in the delineation of an increasing number of distinct loci. Genetic heterogeneity was so far greater than expected on purely clinical grounds. The underlying morbid genes were ultimately uncovered for a number of these traits by conventional positional cloning or by following candidate gene or protein strategies.

In 1995, a new nomenclature of genetic loci was proposed (Bushby and Beckmann, 1995). It distinguished two categories: the *LGMD1* and *LGMD2* loci referring, respectively, to autosomal dominant and recessively inherited diseases, full penetrance being generally assumed. In each category, the suffix numbering with letters (A, B, C, etc.) follows the chronological order of their discovery.

It is now clear that the LGMD acronym lumps together a number of distinct diseases that differ not only genetically but also to a large extent clinically (Ozawa et al., 1998). Even the common clinical denominator – predominance of the muscle wasting in pelvic and shoulder girdle muscles – has been transgressed. Nevertheless, the LGMD acronym has proven useful in the process of cataloguing the multiple loci involved, and it is now applied as a genetic label to an increasing number of distinct morbid loci for autosomally inherited progressive dystrophies (Beckmann et al., 1999).

This chapter deals with the progressive dystrophic muscle diseases that have been assigned to distinct genetic loci. To date, this group comprises eight recessive loci, *LGMD2A* to *LGMD2H* (Table 20.1), and five dominant loci, *LGMD1A* to *LGMD1E* (Table 20.2). These result in changes in a number of muscle proteins (Table 20.3).

Autosomal recessive proximal muscular dystrophies

Limb girdle dystrophy type 2A: calpain 3 deficiency

The discovery of a group of patients in the southern part of the Reunion Island whose age of disease onset, pattern of

Table 20.1. Genetic classification of the recessive limb girdle dystrophies

Locus[a] (MIM number)	Disease[b]	Chromosome	Gene product (symbol)	Remark	Key references
LGMD2A (253600)	LGMD	15q15.1-q21.1	Calpain 3 (CAPN3)		Beckmann et al. (1991)[c]; Richard et al. (1995)[d]
LGMD2B (253601)	Autosomal recessive LGMD	2p13	Dysferlin (DYSF)	Allelic to Miyoshi distal myopathy (254130)	Bashir et al. (1994)[c]; Bashir et al. (1998)[d]; Liu et al. (1998)[d]
LGMD2C (253700)	Autosomal recessive Duchenne-like MD	13q12	Gamma-sarcoglycan (SGCC)		Ben Othmane et al. (1992)[c]; Noguchi et al. (1995)[d]
LGMD2D (600119)	Autosomal recessive MD	17q21	Alpha-sarcoglycan (SGCA)		Roberds et al. (1994)[c,d]
LGMD2E (600900)	Autosomal recessive MD/LGMD	4q12	Beta-sarcoglycan (SGCB)		Bönnemann et al. (1995)[d]; Lim et al. (1995)[d]
LGMD2F (601287)	Autosomal recessive MD	5q33-q34	Delta-sarcoglycan (SGCD)		Passos-Bueno et al. (1996b)[c]; Nigro et al. (1996a,b)[d]
LGMD2G (601954)	Autosomal recessive LGMD	17q11-q12	Telethonin		Moreira et al. (1997[c], 2000[d])
LGMD2H (254110)	Autosomal recessive LGMD	9q31-q34.1	?	Only in a Hutterite isolate	Weiler et al. (1998)[c]

Notes:

LGMD, limb girdle muscular dystrophy; MD, muscular dystrophy.

[a] ENMC nomenclature (Beckmann et al., 1999); MIM number (McKusick, 1998).

[b] Disease named as in key reference.

[c] Key reference giving first linkage.

[d] Key reference giving gene identification.

muscular involvement and rate of disease evolution fitted well with the original description of the juvenile form of LGMD (Erb, 1884) prompted the genetic study of these families (Fardeau et al., 1989). This led eventually to the localization of the first *LGMD* locus, *LGMD2A*, on the long arm of chromosome 15 (Beckmann et al., 1991). As there were neither noticeable chromosomal rearrangements nor known candidate genes, the morbid locus was identified upon the discovery (following a positional cloning strategy) of mutations in the gene coding for a calcium-activated neutral protease, calpain 3 (*CAPN3*) (Richard et al., 1995). Interestingly, this protein was already known and its cDNA cloned since 1989 (Sorimachi et al., 1989), but it had, however, never been considered a priori as a candidate gene.

The gene, the protein and its function

Calpain 3, also called p94, is a 94 kDa nonlysosomal cysteine protease presumed to be specific for skeletal muscles (reviewed in Richard et al., 1999a). Calpain 3 belongs to a family of calcium-dependent neutral proteases the biological functions of which remain unknown. It is the first and so far only member of this family for which a firm association with a disease has been established. Like the other large calpain subunits, it comprises four protein domains, two of which have a known function: the active cysteine protease site (domain II) and the calcium-binding sites (domain IV). It also bears a nuclear translocation signal and a putative anchoring site for binding to titin, an elastic protein associated with thick filaments, which extends over half a sarcomere. During embryonic development, calpain 3 transcription occurs initially in nonskeletal muscle tissues, particularly in the heart (Fougerousse et al., 1998, 1999).

Gene pathology

So far, 118 variants have been detected after screening of *CAPN3* in a total of 188 LGMD2A families from 23 different ethnic or geographic origins (Chou et al., 1999; Richard et al., 1999b). A database of mutations in *CAPN3* and the other LGMD genes is maintained at the Leiden University Medical Centre (Leiden Muscular Dystrophy pages© accessible on the internet: http://www.dmd.nl/). These variants include 101 pathogenic mutations, 12 polymorphisms and five additional unclassified variants.

Table 20.2. Genetic classification of the dominant limb girdle dystrophies

Locus[a] (MIM number)	Disease[b]	Chromosome	Gene product (symbol)	Remark	Key references
LGMD1A (159000)	Autosomal dominant LGMD	5q31	Myotilin		Speer et al. (1992)[c]; Hauser et al. (1999, 2000)[d]
LGMD1B (159001)	Autosomal dominant LGMD with cardiac involvement	1q11-21	Lamin A/C	Allelic to Emery–Dreifuss autosomal dominant: lamin A/C (181350)	van der Kooi et al. (1997)[c]; Bonne et al. (1999); Muchir et al. (2000)
LGMD1C (601253)	Autosomal dominant LGMD	3p25	Caveolin 3 (CAV3)		Minetti et al. (1998)[d]
LGMD1D (602067)	Familial dilated cardiomyopathy with conduction defect and MD (FDC-CDM)	6q23	?		Messina et al. (1997)[c]
LGMD1E (603511)	Autosomal dominant LGMD	7q	?		Speer et al. (1999)[c]
VPDMD (158580)	Vocal cord and pharyngeal weakness with autosomal dominant distal myopathy (VCPDM)	5q31	?	Possibly allelic to LGMD1A	Feit et al. (1998)[c]

Notes:

LGMD, limb girdle muscular dystrophy; MD, muscular dystrophy; VPDMD, velopharyngeal distal muscular dystrophy.

[a] MIM number (McKusick, 1998); ENMC nomenclature (Beckmann et al., 1999).

[b] Disease named as in key reference.

[c] Key reference giving first linkage.

[d] Key reference giving gene identification.

About half of the pathological alleles are null mutations (no protein is expected to be produced from the corresponding alleles) the rest are missense mutations from which an aberrant protein is presumed to be produced. Most mutations represent private variants (71/101), though certain particular mutations were found more frequently (Richard et al., 1999b). Among the latter, 11 mutations are associated with a founder effect: the most notable being seen in the Reunion island (Beckmann et al., 1991), the Amish (Richard et al., 1995) and the Basque (Urtasun et al., 1998) isolates. Mutations are evenly distributed over all 24 exons of *CAPN3*, which spans over 45 kb of genomic DNA, apart from an excess of missense mutations in a cluster of 11 amino acid residues encoded by exon 11 (Richard et al., 1999b).

Clinical pattern

The first symptoms are running and walking difficulties, most often noticed around 10–15 years (range from 2 to over 40 years of age). The pattern of muscular involvement is characterized by a usually very selective, symmetrical weakness and atrophy of limb girdle and trunk muscles. In the early stages of the disease, the weakness predominates in the pelvic girdle, mainly affecting gluteus maximus, thigh adductors and, to a lesser degree, gluteus medius, psoas and posterior thigh muscles. The contrast between the involvement of these muscles and the integrity of quadriceps muscle, in this early stage, is well evidenced on computed tomographic (CT) scans (Fig. 20.1). At the scapular girdle, the deficit predominates on latissimus dorsi, serratus magnus, rhomboid, pectoralis major and, to a lesser degree, on biceps and brachioradialis muscles. Abdominal and spinal muscles are among the first affected muscles. A waddling gait is observed with a slight hyperlordosis; contracture of the Achilles tendon is frequent at this early stage of the disease. Serum creatine kinase is markedly increased in the early phases of the disease; it then decreases to normal values in the late stages.

At a more advanced stage, when the patient is unable to climb up stairs or to rise up from a chair, the weakness extends to quadriceps, tibialis anterior and calf muscles. In the upper limbs, deltoid, triceps, radialis muscles are affected. Contractures may involve not only calf muscles but also hip and knee flexors.

Table 20.3. The molecular basis of the limb girdle muscular dystrophies

Type	Gene Name	Gene Size (kb)	Exons	Protein Name	Size (kDa)	No. residues	Cellular localization	Tissue distribution	Mutations	Inheritance
Calpainopathy										
LGMD2A	CAPN3	>40	24	Calpain-3	94	821	Cytosol + nucleus? (*proteolytic enzyme*)	Skeletal muscle	>100 mutations, mainly sporadic point mutations (null and missense) Founder effect in Reunion, Amish and Basque populations	AR
Sarcoglycanopathies										
LGMD2D	SGCA	10	10	Alpha-sarcoglycan (previously adhalin)	50	387	Sarcolemma (*DGC*)	Skeletal and cardiac muscle	>30: sporadic mutations, mainly point mutations (null and missense) Exon 3 (65%) R77C (42%)	AR
LGMD2E	SGCB	13.5	6	Beta-sarcoglycan	43	318	Sarcolemma (*DGC*)	Ubiquitous	Sporadic mutations	AR
LGMD2C	SGCG	>100	8	Gamma-sarcoglycan	35	291	Sarcolemma (*DGC*)	Skeletal and cardiac muscle	2 founder mutations: del521T (Mediterranean) and C283Y (Gypsies) Various other sporadic rare alleles	AR
LGMD2F	SGCD	100	8	Delta-sarcoglycan	35	290	Sarcolemma (*DGC*)	Ubiquitous	Few sporadic mutations	AR
Dysferlinopathy										
LGMD2B	DYSF	>150	55	Dysferlin	230	2080	Sarcolemma	Ubiquitous	Sporadic mutations Founder effect in Libyan Jews	AR
Caveolinopathy										
LGMD1C	CAV3	~1.5	2	Caveolin 3 (monomer)	22	151	Sarcolemma (*caveolae*)	Skeletal and cardiac muscle		AD (AR?)

Notes:

SG, sarcoglycan; DGC, dystrophin-associated glycoprotein complex; AR, autosomal recessive; AD, autosomal dominant.

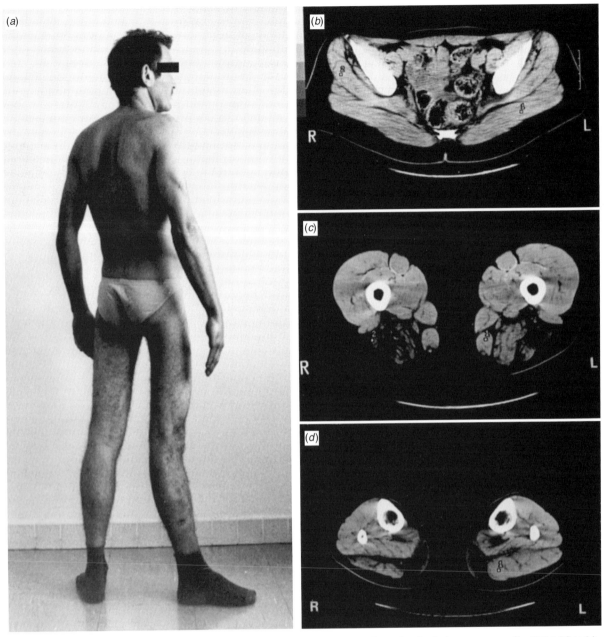

Fig. 20.1. A 27-year-old patient with limb girdle dystrophy type 2A (calpainopathy). The patient had a homozygous splice 946-1 AG to AA mutation in *CAPN*3. (*a*) Notice the moderate bilateral scapular winging and important atrophy of thigh posterior muscles. Computed tomographic scans from the same patient show (*b*) the pelvic girdle with relative preservation of glutei muscles; (*c*) important loss of posterior thigh muscles contrasting with relative preservation of anterior muscles; and (*d*) moderate loss of calf muscles.

The disease is usually progressive, with a great variability in the rate of deterioration (Fardeau et al., 1996a). Most patients become wheelchair bound between 20 and 30 years. The mean time elapsed before loss of ambulation is 17.3 years (range from 5 to over 39 years) (Richard et al., 1999b). Altogether, the disease is never as severe as DMD and, in some cases, it may be very mild (Fardeau et al., 1996a; Topaloglu et al., 1997). When the patient is no longer able to walk without help, the deficit extends to distal muscles, affecting peroneal and posterior tibial muscles, forearm long extensors and palmaris muscles. When the patient is wheelchair bound, contractures increase around elbow, hip, knee and ankle joints. Weakness of neck muscles is only noticed at very late stages. As a rule, there is no involvement of facial muscles, except in severe forms with very early onset. The disease process is purely atrophic. Tendon reflexes are weak, often absent. Heart function is clinically normal. There is no intellectual impairment.

This pattern, initially analysed in detail in Reunion Island patients (Fardeau et al., 1996b), was also found among the Amish population of northern Indiana (C. Jackson and M. Fardeau, unpublished observations), Basque (Urtasun et al., 1998) and Turkish (Dinçer et al., 1997; Topaloglu et al., 1997) calpain 3-deficient patients. Slight variations in the involvement of distal muscle or in the extent of the contractures were observed in French metropolitan families (Fardeau et al., 1996b). Calf hypertrophy was noticed in several occasions in Brazilian families (Passos-Bueno et al., 1999).

Muscle biopsy
Histopathology
Muscle biopsy from patients with calpain 3 deficiency show nonspecific dystrophic features: variation in size of the muscle fibres without group atrophy, increased number of internal nuclei and presence of some necrotic and regenerating fibres. This necrotic–regenerative pattern is not seen in a muscle that is not yet weak or atrophic and is mainly apparent during the evolutive stages of the disease (Fardeau et al., 1996a). These changes are accompanied by a progressive type I fibre predominance and a moderate increase of the endomysial collagen. In the late stages of the process, an abnormal lobulation of the muscle fibres is most often seen in the biopsies, which can be assessed by electron microscopy.

Immunocytochemical studies show normal sarcolemmal labelling with antibodies to dystrophin, utrophin and the different SGs. Preliminary results with polyclonal antibodies to calpain 3 showed that the normal myofibrillar and myonuclear staining is abolished in LGMD biopsies (Baghdiguian et al., 1999).

Immunoblotting
The recently developed monoclonal antibodies (Anderson et al., 1998) visualize calpain 3 on immunoblots from control extracts as a major band of 94 kDa and a smaller 30 kDa derived fragment (see Fig. 20.7, below). In specimens from patients with defined mutations, the intensity of the bands is usually decreased, but there is no simple relationship between the abundance and clinical severity. There are even exceptions in which no quantitative effect is observed on Western blots (Anderson et al., 1998). These

patients are likely candidates for being purely loss-of-function mutants.

Epidemiology
In addition to the initially described Reunion Island patients with LGMD2A, other genetic isolates carrying different CAPN3 mutations were described, such as the Amish (Richard et al., 1995), Basque (Urtasun et al., 1998) and Turkish populations (Dinçer et al., 1997) in which either a predominant allele or a limited number of prevalent alleles were found.

In outbred populations, published figures on prevalence amongst muscular dystrophies vary substantially: 10% in Italy and the USA (Chou et al., 1999), 17% in Brazil (Passos-Bueno et al., 1996a) and close to 40% in a European multicentric study (Richard et al., 1997). These differences reflect the respective genetic histories of these populations and differences in ascertainment conditions. Altogether, these data nevertheless suggest that calpain 3 deficiencies may account for a substantial fraction of the autosomal recessive LGMDs.

Genotype–phenotype correlation
Clinical information based on 163 patients confirmed that the typical relationship described for the Reunion Island patients is found for most calpain 3-deficient patients (Richard et al., 1999b). The study of this large a cohort confirmed the marked heterogeneity in severity but failed to reveal any influence of the patient's gender on age of onset or disease evolution. No obvious correlations between the mutations and the clinical manifestations of LGMD2A could be established, between or even within the families, although as a generality, null mutations result in more severe clinical consequences than missense mutations (Richard et al., 1999b). Some intrafamilial variability was reported (Penisson-Besnier et al., 1998).

Pathophysiology
Little is known about the physiological role of the calpains in general, and there is no current solid hypothesis to explain how defects of calpain 3, a muscle-specific protease, may result in progressive muscular dystrophy.

The incrimination of a protease contrasts with the observations on the pivotal aetiologic role played in most myopathies by structural proteins – all directly or indirectly associated with dystrophin – and raises the issue of whether these pathogenic mechanisms are all part of one pathway or form part of distinct pathophysiological pathways (structuropathy versus enzymopathy) leading to similar phenotypes. The association with titin may provide a structural connection to calpain 3, linking it in this

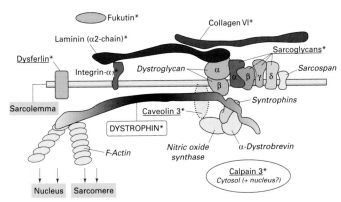

Fig. 20.2. The dystrophin–glycoprotein complex comprises the following known proteins: (i) dystrophin + syntrophin + α-dystrobrevin + nitric oxide synthase; (ii) the dystroglycan complex; (iii) the sarcoglycan complex + sarcospan. Proteins known to be involved in muscle diseases are indicated by *; those proteins involved in limb girdle dystrophies are underlined.

manner to the known genes involved in muscular dystrophy. It was recently suggested that apoptosis may be an early and specific event in the pathogenesis of calpainopathies and that calpain 3 may play a role in the regulation of survival genes (Baghdiguian et al., 1999).

Knock-out mice are currently being investigated. Preliminary observation shows that these fully fertile animals do not manifest gross behavioural or motor anomalies. Histopathological observation reveals the presence in ageing animals of necrosis and centrally located myonuclei (Richard et al., 2000).

Molecular diagnosis

The relatively large size of *CAPN3*, the wide spectrum of *CAPN3* mutations and the fact that most mutations seem to be private and evenly distributed over most exons, all create significant practical problems for diagnosis of calpainopathies (Richard et al., 1999b). Because of all these characteristics, no single mutation detection method appears ideal and the challenge remains. The assessment of calpain 3 in muscle biopsies by Western blot and immunohistochemistry may become an important additional diagnostic tool for calpainopathies (Spencer et al., 1997; Anderson et al., 1998). Ultimately, however, these protein assessments need to be validated by mutation screening.

Muscular dystrophies with sarcoglycan deficiency: sarcoglycanopathies

Sarcoglycanopathy is a collective name for a genetically and phenotypically heterogeneous group of autosomal

recessive muscular dystrophies caused by mutations in any of the four genes encoding the members of the SG complex (Noguchi et al., 1995), namely α-, β-, γ- or δ-SG, linked, respectively, to four morbid loci: *LGMD2D* (chromosome 17), *LGMD2E* (chromosome 4), *LGMD2C* (chromosome 13) and *LGMD2F* (chromosome 5) (Tables 20.1 and 20.3).

Biochemical grounds: the dystrophin connection

Following the milestone discovery of dystrophin and of its role in DMD (see Chapters 4 and 19), biochemical methods were applied to decipher how this protein is attached to the muscle membrane or sarcolemma and what proteins it interacts with (reviewed in Matsumura and Campbell, 1994; Ozawa et al., 1995; Straub and Campbell, 1997). This led eventually to the discovery of a complex network of proteins interacting either directly or indirectly with dystrophin, representing literally a dystrophin connection, with both a physical and a heuristic connotation, linking the extracellular matrix to the cytoplasm (Fig. 20.2).

The core of this network is the dystrophin–glycoprotein complex (DGC), a biochemical supramolecular entity that is resistant to dissociating treatments and is obtained by affinity chromatography fractionation of the glycosylated muscle membrane proteins (Ervasti and Campbell, 1991; Yoshida et al., 1994). The DGC comprises at least 10 sarcolemmal proteins (Fig. 20.2) and can be subdivided into three subcomplexes. The first is a group of intracellular subsarcolemmal proteins comprising *dystrophin*, *syntrophins* (interacting with nitric oxide synthase) and *dystrobrevin*. The second is the *dystroglycan* complex, composed of two closely linked subunits translated from a single mRNA and subsequently processed into two distinct polypeptides. Alpha-dystroglycan is a 156 kDa extracellular protein serving as a receptor for laminin-2, a protein belonging to the extracellular matrix system that is also involved in congenital dystrophies (Chapter 25). Beta-dystroglycan is a 43 kDa transmembrane protein; its proline-rich intracellular tail binds the C-terminal domain of dystrophin. The third subcomplex is sarcolemmal *sarcoglycan*, a detergent-resistant structure composed of four transmembrane monomeric glycoproteins: α-, β-, γ- and δ-SG, with respective masses of 50, 43, 35 and 35 kDa (reviewed in Lim and Campbell, 1998). Each SG is encoded by a different gene (Tables 20.1 and 20.3) that is expressed exclusively (α and γ), or predominantly (β and δ) in skeletal and cardiac muscles. These four SG proteins share common structural features, each having a short intracytoplasmic stretch, a single transmembrane domain and a long extracellular domain. In addition, the SG complex is tightly attached to *sarcospan*, a distinct 25 kDa protein possessing four transmembrane domains. Sarcospan, which is thought to be essential for the stabilization and membrane targeting of the complex, was found to be missing in *mdx* mice (Crosbie et al., 1999). Prior to its incorporation into the sarcolemma, the SG complex is assembled in the intracellular compartment (Holt and Campbell, 1998). The precise assembly mode of the SG complex and its likely interactions with dystroglycan are still unknown. It should be noted that in the smooth muscle α-SG is replaced by ε-SG (Straub et al., 1999), a highly homologous protein coded by a fifth gene mapping on chromosome 7q21 (Ettinger et al., 1997; McNally et al., 1998a); ε-SG is so far not known to be involved in a pathology.

In muscle cells, the DGC appears to provide a structural link between the F-actin cytoskeleton and the extracellular matrix via, respectively, dystrophin and β-dystroglycan (Fig. 20.2). In vivo, this link is believed to be critical for muscle membrane stability during contraction and relaxation. The DGC also interacts with proteins involved in signal transduction (reviewed in Grady et al., 1999). Of all of the above mentioned proteins, dystrophin (Chapter 19), the four members of the SG subcomplex and the α2-chain of laminin-2 (merosin; Chapter 25) are known to be involved in muscle disease. However, only the dystrophinopathies and sarcogylcanopathies result in a disruption of the DGC with loss or decrease of some of its constituents (Ervasti et al., 1990; Matsumura et al., 1992; Lim and Campbell, 1998).

Dystroglycans are required for the attachment of the extracellular matrix to the basal membrane (Henry and Campbell, 1998); inactivation of the corresponding gene is lethal in mice (Williamson et al., 1997). These data are consistent with the lack of reported pathology for this gene in humans.

Discovery of the four sarcoglycanopathies

The discovery of the four sarcoglycanopathies has been reviewed by Ozawa et al. (1998) and Lim and Campbell (1998).

In the early 1980s, interest focused on families with patients exhibiting a progressive muscular dystrophy resembling closely the DMD phenotype but with autosomal recessive inheritance, as described in Tunisia (Ben Hamida and Fardeau, 1980; Ben Hamida et al., 1983) and in Sudan (Salih et al., 1983). This was often referred to under the acronym of SCARMD (severe childhood-onset autosomal recessive muscular dystrophy). In spite of the DMD-like phenotype, the muscles of patients with SCARMD exhibited normal dystrophin levels (Ben Jelloun-Dellagi et al., 1990) but, as observed in DMD, the other proteins of the DGC were defective, with a predominant decrease of the

50 kDa component (Matsumura et al., 1992). This 50 kDa protein was invariably absent in muscle from patients of North-African origin with SCARMD, hence the name initially given to this protein, adhalin after the Arabic word for muscle (Roberds et al., 1993). The defect was also soon found in patients with SCARMD of European origin (Fardeau et al., 1993). When it was demonstrated that adhalin was one of the four components of the SG subcomplex, it was renamed α-SG.

Genetic analysis in Tunisian families showed linkage of the morbid locus to chromosome 13q (Ben Othmane et al., 1992). However this locus (*LGMD2C*) was excluded in Brazilian and French families, demonstrating the genetic heterogeneity of SCARMD (Passos-Bueno et al., 1993; Romero et al., 1994). The gene encoding the 50 kDa component (α-SG) was cloned, mapped to chromosome 17q (McNally et al., 1994; Roberds et al., 1994), and found to be mutated in one of the families, in which the morbid locus was linked to markers of chromosome 17q21 (Roberds et al., 1994). Hence, α-SG deficiency could have different genetic origins, being either primary when the pathogenic mutation affects the chromosome 17q *LGMD2D* locus or secondary, as in patients with the chromosome 13q-linked SCARMD.

With the incrimination of α-SG, the genes of the three other members of the SG subcomplex became strong candidates for the non-17q-linked LGMDs, particularly for those for which a deficit in the SG proteins could be demonstrated. Indeed the subsequent cloning and mapping of the genes for γ-, β-, and δ-SG provided the molecular basis for *LGMD2C* (γ-SG) on chromosome 13 (Noguchi et al., 1995), *LGMD2E* (β-SG) on chromosome 4 (Bönnemann et al., 1995; Lim et al., 1995) and LGMD2F (δ-SG) on chromosome 5 (Table 20.1) (Nigro et al., 1996a and b). The genes for α- to δ-SG were assigned genetic symbols *SGCA* to *SGCD*, respectively. The main molecular characteristics of the genes and their products are summarized in Table 20.3.

Alpha-sarcoglycanopathy (limb girdle dystrophy type 2D)

Gene pathology

Deficiency of α-SG was the first sarcoglycanopathy to be identified (Roberds et al., 1994; Piccolo et al., 1995). Because it is distributed worldwide and is probably the most frequent sarcoglycanopathy, it remains currently the best documented entity, with about 40 mutations already described (Kawai et al., 1995; Ljunggren et al., 1995; Passos-Bueno et al., 1995; Carrié et al., 1997; Duggan et al., 1997a; Higuchi et al., 1997; Angelini et al., 1999; Vainzof et al., 1999). In a series of 64 unrelated patients with primary α-SG deficiency, we found nine null and 23 missense mutations

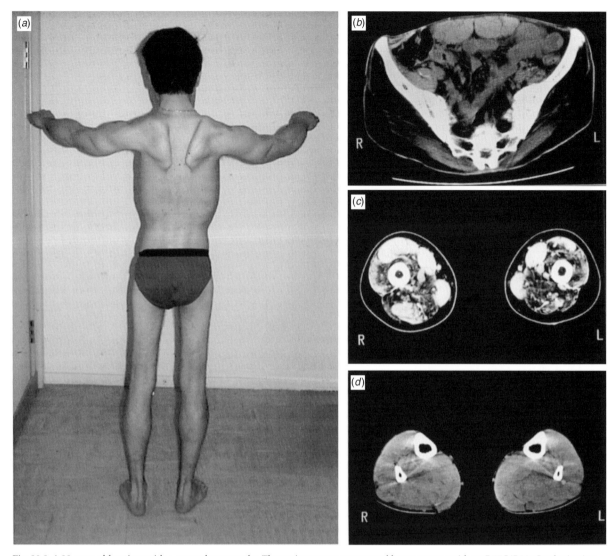

Fig. 20.3. A 28-year-old patient with α-sarcoglycanopathy. The patient was a compound heterozygote with an R77C/R284C substitution resulting from mutations in *SGCA*. (*a*) Notice the bilateral scapular winging and the calf hypertrophy. Computed tomographic scans of the same patient show (*b*) the pelvic girdle with major bilateral loss of glutei; (*c*) the thigh, with irregular loss of muscles in both anterior and posterior compartments; and (*d*) the relative preservation of calf muscle density.

(J.-C. Kaplan, unpublished data). The missense mutations map to the large extracellular domain of the protein, with a striking clustering in exon 3 (two-thirds of the missense mutations) and high predominance of the R77C substitution (42% of the mutated chromosomes). Because the latter is found in unrelated populations and on different haplotype backgrounds, this mutation is believed to result from recurrent mutational events rather than a founder effect (Carrié et al., 1997). As expected for a recessively inherited disease, the patients are either homozygous for a given mutation or compound heterozygotes for two different α-

SG alleles. As in the calpainopathies (Richard et al., 1997), heterozygous siblings, although clinically normal, may have a moderate but significant increase of serum creatine kinase levels (Romero et al., 1994).

Clinical pattern
Clinical onset is usually around 8–10 years of age, with a large range from 3 to 15 years (Fig. 20.3). First complaints are difficulties in running or climbing stairs, after normal early milestones.

The pattern of muscular involvement is roughly similar

in all patients (Carrié et al., 1997; Eymard et al., 1997). In the early stages of the disease, when the patient presents with a waddling gait and a slight hyperlordosis, the weakness predominates in pelvic girdle muscles and glutei and thigh adductors; the quadriceps is affected early, as are the hamstring muscles. Distal muscle involvement, when present, is minimal and affects the tibialis anterior. This proximal muscle involvement is mainly atrophic, but calf hypertrophy is almost consistently present, sometimes associated with a slight hypertrophy of the lower part of the quadriceps. At this early stage of the disease, weakness is also present in the scapular muscles, predominating in serratus magnus, latissimus dorsi, trapezius inferior, rhomboid, subscapularis and infraspinatus muscles. Scapular winging is usual. The deltoid muscle is often markedly involved early on in the disease, as are the biceps and brachioradialis. Other limb muscles are much less affected. Trunk extensors are more affected than abdominal muscles, while neck muscles are relatively spared.

At more advanced stages of the disease, the distribution remains identical but extends to distal muscles: peroneal and posterior tibial muscles in the lower limbs, triceps brachialis, pronator, supinator radii, radialis and palmaris muscles in the upper limbs. Contractures develop in these late stages of the disease, when the patient is wheelchair bound. Kyphoscoliosis may also be present.

There is no involvement of facial, ocular or velopharyngeal muscles; enlargement of the tongue is sometimes noticed. Cardiac function is, as a rule, normal, as are electrocardiographic and echocardiographic examinations. Respiratory function is normal or moderately reduced, even in the late stages of the disease. Intellectual impairment is never observed.

Serum creatine kinase levels are constantly elevated, very high in the early stages of the disease, then decreasing with age. Electromyography is compatible with a dystrophic process.

Muscle imaging may help to differentiate the pattern of muscle involvement from calpain 3-deficient LGMD, showing in the early stage of the disease similar involvement of deep anterior and posterior compartments of femoral muscles with preservation and often hypertrophy of sartorius and gracilis muscles (Fig. 20.3). This pattern is close to that observed in DMD/BMD, and many patients are initially misdiagnosed as having BMD.

The evolution of the disease is progressive, but it shows a marked heterogeneity between and within families. In severe disease, walking may be lost before 15 years of age. But there is also very mild disease with late onset beyond 15 years and slow progression without loss of ambulatory ability. Some patients may even remain asymptomatic or

present for decades with minimal muscle symptoms, such as pain and/or exercise intolerance, or isolated elevation of serum creatine kinase levels (Carrié et al., 1997; Eymard et al., 1997; Angelini et al., 1999; Passos-Bueno et al., 1999). As for calpainopathies, marked intrafamilial variability of severity is observed (Angelini et al., 1998).

Muscle biopsy
Muscle biopsies show nonspecific features of many dystrophic processes, variation in size of the muscle fibres, increased number of internal nuclei and slight endomysial fibrosis. Necrosis and regeneration are predominant in the early stages of the disease. A type I fibre predominance is common.

By immunocytochemistry, dystrophin is normal, and sarcolemmal labelling of α-SG is either completely absent or markedly reduced (Fig. 20.4). Staining of β-, γ- and δ-SG is decreased to a lesser degree (Fig. 20.4). Semiquantitative analysis by Western blots shows normal amounts of dystrophin and reduced α-SG, varying from total absence to substantial residual amounts. The other SGs are usually reduced to a lesser extent (Fig. 20.5).

Epidemiology
Alpha-sarcoglycanopathy has been found on all continents, with variable incidence (Carrié et al., 1997; Duggan et al., 1997a; Fanin et al., 1997; Hayashi and Arahata, 1997; Vainzof et al., 1999). No founder effect has been reported yet.

Genotype–phenotype correlation
The presence of a null mutation on both alleles usually results in a severe clinical course, resembling DMD, with total loss of the α-SG protein on Western blots (Piccolo et al., 1995). Missense mutations are of variable severity in age of onset and progression, ranging from Duchenne-like SCARMD to late-onset minor disability (Piccolo et al., 1995; Morandi et al., 1996; Carrié et al., 1997; Eymard et al., 1997; Angelini et al., 1999). A given substitution, such as the frequent R77C, may result in either a severe or a milder phenotype (Passos-Bueno et al., 1995; Carrié et al., 1997). The R284C substitution, another recurrent change, seems to result only in a mild or very mild form of disease (Carrié et al., 1997; Angelini et al., 1998). This variability is still unexplained. It has been postulated that it might correlate with the amount of residual α-SG expression (Vainzof et al., 1996; Carrié et al., 1997; Eymard et al., 1997; Angelini et al., 1999) and/or with the degree of secondary impairment of the other partners in the SG subcomplex. Exceptions to this rule have, however, also been reported (Higuchi et al., 1998). It should be emphasized that, to date, all reported

Dystrophin   γ-Sarcoglycan   α-Sarcoglycan

Normal

γ-Sarcoglycanopathy

α-Sarcoglycanopathy

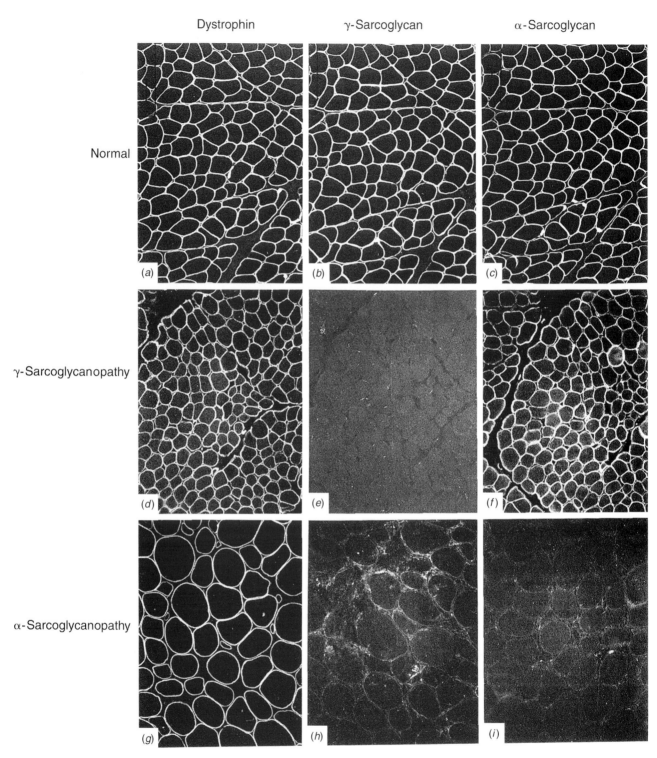

Fig. 20.4. Immunofluorescent analysis of muscle biopsies from patients with α- and γ-sarcoglycanopathy. Serial cryostat sections of muscle biopsies (X160) were stained with monoclonal anti-dystrophin N-terminal region (NCL-DYS3, Novocastra); monoclonal anti-α-sarcoglycan (NCL-a-SARC, Novocastra) and monoclonal anti-γ-sarcoglycan (NCL-g-SARC, Novocastra). Note the complete deficiency of γ-sarcoglycan (e) and relative preservation of α-sarcoglycan (f) in the biopsy from the patient with γ-sarcoglycanopathy (homozygous del 521T). The patient with α-sarcoglycanopathy was a compound heterozygote (Q135/I124T).

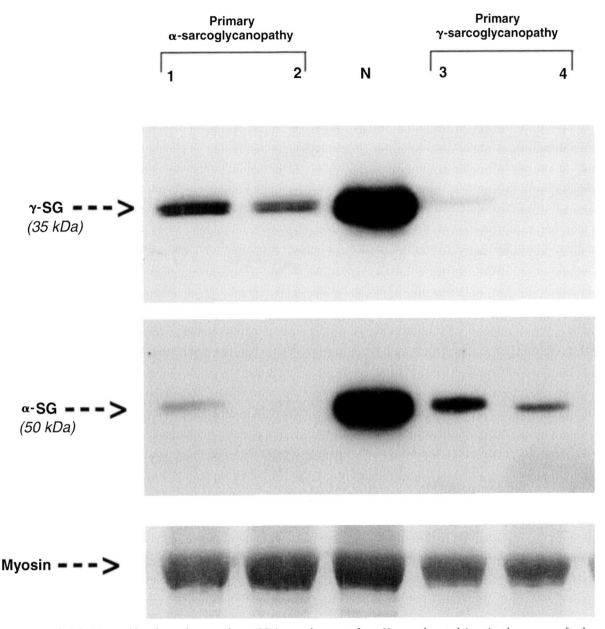

Fig. 20.5. Analysis by Western blot of α- and γ-sarcoglycan (SG) in muscle extracts from: N, normal control; 1, patient homozygous for the mutation in the α-SG gene resulting in an R284C substitution; 2, patient homozygous for a splice mutation in the α-SG gene (AG to AA (-1 exon 7); 3, patient homozygous for the mutation carried by Gypsies in the γ-SG gene (C283Y); and 4, patient homozygous for the 'Tunisian mutation' in the γ-SG gene (del1521T). The method followed that in Nicholson et al. (1989). Reacting antibodies are detected by enhanced chemoluminescence (ECL, Amersham). The antibodies used are anti-α-SG (NCL-a-SARC from Novocastra) and anti-γ-SG (NCL-g-SARC from Novocastra); myosin is used as a marker. (Kindly provided by F. Letweg, Laboratory of Molecular Genetics, Hôpital Cochin, Paris, France.)

missense mutations reside in the area of the gene encoding the extracellular part of the α-SG protein and result in a profound decrease in the amount of this protein and, to a lesser degree, of its partners, an effect that is not a result of a transcriptional event (Carrié et al., 1997). This suggests a variable impact on the assembly of the SG complex. The inter- and intrafamilial variability of phenotype produced by a given mutation is not exceptional in genetic diseases, and the numerous putative factors that may be involved (reviewed in Wolf, 1997) are unknown.

Beta-sarcoglycanopathy (limb girdle dystrophy type 2E)

The identification of the gene coding for the 43 kDa β-SG was accomplished independently by two groups studying patients exhibiting a secondary α-SG deficiency (Bönnemann et al., 1995; Lim et al., 1995). Lim et al. (1995) investigated patients from 11 Amish families from southern Indiana suffering from a mild form of LGMD not linked to the *LGMD2A* locus, thus not attributable to a pathology of calpain 3. This locus was subsequently mapped to 4q12 as defining the *LGMD2E* locus (Allamand et al., 1995) and was shown to contain the gene for β-SG, cloned from partial knowledge of the protein sequence. The role of this candidate gene was ultimately validated by the uncovering in all these patients of a homozygous missense mutation, causing a T151A substitution, carried on a common haplotype (Lim et al., 1995). Independently, Bönnemann et al. (1995) cloned the gene for β-SG and found truncating mutations in a young girl with early-onset severe LGMD. Additional mutations affecting β-SG were later detected: four in Brazil (Bönnemann et al., 1996), one in Tunisia (Bönnemann et al., 1998) and one again in the Amish isolate (Duclos et al., 1998a). Altogether about 20 different point mutations (50% null and 50% missense) have been reported in the Leiden database (web site: http://www.dmd.nl/), 50% of which hit exon 3.

Clinical pattern

Clinical observation of β-SG-deficient patients is still scanty. Eleven Amish patients with the original missense T151A mutation were evaluated in families from southern Indiana. Clinical onset was around 7 years of age (range 4 to 12 years of age). Weakness predominated in proximal limb and trunk muscles. The pattern of muscle involvement is still poorly documented. Calf hypertrophy was present in all these patients. Serum creatine kinase was markedly elevated in the early stages of the disease. There was no evidence of any heart or major respiratory dysfunction. The evolution was progressive, with loss of walking around 26 years, with again a large range from 12 to 38 years (C. Jackson and M. Fardeau, unpublished observations; Beckmann et al., 1999).

Muscle biopsy

Muscle biopsy shows the usual features of dystrophy. Immunostaining with β-SG antibodies is greatly decreased in all patients, and labelling of α-, γ- and δ-SG is reduced to the same extent. Reduced expression of the α-dystroglycan has been described (Duclos et al., 1998a). Dystrophin, β-dystroglycan and laminin α2-chains are usually found at normal levels.

Genotype–phenotype correlation

The relative clinical homogeneity of the Amish patients is likely attributable to their allelic homogeneity (T151A allele; Lim et al., 1995). A second rare missense mutation (resulting in R91C) was, however, uncovered in patients from the same community who presented a milder clinical phenotype (Duclos et al., 1998a). In contrast, most of the mutations affecting β-SG, found in other populations, result in a much more severe disease, with early onset, regardless of the type of mutation (Bönnemann et al., 1995, 1996, 1998).

Gamma-sarcoglycanopathy (limb girdle dystrophy type 2C)

Gamma-sarcoglycanopathy mainly refers to SCARMD, which was initially described in Tunisian families and is characterized by a Duchenne-like clinical phenotype with an autosomal mode of inheritance (Ben-Hamida et al., 1983). It was subsequently also found to be common in other North African countries (Azibi et al., 1993; El Kerch et al., 1994). The SCARMD phenotype was characterized by loss of the 50 kDa component of the DGC (α-SG) (Matsumura et al., 1992) and segregated in these families with chromosome 13q12 markers (Ben Othmane et al., 1992; Azibi et al., 1993), thus defining the *LGMD2C* locus (Bushby and Beckmann, 1995). Ultimately the gene coding for the 35 kDa γ-SG was cloned, mapped to the *LGMD2C* locus and all Tunisian patients were found to carry the same point mutation (del521T), while a Japanese patient harboured an internal deletion (Noguchi et al., 1995).

Clinical pattern

Detailed clinical data for γ-sarcoglycanopathy were reported for the Tunisian patients long before the molecular genetic era (Ben Hamida and Fardeau, 1980; Ben Hamida et al., 1983). This autosomally inherited trait affects equally females and males. Clinical onset is usually between 2 and 12 years of age. Initially, pelvic girdle muscles are more affected, with also some scapular winging. Calf hypertrophy is almost constant. SCARMD boys have a waddling gait, a slight hyperlordosis and difficulties in rising from the floor, a clinical picture that is strikingly similar to that of a patient with DMD. In the intermediate stages of the disease, besides the limb girdle weakness, there is a marked involvement of abdominal and spinal muscles, as well as of neck flexors. Contractures are present and develop rapidly along with kyphoscoliosis once the patient becomes wheelchair dependent. Facial muscles may be slightly involved and tongue enlargement is sometimes noticed. There is no ocular or pharyngeal involvement. Cardiac function is usually normal; however, some anomalies may start in the intermediate stages of the disease, and electrocardiographic and echocardiographic abnormalities may be detected (Ben Hamida et al., 1996). Respiratory muscle weakness is a major problem at a later stage, requiring specific assistance. There is no cognitive impairment (Miladi et al., 1999). Serum creatine kinase levels are very high in the early stages then decline with the progression of the disease. The electromyograph is myopathic. The rate of progression is slower and more variable than in DMD, with patients with severe disease losing their walking ability around 10 years of age, and those with milder forms being wheelchair bound at 30 years. Death, by respiratory insufficiency, may occur after 25/30 years of age. A marked intrafamilial variability is often noticed (Ben Hamida et al., 1983, 1996).

Muscle biopsy
There are marked dystrophic changes in muscle biopsies, with foci of necrotic and regenerating fibres and a moderate increase of endomysial collagen. Type I fibre predominance increases as disease progresses. Upon immunostaining, γ-SG is not seen and the other SG members are usually, but not constantly, decreased (Fig. 20.4). By Western blot, a preferential loss of γ-SG over the other SGs is usually observed (Fig. 20.5). Contrary to the other sarcoglycanopathies, dystrophin is often reduced on sections and on Western blots (Jones et al., 1998; Passos-Bueno et al., 1999).

Gene pathology and genotype–phenotype correlation
There are only seven published γ-SG mutations. Five are frameshifting, thus truncating the protein. These include the del521T mutation, which is prevalent in North Africa and most probably in the Mediterranean area, and is caused by a founder effect, as evidenced by a complete linkage disequilibrium with a rare intragenic allele (Ben Othmane et al., 1995; Noguchi et al., 1995). The del521T mutation results in the DMD/BMD-like phenotype described above. In a series of 40 Algerian patients with the del521T mutation, 30 became wheelchair bound before or around the age of 14 years, without a noticeable gender effect (M. Chaouch and J.-C. Kaplan, unpublished data). There is however, one intriguing Afro-Brazilian family in which three siblings who are homozygous for the del521T

mutation are remarkably paucisymptomatic, exhibiting only calf hypertrophy and elevated serum creatine kinase levels (McNally et al., 1996a).

Only two missense point mutations have been reported in the γ-SG gene. One results in the C283Y substitution, near the C-terminal end of the protein. It is found only in gypsies, who, as a result of inbreeding, are homozygous carriers of this allele (Piccolo et al., 1996). The phenotype is severe, 86% of the patients becoming wheelchair bound before or at 14 years (Merlini et al., 2000). The other missense variant, L193S, reported in five patients of a Dutch consanguineous family, gives rise to a mild disease with onset in childhood but very slow progression (van der Kooi et al., 1998a).

All the reported mutations, apart from the Dutch one abolish (truncating mutations) or perturb (gypsy mutation) the epidermal growth factor (EGF)-like cysteine-containing repeats in the extra-cellular C-terminal region of the protein, which appear to be critical (McNally et al., 1996b).

Epidemiology
A few cases of sporadic diseases caused by rare mutations affecting γ-SG have also been reported in patients from Japan (Noguchi et al., 1995), Italy (McNally et al., 1996b), Turkey (Dinçer et al., 1997) and the Netherlands (van der Kooi et al., 1998a). Gamma-sarcoglycanopathy is, however, frequent in two endogamic populations as a result of the prevalent founder mutations. One is the del521T mutation, which is widespread in North Africa (Noguchi et al., 1995) but is also found in Brazilian patients of African ancestry (Ben Othmane et al., 1995; McNally et al., 1996a). Interestingly, few sporadic cases of patients with LGMD1C carrying one or two del521T alleles have been observed out of Africa, mainly in Mediterranean countries, most of them sharing the Tunisian haplotype (McNally et al., 1996b; J.-C. Kaplan, unpublished data). The second founder mutation results in the C283Y substitution, and is found exclusively in Gypsy patients (Piccolo et al., 1996; Lasa et al., 1998; Merlini et al., 2000). Haplotype analysis in these families suggest that this mutation probably occurred 12 centuries ago, i.e. before the presumed migration of Gypsies out of India (Piccolo et al., 1996).

Delta-sarcoglycanopathy (limb girdle dystrophy type 2F)
Delta-sarcoglycan is the fourth and last member of the SG complex to have been incriminated in LGMD. First, a sixth locus for an autosomal form of LGMD was mapped to chromosome 5q33, *LGMD2F*, in two African-Brazilian families (Passos-Bueno et al., 1996b). Second, because muscle specimens of patients with LGMD2F exhibited a

secondary deficit of α-SG, the candidate gene was likely to be the fourth member of the SG complex. This was demonstrated by positional cloning of the gene for δ-SG in the suspected chromosome region, which coded for a sarcolemmal 35 kDa glycoprotein (Nigro et al., 1996a) and proved to be mutated in these LGMD2F families (Nigro et al., 1996b). Independently the δ-SG cDNA was cloned on the basis of the partial peptide sequence of the non-γ-SG 35 kDa SG (Jung et al., 1996).

Gene pathology and clinical presentation
Delta-sarcoglycanopathy seems to be the rarest of all sarcoglycanopathies with only few cases documented. Four Brazilian families of African descent carry the same frameshifting del656C mutation (Nigro et al., 1996b). Another Brazilian patient, of Caucasian origin, was found to carry a missense mutation resulting in the substitution E262K (Moreira et al., 1998), and two Caucasian patients in the USA carried a stop mutation (Duggan et al., 1997b). Except for the one patient with the missense mutation, all had the severe type of disease, with a DMD-like presentation and progression.

Interestingly there is no mention of specific heart problems in these patients. This is in sharp contrast with the severe cardiomyopathy observed in the spontaneous BIO 14.6 Syrian hamster strain, in which the first exon and upstream region of the gene for the δ-SG are deleted (Nigro et al., 1997).

Muscle biopsy
A typical myopathic pattern is observed in muscle biopsies. In all the reported cases, the complete absence of δ-SG in muscle specimens was always accompanied by complete loss of α-, β- and γ-SG, and a reduction of dystrophin (Nigro et al., 1996b; Passos-Bueno et al., 1999).

General aspects of the sarcoglycanopathies
The SG complex functions as a tetrameric unit that is disrupted by the loss or defect of any of its members. The four sarcoglycanopathies share some clinical features in term of muscle selectivity, absence of intellectual impairment and lack of prominent symptoms of cardiac dysfunction. Indeed, contrary to the dystrophinopathies, where dilated cardiomyopathy is a common feature, overt cardiac symptoms are rare in sarcoglycanopathies (reviewed in van der Kooi et al., 1998b; Melacini et al., 1999).

This is in contrast with animal models of sarcoglycanopathy, which have prominent cardiomyopathy, such as the spontaneous δ-sarcoglycanopathy of the BIO14.6 Syrian hamster (Nigro et al., 1997) and the γ-SG null (Hack et al., 1998) or δ-SG null (Coral-Vazquez et al., 1999) mouse models produced by gene invalidation. It should be noted

that the α-SG null (Duclos et al., 1998b) and β-SG-null (Araishi et al., 1999) mice do not exhibit major heart involvement. In the δ-SG knock-out model, there is a loss of the smooth muscle SG complex also in coronary vasculature, a phenomenon not observed in α-SG null mice (Coral-Vazquez et al., 1999). This difference could be explained at the molecular level by the fact that in smooth muscle α-SG is replaced by a homologous polypeptide encoded by the gene for ε-SG (Straub et al., 1999).

Although striking intra- and interfamilial variation of severity may be observed for a given sarcoglycanopathy and even for the same mutation, it now appears that the β-, γ- and δ-sarcoglycanopathies are usually severe, while the clinical spectrum of α-sarcoglycanopathy is much broader (Eymard et al., 1997; Beckmann et al., 1999; Passos-Bueno et al., 1999).

Becaues the sarcoglycanopathies have only been identified relatively recently, epidemiological data are still scarce. Fanin et al. (1997) estimated the prevalence of primary sarcoglycanopathies in the population to be 5.6 per million. Duggan et al. (1997a) estimated the frequency of sarcoglycanopathy among autosomally inherited dystrophin-positive dystrophies (sampled mostly from Italy) to be 11%.

There are no reliable clinical discriminating features allowing a defect in any specific SG component to be anticipated. A deficit of α-SG, whether primary or secondary, is a hallmark common to all sarcoglycanopathies and is thus of high diagnostic value. Careful protein analysis by semiquantitative Western blot (Anderson and Davison, 1999) may sometimes provide a clue when staining for one of the four SGs is much more severely decreased, indicating a likely candidate gene (Fig. 20.5). A total loss of the four SGC components is indicative of a primary β- or δ-SG defect. Other elements can also be taken into consideration. The population origin may help to decide which gene is a better candidate, either because of the suspicion of founder effects or knowledge on relative prevalence. For example, in a Gypsy with LGMD, the private C283Y substitution in γ-SG should be explored first; North African patients have a very high probability to carry the γ-SG del521T mutation. Mutations in the genes for α-SG and β-SG have, however, also been found in Algerian, Moroccan and Tunisian patients (Carrié et al., 1997; Bönnemann et al., 1998). In nonendogamic populations mutations of the gene for α-SG are prevailing among those with LGMD (Duggan et al., 1997a; Angelini et al., 1999, Passos-Bueno et al., 1999; Vainzof et al., 1999).

Pathophysiology
Function of the SG complex remains still elusive. While the mechanism by which a defect in any of the four SG

components prevents the SG subcomplex from being present at the membrane remains to be established (see review in Lim and Campbell, 1998), there is some evidence that SG mutants abrogate complex assembly, which in turn impairs normal trafficking to sarcolemma (Holt et al., 1998a; Crosbie et al., 1999). Sarcoglycanopathies belong, therefore, to the 'sarcolemmopathies' (Fadic et al., 1997). Indeed a dramatic increase in sarcolemma permeability for dyes, such as Evans blue, that do not penetrate into normal skeletal muscle fibres has been recently documented in mice with either dystrophinopathy or sarcoglycanopathy (Straub et al., 1997; Duclos et al., 1998b; Araishi et al., 1999). Interestingly, this phenomenon was not observed in the *dy/dy* mice with congenital muscular dystrophy caused by a defective laminin $\alpha 2$-chain (merosin; Straub et al., 1997). Sarcospan was also found to be missing from the sarcolemma of β-SG null mice, in which the dystrophin–DGC was reported to be unstable (Araishi et al., 1999). Since the SG complex belongs to the DGC, sarcoglycanopathy is believed to share some common pathophysiology with dystrophinopathy, i.e. the breaking of the structural link between laminin-2 in the extracellular matrix system and dystrophin/F-actin in the intracellular cytoskeleton, resulting in a contraction-induced mechanical damage (Petrof et al., 1993). Interestingly, the amounts of dystrobrevin, a remote intracellular member of the DGC (Fig. 20.2), are severely reduced in the sarcolemma from patients with either DMD or sarcoglycanopathy (Metzinger et al., 1997). A signalling role in skeletal and cardiac muscle has been recently advocated for dystrobrevin and more generally for the DGC complex (Grady et al., 1999). In this situation, a DGC pathology such as sarcoglycanopathy or dystrophinopathy would cause both a structural and a signalling dysfunction.

Proximo-distal muscular dystrophy with dysferlin deficiency

Proximo-distal muscular dystrophy was first described in a large inbred Palestinian family (Mahjneh et al., 1992) and mapped to chromosome 2p13, thereby defining the *LGMD2B* locus (Bashir et al., 1994, 1996). Patients belonging to this family suffered from a mild LGMD that also showed eventually a distal distribution (Mahjneh et al., 1992, 1996; Passos-Bueno et al., 1996a). Muscle biopsies of patients with LGMD2B show no alteration in dystrophin, SG or merosin staining. The causal gene (*DYSF*) was identified upon positional cloning, and mutations in this gene were shown to be responsible for both the LGMD2B and the adult-onset distal muscular dystrophy known as Miyoshi myopathy (Bashir et al., 1998; Liu et al., 1998). This identification settled an important issue as it was demonstrated that the same mutation could lead to either one of these conditions (Liu et al., 1998; Weiler et al., 1999), as initially suspected from genetic analyses of discordant phenotypes among haplo-identical siblings (Illarioshkin et al., 1996; Weiler et al., 1996). It is now established that proximal LGMD2B disease and the Miyoshi myopathy are linked to chromosome 2p and are, in fact, phenotypic extremes of an entity sharing the same genetic aetiology. The chance to develop either may, therefore, depend on the presence of additional as yet unknown genetic or nongenetic factors.

The protein and its function

The dysferlin gene (*DYSF*) is a large gene encompassing over 150 kb containing more than 55 exons and encoding a 230 kDa protein (Table 20.3) (Matsuda et al., 1999). Dysferlin is a newly characterized ubiquitously expressed protein showing no homology to any known mammalian protein (Bashir et al., 1998; Liu et al., 1998), with the exception of the recently identified otoferlin protein, deficiency of which was shown to lead to deafness (Yasunaga et al., 1999). Both proteins show partial homology to the *Caenorhabditis elegans* spermatogenesis factor ferlin-1, which is required for membrane fusion. Using a monoclonal antibody, Anderson et al. (1999) localized dysferlin to the muscle fibre membrane, thus in the same cellular environment as dystrophin, caveolin 3, laminin-α_2 and the SG complex, and showed its early expression in human development at a time when the limbs start to form regional differentiation.

Clinical features

The phenotypes exhibited by dysferlin-deficient patients with proximal (LGMD2B) and distal (Miyoshi) presentation were recently reappraised at the European Neuromuscular Centre (ENMC) workshop on LGMD (Beckmann et al., 1999).

In patients with proximal muscle involvement (e.g. Mahjneh et al., 1992), the weakness predominates on lower limbs, biceps femoris, semimembranous, adductor and medial vastus muscles. Interestingly, the infraclinical involvement of the medial gastrocnemius is evidenced by CT scan imaging (Fig. 20.6). Upper limb weakness appears only at later stages on pectoralis major and biceps brachialis. Even in the late stage of the disease, periscapular muscles were only mildly affected and none of the patients presented with winging of the scapulae.

In patients with a major distal weakness, identified as Miyoshi type myopathy (Bejaoui et al., 1995; Liu et al., 1998), clinical onset begins with an inability to stand on tip toes, caused by an early and predominant involvement of

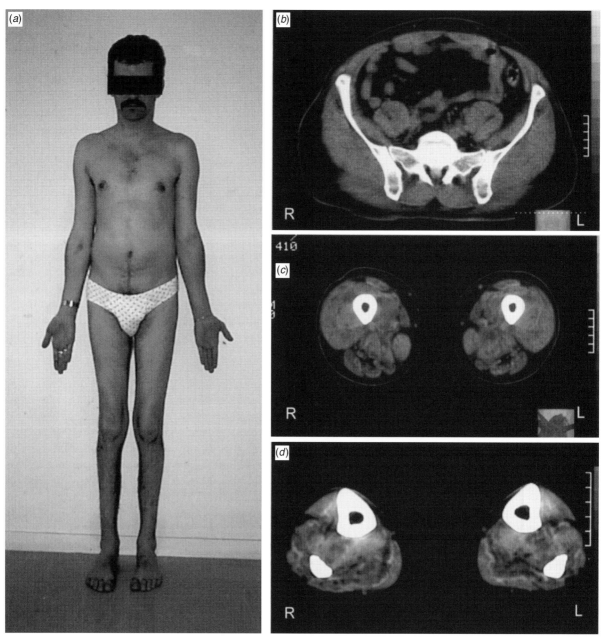

Fig. 20.6. A 30-year-old patient with dysferlinopathy. (*a*) Notice the important atrophy of lower limb distal muscles. Computed tomographic scans from the same patient show (*b*) the pelvic girdle with slight gluteal atrophy; (*c*) the thigh and (*d*) the leg; both (*c*) and (*d*) show diffuse muscle rarefaction, especially in posterior compartments of the leg.

posterior leg muscles while anterior tibial muscles are relatively preserved. This is always well demonstrated on CT scan imaging. A painful 'inflammatory' aspect of the limbs is not exceptional at this early stage of the disease. Weakness extends, after a few years, to hamstrings and quadriceps muscles. Upper limb muscles are preserved for a longer time, except the biceps brachialis, which shows a peculiar 'en boule' atrophy. Axial muscles are affected in late stages while facial, oculomotor and velopharyngeal muscles remain unaffected.

Both phenotypes share many common features: same age of onset (early adulthood) and motor performances, which are often considered as excellent before the first difficulties appear. The clinical course is relatively moderate; use of a wheelchair is required only after at least 10–20 years of duration of the disease. There is never any cardiac, facial or respiratory weakness nor any cognitive impairment. Characteristically, very high serum creatine kinase levels (up to 50 times normal) are observed, even in the advanced stages of the disease.

The electromyograph is myopathic. Muscle biopsies are remarkable by the severity of the necrotic–regenerative pattern in affected muscles, with sometimes rare, small inflammatory infiltrates at the periphery of the necrotic fibres. This explains why a diagnosis of polymyositis is often made in the early stages of this dystrophy. This necrotic–regenerative pattern is always associated with marked 'dystrophic' features of the muscle fibres.

Dystrophin and members of the DGC complex are normal, while dysferlin amounts are specifically and drastically reduced both on immunostaining and on immunoblotting (Anderson et al., 1999). For some dysferlinopathies, a secondary partial deficit in calpain 3 has been reported (Anderson et al., 2000). No 'secondary dysferlinopathy' has been described. Sporadic and familial cases presenting a Miyoshi phenotype that is unlinked to chromosome 2 have been recently described, and a disease locus has been mapped to chromosome 10 (Linssen et al., 1997, 1998).

Epidemiology, gene pathology and genotype–phenotype correlation

The number of null and missense mutations in *DYSF* known so far is still small. These mutations, which are scattered along the entire gene (Bashir et al., 1998; Liu et al., 1998), were found in different populations, either as sporadic cases in Europe (Liu et al., 1998) and in Brazil (Passos-Bueno et al., 1999), or as familial cases with a founder effect in a large Palestinian pedigree (Mahjneh et al., 1992), in the aboriginal Canadian kindred (Weiler et al., 1996, 1999), in the large Avar pedigree of Daghestan (Illarioshkin et al., 1996) and in a more dispersed, yet homogenous isolate of Jews of Libyan origin (Bashir et al., 1998; Argov et al., 2000). Interestingly, within some of these families the same P791R substitution, born by the same haplotype, can lead to either a proximal LGMD2B-like or a distal Miyoshi-type of dystrophy (Weiler et al., 1999).

A naturally occurring mouse model, harbouring an inphase deletion of 171bp, with histopathological dystrophic features compatible with a proximal progressive dystrophy has recently been characterized (Bittner et al., 1999). This mouse is expected to represent a good model of dysferlinopathy.

Other autosomal recessive proximal dystrophies

This group includes familial forms of progressive proximal muscular dystrophy with autosomal recessive mode of inheritance, where, after exclusion of the six already identified *LGMD2* loci (*A* to *F*), a significant linkage to one of two other loci, namely *LGMD2G* and *LGMD2H*, was obtained. The *LGMD2G* locus has recently been identified, but *LGMD2H* awaits identification.

LGMD2G

The *LGMD2G* locus was assigned to 17q11–12 in a nonconsanguineous kindred of Italian ancestry in which six patients were carefully investigated over 20 years (Moreira et al., 1997). The first difficulties in running and climbing stairs were observed around 12 years of age. Progressive atrophy affected proximal muscles in the upper limbs and both proximal and distal muscles in the lower limbs. Foot drop was a common feature. There was no cardiac or intellectual dysfunction. A 3- to 17-fold elevation of serum creatine kinase was observed in the early stages. Muscle biopsies exhibited a necrotic–regenerative pattern and a large number of rimmed vacuoles. Dystrophin and α-SG staining were normal. The disease progression was slow but constant since four of the six patients were confined to a wheelchair in their thirties, about 18 years after onset.

The linkage of *LGMD2G* to a 3cM region on 17q11–12 excludes the gene for α-SG (which also maps to chromosome 17 but to a region 9cM apart) as well as two other diseases showing rimmed vacuoles in muscle, namely the distal myopathy with rimmed vacuoles (DMRV) described by Nonaka et al. (1981), which maps to 9p1 (Mitrani-Rosenbaum et al., 1996; Ikeuchi et al., 1997), and Kugelberg–Welander disease (or spinal atrophy type III), which maps to 5q11-q13 (Lefebvre et al., 1995). In another family with patients presenting similar symptoms and rimmed vacuoles, the disease was found to be linked to the *LGMD2G* region and could, therefore, be allelic (Moreira et al., 1997). While this chapter was in press, *LGMD2G* was identified. It codes for telethonin, a sarcomeric protein (Moreira et al., 2000).

LGMD2H

The *LGMD2H* locus, the eighth in the series of autosomal recessive LGMDs, was localized by a study of a large Hutterite kindred of Manitoba (Weiler et al., 1997). In this inbred community, more than 60 individuals have been found to be affected with a mild form of autosomal recessive LGMD, first described in 1976 (Shokeir and Kobrinsky, 1976).

The disease is characterized by proximal limb weakness, back pain, fatigue and waddling gait, and it starts at approximately 20 years of age (range 8–27 years). Facial involvement was reported in some patients. Evolution is very slow and most patients remain ambulant. Of the numerous patients recorded, only three were wheelchair bound in their forties (Shokeir and Rozdilsky, 1985; Weiler et al., 1997).

Muscle biopsy shows a nonspecific pattern of dystrophy, with normal staining of dystrophin and the DGC proteins (K. Wrogemann, personal communication).

Linkage and haplotype analysis of four large related Hutterite families localized the morbid locus, *LGMD2H*, within a 300 kb interval of the chromosome 9q31-q33 region, distal to the neighbouring Fukuyama locus (Weiler et al., 1997). In this genetic isolate, the ancestry of which could be traced back for 11 generations, it is assumed, based on shared haplotypes, that the disease alleles are identical by descent (Weiler et al., 1997).

Other unmapped *LGMD* loci

As not all autosomal recessive families can be accounted for by these eight genes, other loci are likely to be identified in the future (Moreira et al., 1997). A new locus, *LGMD2I*, mapping on chromosome 19q13.3 has recently been found in a large consanguineous Tunisian family (Driss et al., 2000).

Autosomal dominant proximal muscular dystrophies

Few early reports of familial cases of dominantly inherited muscular diseases without facial involvement, excluding the diagnosis of FSH muscular dystrophy, may qualify as dominant LGMDs (Schneiderman et al., 1969; Bacon and Smith, 1971; De Coster et al., 1974). Even now, discrimination between dominant LGMD and FSH dystrophy on purely clinical grounds may be difficult to achieve. The now possible identification of FSH dystrophy by direct DNA analysis is of great help in dubious cases.

The first proven example of a true dominant LGMD family was the extensive pedigree described by Gilchrist et al. (1988), leading to the mapping by linkage analysis of the first dominant *LGMD* locus, coined *LGMD1A*, to chromosome 5 (Speer et al., 1992). Subsequently four additional *LGMD1* loci have been mapped (Table 20.2), of which only one, *LGMD1C*, has been identified, corresponding to caveolin 3 (McNally et al., 1998b; Minetti et al., 1998). More loci will probably be uncovered in the future. Equally, the qualification as LGMD for some of the entities described below remains questionable until their underlying causative gene is identified. Altogether the assumption that dominant LGMD is much less frequent than the recessively inherited forms (Bushby and Beckmann, 1995) remains valid.

Limb girdle dystrophy type 1A

The *LGDM1A* locus was singularized in an extended multi-generational American family of West Virginia, with 62 affected individuals, originally described by Gilchrist et al. (1988). It was mapped to chromosome 5q22.3-q31.3 (Speer et al., 1992) and subsequently more precisely to a 7 cM region in 5q31-q33 (Yamaoka et al., 1994). The first symptoms appear in adulthood, between 18 and 35 years. Muscle weakness predominates on the upper limb girdle. Occasional Achilles tendon contractures and nasal quality of voice are distinctive features. Serum creatine kinase is slightly elevated (three to four times normal). The disease progresses very slowly without complete loss of ambulation. Anticipation of the age of onset throughout generations suggests a possible unstable triplet expansion pathology (Speer et al., 1998). The corresponding gene is still not identified. However, myotilin, a muscle-specific protein with partial homology to titin and sarcolemmal and sarcomeric localization, has recently been cloned and mapped precisely to the chromosomal region containing the *LGMD1A* locus (Salmikangas et al., 1999). So far, one missense variant has been found to co-segregate with the disease (Hauser et al., 1999), making this a very attractive candidate for this locus.

A different study of a four generation North American pedigree with dominantly inherited distal myopathy characterized by late onset (after 35 years) and velopharyngeal weakness led to the mapping of a morbid locus to chromosome 5q31, in the same region as the *LGMD1A* locus (Feit et al., 1998). In spite of some distinctive features, such as distal distribution of muscle involvement and presence of rimmed vacuoles on biopsy, it has been suggested that this locus, designated *VPDMD* (velopharyngeal distal muscular dystrophy), might be allelic to *LGMD1A*. The question will be solved upon the discovery of the underlying morbid gene(s).

Limb girdle dystrophy type 1B

The *LGMD1B* locus was assigned to 1q11-q21 in three extended unrelated multigenerational families, one from the Netherlands, one from Surinam and one from the Caribbean islands (van der Kooi et al., 1996, 1997). The disease, observed in 35 individuals, is characterized by proximal symmetrical limb weakness, starting in half the patients during childhood (range 4–38 years), beginning at lower limbs and extending very slowly to upper limbs. Little or no contractures are observed. Creatine kinase is normal or slightly elevated. Muscle biopsy shows non-specific signs of a dystrophic process. Cardiac abnormalities are observed in two-thirds of the patients, with dysrhythmias and atrioventricular conduction disturbances appearing after 25 years of age, increasing with age and necessitating pacemaker implantation. Sudden cardiac arrest has been reported. Dilated cardiomyopathy was rarely observed. After the age of 45 years, cardiac dysfunction is present in all patients. In a few, the cardiac symptoms can be predominant (van der Kooi et al., 1996). Another family with similar skeletal and cardiac symptoms, for which mapping data are still unavailable, was reported in Taiwan (Fang et al., 1997).

With its life-threatening conduction disturbances this dystrophy is reminiscent of the autosomal dominant form of Emery–Dreifuss muscular dystrophy, which results from lamin A/C deficiency (Bonne et al., 1999) (see Chapter 23). However, the early contractures of elbows, the Achilles tendons and postcervical muscles – prominent features of autosomal-dominant Emery–Dreifuss dystrophy – are not seen in LGMD1B (van der Kooi et al., 1996). In fact, since the loci for both diseases map to the same region of chromosome 1, it is reasonable to hypothesize that the two conditions are allelic. This was eventually confirmed by the discovery of mutations in the gene for lamin A/C in subjects originally reported with LGMD1B disease (Muchir et al., 2000). Consequently, the two different phenotypes are A/C laminopathies, and should be considered together.

Limb girdle dystrophy type 1C: caveolin 3 deficiency

Caveolin 3 is the muscle-specific member of a family of small transmembrane proteins. Caveolins have both N- and C-termini in the cytoplasm and form oligomers within the caveolae's microdomains of the plasma membrane, where they act as scaffolding proteins to organize and concentrate specific proteins and lipids implicated in G-protein-associated transmembrane signalling events (Song et al., 1996). Although it co-localizes with DGC, caveolin 3 is not an integral component of the DGC (Crosbie et al., 1998).

The gene locus maps at 3p25. To date, only four independent primary defects of caveolin 3 have been uncovered upon a systematic screening of patients with LGMD of unknown aetiology (Minetti et al., 1998; McNally et al., 1998b). The first study found eight patients exhibiting a drastic reduction of sarcolemmal caveolin 3. These patients belong to two different Italian families (Minetti et al., 1998) in which the disease showed autosomal dominant inheritance. The patients exhibited proximal muscle weakness, positive Gowers' sign, calf hypertrophy and high serum creatine kinase, with onset around 5 years of age but slow disease progression to adulthood without loss of ambulation. The patients were found to be heterozygous for mutations perturbing invariant residues in an essential domain of caveolin 3. In one family a missense mutation resulted in P104L, involving the membrane-spanning region. In the other family a 9 bp deletion removed residues

63 to 65 in the conserved scaffolding domain of the protein. Since both domains are essential for homo-oligomerization and interaction with caveolin-associated signalling molecules, heterozygous mutations can be detrimental and may have a dominant negative effect.

In the second study (McNally et al., 1998a), patients' mRNA was systematically screened for the presence of caveolin 3 mutations. Two unrelated patients with mild-to-moderate proximal muscle weakness were found. In the first family, the patient carried a homozygous missense mutation resulting in a G56S substitution. Immunostaining of sarcolemmal caveolin 3 was not diminished, suggesting that the abnormal allele is a recessive functional mutant without quantitative effect. In the second family the patient was a carrier of the missense mutation resulting in a C72W substitution. Since this allele was also found in three other asymptomatic subjects, a recessive mode of inheritance was again suggested (McNally et al., 1998a). The pathogenicity of these variants remains to be established.

Limb girdle dystrophy type 1D

LGMD1D refers to the yet uncharacterized gene involved in a familial dilated cardiomyopathy–conduction disease and myopathy (FDC-CDM) described by Messina et al. (1997) in a large pedigree of French-Canadian ancestry, in which the disease, affecting 25 patients, segregated as an autosomal dominant trait. The proximal skeletal involvement in this family remained moderate and the patients remained ambulatory throughout their lifetime. Serum creatine kinase levels were slightly increased. In contrast, heart involvement resulted in a major and life-threatening disease, manifesting in the second decade and worsening with age, with instances of sudden death. LGMD1D is characterized by a dilated cardiomyopathy with conduction disturbances, sometimes necessitating pacemaker implementation. The locus was mapped to a 3 cM interval on chromosome 6q23, which excludes the five already mapped loci of autosomal dominant familial cardiomyopathy (Messina et al., 1997). Once again, it is unclear whether this entity should be classified under the LGMD umbrella. This will probably be solved upon the identification of its molecular genetic aetiology.

Limb girdle dystrophy type 1E

LGMD1E was mapped to a 9 cM interval on chromosome 7q in two families exhibiting an adult-onset proximal weakness with elevated serum creatine kinase, without any other distinctive feature (Speer et al., 1999). Thompson et al. (1999) suggested recently that *FLN2*, encoding the muscle-specific isoform filamin-2, might be involved in this disease.

Other type 1 limb girdle dystrophies

As for the recessively inherited LGMDs, the five loci *LGMD1A–E* do not account for all dominant proximal muscular dystrophies, and it is expected that additional loci will be uncovered in the future (Speer et al., 1999).

General features of limb girdle dystrophies

Incidence and epidemiology

The LGMDs constitute a genetically and clinically heterogeneous group of diseases of low prevalence, estimated to be approximately 10^{-5} (Emery, 1991). The dominant LGMDs are rare, comprising to date less than a dozen genetically well-documented families affected at one of the six putative loci listed in Table 20.2. In contrast, the recessive LGMDs are much more frequent. In this category the contribution of each locus (Table 20.1) varies from population to population, reflecting their respective genetic history. In endogamous populations, one encounters either a predominant or a limited series of prevalent mutations, depending on the relative weight of founder mutations, as discussed above. These populations represent, however, particular situations. For exogamous populations, there are still too few reports to infer realistic figures. This situation is likely to change rapidly as a result of the deciphering of the genetic aetiology of these clinical entities and the improvement of molecular diagnosis screening tests, based both on gene and protein analyses. Whereas the relative proportions of the different LGMD entities are likely to vary from region to region, preliminary data suggest that some are more frequent than others. For instance, α-SG deficiencies seem to be the most abundant among the sarcoglycanopathies in noninbred populations (Angelini et al., 1999; J.-C. Kaplan et al., unpublished data). Likewise calpain 3 deficiency seems to account for a substantial fraction of the autosomal recessive-LGMDs among Europeans (Richard et al., 1997). In Brazil, however, the two most frequent reported LGMDs are dysferlinopathy and calpainopathy (Passos-Bueno et al., 1999).

The diagnostic problems

General differential diagnosis

As the majority of human muscle disorders tend to predominate upon limb girdle muscles, almost every area of muscle pathology is involved in the differential diagnosis, and many other diseases must be excluded before considering the diagnosis of any of the LGMDs. The following steps ought to be taken. First, it is necessary to exclude any nonhereditary pathological disorder, such as dysendocrinial (hypothyroidism), iatrogenic (such as hypocholesterol drugs) or inflammatory disorders. The last diagnosis may be difficult to make, particularly in dysferlinopathies where the necrotic process in the affected muscles is very severe and may include small inflammatory infiltrates (see above). A scrupulous clinical examination and muscle imaging may help to differentiate these conditions.

Second, it is necessary to exclude other hereditary non-dystrophic disorders. This again may be difficult, as some of these hereditary neuromuscular disorders may present with a selective involvement of skeletal muscles. Late-onset spinal muscular atrophy (type III) is easily excluded by electromyography and, if necessary, by analysis of the SMN gene. A muscle biopsy with all histochemical and ultrastructural analyses is mandatory to differentiate, LGMDs clearly from late-onset congenital myopathies (centronuclear myopathies), mitochondrial myopathies, glycogenosis type III, acid maltase deficiencies, triglyceride storage disease (Chanarin's disease), myopathies with excessive autophagy or desmin-related myopathies.

Finally, it is necessary to differentiate LGMDs from other muscular dystrophies.

- FSH dystrophy is usually clinically characterized by its asymmetrical involvement of skeletal and facial muscles, but these features may be discrete and hard to evaluate. In these patients, DNA analysis of the *FSH* locus is the ultimate proof.
- Emery–Dreifuss dystrophies have their own skeletal and cardiac phenotype and inheritance mode. Emerin deficiency in the X-linked form can be visualized in muscle or skin biopsies. There are early-onset emerinopathies that may present with a LGMD phenotype (Muntoni et al., 1998). In autosomal dominant forms, mutations in lamin A/C can also result in a LGMD phenotype (LGMD1B) (Bonne et al., 1999; Muchir et al., 2000). (See Chapter 19.)
- Most congenital dystrophies are characterized by a very early onset and an early development of severe contractures, with abnormalities of the central nervous system being present in many patients. However, patients with partial merosin deficiencies may be mistaken as LGMDs. Brain imaging is of great diagnostic value in these patients (Tan et al., 1997; Naom et al., 1998).
- Non-Miyoshi distal myopathies, such as those described by Markesbery et al. (1977), Satoyoshi (1990), Udd et al. (1993) and Nonaka et al. (1998), have their own clinical and histological features.

- The most common problem is distinguishing the various LGMDs from dystrophinopathies, e.g. DMD/BMD males or manifesting female carriers, because, as already emphasized, the phenotypes are close if not similar to sarcoglycanopathies. For this reason, dystrophin analysis of muscle biopsy is a mandatory prerequisite.

Positive diagnosis

Ultimately it is also necessary to differentiate the different LGMDs. A scrupulous analysis of clinical data, including imaging (CT scan or magnetic resonance imaging) allows evaluation of the selectivity of affected muscle territories, an important clue to discriminate between the different LGMDs. Additional features, such as calf hypertrophy, macroglossia, contractures and cardiac involvement, are also important. A presentation reminiscent of a DMD/BMD phenotype is suggestive of a sarcoglycanopathy; one close to Erb's description (the so-called Reunion Island phenotype) points to a calpainopathy; a proximo-distal or distal Miyoshi-like myopathy is indicative of a dysferlinopathy. Yet, because of the phenotypic overlap and presence of outliers, such a diagnosis will always need to be supported by independent and objective parameters. The collection of familial data to assess the mode of inheritance is also essential.

The identification of the causative mutation represents the ultimate aetiological diagnosis. It is a prerequisite for accurate genetic counselling and prenatal diagnosis. However, given the number of candidate genes and the often large target size of some of these genes, it is far from being practical as a first step in a diagnostic procedure. Additional information must be gleaned from different sources to enable a hierarchy in the molecular investigations to be established. Detailed flowcharts have been proposed for a stepwise diagnosis of the LGMDs (Bushby and Beckmann, 1995; Anderson, 1996; Jones and North, 1997; Urtasun et al., 1998). At this stage, muscle sampling is mandatory, not only to confirm the dystrophic nature but also to investigate the protein make-up with a panel of relevant antibodies, indicating the possible specific protein defect. In the absence of specific functional assays for each of the proteins involved in muscular dystrophy, current tests rely on the measurement of the amounts of protein present and visualization of their cellular distribution. Specific antibodies recognizing dystrophin, the different SGs, calpain 3, laminin-α_2 and dysferlin provide a powerful means to expedite the diagnosis of the autosomal recessive-LGMD (Fig. 20.7) (Anderson and Davison, 1999b). Whenever a biopsy has been sampled, the use of these antibodies would guide such a diagnosis on a defined path along the decision tree. For instance, the integrity of the dystrophin and merosin staining is a prerequisite in all LGMDs, although some quantitative defects were reported; likewise, SGs are preserved in calpainopathies and dysferlinopathies. Western blots are particularly attractive as they lend themselves to multiplex assays and are semiquantitative (Fig. 20.5 and 20.7) (Anderson and Davison, 1999). It must be kept in mind that the observation of decreased levels of a particular protein in muscle biopsy specimens (visualized by immunofluorescence and/or Western blot) is, until further proof, only indicative of a primary defect in the corresponding gene. This is clearly illustrated by the sarcoglycanopathies, caused by mutations in any one of the four SG genes. Noteworthy is the fact that in about 30% of SG deficiencies, no mutations are identified (Duggan et al., 1997a), either because of insufficient gene exploration or because the primary defect is in another still unidentified gene.

The last word of caution deals with the fact that the currently available protein assays are quantitative, indicating a decrease in protein, but not qualitative, indicating functional impairment. At present, for almost every identified LGMD mutation, the cognate protein is diminished on immunostaining, but this does not need to be a general rule. One must indeed consider the possibility of mutants with functional changes and yet no gross quantitative effects on the amount of mutant protein. Relying exclusively on protein quantification would, in such cases, lead to a bias in the screening, as the presence of 'normal' amounts would induce one to reject diagnosis. A few cases of calpainopathy with defined missense mutations and yet normal amounts of the 94 kDa calpain 3 band on Western blots (Anderson et al., 1998) would fit this category of purely functional mutants.

Muscle biopsies are unfortunately not always available. For those widely expressed proteins, such as dysferlin, the need for muscle biopsy can be bypassed because the corresponding protein can be assessed in other biological samples such as blood, saliva, amniotic fluids, hair or skin biopsies. In the other cases, the need to scan one by one the different candidate genes for the presence of mutations is a formidable task with the present technology. It must be noted that current technologies and strategies are not fully efficient, and in a number of instances only one variant allele will have been recognized. Such cases are not exceptional and pose difficult diagnostic problems. With the emergence of new technologies, e.g. DNA chips, mutation analyses may become more straightforward.

Although clinics are mostly confronted with sporadic cases, which present the most diagnostic difficulties, for familial cases the diagnostic routine can be complemented by studying the segregation of markers bracketing each of

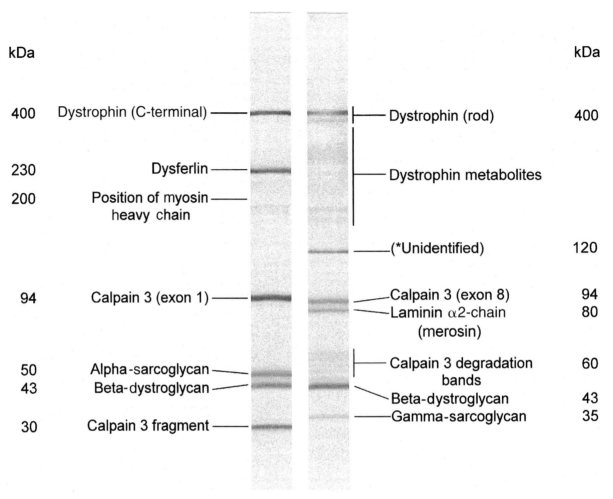

Fig. 20.7. Simultaneous visualization of proteins of interest for the molecular diagnosis of LGMDs by immunoblotting. Photography of two Western blot strips from a normal control human skeletal muscle labelled with cocktails of monoclonal antibodies to the proteins indicated. The position of the large myosin heavy chain (not stained) is indicated at 200 kDa. The unidentified band was detected with antibody 35DAG/21B5 to γ-sarcoglycan. The multiplex method used here was devised and described by Anderson and Davison (1999). Picture kindly provided by Louise V. B. Anderson (Neurobiology Department, University Medical School, Newcastle-upon-Tyne, UK).

the chromosomal *LGMD* loci. A fluorescent marker kit was developed for this purpose using a set of markers bracketing the *LGMD2A–F* disease loci to help to decide which gene should be explored first (Richard et al., 1999c). In some instances, haplotype analyses can be used to infer a common ancestral origin and thus point to specific mutation(s). The geographic or ethnic origin of the patient is another element that can direct the mutation screening (see above). Gross gene alterations (deletions, nonsense or frameshift mutations) are unambiguously pathogenic. Point mutations may pose problems because it is sometimes difficult to discriminate between a 'neutral' polymorphism and a morbid DNA sequence variation. This has

been particularly exemplified in the gene for calpain (Richard et al., 1999b).

The problem of nosography

With the discovery of a growing number of distinct *LGMD* loci, and ultimately the deciphering of the gene defects and the identification of the proteins involved, it is now possible to define a nosology based on molecular grounds. Clearly this aetiological nosology, which is essential for appropriate genetic counselling and further elucidation of the pathophysiology, does not fit the classical clinical and histopathological nosology. This is because (i) defects in several alternative genes may ultimately result in a similar phenotype (one disease, several alternative genes); (ii) defects in a given gene can produce distinct phenotypes without clearcut genotype/phenotype correlation (one gene, several diseases); (iii) even a given allele in a single gene can produce distinct patterns. For instance, α-sarcoglycanopathy can take the form of a severe DMD-like or BMD-like disease, or even of a mild disability; in dysferlinopathy, the same mutant allele can cause a proximal typical LGMD or a distal Miyoshi-type dystrophy.

The uncovering of the genetic aetiology of the dominant dystrophies may force a reappraisal and further simplification of the nosology, as defined entities may be removed from the LGMD cluster into more appropriate entities. This is exemplified by *LGMD1B*, which now coalesces with autosomal dominant Emery–Dreifuss dystrophy to form the laminopathies.

Other criteria of classification can be considered now, based on the cellular compartment affected (pathology of the sarcolemma, cytoskeleton, sarcomere) or on the type of dysfunction (pathology of structural proteins, of enzymes or signalling proteins). Such criteria may become essential for the understanding of pathogenesis and for development of appropriate treatment.

Therapeutic perspectives

We only mention here selected aspects specific to LGMDs, since the general issues will be considered in Chapter 36.

The increasing understanding of the molecular basis of LGMDs combined with the initial glimpses into their pathophysiology raise legitimately hopes and expectations for adequate treatments of these patients. No doubt new, original and imaginative gene-based therapies will emerge. Currently, one of the most favoured approaches is simply to complement the deficit by supplying a correcting version of the missing or defective gene. Initial results on the δ-SG-deficient animal models (Holt et al., 1998; Greelish et al., 1999) are encouraging, as both a dramatic decrease in centralized myonuclei and restoration of the sarcolemmal integrity were observed. Hence, two typical hallmarks of the progression of a sarcoglycanopathy were corrected. However, these represent only the first steps towards such applications. Moreover, most of these protocols will remain, as for DMD therapy, limited as long as they are confined to highly localized areas (the point of injection) and do not resolve the important issue of a systemic delivery.

The attempt to repopulate diseased muscle with normal stem cells is an original and exciting new avenue, still too recent to be discussed here (Gussoni et al., 1999).

Another, yet unexplored, attractive investigative approach would be to decipher the mechanism of muscle selectivity. If one could establish the molecular basis by which some muscle territories are spared at a given time, interesting therapeutic consequences might ensue.

Future prospects

By the years 2000 and 2003, respectively, the first and final draft of the human genome sequence will have been completed. Consequently, all facts, concepts and speculations mentioned in this chapter will evolve and change drastically. Molecular phenotypes will eventually no longer be interpreted in terms of single proteins but in terms of the resulting perturbations of protein–protein and protein–environment networks. It is hard to anticipate at present the impact of this knowledge on nosology, on our understanding of pathophysiology and on therapeutic practice (pharmacogenomics). The more knowledge accrues, the more complex the recapitulation of the different elements may appear. Yet, ultimately, it is hoped that common specific features will emerge, facilitating the recognition, diagnosis, management and eventually treatment of these disorders.

Some may be tempted to replace the current established nosology (clinical and morphological) by emerging new nosological perceptions, such as molecular, cellular or functional forms. Actually none of these is self-sufficient and, hopefully, the next edition of this book will provide an integrated nosology of these intriguing and challenging diseases, and perhaps describe the first successful therapeutic attempts.

Acknowledgements

We thank Louise V. B. Anderson, Norma B. Romero and J. A. Urtizberea for their valuable help in the preparation of this chapter.

References

Allamand, V., Broux, O., Bourg, N. et al. (1995). Genetic heterogeneity of autosomal recessive limb-girdle muscular dystrophy in a genetic isolate (Amish) and evidence for a new locus. *Hum. Mol. Genet.* **4**, 459–463.

Anderson, L. V. (1996). Optimized protein diagnosis in the autosomal recessive limb-girdle muscular dystrophies. *Neuromusc. Disord.* **6**, 443–446.

Anderson, L. V. and Davison, K. (1999). Multiplex Western blotting system for the analysis of muscular dystrophy proteins. *Am. J. Pathol.* **154**, 1017–1022.

Anderson, L., Davison, K., Moss, J. et al. (1998). Characterization of monoclonal antibodies to calpain 3 and protein expression in muscle from patients with limb-girdle muscular dystrophy type 2A. *Am. J. Pathol.* **153**, 1169–1179.

Anderson, L., Davison, K., Moss, J. et al. (1999). Dysferlin is a plasma membrane protein and is expressed early in human development. *Hum. Mol. Genet.* **8**, 855–861.

Anderson, L. V., Harrison, R. M., Pogue, R. et al. (2000). Secondary reduction in calpain 3 expression in patients with limb girdle muscular dystrophy type 2B and miyoshi myopathy (primary dysferlinopathies). *Neuromusc. Disord.* **10**, 553–559.

Angelini, C., Fanin, M., Menegazzo, E., Freda, M. P., Duggan, D. J. and Hoffman, E. P. (1998). Homozygous alpha-sarcoglycan mutation in two siblings: one asymptomatic and one steroid-responsive mild limb-girdle muscular dystrophy patient. *Muscle Nerve* **21**, 769–775.

Angelini, A., Fanin, M., Freda, M., Duggan, D., Siciliano, G. and Hoffman, E. (1999). The clinical spectrum of sarcoglycanopathies. *Neurology* **52**, 176–179.

Araishi, K., Sasaoka, T., Imamura, M. et al. (1999). Loss of the sarcoglycan complex and sarcospan leads to muscular dystrophy in beta-sarcoglycan-deficient mice. *Hum. Mol. Genet.* **8**, 1589–1598.

Argov, Z., Sadeh, M., Mazor, K. et al. (2000). Muscular dystrophy due to dysferlin deficiency in Libyan Jews. Clinical and genetic features. *Brain* **123**, 1229–1237.

Azibi, K., Chaouch, M., Reghis, A. et al. (1991). Linkage analysis of 19 families with Autosomal Recessive (Duchenne-like) muscular dystrophy from Algeria. *Cytogenet. Cell Genet.* **58**, 1907.

Azibi, K., Bachner, L., Beckmann, J. S. et al. (1993). Severe childhood autosomal recessive muscular dystrophy with the deficiency of the 50 kDa dystrophin-associated glycoprotein maps to chromosome 13q12. *Hum. Mol. Genet.* **2**, 1423–1428.

Bacon, P. and Smith, B. (1971). Familial muscular dystrophy of late onset. *J. Neurol. Neurosurg. Psychiatry* **34**, 93–97.

Baghdiguian, S., Martin, M., Richard, I. et al. (1999). Calpain 3 deficiency is associated with myonuclear apoptosis and profound perturbation of the IκBα/NF-κB pathway in limb-girdle muscular dystrophy type 2A. *Nat. Med.* **5**, 503–511.

Bashir, R., Strachan, T., Keers, S. et al. (1994). A gene for autosomal recessive limb-girdle muscular dystrophy maps to chromosome 2. *Hum. Mol. Genet.* **3**, 455–457.

Bashir, R., Keers, S., Strachan, T. et al. (1996). Genetic and physical mapping at the limb-girdle muscular dystrophy locus (*LGMD2B*) on chromosome 2p. *Genomics* **33**, 46–52.

Bashir, R., Britton, S., Strachan, T. et al. (1998). A gene related to *Caenorhabditis elegans* spermatogenesis factor Fer-1 is mutated in limb-girdle muscular dystrophy type 2B. *Nat. Genet.* **20**, 37–42.

Beckmann, J. S., Richard, I., Hillaire, D. et al. (1991). A gene for limb-girdle muscular dystrophy maps to chromosome 15 by linkage. *C. R. Acad. Sci. (Paris) Ser. III*, **312**, 141–148.

Beckmann, J., Brown, R., Muntoni, F., Urtizberea, A., Bonnemann, C. and Bushby, K. (1999). Workshop report: the 66th/67th ENMC sponsored workshop the limb-girdle muscular dystrophies. *Neuromusc. Disord.* **9**, 436–445.

Bejaoui, K., Hirabayashi, K., Hentati, F. et al. (1995). Linkage of Miyoshi myopathy (distal autosomal recessive muscular dystrophy) locus to chromosome 2p12–14. *Neurology* **45**, 768–772.

Ben Hamida, M. and Fardeau, M. (1980). Severe, autosomal recessive, limb-girdle muscular dystrophies frequent in Tunisia. In: *Muscular Dystrophy Research: Advances and New Trends*, eds. C. Angelini, G. A. Danieli and D. Fontanari, pp. 143–146. Amsterdam: Excerpta Medica.

Ben Hamida, M., Fardeau, M. and Attia, N. (1983). Severe childhood muscular dystrophy affecting both sexes and frequent in Tunisia. *Muscle Nerve* **6**, 469–480.

Ben Hamida, M., Ben Hamida, C., Zouari, M., Belal, S. and Hentati, F. (1996). Limb-girdle muscular dystrophy 2C: clinical aspects. *Neuromusc. Disord.* **6**, 493–494.

Ben, Jelloun-Dellagi, S., Chafey, P. et al. (1990). Presence of normal dystrophin in Tunisian severe childhood autosomal recessive muscular dystrophy. *Neurology* **40**, 1903.

Ben Othmane, K., Ben Hamida, M., Pericak-Vance, M. et al. (1992). Linkage of Tunisian autosomal recessive Duchenne-like muscular dystrophy to the pericentromeric region of chromosome 13q. *Nat. Genet.* **2**, 315–317.

Ben Othmane, K., Speer, M. C., Stauffer, J. et al. (1995). Evidence for linkage disequilibrium in chromosome 13–Linked Duchenne-like muscular distrophy (LGMD2C). *Am. J. Hum. Genet.* **57**, 732–734.

Bittner, R., Anderson, L., Burkhard, E. et al. (1999). Dysferlin deletion in SJL mice defines a naturally occurring model for limb girdle muscular dystrophy type 2B. *Nat. Genet.* **23**, 141–142.

Bonne, G. B., Di Barletta, M. R., Varnous, S., et al. (1999). Mutations in the gene encoding lamin A/C cause autosomal dominant Emery–Dreifuss muscular dystrophy. *Nat. Genet.* **21**, 285–288.

Bönnemann, C. G., Modi, R., Noguchi, S. et al. (1995). Beta-sarcoglycan (A3b) mutations cause autosomal recessive muscular dystrophy with loss of the sarcoglycan complex. *Nat. Genet.* **11**, 266–273.

Bönnemann, C. G., Passos-Bueno, M. R., McNally, E. M. et al. (1996). Genomic screening for beta-sarcoglycan gene mutations: missense mutations may cause severe limb-girdle muscular dystrophy type 2E (LGMD2E). *Hum. Mol. Genet.* **5**, 1953–1961.

Bönnemann, C. G., Wong, J., Ben Hamida, C., Hamida, M. B., Hentati, F. and Kunkel, L. M. (1998). LGMD2E in Tunisia is caused by a homozygous missense mutation in beta-sarcoglycan exon 3. *Neuromusc. Disord.* **8**, 193–197.

Brooke, M. (1977). A clinician's view of neuromuscular diseases. Baltimore, MD: Williams and Wilkins.

Bushby, K. and Beckmann, J. (1995). Workshop report: the 30th and 31st ENMC International workshop on the limb-girdle muscular dystrophies, and proposal for a new nomenclature. *Neuromusc. Disord.* **5**, 337–344.

Carrié, A., Piccolo, F., Leturcq, F. et al. (1997). Mutational diversity and hot spots in the alpha-sarcoglycan gene in autosomal recessive muscular dystrophy (LGMD2D). *J. Med. Genet.* **34**, 470–475.

Chou, F., Angelini, C., Daentl, D. et al. (1999). Calpain III mutation analysis of a heterogeneous limb-girdle muscular dystrophy population. *Neurology* **52**, 1015–1020.

Coral-Vazquez, R., Cohn, R., Moore, S. et al. (1999). Disruption of the sarcoglycan-sarcospan complex in vascular smooth muscle: a novel mechanism in the pathogenesis of cardiomyopathy and muscular dystrophy. *Cell* **98**, 465–474.

Crosbie, R. H., Yamada, H., Venzke, D. P., Lisanti, M. P. and Campbell, K. P. (1998). Caveolin-3 is not an integral component of the dystrophin glycoprotein complex. *FEBS Lett.* **427**, 2792–82.

Crosbie, R., Yamada, H., Venzke, D., Lisanti, M. and Campbell, K. (1999). Membrane targeting and stabilization of sarcospan is mediated by the sarcoglycan subcomplex. *J. Cell Biol.* **145**, 153–165.

de Coster, W., de Reuck, J. and Thiery, E. (1974). A late autosomal dominant form of limb-girdle muscular dystrophy; a clinical genetic, and morphological study. *Eur. Neurol.* **12**, 159–172.

Dinçer, P., Leturcq, F., Richard, I. et al. (1997). A biochemical, genetic, and clinical survey of autosomal recessive limb girdle muscular dystrophies in Turkey. *Ann. Neurol.* **42**, 222–229.

Driss, A., Amouri, R., Ben Hamida, C. et al. (2000). A new locus for autosomal recessive limb-girdle muscular dystrophy in a large consanguineous Tunisian family maps to chromosome 19q13.3. *Neuromusc. Disord.* **10**, 240–246.

Duclos, F., Broux, O., Bourg, N. et al. (1998a). Beta-sarcoglycan: genomic analysis and identification of a novel missense mutation in the LGMD2E Amish isolate. *Neuromusc. Disord.* **8**, 30–38.

Duclos, F., Straub, V., Moore, S. A. et al. (1998b). Progressive muscular dystrophy in alpha-sarcoglycan-deficient mice. *J. Cell Biol.* **142**, 1461–1471.

Duggan, D. J., Gorospe, J. R., Fanin, M., Hoffman, E. P. and Angelini, C. (1997a). Mutations in the sarcoglycan genes in patients with myopathy. *N. Eng. J. Med.* **336**, 618–624.

Duggan, D., Manchester, D., Stears, K., Mathews, D., Hart, C. and Hoffmann, E. (1997b). Mutations in the delta sarcoglycan gene are a rare cause of autosomal recessive limb-girdle muscular dystrophy (LGMD2). *Neurogenetics* **1**, 49–58.

El Kerch, F., Sefiani, A., Azibi, K. et al. (1994). Linkage analysis of families with severe childhood autosomal recessive muscular dystrophy (SCARMD) in Morocco indicates genetic homogeneity of the disease in North-Africa. *J. Med. Genet.* **31**, 342–343.

Emery, A. E. H. (1991). Population frequencies of inherited neuromuscular diseases – a world survey (Review). *Neuromusc. Disord.* **1**, 19–29.

Erb, W. (1884). Ueber die 'Juvenile Form' des progressiven Muskelatrophie ihre Beziehungen zur sogennten Pseudohypetrophie der Muskeln. *Dtsch. Arch. Klin. Med.* **34**, 467–519.

Ervasti, J. M. and Campbell, K. P. (1991). Membrane organization of the dystrophin–glycoprotein complex. *Cell* **66**, 1121–1131.

Ervasti, J. M., Ohlendieck, K., Kahl, S. D., Gaver, M. G. and Campbell, K. P. (1990). Deficiency of a glycoprotein component of the dystrophin complex in dystrophic muscle. *Nature* **345**, 315–319.

Ettinger, A. J., Feng, G. and Sanes, J. R. (1997). Epsilon-sarcoglycan, a broadly expressed homologue of the gene mutated in limb-girdle muscular dystrophy 2D. *J. Biol. Chem.* **272**, 32534–32538.

Eymard, B., Romero, N. B., Leturcq, F. et al. (1997). Primary adhalinopathy (alpha-sarcoglycanopathy): clinical, pathological and genetic correlation in twenty patients with autosomal recessive muscular dystrophy. *Neurology* **48**, 1227–1234.

Fadic, R., Waclawik, A. J., Lewandoski, P. J. and Lotz, B. P. (1997). Muscle pathology and clinical features of the sarcolemmopathies. *Pediatr. Neurol.* **16**, 79–82.

Fang, W., Huang, C., Chu, N., Chen, C., Lu, C. and Wang, C. (1997). Childhood onset autosomal dominant limb girdle muscular dystrophy with cardiac conduction block. *Muscle Nerve* **20**, 286–292.

Fanin, M., Duggan, D. J., Mostacciuolo, M. L. et al. (1997). Genetic epidemiology of muscular dystrophies resulting from sarcoglycan gene mutations. *J. Med. Genet.* **34**, 973–977.

Fardeau, M., Matsumura, K., Tomé, F. M. S. et al. (1993). Deficiency of the 50kDa dystrophin associated glycoprotein (adhalin) in severe autosomal recessive muscular dystrophies in children native from European countries. *C. R. Acad. Sci. Paris: Sci.* **316**, 799–804.

Fardeau, M., Hillaire, D., Mignard, C. et al. (1996a). Juvenile limbgirdle muscular dystrophy. Clinical, histopathological and genetic data from a small community living in the Reunion island. *Brain* **119**, 295–308.

Fardeau, M., Eymard, B., Mignard, C., Tomé, F., Richard, I. and Beckmann, J. (1996b). Chromosome15-linked limb girdle muscular dystrophy: clinical phenotypes in Reunion island and French metropolitan communities. *Neuromusc. Disord.* **6**, 447–453.

Feit, H., Silbergleit, A., Schneider, L. et al. (1998). Vocal cord and pharyngeal weakness with autosomal dominant distal myopathy: clinical description and gene localization to 5q31. *Am. J. Hum. Genet.* **63**, 1732–1742.

Fougerousse, F., Durand, M., Suel, L. et al. (1998). Expression of genes (CAPN3, SGCA, SGCB, and TTN) involved in progressive muscular dystrophies during early human development. *Genomics* **48**, 145–156.

Fougerousse, F., Anderson, L., Delezoide, A.-L., Suel, L., Durand, M. and Beckmann, J. S (1999). Calpain expression during human cardiogenesis. *Neuromusc. Disord.* **10**, 251–256.

Gilchrist, J., Pericak-Vance, M., Silverman, L. and Roses, A. (1988). Clinical and genetic investigation in autosomal dominant limbgirdle muscular dystrophy. *Neurology* **38**, 5–9.

Grady, R., Grange, R., Lau, K. et al. (1999). Role for alpha-dystrobrevin on the pathogenesis of dystrophin-dependent muscular dystrophies. *Nat. Cell Biol.* **1**, 215–220.

Greelish, J. P., Su, L. T., Lankford, E. B. et al. (1999). Stable restoration of the sarcoglycan complex in dystrophic muscle perfused with histamine and a recombinant adeno-associated viral vector. *Nat. Med.* **5**, 439–443.

Gussoni, E., Soneoka, Y., Strickland, C. et al. (1999). Dystrophin expression in the *mdx* mouse retored by stem cell transplantation. *Nature* **401**, 390–394.

Hack, A. A., Ly, C. T., Jiang, F. et al. (1998). Gamma-sarcoglycan deficiency leads to muscle membrane defects and apoptosis independent of dystrophin. *J. Cell Biol.* **142**, 1279–1287.

Hauser, M., Salminkangas, P., Horrigan, S. et al. (1999). Positional cloning of the gene responsible for limb girdle muscular dystrophy 1A. *Am. J. Hum. Genet.* **65** (Suppl.), A109.

Hauser, M. A., Horrigan, S. K., Salmikangas, P. et al. (2000). Myotilin is mutated in limb girdle muscular dystrophy 1A. *Hum. Mol. Genet.* **9**, 2141–2147.

Hayashi, Y. K. and Arahata, K. (1997). The frequency of patients with adhalin deficiency in a muscular dystrophy patient population. *Nippon Rinsho* **55**, 3165–3168.

Henry, M. and Campbell, K. (1998). A role for dystroglycan in basement membrane assembly. *Cell* **95**, 859–870.

Higuchi, I., Iwaki, H., Kawai, H. et al. (1997). New missense mutation in the alpha-sarcoglycan gene in a Japanese patient with severe childhood autosomal recessive muscular dystrophy with incomplete alpha-sarcoglycan deficiency. *J. Neurol. Sci.* **153**, 100–105.

Higuchi, I., Kawai, H., Umaki, Y. et al. (1998). Different manners of sarcoglycan expression in genetically proven alpha-sarcoglycan deficiency and gamma-sarcoglycan deficiency. *Acta Neuropathol.* **96**, 202–206.

Holt, K. and Campbell, K. (1998). Assembly of the sarcoglycan complex. Insights for muscular dystrophy. *J. Biol. Chem.* **23**, 34667–34670.

Holt, K. H., Lim, L. E., Straub, V. et al. (1998). Functional rescue of the sarcoglycan complex in the BIO 14.6 hamster using delta-sarcoglycan gene transfer. *Mol. Cell.* **1**, 841–848.

Ikeuchi, T., Asaka, T., Saito, M. et al. (1997). Gene locus for autosomal recessive distal myopathy with rimmed vacuoles maps to chromosome 9. *Ann. Neurol.* **41**, 432–437.

Illarioshkin, S., Ivanova-Smolenskaya, I., Tanaka, H. et al. (1996). Clinical and molecular analysis of a large family with three distinct phenotypes of progressive muscular dystrophy. *Brain* **119**, 1895–1909.

Jackson, C. and Carey, J. (1961). Progressive muscular dystrophy: autosomal recessive type. *Pediatrics* **28**, 77–84.

Jackson, C. and Strehler, D. (1968). Limb-girdle muscular dystrophy: clinical manifestations and detection of preclinical disease. *Pediatrics* **41**, 495–502.

Jones, K. J. and North, K. N. (1997). Recent advances in diagnosis of the childhood muscular dystrophies. *J. Paediatr. Child. Health* **33**, 195–201.

Jones, K. J., Kim, S. S. and North, K. N. (1998). Abnormalities of dystrophin, the sarcoglycans, and laminin alpha2 in the muscular dystrophies. *J. Med. Genet.* **35**, 379–386.

Jung, D., Duclos, F., Apostol, B. et al. (1996). Characterization of delta-sarcoglycan, a novel component of the oligomeric sarcoglycan complex involved in limb-girdle muscular dystrophy. *J. Biol. Chem.* **271**, 32321–32329.

Kawai, H., Akaike, M., Endo, T. et al. (1995). Adhalin gene mutations in patients with autosomal recesssive childhood onset muscular dystrophy with adhalin deficiency. *J. Clin. Invest.* **96**, 1202–1207.

Lasa, A., Piccolo, F., de Diego, C. et al. (1998). Severe limb girdle muscular dystrophy in Spanish gypsies: further evidence for a founder mutation in the gamma-sarcoglycan gene. *Eur. J. Hum. Genet.* **6**, 396–399.

Lefebvre, S., Bürglen, L., Reboullet, S. et al. (1995). Identification and characterization of a spinal muscular atrophy-determining gene. *Cell* **80**, 155–165.

Levison, H. (1951). Dystrophia musculorum progressiva. *Acta Psychiatr. Neurol. Scand.* **76**, 7–17.

Lim, L. and Campbell, K. (1998). The sarcoglycan complex in limb-girdle muscular dystrophy. *Curr. Opin. Neurol.* **11**, 443–452.

Lim, L. E., Duclos, F., Broux, O., et al. (1995). β-Sarcoglycan: characterization and role in limb-girdle muscular dystrophy linked to 4q12. *Nat. Genet.* **11**, 257–285.

Linssen, W., Notermans, N., van der Graaf, Y. et al. (1997). Miyoshi-type distal muscular dystrophy. Clinical spectrum in 24 Dutch patients. *Brain* **120**, 1989–1996.

Linssen, W., de Visser, M., Notermans, N. et al. (1998). Genetic heterogeneity in Miyoshi-type distal muscular dystrophy. *Neuromusc. Disord.* **8**, 317–320.

Liu, J., Aoki, M., Illa, I., et al. (1998). Dysferlin, a novel skeletal muscle gene, is mutated in Miyoshi myopathy and limb girdle muscular dystrophy. *Nat. Genet.* **20**, 31–36.

Ljunggren, A., Duggan, D., McNally, E. et al. (1995). Primary adhalin deficiency as a cause of muscular dystrophy in patients with normal dystrophin. *Ann. Neurol.* **38**, 367–372.

Mahjneh, I., Vannelli, G., Bushby, K. and Marconi, G. (1992). A large inbred Palestinian family with two forms of muscular dystrophy. *Neuromusc. Disord.* **2**, 277–283.

Mahjneh, I., Passos-Bueno, M., Zatz, M. et al. (1996). The phenotype of chromosome 2p-linked limb-girdle muscular dystrophy. *Neuromusc. Disord.* **6**, 483–490.

Markesbery, W. R., Griggs, R. C. and Herr, B. (1977). Distal myopathy: electron microscopic and histochemical studies. *Neurology* **27**, 727–735.

Matsuda, C., Aoki, M., Hayashi, Y. K., Ho, M. F., Arahata, K. and Brown, R. H. Jr (1999). Dysferlin is a surface membrane-associated protein that is absent in Miyoshi myopathy. *Neurology* **53**, 1119–1122.

Matsumura, K. and Campbell, K. P. (1994). Dystrophin-glycoprotein complex: its role in the molecular pathogenesis of muscular dystrophies. *Muscle Nerve* **17**, 2–15.

Matsumura, K., Tomé, F. M. S., Collin, H. et al. (1992). Deficiency of the 50kDa dystrophin-associated glycoprotein in severe childhood autosomal recessive muscular dystrophy. *Nature* **359**, 320–322.

McKusick, V. A. (1998). *Mendelian Inheritance in Man. Catalogs of Human Genes and Genetic Disorders*, 12th edn. Baltimore, MD: Johns Hopkins University Press.

McNally, E. M., Yoshida, M., Mizuno, Y., Ozawa, E. and Kunkel, L. M. (1994). Human adhalin is alternatively spliced and the gene is located on chromosome 17q21. *Proc. Natl. Acad. Sci. USA* **91**, 9690–9694.

McNally, E. M., Passos-Bueno, M. R., Bonnemann, C. G. et al. (1996a). Mild and severe muscular dystrophy caused by a single gamma-sarcoglycan mutation. *Am. J. Hum. Genet.* **59**, 1040–1047.

McNally, E. M., Duggan, D., Gorospe, J. R. et al. (1996b). Mutations that disrupt the carboxyl-terminus of gamma-sarcoglycan cause muscular dystrophy. *Hum. Mol. Genet.* **5**, 1841–1847.

McNally, E. M., Ly, C. T. and Kunkel, L. M. (1998a). Human epsilon-sarcoglycan is highly related to alpha-sarcoglycan (adhalin), the limb girdle muscular dystrophy 2D gene. *FEBS Lett.* **422**, 27–32.

McNally, E., de Sa Moreira, E., Duggan, D. et al. (1998b). Caveolin-3 in muscular dystrophy. *Hum. Mol. Genet.* **7**, 871–877.

Melacini, P., Fanin, M., Duggan, D. et al. (1999). Heart involvement in muscular dystrophies due to sacoglycan gene mutations. *Muscle Nerve* **22**, 473–479.

Merlini, L., Kaplan, J. C., Navarro, C., Barois, A. et al. (2000). Homogeneous phenotype of the Gypsy limb-girdle MD with the gamma-sarcoglycan C283Y mutation. *Neurology*, **54**, 1075–1079.

Messina, D. N., Speer, M. C., Pericak-Vance, M. A. and McNally, E. M. (1997). Linkage of familial dilated cardiomyopathy with conduction defect and muscular dystrophy to chromosome 6q23. *Am. J. Hum. Genet.* **61**, 909–917.

Metzinger, L., Blake, D. J., Squier, M. V. et al. (1997). Dystrobrevin deficiency at the sarcolemma of patients with muscular dystrophy. *Hum. Mol. Genet.* **6**, 1185–1191.

Miladi, N., Bourguignon, J. P. and Hentati, F. (1999). Cognitive and psychological profile of a Tunisian population of limb girdle muscular dystrophy. *Neuromusc. Disord.* **9**, 352–354.

Minetti, C., Sotgia, F., Bruno, C. et al. (1998). Mutations in the caveolin-3 gene cause autosomal dominant limb-girdle muscular dystrophy. *Nat. Genet.* **18**, 365–368.

Mitrani-Rosenbaum, S., Argov, Z., Blumenfeld, A., Seidman, C. E. and Seidman, J. G. (1996). Hereditary inclusion body myopathy maps to chromosome 9p1-q1. *Hum. Mol. Genet.* **5**, 159–163.

Morandi, L., Barresi, R., Di Blasi, C. et al. (1996). Clinical heterogeneity of adhalin deficiency. *Ann. Neurol.* **39**, 196–202.

Moreira, E., Vainzof, M., Marie, S., Sertié, A., Zatz, M. and Passos-Bueno, M. (1997). The seventh form of autosomal recessive limb-girdle muscular dystrophy is mapped to 17q11–12. *Am. J. Hum. Genet.* **61**, 151–159.

Moreira, E., Vainzof, M., Marie, S., Nigro, V., Zatz, M. and Passos-Bueno, M. (1998). A first missense mutation in the delta-sarcoglycan gene associated with a severe phenotype and frequency of limb-girdle muscular dystrophy type 2F (LGMD2F) among Brazilian sarcoglycanopathies. *J. Med. Genet.* **35**, 951–963.

Moreira, E. S., Wiltshire, T. J., Faulkner, G. et al. (2000). Limb-girdle muscular dystrophy type 2G is caused by mutations in the gene encoding the sarcomeric protein telethonin. *Nat. Genet.* **24**, 163–166.

Muchir, A., Bonne, G., van der Kooi, A. J. et al. (2000). Identification of mutations in the genes encoding lamins A/C in autosomal dominant limb-girdle muscular dystrophy with atrioventricular conductance disturbances. *Hum. Mol. Genet.* **9**, 1453–1459.

Muntoni, F., Lichtarowicz-Krynska, E. J., Sewry, C. A. et al. (1998). Early presentation of X-linked Emery–Dreifuss muscular dystrophy resembling limb-girdle muscular dystrophy. *Neuromusc. Disord.* **8**, 72–76.

Naom, I., D'Alessandro, M., Sewry, C. A. et al. (1998). Laminin alpha 2-chain gene mutations in two siblings presenting with limb-girdle muscular dystrophy. *Neuromusc. Disord.* **8**, 495–501.

Nicholson, L. V. B., Davison, K., Falkous, G. et al. (1989). Dystrophin in skeletal muscle I. Western blot analysis using a monoclonal antibody. *J. Neurol. Sci.* **94**, 125–136.

Nigro, V., Piluso, G., Belsito, A. et al. (1996a). Identification of a novel sarcoglycan gene at 5q33 encoding a sarcolemmal 35 kDa glycoprotein. *Hum. Mol. Genet.* **5**, 1179–1186.

Nigro, V., Moreira, E., Piluso, G. et al. (1996b). Autosomal recessive limb-girdle muscular dystrophy, LGMD2F, is caused by a mutation in the delta-sarcoglycan gene. *Nat. Genet.* **14**, 195–198.

Nigro, V., Okazaki, Y., Belsito, A. et al. (1997). Identification of the Syrian hamster cardiomyopathy gene. *Hum. Mol. Genet.* **6**, 601–607.

Noguchi, S., McNally, E., Ben Othmane, K., et al. (1995). Mutations in the dystrophin-associated protein gamma-sarcoglycan in chromosome 13 muscular dystrophy. *Science* **270**, 819–822.

Nonaka, I., Sunohara, N., Ishiura, S. and Satayoshi, E. (1981). Familial distal myopathy with rimmed vacuole and lamellar (myeloid) body formation. *J. Neurol. Sci.* **51**, 141–155.

Nonaka, I., Murakami, N., Suzuki, Y. and Kawai, M. (1998). Distal myopathy with rimmed vacuoles. *Neuromusc. Disord.* **8**, 333–337.

Ozawa, E., Yoshida, M., Suzuki, A., Mizuno, Y., Hagiwara, Y. and Noguchi, S. (1995). Dystrophin-associated proteins in muscular dystrophy. *Hum. Mol. Genet.* **4**, 1711–1716.

Ozawa, E., Noguchi, S., Mizuno, Y., Hagiwara, Y. and Yoshida, M. (1998). From dystrophinopathy to sarcoglycanopathy: evolution of a concept of muscular dystrophy. *Muscle Nerve* **21**, 421–438.

Passos-Bueno, M., Terwillinger, J., Ott, J. et al. (1991). Linkage analysis in families with autosomal recessive limb-girdle muscular. *Am. J. Med. Genet.* **38**, 140–146.

Passos-Bueno, M. R., Oliveira, J. R., Bakker, E. et al. (1993). Genetic heterogeneity for Duchenne-like muscular dystrophy (DLMD) based on linkage and 50 DAG analysis. *Hum. Mol. Genet.* **2**, 1945–1947.

Passos-Bueno, M. R., Moreira, E., Vainzof, M. et al. (1995). A common missense mutation in the adhalin gene in three unrelated Brazilian families with a relatively mild form of autosomal recessive limb-girdle muscular dystrophy. *Hum. Mol. Genet.* **4**, 1163–1167.

Passos-Bueno, M. R., Moreira, E. S., Marie, S. K. N. et al. (1996a). Main clinical features of the three mapped autosomal recessive limb-girdle muscular dystrophies and estimated proportion of each form in 13 Brazilian families. *J. Med. Genet.* **33**, 97–102.

Passos-Bueno, M. R., Moreira, E. S., Vainzof, M., Marie, S. K. and Zatz, M. (1996b). Linkage analysis in autosomal recessive limb-girdle muscular dystrophy (AR LGMD) maps a sixth form to 5q33–34 (LGMD2F) and indicates that there is at least one more subtype of AR LGMD. *Hum. Mol. Genet.* **5**, 815–820.

Passos-Bueno, M., Vainzof, M., Moreira, E. and Zatz, M. (1999). Seven autosomal recessive limb-girdle muscular dystrophies in the Brazilian population: from LGMD2A to LGMD2G. *Am. J. Med. Genet.* **82**, 392–398.

Penisson-Besnier, I., Richard, I., Beckmann, J. and Fardeau, M. (1998). Phenotypic variations of calpain deficiency in two siblings. *Muscle Nerve* **21**, 1078–1080.

Petrof, B. J., Shrager, J. B., Stedman, H. H., Kelly, A. M. and Sweeney, H. L. (1993). Dystrophin protects the sarcolemma from stresses developed during muscle contraction. *Proc. Natl. Acad. Sci. USA* **90**, 3710–3714.

Piccolo, F., Roberds, S. L., Jeanpierre, M. et al. (1995). Primary adhalinopathy: a common cause of autosomal recessive muscular dystrophy of variable severity. *Nat. Genet.* **10**, 243–245.

Piccolo, F., Jeanpierre, M., Leturcq, F. et al. (1996). A founder mutation in the gamma-sarcoglycan gene of Gypsies possibly predating their migration out of India. *Hum. Mol. Genet.* **5**, 2019–2022.

Richard, I., Broux, O., Allamand, V. et al. (1995). Mutations in the proteolytic enzyme calpain 3 cause limb-girdle muscular dystrophy type 2A. *Cell* **81**, 1–20.

Richard, I., Brenguier, L., Dinçer, P. et al. (1997). Multiple independent molecular etiology for limb girdle muscular dystrophy type 2A patients from various geographical origins. *Am. J. Hum. Genet.* **60**, 1128–1138.

Richard, I., Beckmann, J. and Fardeau, M. (1999a). Calpain 3 (p94) in limb-girdle muscular dystrophy type 2A. *Calpain: Pharmacology and Toxicology of Calcium-dependent Protease*, eds. Wang and Yuen, pp. 369–389. London: Taylor & Francis.

Richard, I., Roudaut, C., Saenz, A. et al. (1999b). Calpainopathy: a survey of mutations and polymorphisms. *Am. J. Hum. Genet.* **64**, 1524–1540.

Richard, I., Bourg, N., Marchand, S. et al. (1999c). A diagnostic fluorescent marker kit for six limb-girdle muscular dystrophies. *Neuromusc. Disord.* **9**, 555–563.

Richard, I., Roudaut, C., Marchand, S. et al. (2000). Loss of calpain 3 proteolytic activity leads to muscular dystrophy and to apoptosis-associated IκBα/nuclear factor κB pathway perturbation in Mice. *J. Cell Biol.* **151**, 1583–1590.

Roberds, S. L., Anderson, R. D., Ibraghimov-Beskrovnaya, O. and Campbell, K. P. (1993). Primary structure and muscle-specific expression of the 50-kDa dystrophin-associated glycoprotein (adhalin). *J. Biol. Chem.*, **268**, 23739–23742.

Roberds, S. L., Leturcq, F., Allamand, V. et al. (1994). Missense mutations in the adhalin gene linked to autosomal recessive muscular dystrophy. *Cell* **78**, 625–633.

Romero, N. B., Tomé, F. M. S., Leturcq, F. et al. (1994). Genetic heterogeneity of severe childhood autosomal recessive muscular dystrophy with adhalin (50 kDa dystrophin-associated glycoprotein) deficiency. *C. R. Acad. Sci. Paris: Sci.* **317**, 70–76.

Salih, M. A. M., Omer, M. I. A., Bayoumi, R. A., Karrar, O. and Johnson, M. (1983). Severe autosomal recessive muscular dystrophy in an extended Sudanese kindred. *Dev. Med. Child. Neurol.* **25**, 43–52.

Salmikangas, P., Mykkanen, O. M., Gronholm, M., Heiska, L., Kere, J. and Carpen, O. (1999). Myotilin, a novel sarcomeric protein with two Ig-like domains, is encoded by a candidate gene for limb-girdle muscular dystrophy. *Hum. Mol. Genet.* **8**, 1329–1336.

Satoyoshi, E. (1990). Distal myopathy. *Tohoku J. Exp. Med.* **161**(Suppl.), 1–19.

Schneiderman, L., Sampson, W., Schoene, W. and Haydon, G. (1969). Genetic studies of a family with two unusual autosomal dominant conditions: muscular dystrophy and Pelger–Huet anomaly. Clinical, pathologic and linkage considerations. *Am. J. Med.* **46**, 380–393.

Shokeir, M. and Kobrinsky, N. (1976). Autosomal recessive muscular dystrophy in Manitoba Hutterites. *Clin. Genet.* **9**, 197–202.

Shokeir, M. and Rozdilsky, B. (1985). Muscular dystrophy in Saskatchewan Hutterites. *Am. J. Med. Genet.* **22**, 487–493.

Song, K. S., Li, S., Okamoto, T., Quillam, L. A., Sargiacomo, M. and Lisanti, M. P. (1996). Co-purification and direct activation of Ras with caveolin, an integral membrane protein of caveolae microdomains. Detergent-free purification of caveolae microdomains. *J. Biol. Chem.* **271**, 9690–9697.

Sorimachi, H., Imajoh-Ohmi, S., Emori, Y. et al. (1989). Molecular cloning of a novel mammalian calcium-dependent protease distinct from both m- and mu-type. Specific expression of the mRNA in skeletal muscle. *J. Biol. Chem.* **264**, 20106–2011.

Speer, M. C., Yamaoka, L. H., Gilchrist, J. H. et al. (1992). Confirmation of genetic heterogeneity in limb-girdle muscular dystrophy: linkage of an autosomal dominant form to chromosome 5q. *Am. J. Hum. Genet.* **50**, 1211–1217.

Speer, M. C., Gilchrist, J. M., Stajich, J. M. et al. (1998). Evidence for anticipation in autosomal dominant limb-girdle muscular dystrophy. *J. Med. Genet.* **35**, 305–308.

Speer, M., Vance, J., Grubber, J., et al. (1999). Identification of a new autosomal dominant limb-girdle muscular dystrophy locus on chromosome 7. *Am. J. Hum. Genet.* **64**, 556–562.

Spencer, M. J., Tidball, J. G., Anderson, L. V. et al. (1997). Absence of calpain 3 in a form of limb-girdle muscular dystrophy (LGMD2A). *J. Neurol. Sci.* **146**, 173–178.

Stevenson, A. (1953). Muscular dystrophy in Northern Ireland. *Ann. Eugen.* **18**, 50–91.

Straub, V. and Campbell, K. (1997). Muscular dystrophies and the dystrophin–glycoprotein complex. *Curr. Opin. Neurol.* **10**, 168–175.

Straub, V., Rafael, J., Chamberlain, J. and Campbell, K. (1997). Animal models for muscular dystrophy show different patterns of sarcolemmal disruption. *J. Cell Biol.* **139**, 375–385.

Straub, V., Ettinger, A. J., Durbeej, M. et al. (1999). Epsilon-sarcoglycan replaces alpha-sarcoglycan in smooth muscle to form a unique dystrophin-glycoprotein complex. *J. Biol. Chem.* **274**, 27989–27996.

Tan, E., Topaloglu, H., Sewry, C. et al. (1997). Late onset muscular dystrophy with cerebral white matter changes due to partial merosin deficiency. *Neuromusc. Disord.* **7**, 85–89.

Thompson, T., Watkins, S., Chan, Y. et al. (1999). Filamin 2, a muscle specific form of filamin, interacts with γ-sarcoglycan, a member of the dystrophin glycoprotein complex. *Am. J. Hum. Genet.* **65**(Suppl.), 1113.

Topaloglu, H., Dinçer, P., Richard, I. et al. (1997). Calpain-3 deficiency causes a mild muscular dystrophy in childhood. *Neuropediatrics* **28**, 212–216.

Udd, B., Partanen, J., Halonen, P. et al. (1993). Tibial muscular dystrophy. Late adult-onset distal myopathy in 66 Finnish patients. *Arch. Neurol.* **50**, 604–608.

Urtasun, M., Saenz, A., Roudaut, C. et al. (1998). Limb-girdle muscular dystrophy in Guipuzcoa (Basque country, Spain). *Brain* **121**, 1735–1747.

Vainzof, M., Passos-Bueno, M. R., Canovas, M. et al. (1996). The sarcoglycan complex in the six autosomal recessive limb-girdle muscular dystrophies. *Hum. Mol. Genet.* **5**, 1963–1969.

Vainzof, M., Passos-Bueno, M., Pavanello, S., Oliveira, A. and Zatz, M. (1999). Sarcoglyanopathies are responsible for 68% of severe autosomal recessive limb-girdle muscular dystrophy in the Brazilian population. *J. Neurol. Sci.* **164**, 44–49.

van der Kooi, A., Ledderhof, T., de Voogt, W. et al. (1996). A newly recognized autosomal dominant limb girdle muscular dystrophy with cardiac involvement. *Ann. Neurol.* **39**, 636–642.

van der Kooi, A. J., Meegen, M. V., Ledderhof, T. M., McNally, E. M., de Visser, M. and Bolhuis, P. A. (1997). Genetic localization of a newly recognized autosomal dominant limb-girdle muscular dystrophy with cardiac involvement (LGMD1B) to chromosome 1q11–21. *Am. J. Hum. Genet.* **60**, 891–895.

van der Kooi, A. J., de Visser, M., van Meegen, M. et al. (1998a). A novel gamma-sarcoglycan mutation causing childhood onset, slowly progressive limb girdle muscular dystrophy. *Neuromusc. Disord.* **8**, 305–308.

van der Kooi, A. J., de Voogt, W. G., Barth, P. G. et al. (1998b). The heart in limb girdle muscular dystrophy. *Heart* **79**, 73–77.

Walton, J. N. and Nattrass, F. J. (1954). On the classification , natural history and treatment of the myopathies. *Brain* **77**, 169–231.

Weiler, T., Grennberg, C., Nylen, E. et al. (1996). Limb-girdle musular dystrophy and Miyoshi myopathy in an aboriginal Canadian kindred map to LGMD2B and segregate with the same haplotype. *Am. J. Hum. Genet.* **59**, 872–878.

Weiler, T., Greenberg, C., Nylen, E. et al. (1997). Limb girdle muscular dystrophy in Manitoba Hutterites does not map to any of the known LGMD loci. *Am. J. Med. Genet.* **72**, 363–368.

Weiler, T., Grennberg, C., Zelinski, T. et al. (1998). A gene for autosomal recessive limb-girdle muscular dystrophy in Manitoba Hutterites maps to chromosome region 9q31-q33: evidence for another limb-girdle muscular dystrophy locus. *Am. J. Hum. Genet.* **63**, 140–147.

Weiler, T., Bashir, R., Anderson, L. et al. (1999). Identical mutation in patients with limb girdle muscular dystrophy type 2B or Miyoshi myopathy suggests a role for modifier gene(s). *Hum. Mol. Genet.* **8**, 871–877.

Williamson, R. A., Henry, M. D., Daniels, K. J. et al. (1997). Dystroglycan is essential for early embryonic development: Disruption of Reichert's membrane in Dag1-null mice. *Hum. Mol. Genet.* **6**, 831–841.

Wolf, U. (1997). Identical mutations and phenotypic variations. *Hum. Genet.* **100**, 305–321.

Yamaoka, L. H., Westbrook, C. A., Speer, M. C. et al. (1994). Development of a microsatellite genetic map spanning 5q31-q33 and subsequent placement of the LGMD1A locus between D5S178 and IL9. *Neuromusc. Disord.* **4**, 471–475.

Yasunaga, S., Grati, M., Cohen-Salmon, M., et al. (1999). A mutation in OTOF, encoding otoferlin, a Fer-1-like protein, causes DFNB9, a nonsyndromic form of deafness. *Nat. Genet.* **21**, 363–369 .

Yoshida, M., Suzuki, A., Yamamoto, H., Noguchi, S., Mizuno, Y. and Ozawa, E. (1994). Dissociation of the complex of dystrophin and its associated proteins into several unique groups by n-octyl-β-ᴅ-glucoside. *Eur. J. Biochem.* **222**, 1055–1061.

21

Facioscapulohumeral dystrophy

Rabi Tawil and Robert C. Griggs

Introduction

Facioscapulohumeral muscular dystrophy (FSHD) has an estimated prevalence of 1:20000 and is the third most common form of muscular dystrophy after Duchenne and myotonic muscular dystrophies (Padberg, 1982). It is characterized by a distinctive, initially restricted pattern of muscle weakness. Disease progression is generally slow and, in the absence of respiratory, cardiac or bulbar involvement, life expectancy is unaffected. There is however, extreme variability relative to age of onset, degree of muscle weakness and rate of progression. The spectrum of clinical manifestations ranges from asymptomatic facial or scapular weakness to severe limb weakness with early loss of ambulation in the infantile form. As many as 20% of affected individuals eventually become wheelchair bound.

Genetics

FSHD is an autosomal dominant disorder with a high frequency of sporadic cases (Padberg et al., 1995). Penetrance is virtually complete, with greater than 95% of affected individuals showing clinical signs by the age of 20 years (Padberg, 1982). FSHD is linked to chromosome 4q35, where a subtelomeric rearrangement has been identified (Wijmenga et al., 1992). This rearrangement consists of deletions of an integral number of copies of a 3.3 kb DNA repeat named D4Z4 (van Deutekom et al., 1993). Thus individuals with FSHD have 10 or fewer repeats whereas unaffected individuals have 15 or more repeat elements. It was initially assumed that the deletions disrupted expressed gene sequences and that the gene for FSHD must, therefore, lie within the disrupted 3.3 kb repeats. However, no transcribed gene sequences have been identified within these repeat elements (Tawil and Griggs,

1997). Moreover, analysis of the sequence of the repeats show high homology to L Sau DNA, a family of heterochromatic repeats that is highly compacted and transcriptionally inactive (Winokur et al., 1994). This finding has led to the hypothesis that deletion of a critical number of repeats may influence the expression of a distant gene(s), a mechanism referred to a position effect variegation (Winokur et al., 1994). Since no expressed sequences are known to be present distal to the repeats, current research is focused on identifying genes centromeric to the 3.3 kb repeats that display altered expression in muscle from affected individuals. A case report of an individual with a chromosomal aberration resulting in a single copy (haploinsufficiency) of 4q35 but showing no signs of FSHD suggests that mutations within D4Z4 in FSHD result in a deleterious gain of function (Tupler et al., 1996).

Clinical features

FSHD is characterized by early, usually asymptomatic, facial weakness followed sequentially and in a descending fashion by scapular fixator, humeral, truncal and lower extremity weakness. Progression is usually slow and gradual, although many patients describe a relapsing progressive course. Some patients also describe episodes of rapid loss of function in a particular muscle heralded by severe pain in the affected limb. Individuals with infantile-onset FSHD are severely disabled at an early age (Bakker et al., 1995).

The most common presenting symptom is weakness of scapular fixators resulting in visible winging of the scapulae or difficulty lifting the arms overhead. Further questioning may elicit a long-standing difficulty climbing rope or doing push-ups. Most of these patients have co-existing, at times asymptomatic, facial weakness, with a history of

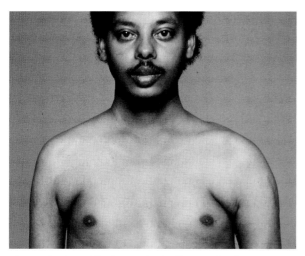

Fig. 21.1. Patient with FSHD and typical myopathic facies, straight clavicles and pectoral wasting with axillary creases.

difficulty whistling and drinking through a straw. They are often observed sleeping with their eyes partially open. Striking bifacial weakness, often misdiagnosed as Mobius syndrome, can be the presenting symptom in infantile FSHD. In some patients, the presenting symptom is tripping or inability to run, secondary to footdrop. These individuals have co-existing, asymptomatic facial and scapular fixator weakness. Although lower extremity involvement is initially distal, proximal lower extremity weakness is present in many patients and can be more severe than distal weakness.

On inspection, patients with FSHD have widened palpebral fissures and decreased facial expression (Fig. 21.1). The lips are pouted and dimples appear at the corners of the mouth. The shoulders are rounded, forward sloping and the clavicles are straight (Fig. 21.1). The scapulae are widely set and may wing even at rest. With more severe upper extremity weakness, the humeral musculature may be atrophic relative to the forearm, producing the 'Popeye' arm appearance (Fig. 21.2). The pectoral muscles may be atrophic and an axillary crease is often evident. The abdomen is often protruberant and there is increased lumbar lordosis (Fig. 21.3).

Examination confirms facial weakness, with an inability to bury lashes, a transverse smile and inability to purse lips. Lower facial (orbicularis oris) weakness is usually more pronounced than weakness of eye closure (orbicularis oculi). Extraocular, eyelid, tongue, masseter and bulbar muscles are normal. Neck flexion is preserved early on relative to extensors. If not present at rest, scapulae wing with arm abduction or forward flexion. Because of preferential weakness of the lower trapezius, the scapulae

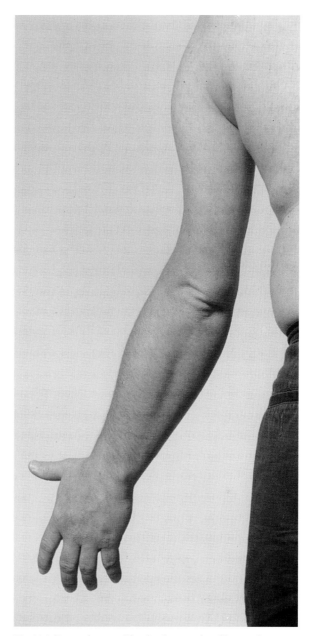

Fig. 21.2. 'Popeye' arms with selective atrophy of humeral muscles and preservation of forearm muscle bulk.

often jut upwards (Fig. 21.4). Manual fixation of the scapulae to the chest wall results in significant improvement in the patient's ability to lift the arm. Even with severe wasting of the scapular fixators and humeral (triceps, biceps) muscles, the deltoids remain intact. Distally, wrist extensors may become involved. Weakness of the abdominal wall musculature results in difficulty sitting up from a supine position. The lower abdominal muscles are selectively affected, resulting in a striking upward movement of

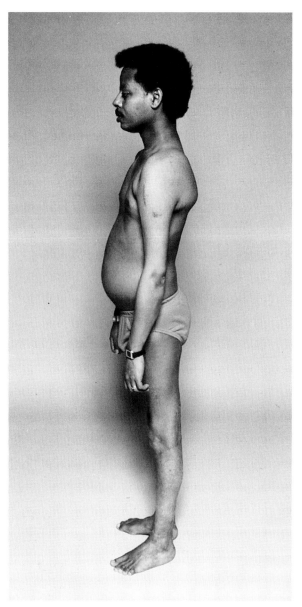

Fig. 21.3. Patient with advanced FSHD demonstrating scapular winging at rest, forward sloping of the shoulders weak abdominal muscles, with resultant protuberant abdomen, and atrophy of the thigh muscles.

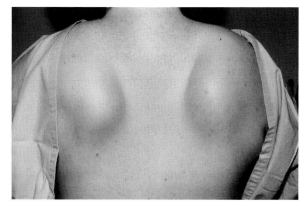

Fig. 21.4. Weakness of the scapular fixators demonstrated on attempted forward flexion of the arm with winging of the scapulae. Note also the upward jutting of the scapulae as a result of preferential involvement of the lower trapezius.

the umbilicus when flexing the neck in a supine position (Beevor's sign). In the distal lower extremities, tibialis anterior muscles are involved sparing the calves. Proximally, the hip girdle is variably involved as are the knee flexors and extensors. Although the classic description of FSHD emphasizes the foot dorsiflexor involvement as the initial manifestation of weakness in the lower extremities, thigh and hip girdle muscle weakness can be

more profound than distal leg weakness in a subpopulation of patients with FSHD (Tawil et al., 1994). Muscle stretch reflexes are often diminished or absent in affected muscles and the sensory examination is intact. Contractures are rarely present in FSHD even in profoundly weak muscle. One of the striking and characteristic findings in FSHD is the degree of side-to-side asymmetry in muscle weakness. Although one study suggested that this was more profound in the dominant limb and thus related to overuse (Brouwer et al., 1992), another study failed to show a relationship of handedness to degree of weakness (Tawil et al., 1994).

Extramuscular manifestations of FSHD are usually asymptomatic and include hearing loss of high frequencies and retinal telengectasias. Screening of affected individuals within an FSHD kindred shows mild high-frequency hearing loss in the majority (Brouwer et al., 1991). Hearing loss can be occasionally severe enough to require the use of hearing aids, especially in infantile FSHD. Similarly, screening an FSHD kindred with fluorescein angiography reveals peripheral retinal telengectasias in a majority of affected individuals (Fitzimons et al., 1987). Rarely, these vascular malformations can result in an exudative retinopathy and retinal detachment (Coat's syndrome) (Desai and Sabates, 1990; Pauleikhoff et al., 1992).

Symptomatic cardiac involvement in FSHD is rare. Atrial abnormalities on surface electrocardiography are evident in 60% of patients as well as atrioventricular nodal or infranodal abnormalities in about 25% (Stevenson et al., 1990). Moreover, in 10 of 12 patients studied electrophysiologically, atrial flutter or fibrillation could be induced (Stevenson et al., 1990). This is confirmed by two reports of typical patients with FSHD who developed atrial tachyarrhythmias (Woelfel et al., 1989; Shen and Madsen, 1991). In a more recent study of molecularly confirmed cases of FSHD, about 5% were estimated to have cardiac involvement, with conduction abnormalities and a predilection for supaventricular tachyarrhythmias (Laforet et al., 1998). Atrial standstill, characteristic of X-linked Emery–Dreifuss dystrophy, was reported in four patients with FSHD (Bloomfield and Sinclair-Smith, 1965; Caponnetto et al., 1968; Baldwin et al., 1973; Woelfel et al., 1989). However, the diagnosis of Emery–Dreifuss dystrophy cannot be excluded based on the clinical description in these reports.

Central nervous system involvement is not typical in FSHD. However, a recent survey of Japanese patients with FSHD showed that 8 of 20 patients with early-onset FSHD were mentally retarded, of whom four also suffered from seizures (Funakoshi et al., 1998).

Pathophysiology

Even though the gene lesion responsible for FSHD is known, the gene product(s) and pathophysiology of FSHD are unknown. Histopathological examination of FSHD muscle shows mostly nonspecific myopathic changes, with up to 30% also demonstrating variable degrees of mononuclear inflammation (Padberg, 1982). The pathological significance of this inflammation, often observed in other dystrophic processes, is unclear. The associated retinal abnormalities and hearing loss suggest that the responsible gene has pleiotropic effects. Another possibility, suggested by the position effect hypothesis of FSHD molecular pathogenesis, is that several adjacent genes are involved.

Diagnosis

Clinical diagnosis

Clinical diagnosis of FSHD is based on the characteristic distribution of weakness, absence of contractures as well as absence of extraocular, bulbar and respiratory muscle weakness. The diagnosis is further aided by the presence of an autosomal dominant family history with similar findings in affected family members. Serum creatine kinase levels are usually three to five times normal levels; a value that is ten or more times normal suggests an alternative diagnosis. Electromyography confirms the presence of a myopathic process and is helpful to rule out a neurogenic process when the clinical features are not typical. Since histophathological changes in FSHD are nonspecific, a

muscle biopsy helps to exclude other conditions with specific pathological changes and clinical presentations that can mimic FSHD. Such conditions include polymyositis, nemaline myopathy, centronuclear myopathy, acid maltase deficiency, scapuloperoneal syndromes and mitochondrial myopathy. A muscle biopsy is necessary only in sporadic cases where the treating clinician has no access to molecular genetic diagnosis or when molecular diagnosis suggests an alternative diagnosis.

Molecular genetic diagnosis

Molecular diagnosis of FSHD has been available in Europe and Canada for a number of years and has recently become commercially available in the USA. Initially, molecular diagnosis of FSHD was performed on leukocyte DNA using probe p13E-11 following digestion with EcoRI. However, p13E-11 also hybridizes to a region on 10q26 homologous to 4q35 and detects fragments in the size range diagnostic for FSHD, potentially complicating molecular diagnosis (Bakker et al., 1995). The accuracy of FSHD molecular diagnosis was significantly improved with the finding of a restriction site (BlnI) that is unique to the 3.3 kb repeats of 10q26 origin (Fig. 21.5) (Deidda et al., 1996). Consequently, double digestion with EcoRI/BlnI results in complete digestion of 10q26 alleles and confirms the 4q35 origin of the remaining alleles. Molecular diagnosis performed using the double digestion technique identifies the FSHD-associated 4q35 deletion in >95% of patients with the disease. In normal individuals restriction fragments of 50–300 kb are apparent whereas affected individuals have fragments ranging from 10 to 35 kb (Fig. 21.5) (Orrell et al., 1999). Detection of the deletion in affected family members or its appearance de novo in sporadic cases confirms the diagnosis of FSHD. The absence of an identifiable deletion in 1–5% of patients who fulfil the clinical criteria of FSHD could be attributed to technical problems with degraded or partially digested DNA, translocation between 4q35 and 10q26 complicating the interpretation of the data, FSHD unlinked to 4q35 or non-FSHD myopathy.

In addition to confirming the clinical diagnosis, determination of deletion size has some prognostic relevance. Several investigators have noted a direct correlation between deletion size and disease severity. The larger the deletion (i.e. the smaller the restriction fragment), the more severe the clinical manifestations (Lunt et al., 1995; Tawil et al., 1996; Ricci et al., 1999). However, since deletion size is the same within an affected kindred, other factors must account for the intrafamilial variability in disease severity.

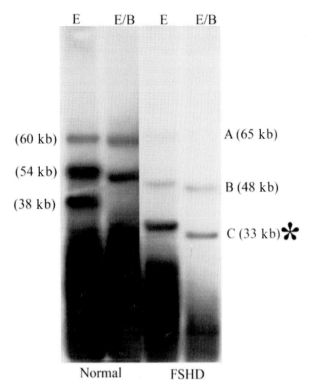

Fig. 21.5. Pulse field gel electropheresis results from a normal individual (left two lanes) and a patient with facioscapulohumeral dystrophy (FSHD) (right two lanes) using single *Eco*RI (E) or double *Eco*RI/*Bln*I (E/B) restriction enzyme digest. The normal individual has a 38 kb (C) allele (in the range diagnostic of FSHD) on single digestion that is not apparent with double digest, proving its 10q26 origin. The affected individual has a 33 kb allele (C) that persists with double digestion, proving its 4q35 origin and confirming the diagnosis.

Management

There is no known effective treatment for the progressive muscle weakness in FSHD. Because of the presence of inflammation in a large percentage of FSHD biopsies, prednisone was tried and reported to be at least transiently effective in individual case reports (Tawil and Griggs, 1997). A three month, open-label trial of prednisone in FSHD failed to show any benefit in either strength or lean body mass. Recently, an open-label, three month trial of slow-release albuterol (Proventil Repetabs; 8 mg/twice daily) in 15 patients with FSHD demonstrated a significant increase in both lean body mass and in strength measured by quantitative isometric myometry (Kissel et al., 1997). The rationale for the use of a β_2-adrenergic agent is based

on numerous studies demonstrating the anabolic potential of such agents in animal models of muscle wasting, including the *mdx* mouse, an animal model for Duchenne dystrophy (Rothwell and Stock, 1985). A one year, randomized controlled trial of albuterol in FSHD in 90 patients was recently completed. The study showed that high-dose, sustained-release albuterol resulted in significant increase in lean body mass. However, this increased muscle mass was not associated with a similar increase in strength (Kissel et al., 2000). More recently, creatine kinase has received much attention in the treatment of muscle-wasting diseases. Two small studies that included a variety of neuromuscular conditions, including FSHD, have demonstrated improvement in overall strength following short-term supplementation with creatine monohydrate (Tarnopolsky and Martin, 1999; Walter et al., 1999). How creatine, which is the immediate source of energy during vigorous muscle contraction, can improve strength in long-standing dystrophic conditions remains unclear. Creatine supplementation in normal athletes slightly enhances, at best, performance during high-intensity, short-term exercise (Williams and Branch, 1998).

Symptomatic treatment of patients with FSHD is limited. Ankle foot orthoses are helpful in patients with foot drop. However, in patients with severe weakness of knee extension, rigid ankle-foot orthoses actually hinder ambulation by preventing patients from hyperextending and locking their knees. Inability to abduct shoulders because of weak scapular fixators is a major limitations in most patients with FSHD. Surgical fixation of the scapulae can significantly improve arm range of motion. However, information about the benefits of scapular fixation in FSHD is sparse (Letournel et al., 1990; Bunch and Siegel, 1993; Jakab and Gledhill, 1993). Many patients learn to adapt to their limitations and opt against surgical scapular fixation. There are several drawbacks to surgical scapular fixation: (i) the wire fixating the scapula to the chest wall can break; (ii) bilateral fixation results in unacceptable loss of mobility of the shoulders; (iii) the benefits of fixation may be short lasting in patients with relatively rapid progression of weakness; and (iv) the prolonged casting required by some techniques results in disuse atrophy, which is often not fully reversible. Our recommendation is that fixation should never be bilateral, should be performed by a surgeon experienced in the technique and should be performed on patients with slowly progressive disease. Moreover, in patients with severe weakness of the humeral muscles, improved shoulder abduction may not translate into a useful functional gain. In patients considering surgery, the amount of improvement that can be expected with fixation can be easily measured by having the examiner manually fixate the scapula as the patient abducts the shoulder.

Prognosis

The long-term prognosis for most patients with FSHD is good. In the absence of respiratory, bulbar or cardiac involvement, life expectancy is normal. Variable degrees of physical limitations arise depending on the extent and severity of muscle involvement. A recent prospective natural history study demonstrated that progression, on average, is slow and steady (The FSH-DY Group, 1997). Most patients adapt remarkably well to their limitation, but eventually about 20% become wheelchair bound (Padberg, 1982).

References

Bakker, E., Wijmenga, C., Vossen, R. H. et al. (1995). The FSHD-linked locus D4F104S1 (p13E-11) on 4q35 has a homologue on 10qter. *Muscle Nerve* **2**, S39–S44.

Baldwin, B. J., Talley, R. C., Johnson. C. et al. (1973). Permanent paralysis of the atrium in a patient with facioscapulohumeral muscular dystrophy. *Am. J. Cardiol.* **31**, 649–653.

Bloomfield, D. A. and Sinclair-Smith, B. C. (1965). Persistent atrial standstill. *Am. J. Med.* **39**, 335–340.

Brouwer, O. F., Padberg, G. W., Ruys, C. J. M. et al. (1991). Hearing loss in facioscapulohumeral muscular dystrophy. *Neurology* **41**, 1878–1881.

Brouwer, O. F., Padberg, G. W. and Van der Ploeg, R. J. (1992). The influence of handedness on the distribution of muscular weakness of the arm in facioscapulohumeral muscular dystrophy. *Brain* **115**, 1587–1598.

Bunch, W. H. and Siegel, I. M. (1993). Scapulothoracic arthrodesis in facioscapulohumeral muscular dystrophy. Review of seventeen procedures with three to twenty-one-year follow up. *J. Bone Joint Surg.* **75**, 372–376.

Caponnetto, S., Pastrioni. C. and Tirelli, G. (1968). Persistent atrial standstill in a patient affected with facioscapulohumeral muscular dystrophy. *Cardiologia* **53**, 341–350.

Deidda, G., Cacurri, S., Piazzo, N. et al. (1996). Direct detection of 4q35 rearrangements implicated in facioscapulohumeral muscular dystrophy (FSHD). *J. Med. Genet.* **33**, 361–365.

Desai, U. R. and Sabates, F. N. (1990). Long-term follow-up of facioscapulohumeral muscular dystrophy and Coat's disease. *Am. J. Ophthalmol.* **110**, 568–569.

Fitzsimons, R. B., Gurwin, E. B. and Bird, A. C. (1987). Retinal vascular abnormalities in facioscapulohumeral muscular dystrophy. *Brain* **110**, 631–684.

Funakoshi, M., Goto, K. and Arahata, K. (1998). Epilepsy and mental retardation in a subset of early onset 4q35-associated facioscapulohumeral muscular dystrophy. *Neurology* **50**, 1791–1794.

Jakab, E. and Gledhill, R. B. (1993). Simplified technique for scapulocostal fusion in facioscapulohumeral dystrophy. *J. Ped. Orthoped.* **13**, 749–751.

Kissel, J., Mendell, J. R., Griggs, R. C. et al. (1997). Open-label clinical trial of albuterol in facioscapulohumeral muscular dystrophy. *Neurology* **48**, A194.

Kissel, J. T., Tawil, R., McDermott, M. et al. (2000). Double-blind, randomized controlled trial of albuterol in FSH dystrophy. *Neurology* **54**, 2350.

Laforet, P., de Toma, C., Eymard. B. et al. (1998). Cardiac involvement in genetically confirmed facioscapulohumeral muscular dystrophy. *Neurology* **51**, 1454–1456.

Letournel, E., Fardeau, M. and Lytle, J. O. (1990). Scapulothoracic arthrodesis for patients who have facioscapulohumeral muscular dystrophy. *J. Bone Joint Surg.* **72**, 78–84.

Lunt, P. W., Jardine, P. E., Koch, M. C. et al. (1995). Correlation between fragment size at D4F104S1 and age of onset or at wheelchair use, with a possible generational effect, accounts for much phenotypic variation in 4q35-facioscapulohumeral muscular dystrophy (FSHD). *Hum. Mol. Genet.* **4**, 951–958.

Orrell, R. W., Tawil, R., Forrester, J. et al. (1999). Definitive molecular diagnosis of facioscapulohumeral dystrophy. *Neurology* **52**, 1822–1826.

Padberg, G. W. (1982). *Facioscapulohumeral Disease.* Leiden, the Netherlands: University of Leiden Thesis.

Padberg, G., Brouwer, O. F., de Keizer, R. J. et al. (1995). On the significance of retinal vascular disease and hearing loss in facioscapulohumeral muscular dystrophy. *Muscle Nerve* **Suppl. 2**, S73–S80.

Pauleikhoff, D., Bornfeld, N. and Bird, A. C. (1992). Severe visual loss associated with retinal telangiectasis and facioscapulohumeral muscular dystrophy. *Graef. Arch. Clin. Exp. Ophthalmol.* **230**, 362–365.

Ricci, E., Galluzzi, G. and Deidda, F. (1999). Progress in the molecular diagnosis of facioscapulohumeral muscular dystrophy and correlation between the number of KpnI repeats a the 4q35 locus and clinical phenotype. *Ann. Neurol.* **45**, 751–757.

Rothwell, N. J. and Stock, M. J. (1985). Modification of body composition by clenbuterol in normal and dystrophic (*mdx*) mice. *Biosci. Rep.* **5**, 755–760.

Shen, E. N. and Madsen, T. (1991). Facioscapulohumeral muscular dystrophy and recurrent pacemaker lead dislodgment. *Am. Heart J.* **122**, 1167–1169.

Stevenson, W. G., Perloff, J. K., Weiss, J. N et al. (1990). Facioscapulohumeral muscular dystrophy: evidence for selective genetic electrophysiologic cardiac involvement. *J. Am. Coll. Cardiol.* **15**, 292–299.

Tarnopolsky, M. and Martin, J. (1999). Creatine monohydrate increases strength in patients with neuromuscular disorders. *Neurology* **52**, 854–857.

Tawil, R. and Griggs, R. C. (1997). Facioscapulohumeral muscular dystrophy. In: *The Molecular and Genetic Basis of Neurological Disease,* ed. R. N. Rosenberg, S. B. Prusiner, S. DiMauro and R. L. Barchi, pp. 931–938. Boston, MA: Butterworth-Heinemann.

Tawil, R., McDermott, M. P., Mendell, J. R. et al. (1994). Facioscapulohumeral muscular dystrophy (FSHD): design of natural history study and results of baseline testing. *Neurology* **44**, 442–446.

Tawil, R., Forrester, J. and Griggs, R. C. et al. (1996). Evidence for anticipation and association of deletion size with severity of facioscapulohumeral muscular dystrophy. *Ann. Neurol.* **39**, 744–748.

The FSH-DY Group (1997). A prospective, quantitative study of the natural history of facioscapulohumeral muscular dystrophy (FSHD): implications for therapeutic trials. *Neurology* **48**, 38–46.

Tupler, R., Berardinelli, A., Barbierato, L. et al. (1996). Monosomy of distal 4q does not cause facioscapulohumeral muscular dystrophy. *J. Med. Genet.* **33**, 366–370.

van Deutekom, J. C. T., Wijmenga, C., van Tienhoven, E. A. E. et al. (1993). FSHD associated DNA rearrangements are due to large deletions of intergral copies of a 3.2 kb tandemly repeated unit. *Hum. Mol. Genet.* **2**, 2037–2042.

Walter, M. C., Lochmuller, H., Hartart, M. et al. (1999). Creatine monohydrate in muscular dystrophies: a double-blind placebo-controlled clinical study. *Neurology* **52**, A543.

Wijmenga, C., Hewitt, J. E., Sandkuijl, L. A. X. et al. (1992). Chromosome 4q DNA rearrangements associated with facioscapulohumeral muscular dystrophy. *Nat. Genet.* **2**, 26–30.

Williams, M. H. and Branch, J. D. (1998). Creatine supplementation and exercise performance: an update. *J. Am. Coll. Nutrit.* **17**, 216–234.

Winokur, S. T., Bengtsson, U., Feddersen, J. et al. (1994). The DNA rearrangement associated with facioscapulohumeral muscular dystrophy involves a heterochromatin-associated repetitive element: implications for a role of chromatin structure in the pathogenesis of the disease. *Chromosome Res.* **2**, 225–234.

Woelfel, A., Cascio, W. and Smith, S. W. (1989). Cerebral embolization in two young patients with facioscapulohumeral muscular dystrophy and atrial dysrhythmias. *Am. Heart J.* **118**, 632–633.

22

Distal myopathies

Richard J. Barohn and Robert C. Griggs

Introduction

Distal myopathies are inherited or sporadic primary muscle disorders characterized clinically by progressive weakness and atrophy beginning in the muscles of the distal limbs and pathologically by myopathic changes in skeletal muscle. This is in contrast to most myopathies, where the earliest and most prominent weakness is in proximal muscles. There are at least six distinct distal myopathies (Table 22.1) based on clinical and molecular characterization of these disorders (Barohn, 1993; Barohn et al., 1998; Barohn and Amato, 1999).

The distal myopathies are uncommon. While incidence and prevalence rates are not available for most of these disorders, some overall idea can be obtained by examining the relative frequency with which such patients are encountered in neuromuscular centres. In the classification of myopathies by Walton and Nattrass (1954), only 2 of 105 consecutively ascertained patients with muscular dystrophy or a myotonic disorder in the UK had a distal myopathy other than myotonic dystrophy. In Germany, Ricker and Mertens (1968) observed only 1 out of 212 patients with muscular dystrophy had a distal predilection for weakness. However, Udd and colleagues believe the autosomal dominant tibial muscular dystrophy is underdiagnosed. They estimate a prevalence of 5/100 000 in Finland (Udd et al., 1998b). Another specific form of distal myopathy, Miyoshi myopathy, is estimated to have a prevalence of 1 in 440 000 in Japan (Bejaoui et al., 1995).

Historical perspective

Gowers has traditionally been credited with providing the first descriptions of distal myopathy in his description of two patients (Gowers, 1902). Subsequently, a number of reports appeared describing myopathic disorders with a distal predilection of weakness (Dejerine and Thomas, 1904; Campbell, 1906; Spiller, 1907; Batten, 1910; Milhorat and Wolff, 1943). These various authors point out the difficulty in differentiating between these cases and Charcot–Marie–Tooth disease. The absence of sensory symptoms or signs, with no pathological change in the spinal cord or peripheral nerves at portmortem, provided the best available evidence supporting a myopathy. S. A. Kinnier Wilson raised the dilemma in this manner (Wilson, 1940): 'The question at issue is simply posed: does a distal *myogenic* type occur, analogous to the known *myelogenic* (neural) form termed **peroneal muscular atrophy**? At present, no definite answer can be returned, but no good reason for denying the possibility has been adduced. Of the genuineness of the type, "I am myself convinced".' [Italics and boldface per Wilson.]

Welander clarified the existence of a true distal myopathy in her 1951 monograph describing a large cohort of Scandinavian patients (Welander, 1951). This paper has been so influential that many physicians continue to describe any case of distal myopathy as Welander myopathy. In a 1980 review, Kratz and Brooke (1980) documented nine publications from the Western literature that were believed to describe definite cases of distal myopathy, and six other probable cases. However, throughout the 1960s and 1970s, a number of reports on distal myopathy were published in the Japanese literature that were rarely recognized elsewhere. With a broader awareness of these disorders by 1986, Markesbery and Griggs (1986) produced a classification system that encompassed three distinct distal myopathies (two of late adult onset and one of early adult onset). In 1991, Barohn et al. (1991) divided the distal myopathies into four major types: Welander myopathy (late adult-onset type I), Markesbery myopathy (late adult-onset type II), Nonaka myopathy (early adult-onset type I)

Table 22.1. Classification of distal myopathies

Type	Inheritance	Gene localization	Gene product	Initial weakness	Serum creatine kinase	Biopsy
Welander: late adult-onset type I	Autosomal dominant	2p13	? Dysferlin	Hands, fingers/ wrist extensors	Normal or slightly increased	Myopathic; vacuoles in some cases
Markesbery– Griggs/Udd: late adult-onset type II	Autosomal dominant	2q31 Other loci	Titin ?	Legs, anterior compartment	Normal or slightly increased	Vacuolar myopathy
Nonaka: early adult-onset type I (familial IBM)[a]	Autosomal recessive or sporadic	9p1-q1	?	Legs, anterior compartment	Slightly to moderately increased, usually <5× normal	Vacuolar myopathy
Miyoshi: early adult-onset type II (LGMD 2B)[b]	Autosomal recessive or sporadic	2p13 10	Dysferlin ?	Legs, posterior compartment	Increased 10–150× normal	Myopathic, usually without vacuoles
Laing: early-onset type III	Autosomal dominant	14	?	Legs, anterior compartment and neck flexors	Slightly increased, <3× normal	Moderate myopathic changes/no vacuoles
Myofibrillar (desmin) myopathy: Onset in childhood to 7th decade	Autosomal dominant or sporadic (?autosomal recessive/ ?X-linked)	11q21–23 2q35 12	$\alpha\beta$-Crystallin Desmin ?	Hands or legs	Moderately increased, <5× normal	Myopathy, occasionally with vacuoles; foci of myofibrillar destruction or cytoplasmic inclusions; accumulations of desmin and other proteins

Notes:

[a] Autosomal recessive familial inclusion body myopathy (IBM), also known as quadriceps sparing myopathy, has been genetically linked with the Nonaka distal myopathy.

[b] Limb girdle muscular dystrophy type 2B and distal myopathy both have mutations in the dysferlin gene on chromosome 2 (p13).

and Miyoshi myopathy (early adult-onset type II). Since that publication, Laing myopathy (early-onset type III) and myofibrillar myopathy have been added to the distal myopathy classification (Table 22.1) and genetic localization has been established for each disorder. The gene and abnormal gene product is now known for Miyoshi myopathy and suggested for myofibrillar myopathy. It is already clear that disorders allelic to the distal myopathies can have a proximal, limb girdle presentation. For example, Miyoshi myopathy and limb girdle muscular dystrophy type 2B (LGMD2B) are both caused by defects in the same protein, dysferlin, encoded by a gene on chromosome 2 (Bashir et al., 1998; Liu et al., 1998). Welander myopathy may result from the same mutation (Åhlberg et al., 1999). Therefore, it is possible that the concept of distal myopathies may become obsolete. Instead, these conditions may become known by their genetic mutation or abnormal gene product, much like Duchenne and Becker dystrophy. How a mutation in the same gene can produce such

strikingly different phenotypes remains to be elucidated. Moreover, it is possible that whether the gene lesion causes distal or proximal myopathy depends on an additional gene or genes that determine(s) the distribution of weakness.

Welander distal myopathy: late adult-onset type I

Clinical features

Welander described 249 cases of distal myopathy in 72 families (Welander, 1951). Of this cohort, 149 were men and 215 had subjective weakness. The pattern of inheritance is autosomal dominant. Most patients develop symptoms in the fifth decade (mean 47 years) but some patients first note symptoms in their seventies. Consequently, Welander myopathy has been classified as a late adult-onset disorder to differentiate from the early adult-onset distal myopathies (Markesbery and Griggs, 1986; Barohn, 1993; Griggs and Markesbery, 1994). Patients nearly always develop weakness first in the distal upper extremities, usually finger and wrist extensors. In 85% of patients, the hand weakness can be asymmetric (Welander, 1951). Distal flexor groups are spared initially; however, of patients who have had symptoms for over 25 years, 73% had weakness in wrist flexors. Gradually, symptoms spread to the distal lower extremities, primarily in toe and ankle extensors. Only rarely do proximal limb muscle symptoms and signs develop, even as the disease progresses. Muscle stretch reflexes are preserved except for ankle reflexes, which may be lost later in the disease. Sensory examination is generally normal, except for impaired vibratory sensation in the feet in 85% of patients with Welander myopathy, but this was considered age appropriate.

Patients with Welander myopathy experience very slow progression of weakness. Many continue to work, and the duration of life is not reduced (Welander, 1951).

Laboratory features

Serum creatine kinase levels are normal or slightly elevated (two to three times normal) in the disorder (Borg et al., 1991b; Lindberg et al., 1991). Needle electromyography (EMG) shows small, brief 'myopathic' motor units, although some authors have reported mixed 'myopathic–neuropathic' patterns (Edström, 1975; Borg et al., 1991a,b; Lindberg et al., 1991). Fibrillations are often but not invariably present, and other involuntary discharges such as myotonia and pseudomyotonia have been reported (Borg et al., 1991a, 1998; Lindberg et al., 1991). Motor and sensory nerve conduction studies are normal despite mild abnormalities on sural nerve biopsy (Borg et al., 1989). Quantitative sensory testing may reveal some deficits on temperature and vibration examination (Borg et al., 1987). Therefore, patients with Welander myopathy also have a length-dependent, predominantly small-fibre, asymptomatic neuropathy.

In a lower extremity investigation using magnetic resonance imaging (MRI) of seven patients with Welander myopathy, signal changes consistent with fatty replacement affected the posterior leg compartment in seven patients and the anterior compartment in three (Åhlberg et al., 1994). The peroneal, posterior tibial and thigh muscles were normal. Therefore, by MRI criteria, there is early selective involvement of the *posterior* leg muscles, contrasting with the clinically observed preference for early ankle and toe dorsiflexor weakness. This paradox may reflect the greater strength of the posterior compartment musculature.

Muscle biopsy showed dystrophic features with fibre size variability, increase in connective tissue, fat, central nuclei and split fibres (Welander, 1951). The severity of changes depended to some extent on disease duration. Edström (1975) reported selective type I fibre atrophy and proliferation of muscle nuclei, often in clumps. Vacuoles, a common feature in several of the distal dystrophies, have been observed by some (Welander, 1951; Borg et al., 1989, 1991b, 1993, 1998) but not all (Dahlgaard, 1960; Barrows and Duemler, 1962; Edström, 1975) authors. In recent reports, rimmed vacuoles were abundant in patients with moderate to severe weakness but absent in those with early disease (Borg et al., 1991a,b, 1993, 1998; Lindberg et al., 1991). Interestingly, in the more recent Scandinavian reports in which rimmed vacuoles have been seen, 15 to 18 nm cytoplasmic and nuclear filaments were observed on electron microscopy (Borg et al., 1991b, 1993, 1998; Lindberg et al., 1991). Therefore, these filaments are not specific to inclusion body myositis (IBM). Indeed, according to Lindberg et al. (1991), the main pathological feature that distinguishes IBM from Welander myopathy is the presence of inflammatory infiltrates in IBM. Groups of small angular fibres can also be seen, suggesting a neurogenic component (Borg et al., 1989). Mild neuropathic features on muscle biopsy, EMG and, occasionally, on nerve biopsy are often seen in a number of the distal myopathic conditions.

Molecular genetics

Åhlberg et al. (1997, 1998b) initially reported that Welander myopathy was not linked to other distal myopathy gene loci on chromosomes 2p, 2q, 9p and 14q. However, the same investigators found linkage to chromosome 2p13 near the genetic loci of Miyoshi myopathy and LGMD2B (Åhlberg et al., 1998a, 1999), suggesting that the dysferlin gene is the primary candidate gene for Welander myopathy.

Markesbery–Griggs/Udd distal myopathy: late adult-onset, type II

Clinical features

In the 1970s, a non-Scandinavian autosomal dominant late-onset distal myopathy was reported by Markesbery et al. in a French–English family (Markesbery et al., 1974). Three of seven affected family members were examined.

The English kindred of Sumner et al. (1971) may represent the same condition. The large pedigrees and several sporadic cases recently reported from Finland by Udd and colleagues (described as 'tibial muscular dystrophy') also fall in this category (Udd, 1991a, 1992, 1993, 1998b,c; Partanen et al., 1994).

Weakness begins in the anterior compartment of the distal lower extremities (ankle dorsiflexors), in contrast to Welander myopathy in which weakness begins in the hands. Markesbery's patients first developed weakness between ages 43 and 51 years and the Scandinavian patients had symptom onset from age 35 to the eighth decade of life. As the disease slowly progresses, distal finger and wrist extensors of the upper extremities can become involved and, much later, proximal weakness can occur. The patients described by Markesbery et al. (1974) appeared to show faster disease progression than did patients with Welander myopathy. Unlike Welander myopathy, the disorder was ultimately disabling; ambulation was lost after 15 to 20 years, with complete incapacitation after 30 years. One of Markesbery's patients also had a cardiomyopathy with heart block and failure requiring a pacemaker. Most of the Finnish patients progressed more slowly than Markesbery's patients and the disease rarely involved the upper extremity or proximal muscles (Partanen et al., 1994). Only 10% of the Finnish patients developed proximal leg weakness in the late stages of the illness, and generally severe disability did not ensue, with preservation of walking throughout the illness. However, 8 of 34 affected family members from the pedigree in Western Finland (Larsmo) exhibited a LGMD phenotype: four severe and four mild (Udd et al., 1991a, 1992, 1993). Udd et al. suggested that the patients with the typical LGMD (Udd et al., 1993) phenotype may be homozygous for the dominant gene. Neither Finnish or non-Finnish families had face, bulbar or neck weakness.

Laboratory features

Serum creatine kinase was normal or slightly elevated (three to four times normal). EMG revealed small, brief myopathic motor units with increased recruitment, particularly in the tibialis anterior muscle. Imaging with computed tomography and MRI of skeletal muscle demonstrated selective fatty degeneration of the tibialis anterior muscle (Udd et al., 1991a,b). Biopsy revealed a dystrophic process. The striking feature in Markesbery's patients was the presence of single or multiple rimmed vacuoles within many muscle fibres. In the Finnish patients, vacuoles were occasionally present (Udd et al., 1991a, 1993; Partanen et al., 1994). Approximately 30% of the Finnish biopsies contained vacuolated fibres, ranging in abundance from 0.6 to 10% of all fibres (Udd et al., 1998c); vacuoles are not essential for diagnoses (Udd et al., 1998b). At postmortem of one patient with a cardiomyopathy (Markesbury et al., 1974), there was severe fibrosis of the left ventricular myocardium, numerous degenerating cardiac muscle fibres and vacuolization within myocardial cells.

The ultrastructural examinations by Markesbery et al. (1977) demonstrated foci of myofibrillar disruption and fragmentation accompanied by Z bodies, contraction clumps of massed myofibrils and other granular masses. These changes are typical of myofibrillar myopathy, but in this early study immunohistochemical stains for desmin were not done. In the Finnish patients, 15–20 nm tubofilaments were occasionally seen in the cytoplasm adjacent to rimmed vacuoles. Immunohistochemical stains were negative for expressions of desmin, dystrophin, laminins, spectrin, tau protein and β-amyloid (Udd et al., 1998c).

Molecular genetics

The genetic defect in Finnish families has been localized to chromosome 2q31 (Haravuori et al., 1998b). Patients from the Larsmo kindred with severe LGMD were, in fact, homozygous for the common core haplotype, but those with the milder LGMD syndrome were heterozygotes, signifying phenotypic heterogeneity. The Markesbery–Griggs kindred also localizes to this region (Haravuori et al., 1998a; Udd et al., 1998a). This confirmed that the Finnish and non-Finnish cases are allelic disorders that may differ only in the extent of progression, degree of disability, frequency of finding vacuoles on muscle biopsy and cardiac involvement. A French kindred with progressive anterior tibial atrophy commencing from age 40 to 50 years has also now been linked to the 2q31 locus (Udd et al., 1998a). A possible candidate gene is that for the muscle protein titin (Udd et al., 1998b). An autosomal dominant distal myopathy resembling Markesbery–Griggs/Udd myopathy has been recently described that did not localize to loci on chromosomes 2, 9 or 14, which are known to be linked with distal myopathy (Felice et al., 1999).

Nonaka distal myopathy: early adult-onset type I

Clinical features

Both forms of early adult-onset autosomal recessive distal muscular dystrophy were first reported in the Japanese literature in the 1960s and 1970s (Murone et al., 1963; Miyoshi et al., 1967, 1975; Sasaki et al., 1969). These reports were not widely known in the West until Nonaka and colleagues published a series of papers on autosomal recessive distal myopathy with rimmed vacuole formation (Nonaka et al., 1981, 1985; Sunohara et al., 1989). These cases are not confined to Japan, as similar cases have been reported from America (Markesbery et al., 1977; Miller et al., 1979; Krendel et al., 1988), South Africa (Isaacs et al., 1988), Spain (Arenas et al., 1995), Brazil (Werneck et al., 1993) and possibly from Italy (Scoppetta et al., 1988), although the exact classification of the Italian family is unclear (Somer, 1995). The two cases reported by Walton and Nattras (1954) may fall into this category.

Men and women are equally affected. Weakness begins late in the second or third decade: average age of onset 26 years (range 0–41) (Nonaka et al., 1998; Satoyoshi et al., 1998). Initial weakness is in the distal leg anterior compartment (ankle dorsiflexors) and toe extensors. Patients present with foot drop and a steppage gait. Early in the disease, the finger and hand muscles can be weak, but not to the extent of the leg weakness. In typical cases, weakness spreads from the anterior leg to the posterior calf, proximal lower limbs and neck flexors over the first few years of the illness. After 10–15 years of illness, the process is generalized, sparing only the ocular, facial, bulbar and respiratory muscles. Most patients become wheelchair dependent 10–15 years (mean 12) from disease onset (Mizusawa et al., 1987a; Nonaka et al., 1998). Complete heart block producing syncope requiring a pacemaker has been reported (Sunohara et al., 1989).

Laboratory features

Serum creatine kinase levels are typically elevated three to four times normal. Muscle computed tomography shows fatty replacement (Mizusawa et al., 1987a; Nonaka et al., 1998). EMG studies reveal myopathic motor units, but neurogenic potentials may be superimposed. Fibrillations are observed in 50% of patients.

The muscle biopsy from both Japanese and non-Japanese patients usually show a striking vacuolar dystrophic myopathy (Fig. 22.1) (Markesbery et al., 1977; Miller et al., 1979; Isaacs et al., 1988; Krendel et al., 1988; Scoppetta et al., 1988). The vacuoles are lined with granular material that is basophilic on staining with haematoxylin and eosin and purple-red with the modified Gomori trichrome stain: so-called rimmed vacuoles. The vacuoles exhibit acid phosphatase activity. On electron microscopy, in addition to autophagic vacuoles, some patients have nuclear or cytoplasmic 15–18 nm filamentous inclusions

(Kumamota et al., 1982; Matsubara and Tanabe 1982; Mizusawa et al., 1987b). These filaments, which were originally believed to be characteristic of IBM (see below), have, therefore, been documented in Welander, Markesbery–Griggs/Udd and Nonaka distal myopathies (Jongen et al., 1995).

Relationship to familial inclusion body myopathy

It is now accepted that the disorders described as both 'vacuolar myopathy sparing the quadriceps' (Sadeh et al., 1993) and autosomal recessive 'hereditary IBM' (Sivakumar and Dalakas, 1996) are the same as Nonaka distal myopathy. The original cases were described in Iranian Jews (Argov and Yarom, 1984; Massa et al., 1991; Sadeh et al., 1993); however, the most recent cases are Caucasian American and Asian Indian (Sivakumar and Dalakas, 1996). Clinically and histologically, these patients are indistinguishable from those with Nonaka distal myopathy. Like Nonaka myopathy, the inheritance pattern of hereditary IBM/quadriceps-sparing myopathy is autosomal recessive. Patients with 'hereditary IBM' develop distal weakness in the lower extremity anterior compartment as young adults (mean age onset 31 years) (Sadeh et al., 1993). The weakness spreads to both proximal and distal muscles in the arms and legs, producing significant disability. A consistent clinical finding is the sparing of quadriceps muscle strength despite profound weakness of other proximal muscles in the later stages. In addition, Mizusawa et al. (1987a) emphasized that the quadriceps were spared when proximal progression had occurred. The pathology is identical in Nonaka myopathy and vacuolar myopathy sparing the quadriceps/familial IBM. In both disorders, there is a vacuolar myopathy, no inflammation and cytoplasmic and intranuclear 15–18 nm filaments.

It should be emphasized that the features that separate all these patients from those with sporadic IBM (see below) are early onset with the initial symptoms in the ankle dorsiflexors, quadriceps sparing, autosomal recessive inheritance and lack of inflammation on muscle biopsy. Otherwise, routine light and electron microscopic findings are similar in all of these disorders.

Molecular genetics

Nonaka distal myopathy and the quadriceps-sparing form of familial IBM have been localized to chromosome 9p1-q1 (Argov et al., 1997; Askanas, 1997; Ikeuchi et al., 1997). Consequently, these disorders are the same and may both be considered early adult-onset distal myopathy type I.

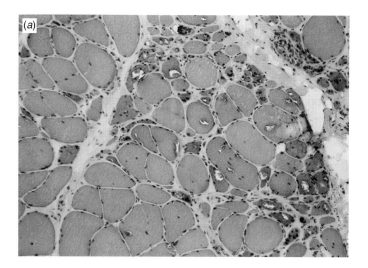

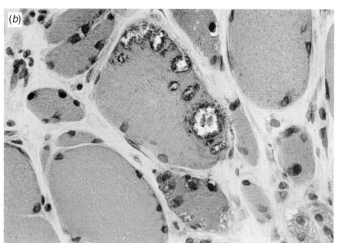

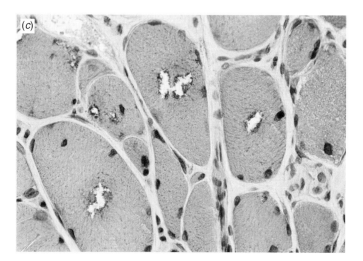

Fig. 22.1. Nonaka distal myopathy (early adult-onset type I). Muscle biopsy stained with haematoxylin and eosin shows (*a*) variability of muscle fibre size, central nuclei, fibre splitting and numerous vacuolated fibres (original magnification ×143); (*b*) multiple rimmed vacuoles at the periphery of the fibres (original magnification ×575); and (*c*) single rimmed vacuoles in the centre of the fibres (original magnification ×575). (With permission from Barohn, 1993.)

Miyoshi distal myopathy: early adult-onset type II

Clinical features

The early reports of Miyoshi distal myopathy (Miyoshi et al., 1967, 1975) were largely unnoticed until the cases were published in the Western literature (Miyoshi et al., 1986). Since then, similar patients have been reported worldwide (Kuhn and Schroder, 1981; Alderson and Ziter, 1985; Galassi et al., 1987; Barohn et al., 1991; Werneck et al., 1993; Arenas et al., 1995; Illarioshkin et al., 1996; Meola et al., 1996; Weiler et al., 1996; Eymard et al., 1997; Flachenecker et al., 1997; Linssen et al., 1997; Cha et al., 1998; Cupler et al., 1998). The largest series to date of Miyoshi myopathy, as it is now called, was published by Linssen and colleagues (1997, 1998) and detail 12 patients with sporadic disease and 12 Dutch patients with familial disease; Miyoshi myopathy occurs with a prevalence of at least 1 in 440 000 in Japan (Bejaoui et al., 1995). As in Nonaka distal myopathy, symptoms develop between the ages of 15 and 25 (mean 20 years) and the disorder is autosomal recessive. However, in classic Miyoshi myopathy, the initial symptoms are in the distal lower extremity posterior compartment (i.e. the gastrocnemius muscles). Patients notice that they cannot walk on their toes or climb stairs. Aching discomfort in the calves can occur. The gastrocnemius muscles become atrophic and ankle muscle stretch reflexes are lost (Fig. 22.2). The anterior compartment muscles of the distal lower extremities remain relatively spared early in the disease; however, eventually they are also affected. The predilection for early involvement of the gastrocnemius muscles is the clinical hallmark of Miyoshi myopathy that distinguishes it from other distal dystrophies. In Miyoshi's cohort, the weakness was always symmetric. In the Dutch series of 24 patients, nearly one-half of the patients had asymmetric involvement of the calves at the time of presentation and in 12.5% (3/24) the disease remained confined to one leg during follow-up (Linssen et al., 1997). Involvement of arms and hands is unusual early

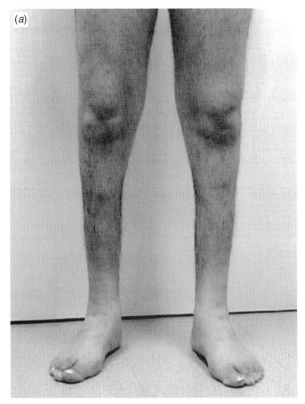

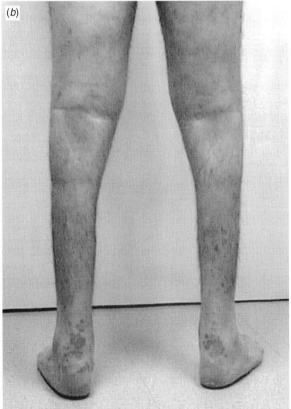

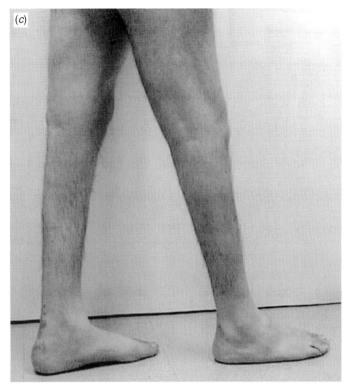

Fig. 22.2. Distal tapering with posterior compartment (gastrocnemius) atrophy in a patient with Miyoshi distal myopathy (early adult-onset type II).

in the disease. After a period of 2–8 years, patients can develop proximal leg and arm weakness to varying degrees. The hamstring muscle group (knee flexors) are weaker than quadriceps muscles (knee extensors), and this may have implications for choice of biopsy site (Barohn et al., 1991). Progression is variable, with some patients remaining fairly stable with distal weakness while others can have a more aggressive pattern involving both proximal and distal muscles (Miyoshi et al., 1986). Overall, Miyoshi myopathy evolves at a slower rate than the Nonaka type. Some patients have preserved upper extremity function throughout the course of the disease. Lower extremity function steadily decreases in the early stages but often stabilizes once assistance is required for standing. Patients affected for 20–45 years have continued to walk (Miyoshi et al., 1986; Meola et al., 1996). However, as many as 13% of patients require wheelchairs for transportation outside the home after 10 years of symptoms (Linssen et al., 1997).

Laboratory features

All Japanese and Western patients have strikingly elevated serum creatine kinase, from 20 to 150 times normal. An extremely high creatine kinase ('asymptomatic hyper-CKaemia') can precede clinical weakness or atrophy (Galassi et al., 1987). Needle EMG reveals brief myopathic motor units and increased recruitment patterns. However, in extremely weak and atrophic gastrocnemius muscles, motor units are very sparse and long duration/polyphasic motor units with a decreased recruitment pattern can be seen. Muscle imaging has confirmed that the posterior compartment muscles of the distal lower extremity are more severely involved than those of the anterior compartment (Meola et al., 1996).

If a weak atrophic gastrocnemius muscle is biopsied, the usual finding is extensive fibrosis and fatty replacement, with loss of the majority of muscle fibres; this is so-called 'end-stage muscle'. By comparison, if a relatively strong quadriceps muscle is biopsied, only minimal myopathic changes may be seen (fibre size variability, central nuclei). Biopsy of an asymptomatic proximal arm muscle may also be relatively uninformative. Therefore, it is useful to biopsy a hamstring muscle (biceps femoris) in these patients; this biopsy may show intermediate histological changes, with striking fibre size variability and numerous necrotic and regenerating fibres (Fig. 22.3). Both dystrophin and dystrophin-associated proteins are expressed normally on the muscle fibres (Yamanouchi et al., 1994). While most patients with Miyoshi myopathy do not have vacuoles in their muscle fibres, two patients have been reported with rare rimmed vacuoles (Shaibani et al., 1997). Therefore, it appears that vacuole formation, while it may be more dramatic in some of the distal myopathies (i.e. Nonaka myopathy), is ultimately a nonspecific histological feature (Jongen et al., 1995; Satoyoshi et al., 1998).

Molecular genetics

Miyoshi myopathy has been linked to chromosome 2p13 (Bejaoui et al., 1995). LGMD2B has also been linked to this locus (Bashir et al., 1994). A family with the mutation has been described in which some members have the typical LGMD clinical phenotype and others have the distal myopathy phenotype (Illarioshkin et al., 1996). In addition, a large Spanish family has been described with distal onset anterior compartment myopathy and linkage to 2p13 (Illa et al., 1998). The mutated gene at this locus has been cloned by two groups and the protein has been named dysferlin (Bashir et al., 1998; Liu et al., 1998). This name stems from the protein's homology to the *Caenorhabditis elegans* spermatogenesis factor Fer-1 (Bashir et al., 1998; Liu et al., 1998). One of these groups of investigators (led by Robert Brown) identified dysferlin as a membrane-located protein of 230 kDa (Matsuda et al., 1999). These same investigators

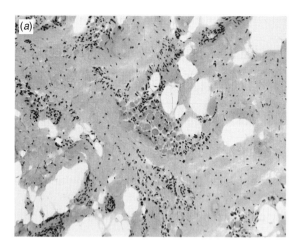

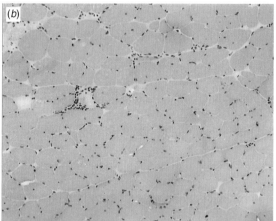

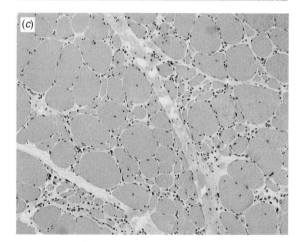

Fig. 22.3. Histology in Miyoshi distal myopathy (early adult-onset type II). (*a*) The lateral gastrocnemius shows extensive fibre loss, with replacement by connective and adipose tissue. (*b*) The vastus lateralis shows slight muscle size variability and a single necrotic fibre undergoing phagocytosis. (*c*) The biceps femoris shows intermediate changes, with variable muscle size, groups of small round fibres and central nuclei. (Haematoxylin and eosin; original magnification ×143). (With permission from Barohn, 1993.)

showed dysferlin was absent in Miyoshi myopathy muscle by both Western immunoblots and direct immunofluorescent studies. The function of dysferlin remains unknown. It is still being determined whether the different phenotypes can be accounted for by identical mutations (Liu et al., 1998) or different frameshift mutations (Bashir et al., 1998).

Finally, there appears to be genetic heterogeneity of the Miyoshi myopathy phenotype. Linssen et al. (1998) reported three families who failed to demonstrate linkage to 2p13. Two of these kinships linked to chromosome 10.

Laing distal myopathy: early-onset type III

Laing et al. (1995a) have reported an Australian family of English/Welsh origin in which weakness began in the anterior compartment of the legs and the neck flexors and was followed by distal finger extensor involvement. Patients developed weakness between 4 and 25 years of age. Inheritance was autosomal dominant. Hand intrinsic finger flexor, facial bulbar and cardiac involvement was absent. Reflexes and sensation were preserved. The disease was only moderately disabling with no incidence of wheelchair dependence. Serum creatine kinase levels were one to three times normal and muscle biopsy showed moderate myopathic changes without vacuoles. EMG revealed occasional fibrillations and small-amplitude, short-durations, polyphasic motor unit potentials in distal more than proximal muscles.

Molecular genetic studies in this family revealed linkage to chromosome 14q11. Hopefully, these findings will be confirmed as additional early adult-onset autosomal dominant families are identified. It is possible that the recent report of autosomal dominant distal myopathy presenting in the first decade of life (Scoppetta et al., 1995) and other early reports of childhood-onset distal myopathy could represent the same disorder (see below).

Myofibrillar myopathy with abnormal foci of desmin

Another new category of distal myopathy has been proposed that is characterized by the pathological finding of excessive desmin accumulation in muscle fibres (Edström et al., 1980; Helliwell et al., 1994; Horowitz and Schmalbruch, 1994; Muntoni et al., 1994; Goebel, 1995; Nakano et al., 1996; Amato et al., 1997, 1998). Desmin is an intermediate filament protein of skeletal, cardiac and some smooth muscle cells (Goebel, 1995). This cytoskeletal protein links Z bands with the plasmalemma and the nucleus. Desmin is

not the only protein that accumulates in this disorder, and Nakano et al. (1996) recommended the term myofibrillar myopathy as this may be a more accurate description of the spectrum of the pathogenic features. This myopathy has been reported as desmin myopathy (Cameron et al., 1995), desmin storage myopathy (Fardeau and Tomé, 1994), spheroid body myopathy (Goebel et al., 1978), cytoplasmic body myopathy (Caron et al., 1995), Mallory body myopathy, intermediate filament myopathy (Fidzianska et al., 1983), familial cardiomyopathy with subsarcolemmal vermiform deposits (Calderon et al., 1987) and myopathy with intrasarcoplasmic accumulation of dense granulofilamentous material (Fardeau et al., 1978). In addition, some patients previously diagnosed with other forms of distal myopathy probably actually have myofibrillar myopathy. Of note is the report of Horowitz and Schmalbruch (1994) of a family with myofibrillar myopathy that was previously reported by Milhorat and Wolff (1943) as a distal myopathy. This family had been considered to have Markesbery myopathy (Barohn, 1993) until the desmin stains were performed.

Clinical features

The clinical features are to some extent heterogeneous and it is unclear if myofibrillar myopathy is a distinct entity. There is a wide clinical spectrum in the myopathies associated with focal desmin accumulation (Helliwell et al., 1994; Goebel, 1995; Amato et al., 1998). Amato et al. (1998) have reviewed the heterogeneous manifestations of myofibrillar myopathy. Most patients develop weakness between 25 and 45 years of age, although there are reports of onset in infancy and later in life. In the Scandinavian cases (Edström et al., 1980), weakness began around 40 years of age in the distal upper extremities. In other patients, the distal lower extremities exhibit weakness first, usually in the anterior compartment (Helliwell et al., 1994; Horowitz and Schmalbruch, 1994). A scapuloperoneal pattern has been reported in a large pedigree (Wilhelmsen et al., 1996). Many of the patients have an associated cardiomyopathy, with heart block, arrhythmias (often requiring a pacemaker) and congestive heart failure. Progression to proximal muscles usually occurs, and some patients develop respiratory involvement requiring mechanical ventilation (Horowitz and Schmalbruch, 1994). Some patients develop cardiac symptoms before skeletal muscle weakness develops. A number of paedriatic cases have been reported, as young as one year of age. Children can have diffuse, primary proximal or distal weakness. Several children have been described with a giant axonal neuropathy associated with desmin accumulation in cardiac and skeletal muscle. The family described by Muntoni et al. (1994), with cardiac/respiratory involvement and distal weakness, also had mental retardation.

Laboratory features

Serum creatine kinase levels are modestly elevated, usually not greater than five times normal. EMG shows myopathic motor units and fibrillations. Complex repetitive discharges are common. Muscle biopsy demonstrated variability in fibre size, fibre splitting, increased central nuclei, increased connective tissue and, occasionally, muscle fibres with rimmed vacuoles. The two major histological abnormalities are nonhyaline lesions consisting of loci of myofibrillar destruction and hyaline lesions composed of compacted and degraded myofibrillar elements (Fig. 22.4) (Nakano et al., 1996). Immunohistochemistry reveals that these lesions react strongly to desmin and numerous other proteins (Fig. 22.4b,c) (DeBleecker et al., 1996; Amato et al., 1998). These deposits are amyloidogenic and stain with Congo red (Amato et al., 1997). Excessive desmin accumulation has also been shown in cardiac muscles in patients with cardiomyopathy (Muntoni et al., 1994). The nonhyaline lesions express desmin, gelsolin, β-amyloid precursor protein, dystrophin and neural cell adhesion molecule but are depleted of actin, α-actinin and myosin (DeBleecker et al., 1996; Amato et al., 1998). The hyaline lesions react variably to antibodies to desmin and strongly react to those for dystrophin, gelsolin, β-amyloid precursor protein, titin, nebulin, actin, myosin and α-actinin. They do not react for neural cell adhesion molecule. Further, both the haline and nonhyaline lesions demonstrate abnormal expression of various cyclic nucleotide-dependent kinases, nuclear matrix protein and lamin B (Nakano et al., 1997; Amato et al., 1998).

Electron microscopy demonstrates two major types of lesion: foci of myofibrillar destruction and hyaline structures that appear as cytoplasmic or spheroid bodies (Amato et al., 1998). The foci of myofibrillar destruction consist of disrupted myofilaments, Z-disc-derived bodies, dappled dense structures of Z-disc origin and streaming of the Z disc (Calderon et al., 1987). The hyaline structures are composed of compacted and degraded remnants of thick and thin filaments (Nakano et al., 1996). Although some authors have demonstrated the accumulation of 8–10nm filaments (Porte et al., 1980), others have not found these intermediate sized filaments despite extensive searching (Nakano et al., 1996). However, 15–18nm filaments have been described (Goebel et al., 1978; Fidzianska et al., 1983; Cameron et al., 1995; Amato et al., 1998).

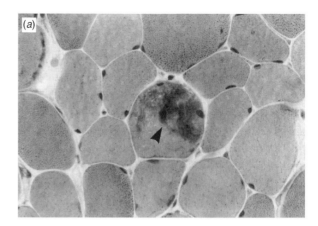

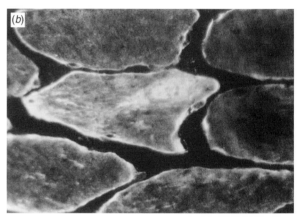

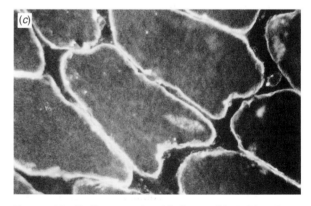

Fig. 22.4. Myofibrillar myopathy with abnormal foci of desmin. (a) Muscle biopsy specimen demonstrates variability in fibre size and dark green irregularly lobulated areas of amorphous material within muscle fibres (nonhyaline lesion) (arrowhead) (modified Gomori, trichrome, ×439). (b) Muscle fibre demonstrates abnormal reactivity to desmin (immunofluorescence stain for desmins, ×571). (c) Ectopic dystrophin expression co-localizes to the area of increased desmin (immunofluorescence stain for dystrophin, ×571). (With permission from Amato et al. 1998. The wide spectrum of myofibrillar myopathy suggests a multifactorial etiology and pathogenesis. *Neurology* **51**, 1646–1655.)

Molecular genetics

Most of the pedigrees are autosomal dominant, although X-linked transmission is suspected in at least one family (Muntoni et al., 1994). There are also reports of sporadic and autosomal recessive inheritance (Helliwell et al., 1994). Desmin is encoded by a single gene on chromosome 2q35 (Goebel, 1995). Mutations in the desmin gene have been identified in at least six families with myofibrillar myopathy and in several sporadic cases (Muñoz-Mármol et al., 1998; Goldfarb et al., 1998; Dalakas et al., 2000). Most of the cases were dominantly inherited adult-onset skeletal myopathies associated with a cardiomyopathy. One family had what was believed to be an autosomal recessive inheritance of an aggressive childhood-onset myopathy and cardiomyopathy (Goldfarb et al., 1998). One patient with sporadic disease with generalized weakness and intestinal pseudo-obstruction was found to have a deletion in the desmin gene (Muñoz-Mármol et al., 1998). Further, in a family with autosomal dominant desmin myopathy, a missense mutation on chromosome 11q21–23 in the gene for αB-crystallin was identified (Vicart et al., 1998). The protein αB-crystallin possesses molecular chaperone activity and is thought to interact with desmin in the assembly of the intermediate filament network. The genetic defect(s) of other kinships and sporadic cases remains to be determined. Finally, a family with autosomal dominant myofibrillar myopathy and scapuloperoneal weakness cardiomyopathy was linked to changes on chromosome 12 (Wilhelmsen et al., 1996).

While it seems clear that some patients with distal myopathy do have abnormal desmin deposits, desmin accumulation can be seen in a variety of neuromuscular conditions including X-linked myotubular myopathy, congenital myotonic dystrophy, spinal muscular atrophy, nemaline rod disease, fetal myotubes and toxic drug-induced myopathy, and in regenerating muscle fibres of any aetiology (Sarnat, 1992; Goebel, 1995; Amato et al., 1998). Consequently, focal accumulation of desmin is a nonspecific finding and while we can tentatively add myofibrillar myopathy with abnormal foci of desmin to our distal myopathy category, we must keep in mind these caveats. Perhaps other previously reported cases of distal myopathy with cardiac abnormalities (Markesbery et al., 1974; Krendel et al., 1988) should be restudied for desmin accumulation. Desmin antibody is commercially available and immunohistochemical staining should probably be done on muscle biopsy specimens from all those with distal myopathy.

Table 22.2. Other myopathies that can have distal weakness

| Childhood-onset distal myopathy |
| Infantile onset (before age 2 years) |
| Juvenile onset (before age 15 years) |
| (? if these are Laing myopathy) |
| Myotonic dystrophy |
| Facioscapulohumeral dystrophy[a] |
| Scapuloperoneal myopathy[a] |
| Oculopharyngeal dystrophy |
| Emery–Dreifuss humeroperoneal dystrophy[a] |
| Inflammatory myopathies |
| Inclusion body myositis |
| Polymyositis |
| Metabolic myopathy |
| Debrancher deficiency |
| Acid maltase deficiency[a] |
| Congenital myopathy |
| Nemaline myopathy[a] |
| Central core myopathy[a] |
| Centronuclear myopathy |

Notes:
[a] Scapuloperoneal distribution of weakness can occur.

Other myopathies with distal weakness

There are a number of other myopathies that can show distal weakness (Table 22.2).

Infantile and juvenile distal myopathy

There are six reports of infantile-onset distal myopathy, including one sporadic case and four autosomal dominant kindreds (Magee and DeJong, 1965; Heyck et al., 1968; van der Does de Willebois et al., 1968; Bautista et al., 1978; Scoppetta et al., 1995; Voit et al., 1998). The clinical picture painted by these studies follows closely Batten's 1910 description of early childhood-onset familial distal myopathy (Batten, 1910). Deficits are first noticed at 12 to 24 months of life when the child begins to walk. Ambulation may be delayed to 18 to 24 months and, when finally achieved, is characterized by 'floppy feet', frequent falling or toe-walking. Weakness involves the anterior leg, sparing the posterior compartment with time; this leads to severe foot drop. Pes cavus and ankle contractures are commonly observed. During the first three decades, weakness spreads to the wrist and finger extensors and intrinsic hand muscles in most patients. The myopathy follows a very slowly progressive to nonprogressive course, with no significant disability; however, a few patients develop more generalized symptoms in the fourth decade. The family reported by Scoppetta et al. in 1995 is atypical because they showed no distal arm weakness, mild facial diparesis and juvenile-onset neck, trunk and proximal limb weakness. No ocular, bulbar or cardiac disturbances occurred. Serum creatine kinase levels were normal except for one anomalous patient who had an 18-fold elevation (Bautista et al., 1978). EMG revealed low-voltage, short-duration motor unit potentials, with no or sparse fibrillation potentials. Muscle biopsies showed myopathic changes with rare vacuoles; two reports documented fibre type disproportion (Bautista et al., 1978; Scoppetta et al., 1995). Immunostaining for dystrophin, α-, β-, γ- and δ-sarcoglycans and the laminins was normal in one patient (Voit et al., 1998).

Infantile-onset distal myopathy shows some resemblance to Laing myopathy but is distinguished by the earlier age of onset, hand intrinsic involvement and lack of neck flexor weakness in most kindreds. Nevertheless, linkage to chromosome 14q11 bears investigation.

One family with so-called juvenile-onset distal myopathy has been described (Biemond, 1955). In this large Dutch pedigree, 19 members developed distal weakness in the hands and feet between the ages of 5 and 15 years. An autosomal dominant inheritance was suspected. Both flexor and extensor distal muscle groups were affected. The disease progressed extremely slowly and the patients remained functional and active during adult life. Both myopathic and neuropathic features were seen on muscle biopsy and autopsy.

Other muscular dystrophies

Weakness of distal muscle groups may be prominent in other muscular dystrophies. In myotonic dystrophy, wrist and finger extensors, and ankle dorsiflexors, are typically weaker than proximal limb muscles, especially early in the disease. Because the prevalence of myotonic dystrophy is 5 per 100 000 (Harper and Rüdel, 1994), it is probably the most commonly seen myopathic condition in which prominent distal weakness is present, especially in the young and middle-age groups. Rare patients with the phenotypic appearance of myotonic dystrophy and distal weakness, but without clinical or electrical myotonia, have been described (Schotland and Rowland, 1964). Patients with fascioscapulohumeral dystrophy may develop weakness of ankle dorsiflexion and wrist/finger extension along with the typical facial and scapular muscle involvement. Rarely, they can present with ankle weakness (Munsat, 1994). Indeed, the presence of foot dorsiflexor weakness is

included in the diagnostic criteria for fascioscapulohumeral dystrophy (Tawil et al., 1994). This dystrophy has been mapped to chromosome 4q35 (Wijmenga et al., 1991). Patients with the so-called myopathic form of the scapuloperoneal syndrome have significant ankle weakness (Thomas et al., 1975; Ricker and Merten, 1968; Todman and Cooke, 1984; Yee et al., 1988). Recently, a large family with a scapuloperoneal myopathy was found to have genetic linkage to chromosome 12 (Wilhelmsen et al., 1996). Histologically, there was evidence of abnormal desmin expression, as noted above. Patients with the X-linked Emery–Dreifuss disease, also known as humeroperoneal muscular dystrophy, present with ankle dorsiflexion, triceps and biceps weakness, and with contraction at the elbow and ankle (Rowland et al., 1979). Some pedigrees of oculopharyngeal muscular dystrophy also have significant distal extremity weakness (Satoyoshi and Kinoshita, 1977; Fukuhara et al., 1982; Vita et al., 1983; Amato et al., 1995; Satoyoshi et al., 1998).

Inflammatory myopathies

Rarely, cases of polymyositis have been described in which patients first develop weakness of the hands and ankles (Hollinrake, 1969; van Kasteren, 1979). Biopsy of proximal muscles revealed an inflammatory myopathy and patients improved with steroid therapy.

A more frequent situation in which an inflammatory myopathy presents with early distal weakness occurs with sporadic cases of IBM (Lotz et al., 1989; Griggs et al., 1995; Amato et al., 1996; Amato and Barohn, 1997). Sporadic IBM accounts for approximately one-third of all inflammatory myopathies and is the most common distal myopathy in elderly patients. Patients with sporadic IBM develop slowly progressive weakness, usually after the age of 50 years. The pattern of weakness in IBM is unique in that the clinical hallmark is early weakness and atrophy of wrist and finger flexors, quadriceps and ankle dorsiflexors. Toe flexors are also frequently weak, sometimes producing a position of chronic great toe extension, or a pseudo-Babinski sign. Some degree of asymmetry in muscle weakness is the rule. Because of the dramatic knee extensor involvement, it is not exclusively a distal myopathy, although distal upper extremity flexor weakness is an invariable component of the disease. Both knee extensor and forearm/finger flexor weakness are included in the clinical diagnostic criteria for IBM (Griggs et al., 1995). Severe weakness in these muscle groups is so characteristic of IBM that even if the classic histological findings are not present on muscle biopsy a presumptive diagnosis of 'possible' IBM should be considered (Amato et al., 1996).

Classic light microscopy features are endomysial inflammation with invasion of non-necrotic muscle fibres, eosinophilic cytoplasmic inclusions and rimmed vacuoles containing amyloid deposits within the muscle fibres (Mendell, 1991; Griggs et al., 1995). On electron microscopy, there is an accumulation of cytoplasmic and intranuclear 15–21 nm filaments. Despite the presence of inflammation in IBM, the disease is typically refractory to immunosuppressive therapy (Barohn et al., 1995).

Autosomal recessive hereditary IBM (Sivakumar and Dalakas, 1996) was described above with Nonaka distal myopathy as recent molecular genetic studies indicate that they are the same myopathic disorder (Argov et al., 1997; Ikeuchi et al., 1997).

Metabolic and congenital myopathies

Debrancher enzyme deficiency has been reported with severe distal leg weakness (DiMauro et al., 1979). We have observed a 30-year-old male with adult-onset acid maltase deficiency who presented with a scapuloperoneal pattern of weakness (Barohn et al., 1993).

Patients with nephropathic cystinosis develop a distal myopathy as a late complication of the disease. This is an autosomal recessive lysosomal storage disorder in which cystine accumulates and leads to renal failure. Patients who survive childhood because they receive a kidney transplant develop weakness and wasting in the hand muscles. Electrodiagnostic studies are consistent with a myopathic process, and muscle biopsy of hand muscles shows a vacuolar myopathy (Charnas et al., 1994).

Nonprogressive congenital muscle diseases such as nemaline rod (Hausmanowa-Petrusewicz et al., 1992; Laing et al., 1992; Laing et al., 1995b), central core (Kratz and Brooke, 1980) and centronuclear (Moxley et al., 1978) myopathy can have significant involvement of distal muscles. One family with autosomal dominant nemaline myopathy has been shown to have a mutation of the gene for α-tropomyosin on chromosome 1 (Laing et al., 1992, 1995b). In this Australian pedigree, patients first develop symptoms in late childhood, and ankle dorsiflexion weakness is the initial and most significant manifestation of the disease (Laing et al., 1992, 1995b).

References

Åhlberg, G., Jakobsson, F., Fransson, A., Moritz, A., Borg, K. and Edström, L. (1994). Distribution of muscle degeneration in Welander distal myopathy – a magnetic resonance imaging and muscle biopsy study. *Neuromusc. Disord.* **4**, 55–62.

Åhlberg, G., Borg, J., Edström, L. and Anvent, M. (1997). Welander distal myopathy is not linked to other defined distal myopathy gene loci. *Neuromusc. Disord.* **7**, 256–260.

Åhlberg, G., Borg, J., Ansved, L., Edström, L. and Anvent, M. (1998a). Welander distal myopathy: genetic linkage and candidate genes on chromosome 2p. *Muscle Nerve* **21** (Suppl. 7), S6.

Åhlberg, G., Borg, J., Edström, L. and Anvent, M. (1998b). Welander hereditary distal myopathy, a molecular genetic comparison to hereditary myopathies with inclusion bodies. *Neuromusc. Disord.* **8**, 111–114.

Åhlberg, G., von Tell, D., Borg, K., Edström, L. and Anvert, M. (1999). Genetic linkage of Welander distal myopathy to chromosome 2p13. *Ann. Neurol.* **46**, 399–404.

Alderson, M. K. and Ziter, F. A. (1985). Distal muscular dystrophy. *Muscle Nerve* **8**, 723.

Amato, A. A. and Barohn, R. J. (1997). Idiopathic inflammatory myopathies. *Neurol. Clin.* **15**, 615–648.

Amato, A. A., Jackson, C. E., Ridings, L. and Barohn, R. J. (1995). Childhood-onset oculopharyngodistal myopathy with chronic intestinal pseudo-obstruction. *Muscle Nerve* **18**, 842–847.

Amato, A. A., Gronseth, G. S., Jackson, C. E. et al. (1996). Inclusion body myositis: clinical and pathologic boundaries. *Ann. Neurol.* **40**, 581–586.

Amato, A. A., Ferrante, M., Kagan-Hallet, K. and Barohn, R. J. (1997). The spectrum of myofibrillar myopathy with accumulation of excess desmin. *J. Child Neurol.* **12**, 131.

Amato, A. A., Kagan-Hallet, K., Jackson, C. E. et al. (1998). The wide-spectrum of myofibrillar myopathy suggests a multifactorial etiology and pathogenesis. *Neurology* **51**, 1646–1655.

Arenas, C., Bautista, J., Galan, J. et al. (1995). Miopatias distales recesivas. Aportacion de cinco casos. *Neurologia* **10**, 1–6.

Argov, Z. and Yarom, R. (1984). 'Rimmed vacuole myopathy' sparing the quadriceps: a unique disorder in Iranian Jews. *J. Neurol. Sci.* **64**, 33–43.

Argov, Z., Tiram, E., Eisenberg, I. et al. (1997). Various types of hereditary inclusion body myopathy maps to chromosome 9p1-q1. *Ann. Neurol.* **41**, 548–551.

Askanas, V. (1997). New developments in hereditary inclusion body myopathies. *Ann. Neurol.* **41**, 421–422.

Barohn, R. J. (1993). Distal myopathies and dystrophies. *Semin. Neurol.* **13**, 247–255.

Barohn, R. J. and Amato, A. A. (1999). Distal myopathies. *Semin. Neurol.* **19**, 45–58.

Barohn, R. J., Miller, R. G. and Griggs, R. C. (1991). Autosomal recessive distal dystrophy. *Neurology* **41**, 1365–1370.

Barohn, R. J., McVey, A. L. and DiMauro, S. (1993). Adult acid maltase deficiency. *Muscle Nerve* **16**, 672–676.

Barohn, R. J., Amato, A. A., Sahenk, Z., Kissel, J. T. and Mendell, J. R. (1995). Inclusion body myositis: explanation for poor response to immunosuppressive therapy. *Neurology* **45**, 1302–1304.

Barohn, R. J., Amato, A. A. and Griggs, R. C. (1998). Overview of distal myopathies: from the clinical to the molecular. *Neuromusc. Disord.* **8**, 309–316.

Barrows, H. S. and Duemler, L. P. (1962). Late distal myopathy. Report of a case. *Neurology* **12**, 547–550

Bashir, R., Strachan, T., Keers, S. et al. (1994). A gene for autosomal recessive limb-girdle muscular dystrophy maps to chromosome 2p. *Hum. Mol. Genet.* **3**, 455–457.

Bashir, R., Britton, S., Strachan, T. et al. (1998). A gene related to *Caenorhabditis elegans* spermatogenesis factor *fer-1* is mutated in limb-girdle muscular dystrophy type 2B. *Nat. Genet.* **20**, 37–42.

Batten, F. E. (1910). Distal type of myopathy in several members of a family. *Proc. Roy. Soc. Med.* **3**, 93–95.

Bautista, J., Rafel, E., Castilla, J. and Alberca, R. (1978). Hereditary distal myopathy with onset in early infancy. *J. Neurol. Sci.* **37**, 149–158.

Bejaoui, K., Hirabayashi, K., Hentati, F., Haines, J. L., Ben Weissenbach, J. and Rowland, L. P. (1995). Linkage of Miyoshi myopathy (distal autosomal recessive muscular dystrophy) locus to chromosome 2p12–14. *Neurology* **45**, 768–772.

Biemond, A. (1955). Myopathia distalis juvenilis hereditaria. *Acta Psychiatr. Neurol. Scand.* **30**, 25–38.

Borg, K., Borg, J. and Lindblom, U. (1987). Sensory involvement in distal myopathy (Welander). Histochemical and morphological observations on muscle and nerve biopsies. *J. Neurol. Sci.* **80**, 323–332.

Borg, K., Solders, G., Borg, J., Edström, L. and Kristersson, K. (1989). Neurogenic involvement in distal myopathy (Welander). *J. Neurol. Sci.* **91**, 53–70.

Borg, K., Åhlberg, G., Borg, J. and Edström, L. (1991a). Welander's distal myopathy: clinical, neurophysiological and muscle biopsy observations in young and middle aged adult with early symptoms. *J. Neurol. Neurosurg. Psychiatry* **54**, 494–498.

Borg, K., Tomé, F. and Edström, L. (1991b). Intranuclear and cytoplasmic filamentous inclusions in distal myopathy (Welander). *Acta Neuropathol.* **82**, 102–106.

Borg, K., Åhlberg, G., Hedberg, B. and Edström, L. (1993). Muscle fibre degeneration in distal myopathy (Welander) – ultrastructure related to immunohistochemical observations on cytoskeletal proteins and leu-19 antigen. *Neuromusc. Disord.* **3**, 149–155.

Borg, K., Åhlberg, G., Anvret, M. and Edström, L. (1998). Welander distal myopathy: clinical pathophysiologic, and molecular aspects. In: *Inclusion-body Myositis and Myopathies*, ed. V. Askanas, G. Serratrice and W. K. Engel, pp. 221–231. Cambridge, UK: Cambridge University Press.

Campbell, C. M. (1906). A case of muscular dystrophy affecting hand and feet. *Rev. Neurol. Psychiatry* **4**,192–202.

Cameron, C. H. S., Mirakhur, M. and Allen, I. V. (1995). Desmin myopathy with cardiomyopathy. *Acta Neuropathol.* **89**, 560–566.

Calderon, A., Becker, L. E. and Murphy, E. G. (1987). Subsarcolemmal vermiform deposits in skeletal muscle associated with familial cardiomyopathy: Report of two cases of a new entity. *Ped. Neurosci.* **13**, 108–112.

Caron, A., Viader, F., Lechevalier, B. and Chapon, F. (1995). Cytoplasmic body myopathy: familial cases with accumulation of desmin and dystrophin. An immunohistochemical, immunoelectron microscopic and biochemical study. *Acta Neuropathol.* **90**, 150–157.

Cha, C., Wolfe, G. I., Bryan, W. W., Burns, D. K. and Barohn, R. J. (1998). Miyoshi myopathy in Hispanic siblings. *J. Child Neurol.* **13**, 134.

Charnas, L. R., Luciano, C. A., Dalakas, M. et al. (1994). Distal vacuolar myopathy in nephropathic cystinosis. *Ann. Neurol.* **35**, 181–188.

Cupler, E. J., Bohlega, S., Hessler, R., McLean, D., Stigsby, B. and Ahmad, J. (1998). Miyoshi myopathy in Saudi Arabia: clinical, electrophysiological, histopathological and radiological features. *Neuromusc. Disord.* **8**, 321–326.

Dahlgaard, E. (1960). Myopathia distalis tarda hereditaria. *Acta Psychiatr. Neurol. Scand.* **35**, 440–447.

Dalakas, M. C., Park, K.-Y., Semino-Mora, C., Lee, H. S., Sivakumar, K. and Goldfarb, L. G. (2000). Desmin myopathy, a skeletal myopathy with cardiomyopathy caused by mutations in the desmin gene. *N. Eng. J. Med.* **342**, 770–780.

DeBleecker, J. L., Engel, A. G. and Ertl, B. B. (1996). Myofibrillar myopathy with abnormal foci of desminpositivity. II. Immunocytochemical analysis reveals accumulation of multiple other proteins. *J. Neuropathol. Exp. Neurol.* **55**, 563–577.

Dejerine, J. and Thomas, A. (1904). Un cas de myopathie a topographie type Aran-Duchenne suivi d'autopsie. *Rev. Neurol.* **12**, 1187–1190.

DiMauro, S., Hartwig, G., Hays, A. et al. (1979). Debrancher deficiency: neuromuscular disorder in 5 adults. *Ann. Neurol.* **5**, 422–436.

Edström, L. (1975). Histochemical and histopathological changes in skeletal muscle in late-onset hereditary distal myopathy (Welander). *J. Neurol. Sci.* **26**, 147–157.

Edström, L., Thornell, L. E. and Eriksson, A. (1980). A new type of hereditary distal myopathy with characteristic sarcoplasmic bodies and intermediate (Skeletin) filaments. *J. Neurol. Sci.* **47**, 171–190.

Eymard, B., Laforet, P., Tomé, F. M. S. et al. (1997). Distal myopathy of Miyoshi type: report of 21 French cases. *Neuromusc. Disord.* **7**, 461.

Fardeau, M. and Tomé, F. M. S. (1994). Congenital myopathies. In: *Myology*, 2nd edn, eds. A. G. Engel and C. Fanzini-Armstron, pp. 522–526. New York: McGraw-Hill.

Fardeau, M., Godet-Guillain, J., Tomé, F. et al. (1978). Une nouvelle affection musculaire familiale, de finie par l'accumulation intra-sarcoplasmique d'un materiel graunulofilmentaire dense en microscopie electronique. *Rev. Neurol.* **134**, 411–425.

Felice, K. J., Meredith, C., Binz, N. et al. (1999). Autosomal dominant distal myopathy not linked to the known distal myopathy loci. *Neuromusc. Disord.* **9**, 59–65.

Fidzianska, A., Goebel, H. H., Osborn, M., Lenard, H. G., Osse, G. and Langenbeck, U. (1983). Mallory body-like inclusions in a hereditary congenital neuromuscular disease. *Muscle Nerve* **6**, 195–200,

Flachenecker, P., Kiefer, R., Naumann, M., Handwerker, M. and Reichmann, H. (1997). Distal muscular dystrophy of Miyoshi type. Report of two cases and review of the literature. *J. Neurol.* **244**, 23–29.

Fukuhara, N., Kumamoto, T., Tsubaki, T., Mayuzumi, T. and Nitta, H. (1982). Oculopharyngeal muscular dystrophy and distal myopathy: intrafamilial difference in the onset and distribution of muscular involvement. *Acta Neurol. Scand.* **65**, 458–467.

Galassi, G., Rowland, L. P., Hays, A. P., Hopkins, L. C. and DiMauro, S. (1987). High serum levels of creatine kinase: asymptomatic prelude to distal myopathy. *Muscle Nerve* **10**, 346–350.

Goebel, H. H. (1995). Desmin-related neuromuscular disorders. *Muscle Nerve* **18**, 1306–1320.

Goebel, H. H., Muller, J., Gillen, H. W. and Merrit, A. D. (1978). Autosomal dominant 'spheroidal body myopathy'. *Muscle Nerve* **1**, 14–26.

Goldfarb, L. G., Park, K.-Y., Cervenaková, L. et al. (1998). Missense mutations in desmin associated with familial cardiac and skeletal myopathy. *Nat. Genet.* **19**, 402–403.

Gowers, W. R. (1902). A lecture on myopathy and a distal form. *Br. Med. J.* **2**, 89–92.

Griggs, R. C. and Markesbery, W. R. (1994). Distal myopathies. In: *Myology*, 2nd edn, eds. A. Engel and C. Franzini-Armstrong, pp. 1246–1257. New York: McGraw Hill.

Griggs, R. C., Askanas, V., DiMauro, S. et al. (1995). Inclusion body myositis and myopathies. *Ann. Neurol.* **38**, 705–713.

Haravuori, H., Mäkelä-Bengs, P., Figlewicz, D. A. et al. (1998a). Tibial muscular dystrophy and late-onset distal myopathy are linked to the same locus on chromosome 2q. *Neurology* **50**, A186.

Haravuori, H., Mäkelä-Bengs, P., Udd, B. et al. (1998b). Assignment of the dystrophy locus to chromosome 2q31. *Am. J. Hum. Genet.* **62**, 620–626.

Harper, P. S. and Rüdel, R. (1994). Myotonic dystrophy. In: *Myology*, 2nd edn, eds. A. Engel and C. Franzini-Armstrong, pp. 1192–1219. New York: McGraw Hill.

Hausmanowa-Petrusewicz, I., Fidzianska, A. and Badurska, B. (1992). Unusual course of nemaline myopathy. *Neuromusc. Disord.* **2**, 413–418.

Helliwell, T. R., Green, A. R. T., Green, A. and Edwards, R. H. (1994). Hereditary distal myopathy with granulo-filamentous cytoplasmic inclusions containing desmin, dystrophin and vimentin. *J. Neurol. Sci.* **124**, 174–187.

Heyck, H., Luders, C. J. and Wolter, M. (1968). Uber eine kongenitale distale Muskeldystrophie mit benigner Progredienz. *Nervenartz* **39**, 549–552.

Hollinrake, K. (1969). Polymyositis presenting as a distal muscle weakness – a case report. *J. Neurol. Sci.* **8**, 479–484.

Horowitz, S. and Schmalbruch, H. (1994). Autosomal dominant distal myopathy with desmin storage: a clinicopathologic and electrophysiologic study of a large kinship. *Muscle Nerve* **17**, 151–160.

Ikeuchi, T., Asaka, T., Saito, M. et al. (1997). Gene locus for autosomal recessive distal myopathy with rimmed vacuoles maps to chromosome 9. *Ann. Neurol.* **41**, 432–437.

Illa, I., Serrano, C., Gallardo, E. et al. (1998). Distal anterior compartment myopathy: a new severe dystrophic phenotype linked to chromosome 2p13. *Neurology* **50**, A186.

Illarioshkin, S. N., Ivanova-Smoleskaya, I. A., Tanaka, H. et al. (1996). Clinical and molecular analysis of a large family with 3 distinct phenotypes of progressive muscular dystrophy. *Brain* **119**, 1895–1909.

Isaacs, H., Badenhorst, M. E. and Whistler, T. (1988). Autosomal recessive distal myopathy. *J. Clin. Pathol.* **41**, 188–194.

Jongen, P. J. H., Laak, H. J. T. and Stadhouders, A. M. (1995). Rimmed basophilic vacuoles and filamentous inclusions in neuromuscular disorders. *Neuromusc. Disord.* **5**, 31–38.

Kratz, R. and Brooke, M. H. (1980). Distal myopathy. In: *Handbook of Clinical Neurology*, Vol. 40, eds. P. J. Vinken and G. W. Bruyn, pp. 471–483. Amsterdam: North-Holland.

Krendel, D. A., Gilchrist, J. M. and Bossen, E. H. (1988). Distal vacuolar myopathy with complete heart block. *Arch. Neurol.* **45**, 698–699.

Kuhn, E. and Schroder, M. (1981). A new type of distal myopathy in two brothers. *J. Neurol.* **226**, 181–185.

Kumamota, T., Fukuhara, N., Nagashima, M., Kanda, T. and Wakabayashi, M. (1982). Distal myopathy: histochemical and ultrastructural studies. *Arch. Neurol.* **39**, 367–371.

Laing, N. G., Majda, B. T., Akkari, P. A. et al. (1992). Assignment of a gene (*NEM1*) for autosomal dominant nemaline myopathy to chromosome 1. *Am. J. Hum. Genet.* **50**, 576–583.

Laing, N. G., Laing, B. A., Meredith, C. et al. (1995a). Autosomal dominant distal myopathy: linkage to chromosome 14. *Am. J. Hum. Genet.* **56**, 422–427.

Laing, N. G., Wilton, S. D., Akkari, P. A. et al. (1995b). A mutation in the α-tropomyosin gene TPM3 associated with autosomal dominant nemaline myopathy. *Nat. Genet.* **9**, 75–79.

Lindberg, C., Borg, K., Edström, L., Hedstrom, A. and Oldfors, A. (1991). Inclusion body myositis and Welander distal myopathy: a clinical, neurophysiological and morphological comparison. *J. Neurol. Sci.* **103**, 76–81.

Linssen, W. H. J. P., Notermans, N. C., van der Graaf, Y. et al. (1997). Miyoshi-type distal muscular dystrophy. Clinical spectrum in 24 Dutch patients. *Brain* **120**, 1989–1996.

Linssen, W. H. J. P., de Visser, M., Notermans, N. C. et al. (1998). Genetic heterogeneity in Miyoshi-type distal muscular dystrophy. *Neuromusc. Disord.* **8**, 317–320.

Liu, J., Aoki, M., Illa, I. et al. (1998). Dysferlin, a novel skeletal muscle gene, is mutated in Miyoshi myopathy and limb girdle muscular dystrophy. *Nat. Genet.* **20**, 31–36.

Lotz, B. P., Engel, A. G., Nishino, H., Stevens, J. C. and Litchy, W. J. (1989). Inclusion body myositis: observations in 40 patients. *Brain* **112**, 727–747.

Magee, K. R and DeJong, R. N. (1965). Hereditary distal myopathy with onset in infancy. *Arch. Neurol.* **13**, 387–390.

Markesbery, W. R. and Griggs, R. C. (1986). Distal myopathies. In: *Myology*, eds. A. Engel and B. Q. Banker, pp. 1313–1325. New York: McGraw-Hill.

Markesbery, W. R., Griggs, R. C., Leach, R. P. and Lapham, L. W. (1974). Late onset hereditary distal myopathy. *Neurology* **23**, 127–134.

Markesbery, W. R., Griggs, R. C. and Herr, B. (1977). Distal myopathy: electron microscopic and histochemical studies. *Neurology* **27**, 727–735.

Massa, R., Weller, B., Karpati, G., Shoubridge, E. and Carpenter, S. (1991). Familial inclusion body myositis among Kurdish-Iranian Jews. *Arch. Neurol.* **48**, 519–522.

Matsubara, S. and Tanabe, H. (1982). Hereditary distal myopathy with filamentous inclusions. *Acta Neurol. Scand.* **65**, 363–368.

Matsuda, C., Aoki, M., Hayashi, Y. K., Hom, M. F., Arahata, K. and Brown, R. H. (1999). Dysferlin is a membrane-associated protein that is absent in Miyoshi myopathy. *Neurology* **53**, 1119–1122.

Mendell, J. R., Sahenk, Z., Gales, T. and Paul, L. (1991). Amyloid filaments in inclusion body myositis: novel findings provide insight into nature of filaments. *Arch. Neurol.* **48**, 1229–1234.

Meola, G., Sansone, V., Rotondo, G. and Jabbour, A. (1996). Computerized tomography and magnetic resonance muscle imaging in Miyoshi's myopathy. *Muscle Nerve* **19**, 1476–1480.

Milhorat, A. T. and Wolff, H. G. (1943). Studies in diseases of muscle. XII. Progressive muscular dystrophy of atrophic distal type; report on a family; report of an autopsy. *Arch. Neurol. Psychiatry* **49**, 655–664.

Miller, R. G., Blank, N. K. and Layzer, R. B. (1979). Sporadic distal myopathy with early adult onset. *Ann. Neurol.* **5**, 220–227.

Miyoshi, K., Saijo, K., Kuryu, Y. et al. (1967). Four cases of distal myopathy in two families [abstract in Japanese]. *Jap. J. Hum. Genet.* **12**, 113.

Miyoshi, K., Tada, Y., Iwasa, M. et al. (1975). Autosomal recessive distal myopathy observed characteristically in Japan [Japanese with abstract in English]. *Jap. J. Hum. Genet.* **20**, 62–63.

Miyoshi, K., Kawai, H., Iwasa, M., Kusaka, K. and Nishino, H. (1986). Autosomal recessive distal muscular dystrophy: as a new type of progressive muscular dystrophy. *Brain* **109**, 31–54.

Mizusawa, H., Kurisaki, H., Takatsu, M. et al. (1987a). Rimmed vacuolar distal myopathy: a clinical, electrophysiological, histopathological and computed tomographic study of seven cases. *J. Neurol.* **234**, 129–136.

Mizusawa, H., Kurisaki, H., Takatsu, M., Inone, K., Toyokura, Y. and Nakanishi, T. (1987b). Rimmed vacuolar distal myopathy. An ultrastructural study. *J. Neurol.* **234**, 137–145.

Moxley, R. T., Griggs, R. C., Markesbery, W. R. and Vangelder, V. (1978). Metabolic implications of distal atrophy. Carbohydrate metabolism in centronuclear myopathy. *J. Neurol. Sci.* **39**, 247–259.

Muñoz-Mármol, A. M., Strasser, G., Isamat, M. et al. (1998). A dysfunctional desmin mutation in a patient with severe generalized myopathy. *Proc. Natl. Acad. Sci. USA* **95**, 11312–11317.

Munsat, T. L. (1994). Fascioscapulohumeral dystrophy and the scapuloperoneal syndrome. In: *Myology*, 2nd edn, eds. A. Engel and C. Franzini-Armstrong, pp. 1220–1232. New York: McGraw-Hill.

Muntoni, F., Catani, G., Mateddu, A. et al. (1994). Familial cardiomyopathy, mental retardation and myopathy associated with desmin-type intermediate filaments. *Neuromusc. Disord.* **4**, 233–241.

Murone, I., Sato, T., Shirakawa, K. et al. (1963). Distal myopathy – a case of non-hereditary distal myopathy [Japanese with English abstract]. *Clin. Neurol. (Tokyo)* **3**, 378–386.

Nakano, S., Engel, A. G., Waclawik, A. J., Emslie-Smith, A. M. and Busis, N. A. (1996). Myofibrillar myopathy with abnormal foci of desmin postivity. I. Light and electron microscopy analysis of 10 cases. *J. Neuropathol. Exp. Neurol.* **55**, 549–562.

Nakano, S., Engel, A. G., Akiguschi, I. and Kimura, J. (1997). Myofibrillar myopathy III. Abnormal expression of cyclin-dependent kinases and nuclear proteins. *J. Neuropathol. Exp. Neurol.* **56**, 850–856.

Nonaka, I., Sunohara, N., Ishiura, S. and Satoyoshi, E. (1981). Familial distal myopathy with rimmed vacuole and lamellar (myeloid) body formation. *J. Neurol. Sci.* **51**, 141–155.

Nonaka, I., Sunohara, N., Satoyoshi, E., Terasawa, K. and Yonemoto, K. (1985). Autosomal recessive distal muscular dystrophy: a comparative study with distal myopathy with rimmed vacuole formation. *Ann. Neurol.* **17**, 51–59.

Nonaka, I., Murakami, N., Suzuki, Y. and Kawai, M. (1998). Distal myopathy with rimmed vacuoles. *Neuromusc. Disord.* **8**, 333–337.

Partanen, J., Laulumaa, V., Paljärve, L., Partanen, K. and Naukkarinen, A. (1994). Late onset foot-drop muscular dystrophy with rimmed vacuoles. *J. Neurol. Sci.* **125**, 158–167.

Porte, A., Stoeckel, M. E., Sacrez, A. and Batzenschager, A. (1980). Unusual familial cardiomyopathy with storage of intermediate filaments in the cardiac muscular cells. *Virchows Arch. A, Pathol. Anat. Histol.* **386**, 43–58.

Ricker, K. and Mertens, H. G. (1968). The differential diagnosis of the myogenic (facio)-scapuloperoneal-syndrome. *Eur. Neurol.* **1**, 275–307.

Rowland, L. P., Fetell, M., Olarte, M., Hays, A., Singh, N. and Wanat, F. E. (1979). Emery–Dreifuss muscular dystrophy. *Ann. Neurol.* **5**, 111–117.

Sadeh, M., Gadoth, N., Hadar, H. and Ben-David, E. (1993). Vacuolar myopathy sparing the quadriceps. *Brain* **116**, 217–232.

Sarnat, H. B. (1992). Vimentin and desmin in maturing skeletal muscle and developmental myopathies. *Neurology* **42**, 1616–1624.

Sasaki, K., Mori, H., Takahashi, K. et al. (1969). Distal myopathy – report of four cases [Japanese with English abstract]. *Clin. Neurol. (Tokyo)* **9**, 627–637.

Satoyoshi, E. and Kinoshita, M. (1977). Oculopharyngodistal myopathy. *Arch. Neurol.* **34**, 89–92.

Satoyoshi, E., Sunohara, N. and Nonaka, I. (1998). Distal myopathy with rimmed vacuoles, inclusion-body myositis, and related disorders in Japan. In: *Inclusion-body Myositis and Myopathies*, eds. V. Askanas, G. Serratrice and W. K. Engel, pp. 244–251. Cambridge, UK: Cambridge University Press.

Schotland, D. and Rowland, L. (1964). Muscular dystrophy: features of ocular myopathy, distal myopathy, and myotonic dystrophy. *Arch. Neurol.* **10**, 433–445.

Scoppetta, C., Vaccario, M. L., Casali, C., Di Trapani, G. and Mennuni, G. (1988). Distal muscular dystrophy with autosomal recessive inheritance. *Muscle Nerve* **7**, 478–481.

Scoppetta, C., Casali, C., La Cesa, I. et al. (1995). Infantile autosomal dominant distal myopathy. *Acta Neurol. Scand.* **92**, 122–126.

Shaibani, A., Harati, Y., Amato, A. and Ferrante, M. (1997). Miyoshi myopathy with vacuoles. *Neurology* (Suppl.) **47**, A195.

Sivakumar, K. and Dalakas, M. C. (1996). The spectrum of familial inclusion body myopathies in 13 families and a description of a quadriceps-sparing phenotype in non-Iranian Jews. *Neurology* **47**, 977–984.

Somer, H. (1995). Workshop report: the 25th ENMC international workshop on distal myopathies. *Neuromusc. Disord.* **5**, 249–252.

Spiller, W. G. (1907). Myopathy of a distal type and its relation to the neural form of muscular atrophy (Charcot–Marie–Tooth type). *J. Nerv. Mental Dis.* **34**, 14–30.

Sumner, D., Crawfurd, M. d'A. and Harriman, D. G. F. (1971). Distal muscular dystrophy in an English family. *Brain* **94**, 51–60.

Sunohara, N., Nonaka, I., Kamei, N. and Satoyoshi, E. (1989). Distal myopathy with rimmed vacuole formation: a follow-up study. *Brain* **112**, 65–83.

Tawil, R., McDermott, M. P., Mendell, J. R., Kissel, J. and Griggs, R. C. (1994). Fascioscapulohumeral muscular dystrophy (FSHMD): design of natural history study and results of baseline testing. *Neurology* **44**, 442–446.

Thomas, P. K., Schott, G. D. and Morgan-Hughes, J. A. (1975). Adult onset scapuloperoneal myopathy. *J. Neurol. Neurosurg. Psychiatry* **38**, 1008–1015.

Todman, D. H. and Cooke, R. A. (1984). Scapuloperoneal myopathy. *Clin. Exp. Neurol.* **20**, 169–174.

Udd, B., Kääriänen, H. and Somer, H. (1991a). Muscular dystrophy with separate clinical phenotypes in a large family. *Muscle Nerve* **14**, 1050–1058.

Udd, B., Lamminen, A. and Somer, H. (1991b). Imaging methods reveal unexpected patchy lesions in late onset distal myopathy. *Neuromusc. Disord.* **1**, 279–285.

Udd, B., Rapola, J., Nokelainen, P., Arikawa, E. and Somer, H. (1992). Non-vacuolar myopathy in a large family with both late adult onset distal myopathy and severe proximal muscular dystrophy. *J. Neurol. Sci.* **113**, 214–221.

Udd, B., Partanen, J., Halonen, P. et al. (1993). Tibial muscular dystrophy: late adult-onset distal myopathy in 66 Finnish patients. *Arch. Neurol.* **50**, 604–608.

Udd, B., Haravuori, H., Griggs, R. et al. (1998a). Tibial muscular dystrophy (TMD)/late onset distal myopathy (LODM, Markesbery and Griggs) – an update. *Muscle Nerve* **21** (Suppl. 7), S6.

Udd, B., Haravuori, H., Kalimo, H. et al. (1998b). Tibial muscular dystrophy – from clinical description to linkage on chromosome 2q31. *Neuromusc. Disord.* **8**, 327–332.

Udd, B., Kalimo, H., Nokelainen, P. and Somer, H. (1998c). Tibial muscular dystrophy: clinical, genetic and morphoogic characteristics. In: *Inclusion-body Myositis and Myopathies*, eds. V. Askanas, G. Serratrice and W. K. Engel, pp. 232–241. Cambridge, UK: Cambridge University Press.

van der Does de Willebois, A. E., Meyer, A. E., Simons, A. J. and Bethlem, J. (1968). Distal myopathy with onset in early infancy. *Neurology* **18**, 383–390.

van Kasteren, B. J. (1979). Polymyositis presenting with chronic progressive distal muscular weakness. *J. Neurol. Sci.* **41**, 307–310.

Vicart, P., Caron, A., Guicheney, P. et al. (1998). A missense mutation in the α_B-crystallin chaperone gene causes a desmin-related myopathy. *Nat. Genet.* **20**, 92–95.

Vita, G., Dattola, R., Santoro, M. and Messina, C. (1983). Familial oculopharyngeal muscular dystrophy with distal spread. *J. Neurol.* **230**, 57–64.

Voit, T., Herrmann, R., Neuen-Jacob, E. and Cohn, R. D. (1998). Autosomal dominant infantile onset tibial myopathy. *Neuromusc. Disord.* **8**, 251.

Walton, J. N. and Nattrass, F. J. (1954). On the classification, natural history and treatment of the myopathies. *Brain* **77**, 169–231.

Weiler, T., Greenberg, C. R., Nylen, E. et al. (1996). Limb-girdle muscular atrophy and Miyoshi myopathy in an aboriginal Canadian kindred map to LGMD2B and segregate with the same haplotype. *Am. J. Hum. Genet.* **59**, 872–878.

Welander, L. (1951). Myopathia distalis tarda hereditaria. *Acta Med. Scand.* **141** (Suppl. 265), 1–124.

Welander, L. (1957). Homozygous appearance of distal myopathy. *Acta Genet.* **7**, 321–325.

Werneck, L. C., Marrone, C. D. and Scola, R. H. (1993). Miopatias distais: analise clinica, laboratorial, electromiografica, histologico-histoquimica de oito casos. *Arq. Neuropsiquiatr.* **51**, 475–486.

Wijmenga, C., Padberg, G. W., Moerer, P. et al. (1991). Mapping of fascioscapulohumeral muscular dystrophy gene to chromosome 4q35-qter by multipoint linkage analysis and in situ hybridization. *Genomics* **9**, 570–575.

Wilhelmsen, K. C., Blake, D. M., Lynch, T. et al. (1996). Chromosome 12-linked autosomal dominant scapuloperoneal muscular dystrophy. *Ann. Neurol.* **39**, 507–520.

Wilson, S. A. K. (1940). *Neurology*, Vol. 2, pp. 982–983. London: Edward Arnold.

Yamanouchi, Y., Ozawa, E. and Nonaka, I. (1994). Autosomal recessive distal muscular dystrophy: normal expression of dystrophin, utrophin and dystrophin-associated proteins in muscle fibres. *J. Neurol. Sci.* **126**, 70–76.

Yee, W. C., Hahn, A. F. and Gilbert, J. J. (1988). Adult onset scapuloperoneal myopathy: diagnostic value of nerve morphometry and multiple muscle biopsies. *J. Neurol. Neurosurg. Psychiatry* **51**, 808–813.

23

Emery–Dreifuss dystrophy

Kiichi Arahata[†]

Introduction

Emery–Dreifuss muscular dystrophy (EDMD) is a genetically heterogeneous disorder caused by at least two genes (the X-linked gene for emerin (X-EDMD) and the 1q-linked gene for lamin A/C (AD-EDMD)). EDMD is characterized by the clinical triad of early-onset contractures, slowly progressive weakness in humeroperoneal muscles, and cardiomyopathy with conduction block that has a high risk of sudden death. The disease may have been described by Cestan and Lejonne in 1902, and later on by Schenk and Mathias in 1920. In 1966, Emery did a detailed and careful study of a large Virginian family affected by an X-linked muscular dystrophy, which was previously reported by Dreifuss and Hogan (1961) as a benign form of Duchenne muscular dystrophy (Emery and Dreifuss, 1966). The disease observed in the family was quite distinct from both Duchenne and Becker muscular dystrophy because of the unusual early contractures in elbows and Achilles tendons, cardiac abnormalities and absence of muscle hypertrophy and intellectual impairment. After 25 years, Emery reinvestigated the original family and also found anterior tibial and peroneal muscle weakness in severely affected individuals (Emery, 1987; Emery and Emery, 1995). Thomas et al. (1972) described a large family with X-linked recessive early-onset scapuloperoneal syndrome resembles Emery's family and emphasized this type of myopathy as a distinct clinical entity. Other families with an X-linked humeroperoneal syndrome were described by Waters et al. (1975). The X-linked disorder was termed Emery–Dreifuss muscular dystrophy by Rowland et al. (1979). Indeed, patient Y1 from Emery's and a patient from Thomas' original families have subsequently had in-frame deletions of the emerin gene (878 del 15 bp in exon 4; 1763 del 18 bp in exon 6, respectively) (Ellis et al., 1998; Yates et al., 1999).

[†]deceased.

The term Emery–Dreifuss syndrome (EDS) has been proposed because of the striking similarity of symptoms of X-linked and autosomal dominant EDMD (X-EDMD and AD-EDMD) (Witt et al., 1988; Emery, 1989, 1993). Early recognition of EDS is important, because the disease is often associated with life-threatening heart block that can be managed by cardiac pacemaker implantation. The causes of EDS presumably share a common pathological background. Indeed, both the gene products for X-EDMD (emerin) and AD-EDMD (lamin A/C) are localized at the nuclear envelope (Nagano et al., 1996; Manilal et al., 1996; Bonne et al., 1999).

Inheritance

Most families with EDMD show X-linked recessive inheritance (X-EDMD; Online Mendelian Inheritance in Man (OMIM) database 310300) and the gene locus for X-EDMD has been mapped to Xq28. A rare autosomal dominant form (AD-EDMD; OMIM 181350) has been mapped to 1q11-q23. It has been suggested that there is an autosomal recessive form (AR-EDMD) and a few sporadic cases have been reported (EDMD Mutation Database: http://www.path.cam.ac.uk/emd/mutation.html).

X-EDMD is inherited as a recessive disorder that usually manifests by the second–third decade of life, although rare cases have remained asymptomatic even in the fourth decade of life. However, there is a considerable intra- and interfamilial phenotypic variability (Wehnert and Muntoni, 1999). By demonstration of linkage with the gene for factor VIII and the marker DXS15 at Xq28, the gene for EDMD was placed distal to DXS15 (Thomas et al., 1986), and Kress et al. (1992) refined the linkage to a region of about 2 Mb between the marker DXS15 and the factor VIII gene. These data confirmed an earlier finding of a large family in which 'a scapuloperoneal syndrome' segregated with colour blindness (Thomas et al., 1972).

The locus for the AD-EDMD gene was placed distal in an 8 cM interval between D1S2346 and D1S2125 (1q11-q23) in a large French pedigree (Bonne et al., 1999) by demonstration of linkage with the markers between D1S2346 and D1S2624. However, there is also evidence of genetic heterogeneity in AD-EDMD. The gene locus for autosomal recessive EDMD has not been mapped.

Clinical features

X-linked Emery–Dreifuss dystrophy

Based on 25 years of investigation of a large Virginian family, Emery summarized the clinical triad of X-EDMD as follows: (i) early contractures of the elbows, Achilles tendons and posterior neck (with limitation initially of neck flexion but later of forward flexion of the entire spine); (ii) slowly progressive muscle wasting and weakness with a humeroperoneal distribution early in the course of the disease (Fig. 23.1a–d, colour plate) (later, weakness also affects the proximal limb girdle musculature); and (iii) a cardiomyopathy usually presenting as an atrioventricular (AV) conduction block ranging from sinus bradycardia, to prolongation of the PR interval to complete heart block (Emery 1987, 1997; Emery and Emery, 1995). In most patients with EDMD, cardiac abnormalities are noted after the second or third decade of life (Emery and Dreifuss, 1966; Rowland et al., 1979; Merlini et al., 1986; Voit et al., 1988; Funakoshi et al., 1999).

As expected in an X-linked recessive disorder, most heterozygous females show no indication of skeletal muscle disorder. However, female carriers occasionally have conduction abnormalities without muscle weakness, and therefore careful cardiological follow-up examinations are recommended (Merlini et al., 1986; Bialer et al., 1991; Fishbein et al., 1993; Manilal et al., 1998). Serum creatine kinase levels are moderately increased in affected male patients, but carriers are often normal (Merlini et al., 1986; Bialer et al., 1990). The serum creatine kinase activity decreases with age.

Skeletal muscle biopsy shows dystrophic changes with a few scattered necrotic and regenerating fibres, increased internal nuclei, variation in fibre diameter, fibre splitting, and increased perimysial and endomysial connective tissue (Fig. 23.1c, colour plate) (Thomas et al., 1972; Hopkins et al., 1981; Dubowitz 1985; Merlini et al., 1986). The intermyofibrillary network is often disorganized, with a moth-eaten appearance. Both type I and type II fibres are affected. Fibre type grouping is not observed in most patients, although either type I (Merlini et al., 1986) or type II (Rowland et al., 1979; Hopkins et al., 1981) fibre type disproportion has been reported.

Autosomal dominant Emery–Dreifuss dystrophy

AD-EDMD (Fenichel et al., 1982; Miller et al., 1985; Becker, 1986; Witt et al., 1988; Bonne et al., 1999) usually differs little clinically from X-EDMD (Witt et al., 1988; Emery, 1989, 1993). The diagnostic criteria for the EDMD phenotype previously established for X-EDMD were adopted for AD-EDMD by the 60th European Neuromuscular Centre (ENMC) International Workshops on non-X-EDMD (Yates 1991, 1997). In addition, a few characteristic features were added to the diagnostic criteria for AD-EDMD (Wehnert and Muntoni, 1999); in AD-EDMD, isolated cardiac involvement is observed more frequently and impaired left ventricular function is not uncommon at a later stage. Molecular genetic analysis is essential in distinguishing the AD-EDMD from X-EDMD.

Autosomal recessive Emery–Dreifuss dystrophy

A possible autosomal recessive form (Takamoto et al., 1984; Taylor et al., 1998) has been reported. Takamoto et al. (1984) described a 38-year-old woman without a family history of disease who showed early-onset contractures in the neck (flexion) and elbow, associated with humeropelvic muscular weakness and complete AV block. She lost ambulation by 27 years of age and required a cardiac pacemaker at 34 years. Taylor's patients (three boys and two girls) also showed rapid progression of weakness and lost ambulation before the age of 8 years, although the cardiac function was normal.

Joint contractures

The nature of the early-onset joint contractures in the elbows, Achilles tendons, and posterior neck are not well characterized (Fig. 23.1a,b, colour plate). Whether the contractures occur as a result of a primary abnormality of tissues that surround the joints or are secondary to primary dystrophic changes in skeletal muscle remains to be clarified. Merlini et al. (1986) pointed out the early role of the primary muscular atrophy, which may precede the contracture (as detected by computed tomography), as well as the value of computed tomographic scanning to confirm the pattern of selective muscle involvement, particularly of the biceps, cervical and lumbar paravertebral muscles, and posterior thigh and leg muscles (Yates, 1997). However, in EDMD, contractures often occur very early in the childhood (in most patients before 10 years of age) and prior to major weakness of muscle.

Cardiomyopathy

Conduction defects are the main and early cardiac features in both X-EDMD and AD-EDMD (Wehnert and Muntoni, 1999). Voit et al. (1988) performed a detailed cardiological follow-up study in patients with EDMD and found four main features: (i) impairment of impulse-generating cells; (ii) conduction defects with atrial preponderance; (iii) increased atrial and ventricular ectopy; and (iv) functional impairment of ventricular myocardium. Surprisingly, 33% of the well-documented 109 cases of total permanent auricular paralysis were associated with EDMD (Bensaid et al., 1995). These atrial abnormalities were pointed out clearly by Emery and Dreifuss in their original paper (1966) as being a part of the dystrophic process. Rowland et al. (1979) also reported a man who developed permanent atrial paralysis at age 25 years. Consequently, atrial conduction defects are considered to be a hallmark of EDMD cardiomyopathy, although rare ventricular involvement has also occurred (Voit et al., 1988; Bialer et al., 1991).

Importantly, the cardiac conduction defects often cause unpredictable sudden death ($\sim$50%), without prior cardiac symptoms, and therefore, an appropriate insertion of cardiac pacemaker is recommended (ul Hassan et al., 1979; Hopkins et al., 1981; Merlini et al., 1986; Oswald et al., 1987; Wyse et al., 1987; Voit et al., 1988; Emery, 1989; Yoshioka et al., 1989; Bialer et al., 1991; Fishbein et al., 1993; Graux et al., 1993; Rakopvec et al., 1995). However, the pacemaker only treats bradycardia, and other symptoms can occur after its insertion (Yoshioka et al., 1989; Bialer et al., 1991; Graux et al., 1993; Rakovec et al., 1995). Indeed the cardiomyopathy worsens with age (Hara et al., 1987; Yoshioka et al., 1989; Fishbein et al., 1993). Lethal cardiac involvement may also occur in female carriers.

Histological changes of cardiac muscle in EDMD have been reported in a few patients for whom biopsy and postmortem samples were available. Yoshioka et al. (1989) found myocardial changes with focal degeneration and increased endomysial fatty and fibrous connective tissues in a male patient. Marked enlargement of the atria with extremely thin right atrium and replacement of adipose/fibrous connective tissues was observed, together with interstitial fibrosis in the ventricular myocardium (Hara et al., 1987; Fishbein et al., 1993). However, rare patients with EDMD show neither gross cardiac changes nor abnormality in the AV node or bundle of His.

Differential diagnosis

Since EDMD shows considerable phenotypic variability, other diseases can have similar features: rigid spine syndrome (Dubowitz, 1965; Serratrice et al., 1984; Powe et al., 1985; Goto et al., 1986; Kubo et al., 1998), congenital muscular dystrophies with rigidity of the spine and joint contractures (Moghadaszadeh et al., 1998), adult-onset autosomal dominant scapuloperoneal syndrome (Thomas et al., 1975; Emery, 1989), facioscapulohumeral muscular dystrophy (Kazakov et al., 1976), Bethlem myopathy (Taylor et al., 1998) and other X-linked muscular dystrophies. Molecular genetic diagnosis is often needed for definite diagnosis of EDMD.

Although a family with scapuloperoneal spinal muscular atrophy with cardiomyopathy has been reported (Mawatari and Katayama, 1973), there are no postmortem data from EDMD showing morphological abnormalities in the brain, spinal anterior horn cells and myelinated nerve fibres in the ventral roots or sciatic nerve (Thomas et al., 1972; Hara et al., 1987).

Molecular genetics

X-linked form and emerin

In 1994 Bione et al. identified a gene (*STA*) and its mutations in patients with X-EDMD. The gene is very small (2.1 kb) and contains only six exons, with a mRNA of 1.3 kb that is expressed ubiquitously in different tissues (Bione et al., 1994, 1995) as it is in mice (Small et al., 1997a). The human mRNA encodes a novel serine-rich protein named emerin that has 254 amino acid residues with a single hydrophobic domain at the C-terminus (Fig. 23.2). Emerin was identified as a 34 kDa protein (Fig. 23.1*i*, colour plate) (Manilal et al., 1996; Nagano et al., 1996; Mora et al., 1997). There are several consensus phosphorylation sites in the emerin molecule (Cartegni et al., 1997; Tsuchiya and Arahata, 1997; Ellis et al., 1998), and mutant forms of emerin exhibit aberrant phosphorylation (Ellis et al., 1998). Although the function of emerin is not known, the clinical, physiological and pathological changes in X-EDMD are certainly caused by the deficiency of emerin.

To date, more than 90 mutations in the gene for emerin have been submitted in the EDMD Mutation Database (http://www.path.cam.ac.uk/emd/mutation.html) (Yates, 1997). The distribution of the mutations is homogeneous along the gene with no evidence of hot spots; most of the mutations are null alleles (Fig. 23.2). Point mutations (47%) or small deletions (36%) or insertions (10%) are the most common; in nine patients (10%) point mutations were found in splice junctions. Importantly, most mutations (64%) introduced premature STOPs in the open reading frame. Seven mutations (8%) occurred in the starting

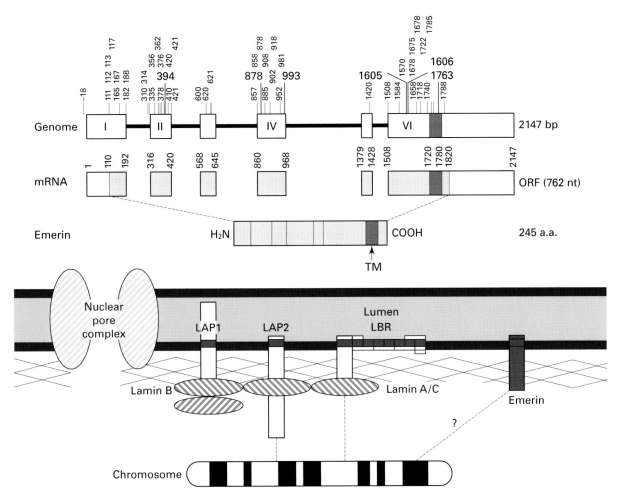

Fig. 23.2. Schematic representation of the emerin gene structure and relative position of the mutations (upper panel). Six exons are represented as boxes. Larger bold numbers are missense or in-frame mutations. Numbering above the mRNA is based on the emerin genomic sequence (Bione et al., 1995). TM is a hydrophobic transmembrane domain. Lower panel shows schematic illustration of nuclear membrane structure. Emerin and lamin A/C localizes on the nucleoplasmic surface of the inner nuclear membrane, but not on the nuclear pore. Emerin and other integral inner nuclear membrane proteins bind to lamins and/or chromosomes. LAP1 and 2, lamina-associated polypeptide 1 and 2; LBR, lamin B receptor; ORF, open reading frame.

codon (ATG) and probably prevented initiation of translation. A deletion of 22 bp was identified in the promoter region (Wulff et al., 1997). Entire gene deletions were reported in five patients (6%) (Small et al., 1997b, Small and Warren, 1998; see also the Mutation Database, 1998). Of special interest, 27 patients (30%) were described as carrying point mutations or deletions/insertions in the last exon. In such patients, emerin lacks the C-terminal part of the protein containing the transmembrane domain. Some patients of this group were shown to lack emerin completely (Nagano et al., 1996; Mora et al., 1997; Manilal et al., 1998), thus demonstrating the importance of the hydrophobic C-terminal domain for membrane insertion and protein stability. Only four missense mutations (4%) and three in-frame deletions (3%) were described. Reduced amounts of emerin were found in three reported patients (one missense and two in-frame deletions) (Funakoshi et al., 1999; Yates et al., 1999). However, an in-frame deletion that removed six amino acid residues from the C-terminal transmembrane domain caused complete loss of emerin from muscle, indicating the importance of proper localization of emerin at the nuclear membrane (Manilal et al., 1998; Tsuchiya et al., 1999). N-terminal residues may also have fundamental functions (Ostlund et al., 1999). The relative low abundance of missense mutations suggests that complete lack of emerin is the usual pathogenesis.

Emerin localizes at the nuclear membrane in skeletal, cardiac and smooth muscle cells (Fig. 23.1*e,g*, colour plate) (Manilal et al., 1996; Nagano et al., 1996; Mora et al., 1997), skin epidermal cells (Manilal et al., 1997; Mora et al., 1997; Toniolo et al., 1998), peripheral blood cells (Manilal et al., 1997; Mora et al., 1997), and exfoliated oral cells (Sabatelli et al., 1998). A majority of patients with X-EDMD show no detectable emerin at the nuclear membrane of these cells (Fig. 23.1*f,h*, colour plate). Most female carriers remain asymptomatic and exhibit either normal or reduced (50% level) emerin protein, but a cardiomyopathy with undetectable emerin levels (<5% of normal) occurs, possibly as a result of skewed X-inactivation (Manilal et al., 1998).

At the ultrastructural level, emerin labelling was found at the nucleoplasmic surface of the inner nuclear membrane but not on nuclear pore complexes (Yorifuji et al., 1997). It is reasonable to suggest that emerin is anchored to the inner nuclear membrane in some way, through its hydrophobic domain, and that its hydrophilic region protrudes into the nucleoplasm (Fig. 23.2). The interaction between emerin and nucleoplasmic components such as nuclear lamina and chromosomes must be important, since loss of the protein causes the disease (Yorifuji et al., 1997; Squarzoni et al., 1998). Indeed, irregular thickening of the nuclear lamina and disorganization of lamina-associated heterochromatin were observed in the skeletal muscle and skin fibroblasts from a patient with X-EDMD (Ognibene et al., 1999). Nuclear abnormalities (condensation of chromatin and extrusion of nuclear chromatin into the sarcoplasm as a consequence of nuclear membrane disintegration) has been observed in biopsied muscles from emerin-deficient patients with X-EDMD (Fidzianska et al., 1998).

Possible emerin localization at the cardiac intercalated discs in addition to the specific localization at the inner nuclear membrane has been reported (Cartegni et al., 1997). However, a panel of 16 monoclonal antibodies against different emerin epitopes did not confirm the intercalated disc localization (Manilal et al., 1999). Therefore, emerin localization at cardiac desmosomes remains to be clarified.

Autosomal dominant form and lamin A/C

Bonne et al. (1999) identified mutations in a lamin A/C gene (*LMNA*) at chromosome 1q11–23 in a large French family and in four other small families with AD-EDMD. Lamin A and C are intermediate filament proteins of the nuclear lamina (a lattice structure localizing between chromatin and inner nuclear membrane) (Fig. 23.2) produced by alternative splicing of *LMNA*, which spans

24kb of genomic DNA containing 12 exons (Lin and Worman, 1993). The lamin A/C mRNA is highly expressed in heart, skeletal muscle and placenta, but not in brain.

In patients with AD-EDMD, lamin A/C and emerin were immunostained normally at the nuclear membrane of skeletal and cardiac muscles. However, in the targeted mouse model for lamin A gene (*lmna* −/−), complete loss of lamin A occurred at the nuclear envelope in association with drastic reduction of emerin expression and focal loss of nuclear envelope proteins such as lamin B and LAP2 (lamina associated polypeptide 2) (Sullivan et al., 1999). It is unclear whether mutations in *LMNA* cause dominant-negative effects or haploinsufficiency.

Mutant lamin A/C and dilated cardiomyopathy

A subset of the autosomal dominant form of dilated cardiomyopathy (CMD1A), with or without skeletal muscle involvement, has been reported to have mutations of *LMNA* (Fatkin et al., 1999; Brodsky et al., 2000). Most had missense mutations in the rod domain of lamin A/C. These results imply the crucial role for this intermediate filament in cardiac conduction and contractility.

Pathomechanism

Nuclear envelopathy?

One plausible clue to the pathomechanism for EDMD and CMD1A is the presence of specific abnormalities of the inner nuclear envelope proteins emerin and lamin A/C. It should be noticed that mutations of *LMNA* are also known to cause Dunnigan-type familial partial lipodystrophy (FPLD) (Cao and Hegele, 2000). Therefore, a group of extremely heterogenous inherited disorders are caused by closely associated nuclear envelope proteins.

Despite the recent progress in clinical and molecular genetic analysis of EDMD, several unresolved issues remain. It is not clear why loss of the ubiquitous inner nuclear envelope proteins emerin (X-EDMD) and lamin A/C (AD-EDMD) selectively affects cardiac and skeletal muscles and causes joint contractures. Does additional absence of lamin B$_1$ from normal skeletal and cardiac myonuclei explain why these tissues are preferentially affected (Manilal et al., 1999)? We still do not know what additional genetic and environmental factors cause phenotypic variability (Muntoni et al., 1998; Hoeltzenbein et al., 1999; Wehnert and Muntoni, 1999). We also do not know how adipocytes and insulin functions are affected as a result of *LMNA* mutation in FPLD. Identification of cell type-specific molecules that interact with emerin and lamins in muscle is essential.

Mutant forms of emerin in lymphoblastoid cell lines, COS cells and myogenic cells exhibit increased solubility and random subcellular localization (Cartegni et al., 1997; Ellis et al., 1998; Tsuchiya et al., 1999) and show aberrant cell cycle-dependent phosphorylated forms (Ellis et al., 1998). These observations imply a possible role for emerin during the process of regeneration of muscle fibres where active proliferation of muscle satellite cells occurs.

If emerin anchors to or binds chromosomes, either directly or indirectly, as a functional molecule, it may participate in the regulation of gene expression and chromosome organization (Lamond and Earnshaw, 1998). In fact, disorganization of the heterochoromatin was reported in the skeletal muscle and skin fibroblasts in a patient with X-EDMD (Ognibene et al., 1999), as well as in the targeted mouse model for *lmna* (Sullivan et al., 1999).

Finally, since skeletal and cardiac muscles and tissues surrounding joints are subject to rigorous movements, the mechanical stability of the nuclear membrane must be necessary. In patients with X-EDMD, nuclear envelope disintegration occurs (Fidzianska et al., 1998; Ognibene et al., 1999). In this context, it should be pointed out that lamins are known to participate not only in anchorage of nuclear envelope proteins and chromatin organization but also in forming a skeletal framework within the nucleus. Several integral inner nuclear membrane proteins, such as LAP2 and LBR (lamin B receptor), are known to interact with lamins (Foisner and Gerace, 1993). Mechanical connections between surface membrane integrins, cytoskeletal filaments and nucleoplasm are suggested to stabilize nuclear structure and thereby may contribute to cellular survival (Maniotis et al., 1997).

Treatment and prevention

Although no specific treatment is available, physical therapy is recommended to reduce contractures. Surgical tendon lengthening may help to some extent. Early diagnosis of EDMD can be life saving as the implantation of a pacemaker can correct cardiac conduction defects. However, the pacemaker only treats bradycardia, and other symptoms, such as cardiac failure owing to progressive cardiomyopathy, can occur after insertion of the pacemaker. In patients with severe cardiomyopathy where skeletal muscles are minimally affected, heart transplantation can be considered. Anaesthetic considerations for EDMD are of note. Patients have difficulties with tracheal intubation, spinal anaesthetic and have a susceptibility to malignant hyperthermia (Jensen, 1996). Western blot and immunocytochemical tests for emerin help to achieve accurate diagnosis of X-EDMD (Nagano et al., 1996; Manilal et al., 1997; Mora et al., 1997; Sabatelli et al., 1998). In X-EDMD, carriers show mosaic pattern of the nuclear immunostaining for emerin in both skin biopsy and oral exfoliative cytology. Molecular diagnosis is necessary for accurate genetic counselling for both X-EDMD and AD-EDMD. Availability of animal models such as the mouse model for targeted disruption of *lmna* (Sullivan et al., 1999) will provide an area in which to explore treatment of EDMD.

Acknowledgements

The author expresses sincere thanks to Dr Hideo Sugita (President Emeritus, NCNP, Japan) for his suggestions and encouragement. This study has been supported in part by grants-in-aid from the Japan Foundation for Aging and Health, Ministry of Health and Welfare, and CREST from JST, Japan.

References

Becker, P. (1986). Dominant autosomal muscular dystrophy with early contractures and cardiomyopathy (Hauptmann–Thannheuser). *Hum. Genet.* **74**, 184.

Bensaid, J., Vallat, J. M., Amsallem, D., Bernard, Y., Rauscher, M. and Borsotti, J. P. (1995). Total permanent auricular paralysis. Review of the literature apropos of 109 cases. *Ann. Cardiol. Angeiol. (Paris)* **44**, 139–145.

Bialer, M. G., Bruns, D. E. and Kelly, T. E. (1990). Muscle enzymes and isoenzyme in Emery–Dreifuss muscular dystrophy. *Clin. Chem.* **36**, 427–430.

Bialer, M. G., McDaniel, N. G. and Kelly, T. E. (1991). Progression of cardiac disease in Emery–Dreifuss muscular dystrophy. *Clin. Cardiol.* **14**, 411–416.

Bione, S., Maestrini, E., Rivella, S. et al. (1994). Identification of a novel X-linked gene responsible for Emery–Dreifuss muscular dystrophy. *Nat. Genet.* **8**, 323–327.

Bione, S., Small, K., Aksmanovic, V. M. A. et al. (1995). Identification of new mutations in the Emery–Dreifuss muscular dystrophy gene and evidence for genetic heterogeneity of the disease. *Hum. Mol. Genet.* **4**, 1859–1863.

Bonne, G., Di Barletta, M. R., Varnous, S. et al. (1999). Mutations in the gene encoding lamin A/C cause autosomal dominant Emery–Dreifuss muscular dystrophy. *Nat. Genet.* **21**, 285–288.

Brodsky, G. L., Muntoni, F., Miocic, S. et al. (2000). Lamin A/C gene mutation associated with dilated cardiomyopathy with variable skeletal muscle involvement. *Circulation* **101**, 473–476.

Cao, H. and Hegele, R. A. (2000). Nuclear lamin A/C R482Q mutation in Canadian kindreds with Dunnigan-type familial partial lipodystrophy. *Hum. Mol. Genet.* **9**, 109–112.

Cartegni, L., Raffaele di Barletta, M., Barresi, R. et al. (1997). Heart-specific localization of emerin: new insights into Emery–Dreifuss muscular dystrophy. *Hum. Mol. Genet.* **6**, 2257–2264.

Cestan, R. and Lejonne, P. (1902). Une myopathie avec retractions families. *Nouvelle Iconographie de la Salpetriere* **15**, 38–52.

Dreifuss, F. E. and Hogan, G. R. (1961). Survival in X-chromosomal muscular dystrophy. *Neurology* **11**, 734–737.

Dubowitz, V. (1965). Pseudo-muscular dystrophy in research in muscular dystrophy. In: *Proceedings of the Third Symposium. Research Committee of the Muscular Dystrophy Group of Great Britain*, pp. 57–73. London: Pitman Medical.

Dubowitz, V. (1985). *Muscle Biopsy. A Practical Approach*, 2nd edn. London: Ballière Tindall.

Ellis, J. A., Craxton, M., Yates, J. R. W. and Kendric-Jones, J. (1998). Aberrant intracellular targeting and cell cycle-dependent phosphorylation of emerin contribute to the Emery–Dreifuss muscular dystrophy phenotype. *J. Cell Sci.* **111**, 781–792.

Emery, A. E. H. (1987). X-linked muscular dystrophy with early contractures and cardiomyopathy (Emery–Dreifuss type). *Clin. Genet.* **32**, 360–376.

Emery, A. E. H. (1989). Emery–Dreifuss muscular dystrophy and other related disorders. *Brit. Med. Bull.* **45**, 772–787.

Emery, A. E. H. (1993). Emery–Dreifuss syndrome. *J. Med. Genet.* **26**, 637–641.

Emery, A. E. H. (1997). Duchenne and other X-linked muscular dystrophies. In: *Principles and Practice of Medical Genetics*, 3rd edn, eds. A. E. H. Emery and D. L. Primoin, pp. 2337–2354.

Emery, A. E. H. and Dreifuss, F. E. (1966). Unusual type of benign X-linked muscular dystrophy. *J. Neurol. Neurosurg. Psychiatry* **29**, 338–342.

Emery, A. E. H. and Emery, M. L. H. (1995). Emery–Dreifuss muscular dystrophy. In: *The History of a Genetic Disease; Duchenne Muscular Dystrophy or Meryon's Disease*, ed. A. E. H. Emery, pp. 127–146. London: Royal Society of Medicine Press.

Fatkin, D., MacRae, C., Sasaki, T. et al. (1999). Missense mutations in the rod domain of the lamin A/C gene as causes of dilated cardiomyopathy and conduction-system disease. *N. Eng. J. Med.* **341**, 1715–1724.

Fenichel, G. M., Yi, C.-S., Kilroy, A. W. and Blouin, R. (1982). An autosomal dominant dystrophy with humeropelvic distribution and cardiomyopathy. *Neurology* **32**, 1399–1401.

Fidzianska, A., Toniolo, D. and Hausmanowa-Petrusewicz, I. (1998). Ultrastructural abnormality of sarcolemmal nuclei in Emery–Dreifuss muscular dystrophy (EDMD). *J. Neurol. Sci.* **159**, 88–93.

Fishbein, M. C., Siegel, R. J., Thompson, C. E. and Hopkins, L. C. (1993). Sudden death of a carrier of X-linked Emery–Dreifuss muscular dystrophy. *Ann. Inter. Med.* **119**, 900–905.

Foisner, R. and Gerace, L. (1993). Integral membrane proteins of the nuclear envelope interact with lamins and chromosomes, and binding is modulated by mitotic phosphorylation. *Cell* **73**, 1267–1279.

Funakoshi, M., Tsuchiya, Y. and Arahata, K. (1999). Emerin and cardiomyopathy in Emery–Dreifuss muscular dystrophy. *Neuromusc. Disord.* **9**, 108–114.

Goto, I., Ishimoto, S., Yamada, T., Hara, H. and Kuroiwa, Y. (1986). The rigid spine syndrome and Emery–Dreifuss muscular dystrophy. *Clin. Neurol. Neurosurg.* **88**, 293–298.

Graux, P., Carlioz, R., Mekerke, W., Camilleri, G. and Dutoit, A. (1993). Emery–Dreifuss muscular dystrophy with major conduction disorders and cardiac excitability. *Ann. Cardiol. Angeilo (Paris)* **42**, 554–560.

Hara, H., Nagata, H., Mawatari, S., Kondo, A. and Sato, H. (1987). Emery–Dreifuss muscular dystrophy. An autopsy case. *J. Neurolog. Sci.* **79**, 23–31.

Hoeltzenbein, M., Karow, T., Zeller, J. A. et al. (1999). Severe clinical expression in X-linked Emery–Dreifuss muscular dystrophy. *Neuromusc. Disord.* **9**, 166–170.

Hopkins, L. C., Jackson, J. A. and Elsas, L. J. (1981). Emery-Dreifuss humeroperoneal muscular dystrophy: an X-linked myopathy with unusual contractures and bradycardia. *Ann. Neurol.* **10**, 230–237.

Jensen, V. (1996). The anesthetic management of a patient with Emery Dreifuss muscular dystrophy. *Can. J. Anaesthesiol.* **43**, 968–971.

Kazakov, V. M., Bogorodinski, D. K. and Skorometz, A. A. (1976). The myogenic scapulo-peroneal syndrome. Muscular dystrophy in the K. kindred: clinical study and genetics. *Clin. Genet.* **10**, 41–50.

Kress, W., Muller, E., Kausch, K. et al. (1992). Multipoint linkage mapping of the Emery–Dreifuss muscular dystrophy gene. *Neuromusc. Disord.* **2**, 111–115.

Kubo, S., Tsukahara, T., Takemitsu, M. et al. (1998). Presence of emerinopathy in cases of rigid spine syndrome. *Neuromusc. Disord.* **8**, 502–507.

Lamond, A. I. and Earnshaw, W. C. (1998). Structure and function in the nucleus. *Science* **280**, 547–553.

Lin, F. and Worman, H. J. (1993). Structural organization of the human gene encording nuclear lamin A and nuclear lamin C. *J. Biol. Chem.* **268**, 16321–16326.

Manilal, S., Nguyen, T. M., Sewry, C. A. and Morris, G. E. (1996). The Emery–Dreifuss muscular dystrophy protein, emerin, is a nuclear membrane protein. *Hum. Mol. Genet.* **5**, 801–808.

Manilal, S., Sewry, C. A., Nguyen, T. M., Muntoni, F. and Morris, G. E. (1997). Diagnosis of X-linked Emery–Dreifuss muscular dystrophy by protein analysis of leukocytes and skin with monoclonal antibodies. *Neuromusc. Disord.* **7**, 63–66.

Manilal, S., Recan, D., Sewry, C. A. et al. (1998). Mutations in Emery–Dreifuss muscular dystrophy and their effects on emerin protein expression. *Hum. Mol. Genet.* **7**, 855–864.

Manilal, S., Sewry, C. A., Pereboev, A. et al. (1999). Distribution of emerin and lamins in the heart and implications for Emery–Dreifuss muscular dystrophy. *Hum. Mol. Genet.* **8**, 353–359.

Maniotis, A. J., Chen, C. S. and Ingber, D. E. (1997). Demonstration of mechanical connections between integrins, cytoskeletal filaments, and nucleoplasm that stabilize nuclear structure. *Proc. Natl. Acad. Sci. USA* **94**, 849–854.

Mawatari, S. and Katayama, K. (1973). Scapuloperoneal muscular atrophy with cardiopathy. *Arch. Neurol.* **28**, 55–59.

Merlini, L., Granata, C., Dominici, P. and Bonfiglioli, S. (1986). Emery–Dreifuss muscular dystrophy: report of five cases in a family and review of the literature. *Muscle Nerve* **9**, 481–485.

Miller, R. G., Layzer, R. B., Mellenthin, M. A., Golabi, M., Francoz, R. A. and Mall, J. C. (1985). Emery–Dreifuss muscular dystrophy with autosomal dominant transmission. *Neurology* **35**, 1230–1233.

Moghadaszadeh, B., Desguerre, I., Topaloglu, H. et al. (1998). Identification of a new locus for a peculiar form of congenital muscular dystrophy with early rigidity of spine, on chromosome 1p35–36. *Am. J. Hum. Genet.* **62**, 1439–1445.

Mora, M., Cartegni, L., Di Blasi, C. et al. (1997). X-linked Emery–Dreifuss muscular dystrophy can be diagnosed from skin biopsy or blood sample. *Ann. Neurol.* **42**, 249–253.

Muntoni, F., Lichtarowicz-Krynska, E. J., Sewry, C. et al. (1998). Early presentation of X-linked Emery–Dreifuss muscular dystrophy resembling limb-girdle muscular dystrophy. *Neuromusc. Disord.* **8**, 72–76.

Nagano, A., Koga, R., Ogawa, M. et al. (1996). Emerin deficiency at the nuclear membrane in patients with Emery–Dreifuss muscular dystrophy. *Nat. Genet.* **12**, 254–259.

Ognibene, A., Sabatelli, P., Petrini, S. et al. (1999). Nuclear changes in a case of X-linked Emery–Dreifuss muscular dystrophy. *Muscle Nerve* **22**, 864–869.

Ostlund, C., Ellenberg, J., Hallberg, E., Lippincott-Schwartz, J. and Worman, J. (1999). Intracellular trafficking of emerin, the Emery–Dreifuss muscular dystrophy protein. *J. Cell Sci.* **112**, 1709–1719.

Oswald, A. H., Goldblatt, J., Horak, A. R. and Town, R. S. A. (1987). Lethal cardiac conduction defects in Emery–Dreifuss muscular dystrophy. *S. Afr. Med. J.* **72**, 567–570.

Powe, W., Willeit, E., Sluga, E. and Mayr, U. (1985). The rigid spine syndrome – a myopathy of uncertain nosological position. *J. Neurol. Neurosurg. Psychiatry* **48**, 887–893.

Rakovec, P., Zidar, J., Sinkovec, M., Zupan, I. and Brecelj, A. (1995). Cardiac involvement in Emery–Dreifuss muscular dystrophy: role of a diagnostic pacemaker. *Pacing Clin. Electrophysiol.* **18**, 1721–1724.

Rowland, L. P., Fetell, M., Olarte, M., Hays, A., Singh, N. and Wanat, F. E. (1979). Emery–Dreifuss muscular dystrophy. *Ann. Neurol.* **5**, 111–117.

Sabatelli, P., Squarzoni, S., Petrini, S. et al. (1998). Oral exfoliative cytology for the non-invasive diagnosis in X-linked Emery–Dreifuss muscular dystrophy patients and carriers. *Neuromusc. Disord.* **8**, 67–71.

Schenk, P. and Mathias, E. (1920). Zur Kasuistik der Dystrophia musculorum progressiva retrahens. *Ber. Klin. Wochensch.* **24**, 557–558.

Serratrice, G., Pellissier, J. F., Pouget, J. and Gastaut, J. L. (1984). The rigid spine syndrome and its nosological borders: 2 cases. *Presse Med.* **13**, 1129–1132.

Small, K. and Warren, S. T. (1998). Emerin deletions occurring on both Xq28 inversion backgrounds. *Hum. Mol. Genet.* **7**, 135–139.

Small, K., Wagener, M. and Warren, S. T. (1997a). Isolation and characterization of the complete mouse emerin gene. *Mamm. Genome* **8**, 337–341.

Small, K., Iber, J. and Warren, S. T. (1997b). Emerin deletion reveals a common X-chromosome inversion mediated by inverted repeats. *Nat. Genet.* **16**, 96–99.

Squarzoni, S., Sabatelli, P., Ognibene, A. et al. (1998). Immunocytochemical detection of emerin within the nuclear matrix. *Neuromusc. Disord.* **8**, 338–344.

Strom, E. H., Skjorten, F. and Stokke, E. S. (1993). Polycystic tumor of the atrioventricular nodal region in a man with Emery–Dreifuss muscular dystrophy. *Pathol. Res. Pract.* **189**, 960–964.

Sullivan, T., Escalante-Alcalde, D., Bhatt, H. et al. (1999). Loss of A-type lamin expression compromises nuclear envelope integrity leading to muscular dystrophy. *J. Cell Biol.* **147**, 913–920.

Takamoto, K., Hirose, K., Uono, M. and Nonaka, I. (1984). A genetic variant of Emery Dreifuss muscular dystrophy with humeropelvic distribution, early joint contracture, and permanent atrial paralysis. *Arch. Neurol.* **41**, 1292–1293.

Taylor, J., Sewry, C. A., Dubowitz, V. and Muntoni, F. (1998). Early onset, autosomal recessive muscular dystrophy with Emery–Dreifuss phenotype and normal emerin expression. *Neurology* **51**, 1116–1120.

Thomas, N. S. T., Williams, H., Elsas, L. J., Sarfarazi, M. and Harper, P. S. (1986). Localization of the gene for Emery–Dreifuss muscular dystrophy to the distal long arm of the X-chromosome. *J. Med. Genet.* **23**, 596–598.

Thomas, P. K., Calne, D. B. and Elliott, C. F. (1972). X-linked scapuloperoneal syndrome. *J. Neurol. Neurosurg. Psychiatry* **35**, 208–215.

Thomas, P. K., Schott, G. D. and Morgan-Hughes, J. A. (1975). Adult onset scapuloperoneal myopathy. *J. Neurol. Neurosurg. Psychiatry* **38**, 1008–1015.

Toniolo, D., Bione, S. and Arahata, K. (1998). Emery–Dreifuss muscular dystrophy. In: *Neuromuscular Disorders: Clinical and Molecular Genetics*, ed. A. E. H. Emery, pp. 87–103. New York: John Wiley.

Tsuchiya, Y. and Arahata, K. (1997). Emery–Dreifuss syndrome. *Curr. Opin. Neurol.* **10**, 421–425.

Tsuchiya, Y., Hase, A., Ogawa, M., Yorifuji, H. and Arahata, K. (1999). Distinct regions specify the nuclear membrane targeting of emerin, the responsible protein for Emery–Dreifuss muscular dystrophy. *Eur. J. Biochem.* **259**, 859–865.

ul Hassan, Z., Fastabend, C. P., Mohanty, P. K. and Isaacs, E. R. (1979). Atrioventricular block and supraventricular arrhythmias with X-linked musculardystrophy. *Circulation* **60**, 1365–1369.

Voit, T., Krogmann, O., Lenard, H. G. et al. (1988). Emery–Dreifuss muscular dystrophy: disease spectrum and differential diagnosis. *Neuropaediatrics* **19**, 62–71.

Waters, D. D., Nutter, D. O., Hopkins, L. C. and Dorney, E. R. (1975). Cardiac features of an unusual X-linked humeroperoneal neuromuscular disease. *N. Eng. J. Med.* **293**, 1017–1022.

Wehnert, M. and Muntoni, F. (1999). Workshop report: the 60th ENMC international workshop on non-X-linked Emery–Dreifuss muscular dystrophy. *Neuromusc. Disord.* **9**, 115–121.

Witt, T. N., Graner, C. G., Pongratz, D. and Baur, X. (1988). Autosomal dominant Emery–Dreifuss syndrome: evidence of a neurogenic variant of the disease. *Eur. Arch. Psychiatric Neurol. Sci.* **273**, 230–236.

Wulff, K., Parrish, J. E., Herrmann, F. H. and Wehnert, M. (1997). Six novel mutations in the emerin gene causing X-linked Emery–Dreifuss muscular dystrophy. *Hum. Mutat.* **9**, 526–530.

Wyse, D. G., Nath, F. C. and Browell, A. K. (1987). Benign X-linked (Emery–Dreifuss) muscular dystrophy is not benign. *Pacing Clin. Electrophysiol.* **10**, 533–537.

Yates, J. R. W. (1991). Workshop report: the European workshop on Emery–Dreifuss muscular dystrophy. *Neuromusc. Disord.* **1**, 393–396.

Yates, J. R. W. (1997). Workshop report: the 43rd ENMC international workshop on Emery–Dreifuss muscular dystrophy. *Neuromusc. Disord.* **7**, 67–69.

Yates, J. R. W., Bagshaw, J., Aksmanovic, V. M. A. et al. (1999). Genotype-phenotype analysis on X-linked Emery–Dreifuss muscular dystrophy and identification of a missense mutation associated with a milder phenotype. *Neuromusc. Disord.* **9**, 159–165.

Yorifuji, H., Tadano, Y., Tsuchiya, Y. et al. (1997). Emerin, deficiency of which causes Emery–Dreifuss muscular dystrophy, is localized at the inner nuclear membrane. *Neurogenetics* **1**, 135–140.

Yoshioka, M., Saida, K., Itagaki, Y. and Kamiya, T. (1989). Follow up study of cardiac involvement in Emery–Dreifuss muscular dystrophy. *Arch. Dis. Child.* **64**, 713–715.

24

Oculopharyngeal muscular dystrophy

Bernard Brais

Introduction

The mutations responsible for oculopharyngeal muscular dystrophy (OPMD) have been identified using a positional cloning approach (Brais et al., 1998). This disease, which appeared to be clinically homogeneous, was shown also to be genetically homogenous. Dominant and recessive OPMD are caused by stable short $(GCG)_{7-13}$ triplet repeat expansions in the gene for polyadenylation binding protein 2 (*PABP2*). OPMD is the first disease described to be caused by the expansions of a short $(GCG)_n$ triplet repeat coding for polyalanine (Brais et al., 1998).

Autosomal dominant OPMD was first clearly reported in a Bostonian family of French-Canadian descent (Taylor, 1915). OPMD was acknowledged as a distinct muscular dystrophy in 1962 (Victor et al., 1962). It was described as causing a selective progressive ptosis and dysphagia that usually commenced after the age of 50 years. The essentially myopathic nature of the condition was underlined. André Barbeau established the existence of a large French-Canadian cluster caused probably by a founder effect (Barbeau, 1966, 1969; Bouchard, 1997). He also established that proximal limb weakness, particularly of the lower extremities, was a common finding late in the course of the disease and in some patients could be quite incapacitating. In 1980, Tomé and Fardeau identified by electron microscopy unique filamentous intranuclear inclusions (INI) in deltoid muscles biopsies from three unrelated patients with OPMD. Theses INI are now considered to be the specific histological marker of OPMD (Tomé et al., 1997).

Dominant OPMD has a worldwide distribution, with cases described in 30 countries: Armenia, Australia, Brazil, Belgium, Canada, Denmark, France, Germany, Holland, Hungary, Israel, Ireland, Italy, Japan, Lebanon, Malaysia, Mexico, New Zealand, Norway, Portugal (also in the Azores), Russia, Spain (also in the Canaries), Sweden, Switzerland, Taiwan, UK, USA, Uzbekistan, Uruguay and Yugoslavia. Only in three populations has the prevalence of OPMD been estimated. In France it is in the order of 1 : 200 000 (Brunet et al., 1990). It is particularly prevalent in the French-Canadian population of the province of Quebec (1 : 1000) and in Bukhara Jews living in Israel (1 : 600) (Brais et al., 1995; Blumen et al., 1997). In the USA, the vast majority of patients are of French-Canadian extraction. The predicted prevalence of the recessive form should be in the order of 1 : 10 000 in France, Quebec and Japan based on the allele frequency of the $(GCG)_7$ recessive mutation in these populations (Brais et al., 1998). The less-frequent diagnosis of recessive OPMD may reflect the milder and later onset of this condition.

The age of onset of autosomal dominant OPMD is variable and often difficult to pinpoint. A study of 72 French-Canadian symptomatic carriers of a $(GCG)_9$ mutation established a mean age of onset for ptosis of 48.1 years (26–65) and for dysphagia of 50.7 years (40–63) (Bouchard et al., 1997). Ptosis appears to be the most common presenting symptom in female patients, probably for aesthetic reasons, while dysphagia is more often the initial symptom in males. Early symptoms that are more suggestive of a dysphagia caused by OPMD are an increasing time required for a meal and an acquired avoidance of dryer foods. The other signs observed as the disease progresses are proximal upper extremity weakness (38%), facial muscle weakness (43%), limitation of upper gaze (61%), dysphonia (67%), proximal lower extremity weakness (71%) and tongue atrophy and weakness (82%) (Bouchard et al., 1997). Mutation analysis has also established three subgroups of patients with more severe phenotypes (Brais et al., 1998). The most severe form is observed in patients homozygous for two dominant mutations (Blumen et al., 1999). In these children of two affected parents, symptoms start in the twenties and progress to include leg weakness in the

PABP2 genomic (GCG)ₙ dominant mutations

Normal: ATG GCG GCG GCG GCG GCG GCG GCA GCA GCA GCG

Dominant: ATG GCG GCG GCG GCG GCG GCG **(GCG)₂₋₇** GCA GCA GCA GCG

Expansions in the PABP2 N-terminal polyalanine domain in OPMD

Normal: M A A A A A A A A A A G A A G G R G S

Dominant: M A A A A A A A A A A **(A)₂₋₇** G A A G G R G S

Fig. 24.1. Mutations in *PABP2* and polyalanine expansions of the homopolymeric polyalanine domain of the polyadenylation binding protein 2 (PABP2) in oculopharyngeal muscular dystrophy (OPMD).

thirties. Patients that are compound heterozygotes for a dominant mutation and a $(GCG)_7$ recessive mutation also have a more severe phenotype, with symptoms starting in the late thirties or early forties and symptomatic leg weakness before the age of 55 years (Brais et al., 1998). Lastly, 18% of patients will have a similar phenotype to that of the compound heterozygotes but are only carriers of a dominant mutation. These cases usually cluster in families, suggesting that other genetic factors can influence the severity of OPMD. Unfortunately, these three forms of severe OPMD will lead much earlier to surgical treatment and often to the use of a wheelchair. The size of the *PABP2* $(GCG)_n$ mutation may also influence the severity of the condition, but this still needs to be confirmed. The recessive OPMD clinical phenotype appears to be similar to the dominant though possibly milder and with an older age of onset (Fried et al., 1975). Intranuclear inclusions are also observed in muscle of patients with recessive disease (Brais et al., 1998). Children with an OPMD-like phenotype have been described but their symptoms do not appear to be caused by mutation in *PABP2* (Lacomis et al., 1991).

Pathophysiology

How mutations in *PABP2* lead to myofibre loss that is more serious in certain muscle types is still unknown. However, a polyalanine nuclear toxicity model has been proposed (Brais et al., 1998, 1999). This hypothesis is based on PABP2 being a nuclear protein which has lengthening of the N-terminus polyalanine domain by the OPMD mutations (Fig. 24.1). The 918 bp sequence of the *PABP2* cDNA codes for a protein of 306 amino acid residues of 33 kDa in its monomeric form. It is involved in the polyadenylation of all mRNA (Wahle, 1991; Bienroth et al., 1993, Wahle et al.,

1993; Krause et al., 1994; Nemeth et al., 1995). This process is biphasic. Polyadenylation depends for its first step on poly(A) polymerase and the cleavage and polyadenylation specificity factor (CPSF), while the rapid final elongation of the mRNA poly(A) tails is dependent on the addition of PABP2 to the polyadenylation complex (Bienroth et al., 1993). PABP2 is ubiquitously expressed but occurs at higher levels in skeletal muscle (Brais et al., 1998). The polyalanine nuclear toxicity gain-of-function hypothesis proposes that PABP2 is a passive carrier protein of a pathogenic expanded polyalanine domain to nuclei. It is analogous to a carrier model proposed in CAG repeat diseases (Sisodia, 1998). Different lines of evidence suggest that polyalanine oligomers could form resistant macromolecules. Polyalanine oligomers are known to be very resistant to protease digestion or chemical degradation (Forood et al., 1995). They form β-sheet structure in vitro (Forood et al., 1995). Furthermore, polyalanine oligomers containing more than eight alanines in a row form fibrils spontaneously (Billingsley et al., 1994). It is proposed that beyond 10 alanines, the normal number of alanines in PABP2, the polyalanine domains polymerize to form stable β-sheets that are resistant to nuclear degradation. The polyalanine macromolecules would grow with time to form the OPMD intranuclear filaments that are seen on electron microscopy. Preliminary evidence does suggest that mutated PABP2 is an integral part of INI. Nuclear dysfunction would ensue when a significant part of a nucleus is occupied by the PABP2 aggregates. One of the variables that may influence the differential involvement of certain muscles may be the level of PABP2 expression. Two lines of pathological evidence support this. First, the proportion of nuclei with INI was found to be 8% in the more affected cricothyroid pharyngeal muscle compared with 4% in the deltoid muscle of the same patient (Coquet et al., 1990). Second, in muscle biopsies from patients with homozygous OPMD twice as many nuclei showed INI than usually observed in heterozygous patients (9.4% versus 4.9%; $p < 0.02$) (Blumen et al., 1999).

Histopathology

Rimmed vacuoles and INI are the two main morphological changes observed in OPMD (Fig. 24.2). (Tomé et al., 1997). Rimmed vacuoles are readily detected by light microscopy. They were first described in OPMD but have been observed since in other myopathies, in particular in inclusion body myositis (Dubowitz and Brooke, 1973; Askanas and Engel, 1995). The rimmed vacuoles are not membrane bound and are believed to be of an autophagic nature. They are found in 90% of biopsies in both normal and atrophied fibres but are not specific for OPMD (Tomé et al., 1997). On semithin sections, INI can be observed as clear zones in 2 to 5% (mean 4%) of heterozygote deltoid muscle nuclei (Fig. 24.2a). The percentage of nuclei observed with INI is believed to correlate with the limited volume occupied by the filaments (Tomé et al., 1997). The INI in OPMD consisted of tubular filaments, often arranged in palisades or tangles (Fig. 24.2b) (Tomé and Fardeau, 1980). The filaments are up to 0.25 μm in length with 8.5 nm external diameter and 3 nm internal diameter. These filaments are exclusively nuclear and have not been found in the nuclei of other tissues. They are different from the nuclear and cytoplasmic filaments of 15–18 nm diameter seen in inclusion body myositis. However, filaments of the inclusion body myositis type are seen in the cytoplasm and, more rarely, in the nucleus in OPMD (Tomé et al., 1997). Other nonspecific pathological changes observed in OPMD include atrophied small angulated muscle fibres and predominance of type I fibres. Necrotic fibres are only rarely seen (Tomé et al., 1997).

Molecular biology

The dominant OPMD locus was mapped to chromosome 14q11 in three large French-Canadian families (Brais et al., 1995). Linkage to the same markers was confirmed by four other groups (Porschke et al., 1997; Stajich et al., 1997; Teh et al., 1997; Grewal et al., 1998). Linkage studies further supported the genetically homogeneous nature of dominant OPMD. A positional cloning strategy relying on the French-Canadian founder effect led to the identification of short $(GCG)_{8-13}$ expansions in *PABP2* in all patients with dominant OPMD (Brais et al., 1998). These expanded repeats are mitotically and meiotically stable. Based on the study of a large group of French-Canadian families, the estimated rate of a second expansion of an existent OPMD mutation is in the order of 1 : 500 meioses (Brais et al., 1998). The normal $(GCG)_6$ repeat in the first exon of the gene immediately follows the ATG start codon (Fig. 24.1). The normal 10 alanine homopolymeric domain is coded by a $(GCG)_6$ repeat followed by four other different alanine codons. Dominant mutations consist of the addition of two to seven (GCG) repeats to the $(GCG)_6$ stretch. These will cause the lengthening of the polyalanine stretch from 10 to 12–17 alanines. The study of 81 non-French-Canadian families originating from 17 countries documented the existence of six different mutation sizes (Table 24.1). All the different mutation sizes have been observed in North America and Europe except for the $(GCG)_{13}$ muta-

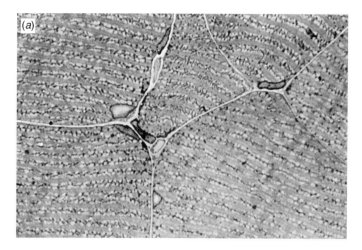

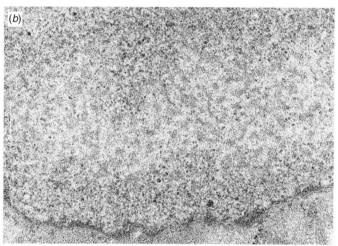

Fig. 24.2. Intranuclear inclusions (INI) in oculopharyngeal muscular dystrophy. (a) Clear zones occupied by INI can be seen in two nuclei (arrows) on a semithin section (×1600). (b) By electron microscopy, the INI can be seen to comprise palisading tubulas filaments, which often form tangles (×63 000). (Photographs kindly provided by F. M. S. Tomé.)

tion, which has been found only in one North American family of Russian origin. In French-Canadians and Bukhara Jews, OPMD is caused by two historically distinct $(GCG)_9$ founder mutations (Brais et al., 1998).

As discussed above, the dominant OPMD phenotype varies in severity (Bouchard et al., 1997). Whether the size of the repeat influences severity still needs to be established. However, the molecular basis for two more severe presentations has been elucidated. More severe disease is defined as having an onset of ptosis and dysphagia before the age of 45 years and of symptomatic proximal leg weakness before age 55. Patients with more severe disease by

Table 24.1. Percentage of families that share the different sizes of PABP2 (GCG)$_n$ mutations in oculopharyngeal dystrophy

Mutations	No. alanine residues[a]	Percentage[b]
$(GCG)_8$	12	5%
$(GCG)_9$	13	40%
$(GCG)_{10}$	14	26%
$(GCG)_{11}$	15	21%
$(GCG)_{12}$	16	7%
$(GCG)_{13}$	17	1%

Notes:

[a] Normal polyadenine binding protein 2 (PABP2) has 10 alanine residues.

[b] Percentage based on the study of 81 non-French-Canadian families.

this definition represent 21% of heterozygote cases in the French-Canadian population. The most severely affected individuals are homozygotes for a dominant OPMD mutation (Blumen et al., 1996; Brais et al., 1998); 23% of the more severe heterozygotes have inherited, beside the dominant mutation, a recessive $(GCG)_7$ mutation from their unaffected parent (Brais et al., 1998). This mutation has a 1–2% prevalence in North America, France and Japan. The molecular basis of autosomal recessive OPMD is the homozygous state for the $(GCG)_7$ mutation. Patients with this form may be underdiagnosed because of a milder phenotype and the absence of clear family history. Therefore, the $(GCG)_7$ mutation is an example of a polymorphism that can act either as a modifier of a dominant phenotype or as a recessive mutation.

Diagnosis

The following strict clinical diagnostic criteria for dominant OPMD have been proposed: (i) a positive family history of OPMD, (ii) at least one palpebral fissure at rest smaller than 8 mm (or previous blepharoplasty) and (iii) a swallowing time greater than 7 seconds when asked to drink 80 ml ice-cold water (Brais et al., 1995). The decade-specific penetrances for carriers of a dominant $(GCG)_9$ mutation are 1% (<40), 6% (40–49), 31% (50–59), 63% (60–69), 99% (>69) (Brais et al., 1997). Though dominant OPMD is fully penetrant past the age 70, a third of patients in their sixties will not meet the strict clinical diagnostic criteria. The clinical diagnosis of recessive OPMD is more problematic. Late-onset ptosis and

dysphagia without a clear family history should raise this diagnostic possibility.

Until the identification of the OPMD *PABP2* mutations, definitive diagnosis relied on the electron microscopy observation of INI (Tomé and Fardeau, 1994). This approach has now been replaced by DNA testing (Brais et al., 1998). Autosomal dominant and recessive OPMD being allelic, the molecular diagnosis of both conditions is quite straightforward. A single polymerase chain reaction (PCR) is required to establish the carrier status of an individual (Brais et al., 1998). The region of the gene that is mutated is amplified by PCR, the DNA products are subsequently separated on a denaturing polyacrylamide gel and size differences are established. The test has a 100% sensitivity and specificity and is available through commercial and research laboratories. The major indications for DNA testing of a symptomatic individuals are (i) confirmation of the diagnosis in a family never tested, (ii) the clinical picture presents a diagnostic dilemma, (iii) the patient has a severe earlier onset form of the disease, and (iv) the patient may suffer from recessive OPMD. However, much thought should be taken before requesting the predictive testing of an asymptomatic individual. It is unclear if these individuals will benefit from the test, considering that there is no medical therapy or prevention for this disease. Presymptomatic testing should be performed in a context in which genetic counselling and psychological support can be offered.

Management

There is no medical treatment yet available for OPMD. A high-protein diet is recommended. This is particularly important as the dysphagia becomes severe and patients shy away from sources of animal proteins such as meats. Special attention should be made to prevent the frequent social withdrawal of patients as their dysphagia progresses. They should be told to eat prior to or after social gatherings. They should be reassured about the risk of fatal choking, which is extremely small. Aspiration pneumonia is a frequent cause of death, and the patient should be advised to consult early on if they have a productive cough accompanied by fever. Exercises that maintain a good cardiovascular condition should be encouraged, but strenuous exercises should not be promoted. A wheelchair will be needed by those more severely affected. An even larger percentage of patients will use either a cane or a walker late in the course of the disease. Prevention of traumatic fractures from falls is paramount.

The surgical treatments presently available are used to

correct the eyelid ptosis and improve swallowing in moderately or severely affected individuals. Two types of operation are used to correct the ptosis, with overall good results: resection of the levetor palpebral aponeurosis and frontal suspension of the eyelids (Codère, 1993). Resection of aponeurosis is easily done but usually needs to be repeated once or twice (Rodrigue and Molgat, 1997). Frontal suspension of the eyelids involves using a thread of skeletal muscle fascia as a sling, which is inserted in the tarsal plate of the upper eyelid and attached at its ends in the frontalis muscle, which is relatively preserved in OPMD (Codère, 1993). Its major advantage is that it is permanent, but it requires a general anesthetic for insertion. Surgery is recommended when the ptosis interferes with vision, or cervical pain appears secondary to the constant dorsiflexion of the neck. Contraindications to blepharoplasty are marked ophthalmoplegia, a dry-eye syndrome or a poor orbicularis function. Surgical evaluation of symptomatic dysphagia should be prompted by severe dysphagia, marked weight loss, near-fatal choking or recurrent pneumonia. Cricopharyngeal myotomy will alleviate symptoms in most patients. Unfortunately, dysphagia will slowly reappear. Severe dysphonia and lower oesophageal sphincter incompetence are contraindications to surgery (Duranceau, 1997). Repetitive dilatations of the upper-oesophageal sphincter with bougies is still at the experimental stage (Mathieu et al., 1997).

Prevention

They are no means to prevent or delay the onset of OPMD.

Prognosis

The severity of OPMD is variable. The individuals that fall in the severe OPMD subgroups, as defined above, will unfortunately suffer greatly from their condition. The suspicion of a severe form of the disease should prompt DNA testing to establish if the individual has inherited, beside a dominant mutation, a recessive $(GCG)_7$ mutation. If this proven modulator of severity is present, the patient should be informed of the greater impact of OPMD on future life.

References

Askanas, V. and Engel, W. K. (1995). New advances in the understanding of sporadic inclusion-body myositis and hereditary inclusion-body myositis, *Curr. Opin. Rheumatol.* **7**, 486–496.

Barbeau, A. (1966). The syndrome of hereditary late onset ptosis and dysphagia in French Canada. In: *Symposium über progressive Muskeldystrophie*, ed. E. Kuhn, pp. 102–109. Berlin: Springer-Verlag.

Barbeau, A. (1969). Oculopharyngeal muscular dystrophy in French Canada. In: *Progress in Neuro-ophthalmology*, Vol. 2, eds. J.-R. Brunette and A. Barbeau, p. 3. Amsterdam: Excerpta Medica.

Bienroth, S., Keller, W. and Wahle, E. (1993). Assembly of a processive messenger RNA polyadenylation complex. *EMBO J.* **12**, 585–594.

Billingsley, G. D., Cox, D. W., Duncan, A. M. V., Googfellow, P. J. and Grzeschil, K.-H. (1994). Regional localization of loci on chromosome 14 using somatic cell hybrids. *Cytogenet. Cell Genet.* **66**, 33–38.

Blumen, S. C., Sadeh, M., Korczyn, A. D. et al. (1996). Intranuclear inclusions in oculopharyngeal muscular dystrophy among Bukhara Jews. *Neurology* **46**, 1324–1328.

Blumen, S. C., Nisipeanu, P., Sadeh, M. et al. (1997). Epidemiology and inheritance of oculopharyngeal muscular dystrophy in Israel, *Neuromusc. Disord.* **7**, S38–S40.

Blumen, S. C., Brais, B., Korczyn, A. D. et al. (1999). Homozygotes for oculopharyngeal muscular dystrophy have a severe form of the disease. *Ann. Neurol.* **46**, 115-118.

Bouchard, J.-P. (1997). André Barbeau and the oculopharyngeal muscular dystrophy in French Canada and North America. *Neuromusc. Disord.* **7**, S5–S11.

Bouchard, J.-P., Brais, B., Brunet, D., Gould, P. V. and Rouleau, G. A. (1997). Recent studies on oculopharyngeal muscular dystrophy in Quebec. *Neuromusc. Disord.* **7**, S22–S29.

Brais, B., Xie, Y.-G., Sanson, M. et al. (1995). The oculopharyngeal muscular dystrophy locus maps to the region of the cardiac α and β myosin heavy chain genes on chromosome 14q11.2-q13. *Hum. Mol. Genet.* **4**, 429–434.

Brais, B., Bouchard, J.-P., Ya-Gang, X. et al. (1997). Using the full power of linkage analysis in 11 French Canadian families to fine map the oculopharyngeal muscular dystrophy gene. *Neuromusc. Disord.* **7**, S70–S75.

Brais, B., Bouchard, J.-P., Xie, Y.-G. et al. (1998). Short GCG expansions in the PABP2 gene cause oculopharyngeal muscular dystrophy. *Nat. Genet.* **18**, 164–167.

Brais, B., Rouleau, G. A., Bouchard, J.-P., Fardeau, M. and Tomé, F. (1999). Oculopharyngeal muscular dystrophy, *Semin. Neurol.* **19**, 59–66.

Brunet, G., Tomé, F. M. S., Samson, F., Robert, J. M. and Fardeau, M. (1990). Dystrophie musculaire oculo-pharyngée. Recensement des familles françaises et étude généalogique. *Rev. Neurolog.* **146**, 425–429.

Codère, F. (1993), Oculopharyngeal muscular dystrophy. *Can. J. Ophthalmol.* **28**, 1–2.

Coquet, M., Vital, C. and Julien, J. (1990). Presence of inclusion body myositis-like filaments in oculopharyngeal muscular dystrophy: ultrastructural study of 10 cases. *Neuropathol. Appl. Neurobiol.* **16**, 393.

Dubowitz, V. and Brooke, M. H. (1973). *Muscle Biopsy. A Modern Approach*, Philadelphia, PA: Saunders.

Duranceau, A. (1997). Cricopharyngeal myotomy in the management of neurogenic and muscular dysphagia. *Neuromusc. Disord.* **7**, S85–S89.

Forood, B., Pérez-Payá, E., Houghten, R. A. and Blondelle, S. E. (1995). Formation of an extremely stable polyalanine β-sheet macromolecule, *Biochem. Biophys. Res. Commun.* **211**, 7–13.

Fried, K., Arlozorov, A. and Spira, R. (1975). Autosomal recessive oculopharyngeal muscular dystrophy. *J. Med. Genet.* **12**, 416–418.

Grewal, R. P., Cantor, R., Turner, G., Grewal, R. K. and Detera-Wadleigh, S. D. (1998). Genetic mapping and haplotype analysis of oculopharyngeal muscular dystrophy. *Neuroreport* **9**, 961–965.

Krause, S., Fakan, S., Weis, K. and Wahle, E. (1994). Immunodetection of poly(A) binding protein II in cell nucleus. *Exp. Cell Res.* **214**, 75–82.

Lacomis, D., Kupsky, W. J., Kuban, K. K. and Specht, L. A. (1991). Childhood onset oculopharyngeal muscular dystrophy. *Ped. Neurol.* **7**, 382–384.

Mathieu, J., Lapointe, G., Brassard, A., Tremblay, C., Brais, B., Rouleau, G. A. and Bouchard, J. P. (1997). A pilot study on upper oesophageal sphincter dilatation for the treatment of dysphagia in patients with oculopharyngeal muscular dystrophy. *Neuromusc. Disord.* **7**, S100–104.

Nemeth, A., Krause, S., Blank, D., Jenny, A., Jenö, P., Lustig, A. and Wahle, E. (1995). Isolation of genomic and cDNA clones encoding bovine poly(A) binding protein II. *Nucl. Acids Res.* **23**, 4034–4041.

Porschke, H., Kress, W., Reichmann, H., Goebel, H. H. and Grimm, T. (1997). Oculopharyngeal muscular dystrophy in a Northern German family linked to chromosome 14q, and presenting carnitine deficiency. *Neuromusc. Disord.* **7**, S57–S62.

Rodrigue, D. and Molgat, Y. M. (1997). Surgical correction of blepharoptosis in oculopharyngeal muscular dystrophy. *Neuromusc. Disord.* **7**, S82–S84.

Sisodia, S. S. (1998). Nuclear inclusions in glutamine repeat disorders: are they pernicious, coincidental, or beneficial? *Cell* **95**, 1–4.

Stajich, J. M., Gilchrist, J. M., Lennon, F. et al. (1997). Confirmation of linkage of oculopharyngeal muscular dystrophy to chromosome 14q11.2-q13. *Ann. Neurol.* **40**, 801–804.

Taylor, E. W. (1915). Progressive vagus-glossopharyngeal paralysis with ptosis: a contribution to the group of family diseases. *J. Nerv. Mental Dis.* **42**, 129–139.

Teh, B. T., Sullivan, A. A., Farnebo, F. et al. (1997). Oculopharyngeal muscular dystrophy; report and genetic studies of an Australian kindred. *Clin. Genet.* **51**, 52–55.

Tomé, F. M. S. and Fardeau, M. (1980). Nuclear inclusions in oculopharyngeal muscular dystrophy. *Acta Neuropathol.* **49**, 85–87.

Tomé, F. M. S. and Fardeau, M. (1994). Oculopharyngeal muscular dystrophy. In: *Myology*, Vol. 2, eds. A. G. Engel and C. Franzini-Armstrong, pp. 1233–1245. New York: McGraw-Hill.

Tomé, F. M. S., Chateau, D., Helbling-Leclerc, A. and Fardeau, M. (1997). Morphological changes in muscle fibres in oculopharyngeal muscular dystrophy. *Neuromusc. Disord.* **7**, S63–S69.

Victor, M., Hayes, R. and Adams, R. D. (1962). Oculopharyngeal muscular dystrophy: a familial disease of late life characterized by dysphagia and progressive ptosis of the eyelids. *N. Eng. J. Med.* **267**, 1267–1272.

Wahle, E. (1991). A novel poly(A)-binding protein acts as a specificity factor in the second phase of messenger RNA polyadenylation. *Cell* **66**, 759–768.

Wahle, E., Lustig, A., Jenö, P. and Maurer, P. (1993). Mammalian poly(A)-binding protein II: physical properties and binding to polynucleotides. *J. Biol. Chem.* **268**, 2937–2945.

25

Congenital muscular dystrophies

Thomas Voit

Introduction

Congenital muscular dystrophy (CMD) was first described in a series of lucid articles by Frederick Eustace Batten in London between 1903 and 1910. In 1903 he reported three children with 'myopathy, infantile type' (Batten, 1903a) and another case under the label of myositis fibrosa (Batten, 1903b). The term muscular dystrophy (dystrophia muscularis congenita) was introduced by Howard in 1908 when he described a twin child who was born with bilateral talipes equino varus and died after 7 days. Howard thought that there was a 'primary degeneration of the muscles occuring before birth'. In 1904, Batten had already provided photographic documentation of an affected child plus a detailed drawing of the histological changes in the affected muscle, including variation of fibre sizes, considerable fibrosis and lipomatosis (Batten, 1904). Finally, he summed up the characteristics of the disease he called 'muscular dystrophy, simple atrophic type' (Batten, 1909/10).

The disease is congenital or starts in early infancy, and is characterized by smallness, lack of power and loss of tone in all the muscles of the body without localized atrophy or hypotrophy of individual muscles or groups of muscles . . . The disease is but slowly progressive for the child may as development takes place, learn to sit up, and possibly to stand with support. The child usually learns to talk at the normal age, and intellectually is often in advance of his years. As a rule these children never learn to walk but adopt some strange method of getting about. . . . In the later stages of the disease, some contraction of the flexors usually takes place, so that the legs cannot be fully extended.

Over the next 80 years, many different conditions were reported under the diagnostic label of CMD but also under such different terms as myotonia congenita, amyotonia congenita, congenital myositis, arthrogryposis multiplex or rigid spine syndrome (for review see Tomé, 1999). Most of these conditions shared a number of clinical and laboratory features that are still useful as a working definition of CMD (Table 25.1). Several milestone papers influenced the nosological concept of what we now call CMD. Arthrogryposis multiplex caused by CMD was first described by Banker and coworkers in 1957. Zellweger et al. (1967a,b) distinguished severe and milder forms of CMD, thereby enlarging the spectrum of these conditions beyond the first year of life. In addition, four distinct phenotypes were reported, which were later confirmed by molecular studies. In Japan, Fukuyama et al. (1960) described a form of CMD that is endemic in Japan and characterized by a combination of muscular dystrophy and brain involvement with micropolygyria, alterations of the cerebellum and eyes (Fukuyama CMD (FCMD)). In Finland, Santavuori and coworkers (1977) also described a CMD with a combination of pachygyria and polymicrogyria, brainstem hypoplasia, cerebellar dysgenesis and eye involvement, which they called muscle–eye–brain disease (MEB). Similar eye changes with a combination of congenital retinal detachment and hydrocephalus had been described by Walker in 1942 and by Warburg in 1978. Subsequently, Williams et al. (1984) and Dobyns et al. (1985) recognized that this combination of ocular dysgenesis and type 2 lissencephaly with muscular dystrophy was a specific syndrome, which they eponymously labelled Walker Warburg syndrome (WWS).

Another congenital muscle disorder characterized by early contractures and, in particular, rigidity of the spine was first recognized by Dubowitz in 1971 (Dubowitz, 1971, 1973). However, phenotypic overlap between these disorders with regard to the degree of brain involvement, the occurrence of contractures or the severity of muscle involvement led to a tangle that could only be solved by molecular techniques. From 1993 to 1999 an international consortium convened under the auspices of the European

Table 25.1. Working definition of congenital muscular dystrophy

Muscle weakness and hypotonia present from birth or first months of life
Congenital or early contractures, often involving the spine
Histological changes compatible with a 'dystrophic' process combining active de- and regeneration, fibrosis, and lipomatosis
Serum creatine kinase levels normal or elevated
Intellect normal or impaired
Brain on imaging/postmortem normal or evidence of white matter changes, disorders of migration and cerebellar or brainstem abnormalities

Neuromuscular Centre (ENMC) in a series of workshops. Ongoing collaboration among the international groups of scientists involved has led to a completely new classification of CMDs. To date, five conditions have been defined at the molecular level and many more have been thoroughly delineated in terms of nosology and pattern of inheritance (Table 25.2).

Group I: congenital muscular dystrophy with primary deficiency of laminin-α2

Laminin-α2-deficient CMD is the most common form of CMD worldwide and accounts for roughly 50% of patients with CMD in the Caucasian population (Dubowitz and Fardeau, 1995; Dubowitz, 1996). In 1994, F. Tomé and colleagues discovered a complete lack of the heavy α2-chain of laminin in 13 patients with CMD. The same group subsequently localized this form of CMD to chromosome 6q2 (Hillaire et al., 1994; Helbling-Leclerc et al., 1995a) and finally described the first mutations of the gene for α2-chain of laminin, *LAMA-2*, in two families (Helbling-Leclerc et al., 1995b).

Aetiology and pathogenesis

Laminins are a family of glycoproteins that are abundant in basement membranes. They are most commonly assembled as a central heavy chain (α-chain) and two light chains (β- and γ-chain) to form a cross-shaped heterotrimer (Fig. 25.1). In skeletal muscle, the prevailing variant is the 120 nm long 600 kDa laminin-2 (α2, β1, γ1), also called merosin (for review see Wewer and Engvall, 1996). The laminin-α2-heavy chain is also associated with the light chains β2 and γ1 in skeletal muscle to form laminin-4 (α2,

β2, γ1). In developing muscle, laminin-10 (α5, β1, γ1) is strongly expressed (Sewry et al., 1995; Tiger and Gullberg, 1997). Laminin-8 (α4, β1, γ1) is expressed in skeletal muscle basement membranes but is less abundant (Iinvanainen et al., 1995).

The laminin heavy and light chains are composed of partially homologous domains labelled, from the C-terminal end, G, I, B (α), II, III, IV, IV', V and VI (Fig. 25.1). The function of the G-domain is to bind heparin, perlecan, integrin, α-dystroglycan and other cellular receptors. Domains I and II are important for intermolecular assembly and form possible cell adhesion sides. Domain III is important for entactin/nidogen binding and also possibly for cell adhesion. The functions of domains IV, IV' and V are not clearly understood. Domain VI is involved in laminin polymerization and integrin binding (Engvall and Wewer, 1996; Wewer and Engvall, 1996). Laminins are expressed very early in development. Initially, $\beta\gamma$-dimers are formed in the cell to which an α-chain is added as the rate-limiting step. This heterotrimer is secreted by the cell, and, once outside, spontaneously polymerizes. The heterotrimer with entactin/nidogen, perlecan and collagen IV, form the basement membrane sheet. In skeletal and cardiac muscle, laminin-2 is tightly linked via α-dystroglycan to the dystrophin–glycoprotein complex, which connects the actin cytoskeleton to the extracellular matrix (Fig. 25.1). Laminin-2 is also expressed in numerous other tissues, notably in placenta, skin, Schwann cells, in the basement membrane of blood vessels of the central nervous system (CNS) and in the glia limitans of the brain (Ehrig et al., 1990; Vuolteenaho et al., 1994; Sewry et al., 1996a; Villanova et al., 1996). This tissue distribution can be used for prenatal (placenta) or in vivo (skin) diagnosis but also contributes to the clinical phenotype through peripheral nerve and CNS involvement.

In skeletal muscle, the laminins contribute to myogenesis by regulating cell-matrix attachment and by contributing to synaptogenesis (Patton et al., 1997). They are probably also involved in maintaining tissue integrity as there is ongoing muscle fibre degeneration in the laminin-α2-deficient CMD muscle. The pathogenetic cascade that results from laminin-α2 deficiency in skeletal muscle is not fully understood. In the basement membrane, loss of laminin-α2 is accompanied by overexpression of laminin-α4 and laminin-α5 as well as by reduction of the light β2-chain (Tomé et al., 1994; Sewry et al., 1995, 1996b; Cohn et al., 1997, 1998; Tiger and Gullberg, 1997; Ringelmann et al., 1999). In the plasma membrane, the laminin receptor α_7-integrin also becomes reduced as a secondary change (Hodges et al., 1997; Cohn et al., 1999). The expression of dystrophin, β-dystroglycan and the sarcoglycans are usually unchanged, which is also important from a

Table 25.2. A working classification of congenital muscular dystrophies (CMDs)

Group	Disorders	Gene	Protein	Characteristics
I	Primary laminin-α2-deficient CMD	6q2	Laminin-α2	Approximately 50% of Caucasians with CMD
II	Fukuyama CMD (FCMD)	9q31	Fukutin	Combination of CMD and a cerebral
	Muscle–eye–brain disease (MEB)	1p32–34	?	and cerebellar migration disorder
	Walker Warburg syndrome (WWS)	excl. 1p32–34	?	
III	CMD with rigid spine syndrome	1p35–36	?	Prominent and early rigidity of the
III	CMD with rigid spine syndrome	excl. 1p35	?	spine
IV	CMD with secondary reduction in laminin-α2	1q42	?	At least three forms exist; may be more
IV	CMD with secondary reduction in laminin-α2	excl. 1q42	?	
IV	CMD with secondary reduction in laminin-α2 and mental retardation	?	?	
V	'Pure' CMD with normal laminin-α2 expression	?	?	Only, or mainly, muscle is affected;
V	CMD with laminin-α2 expression and mental retardation	?	?	expression of laminin-α_2 is unchanged
V	CMD with laminin-α2 expression and cerebellar hypoplasia	?	?	
VI	Rare forms of CMD	?	?	Described in single families or isolated patients

Notes:
This working classification uses clinical, protein biochemical and molecular tools for subdivision of the disorders and is bound to change substantially over the next years.

diagnostic point of view. However, in contrast to primary deficiency of dystrophin or components of the sarcoglycan complex, no general 'impairment' of plasma membrane permeability for molecules like Evans blue (960 Da) or albumin (65 kDa) results from laminin-α2 deficiency. This indicates that there are differences in the pathogenetic process between these forms of muscular dystrophy (Straub et al., 1997).

A secondary deficiency of laminin-α2 has been described in FCMD (Hayashi et al., 1993), in MEB (Haltia et al., 1997) and in at least three other nosologically distinct forms of CMD unlinked to the gene loci for laminin-α2, FCMD or MEB (Muntoni et al., 1998; Topaloglu et al., 1998; Brockington et al., 2000; Mercuri et al., 2000). This further suggests that the molecular interactions of the basement membrane are of vital importance for skeletal muscle integrity and that laminin-interacting proteins are strong candidates for other forms of CMD.

Clinical phenotype in complete laminin-α2 deficiency

The child will typically present at birth or shortly thereafter with profound general hypotonia. In utero movements may already have been reduced. The muscle weakness affects the face, the trunk and the extremities quite symmetrically. The muscle bulk may be thin or normal but hypertrophy is uncommon. Sucking and swallowing may be impaired and the child may require tube feeding (Fig. 25.2). Contractures of single or multiple joints, involving mainly elbows knees, hips or ankles, are already present in approximately 50% of these children at birth (Fig. 25.2) (Philpot et al., 1995a; Fardeau et al., 1996; Herrmann et al., 1996). Respiratory insufficiency may occur in conjunction with bronchopulmonary infections and be fatal even in the first year of life. Serum creatine kinase (CK) levels are grossly elevated to 1000–15 000 IU/l. After 6 to 12 months, the weakness generally improves and most children will be able to sit unsupported by two or three years of age but cannot sit up by themselves. The maximum motor capacity in completely laminin-α2-deficient patients is usually to be able to sit or stand with support; a few will be able to support their body weight or even take some steps. As the children become older, limited movements of the extraocular muscles may become apparent in some patients (Philpot and Muntoni, 1999). During the growth spurt, development of skoliosis is common and may require spinal fusion. Nocturnal hypoventilation is not infrequent

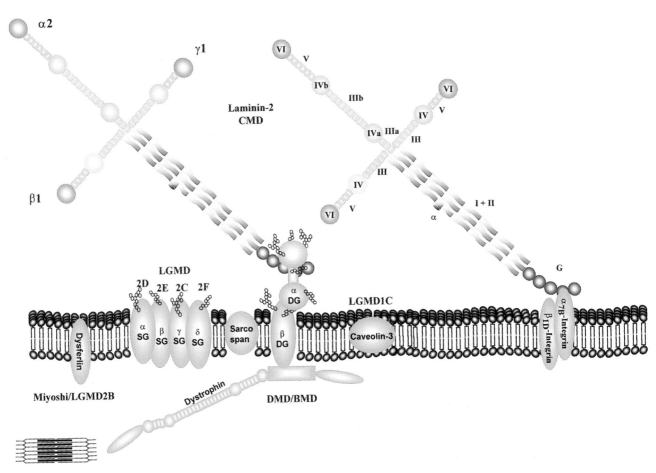

Fig. 25.1. Schematic representation of the laminin heterotrimer and its functional domains in relation to other proteins of the membrane cytoskeleton. Laminin-2 is composed of a central α2-heavy chain and two light chains, β1 and γ1. It binds through the G-domain to α-dystroglycan and α_{7B}-integrin. Through dystroglycan, laminin-2 is connected to the dystrophin–glycoprotein complex. CMD, congenital muscular dystrophy; SG,sarcoglycan; DG, dystroglycan; LGMD, limb girdle muscular dystrophy; DMD/BMD, Duchenne/Becker muscular dystrophy.

and may occur already in the first years. It is usually heralded by morning drowsiness, headaches, weight loss and daytime sleepiness. Weight loss may also, or in addition, be caused by a combination of gastro-oesophageal reflux, a delayed swallowing reflex or frank aspiration (Philpot et al., 1999a). Nocturnal hypoventilation and weight loss usually facilitate and aggravate cardiopulmonary complications and are probably responsible for most of the deaths reported in up to 30% of patients in the first decade of life (Philpot et al., 1995a; Vainzof et al., 1995; Fardeau et al., 1996; Herrmann et al., 1996). In contrast to Duchenne muscular dystrophy or severe sarcoglycan deficiency, muscle power tends to remain quite stable at school age, with some mild deterioration during weight gain and growth spurt. Life expectancy very much depends on the support and care. It is now clear that many children will

survive into the second and third decade, but no formal studies have addressed this question so far.

Central nervous system involvement

Cerebral white matter changes characterized by abnormally high T_2 signals on magentic resonance imaging (MRI) are the hallmark of brain involvement and are present in all patients with severe laminin-α2 deficiency (Dubowitz and Fardeau, 1995; Mercuri et al., 1995a, 1996; Herrmann et al., 1996; van der Knaap et al., 1997). Laminin-α2 is expressed in the basal lamina of all cerebral blood vessels with the exception of the blood vessels of the meninges and choroid plexus. Because capillaries of the CNS show distinct ultrastructural features with presumed function for the blood-brain barrier, it has been speculated that laminin-α2 deficiency will lead to an impairment of

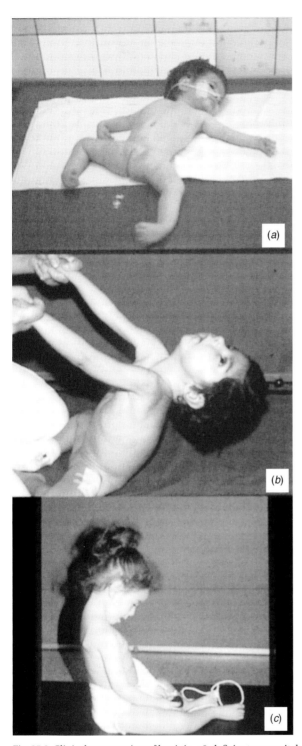

Fig. 25.2. Clinical presentation of laminin-α2-deficient congenital muscular dystrophy (*a*) A neonate presenting with hypotonia, contractures of the wrist and ankles and requiring tube feeding. (*b*) During the first two years there is prominent head lag. (*c*) Head control frequently remains impaired even if the child learns to sit between two and four years.

the selective filtration capacity of the blood–brain barrier, (Villanova et al., 1996, 1997). Lack of laminin-α2 expression in meningeal and choroid plexus vessels, which do not have a blood–brain barrier function, is in keeping with this concept. MRI detects changes in the brain from six months of age onwards (Mercuri et al., 1996). The degree of T_2 signal changes of the CNS white matter varies from individual to individual but is consistant between siblings (Philpot et al., 1995b). The changes may increase in severity during the first years but then persist over time (Philpot et al., 1995b, 1999b; Herrmann et al., 1996; Mercuri et al., 1996). To date, only one postmortem study is available and this is for a four-month-old child. The pattern of myelination was normal (Tarantuto et al., 1999). However, because MRI changes are not necessarily detectable at that age it remains an open question if myelin degeneration occurs in laminin-α2-deficient CMD. Earlier postmortem reports on older patients with CMD and a clinical and pathological picture suggestive of laminin-α2 deficiency showed degeneration of myelin sheaths with unevenness, ballooning and fragmentation (e.g. case 3 in Egger et al., 1983). Further postmortem studies are needed to answer this question.

In addition to the uniform presence of white matter changes, MRI also showed other structural abnormalities of the brain in completely laminin-α2-deficient patients, such as ventricular dilatation, occipital agyria and cerebellar hypoplasia with variable involvement of the pons (Sunada et al., 1995; Mercuri et al., 1996; Pini et al., 1996; van der Knaap et al., 1997; Philpot et al., 1999b). Furthermore, the postmortem brain study (Tarantuto et al., 1999) showed focal folding abnormalities of the grey matter with partial fusion of gyri and irregular cortical lamination as well as multifocal glioneuronal leptomeningeal heterotopias. One might speculate that the expression of laminin-α2 in the glia limitans (Villanova et al., 1997) has a role in regulating neuronal migration. However, laminin-α2 immunoreactivity has also been associated with neuronal fibres and punctate potentially synaptic structures of limbic brain regions in animal studies (Hagg et al., 1997). Furthermore, laminin-α2 in vitro mediated the attachment and spreading of several types of cell and promoted neurite outgrowth from neuronal cells (Engvall et al., 1992). These results make it likely that laminin-2 has a complex role during neuronal migration and development. Clinically, laminin-α2-deficient children with structural brain changes may be mentally retarded, particularly when there is gross occipital agyria (Fig. 25.3) (Pini et al., 1996) but most are of normal intelligence even if there is cerebellar hypoplasia (Philpot et al., 1999b). However, minor perceptuo–motor deficits have been documented using different test systems (Mercuri et al., 1995b). Functional changes of

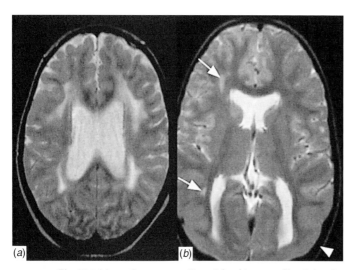

Fig. 25.3. Magnetic resonance T_2-weighted images of laminin-α2-deficient congenital muscular dystrophy. (*a*) Widespread white matter abnormalities and mild ventricular dilatation in the presence of a normal gyral pattern is seen in an eight-year-old patient. (*b*) Other patients show much milder T_2-weighted abnormalities (arrows) but partial occipital agyria (arrowhead) (10-year-old patient).

the cerebral white matter can also be detected using visual evoked potentials (Mercuri et al., 1996).

Epilepsy with complex partial seizures, atypical absences and grand mal seizures occurs in up to 30% of patients (Herrmann et al., 1996; Philpot et al., 1999b). It may be difficult to treat and even lead to a mental handicap secondary to the epilepsy.

The peripheral nervous system

Lack of laminin-α2 in the basement membrane of Schwann cells causes demyelinating peripheral neuropathy (Shorer et al., 1995). This may be difficult to detect in the first months of life when the motor nerve conduction velocity is still in the low normal range but usually gives rise to mild delay of motor and sensory conduction velocity values at later stages (Mercuri et al., 1995b; Mora et al., 1996).

Nerve biopsy has shown a marked reduction in the numbers of myelinated axons and the presence of naked axons and increased intrafibre collagen deposition in affected individuals (Brett et al., 1998).

Peripheral neuropathy can also be found in milder, partially laminin-α2-deficient patients (Mora et al., 1996; T. Voit, personal observations).

The skin

Laminin-α2 occurs in skin in the cytoplasm of epidermal keratinocytes, the basement membrane at the junction of epidermis and dermis, and the epithelial cells of the hair follicles (Sewry et al., 1996a; Squarzoni et al., 1997). This can be used diagnostically in patients with complete or partial laminin-α2 deficiency (Sewry et al., 1996a; Squarzoni et al., 1997). No clinical symptoms seem to result from this deficiency and wound healing appears normal.

The heart

Laminin-α2 is expressed in the basement membrane of cardiomyocytes. In a study of cardiac function, Spyrou et al. (1998) detected an ejection fraction less than 40% of normal in two out of six merosin-deficient children. The average ejection fraction was also lower than in the normal controls. They concluded that laminin-α2 deficiency might give rise to dilated cardiomyopathy. So far, dilated cardiomyopathy has been observed in a single partially laminin-α2-deficient patient (Poppe et al., 1998). More data are needed to understand the functional importance of laminin-α2 deficiency for the heart.

Clinical features of partial laminin-α2 deficiency

Several patients with a milder phenotype and partial expression of laminin-α2 have been described. The clinical spectrum ranges from onset with hypotonia in the first months of life and delayed motor milestones to near-normal adults with a limb girdle type of weakness and mild MRI-detected changes of the brain (Fig. 25.4). Serum creatine kinase levels may range from 300 to 2000 IU/l and do not necessarily correlate well with the severity of the clinical picture. Ambulation may be possible for only a few years or for several decades (Herrmann et al., 1996; Mora et al., 1996; Allamand et al., 1997; Tan et al., 1997). Delayed walking is not necessarily prognostic for a short ambulation period, as 30 years of ambulation have been reported in a patient who only achieved independent ambulation at the age of six years (Dubowitz, 1996). Some patients may develop contractures of the ankles and elbows and rigidity of the spine. This clinical picture may easily be mistaken for an Emery–Dreifuss type of muscular dystrophy (Fig. 25.4) (Herrmann et al., 1996; Mora et al., 1996). Muscle pain on exercise may inhibit the patient's acitivity as much as muscle weakness. Epilepsy, with subsequent mental deterioration, may occur during later stages of the disease. The peripheral nervous system can also be affected. Interestingly, Hayashi et al. (1997) documented complete lack of laminin-α2 expression in peripheral nerve Schwann cells but only partial deficiency in skeletal muscle in a 40-year-old man who was ambulant from age 6 to 35 years. This indicates that some mutations may affect laminin-α2 expression in a tissue-specific manner.

To date, no significant heart involvement has been reported in patients with partial deficiency. However, in view of its occurrence in patients with complete deficiency, cardiac function should be carefully monitored.

Histopathological and molecular diagnosis of laminin-α2 deficiency

Histopathological analysis of skeletal muscle biopsies in complete or partial laminin-α2 deficiency shows changes that are compatible with a dystrophic process. There is increased variation of fibre size, ongoing degeneration and regeneration and, already at early stages, a significant amount of endomysial and perimysial fibrosis. In addition, mononuclear cell infiltration may be a prominent feature, especially in the first months of life, and has in the past given rise to descriptions under the heading of 'infantile myositis'. In general, the morphological picture is clearly indicative of a muscular dystrophy but is not sufficiently specific to allow distinction from other forms. A more chronic myopathic picture with rimmed vacuoles and cytoplasmic and intranuclear tubulofilamentous inclusions has been reported in a patient with partial laminin-α2 deficiency that resulted from two novel compound heterozygous mutations of *LAMA-2* (Dubowitz, 1999). This emphasizes that the morphological picture usually seen in hereditary inclusion body myositis can also result from a mutation in *LAMA-2*.

Complete or partial deficiency of the heavy α2-chain of laminin is readily detected by immunofluorescence or Western blot in skeletal muscle or skin biopsies. The most common diagnostic approach involves immunofluorescence detection of laminin-α2 using a panel of antibodies directed against various domains of the molecule (Tomé et al., 1994; Sewry et al., 1995, 1997; Fardeau et al., 1996; Cohn et al., 1998). While initial studies relied on the commercially available monoclonal antibody that recognized the C-terminal 80 kDa fragment only, subsequent studies using multiple antibodies clearly showed that partial deficiency of laminin-α2 is readily missed if only a C-terminus-directed antibody is used (Sewry et al., 1997; Cohn et al., 1998). Most patients with a severe phenotype show a complete lack of laminin-2 expression with all antibodies (Fig. 25.5). In contrast, most patients with partial deficiency show preserved or minimally reduced expression of the C-terminal portion of the laminin-α2-chain but a marked reduction of the N-terminal 300 kDa fragment (Allamand et al., 1997; Sewry et al., 1997; Cohn et al., 1998). However, occasional patients have been documented in whom a severe clinical phenotype is associated with preserved expression of the C-terminal part of the protein (Cohn et al., 1998).

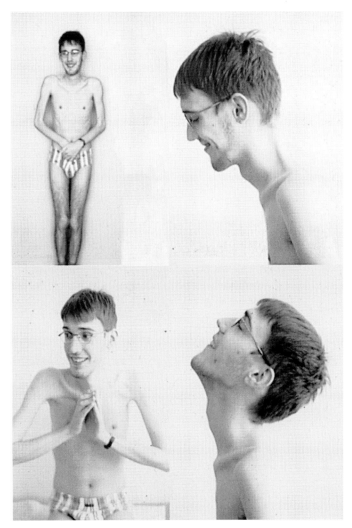

Fig. 25.4. A 16-year-old patient with partial laminin-α2 deficiency. Note the prominent contractures of elbows and also interphalangeal joints. There is also stiffness of the spine with limited anterior flexion.

Western blotting has also been used successfully to document abnormal laminin-α2 expression or to detect a protein of abnormal molecular weight (Vainzof et al., 1995; Allamand et al., 1997; Bushby et al., 1998).

Laminin-α2 deficiency is accompanied by a characteristic pattern of secondary protein changes, which can be used for diagnostic purposes. While the expression of the laminin β1- and γ1-chains is unchanged, the laminin heavy α5- and α4-chains are characteristically overexpressed and the laminin light β2-chain is reduced in laminin-α2 deficient muscle (Sewry et al., 1995, 1997; Cohn et al., 1997, 1998; K. Trygvarsson and T. Voit, unpublished). In particular, quantification showed that the decrease of

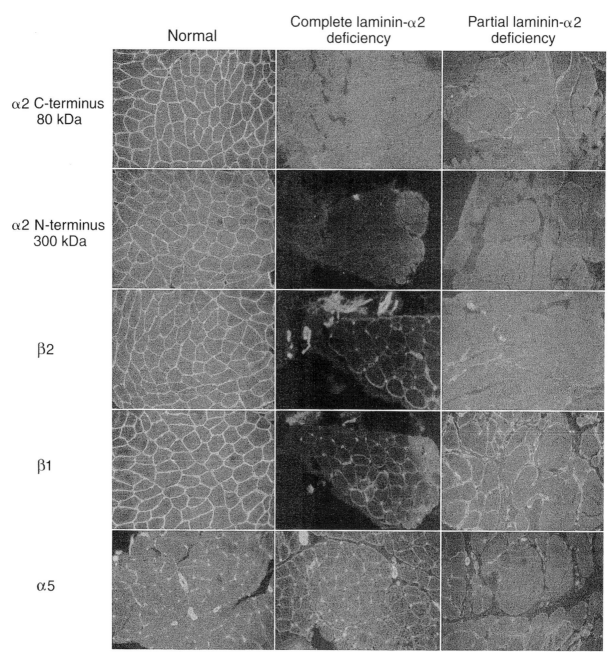

Fig. 25.5. Comparative immunolabelling of normal muscle, laminin-α2-deficient muscle in congenital muscular dystrophy (CMD) and partial laminin-α2 deficiency using an antibody against the 80 kDa C-terminus and one against the 300 kDa N-terminal portion of laminin-α2. There is complete lack of labelling of laminin-α2 in laminin-α2-deficient CMD and partial irregular labelling for both antibodies in partial laminin-α2 deficiency. Laminin β2-chain labelling is also variably reduced in both. In contrast, there is normal labelling of the laminin β1-chain and overexpression of the laminin α5-chain in both complete and partial laminin-α2 deficiency.

laminin-β2 expression was correlated with the amount of C-terminal but not with the amount of N-terminal laminin-α2 expressed (Cohn et al., 1998). In addition to the laminins, expression of the laminin receptor α_7-integrin is also reduced in laminin-α2 deficient muscle (Hodges et al., 1997; Cohn et al., 1999). It is important to note that the expression of α_7-integrin is developmentally regulated in skeletal muscle. Therefore, the isoform recognized by the specific antibody and the age of the individual assessed have to be taken into account when assessing apparent failure of expression of α_7-integrin. However, primary deficiency of α_7-integrin as a result of mutations in the gene for α_7-integrin were reported by Hayashi et al. (1998) in three unrelated children with a congenital myopathy with delayed motor milestones.

A number of mutations in *LAMA-2* resulting in both complete and partial laminin-α2 deficiency have been described (Helbling-Leclerc et al., 1995b; Nissinen et al., 1996; Guicheney et al., 1997, 1998; Naom et al., 1998; Pegoraro et al., 1998). In contrast to *dystrophin* no simple pattern emerges for *LAMA-2*. The gene exceeds 260 000 bp in size and contains 64 exons (Zhang et al., 1996). A total of 14 mutations were found on 19 chromosomes from 14 families (nine consanguineous, five nonconsanguineous) in a recent study by Guicheney et al. (1998). Only 60–70% of the mutations could be identified by mutation screening using single-stranded conformational polymorphisms in the polymerase chain reaction. In patients with complete merosin deficiency, small deletions of 1 or 2 bp, nonsense or splice mutations leading to trunkated proteins were identified. In patients with partial merosin deficiency a homozygous splice site mutation, an insertion mutation and a number of missense mutations spread over the gene have been described (Allamand et al., 1997; Guicheney et al., 1997, 1998; Hayashi et al., 1997). Loss-of-function mutations were detected in 21 out of 22 chromosomes from patients negative for the laminin-α2 C-terminus (Pegoraro et al., 1998). Interestingly, a single patient has been described by Morandi with a missense mutation in exon 54 in the C-terminal G-domain, which induced the loss of immunofluorescence labelling for the C-terminal Chemicon antibody (in Dubowitz, 1999). In contrast, antibodies directed against more N-terminal portions of the molecule showed partial α2-chain expression. Disease in this patient followed a milder course whereas all other patients with complete lack of the C-terminus to date have shown a severe clinical phenotype. Further study of single mutations may yield important information about functional domains of the laminin-α2-chain and be helpful for prenatal counselling of individual families. At present, mutation analysis must still be

considered a research tool rather than a regular diagnostic service in view of the many experimental difficulties and the high costs.

Prenatal diagnosis

Prenatal diagnosis of laminin-α2-deficient CMD can be reliably achieved through a combination of haplotype analysis, immunofluorescence study of the fetal trophoblast tissue in all, and mutation analysis in some families (Voit et al., 1994; Muntoni et al., 1995; Guicheney et al., 1997; Naom et al., 1997). Mutation analysis will be reserved for those where a mutation in the homozygous state or two mutations in a compound heterozygous state have been unequivocally shown in the index patient. For all other patients, a combination of haplotype analysis and fetal trophoblast immunocytochemistry from a chorionic villus sample is recommended. Study of the fetal trophoblast will avoid the potential hazard of double crossovers occurring when haplotype analysis only is performed and the precise locality of the causative mutation is unknown. To date, more than 20 prenatal diagnoses have been made with this combination. Where complete absence of laminin-α2 expression was detected in the trophoblast, the fetus was affected and when normal amounts occurred the fetus was always unaffected (Naom et al., 1997; M. Fardeau et al., personal communication; T. Voit, unpublished data). In a single patient where there was partial labelling of the trophoblast tissue, the fetus was subsequently found to be a carrier of the disease (Naom et al., 1997) but it is not yet clear how reliable trophoblast labelling is in patients with partial laminin-α2 deficiency.

Therapy

As long as no direct therapy for the disease itself is available efforts should be directed towards achieving and maintaining a good quality of life. In completely laminin-α2 deficient CMD, early release of contractures is frequently necessary in order to mobilize patients in callipers or other orthotic devices (Fig. 25.6). The development of skoliosis may require bracing and eventually spinal fusion, sometimes by as early as five to ten years of age. Feeding problems and weight loss can be effectively counteracted by gastrostomy (Philpot et al., 1999a; T. Voit, personal observations). Noctural hypoventilation can be effectively treated by night-time bilevel positive airway pressure ventilation even in children younger than two years of age. The risk for epilepsy requires electroencephalographic monitoring. Similarly, the cardiac function should be assessed at intervals. With appropriate support, most children with laminin-α2 deficient CMD will be able to follow regular

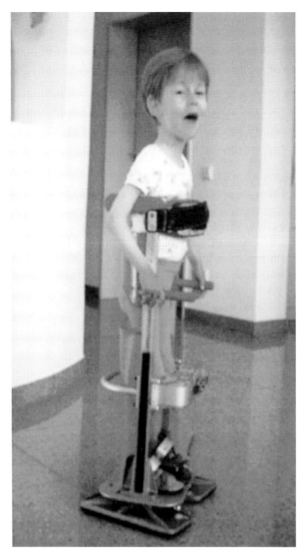

Fig. 25.6. A five-year-old girl with complete laminin-α2 deficiency is ambulant in a swivel walker.

schooling schemes, and patients with partial laminin-α2 deficiency have followed successful academic careers.

Animal models

Laminin-α2 deficiency was detected in a muscular dystrophy mouse model, the *dy/dy* mouse (Arahata et al., 1993; Xu et al., 1994a,b). An allelic mouse strain dy^{2J}/dy^{2J} with milder disease is caused by a splice site mutation resulting in a deletion in domain VI (Xu et al., 1994a). Homozygous *dy/dy* mice have a severe phenotype. They are smaller than their littermates and after two to four weeks develop progressive weakness and paralysis first of the hind legs and then spreading to the axial and forelimb muscles. They die at four to six months and are unable to breed, whereas the milder dy^{2J}/dy^{2J} mice are able to breed. Partial restoration of laminin-α2 expression has been achieved by transplantation of a primary muscle cell culture (Vilquin et al., 1996).

Group II: congenital muscular dystrophy with a cerebral and cerebrellar migration disorder

Fukuyama congenital muscular dystrophy

FCMD was first described by Fukuyama and colleagues in 1960 and in many subsequent papers of his group (Kamoshita et al., 1976; Fukuyama et al., 1981; Osawa et al., 1991). The disease is endemic in Japan with an incidence of approximately 1:100 000 of the population; it is, therefore, the second most common muscular dystrophy after Duchenne dystrophy in Japan (Sugita et al., 1995). A single patient of Japanese descent has been documented outside Japan (McMenamin et al., 1982) and a possible but not proven case has been reported from Korea (Huh et al., 1992). The gene of this autosomal recessive disorder has been linked to chromosome 9q31 (Toda et al., 1993, 1994) and has been cloned (Kobayashi et al., 1998a). The high incidence of the disorder in the Japanese population is caused by a founder mutation, which gives rise to a mild phenotype (Kobayashi et al., 1998b). FCMD is characterized by a combination of CNS malformation and muscular dystrophy. To a lesser degree, the eyes are also involved. This pattern of changes shows considerable overlap with features observed in MEB and WWS.

Clinical features

Newborns with FCMD present with general muscle hypotonia and weakness, which is most prominent in the legs. In some patients, lack of visual pursuit movements was the initial complaint. Sometimes in utero movements were reduced, and poor sucking and a weak cry are present in about 50%. Some patients may show congenital nystagmus or cortical blindness. The face usually shows prominent myopathic weakness but also frequently protruding 'pseudo-hypertrophic' cheeks. The subsequent motor development varies considerably. Severely affected patients never develop head control and are profoundly mentally retarded (Fig. 25.7, colour plate). However, most patients will learn to sit unaided and obtain a peak motor function of shuffling on their buttocks. A few patients learn to stand with support or even walk some steps. Clinical improvement of motor function occurs until six years of age and the maximum motor capacity can usually be maintained until eight years, when it starts to decline again (Osawa et al., 1997). Some patients develop muscle hypertrophy of the forearms and calves. Serum creatine kinase is usually elevated 10–50 times; it increases up to the time of peak motor function at about six years and later declines again. All patients are moderately to profoundly mentally retarded and at best will be able to speak up to 20 words. Joint contractures at birth are rare and joints are rather hyperextensible in infants. However, most children develop joint contractures of the hips, knees, ankles, and later elbows and even interphalangeal finger joints, between five months and six years (Fig. 25.7, colour plate). Skoliosis and rigidity of the spine may follow. The average life expectancy is around 15 years but varies from 2 to 27 years (Mukuyama et al., 1993, cited in Osawa et al., 1997). Of those patients with FCMD who died early, most seem to have suffered from a common cold and died suddenly at night. It is tempting to speculate that death might have been brought about by respiratory insufficiency. This becomes even more likely in view of the interesting observation that transient exacerbations of muscle weakness after a febrile illness, with concomitant increases in serum creatine kinase to two to six times the usual level have been documented in 16 patients with FCMD (Osawa et al., 1997). Two of these patients required artificial ventilation because of transient respiratory muscle weakness during such episodes. They subsequently almost recovered to their previous peak motor function.

Central nervous system
Patients with FCMD are mentally retarded, but even the most severely affected will usually be able to recognize their immediate relatives and achieve some primitive forms of communication. Seizures occur in approximately 60%, most frequently as febrile seizures during the first year of life followed by afebrile tonic clonic seizures later in life. Almost 10% suffer a status epilepticus at some stage (Osawa et al., 1997). Neuropathological examinations showed a combination of micropoligyria, pachygyria and minor alterations of the cerebellar hemispheres (Kamoshita et al., 1976; Fukuyama and Osawa, 1982; Yoshioka et al., 1991; Osawa et al., 1997). Additional findings were hemispheric fusion, hypoplastic pyramidal tracts and mild-to-moderate ventricular dilatation. Studies of fetal brain in FCMD revealed widespread abnormality of the neurogliomesenchymal tissue of the cerebral cortex. There was massive overmigration of neurons into and beyond the glia limitans, suggesting that breaches in the glia limitans or incapacity of the glia limitans to stop neuronal migration might be underlying the diffuse micropolygyria in FCMD (Takada et al., 1987; Nakano et al., 1996). In patients with

severe FCMD extensive agyria and polymicrogyria can occur.

Neuroimaging usually detects abnormally high T_2-weighted signals from the periventricular white matter in addition to the abnormalities of neuronal migration (Osawa et al., 1991). However, follow-up MRI studies after the age of six years will frequently show normalization of the previously abnormal periventricular T_2-weighted abnormalities (M. Osawa, personal communication).

The eyes
Ocular findings in FCMD show abnormalities and evidence of visual disturbance in all patients (Tsutsumi et al., 1989; Osawa et al., 1997). Myopia is present in more than 80%, most frequently in combination with glaucoma (60%) and, in particular, retinal dysplasia (90%), which is most frequently characterized as 'sharply defined ring atrophic patches' in the more severely affected and as 'uneven and grayish mottling of the retina' in milder disease (Fig. 25.7, colour plate). Cataracts occur in about 25%.

The heart
The heart is affected in FCMD, and cardiomyopathy may contribute significantly to the fatal outcome of the disorder during the second decade. In patients older than 10 years, fibrosis of the myocardium has been documented on postmortem studies (Osawa et al., 1993). Dilated cardiomyopathy has been reported exceptionally (Yoshikawa et al., 1991).

The skin
Skin changes with dry, hyperlucent skin with progressive firmness have been noted as an epiphenomenon. As FCMD progresses, the skin eventually becomes more and more adherent to the underlying tissue until lifting off of folds becomes difficult or impossible (Osawa et al., 1997).

Molecular pathology
Histopathology of skeletal muscles shows changes of progressive degeneration and regeneration, resulting in a marked variation of fibre size and conspicuous endo-, peri- and epimysial fibrosis. At later stages, lipomatosis occurs. Hayashi et al. (1993) were the first to show significant reduction of laminin-α2 expression in FCMD muscle and this study stimulated the subsequent discovery of laminin-α2 deficiency in laminin-α2-deficient CMD. Decreased expression of laminin-α2 and β-dystroglycan were also observed on the spinal cord surface of a fetus with FCMD (Yamamoto et al., 1997a,b). Electron microscopic analysis of FCMD muscle further indicated that the basal lamina in FCMD is disrupted similar to the changes

observed in laminin-α2 deficient CMD (Ishii et al., 1997). However, it was not until the gene was cloned and the protein product, fukutin, described that the pathogenetic process underlying FCMD could be better understood. The FCMD gene encodes a new 161 amino acid residue protein without significant homology to hitherto known proteins (Kobayashi et al., 1998a). Northern blot studies showed expression of the gene in heart, brain, skeletal muscle and pancreas. The protein fukutin contains an N-terminal signal sequence and, according to the results of transfection studies, is secreted by the cells. At present, it is uncertain if and how fukutin interacts with other basement membrane proteins and, in consequence, how deficiency of fukutin leads to FCMD. Ellucidation of the gene also detected an ancient retrotransposal insertion as the underlying founder mutation present in the chromosomes of 87% of the Japanese patients with FCMD (Kobayashi et al., 1998a,b). This retrotransposal insertion is probably a mild mutation that primarily affects mRNA stability. Patients with FCMD homozygous for the founder mutation usually show the milder FCMD phenotype, whereas patients with a severe FCMD phenotype display a combination of the founder mutation on one allele plus a second missense mutation on the second chromosome. This observation might account for the rarity of FCMD outside Japan, because one might speculate that a homozygous situation for two null alleles might be lethal in utero. In two patients with a severe FCMD phenotype, one of the parents was of Caucasian origin and carried a missense mutation (M. Osawa, personal communication).

Muscle–eye–brain disease

MEB was first described by Santavuori et al. in 1977, and over 20 patients have been reported from Finland in the period to 1998 (Santavuori et al., 1998). For a long time, the considerable overlap of clinical and neuropathological features in MEB and WWS gave rise to confusion regarding whether the two disorders are allelic or represent genetically distinct diseases (Santavuori et al., 1990; Dubowitz, 1994; Voit, 1998). Following the localization of the gene for MEB on chromosome 1p32–p34 in seven Finnish families and one Turkish family (Cormand et al., 1999), it is becoming increasingly clear that MEB is not uncommon outside Finland and accounts for many, if not most, of the cases that had previously been reported as milder WWS.

It is of interest that no major common haplotype was observed in Finnish MEB patients (Cormand et al., 1999). The precise nosological borders of the disease remain to be defined. It is possible that much milder variants with preserved speech and normal vision exist (Voit et al., 1999).

Clinical features

Patients with MEB usually present as floppy infants with suspected blindness. General hypotonia and weakness usually persist beyond the first year of life, and contractures may occur during the first years. The maximum motor capacity in MEB is quite variable. Some patients never learn to sit unaided whereas, in a recent study, 3 out of 24 patients were able to take a few steps without support (Santavuori et al., 1998). Additional movement abnormalities such as spasticity or dystonia develop in the majority of patients with MEB to a variable degree. Serum creatine kinase is elevated to as much as 4000 IU/l (Santavuori et al., 1989). Psychomotor development is always slow and depends on the degree of CNS changes. Those patients who smile and show social reactions early may go on to show some social interaction, being able to point to objects they desire or even in exeptional cases speak a few single words (Santavuori et al., 1989, 1998). The peak of psychomotor development is usually between 5 and 25 years and patients may lose their mental and motor abilities thereafter (Santavuori et al., 1989). However, MEB is compatible with survival into the fourth decade and beyond.

Central nervous system

The brain in MEB always shows extensive signs of a neuronal migration disorder. MRI usually shows pachygyria and polymicrogyria with slightly more gyration over the frontal parts of the brain and more agyria over the occipital parts (Fig. 25.8b) (Santavuori et al., 1998). In addition, partial absence of the septum pellucidum and dysplasia of the corpus callosum and hydrocephalus, sometimes even requiring a shunt, are frequent findings. White matter abnormalities detectable as abnormally high T_2 signals of the periventricular white matter are common in younger patients but may also persist beyond the third decade (Valanne et al., 1994). The infratentorial parts of the brain characteristically show almost complete absence of the pontine bulge and extensive abnormalities of the cerebellum, with hypoplastic inferior vermis and tonsils and, characteristically, small cysts in the cerebellar hemispheres (Valanne et al., 1994). Neuropathological examination has shown total disorganization of the cerebral and cerebellar cortices without horizontal lamination. The surface characteristically shows a cobblestone appearance with irregular clusters or islands of cortical neurons separated by gliovascular strands (Haltia et al., 1997). The spinal cord may also be abnormal, with an abnormally thick and adherent pia-arachnoid.

Epilepsy is common and occurred in 17 out of the 19 patients described by Santavuori et al. (1989). Infantile spasms, myoclonic jerks and generalized tonic clonic seizures precipitated by fever were reported.

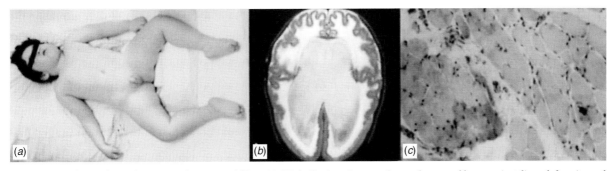

Fig. 25.8. Muscle–eye–brain disease in a four-year-old boy. (*a*) Clinically there is muscular weakness and hypotonia, talipes deformity and lack of psychomotor development. (*b*) Brain MRI shows pachygyria over the frontal and agyria over the occipital parts of the cortex as well as ventricular dilatation and diffuse abnormality of periventricular white matter (*c*) Skeletal muscle shows a dystrophic process with increased variation of fibre size and foci of active necrosis (haematoxylin and eosin).

It is noteworthy that to date none of the Finnish patients with MEB or of the other patients where linkage is compatible with MEB has shown complete lissencephaly or an encephalocoele.

The eyes

Ocular symptoms typically show a combination of anterior and posterior chamber alterations. There is severe myopia ranging from −6 to −27 dioptre, usually combined with pale retina, optic atrophy and, in approximately 30%, glaucoma (Raitta et al., 1978). Glaucoma may be caused by defective cleavage of the chamber angle with persistent membranes and synechiae. Cataracts may also develop in some patients (Raitta et al., 1978). The electroretinogram may be normal in young patients but becomes unrecordable later on. Giant amplitudes (>50 μV) of the visual evoked potentials have been described as a characteristic finding in 70% of patients with MEB (Santavuori et al., 1998). Neuropathological examination has shown moderate-to-severe generalized loss of ganglion cells and nerve fibres in the retina and retinocoroidal scars (Haltia et al., 1997). In addition, there was an unusually pronounced preretinal glial membrane that was almost as thick as the neuroretina itself.

Clinically the patients may show megalocornea (T. Voit, personal observation), nystagmus or completely uncontrolled eye movements. The majority of patients will suffer from a severe visual handicap but some can fixate and follow large colourful objects.

Skeletal muscle

Muscle changes in MEB can be very variable and range from slightly abnormal variation in muscle fibre diameter and an increased number of central nuclei on one hand to severe, full-blown muscular dystrophy with ongoing necrosis, regeneration and prominent fibrosis on the other

(Haltia et al., 1997; Santavuori et al., 1998). Laminin-$\alpha2$ expression was reported as decreased in four patients with MEB (Haltia et al., 1997) but was clearly normal in two patients who were previously reported as having WWS but whose linkage data are compatible with linkage to the MEB locus (cases 3 and 4 in Voit et al., 1995). As in FCMD, the combination of neuronal overmigration in the brain, prominent abnormalities of the glial preretinal membrane in the eye and basement membrane abnormalities in skeletal muscle make it seem likely that a protein interacting with the basement membrane is underlying the pathological processes in MEB.

Walker Warburg syndrome

Warburg in 1978 described a combination of congenital retinal detachment with hydrocephalus. Already in 1942, Walker had described a four-month-old female with lissencephaly, extreme communicating hydrocephalus, absence of the corpus callossum and hypoplasia of the cerebellum. One eye was microphthalmic with congenital retinal detachment, coloboma of the optic disc, congenital cataract and posterior synechiae. Probably the patient reported by Bernheimer in 1894 had suffered from the same disorder.

However, it was only when Williams et al. (1984) reported three patients with almost complete lissencephaly and microphthalmy with persistence of hyaloid vasculature, in combination with a muscular dystrophy in one, that the full spectrum of WWS emerged. This was reviewed by Dobyns et al. in 1985. These authors clearly focused on the combination of lissencephaly and pontocerebellar dysplasia with severe eye changes characterized by congenital retinal detachment and persistent hypoplastic primary vitrous. In a further extensive review, Dobyns et al. (1989) revised the diagnostic criteria for WWS and described cephalocoele in 5/21, microphthalmia in 8/21, ocular colobomas in 3/15, congenital cataracts in 7/20, genital abnormalities in 5/8 males and cleft lip and/or palate in 4/21 patients with WWS. The association of WWS with cleft lip or palate has also been described in siblings, who also suffered from encephalocoele and cataracts, suggesting that this may be a further feature identifying patients with severe WWS (Burton et al., 1987).

From what we know today it is clear that several patients affected by complete or near-complete lissencephaly type 2, severe eye changes with congenital microphthalmy and, in particular, an occipital encephalocoele are excluded by linkage analysis from both the FCMD and the MEB gene loci (Fig. 25.9, colour plate). (Cormand et al., 2001). Equally, many patients previously reported under the label of WWS may have suffered from MEB. Therefore, the precise nosological boundaries of both WWS and MEB have to be redefined using linkage analysis and, eventually, gene analysis. It is highly likely that extreme prenatal-onset hydrocephalus, which was detected in a number of fetal patients and not described in MEB so far, is also typical of WWS (Crowe et al., 1986; Squier et al., 1993). Microscopical examination of the fetal brain showed that there were irregular clusters of neurons in the primitive cortical plate and many cells appeared to be migrating through gaps in the pia mater into the leptomeninges. Groups of neurons extending into the leptomeninges were also found over the cerebellum. This points to the fact that in WWS, as in MEB and FCMD, neuronal overmigration beyond the glia limitans is the pathological process underlying lissencephaly type 2.

Muscle changes in WWS may be severe, with serum creatine kinase levels over 2000 IU/l and a dystrophic picture with ongoing degeneration and regeneration (Fig. 25.9, colour plate). We have observed normal expression of laminin α2-, β1-, γ1- and β2-chains in WWS including fetal muscle (Voit et al., 1995; Cohn et al., 1997). However, deficiency of laminin-β2-chain and reduction in expression of α-sarcoglycan have also been reported in two patients with WWS (Wewer et al., 1995). It is obvious that a molecular classification of patients with WWS is needed in order to interpret these findings further. It is also possible that WWS in itself is heterogeneous.

Group III: congenital muscular dystrophy with early rigidity of the spine

The group III CMDs contain the first disorder that has been identified as a laminin-α2-positive form of muscular dystrophy (see below). As a group, the patients differ from those described in groups I, II and IV in that serum creatine kinase levels and the immunocytochemical markers of the basal and plasma membrane are normal. This strongly suggests that the underlying, and as yet unknown, pathogenetic mechanism is profoundly different from that in patients with primary or secondary laminin-α2 deficiency or the syndromes in group II. Dubowitz was the first to recognize a group of patients in whom the dominant clinical feature was a marked limitation in flexion of the dorsolumbar and cervical spine (Dubowitz, 1971, 1973, 1978). He described these patients as having difficulty walking and going upstairs and that the condition somewhat resembled CMD. The biopsy changes were described as marked fibrosis and replacement of muscle by connective tissue, variation in fibre size and associated cellularity. Serum creatine kinase levels were normal or slightly elevated, up to 380 IU/l. While it has since become clear that a phenotypically comparable picture may be caused by Emery–Dreifuss muscular dystrophy or partial laminin-α2 deficiency, these patients usually have higher levels of serum creatine kinase and later onset of the spinal rigidity, during or after the second decade.

Congenital muscular dystrophy with early rigidity of the spine linked to chromosome 1p35-36

In 1998, Moghadaszadeh et al. (1998a,b) reported five patients from three informative families with a recognizable and clinically rather homogeneous picture of a CMD. Children were hypotonic at birth or during the first year of life. The maximum motor capacity varied in the three siblings from one family and ranged from walking unaided at 11 months to inability to walk. When ambulant, the patients showed a waddling gait and difficulties in climbing stairs, but the motor ability was preserved over the first decade and beyond. The hallmark of the disorder was early rigidity of the spine, combined with a progressive restrictive respiratory syndrome, which resulted in nocturnal hypoventilation and required ventilatory support at night. Serum creatine kinase was normal in all five children. In addition, two possibly affected relatives of index patients died because of respiratory failure at age 14 and 21 years. The disease was localized to chromosome 1p35-36 with a LOD (logarithm of odds) score of 4.48. Several patients have been identified since with a similar clinical picture and a haplotype pattern compatible with linkage to chromosome 1p35-36 (Fig. 25.10, colour plate).

Moghadaszadeh et al. (1999) reported nine patients from seven families showing linkage to the MDRS1 locus on chromosome 1p35-36. A further family with four affected children was reported by Flanigan et al. (2000). All children were affected by hypotonia and prominent neck weakness in infancy. The spinal rigidity developed between 5 and 12 years. Three of the patients required night-time ventilation, one of them already at age 2 years (Dubowitz, 1999; Flanigan et al., 2000).

Congenital muscular dystrophy with rigidity of the spine excluded from chromosome 1p35

At the CMD workshop, Moghadaszadeh et al. also presented data excluding the MDRS1 locus in 12 families with patients presenting clinical features suggestive of rigid spine syndrome. Exclusion of this locus was also reported by Naom et al. in four out of eight families with a picture of CMD and early rigidity of the spine (Moghadaszadeh et al., 1998b; Naom et al., 1998b; Dubowitz, 1999). The clinical features of the patients from these families were heterogeneous, suggesting that more than one gene can give rise to such a clinical phenotype. However, the overall clinical picture allowed these patients to be distinguished from those with primary or secondary laminin-α2 deficiency and from those with one of the muscle and brain syndromes of group II.

Group IV: congenital muscular dystrophies with secondary deficiency of laminin-α2

Group IV is a new emerging group of CMDs in which patients were identified in addition to the clinical picture by uneven and irregular staining for laminin-α2 in several families. Linkage analysis allowed exclusion from the *LAMA-2* locus on chromosome 6q2. Recently, the first gene locus within this group of disorders was localized on chromosome 1q42, but other families were excluded from this new locus. So far all patients described suffered from a muscular dystrophy with active muscle degeneration, serum creatine kinase levels above 1000 IU/l and a progressive course. Together with the immunohistochemical abnormality of laminin-α2, this very strongly suggests that laminin-interacting proteins affecting the stability or metabolism of the basement membrane are underlying these disorders. For future classification, it is possible that groups I and IV will fuse as primary disorders of the basal lamina.

Congenital muscular dystrophy with secondary deficiency of laminin-α2 linked to chromosome 1q42

In 1998 Muntoni et al. described four affected children from one family with an early-onset Duchenne-like muscular dystrophy. The patients were noted to be weak in the first months of life and had prominent calf muscles. The children showed mild facial weakness, prominent neck weakness with selective wasting of the sternomastoid muscles and developed rigidity of the spine and contractures of the Achilles tendon in the first decade. Ambulation was

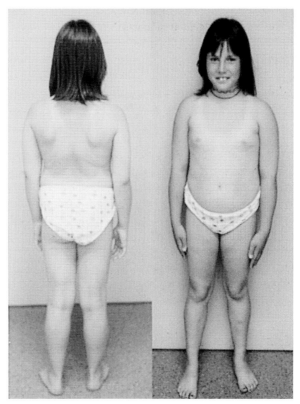

Fig. 25.11. A 10-year-old girl with congenital muscular dystrophy, secondary reduction of laminin-α2 and haplotype analysis compatible with linkage to chromosome 1q42. Mental status and brain MRI were normal. The weakness was Duchenne-like but followed a more static course.

achieved in the third year of life and there was little or no loss of motor capacity over the first ten years. However, all four children developed early respiratory failure as a result of severe diaphragmatic involvement. Two died at age four and seven years and the other two remained dependent on night-time ventilation. Intellect and MRI of the brain were normal. Creatine kinase levels were grossly elevated (2270–7650 IU/l), the biopsy was compatible with a dystrophic process and immunolabelling for the C-terminus and the 300 kDa antibody directed against laminin-α2 showed irregular and partially reduced staining. This family was initially excluded from the *LAMA-2* gene locus on chromosome 6q2 (Muntoni et al., 1998). Recently, the putative gene has been mapped to chromosome 1q42, and a second family from Germany has been identified with similar clinical and immunohistochemical features, who are also compatible with linkage to this locus (Dubowitz, 1999; Brockington et al., 2000). The only difference between the two families was that hypoventilation was not detected in the two affected siblings from the German family, who were 11 and 5 years of age in 1998 (Fig. 25.11).

Congenital muscular dystrophy with secondary deficiency of laminin-α2 excluded from chromosome 1q42

We have recently seen a three-year-old girl born to consanguinous Turkish parents. She was noted to be very hypotonic at three months. She walked at 14 months when put to her feet and learned to rise with a Gowers' manoeuvre at age two years. Her serum creatine kinase was 2000 IU/l. Both the brain MRI scan and motor nerve conduction velocity were normal. The intellect was normal. Her cousin, who is related through the maternal and paternal side, was similarly affected. Both children suffered a bout of rhabdomyolysis during an infection. The muscle biopsy showed an active muscular dystrophy. Immunocytochemistry of the quadriceps muscle showed partial deficiency of laminin-α2, and staining for laminin-β2 was concomitantly reduced. The gene loci for *LAMA-2* on 6q2 and for CMD with secondary laminin-α2 deficiency on 1q42 were excluded by haplotype analysis (T. Voit and F. Muntoni, unpublished data; Dubowitz, 1999). A similar family was reported by Mercuri et al. (2000).

Congenital muscular dystrophy with secondary deficiency of laminin-α2, mental retardation and normal cranial scans

In 1998 Topaloglu et al. published details of two affected siblings from a large consanguinous family. Both children were noted to be floppy immediately after birth. Serum creatine kinase was grossly elevated (1881–2228 IU/l). Motor and mental development were profoundly delayed, and the intelligence quotient was less than 50 in both. The maximum motor capacity was sitting unaided at age four and 10 years. Brain MRI did not show structural or white matter changes and also showed normal structures of the posteria fossa. Muscle biopsy was compatible with a dystrophic process with prominent endo- and perimysial fibrosis. The gene loci *LAMA-2* on 6q2 and for FCMD on 9q31 were excluded by linkage analysis. A combination of a distinct clinical picture with mental retardation and secondary deficiency of laminin-α2 in the muscle biopsy, together with the linkage results, suggests a form of CMD in its own right.

Group V: congenital muscular dystrophy with normal expression of laminin-α2

Group V harbours a number of heterogenous disorders with normal laminin-α2 expression; these are awaiting further definition at the clinical and molecular level.

'Pure' congenital muscular dystrophy with normal expression of laminin-α2 and normal intellect

The group of 'pure' CMD and normal laminin-α2 expression should be reserved for children who conform to the diagnostic criteria of CMD (Table 25.1) and are mentally normal. Preliminary estimates from ongoing linkage studies suggest that 10 to 20% of the children in this group will be reclassified as suffering from CMD with rigid spine syndrome (group III) (Dubowitz, 1999). For further definition of children within this group, it is important not to use abnormalities of myelination or cerebellar structure by MRI as criteria because such abnormalities are not necessarily associated with mental dysfunction. Other forms of muscular dystrophy such as dystrophinopathy, which may give rise to very early onset in occasional patients, must also be excluded.

If these exclusion criteria are fulfilled, a substantial number of patients with CMD remain who may be assigned to this group and may account for up to 30–50% of Caucasian patients with CMD. In several large series, the major differences between laminin-α2-negative and laminin-α2-positive patients were that the latter overall achieved a better maximum motor function, usually became ambulant and showed overall lower creatine kinase levels than the former (Fig. 25.12) (Philpot et al., 1995a; Vainzof et al., 1995; Fardeau et al., 1996; Herrmann et al., 1996; Kobayashi et al., 1996). Although the maximum motor capacity is usually better in patients who are laminin-α2-positive, the long-term prognosis is not necessarily so favourable. Hypoventilation symptoms are common and even death from respiratory insufficiency has been described in the first year of life (Fardeau et al., 1996).

A single family with severe hypotonia at birth, proximal muscle weakness, elevated serum creatine kinase (300–824 IU/l) with relatively mild muscle changes and normal laminin-α2 expression was reported by Salih et al. (1998). One of the two affected siblings had ptosis. Both affected siblings became ambulant at two and four years and were still ambulant at age 15 and 12 years. The older one developed signs of dilated cardiomyopathy. A further large family with a relatively benign clinical course of laminin-α2-positive 'pure' CMD with normal or moderately increased serum creatine kinase was reported by Mahjneh et al. from Palestine (1999). Haplotype analysis in this family excluded the candidate genes on chromosomes 6q2, 9q3,12q13 (α_7-integrin locus) and 1p35–36.

It is possible that the disorder previously reported as CMD with distal joint laxity (Ullrich disease) may belong in this group. In 1930, Ullrich described two patients who were born with contractures of proximal joints and showed

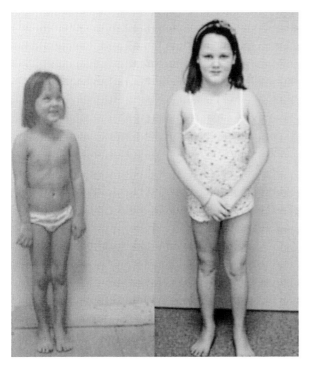

Fig. 25.12. A girl with 'pure' laminin-α2-positive congenital muscular dystrophy at age 4 and 10 years. Surgical release of heel cords was necessary at age 5 years. At age 10, she had developed elbow contractures and needed night-time ventilatory support.

Table 25.3. Rare forms of congenital muscular dystrophy (group VI)

Form described by	Special features	Affected siblings
Wargowski et al. (1991)	Cataracts plus minor brain abnormality	No
Mandel et al. (1993)	Hirschsprung disease	No
Parano et al. (1994)	Syringomyelia	No
Seidhamed et al. (1996)	Lethal form with arthrogryposis and type 2 lissencephaly	Yes
Leyten et al. (1996)	Abdominal wall and genital hypoplasia	No
Sztriha et al. (1999)	Micrencephaly, abnormal myelination, arthrogryposis	Yes

striking hyperelasticity of the distal joints, particularly the wrists and ankles (Ullrich, 1930a,b). Their intelligence was normal and one of two became ambulant (Stoeber, 1939). A total of some 20 patients have been described since who showed this combination of features (Nonaka et al., 1981; de Paillette et al., 1989). Several of these patients achieved ambulation between two and six years but lost ambulation again later on. Intelligence was consistently normal and so was laminin-α2 status where it was assessed (Fardeau et al., 1996; Herrmann et al., 1996). It remains to be shown by molecular techniques if the prominent hyperelasticity of the distal joints, which tends to disappear during the later course of disease, is a distinguishing feature of a form of CMD in its own right.

Laminin-α2-positive congenital muscular dystrophy with mental retardation

A subset of approximately 20% of laminin-α2-positive patients with CMD are mentally retarded (Fardeau et al., 1996; Herrmann et al., 1996). This group should be reserved for those patients without structural brain changes such as pachygyria or pontocerebellar abnormality on MRI. Topaloglu et al. (1997) reported the combina-

tion of laminin-α2-positive CMD with mental retardation and cataracts but without evidence of structural brain changes in three patients, two of them siblings born to consanguineous parents, suggesting that this might be a form of CMD in its own right. No comprehensive linkage studies are available for this group so far.

Laminin-α2-positive congenital muscular dystrophy with cerebellar hypoplasia

At least four patients with the combination of CMD, normal appearing supratentorial brain but the presence of cerebellar hypoplasia have been reported (Arancio et al., 1988; Knubley and Bertorini, 1988; Voit, 1998). These patients had elevated serum creatine kinase levels (300–1500 IU/l), normal or slightly retarded mental status and cerebellar symptoms such as dysarthria and saccadic pursuit movements. Of course, these patients could represent mild allelic variants of any of the disorders present in group II, but as their clinical appearance is very different they should be grouped separately until a molecular definition becomes possible.

Group VI: other rare forms of congenital muscular dystrophy

Several patients with CMD and other associated features have been reported who do not fit into any of the larger groups within the present classification scheme (Table 25.3). It is noteworthy that several of the conditions reported show a combination of muscle dysgenesis commencing in utero and structural abnormality of the CNS. The distinct occurrence of such a pattern in siblings in some families (Seidhamed et al., 1996; Sztriha et al., 1999) strongly argues in favour of distinct genetic conditions.

References

Allamand, V., Sunada, Y., Salih, M. A. et al. (1997). Mild congenital muscular dystrophy in two patients with an internally deleted laminin alpha2-chain. *Hum. Mol. Genet.* **6**, 747–752.

Arahata, K., Hayashi, Y. K., Koga, R. et al. (1993). Laminin in animal models for muscular dystrophy: a defect of laminin M in skeletal and cardiac muscles and peripheral nerve of the homozygous dystrophic *dy/dy* mice. *Proc. Jpn. Acad.* **69**, 259–264.

Arancio, O., Bongiovanni, L. G., Bonadonna, G., Tomélleri, G. and de Grandis, D. (1988). Congenital muscular dystrophy and cerebellar vermis agenesis in two brothers. *Ital. J. Neurol. Sci.* **9**, 485–489.

Banker, B. Q., Victor, M. and Adams, R. D. (1957). Arthrogryposis multiplex due to congenital muscular dystrophy. *Brain* **86**, 319–334.

Batten, F. E. (1903a). Three cases of myopathy, infantile type. *Brain* **26**, 147–148.

Batten, F. E. (1903b). Myositis fibrosa. *Br. Med. J.* **2**, 1333.

Batten, F. E. (1904). Case of myositis fibrosa, with pathological examination. *Trans. Soc. Lond.* **37**, 12–22.

Batten, F. E. (1909/10). The myopathies or muscular dystrophies. *Q. J. Med.* **3**, 313–328.

Bernheimer, S. (1894). Ein Beitrag zur Kenntnis der Missbildungen des Auges. *Arch. Augenheilk.* **28**, 241–263.

Brett, F. M., Loring, P., Caesar, A. et al. (1998). Immunohistochemical evaluation of merosin deficiency in congenital muscular dystrophies. *Arch. Pathol. Lab. Med.* **122**, 69–71.

Brockington, M., Sewry, C. A., Herrmann, R. et al. (2000). Assignment of a form of congenital muscular dystrophy wity secondary merosin deficiency to chromosome 1q42. *Am. J. Hum. Genet.* **66**, 428–435.

Burton, B. K., Dillard, R. G. and Weaver, R. G. (1987). Walker–Warburg syndrome with cleft lip and cleft palate in two sibs. *Am. J. Med. Genet.* **27**, 537–541.

Bushby, K., Anderson, L. V., Pollitt, C., Naom, I., Muntoni, F. and Bindoff, L. (1998). Abnormal merosin in adults. A new form of late onset muscular dystrophy not linked to chromosome 6q2. *Brain* **121**, 581–588.

Cohn, R. D., Herrmann, R., Wewer, U. M. and Voit, T. (1997). Changes of laminin beta 2 chain expression in congenital muscular dystrophy. *Neuromusc. Disord.* **7**, 373–378.

Cohn, R. D., Herrmann, R., Sorokin, L. and Voit, T. (1998). Laminin alpha2 chain-deficient congenital muscular dystrophy: variable epitope expression in severe and mild cases. [See comments] *Neurology* **51**, 94–100

Cohn, R. D., Mayer, U., Saher, G. et al. (1999). Secondary reduction of alpha7B integrin in laminin alpha2 deficient congenital muscular dystrophy supports an additional transmembrane link in skeletal muscle. *J. Neurol. Sci.* **163**, 140–152.

Cormand, B., Avela, K., Pihko, H. et al. (1999). Assignment of the muscle–eye–brain disease gene to 1p32–p34 by linkage analysis and homozygosity mapping. *Am. J. Hum. Genet.* **64**, 126–135.

Cormand, B., Pihko, H., Bayes, M. et al. (2001). Clinical and genetic delineation of Walker–Warburg syndrome and muscle–eye–brain disease. *Neurology*, in press.

Crowe, C., Jassani, M. and Dickerman, L. (1986). The prenatal diagnosis of the Walker–Warburg syndrome. *Prenat. Diagn.* **6**, 177–185.

de Paillette, L., Aicardi, J. and Goutieres, F. (1989). Ullrich's congenital atonic sclerotic muscular dystrophy. A case report. *J. Neurol.* **236**, 108–110.

Dobyns, W. B., Kirkpatrick, J. B., Hittner, H. M., Roberts, R. M. and Kretzer, F. L. (1985). Syndromes with lissencephaly. II: Walker–Warburg and cerebro-oculo-muscular syndromes and a new syndrome with type II lissencephaly. *Am. J. Med. Genet.* **22**, 157–195.

Dobyns, W. B., Pagon, R. A., Armstrong, D. et al. (1989). Diagnostic criteria for Walker–Warburg syndrome. [See comments] *Am. J. Med. Genet.* **32**, 195–210.

Dubowitz, V. (1971). Recent advances in neuromuscular disorders. *Rheumatol. Phys. Med.* **11**, 126–130.

Dubowitz, V. (1973). Rigid spine syndrome: a muscle syndrome in search of a name. *Proc. R. Soc. Med.* **66**, 219–220.

Dubowitz, V. (1978). *Muscle Disorders in Childhood.* London: Saunders .

Dubowitz, V. (1994). Workshop report: the 22nd ENMC sponsored workshop on congenital muscular dystrophy. *Neuromusc. Disord.* **4**, 75–81.

Dubowitz, V. (1996). Workshop report: the 41st ENMC international workshop on congenital muscular dystrophy. *Neuromusc. Disord.* **6**, 295–306.

Dubowitz, V. (1999). Workshop report: the 68th ENMC international workshop on congenital muscular dystrophy. *Neuromusc. Disord.* **9**, 446–454.

Dubowitz, V. and Fardeau, M. (1995). Workshop report: the 27th ENMC sponsored workshop on congenital muscular dystrophy. *Neuromusc. Disord.* **3**, 253–258.

Egger, J., Kendall, B. E., Erdohazi, M., Lake, B. D., Wilson, J. and Brett, E. M. (1983). Involvement of the central nervous system in congenital muscular dystrophies. *Dev. Med. Child. Neurol.* **25**, 32–42.

Ehrig, K., Leivo, I., Argraves, W. S., Ruoslahti, E. and Engvall, E. (1990). Merosin, a tissue-specific basement membrane protein, is a laminin-like protein. *Proc. Natl. Acad. Sci. USA* **87**, 3264–3268.

Engvall, E. and Wewer, U. M. (1996). Domains of laminin. *J. Cell. Biochem.* **61**, 493–501.

Engvall, E., Earwicker, D., Day, A., Muir, D., Manthorpe, M. and Paulsson, M. (1992). Merosin promotes cell attachment and neurite outgrowth and is a component of the neurite-promoting factor of RN22 schwannoma cells. *Exp. Cell. Res.* **198**, 115–123.

Fardeau, M., Tomé, F. M., Helbling-Leclerc, A. et al. (1996). Congenital muscular dystrophy with merosin deficiency: clinical, histopathological, immunocytochemical and genetic analysis. *Rev. Neurol. (Paris)* **152**, 11–19.

Flanigan, K. M., Kerr, L., Bromberg, M. B. et al. (2000). Congenital muscular dystrophy with rigid spine syndrome: a clinical, pathological, radiologic and genetic study. *Ann. Neurol.* **47**, 152–161.

Fukuyama, Y. and Osawa, M. (1982). Congenital muscular dystrophy: clinico-nosological aspects. In: *Proceedings of the International Symposium of Muscular Dystrophy*, 1980 Tokyo, ed. S. Ebashi, pp. 399–424. Tokyo: University of Tokyo Press.

Fukuyama, Y., Kwazura, M. and Haruna, H. (1960). A peculiar form of congenital muscular dystrophy. *Paediatr. Univ. Tokyo* **4**, 5–8.

Fukuyama, Y., Osawa, M. and Suzuki, H. (1981). Congenital progressive muscular dystrophy of the Fukuyama type – clinical, genetic and pathological considerations. *Brain Dev.* **3**, 1–29.

Guicheney, P., Vignier, N., Helbling-Leclerc, A. et al. (1997). Genetics of laminin alpha 2 chain (or merosin) deficient congenital muscular dystrophy: from identification of mutations to prenatal diagnosis. *Neuromusc. Disord.* **7**, 180–186.

Guicheney, P., Vignier, N., Zhang, X. et al. (1998). PCR based mutation screening of the laminin alpha2 chain gene (LAMA2): application to prenatal diagnosis and search for founder effects in congenital muscular dystrophy. *J. Med. Genet.* **35**, 211–217.

Hagg, T., Portera-Cailliau, C., Jucker, M. and Engvall, E. (1997). Laminins of the adult mammalian CNS; laminin-alpha2 (merosin M-) chain immunoreactivity is associated with neuronal processes. *Brain Res.* **764**, 17–27.

Haltia, M., Leivo, I., Somer, H.. et al. (1997). Muscle-eye-brain disease: a neuropathological study. *Ann. Neurol.* **41**, 173–180.

Hayashi, Y. K., Engvall, E., Arikawa-Hirasawa, E. et al. (1993). Abnormal localization of laminin subunits in muscular dystrophies. *J. Neurol. Sci.* **119**, 53–64.

Hayashi, Y. K., Ishihara, T., Domen, K., Hori, H. and Arahata, K. (1997). A benign allelic form of laminin alpha 2 chain deficient muscular dystrophy. [Letter] *Lancet* **349**, 1147.

Hayashi, Y. K., Chou, F. L., Engvall, E. et al. (1998). Mutations in the integrin alpha7 gene cause congenital myopathy. *Nat. Genet.* **19**, 94–97.

Helbling-Leclerc, A., Topaloglu, H., Tomé, F. M. et al. (1995a). Readjusting the localization of merosin (laminin alpha 2-chain) deficient congenital muscular dystrophy locus on chromosome 6q2. *C. R. Acad. Sci. Ser. III* **318**, 1245–1252.

Helbling-Leclerc, A., Zhang, X., Topaloglu, H. et al. (1995b). Mutations in the laminin alpha 2-chain gene (LAMA2) cause merosin-deficient congenital muscular dystrophy. *Nat. Genet.* **11**, 216–218.

Herrmann, R., Straub, V., Meyer, K., Kahn, T., Wagner, M. and Voit, T. (1996). Congenital muscular dystrophy with laminin alpha 2 chain deficiency: identification of a new intermediate phenotype and correlation of clinical findings to muscle immunohistochemistry. *Eur. J. Pediatr.* **155**, 968–976.

Hillaire, D., Leclerc, A., Faure, S. et al. (1994). Localization of merosin-negative congenital muscular dystrophy to chromosome 6q2 by homozygosity mapping. *Hum. Mol. Genet.* **3**, 1657–1661.

Hodges, B. L., Hayashi, Y. K., Nonaka, I., Wang, W., Arahata, K. and Kaufman, S. J. (1997). Altered expression of the alpha7beta1 integrin in human and murine muscular dystrophies. *J. Cell. Sci.* **110**, 2873–2881.

Howard, R. A. (1908). A case of congenital defect of the muscular system (dystrophia muscularis congenita) and its association with congenital talipes equino-varus. *Proc. R. Soc. Med.* **1**, 157–166.

Huh, J., Kim, K. J., Ko, T. S., Kim, D. W., Hwang, S. H. and Hwang, Y. S. (1992). A case of Fukuyama congenital muscular dystrophy. [In Korean] *Korean J. Neurol.* **10**, 388–394.

Iivanainen, A., Sainio, K., Sariola, H. and Tryggvason, K. (1995). Primary structure and expression of a novel human laminin alpha 4 chain. *FEBS Lett.* **365**, 183–188.

Ishii, H., Hayashi, Y. K., Nonaka, I. and Arahata, K. (1997). Electron microscopic examination of basal lamina in Fukuyama congenital muscular dystrophy. *Neuromusc. Disord.* **7**, 191–197.

Kamoshita, S., Konishi, Y., Segawa, M. and Fukuyama, Y. (1976). Congenital muscular dystrophy as a disease of the central nervous system. *Arch. Neurol.* **33**, 513–516.

Knubley, W. A. and Bertorini, T. (1988). Congenital muscular dystrophy with cerebellar atrophy. *Dev. Med. Child Neurol.* **30**, 378–383.

Kobayashi, O., Hayashi, Y., Arahata, K. Ozawa, E. and Nonaka, I. (1996). Congenital muscular dystrophy: Clinical and pathologic study of 50 patients with the classical (Occidental) merosin-positive form. *Neurology* **46**, 815–818.

Kobayashi, K., Nakahori, Y., Miyake, M. et al. (1998a). An ancient retrotransposal insertion causes Fukuyama-type congenital muscular dystrophy. *Nature* **394**, 388–392.

Kobayashi, K., Nakahori, Y., Mizuno, K. et al. (1998b). Founder-haplotype analysis in Fukuyama-type congenital muscular dystrophy (FCMD). *Hum. Genet.* **103**, 323–327.

Leyten, Q. F., Renier, W. O., Gabreels, F. J., Brunner, H. G., ter Laak, H. J. and Mullaart, R. A. (1996). Association of congenital muscular dystrophy with hypoplasia of the abdominal wall musculature and hypoplasia of the exeternal genitalia. *Neuropediatrics* **27**, 108–110.

Mahjneh, I., Bushby, K., Anderson, L. et al. (1999). Merosin-positive congenital muscular dystrophy: a large inbred family. *Neuropediatrics* **30**, 22–28.

Mandel, H., Brik, R., Ludatscher, R., Braun, J. and Berant, M. (1993). Congenital muscular dystrophy with neurological abnormalities: association with Hirschsprung disease. *Am. J. Med. Genet.* **47**, 37–40.

McMenamin, J. B., Becker, L. E. and Murphy, E. G. (1982). Fukuyama-type congenital muscular dystrophy. *J. Pediatr.* **101**, 580–582.

Mercuri, E., Muntoni, F., Berardinelli, A. et al. (1995a). Somatosensory and visual evoked potentials in congenital muscular dystrophy: correlation with MRI changes and muscle merosin status. *Neuropediatrics* **26**, 3–7.

Mercuri, E., Dubowitz, L., Berardinelli, A. et al. (1995b). Minor neurological and perceptuo-motor deficits in children with congenital muscular dystrophy: correlation with brain MRI changes. *Neuropediatrics* **26**, 156–162.

Mercuri, E., Pennock, J., Goodwin, F., Sewry, C., Cowan, F., Dubowitz, L. et al. (1996). Sequential study of central and peripheral nervous system involvement in an infant with merosin-deficient congenital muscular dystrophy. *Neuromusc. Disord.* **6**, 425–429.

Mercuri, E., Sewry, C. A., Brown, S. C. et al. (2000). Congenital muscular dystrophy with secondary merosin deficiency and normal brain MRI. *Neuropediatrics* **31**, 186–189.

Moghadaszadeh, B., Desguerre, I., Topaloglu, H. et al. (1998a). Identification of a new locus for a peculiar form of congenital muscular dystrophy with early rigidity of the spine, on chromosome 1p35– 36. *Am. J. Hum. Genet.* **62**, 1439–1445.

Moghadaszadeh, B., Desguerre, I., Topaloglu, H. et al. (1998b). Genetic heterogeneity of rigid spine syndrome. *Muscle Nerve* **7**, 107.

Moghadaszadeh, B., Topaloglu, H., Merlini, L. et al. (1999). Genetic heterogeneity of congenital muscular dystrophy with rigid spine syndrome. *Neuromusc. Disord.* **9**, 376–382.

Mora, M., Moroni, I., Uziel, G. et al. (1996). Mild clinical phenotype in a 12-year-old boy with partial merosin deficiency and central and peripheral nervous system abnormalities. *Neuromusc. Disord.* **6**, 377–381.

Muntoni, F., Sewry, C., Wilson, L. et al. (1995). Prenatal diagnosis in congenital muscular dystrophy. [Letter] *Lancet* **345**, 591.

Muntoni, F., Taylor, J., Sewry, C. A., Naom, I. and Dubowitz, V. (1998). An early onset muscular dystrophy with diaphragmatic involvement, early respiratory failure and secondary alpha2 laminin deficiency unlinked to the LAMA2 locus on 6q22. *Eur. J. Ped. Neurol.* **1**, 19–26.

Nakano, I., Funahashi, M., Takada, K. and Toda, T. (1996). Are breaches in the glia limitans the primary cause of the micropolygyria in Fukuyama-type congenital muscular dystrophy (FCMD)? Pathological study of the cerebral cortex of an FCMD fetus. *Acta Neuropathol.* **91**, 313–321.

Naom, I., D'Alessandro, M., Sewry, C. et al. (1997). The role of immunocytochemistry and linkage analysis in the prenatal diagnosis of merosin-deficient congenital muscular dystrophy. *Hum. Genet.* **99**, 535–540.

Naom, I., D'Alessandro, M., Sewry, C. A. et al. (1998a). Laminin alpha 2-chain gene mutations in two siblings presenting with limb-girdle muscular dystrophy. *Neuromusc. Disord.* **8**, 495–501.

Naom, I., Brockington, M., Lolli, G. et al. (1998b). The prevalence of chromosome 1p-linked merosin positive congenital muscular dystrophy. *Muscle Nerve* **7**, 107.

Nissinen, M., Helbling-Leclerc, A., Zhang et al. (1996). Substitution of a conserved cysteine-996 in a cysteine-rich motif of the laminin alpha2-chain in congenital muscular dystrophy with partial deficiency of the protein. *Am. J. Hum. Genet.* **58**, 1177–1184.

Nonaka, I., Une, Y., Ishihara, T., Miyoshino, S., Nakashima, T. and Sugita, H. (1981). A clinical and histological study of Ullrich's disease (congenital atonic-sclerotic muscular dystrophy). *Neuropediatrics* **12**, 197–208.

Osawa, M., Arai, Y., Ikenaka, H., Murasugi, H. et al. (1991). Fukuyama type congenital progressive muscular dystrophy. *Acta Paediatr. Jpn.* **33**, 261–269.

Osawa, M., Suzuki, N., Arai, Y. et al. (1993). Fukuyama type congenital progressive muscular dystrophy (FCMD) – special comment on the relationship between the case report by Nakayama et al. and FCMD. *Neuropathology (Tokyo)* **13**, 259–268.

Osawa, M., Sumida, S., Suzuki, N. et al. (1997). Fukuyama type congenital muscular dystrophy. In: *Congenital Muscular Dystrophies*, eds. Y. Fukuyama, M. Osawa and K. Saito, pp. 31–68. Amsterdam: Elsevier.

Parano, E., Falsaperla, R., Pavone, V. and Trifiletti, R. R. (1994). Congenital muscular dystrophy with syringomyelia. *Pediatr. Neurol.* **11**, 263–265.

Patton, B. L., Miner, J. H., Chiu, A. Y. and Sanes, J. R. (1997). Distribution and function of laminins in the neuromuscular system of developing, adult, and mutant mice. *J. Cell Biol.* **139**, 1507–1521.

Pegoraro, E., Marks, H., Garcia, C. A. et al. (1998). Laminin alpha2 muscular dystrophy: genotype/phenotype studies of 22 patients [see comments]. *Neurology* **51**, 101–110.

Philpot, J. and Muntoni, F. (1999). Limitation of eye movement in merosin-deficient congenital muscular dystrophy. [Letter] *Lancet* **353**, 297–298.

Philpot, J., Sewry, C., Pennock, J. and Dubowitz, V. (1995a). Clinical phenotype in congenital muscular dystrophy: correlation with expression of merosin in skeletal muscle. *Neuromusc. Disord.* **5**, 301–305.

Philpot, J., Topaloglu, H., Pennock, J. and Dubowitz, V. (1995b). Familial concordance of brain magnetic resonance imaging changes in congenital muscular dystrophy. *Neuromusc. Disord.* **5**, 227–231.

Philpot, J., Bagnall, A., King, C., Dubowitz, V. and Muntoni, F. (1999a). Feeding problems in merosin deficient congenital muscular dystrophy. *Arch. Dis. Child.* **80**, 542–547.

Philpot, J., Cowan, F., Pennock, J., Sewry, C. et al. (1999b). Merosin-deficient congenital muscular dystrophy: the spectrum of brain involvement on magnetic resonance imaging. *Neuromusc. Disord.* **9**, 81–85.

Pini, A., Merlini, L., Tomé, F. M., Chevallay, M. and Gobbi, G. (1996). Merosin-negative congenital muscular dystrophy, occipital epilepsy with periodic spasms and focal cortical dysplasia. Report of three Italian cases in two families. *Brain Dev.* **18**, 316–322.

Poppe, M., van Landeghem, F., Herrmann, R. et al. (1998). White matter abnormalities on brain MRI in a patient with congenital muscular dystrophy (CMD) and acute dilative cardiomyopathy. *Neuropediatrics* **29**, A1.

Raitta, C., Lamminen, M., Santavuori, P. and Leisti, J. (1978). Ophthalmological findings in a new syndrome with muscle, eye and brain involvement. *Acta Ophthalmol.* **56**, 465–472.

Ringelmann, B., Roder, C., Hallmann, R. et al. (1999). Expression of laminin alpha1, alpha2, alpha4, and alpha5 chains, fibronectin, and tenascin-C in skeletal muscle of dystrophic 129ReJ *dy/dy* mice. *Exp. Cell. Res.* **246**, 165–182.

Salih, M. A., Al Rayess, M., Cutshall, S. et al. (1998). A novel form of familial congenital muscular dystrophy in two adolescents. *Neuropediatrics* **29**, 289–293.

Santavuori, P., Leisti, J. and Kruus, S. (1977). Muscle, eye and brain disease: a new syndrome. *Neuropädiatrie* **8**(Suppl.), 550.

Santavuori, P., Somer, H., Sainio, K. et al. (1989). Muscle–eye–brain disease (MEB). [See comments] *Brain Dev.* **11**, 147–153.

Santavuori, P., Pihko, H., Sainio, K.et al. (1990). Muscle–eye–brain disease and Walker–Warburg syndrome. [Letter; comment] *Am. J. Med. Genet.* **36**, 371–374.

Santavuori, P., Valanne, L., Autti, T., Haltia, M., Pihko, H. and Sainio, K. (1998). Muscle–eye–brain disease. *Eur. J. Ped. Neurol.* **1**, 41–47.

Seidhamed, M. Z., Sunada, Y., Ozo, C. O., Hamid, F., Campbell, K. P. and Salih, M. A. (1996). Lethal congenital muscular dystrophy in two sibs with arthrogryposis multiplex: new entity or variant of cobblestone lissencephaly syndrome? *Neuropediatrics* **27**, 305–310.

Sewry, C. A., Philpot, J., Mahony, D., Wilson, L. A., Muntoni, F. and Dubowitz, V. (1995). Expression of laminin subunits in congenital muscular dystrophy. *Neuromusc. Disord.* **5**, 307–316.

Sewry, C. A., Philpot, J., Sorokin, L. M. et al. (1996a). Diagnosis of merosin (laminin-2) deficient congenital muscular dystrophy by skin biopsy. *Lancet* **347**, 582–584.

Sewry, C. A., Naom, I., D'Alessandro, M. et al(1996b). The protein defect in congenital muscular dystrophy. *Biochem. Soc. Trans.* **24**, 281S.

Sewry, C. A., Naom, I., D'Alessandro, M. et al. (1997). Variable clinical phenotype in merosin-deficient congenital muscular dystrophy associated with differential immunolabelling of two fragments of the laminin alpha 2 chain. *Neuromusc. Disord.* **7**, 169–175.

Shorer, Z., Philpot, J., Muntoni, F., Sewry, C. and Dubowitz, V. (1995). Demyelinating peripheral neuropathy in merosin-deficient congenital muscular dystrophy. *J. Child Neurol.* **10**, 472–475.

Spyrou, N., Philpot, J., Foale, R., Camici, P. G. and Muntoni, F. (1998). Evidence of left ventricular dysfunction in children with merosin-deficient congenital muscular dystrophy. *Am. Heart J.* **136**, 474–476.

Squarzoni, S., Villanova, M., Sabatelli, P. et al. (1997). Intracellular detection of laminin alpha 2 chain in skin by electron microscopy immunocytochemistry: comparison between normal and laminin alpha 2 chain deficient subjects. *Neuromusc. Disord.* **7**, 91–98.

Squier, M. V. (1993). Fetal type II lissencephaly: a case report. *Childs Nerv. Syst.* **9**, 400–402.

Stoeber, E. (1939). Über atonisch-sklerotische Muskeldystrophie (Typ Ullrich). *Z. Kinderheilkd.* **60**, 279–284.

Straub, V., Rafael, J. A., Chamberlain, J. S. and Campbell, K. P. (1997). Animal models for muscular dystrophy show different patterns of sarcolemmal disruption. *J. Cell Biol.* **139**, 375–385.

Sugita, H., Hayashi, Y. K., Arikawa-Hirasawa, E., Nonaka, I. and Arahata, K. (1995). The molecular pathogenesis of Fukuyama type congenital muscular dystrophy. *Acta Cardiomyol.* **1**, 3–9.

Sunada, Y., Edgar, T. S., Lotz, B. P., Rust, R. S. and Campbell, K. P. (1995). Merosin-negative congenital muscular dystrophy associated with extensive brain abnormalities. *Neurology* **45**, 2084–2089.

Sztriha, L., Al-Gazali, L. I., Varady, E. Goebel, H. H. and Nork, M. (1999). Autosomal recessive micrencephaly with simplified gyral pattern, abnormal myelination and arthrogryposis. *Neuropediatrics* **30**, 141–145.

Takada, K., Nakamura, H., Suzumori, K., Ishikawa, T. and Sugiyama, N. (1987). Cortical dysplasia in a 23-week fetus with Fukuyama congenital muscular dystrophy (FCMD). *Acta Neuropathol.* **74**, 300–306.

Tan, E., Topaloglu, H., Sewry, C. et al. (1997). Late onset muscular dystrophy with cerebral white matter changes due to partial merosin deficiency. *Neuromusc. Disord.* **7**, 85–89.

Tarantuto, A. L., Lubieniecki, F., Diaz, D. et al. (1999). Merosin-deficient congenital muscle dystrophy associated with abnormal cerebral cortical gyration: an autopsy study. *Neuromusc. Disord.* **9**, 86–94.

Tiger, C. F. and Gullberg, D. (1997). Abscence of laminin alpha1 chain in the skeletal muscle of dystrophic dy/dy mice. *Muscle Nerve* **20**, 1515–1524.

Toda, T., Segawa, M., Nomura, Y. et al. (1993). Localization of a gene for Fukuyama type congenital muscular dystrophy to chromosome 9q31–33. [Published erratum appears in *Nat. Genet.* 1994, 113] *Nat. Genet.* **5**, 283–286.

Toda, T., Ikegawa, S., Okui, K. et al. (1994). Refined mapping of a gene responsible for Fukuyama-type congenital muscular dystrophy: evidence for strong linkage disequilibrium. *Am. J. Hum. Genet.* **55**, 946–950.

Tomé, F. M. (1999). The Peter Emil Becker Award lecture 1998. The saga of congenital muscular dystrophy. *Neuropediatrics* **30**, 55–65.

Tomé, F. M., Evangelista, T., Leclerc, A., Sunada, Y., Manole, E., Estournet, B. et al. (1994). Congenital muscular dystrophy with merosin deficiency. *C. R. Acad. Sci. Ser. III* **317**, 351–357.

Topaloglu, H., Muruvet, Y., Talim, B. and Alcoren, Z. (1997). Merosin-positive congenital muscular dystrophy with mental retardation and cataracts: A new entity in two families. *Eur. J. Ped. Neurol.* **4**, 127–131.

Topaloglu, H., Talim, B., Vignier, N. et al. (1998). Merosin-deficient congenital muscular dystrophy with severe mental retardation and normal cranial MRI: a report of two siblings. *Neuromusc. Disord.* **8**, 169–174.

Tsutsumi, A., Uchida, Y., Osawa, M. and Fukuyama, Y. (1989). Ocular findings in Fukuyama type congenital muscular dystrophy. *Brain Dev.* **11**, 413–419.

Ullrich, O. (1930a). Kongenitale, atonisch-sklerotische Muskeldystrophie. *Monatsschr. Kinderheilkd.* **47**, 502–510.

Ullrich, O. (1930b). Kongenitale, atonisch-sklerotische Muskeldystrophie, ein weiterer Typus der heredodegenerativen Erkrankung des neuromuskulären Systems. *Z. Ges. Neurol. Psychiatr.* **126**, 171–201.

Vainzof, M., Marie, S. K., Reed, U. C. et al. (1995). Deficiency of merosin (laminin M or alpha 2) in congenital muscular dystrophy associated with cerebral white matter alterations. *Neuropediatrics* **26**, 293–297.

Valanne, L., Pihko, H., Katevuo, K., Karttunen, P., Somer, H. and Santavuori, P. (1994). MRI of the brain in muscle–eye–brain (MEB) disease. *Neuroradiology* **36**, 473–476.

van der Knaap, M. S., Smit, L. M. et al. (1997). Magnetic resonance imaging in classification of congenital muscular dystrophies with brain abnormalities. *Ann. Neurol.* **42**, 50–59.

Villanova, M., Malandrini, A., Toti, P. et al. (1996). Localization of merosin in the normal human brain: implications for congenital muscular dystrophy with merosin deficiency. *J. Submicrosc. Cytol. Pathol.* **28**, 1–4.

Villanova, M., Malandrini, A., Sabatelli, P., Sewry, C. A., Toti, P., Torelli, S. et al. (1997). Localization of laminin alpha 2 chain in normal human central nervous system: an immunofluorescence and ultrastructural study. *Acta Neuropathol. (Berlin)* **94**, 567–571.

Vilquin, J. T., Kinoshita, I., Roy, B. et al. (1996). Partial laminin alpha2 chain restoration in alpha2 chain-deficient *dy/dy* mouse by primary muscle cell culture transplantation. *J. Cell Biol.* **133**, 185–197.

Voit, T. (1998). Congenital muscular dystrophies: 1997 update. *Brain Dev.* **20**, 65–74.

Voit, T., Fardeau, M. and Tomé, F. M. (1994). Prenatal detection of merosin expression in human placenta. [Letter] *Neuropediatrics* **25**, 332–333.

Voit, T., Sewry, C. A., Meyer, K. et al. (1995). Preserved merosin M-chain (or laminin-alpha 2) expression in skeletal muscle distinguishes Walker–Warburg syndrome from Fukuyama muscular dystrophy and merosin-deficient congenital muscular dystrophy. [See comments] *Neuropediatrics* **26**, 148–155.

Voit, T., Cohn, R. D., Sperner, J. et al. (1999). Merosin-positive congenital muscular dystrophy with transient brain dysmyelination, pontocerebellar hypoplasia and mental retardation. *Neuromusc. Disord.* **9**, 95–101.

Vuolteenaho, R., Nissinen, M., Sainio, K. et al. (1994). Human laminin M chain (merosin): complete primary structure, chromosomal assignment, and expression of the M and A chain in human fetal tissues. *J. Cell Biol.* **124**, 381–394.

Walker, A. E. (1942). Lissencephaly. *Arch. Neurol. Psychol.* **48**, 13–29.

Warburg, M. (1978). Hydrocephaly, congenital retinal nonattachment, and congenital falciform fold. *Am. J. Ophthalmol.* **85**, 88–94.

Wargowski, D. S., Chitayat, D., Tyson, R. W., Norman, M. G. and Friedman, J. M. (1991). Lethal congenital muscular dystrophy with cataracts and a minor brain anomaly: new entity or variant of Walker–Warburg syndrome? *Am. J. Med. Genet.* **39**, 19–24.

Wewer, U. M. and Engvall, E. (1996). Merosin/laminin-2 and muscular dystrophy. *Neuromusc. Disord.* **6**, 409–418.

Wewer, U. M., Durkin, M. E., Zhang, X. et al. (1995). Laminin beta 2 chain and adhalin deficiency in the skeletal muscle of Walker–Warburg syndrome (cerebro-ocular dysplasia-muscular dystrophy). *Neurology* **45**, 2099–2101.

Williams, R. S., Swisher, C. N., Jennings, M., Ambler, M. and Caviness, V. S. Jr (1984). Cerebro-ocular dysgenesis (Walker–Warburg syndrome): neuropathologic and etiologic analysis. *Neurology* **34**, 1531–1541.

Xu, H., Wu, X. R., Wewer, U. M. and Engvall, E. (1994a). Murine muscular dystrophy caused by a mutation in the laminin alpha 2 (*LAMA2*) gene. *Nat. Genet.* **8**, 297–302.

Xu, H., Christmas, P., Wu, X. R., Wewer, U. M. and Engvall, E. (1994b). Defective muscle basement membrane and lack of M-laminin in the dystrophic dy/dy mouse. *Proc. Natl. Acad. Sci. USA* **91**, 5572–5576.

Yamamoto, T., Shibata, N., Kanazawa, M. et al. (1997a). Localization of laminin subunits in the central nervous system in Fukuyama congenital muscular dystrophy: an immunohistochemical investigation. *Acta Neuropathol. (Berlin)* **94**, 173–179.

Yamamoto, T., Shibata, N., Kanazawa, M. et al. (1997b). Early ultrastructural changes in the central nervous system in Fukuyama congenital muscular dystrophy. *Ultrastruct. Pathol.* **21**, 355–360.

Yoshikawa, H., Hirayama, Y., Kurokowa, T., Houdo, S. (1991). A case of Fukuyama type congenital muscular dystrophy presenting with rapidly progressive heart failure. [In Japanese] *Iryo (Tokyo)* **45**, 898–902.

Yoshioka, M., Saiwai, S., Kuroki, S. and Nigami, H. (1991). MR imaging of the brain in Fukuyama-type congenital muscular dystrophy. *Am. J. Neuroradiol.* **12**, 63–65.

Zellweger, H., Afifi, A., McCormick, W. F. and Mergner, W. (1967a). Benign congenital muscular dystrophy: a special form of congenital hypotonia. *Clin. Pediatr. (Phil.)* **6**, 655–663.

Zellweger, H., Afifi, A., McCormick, W. F. and Mergner, W. (1967b). Severe congenital muscular dystrophy. *Am. J. Dis. Child.* **114**, 591–602.

Zhang, X., Vuolteenaho, R. and Tryggvason, K. (1996). Structure of the human laminin alpha2-chain gene (*LAMA2*), which is affected in congenital muscular dystrophy. *J. Biol. Chem.* **271**, 27664–27669.

26

Congenital myopathies

Hans H. Goebel

Introduction

The era of congenital myopathies, also called 'new myopathies' (Dubowitz, 1969) was ushered in when, based on the modern myopathological techniques of electron microscopy and enzyme histochemistry, central core disease and nemaline myopathy were described by Shy and Magee in 1956 and Shy et al. in 1963, respectively. Since then, congenital myopathies have been accepted by myologists as a nosological category among other groups of neuromuscular disorders and have been described both in textbooks and in innumerable individual articles. The congenital myopathies have been well defined, with some areas of uncertainty, as occurs with other groups of neuromuscular disorders. For example the muscular dystrophies include those that are not dystrophic in nature such as Emery–Dreifuss or oculopharyngeal muscular dystrophies; the metabolic myopathies include myoadenylate deaminase deficiency, which is still being debated as a nosological entity, and the inflammatory myopathies include inclusion body myositis, which is still being assessed both as a primary inflammatory process and in its relationship with hereditary inclusion body myopathy.

Congenital myopathies are neuromuscular disorders that are often mild, and slowly or nonprogressive in children. They are often inherited and characterized by particular morphological features such as inclusion bodies (Goebel, 1998a). These morphological features occur frequently in a biopsied muscle specimen and have been classified as 'structured' and 'unstructured' entities (Goebel, 1986, 1996; Goebel and Lenard, 1992; Goebel and Fidzianska, 1996). Exclusion of other nosologically well-defined neuromuscular disorders may also be incorporated into this definition. There are exceptions to this definition in that some patients may have a clinically late onset of their congenital myopathies while others may die early from their congenital myopathies, the latter occurring almost always with the early-infantile or neonatal form of nemaline myopathy or with myotubular myopathy. Some morphological features that are considered characteristic of certain congenital myopathies may also be observed in other neuromuscular disorders, such as nemaline bodies or rods, cytoplasmic bodies, tubular aggregates or minicores. Conversely, some well-defined morphological features are not seen in certain congenital myopathies, for instance concentric laminated and filamentous bodies. There are other neuromuscular conditions that display unique morphological structures but are not necessarily congenital myopathies. For example, Marinesco–Sjögren syndrome has distinct perinuclear cisternae within muscle fibres and oculopharyngeal muscular dystrophy has aggregated 8–10 nm intranuclear filaments.

The congenital myopathies may encompass more conditions than those actually characterized by special morphological features; these other conditions have been called 'benign congenital myopathies' (Gardner-Medwin, 1994) or 'minimal change myopathy' (Dubowitz, 1985). This uncertainty in defining the congenital myopathies as a group has influenced classification (Goebel and Fidzianska, 1996) and acceptance of individual congenital myopathies as nosological entities. Classification may be based on morphological features alone (Goebel and Lenard, 1992), on type of lesion, or on their frequency and history. The last gives rise to three categories: well-recognized classic conditions, sporadic rarely reported but established conditions and questionable rarely reported conditions (Goebel, 1996). The European Neuromuscular Centre (ENMC) has been clarifying the congenital myopathies by holding workshops and establishing consortia on nemaline myopathy (Wallgren-Pettersson and Laing, 1996; Wallgren-Pettersson et al., 1998), myotubular myopathy

(Wallgen-Pettersson and Thomas, 1994, 1997; Thomas and Wallgren-Pettersson, 1996; Wallgren-Pettersson, 1998), desmin-related congenital myopathies (Goebel and Fardeau, 1995, 1996) and structural congenital myopathies (Goebel and Anderson, 1999), the last dealing with rarer forms that may or may not be distinct nosological entities. These steps are intended to provide diagnostic criteria for certain congenital myopathies (Emery, 1997) and to form a basis from which further genetic studies may be undertaken to corroborate and possibly modify current classification of the congenital myopathies. At present this classification varies among textbooks and review articles, a situation that occurred at one point with the muscular dystrophies before molecular genetic data became available.

The overall incidence of congential myopathies among the spectrum of neuromuscular diseases is unknown, as is the frequency of individual congenital myopathies. This lack of epidemiological data may result from variation in the patient populations seen by different neuromuscular centres, the requirement for muscle biopsy and suitable preparative workup or the poor characterization of some congenital myopathies.

This chapter will address congenital myopathies from a neuropathological perspective, according to the author's profession, and incorporate progress in the genetics of certain congenital myopathies. Muscle biopsy is often required to identify the particular congenital myopathy affecting a patient because the clinical features are often nonspecific, although occasionally they are quite distinct; the electromyogram is usually myopathic, and serum creatine kinase values are only mildly elevated or not at all. As a result, identification of the disease involved is achieved by myopathological findings and, in the future, by genetic.

Central core disease

Central core disease was the first congenital myopathy described (Shy and Magee, 1956), when electron microscopy and enzyme histochemistry were still in their infancy, because recognition of the characteristic cores, centrally located derangements of sarcomeres along the myofibres, did not require these sophisticated techniques but could be achieved with processed paraffin sections.

Clinically, central core disease is slowly progressive or nonprogressive (perhaps some progress only in later years (Lamont et al., 1998)). An affected parent occasionally is only found to have the disorder when the more severely affected child develops muscle weakness and hypotonia. There may be associated skeletal involvement such as hip dislocation or contractures, scoliosis or talipes (Nagai et

al., 1994). Respiratory insufficiency and cardiomyopathy are not a regular feature. Only rarely is the disease more severe (Manzur et al., 1998).

In central core disease, cytoplasmic organization is abnormal; the cores resemble the target and targetoid fibres associated with denervation and the lesions induced by tenotomy. The cores form either an elongated area extending along the long axis of the muscle fibre with condensed sarcomeres out of register with neighbouring sarcomeres or they may result in complete disruption of the sarcomeres with smearing of Z disc material along the sarcomeres. Both types of lesion, called structured and unstructured cores, respectively, lack mitochondria, giving rise to a focal deficiency of oxidative enzymes. Both structured and unstructured cores may appear in the same patient, the same muscle specimen and the same muscle fibre (Goebel and Lenard, 1992). Immunohistochemically, unstructured cores express increased amounts of dystrophin, actin, α-actinin, gelsolin, neural cell adhesion molecule (NCAM), nebulin, desmin, β_2-microglobulin and α_1-antichymotrypsin as an apparently nonspecific feature, similar to central zones in target fibres (de Bleecker et al., 1996a). The cores may be single or multiple, centrally or peripherally located. They usually occur in type I fibres but not infrequently the entire biopsy population consists only of type I fibres. During the course of the disease, the number of cores may grow, which explains why cores and type I fibre uniformity may be seen in a parent when an affected child has type I fibre uniformity but no cores (Fig. 26.1) (Morgan-Hughes et al., 1973) or cores in uniformly type I fibres of a limb muscle and a type I fibre uniformity without cores in paraspinal muscle (Nagai et al., 1994). The immunological basis of the morphogenesis, pathogenesis and aetiology of the cores is still unexplained.

The autosomal dominant mode of inheritance is a definite feature of central core disease with male-to-male transmission. Recently, a severe form suggested an autosomal recessive mode of inheritance (Manzur et al., 1998). In a few families, linkage studies have assigned a locus on chromosome 19q13.1 (Haan et al., 1990; Kausch et al., 1991) and in certain families, a linkage with malignant hyperthermia. Patients and families with both central core disease and malignant hyperthermia do exist, but others do not share both conditions. The gene product of the locus on 19q13.1 has not been identified for central core disease, but candidate genes at this area coding for a mitochondrial cytochrome c oxidase subunit and a regulatory subunit of calpain show no sequence change in central core disease (Goebel and Anderson, 1999). The ryanodine receptor 1, which is located between the sarcoplasmic reticulum and transverse tubules, is encoded be a gene on

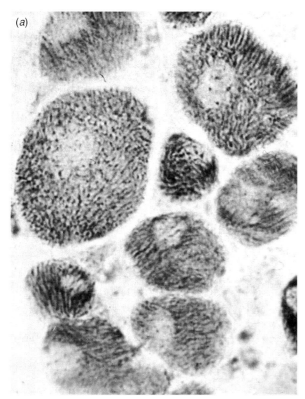
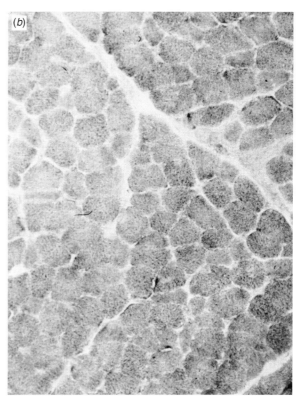

Fig. 26.1. Central core disease in siblings with type I fibre uniformity (biopsied muscle preparations stained with NADH tetrazolium reductase). (*a*) Central and excentric cores occur in the older sister (and in the father) (×920). (*b*) No cores can be seen in muscle from the clinically affected younger brother (×320).

19q13.1 and has been found to carry at least 20 mutations in patients with malignant hyperthermia, several of which are missense mutations (Quane et al., 1993; Zhang et al., 1993). No mutations have been identified in families or patients with central core disease (Goebel and Anderson, 1999).

Centronuclear and myotubular myopathies

The centronuclear and myotubular myopathies are a heterogeneous group with confusion regarding nomenclature. The first patient described with a neuromuscular disorder of this type (Spiro et al., 1966) was an adolescent boy with severe muscle weakness without any aparent X linkage. Subsequently, children with similar morphological features were described as having centronuclear myopathy (Sher et al., 1967). The first family with a severe X-linked form was described in 1969 (van Wijngaarden et al., 1969) and their neuromuscular condition was termed familial myotubular myopathy. A further family in the Netherlands was identified with the same X-linked myotu-

bular myopathy (Barth et al., 1975). The occurrence of a mostly fatal early-onset X-linked myotubular myopathy was established and it was suggested that the term myotubular myopathy should be restricted to this X-linked form, a designation I chose to follow. Patients and families with sporadic centronuclear myopathy or autosomal recessive or autosomal dominant forms were then said to have centronuclear myopathy. However the two terms, myotubular and centronuclear myopathy, have still been used interchangeably (de Angelis et al., 1991; Wallgren-Pettersson et al., 1995a). Based on modes of inheritance and clinical findings, at least three genetically different forms seem to exist.

Myotubular myopathy

Myotubular myopathy is X-linked and is apparent at birth or shortly after. It is marked by floppiness as well as severe respiratory insufficiency which is, frequently, the cause of death. Only a few boys with proven myotubular myopathy have survived and outgrown the necessity for artificial ventilation (de Angelis et al., 1991; de Gouyon et al., 1997;

Barth and Dubowitz, 1998). Morphologically, muscle fibres resemble myotubes, appearing immature with centrally located large nuclei surrounded by a perinuclear halo devoid of myofilaments. Immaturity of these muscle fibres is underscored by the diffuse presence of desmin, vimentin (Sarnat, 1990), and the fetal isoform of myosin heavy chain (MHC) (Sawchak et al., 1991). Vimentin and fetal MHC are usually only found in fetal and regenerating fibres. Transmitting mothers may show an increase in internal nuclei in muscle fibres and may even have central nuclei and fibres resembling myotubes (Wallgren-Pettersson et al., 1995a) or variation in fibre diameters (Goebel and Lenard, 1992).

Myotubular myopathy may be difficult to distinguish from infantile or congenital dystrophic myotonia; in the latter the muscle fibres contain desmin but not vimentin. In addition, mothers of these infants almost always have – even subtle – dystrophic myotonia, which can be confirmed by identification of enhanced CTG trinucleotide repeats.

The gene involved in myotubular myopathy, called *MTM-1*, encodes a protein myotubularin; the gene is located at Xq28 (Laporte et al., 1996) and consists of 15 exons (de Gouyon et al., 1997). A number of mutations, including missense and nonsense mutations and small and large deletions (Laporte et al., 1996; de Gouyon et al., 1997) have been identified in *MTM-1*. Among the missense mutations the C259T in exon 4 is apparently related to a mild phenotype whereas the other mutations result in severe disease. A 'common' mutation does not seem to exist as no single mutation has been identified in more than 10% of all patients screened (de Gouyon et al., 1997). Carrier testing revealed that almost all patients with sporadic disease had inherited the mutation from their mothers; only one of eight mothers with an affected child did not share the mutation with her son (de Gouyon et al., 1997).

Both the wealth and diversity of mutations of *MTM-1* have recently been demonstrated: almost 100 have been identified, including large deletions, nonsense, frameshift, missense and splice-site mutations, together with two intron variants related to partial exon skipping (Tanner et al., 1999). Consequently, mutation screening allows genetic counselling, prenatal diagnosis and carrier ascertainment in X-linked myotubular myopathy.

The normal protein product, called myotubularin, is a tyrosine phosphatase belonging to a larger group of tyrosine phosphatases that are involved in signal transduction (Laporte et al., 1996). A 3.9 kb transcript is present in adult and fetal tissues, but a second 2.4 kb transcript is only seen in skeletal muscle and testis (Laporte et al., 1996). Phosphatases of the myotubularin type are apparently related to fetal signalling pathways linked to SET (Suvar 3–9 Enhancer-of-zeste Trithorax). This SET domain is associated with a motif of unknown function in enzymatic mechanisms of gene regulation (Cui et al., 1998). Data on the role of myotubularin supports the belief that myotubular myopathy is a developmental neuromuscular disorder, which gives rise to myotube-like muscle fibres and the continued presence of both desmin and vimentin, which are usually seen only in fetal and regenerating fibres.

Centronuclear myopathy

Centronuclear myopathy may clinically appear as a childhood disorder, often with bilateral ptosis and skeletal abnormalities (i.e. scoliosis and a high-arched palate; Zanoteli et al., 1998). Rarely, centronuclear myopathy may be associated with cardiomyopathy (Verhiest et al., 1976; Gospe et al., 1987). Fetal immobility, polyhydramnion and perinatal hypoxia may occur (Zanoteli et al., 1998). While the delayed-onset or adult type of centronuclear myopathy often appears to be sporadic, childhood forms may follow an earlier autosomal recessive or later autosomal dominant mode of inheritance (Wallgren-Pettersson et al., 1995a). Prognosis is favourable because of the slow progression, or no progression, of the disease (Wallgren-Pettersson et al., 1995a).

Both the childhood and adult types have muscle fibres with central nuclei, not necessarily solitary but small in size (Fig. 26.2*a*). A morphological pattern of fibre type disproportion results from type I predominance and hypotrophy. Sequential biopsies in the same patient indicated that this fibre proportion change preceded the centronuclear morphology (Danon et al., 1997). However, these biopsies were obtained from one of male dizygotic twins, the other dying from respiratory failure during the first year of life. Consequently, without molecular genetic data, which were not reported, the possibility cannot be excluded that this surviving male patient had a milder form of myotubular myopathy (Danon et al., 1997). Fat cells may be seen within muscle fascicles. Additional circumscribed sarcomeric lesions resembling minicores or focal loss of cross-striation (Fig. 26.2*b*) may be present in affected family members and in different muscles of the same patient (Goebel et al., 1984; Goebel, 1986). The morphological pattern of fibre type disproportion may also be encountered in mini/multicore disease; consequently, a precise separation on morphological grounds of centronuclear myopathy and minicore disease may occasionally be difficult. Muscle fibres in centronuclear myopathy have also been shown to express increased amounts of desmin (Figarella-Branger et al., 1992; Misra et al., 1992). Even in

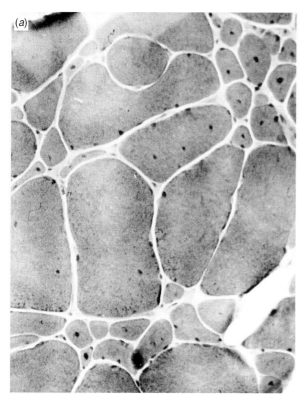
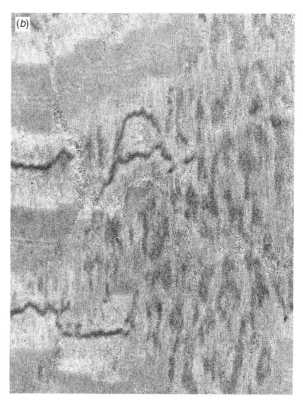

Fig. 26.2. Centronuclear myopathy. (*a*) Small muscle fibres have central nuclei (modified trichrome stain, ×368). (*b*) Fibre showing minicore (×19200).

adult-onset centronuclear myopathy, a few muscle fibres express fetal MHC and embryonic NCAM (Figarella-Branger et al., 1992).

Morphologically, dystrophic myotonia (infantile, childhood and adult) is a differential diagnosis that can only be excluded by genetic analysis for the CTG trinucleotide expansions of dystrophic myotonia.

No gene locus has been mapped in centronuclear myopathy. Such an achievement would be useful in differentiation of centronuclear myopathy from mild myotubular myopathy in a young boy.

Nemaline myopathies

Nemaline, or rod, myopathies are among the most frequent congenital myopathies and may exist in at least two different genetic forms, autosomal dominant and autosomal recessive. There are three different clinical variants, a rapidly progressive malignant early-onset form, a slowly progressive benign form of childhood and an adult form. There may also be a morphological variant marked by intranuclear rods with or without sarcoplasmic rods.

Clinically, the classic type of nemaline myopathy is the one occurring in childhood. This is slowly progressive and marked by proximal or generalized weakness including that of the face, which may be associated with a high-arched palate. Pes cavus and scoliosis are further skeletal abnormalities that may occur and familial rigid spine syndrome has been encountered in nemaline myopathy (Topaloglu et al., 1994). Respiratory insufficiency and pulmonary complications following colds may pose serious clinical problems.

A clinically very severe form of nemaline myopathy may be present at birth and is marked by extreme floppiness and respiratory insufficiency requiring artificial ventilation. Multiple contractures or arthrogryposis may also be characteristic features. The prognosis is often poor, with early death. Prenatal onset of nemaline myopathy may result in the typical fetal akinesia sequence (Lammens et al., 1997). A number of such severely affected infants had intranuclear rods in addition to sarcoplasmic ones, suggesting that the presence of intranuclear rods may be evidence of an unfavourable prognosis (Goebel et al., 1997a).

A third form of nemaline myopathy becomes apparent

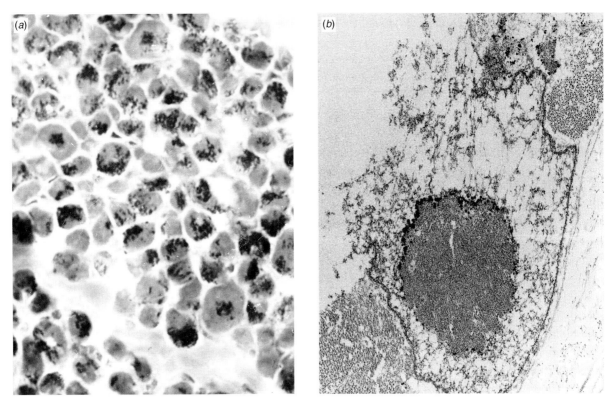

Fig. 26.3. Nemaline myopathy. (*a*) A large number of rods can be seen in small and large fibres (modified trichrome stain; ×382).
(*b*) Electron microscopy demonstrates an intranuclear rod labelled with antibody against α-actinin (×35 200).

in adulthood and is marked by muscle weakness and respiratory problems, the latter occasionally being life threatening.

Occasionally, a cardiomyopathy may be associated with the skeletal myopathy (Meier et al., 1984; Stoessl et al., 1985; van Antwerpen et al., 1988). The electromyogram is usually myopathic; serum creatine kinase activity may be normal or mildly elevated.

Morphologically, the nemaline or rod body is the crucial structural abnormality; it may be seen in a wide range of muscle fibres and has the same structure in all the different clinical forms (Fig. 26.3a). It was first observed in 1958 by Dr R. D. K. Reye at the Royal Alexandra Hospital for Children, Sydney, in paraffin sections (Goebel and Lenard, 1992), before the first publication on nemaline myopathy (Shy et al., 1963). The nemaline rod has features of the Z disc both in its structure and in its protein content; immunohistochemistry demonstrates the presence of α-actinin, an intrinsic component of the Z disc. Small rods may still be in contact with the original Z discs but, more often, rods of various size and shape may cluster in the subsarcolemmal area of the muscle fibre or be scattered across the fibre. When the rods are in clusters, the regular sarcomeres

are not in evidence, but often actin or thin filaments are still attached to the rods. Nemaline bodies may ubiquitously be present in muscle fibres, including those of the diaphragm, and they may increase during the course of the disease (Bergmann et al., 1995). In cardiac muscle, dark inclusions have been encountered in patients with nemaline myopathy and cardiomyopathy (Meier et al., 1984; Bergmann et al., 1995), but their Z disc nature, both structurally and immunohistochemically, has not convincingly been demonstrated. In a few instances, rods and cores have been seen within the same biopsied muscle specimen and even within the same muscle fibre (Pallagi et al., 1998).

Intranuclear rods have been observed in both the childhood and adult forms of nemaline myopathy, mostly as isolated rods, but occasionally as multiple inclusions (Goebel and Warlo, 1997; Goebel et al., 1997a). These rods contain α-actinin, as shown by immunoelectron microscopy (Fig. 26.3b), and are often much larger than sarcoplasmic rods. Occasionally, there might be sarcoplasmic invagination into the nuclei, which often appears lobulated or crenated around the sarcoplasmic rods, suggesting that one way intranuclear rods develop may be by sarcoplasmic

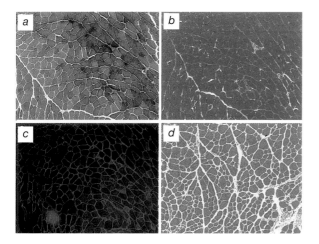

Fig. 19.25. Biochemical and histological rescue of *mdx* mouse muscle by delivery of the full-length dystrophin protein using third-generation adenoviral vectors. Sections are shown from a gastrocnemius muscle of an *mdx* mouse that had an intramuscular injection of an adenoviral construct at six days of age (AdDYSbeta-gal) (Clemens et al. 1996). (*a–c*) Muscle injected with the recombinant adenoviral construct. (*d*) Sham-injected muscle shows typical *mdx* histopathology. (*a*) Blue β-galactosidase staining is evident in the majority of muscle fibres, indicating successful delivery of the transgenes. (*c*) Dystrophin immunostaining shows the large majority of myofibres have biochemical rescue of dystrophin deficiency by the virus. (*b*) The histopathology of the virus-treated muscle shows nearly complete restoration of normal histology (compare with the contralateral sham leg (*d*)). (Taken from Clemens et al. (1996) with permission.)

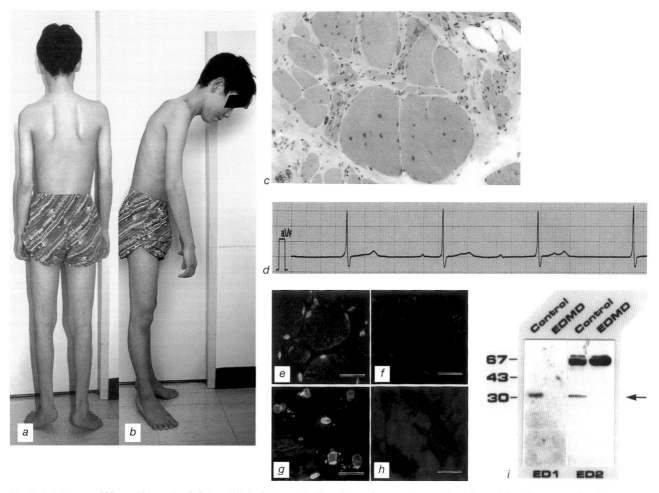

Fig. 23.1. A 14-year-old boy with emerin-deficient X-linked Emery–Dreifuss dystrophy (X-EDMD). (*a,b*) He has mild weakness atrophy of shoulder girdle and proximal part of the arms, and bilateral weakness of the anterior tibial and peroneal muscles, with normal strength of forearm, hand and proximal leg muscles. Note the limitation of his neck and spine flexion (*b*), and flexion contractures of the elbows. He shows toe-walking and cannot place his heels on the floor because of contractures in the Achilles tendons. (*c*) Skeletal muscle shows dystrophic changes with variation in fibre diameter, fibre splitting, increased connective tissue elements and internal nuclei. (*d*) The electrocardiograph shows a third-degree atrioventricular conduction block. (*e–h*) Emerin localizes at the nuclear membrane of control skeletal (*e*) and cardiac (*g*) muscle but is absent in X-EDMD skeletal (*f*) and cardiac (*h*) muscle. (*i*) Western blot test also shows deficiency of 34 kDa emerin in muscle.

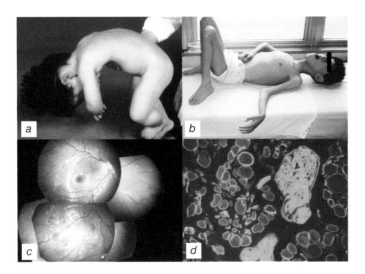

Fig. 25.7. Clinical appearance of Fukuyama congenital muscular dystrophy. (*a*) A one-year-old child with severe hypotonia. (*b*) An eight-year-old child with atrophy and contractures. (*c*) Examination of the fundus shows the irregular mottled grey appearance of the retina. (*d*) Skeletal muscle shows uneven and patchy staining for laminin-α2. (With permission from Dr M. Osawa (*a–c*) and Dr K. Arahata (*d*).)

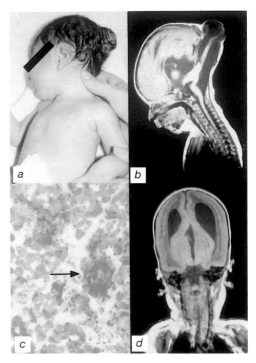

Fig. 25.9. A neonate with Walker Warburg syndrome. (*a,b*) There is an occipital encephalocoele (*a*), which contains rudimental cerebellar structures (*b*). (*c*) Skeletal muscle shows marked variation of fibre size and active muscle degeneration (stain for acid phosphatase). (*d*) Coronal MRI shows complete type II lissencephaly with irregular interdigitation of grey and white matter and hypoplasia of the pons.

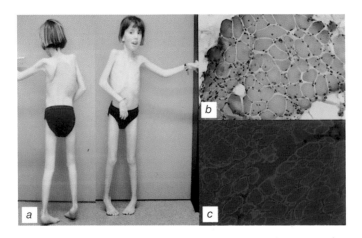

Fig. 25.10. A 10-year-old girl with congenital muscular dystrophy and rigid spine syndrome. Haplotype analysis was compatible with linkage to chromosome 1b35–36. (*a*) Note the contractures of ankles and elbows. Serum creatine kinase levels were normal. (*b*) Muscle biopsy was compatible with a dystrophic process without evidence of active necrosis (haematoxylin and eosin). (*c*) Laminin-α2 expression was normal.

Gomori-Trichrome

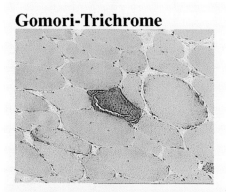

Succinate Dehydrogenase

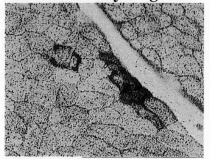

Cytochrome *c* Oxidase

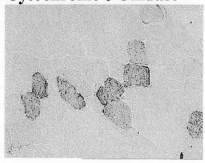

Fig. 29.2. Histochemical stains important in the diagnosis of diseases of oxidative phosphorylation. Ragged-red fibres are observed using the Gomori-Trichrome stain. The succinate dehydrogenase (SDH) reaction and the cytochrome *c* oxidase (COX) reaction are sensitive indicators of mitochondrial dysfunction. Abnormal myofibre segments are detected by focal increases in the SDH reaction and decreases in the COX reaction (COX-deficient fibres).

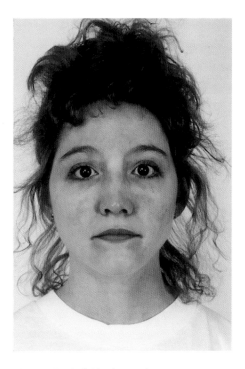

Fig. 31.1. Typical skin changes in a young woman with dermatomyositis. The heliotrope rash is prominent around the eyelids, forehead, bridge of the nose and cheeks. The 'misery' is clear in her expression.

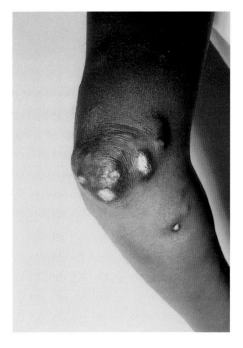

Fig. 31.4. Prominent subcutaneous calcification extends to the surface, with ulcerations and infection in a 26-year-old woman with dermatomyositis.

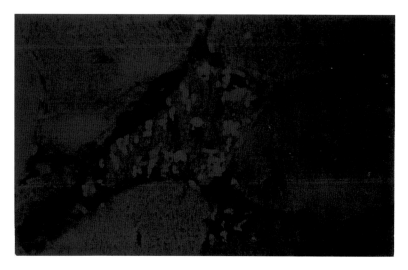

Fig. 31.11. Sporadic inclusion body myositis. A muscle fibre contains numerous congophylic fluorescent masses positive with Texas red optics. (Congo red, ×520.)

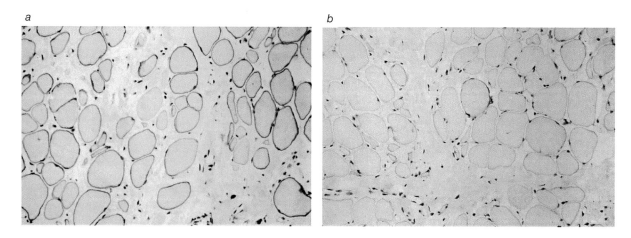

Fig. 35.9. Immunocytochemical analysis with dystrophin antibody (*a*) and α-sarcoglycan antibody (*b*) in a young girl with muscular dystrophy. Initial dystrophin immunostaining led to the provisional diagnosis of manifesting carrier of dystrophinopathy as the staining was patchy and reduced. Subsequent use of the α-sarcoglycan antibody showed much more complete loss of immunostaining and two α-sarcoglycan mutations were subsequently identified. This revised diagnosis was critical for genetic counselling.

invagination. However, crossing of the nuclear envelope by a rod body has never been documented.

The pathogenesis of rods is still unknown. Experimentally, rods have been produced – together with core-like features – after tenotomy (Shafiq et al., 1969; Karpati et al., 1972).

In addition to rods within the muscle fibres, type I fibre atrophy and type I fibre predominance, resembling fibre type disproportion, may be a typical histochemical feature. This fibre type disproportion pattern may also occur regionally without the presence of rods.

The aetiology of nemaline myopathy is still unclear. Genetically, an autosomal dominant form has been assigned to chromosome 1q21–23 (*NEM1*) marked by a mutation in the gene for α-tropomyosin (*TPM3*) (Laing et al., 1992, 1995). However, this has, so far, only been observed in one Australian family (Laing et al., 1992) and separately in one child (Beggs et al., 1998). In this Australian family, clinical symptoms developed during adolescence and progressed into adulthood. However, the majority of adult patients with late-onset nemaline myopathy appear to have sporadic rod myopathy (Palmucci et al., 1993).

The classic childhood form of nemaline myopathy, with little or no progression, appears to be an autosomal recessive trait and the gene locus has been assigned to chromosome 2q21.2–22 (Wallgren-Pettersson et al., 1995b), where mutations in the gene for nebulin have been documented (Pelin et al., 1999). A third gene at 1q42, *ACTA 1*, has shown several missense mutations in other patients with nemaline myopathy (Nowak et al., 1999).

Several workshops sponsored by ENMC (Wallgren-Pettersson and Laing, 1996; Wallgren-Pettersson et al., 1998) have defined diagnostic inclusion and exclusion criteria for nemaline myopathy. The ENMC has also formed a consortium to study the genetics of nemaline myopathy and a global registry for affected patients and families as the basis for future research.

Surplus protein myopathies

Mutation-related muscular dystrophies, the most intensely studied group of hereditary neuromuscular disorders, are marked by reduction or absence of specific proteins, for example dystrophin, sarcoglycans, merosin (laminin-2) or plectin. However, some hereditary and sporadic myopathies are characterized by an accumulation of excess protein within muscle fibres. It is not always clear whether the excess protein is a primary or secondary event in the myopathy.

Desmin-related myopathies

Several of the myopathies marked by a surplus of proteins, including the congenital myopathies of the cytoplasmic body type (Goebel et al., 1981), the spheroid body type (Goebel et al., 1978, 1997b), the sarcoplasmic body type (Edström et al., 1980), the granulofilamentous type (Fardeau et al., 1978) and a Mallory body-like inclusion type (Fidzianska et al., 1983), have been summarily termed 'myofibrillar myopathy' (de Bleecker et al., 1996b; Nakano et al., 1996). Clinically, affected patients and families show a wide spectrum of symptoms and of time of disease onset (Amato et al., 1998). Some forms become apparent in childhood and others in adulthood. Inheritance can be autosomal dominant or autosomal recessive and they can also occur sporadically. Three different groups can be distinguished on morphological, clinical and hereditary grounds (Goebel and Fardeau, 1997): (i) the inclusion body type comprising cytoplasmic bodies, spheroid bodies and sarcoplasmic bodies; (ii) the granulofilamentous type, and (iii) the type with Mallory body-like inclusions or hyaline plaques (Fidzianska et al., 1995). Clinically, the inclusion body type is rarely associated with a cardiomyopathy, whereas the granulofilamentous type appears almost always with an often life-threatening cardiomyopathy. The hyaline plaque type lacks cardiac involvement but shows severe respiratory dysfunction.

Morphologically, the inclusions show a diverse pattern ranging from distinct cytoplasmic bodies; comprising a granular amorphous core surrounded by a halo of intermediate-size filaments of desmin, to spheroid bodies, which are less distinctly separated into two components and tend to be larger (Fig. 26.4*a*), and even to cytoplasmic spheroid complexes (Halbig et al., 1991). These inclusions were also labelled hyaline lesions (de Bleecker et al., 1996b; Nakano et al., 1996; Amato et al., 1998). The granulofilamentous pattern, also described as nonhyaline or 'dappled' lesions (Nakano et al., 1996), is marked by a subsarcolemmal and intracellular mixture of granular material and filaments, which can be seen on cross- or longitudinal sections to traverse the muscle fibre in an irregular garland-type fashion. Not infrequently, both inclusions and granulofilaments occur together, prompting Nakano et al. (1996) and de Bleecker et al. (1996b) to apply the rather generic term myofibrillar myopathy (Sarnat, 1997; Amato et al., 1998) as regular sarcomeres are absent where these lesions appeared. Sometimes, filaments of the intermediate type are not very obvious, but numerous investigators have used immunostaining to show that desmin is an intrinsic component of the lesions. Desmin is a normal component of the intermediate filaments in skeletal and

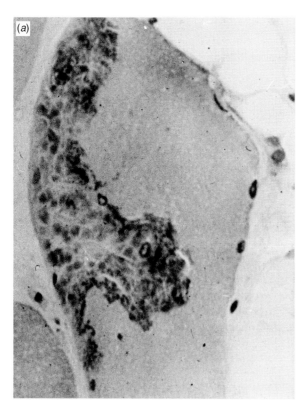

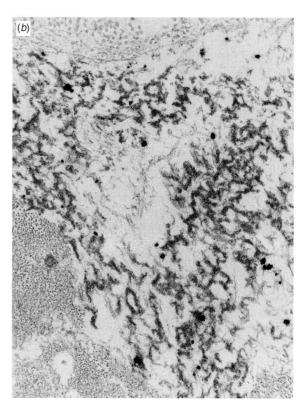

Fig. 26.4. Desmin-related myopathy. (*a*) A large cluster of spheroid bodies can be seen (modified trichrome stain, ×750). (*b*) The granulofilamentous material is demonstrated by labelling with antibody against dystrophin (×42000).

cardiac muscle as well as in certain smooth muscle cells. The consistent presence of desmin in these lesions led to terms such as desmin myopathy (Navarro et al., 1994; Ariza et al., 1995; Cameron et al., 1995; Baeta et al., 1996), desmin-related myopathy (Goebel, 1997) or desminopathy (Vajsar et al., 1993; Pellissier et al., 1996). In addition, a large number of other proteins has been localized to these lesions, including actin, vimentin and dystrophin (Fig. 26.4*b*) and proteins that are considered chaperone proteins (i.e. αB-crystallin and ubiquitin). In addition, proteins that are not considered to be regular components of normal muscle fibres, gelsolin, α_1-antichymotrypsin and several epitopes of the amyloid precursor protein, have been identified in these lesions (Table 26.1) (de Bleecker et al., 1996b; Goebel, 1998b).

With regard to the morphogenesis and pathogenesis of these lesions, it is worth noting that lesions comprising a granular component and cell type-specific intermediate filament are well known in other tissues and diseases. Rosenthal fibres of astrocytes comprise densely packed glial fibrillary acid protein-rich intermediate glial filaments and patches of granular material, the former containing the astrocyte-specific glial fibrillary acidic protein,

and αB-crystallin and even epitopes of β_{A4}-amyloid, α_1-antichymotrypsin and ubiquitin. Another such lesion is the intraneuronal Lewy body, which is marked by a granular core and a halo of intermediate filaments representing neurofilaments. Again, a spate of proteins has been documented in these Lewy bodies, including α-synuclein, which may be mutated in familial Parkinson disease (Polymeropoulos et al., 1997).

When skeletal muscle marked by 'myofibrillar myopathy' was found to contain a diverse number of proteins in structures that differed widely both morphologically and biochemically, impaired extralysosomal degradation of these proteins was suggested as a nonspecific or epiphenomenal cause. However, mutations in the gene for desmin have been found in patients with myopathies marked by desmin accumulation, both missense mutations (Goldfarb et al., 1998) and deletions (Muñoz-Mármol et al., 1998). These results were supported by studies showing the occurrence of an abnormal hyperphosphorylated desmin in a familial myopathy (Rappaport et al., 1988) and by studies showing two distinct desmin forms, a 49 kDa one in addition to the physiological 53 kDa form, in a distal myopathy (Lobrinus et al., 1998). Consequently,

Table 26.3. Proteins found in hereditary inclusion body myopathy

Ubiquitin
β-Amyloid precursor protein
Phosphorylated tau with antibodies: SM1-31, AT8
Prion protein
Neuronal nitric oxide synthase
Inducible nitric oxide synthase
Apolipoprotein
Nitrotyrosine
Presenilin 1 (residues detected with six antibodies)

Source: Askanas and Engel (1998) and Askanas et al. (1998).

desmin-related myopathy, for example β_{A4}-amyloid and α_1-antichymotrypsin.

A further disease in which a physiological protein occurs in excess is oculopharyngeal muscular dystrophy, where nuclear polyA-binding protein accumulates in muscle fibre nuclei as a result of expansion of GCG triplets in its gene (Brais et al., 1998).

Other congenital myopathies

At a recent ENMC workshop on structural congenital myopathies (Goebel and Anderson, 1999), a consortium was formed to deal with rarer congenital myopathies excluding those discussed above. This includes some 12 entities varying from probable to doubtful as nosological entities. Hyaline body myopathy and actin filament myopathy are included in this consortium but have been discussed already above. Doubtful or questionable congenital myopathies largely described by single observers are lamellar body myopathy (Goebel and Anderson, 1999), broad A-band myopathy (Mrak et al., 1993, 1996) and Zebra body myopathy (Lake and Wilson, 1975) whereas several sporadic cases have been studied for cap disease (Fidzianka et al., 1981; Goebel and Anderson, 1999) and reducing body myopathy (Kiyomoto et al., 1995).

Although small cores resembling multicores or minicores may occur in central core disease, multicore or minicore disease is considered a separate condition marked by small morphologically similar lesions within muscle fibres that resemble nonstructured cores and are devoid of mitochondria. The disorder is characterized by proximal weakness, including the face and neck muscles and extraocular muscles, and by ptosis. It is usually observed in children, but it has been documented in adulthood (Bonnette et al., 1974) and associated with respiratory failure (Zeman

et al., 1997). Histopathologically, type I fibre predominance and type I fibre hypotrophy may also be present. When there are increased numbers of central nuclei, it may be difficult to differentiate multi/minicore disease from centronuclear myopathy; both conditions clinically can involve ptosis and cardiomyopathy has been found associated with multi/minicore disease (Shuaib et al., 1988; Tein et al., 1999) and centronuclear myopathy (Verhiest et al., 1976; Gospe et al., 1987). The association of minicore disease with a defect in short-chain acyl-CoA dehydrogenase may represent a unique observation (Tein et al., 1999).

Cylindrical spirals myopathy may occur at all ages, having been observed in children (Goebel et al., 1995a) and adults (Rapuzzi et al., 1995). It has an autosomal dominant mode of inheritance (Tarantuto et al., 1991) and often gives rise to myalgia or cramps; there may also be central nervous system association (Goebel et al., 1995a; Baker et al., 1997). Cylindrical spirals, aggregating subsarcolemmally, are concentrically arranged lamellae, sometimes resembling tubular aggregates, which suggests origin from the sarcotubular system. As aggregates, they appear bright red in colour in the modified trichrome-stained preparation, but they lack oxidative and myofibrillar ATPase activities. Immunohistochemically no specific protein has been found enriched in this condition (Table 26.4).

While tubular aggegates may occur together with cylindrical spirals in cylindrical spirals myopathy (Danon et al., 1989), the same association has not been seen in tubular aggregate myopathies, which may show an autosomal mode of inheritance (Rohkamm et al., 1983; Goebel and Anderson, 1999) and are marked by slowly progressive weakness that originates in childhood. Tubular aggregates were seen in up to 98% of muscle fibres. Myalgia may be a clinical symptom in some patients with this condition, but tubular aggregates may also be a nonspecific feature in a variety of neuromuscular disorders including hyperkalaemic periodic paralysis, congenital neuromuscular transmission disorders or myasthenic syndromes.

A further peculiar disorder has been observed in young males and is marked by mental retardation, cardiomyopathy and vacuoles within muscle fibres (Muntoni et al., 1994; Goebel and Anderson, 1999). These vacuoles actually represented extracellular space within muscle fibres lined by sarcolemma, with positive immunostaining for the sarcolemmal proteins dystrophin, spectrin, α-sarcoglycan and β-dystroglycan as well as for the extracellular matrix protein laminin as the $\alpha2$-, $\beta1$- and $\gamma1$-chains. The possible X-linked inheritance (although the gene locus has not yet

Table 26.4. Proteins not detected by immunostaining in rare myopathies

Condition	Proteins not detectable by immunostaining	Reference
Cylindrical spirals myopathy	Actin, α-actinin, desmin, dystrophin, laminin, nebulin, α- and β-spectrin, subunits of cytochrome c oxidase, tropomyosin, troponin T, α- and β-tubulin, utrophin, vimentin, vinculin	Rapuzzi et al. (1995)
Reducing body myopathy	α-Actinin, nuclear antigens (as detected by antinuclear antibodies), chromosomal proteins, desmin, dystrophin, laminin, spectrin, ubiquitin (10% of fibres positive), vimentin	Kiyomoto et al. (1995)

been identified) and clinical features strongly resemble lysosomal glycogen storage disease without acid maltase deficiency, also called Danon disease (Danon et al., 1981; Usuki et al., 1994). However, in the latter condition the vacuoles are membrane bound, contain glycogen and are truely located intracellularly.

Other morphological features seen in myopathies are of undetermined origin. Fingerprint bodies are parallel concentrically arranged lamellae that are seen in familial fingerprint body myopathy (Goebel and Anderson, 1999) and, nonspecifically, in other neuromuscular disorders. Zebra bodies have also been described in a myopathy. These are parallel alternating bands of light filamentous and dark granular material somewhat resembling Z discs, with adjacent actin or thin filaments but without A bands and thick or myosin filaments. The nosological significance of zebra bodies is still unclear as they are seen nonspecifically in other well-defined neuromuscular disorders in addition to being normal constituents of extraocular muscles and the myotendinous junctions of skeletal muscles. Both fingerprint bodies and zebra bodies can only be identified by electron microscopy.

A reducing body myopathy has been identified by the occurrence of non-membrane-bound granular bodies, reducing bodies, that are strongly positive with the menadione-linked α-glycerophosphate dehydrogenase reaction even without the substrate in the preparation, giving reduction of tetrazolium nitroblue. These bodies are often found close to and even encircling the muscle fibre nucleus are of completely unknown origin. Immunostain analysis has failed to detect a range of muscle proteins in these reducing bodies (Table 26.4) (Kiyomoto et al., 1995). They have been seen in muscle tissues of children suffering from a rapidly progressive fatal myopathy but are also found in benign myopathic conditions. Moreover, they have not infrequently been seen in conjunction with cytoplasmic bodies in a so-called mixed congenital myopathy (Bertini et al., 1994; Goebel et al., 1995b; Goebel, 1998b).

Nonstructural congenital myopathies

Fibre type disproportion is a morphological pattern characterized by type I fibre predominance and type I fibre atrophy/hypotrophy. It may occur as a nonspecific feature in a variety of neuromuscular disorders (Schröder, 1996), particularly in early myotonic dystrophy, in globoid cell and metachromatic leukodystrophies (indicating subtle impaired innervation) and in certain structural congenital myopathies including nemaline myopathy, mini/multicore disease and centronuclear myopathy. It is the hallmark in a condition that has been dubbed congenital fibre type disproportion which is usually observed as a benign, but sometimes more severe, disorder marked by respiratory problems in childhood. Congenital fibre type disproportion has been transmitted in an autosomal dominant (Fardeau et al., 1975) and recessive (Jaffe et al., 1988) manner. In one child, fibre type disproportion as a component of an unstructured congenital myopathy was associated with a t(10;17) translocation (Gerdes et al., 1994). Some children who were originally diagnosed clinically as well as by biopsy as having congenital fibre type disproportion later were found to have other neuromuscular diseases, for example centronuclear myopathy (Danon et al., 1997). Fibre type disproportion may also be a nonspecific finding in denervation of early infancy, for example in infantile spinal muscular atrophy. Consequently, at present, the concept of congenital fibre type disproportion as a separate nosological entity appears somewhat tenuous.

Other nonstructured abnormalities within muscle biopsy specimens marked by histochemical abnormalities may be selective type I fibre hypotrophy, with or without central nuclei, type II fibre hypotrophy (Yoshioka et al., 1987) or lack of fibre type differentiation presenting as fibre type uniformity (Jung et al., 1997). Just as fibre type disproportion can occur in nemaline myopathy in certain muscles with or without focal rod formation, fibre type uniformity, usually of type I, may occur in central core disease in individual biopsy specimens that do not have cores (Fig. 26.1*b*).

Acknowledgement

Support by the Deutsche Gesellschaft für Muskelkranke, Freiburg/Germany, the European Neuromuscular Center (ENMC), Baarn/the Netherlands and the 'MAIFOR' programme, Johannes Gutenberg University, Mainz/Germany as well as photographic aid by Mrs I. Warlo and editorial assistance by Mrs A. Wöber are gratefully acknowledged.

References

Amato, A. A., Kagan-Hallet, K., Jackson, C. E. et al. (1998). The wide spectrum of myofibrillar myopathy suggests a multifactorial etiology and pathogenesis. *Neurology* **51**, 1646–1655.

Ariza, A., Coll, J., Fernández-Figueras, M. T. et al. (1995). Desmin myopathy: a multisystem disorder involving skeletal, cardiac, and smooth muscle. *Hum. Pathol.* **26**, 1032–1037.

Askanas, V. and Engel, W. K. (1998). Sporadic inclusion-body myositis and hereditary inclusion-body myopathies: current concepts of diagnosis and pathogenesis. *Curr. Opin. Rheumatol.* **10**, 520–542.

Askanas, V., Engel, W. K., Yang, C.-C., Alvarez, R. B., Lee, V. M.-Y. and Wisniewski, T. (1998). Light and electron microscopic immunolocalization of presenilin 1 in abnormal muscle fibers of patients with sporadic inclusion-body myositis and autosomal-recessive inclusion-body myopathy. *Am. J. Pathol.* **152**, 889–895.

Baeta, A. M., Figarella-Branger, D., Bille-Turc, F., Lepidi, H. and Pellissier, J.-F. (1996). Familial desmin myopathies and cytoplasmic body myopathies. *Acta Neuropathol. (Berlin)* **92**, 499–510.

Baker, N. S., Sarnat, H. B., Jack, R. M., Patterson, K., Shaw, D. W. and Herndon, S. P. (1997). D-2-Hydroxyglutaric aciduria: hypotonia, cortical blindness, seizures, cardiomyopathy, and cylindrical spirals in skeletal muscle. *J. Child Neurol.* **12**, 31–36.

Barohn, R. J., Brumback, R. A. and Mendell, J. R. (1994). Hyaline body myopathy. *Neuromusc. Disord.* **4**, 257–262.

Barth, P. G. and Dubowitz, V. (1998). X-linked myotubular myopathy – a long-term follow-up study. *Eur. J. Ped. Neurol.* **1**, 49–56.

Barth, P. G., van Wijngaarden, G. K. and Bethlem, J. (1975). X-linked myotubular myopathy with fatal neonatal asphyxia. *Neurology* **25**, 531–536.

Beggs, A. H., Wattanasirichaigoon, D., Swoboda, K. J. et al. (1998). Mutation analysis in nemaline myopathy. *Muscle Nerve* **Suppl. 7**, S80.

Bergmann, M., Kamarampaka, M., Kuchelmeister, K., Klein, H. and Koch, H. (1995). Nemaline myopathy: two autopsy reports. *Childs Nerv. Syst.* **11**, 610–615.

Bertini, E., Salviati, G., Apollo, F. et al. (1994). Reducing body myopathy and desmin storage in skeletal muscle: morphological and biochemical findings. *Acta Neuropathol. (Berlin)* **87**, 106–112.

Bonnette, H., Roelofs, R. and Olson, W. H. (1974). Multicore disease: report of a case with onset in middle age. *Neurology* **24**, 1039–1044.

Bornemann, A., Bloch, P., Petersen, M. and Schmalbruch, H. (1996). Fatal congenital myopathy with actin filament deposits. *Acta Neuropathologica (Berlin)* **92**, 104–108.

Brais, B., Bouchard, J.-P., Xie, Y.-G. et al. (1998). Short GCG expansions in the PABP2 gene cause oculopharyngeal muscular dystrophy. [Letter] *Nat. Genet.* **18**, 164–167.

Cameron, C. H. S., Mirakhur, M. and Allen, I. V. (1995). Desmin myopathy with cardiomyopathy. *Acta Neuropathol. (Berlin)* **89**, 560–566.

Cancilla, P. A., Kalyanaraman, K., Verity, M. A., Munsat, T. and Pearson, C. M. (1971). Familial myopathy with probable lysis of myofibrils in type I fibres. *Neurology* **21**, 579–585.

Ceuterick, C., Martin, J.-J. and Martens, C. (1993). Hyaline bodies in skeletal muscle of a patient with a mild chronic nonprogressive congenital myopathy. *Clin. Neuropathol.* **12**, 79–83.

Cui, X., de Vivo, I., Slany, R., Miyamoto, A., Firestein, R. and Cleary, M. L. (1998). Association of SET domain and myotubularin-related proteins modulates growth control. *Nat. Genet.* **18**, 331–337.

Danon, M. J., Oh, S. J., DiMauro, S. et al. (1981). Lysosomal glycogen storage disease with normal acid maltase. *Neurology* **31**, 51–57.

Danon, M. J., Carpenter, S. and Harati, Y. (1989). Muscle pain associated with tubular aggregates and structures resembling cylindrical spirals. *Muscle Nerve* **12**, 265–272.

Danon, M. J., Giometti, C. S., Manaligod, J. R. and Swisher, C. (1997). Sequential muscle biopsy changes in a case of congenital myopathy. *Muscle Nerve* **20**, 561–569.

de Angelis, M. S., Palmucci, L., Leone, M. and Doriguzzi, C. (1991). Centronuclear myopathy: clinical, morphological and genetic characters. A review of 288 cases. *J. Neurolog. Sci.* **103**, 2–9.

de Bleecker, J. L., Ertl, B. B. and Engel, A. G. (1996a). Patterns of abnormal protein expression in target formations and unstructured cores. *Neuromusc. Disord.* **6**, 339–349.

de Bleecker, J. L., Engel, A. G. and Ertl, B. B. (1996b). Myofibrillar myopathy with abnormal foci of desmin positivity. II. Immunocytochemical analysis reveals accumulation of multiple other proteins. *J. Neuropathol. Exp. Neurol.* **55**, 563–577.

de Gouyon, B. M., Zhao, W., Laporte, J., Mandel, J.-J., Metzenberg, A. and Herman, G. E. (1997). Characterization of mutations in the myotubularin gene in twenty six patients with X-linked myotubular myopathy. *Hum. Mol. Genet.* **6**, 1499–1504.

Dubowitz, V. (1969). The 'new' myopathies. *Neuropediatrics* **1**, 137–148.

Dubowitz, V. (1985). *Muscle Biopsy: A Practical Approach.* London: Baillière Tindall.

Edström, L., Thornell, L.-E. and Eriksson, A. (1980). A new type of hereditary distal myopathy with characteristic sarcoplasmic bodies and intermediate (skeletin) filaments. *J. Neurolog. Sci.* **47**, 171–190.

Emery, A. E. H. (1997). *Diagnostic Criteria for Neuromuscular Disorders.* London: Royal Society of Medicine Press.

Fardeau, M., Harpey, J.-P., Caille, B. and Lafourcade, J. (1975). Hypotonies neo-natales avec disproportion congenitale des differents types de fibre musculaire, et petitesse relative des fibres de type I. *Arch. Franç. Ped.* **32**, 901–914.

Fardeau, M., Godet-Guillain, J., Tomé, F. S. M. et al. (1978). Une nouvelle affection musculaire familiale, définie par l'accumulation intra-sarco-plasmique d'un matériel granulo-filamenteux dense en microscopie électronique. *Rev. Neurolog. (Paris)* **134**, 411–425.

Fidzianska, A., Badurska, B., Ryniewicz, B. and Dembek, I. (1981). 'Cap disease': new congenital myopathy. *Neurology* **31**, 1113–1120.

Fidzianska, A., Goebel, H. H., Osborn, M., Lenard, H. G., Osse, G. and Langenbeck, U. (1983). Mallory body-like inclusions in a hereditary congenital neuromuscular disease. *Muscle Nerve* **6**, 195–200.

Fidzianska, A., Ryniewicz, B., Barcikowska, M. and Goebel, H. H. (1995). A new familial congenital myopathy in children with desmin and dystrophin reacting plaques. *J. Neurolog. Sci.* **131**, 88–95.

Figarella-Branger, D., Calore, E. E., Boucraut, J., Bianco, N., Rougon, G. and Pellissier, J. F. (1992). Expression of cell surface and cytoskeleton developmentally regulated proteins in adult centronuclear myopathies. *J. Neurolog. Sci.* **109**, 69–76.

Gardner-Medwin, D. (1994). Neuromuscular disorders in infancy and childhood. In: *Disorders of Voluntary Muscle*, 6th edn, Ch. 21, eds. J. Walton, G. Karpati, and D. Hilton-Jones, pp. 781–835. Edinburgh: Churchill Livingstone.

Gerdes, A. M., Petersen, M. B., Schrøder, H. D., Wulff, K. and Brøndum-Nielsen, K. (1994). Congenital myopathy with fibre type disproportion: a family with a chromosomal translocation t(10;17) may indicate gene regions. *Clin. Genet.* **45**, 11–16.

Goebel, H. H. (1986). Neuropathological aspects of congenital myopathies. *Prog. Neuropathol.* **6**, 231–262.

Goebel, H. H. (1996). Congenital myopathies. *Semin. Ped. Neurol.* **3**, 152–161.

Goebel, H. H. (1997). Desmin-related myopathies. *Curr. Opin. Neurol.* **10**, 426–429.

Goebel, H. H. (1998a). Congenital myopathies with inclusion bodies: a brief review. *Neuromusc. Disord.* **8**, 162–168.

Goebel, H. H. (1998b). Desminopathies. In *Neuromuscular Disorders: Clinical and Molecular Genetics*, ed. A. E. H. Emery, pp. 217–246. New York: John Wiley and Sons.

Goebel, H. H. and Anderson, J. (1999). Workshop report: the 56th European Neuromuscular Centre (ENMC)-sponsored international workshop – structural congenital myopathies (excluding nemaline myopathy, myotubular myopathy and desminopathies). *Neuromusc. Disord.* **9**, 50–57.

Goebel, H. H. and Fardeau, M. (1995). Desmin in myology. *Neuromusc. Disord.* **5**, 161–166.

Goebel, H. H. and Fardeau, M. (1996). Workshop report: the 36th ENMC sponsored international workshop – familial desmin-related myopathies and cardiomyopathies – from myopathology to molecular and clinical genetics. *Neuromusc. Disord.* **6**, 383–388.

Goebel, H. H. and Fardeau, M. (1997). Desminopathies. In: *Diagnostic Criteria for Neuromuscular Disorders*, ed. A. E. H. Emery, pp. 75–79. London: Royal Society of Medicine Press.

Goebel, H. H. and Fidzianska, A. (1996). Classification of congenital myopathies. In *Handbook of Muscle Disease*, Ch. 14, ed. R. J. M. Lane, pp. 165–176. New York: Marcel Dekker.

Goebel, H. H. and Lenard, H. G. (1992). Congenital myopathies. In: *Handbook of Clinical Neurology*, Vol. 18/62, eds. L. P. Rowland and S. DiMauro, pp. 331–367. Amsterdam: Elsevier Science.

Goebel, H. H. and Warlo, I. (1997). Nemaline myopathy with intranuclear rods – intranuclear rod myopathy. *Neuromusc. Disord.* **7**, 13–19.

Goebel, H. H., Muller, J., Gillen, H. W. and Merritt, A. D. (1978). Autosomal dominant 'spheroid body myopathy'. *Muscle Nerve* **1**, 14–26.

Goebel, H. H., Schloon, H. and Lenard, H. G. (1981). Congenital myopathy with cytoplasmic bodies. *Neuropediatrics* **12**, 166–180.

Goebel, H. H., Meinck, H. M., Reinecke, M., Schimrigk, K. and Mielke, U. (1984). Centronuclear myopathy with special consideration of the adult form. *Eur. Neurol.* **23**, 425–434.

Goebel, H. H., Meier, W. and Rellensmann, G. (1995a). The nosological connotation of cylindrical spiral myopathy. *Electron. J. Pathol. Histol.* **1.3**, 953–08.txt.

Goebel, H. H., Voit, T. and Schober, R. (1995b). Combined cytoplasmic body and reducing body myopathy – a mixed congenital myopathy. *J. Neuropathol. Exp. Neurol.* **54**, 453.

Goebel, H. H., Piirsoo, A., Warlo, I., Schofer, O., Kehr, S. and Gaude, M. (1997a). Infantile intranuclear rod myopathy. *J. Child Neurol.* **12**, 22–30.

Goebel, H. H., D'Agostino, A. N., Wilson, J. et al. (1997b). Spheroid body myopathy – revisited. *Muscle Nerve* **20**, 1127–1136.

Goebel, H. H., Anderson, J. R., Hübner, C., Oexle, K. and Warlo, I. (1997c). Congenital myopathy with excess of thin myofilaments. *Neuromusc. Disord.* **7**, 160–168.

Goldfarb, L. G., Park, K.-Y., Cervenáková, S. et al. (1998). Missense mutations in desmin associated with familial cardiac and skeletal myopathy. [Letter] *Nat. Genet.* **19**, 402–403.

Gospe, S. M., Jr, Armstrong, D. L., Gresik, M. V. and Hawkins, H. K. (1987). Life-threatening congestive heart failure as the presentation of centronuclear myopathy. *Pediatr. Neurol.* **3**, 117–120.

Haan, E. A., Freemantle, C. J., McCure, J. A., Friend, K. L. and Mulley, J. C. (1990). Assignment of the gene for central core disease to chromosome 19. *Hum. Genet.* **86**, 187–190.

Halbig, L., Goebel, H. H., Hopf, H. C. and Moll, R. (1991). Spheroid-cytoplasmic complexes in a congenital myopathy. *Rev. Neurolog. (Paris)* **147**, 300–307.

Jaffe, M., Shapira, J. and Borochowitz, Z. (1988). Familial congenital fibre type disproportion (CFTD) with an autosomal recessive inheritance. *Clin. Genet.* **33**, 33–37.

Jung, E.-Y., Hattori, H., Higuchi, Y., Mitsuyoshi, I. and Kanda, T. (1997). Brain atrophy in congenital neuromuscular disease with uniform type 1 fibers. *Pediatr. Neurol.* **16**, 56–58.

Karpati, G., Carpenter, S. and Eisen, A. A. (1972). Experimental core-like lesions and nemaline rods: a correlative morphological and physiological study. *Arch. Neurol.* **27**, 237–251.

Kausch, K., Lehmann-Horn, F., Janka, M., Wieringa, B., Grimm, T. and Müller, C. R. (1991). Evidence for linkage of the central core disease locus to the proximal long arm of human chromosome 19. *Genomics* **10**, 765–769.

Kiyomoto, B. H., Murakami, N., Kobayashi, Y. et al. (1995). Fatal reducing body myopathy: ultrastructural and immunohistochemical observations. *J. Neurolog. Sci.* **128**, 58–65.

Laing, N. G., Majda, B. T., Akkari, P. A. et al. (1992). Assignment of a gene (*NEM1*) for autosomal-dominant nemaline myopathy to chromosome 1. *Am. J. Hum. Genet.* **50**, 576–583.

Laing, N. G., Wilton, S. D., Akkari, P. A. et al. (1995). A mutation in the alpha-tropomyosin gene *TPM3* associated with autosomal dominant nemaline myopathy. *Nat. Genet.* **9**, 75–79.

Lake, B. D. and Wilson, J. (1975). Zebra body myopathy. *J. Neurolog. Sci.* **24**, 437–446.

Lammens, M., Moerman, P., Fryns, J. P. et al. (1997). Fetal akinesia sequence caused by nemaline myopathy. *Neuropediatrics* **28**, 116–119.

Lamont, P. J., Dubowitz, V., Landon, D. N., Davis, M. and Morgan-Hughes, J. A. (1998). Fifty year follow-up of a patient with central core disease shows slow but definite progression. *Neuromusc. Disord.* **8**, 385–391.

Laporte, J., Hu, L. J., Kretz, C. et al. (1996). A gene mutated in X-linked myotubular myopathy defines a new putative tyrosine phosphatase family conserved in yeast. *Nat. Genet.* **13**, 175–182.

Lobrinus, J. A., Janzer, R. C., Kuntzer, T. et al. (1998). Familial cardiomyopathy and distal myopathy with abnormal desmin accumulation and migration. *Neuromusc. Disord.* **8**, 77–86.

Manzur, A. Y., Sewry, C. A., Zirpin, J., Dubowitz, V. and Muntoni, F. (1998). A severe clinical and pathological variant of central core disease with possible autosomal recessive inheritance. *Neuromusc. Disord.* **8**, 467–473.

Masuzugawa, S., Kuzuhara, S., Narita, Y., Naito, Y., Taniguchi, A. and Ibi, T. (1997). Autosomal dominant hyaline body myopathy presenting as scapuloperoneal syndrome: clinical features and muscle patholoy. *Neurology* **48**, 253–257.

Meier, C. W., Voellmy, W., Gertsch, M., Zimmermann, A. and Geissbühler, J. (1984). Nemaline myopathy appearing in adults as cardiomyopathy: a clinicopathologic study. *Arch. Neurol.* **41**, 443–445.

Melberg, A., Oldfors, A., Blomström-Lundqvist, C. et al. (1999). Autosomal dominant myofibrillar myopathy with arrhythmogenic right ventricular cardiomyopathy linked to chromosome 10q. *Ann. Neurol.* **46**, 684–692.

Misra, A. K., Menon, N. K. and Mishra, S. K. (1992). Abnormal distribution of desmin and vimentin in myofibers in adult onset myotubular myopathy. *Muscle Nerve* **15**, 1246–1252.

Morgan-Hughes, J. A., Brett, E. M., Lake, B. D. and Tomé, F. M. S. (1973). Central core disease or not? Observations on a family with non-progressive myopathy. *Brain* **96**, 527–536.

Mrak, R. E., Lange, B. and Brodsky, M. C. (1993). Broad A bands of striated muscle in Leber's congenital amaurosis: a new congenital myopathy? *Neurology* **43**, 838–841.

Mrak, R. E., Griebel, M. and Brodsky, M. C. (1996). Broad A band disease: a new, benign congenital myopathy. *Muscle and Nerve* **19**, 587–594.

Muñoz-Mármol, A. M., Strasser, G., Isamat, M. et al. (1998). A dysfunctional desmin mutation in a patient with severe generalized myopathy. *Proc. Natl. Acad. Sci. USA* **95**, 11312–11317.

Muntoni, F., Catani, G., Mateddu, A. et al. (1994). Familial cardiomyopathy, mental retardation and myopathy associated wtih desmin-type intermediate filaments. *Neuromusc. Disord.* **4**, 233–241.

Nagai, T., Tsuchiya, Y., Maruyama, A., Takemitsu, M. and Nonaka, I. (1994). Scoliosis associated with central core disease. *Brain Dev.* **16**, 150–152.

Nakano, S., Engel, A. G., Waclawik, A. J., Emslie-Smith, A. M. and Busis, N. A. (1996). Myofibrillar myopathy with abnormal foci of desmin positivity. I. Light and electron microscopy analysis of 10 cases. *J. Neuropathol. Exp. Neurol.* **55**, 549–562.

Navarro, C., Teijeira, S., Fernández, J. M., Gámez, J. and Cervera, C. (1994). Desmin myopathy. Report of two cases with different clinical phenotype and review of literature. *Clin. Neuropathol.* **13**, 105.

Nowak, K. J., Wattanasirichaigoon, D., Goebel, H. H. et al. (1999). Mutations in the skeletal muscle α-actin gene in patients with actin myopathy and nemaline myopathy. *Nat. Genet.* **23**, 208–212.

Pallagi, E., Molnár, M., Molnár, P. and Diószeghy, P. (1998). Central core and nemaline rods in the same patient. *Acta Neuropathol. (Berlin)* **96**, 211–214.

Palmucci, L., Doriguzzi, C., Mongini, T. and Chiadò-Piat, L. (1993). Adult onset nemaline myopathy: a distinct nosologic entity? *Clin. Neuropathol.* **12**, 153–155.

Pelin, K., Hipelä, P., Sewry, C. et al. (1999). Mutations in the nebulin gene associated with autosomal recessive nemaline myopathy. *Proc. Natl. Acad. Sci. USA* **96**, 2305–2310.

Pellissier, J. F., Baeta, A. M., Cassote, E. and Figarella-Branger, D. (1996). Familial desmin myopathies. *Neuropathol. Appl. Neurobiol.* **22**(Suppl. 1), 109.

Polymeropoulos, M. H., Levedan, C., Leroy, E. et al. (1997). Mutation in the alpha-synuclein gene identified in families with Parkinson's disease. *Science* **276**, 2045–2047.

Quane, K. A., Healy, J. M. S., Keating, K. E. et al. (1993). Mutations in the ryanodine receptor gene in central core disease and malignant hyperthermia. *Nat. Genet.* **5**, 51–55.

Rappaport, L., Contard, F., Samuel, J. L. et al. (1988). Storage of phosphorylated desmin in a familial myopathy. *FEBS Lett.* **231**, 421–425.

Rapuzzi, S., Prelle, A., Moggio, M. et al. (1995). High serum creatine kinase levels associated with cylindrical spirals at muscle biopsy. *Acta Neuropathol. (Berlin)* **90**, 660–664.

Rohkamm, R., Boxler, K., Ricker, K. and Jerusalem, F. (1983). A dominantly inherited myopathy with excessive tubular aggregates. *Neurology* **33**, 331–336.

Sarnat, H. B. (1990). Myotubular myopathy: arrest of morphogenesis of myofibres associated with persistence of fetal vimentin and desmin. *Can. J. Neurolog. Sci.* **17**, 109–123.

Sarnat, H. B. (1997). Myofibrillar myopathy in infancy and childhood: five cases in two families of an unclassified congenital myopathy. *J. Child Neurol.* **12**, 132–133.

Sawchak, J. A., Sher, J. H., Norman, M. G., Kula, R. W. and Shafiq, S. A. (1991). Centronuclear myopathy heterogeneity: distinction of clinical types by myosin isoform patterns. *Neurology* **41**, 135–140.

Schröder, J. M. (1996). Congenital fibre type disproportion. In: *Handbook of Muscle Disease*, Ch. 16, ed. R. J. M. Lane, pp. 195–200. New York: Marcel Dekker.

Sciot, R., Ceuterick, C., Lammens, M., Dubois, B., Robbenrecht, W. and Dom, R. (1997). Hyaline body myopathy. *Acta Neurolog. Belg.* **97**, 54.

Shafiq, S. A., Gorycki M. A., Asiedu, S. A. and Milhorat, A. T. (1969). Tenotomy: effect on the fine structure of the soleus of the rat. *Arch. Neurol.* **20**, 625–633.

Sher, J. H., Rimalovski, A. B., Athanassiades, T. J. and Aronson, S. M. (1967). Familial centronuclear myopathy: a clinical and pathological study. *Neurology* **17**, 727–742.

Shuaib, A., Martin, J. M. E., Mitchell, B. and Brownell, K. W. (1988). Multicore myopathy: not always a benign entity. *Can. J. Neurolog. Sci.* **15**, 10–14.

Shy, G. M. and Magee, K. R. (1956). A new congenital non-progressive myopathy. *Brain* **79**, 610–621.

Shy, G. M., Engel, W. K., Somers, J. E. and Wanko, T. (1963). Nemaline myopathy. A new congenital myopathy. *Brain* **79**, 793–810.

Spiro, A. J., Shy, G. M. and Gonatas, N. K. (1966). Myotubular myopathy. *Arch. Neurol.* **14**, 1–14.

Stoessl, A. J., Hahn, A. F., Malott, D., Jones, D. T. and Silver, M. D. (1985). Nemaline myopathy with associated cardiomyopathy. *Arch. Neurol.* **42**, 1084–1086.

Tanner, S. M., Schneider, V., Thomas, N. S. T., Clarke, A., Lazarou, L. and Liechti-Gallati, S. (1999). Characterization of 34 novel and six known *MTM1* gene mutations in 47 unrelated X-linked myotubular myopathy patients. *Neuromusc. Disord.* **9**, 41–49.

Tarantuto, A. L., Matteucci, M., Barreiro, C., Saccolitti, M. and Sevlever, G. (1991). Autosomal dominant neuromuscular disease with cylindrical spirals. *Neuromusc. Disord.* **1**, 433–441.

Tein, I., Haslam, R. H. A., Rhead, W. J., Bennett, M. J., Becker, L. E. and Vockley, J. (1999). Short-chain acyl-CoA dehydrogenase deficiency. A cause of ophthalmoplegia and multicore myopathy. *Neurology* **52**, 366–372.

Thomas, N. and Wallgren-Pettersson, C. (1996). Workshop report; the 33rd ENMC sponsored international workshop – X-linked myotubular myopathy. *Neuromusc. Disord.* **6**, 129–132.

Topaloglu, H., Gögüs, S., Yalaz, K., Kücükali, T. and Seradoglu, A. (1994). Two siblings with nemaline myopathy presenting with rigid spine syndrome. *Neuromusc. Disord.* **4**, 263–267.

Usuki, F., Takenaga, S., Higuchi, I., Kashio, N., Nakagawa, M. and Osame, M. (1994). Morphologic findings in biopsied skeletal muscle and cultured fibroblasts from a female patient with

Danon's disease (lysosomal glycogen storage disease without acid maltase deficiency). *J. Neurolog. Sci.* **127**, 54–60.

Vajsar, J., Becker, L. E., Freedom, R. M. and Murphy, E. G. (1993). Familial desminopathy: myopathy with accumulation of desmin-type intermediate filaments. *J. Neurol. Neurosurg. Psychiatry* **56**, 644–648.

van Antwerpen, C. L., Gospe, S. M. Jr, and Dentinger, M. P. (1988). Nemaline myopathy associated with hypertrophic cardiomyopathy. *Pediatr. Neurol.* **4**, 306–308.

van Wijngaarden, G. K., Fleury, P., Bethlem, J. and Meijer, H. A. E. F. (1969). Familial myotubular myopathy. *Neurology* **19**, 901–908.

Verhiest, W., Brucher, J. M., Goddeeris, P., Lauweryns, J. and de Geest, H. (1976). Familial centronuclear myopathy associated with 'cardiomyopathy'. *Br. Heart J.* **38**, 504–509.

Vicart, P., Caron, A., Guicheney, P., Li, Z. et al. (1998). A missense mutation in the alpha-B crystallin chaperone gene causes a desmin-related myopathy. *Nat. Genet.* **20**, 92–95.

Wallgren-Pettersson, C. (1998). Workshop report: the 50th ENMC sponsored international workshop – myotubular myopathy. *Neuromusc. Disord.* **8**, 521–525.

Wallgren-Pettersson, C. and Laing, N. G. (1996). Workshop report: the 40th ENMC sponsored international workshop – nemaline myopathy. *Neuromusc. Disord.* **6**, 389–391.

Wallgren-Pettersson, C. and Thomas, N. (1994). Workshop report: the 20th ENMC sponsored international workshop – myotubular/centronuclear myopathy. *Neuromusc. Disord.* **4**, 71–74.

Wallgren-Pettersson, C. and Thomas, N. (1997). Workshop report: the 45th ENMC sponsored international workshop – myotubular myopathy. *Neuromusc. Disord.* **7**, 268–271.

Wallgren-Pettersson, C., Clarke, A., Samson, F. et al. (1995a). The myotubular myopathies: differential diagnosis of the X-linked recessive, autosomal dominant, and autosomal recessive forms and present state of DNA studies. *J. Med. Genet.* **32**, 673–679.

Wallgren-Pettersson, C., Avela, K., Marchand, S. et al. (1995b). A gene for autosomal recessive nemaline myopathy assigned to chromosome 2q by linkage analysis. *Neuromusc. Disord.* **5**, 441–443.

Wallgren-Pettersson, C., Beggs, A. H. and Laing, N. G. (1998). Workshop report: the 51st ENMC sponsored international workshop – nemaline myopathy. *Neuromusc. Disord.* **8**, 53–56.

Yoshioka, M., Kuroki, S., Ohkura, K., Itagaki, Y. and Saida, K. (1987). Congenital myopathy with type II muscle fiber hypoplasia. *Neurology* **37**, 860–863.

Zanoteli, E., Oliveira, A. S. B., Schmidt, B. and Gabbai, A. A. (1998). Centronuclear myopathy: clinical aspects of ten Brazilian patients with childhood onset. *J. Neurolog. Sci.* **158**, 76–82.

Zeman, A. Z. J., Dick, D. J., Anderson, J. R., Watkin, S. W., Smith, I. E. and Shneerson, J. M. (1997). Multicore myopathy presenting in adulthood with respiratory failure. *Muscle Nerve* **20**, 367–369.

Zhang, Y., Chen, H. S., Khanna, V. K. et al. (1993). A mutation in the human ryanodine receptor gene associated with central core disease. *Nat. Genet.* **5**, 46–50.

27

Myotonic dystrophy

Peter S. Harper

Introduction

Myotonic dystrophy is the most common muscular dystrophy of adult life and is also an important disorder of childhood and the newborn period. It is distinguished from other primary muscular dystrophies by the occurrence of myotonia and by a wide but distinctive range of abnormalities in other body systems. The disorder is frequently encountered not only by neurologists but by other clinical specialties.

The extreme clinical variability and unusual genetic features of myotonic dystrophy have puzzled both clinicians and geneticists for many years, but since the isolation of the myotonic dystrophy protein kinase (DMPK) gene in 1992 and the recognition that the mutation and mechanism causing myotonic dystrophy involved the expansion of a specific trinucleotide repeat, the understanding of these aspects has been completely transformed and to a large extent clarified. These same advances have also provided important practical benefits in the form of molecular diagnostic testing, presymptomatic detection and prenatal diagnosis. By contrast, the function of the gene and the way in which the myotonic dystrophy mutation disrupts this and the function of neighbouring genes to cause the disease is proving to be highly complex. It is here that our understanding needs to increase considerably before any applications to therapy are likely to be effective.

Myotonic dystrophy is one of the myotonic disorders, (Table 27.1), most of which are nonprogressive; these are considered separately in Chapter 25 and by Rüdel and Lehmann-Horn (1996). Other myotonic disorders are rare, and even when added together are considerably less frequent than myotonic dystrophy alone. The molecular basis of these other disorders has also been largely clarified during the 1990s and this has helped to provide a frame-

work for our understanding of the normal physiology and the ways in which myotonia may occur. One other disorder that is progressive, however, and which is considered in this chapter, is the newly recognized condition proximal myotonic myopathy (PROMM), which closely resembles myotonic dystrophy, even though its genetic basis is distinct.

The orientation of this chapter is deliberately clinical to complement the more basic earlier chapters of this book. Those who wish to explore in detail the molecular and physiological aspects of myotonic dystrophy can find more information in a number of reviews and books, including Winchester and Johnson (1998), Harper and Johnson (2000), Harper (2001) and Chapter 30.

Clinical aspects

Myotonic dystrophy has been recognized as a specific disorder since 1909, when Steinert and also Batten and Gibb independently described its main features and recognized that it was distinct from the previously reported myotonia congenita (Thomsen, 1876). The systemic features were documented surprisingly early, with testicular atrophy being noted in Steinert's initial description, while cataract was associated with the disorder by Greenfield (1911). Therefore, from the outset myotonic dystrophy has been recognized as a systemic disorder, involving not only voluntary, smooth and cardiac muscle but also the eye, brain and endocrine systems among others. The remarkable variability of clinical severity was also described at an early stage, with the ophthalmologist Fleischer (1918) making the notable observation that in some patients cataract might be the only feature and that branches of an affected family could be linked through individuals showing cataract alone.

Table 27.1. The inherited myotonic disorders

Disorder	Inheritance	Primary defect
Myotonic dystrophy	AD	Unstable trinucleotide (CTG) repeat in the gene for a specific protein kinase (DMPK)
Proximal myotonic myopathy (PROMM)	AD	Gene locus on chromosome 3q (some families)
Myotonia congenita		Mutations in skeletal muscle chloride channel
Dominant (Thomsen)	AD	
Recessive (Becker)	AR	
Paramyotonia congenita		Mutations in adult muscle sodium channel
Myotonic periodic paralysis (adynamia episodica)	AD	Mutations in adult muscle sodium channel
Chondrodystrophic myotonia (Schwartz–Jampel syndrome)	AR	Locus mapped to chromosome 1p 34–36 (some families)

Notes:
AD, autosomal dominant; AR, autosomal recessive.

Table 27.2. The distribution of skeletal muscle involvement in myotonic dystrophy

Involvement	Muscles
Muscles most prominently affected	Superficial facial muscles
	Levator palpebrae superioris
	Temporalis and masseters
	Sternocleidomastoids
	Distal muscles of forearm
	Dorsiflexors of foot
Other muscles commonly affected	Quadriceps
	Diaphragm and intercostals
	Intrinsic muscles of hand and feet
	Palate and pharyngeal muscles
	External ocular muscles
Muscles frequently spared	Pelvic girdle
	Hamstrings
	Soleus and gastrocnemius

Neuromuscular involvement

Muscle weakness is the most frequent symptom leading to the diagnosis of myotonic dystrophy, though its interpretation as nonspecific 'tiredness' may delay its recognition. On examination, the degree of muscle weakness may often be more marked than the history might suggest, while its distribution is frequently characteristic, differing from most other neuromuscular disorders. Table 27.2 summarizes the main features, while Fig. 27.1 illustrates some of the features in a series of adult patients seen by the author.

The facial appearance often suggests the diagnosis even before formal examination has been undertaken, with ptosis a prominent feature at an early stage, as may be documented from old photographs taken years before the individual was symptomatic. More general facial weakness and wasting of temporal muscles may be evident, while dysarthria may indicate involvement of a varying combination of jaw, facial and palate weakness, along with myotonia. Recognition of these facial features is often extremely helpful in alerting the interviewer seeing family members for genetic counselling.

When the neuromuscular features of myotonic dystrophy are being considered in relation to other primary muscular dystrophies of adult life, in a patient with a family history of neuromuscular disease, the distinguishing features are even more marked. The mainly proximal muscle involvement of Duchenne, Becker and limb girdle dystrophies is a clear difference, while the absence of myotonia will help to distinguish facioscapulohumeral and oculopharyngeal dystrophies (Chapters 21 and 24).

Detailed examination will commonly confirm the above features and will generally show prominent weakness and wasting of the sternomastoids, which may be marked at a time when the posterior neck muscles are still strong. In the limbs, the weakness is predominantly distal in both upper and lower limbs, and it is this combination of distal limb weakness with facial, jaw and sternomastoid involvement that is characteristic of myotonic dystrophy, even before the presence of myotonia has been elicited.

Despite these often characteristic and obvious features,

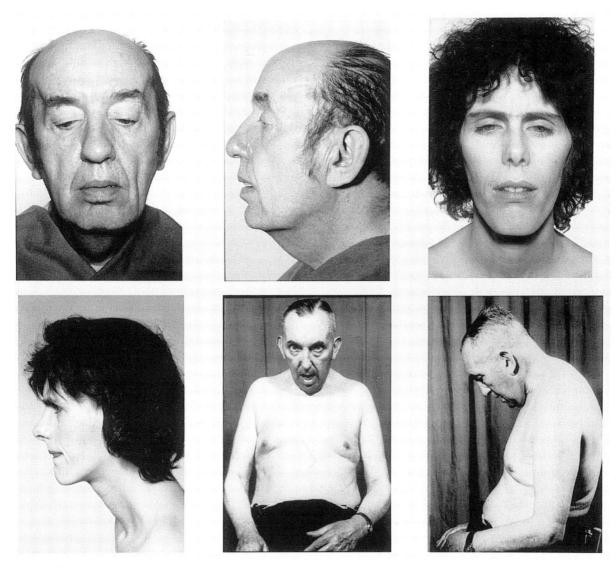

Fig. 27.1. Clinical features of myotonic dystrophy, as shown by a range of patients with adult onset of the disorder. Note particularly the facial weakness, ptosis, and weakness of the jaw and sternomastoid.

there are several factors that may delay or prevent the correct diagnosis being made. Some patients may be reluctant to mention their weakness until a surprisingly advanced stage; if referred to other specialists who are not thinking of a neurological disorder, obvious weakness may be overlooked. Likewise, if no family history is known, or volunteered, the possibility of myotonic dystrophy may not be considered. Most importantly the variability of the condition may mean that neuromuscular abnormalities are atypical, minimal or even entirely absent.

Prominent proximal limb muscle involvement in a patient suspected of myotonic dystrophy should raise the suspicion of the allied disorder PROMM discussed more

fully below, but is not rare in myotonic dystrophy itself.

Two important areas of involvement that have a major influence on prognosis are swallowing abnormalities and respiratory muscle weakness. Although the primary cause of both is neurological, they are considered with the systemic aspects, since their effects are generally manifested as systemic symptoms.

Myotonia in myotonic dystrophy

The finding of myotonia in a patient with a progressive neuromuscular disorder makes it extremely likely that the diagnosis is indeed myotonic dystrophy. Most affected individuals with significant neuromuscular involvement will show myotonia, though it was the presenting symptom in only 20% of the author's early series (Harper, 1989). It is generally obvious as delayed relaxation of grip or following percussion of the thenar muscles, but this presumes that it is looked for. Many patients will refer to their myotonia as stiffness, will have come to terms with it and indeed may not consider it abnormal; consequently, the clinician may not be aware of the feature.

Conversely, the presence of severe symptomatic myotonia, especially with onset in childhood, should raise the question of whether the diagnosis is one of the nonprogressive myotonias (see Chapter 30), which may on occasion be accompanied by mild weakness.

The finding of clinical myotonia is readily confirmed by electromyography (EMG), which shows the characteristic repetitive action potentials after stimulation or voluntary contraction. EMG is valuable only when the patient is not from a known family, or if clinical myotonia is equivocal.

The physiological basis of myotonia is discussed fully in Chapter 10 and also by Harper and Rüdel (1993) and Rüdel and Lehmann-Horn (1996). Even at an early stage, these physiological features were found to differ in myotonic dystrophy from those in myotonia congenita and models such as the myotonic goat, which appeared to represent a more 'pure' disturbance of ion conduction across the muscle membrane (Bryant, 1977). This situation has been confirmed by the molecular characterization of nonprogressive myotonias as the result of specific ion channel defects, involving either the chloride (myotonia congenita) or sodium (paramyotonia) channels (see Chapter 30), while the effects on such channels in myotonic dystrophy is likely to be secondary to the primary DMPK defect or to involvement of ion channels as the result of RNA dysfunction (see below).

Cardiac involvement

Cardiac and respiratory complications are the main cause of death in myotonic dystrophy. Since cardiac problems are in part preventable and treatable and since they may occur in individuals whose neuromuscular problems are relatively mild, or even unrecognized, this is an important aspect for clinicians (and patients themselves) to be familiar with (Phillips and Harper, 1997).

Table 27.3 summarizes the main associated cardiac problems and also indicates forms of cardiovascular disease that are only rarely associated, or not at all. By far, the most prominent area relates to disturbances of cardiac rhythm, and it is here that regular surveillance and careful attention to management are most important.

Table 27.3. Myotonic dystrophy: cardiac aspects

Frequency	Cardiac aspects
Serious or relatively frequent problems	Sudden death (presumed arrhythmic)
	Conduction delay (progressive)
	Tachyarrhythmias (especially atrial flutter and fibrillation)
Infrequent and unassociated problems	Cardiomyopathy (rare)
	Coronary heart disease (not increased)
	Hypertension (blood pressure commonly low)

Abnormalities of the atrioventricular conduction tissues are well documented both electrophysiologically and pathologically (Nguyen et al., 1988; Phillips and Harper, 1997). It is important to recognize that the process is progressive, with a prolongation of QT interval usually demonstrable by electrocardiography (ECG) for a considerable period before symptomatic abnormalities occur. Although cardiac pacemaker insertion has been recommended presymptomatically (Prystowsky et al., 1979), most centres advise a policy of regular ECG monitoring and active enquiry into symptoms (Fragola et al., 1994; Phillips and Harper, 1997), with more detailed investigation and surgical intervention only if there are symptoms or potentially hazardous conduction defects present.

Tachyarrhythmias, commonly atrial flutter and fibrillation, commonly lead to cardiological referral, even before any underlying neurological disorder is recognized. Ventricular arrhythmias are less frequent but potentially more lethal. Abnormal late potentials on ECG have been found to indicate predisposition to these (Olofsson et al., 1988). Familial aggregation of cardiac problems seems likely, at least in some kindreds (Hawley et al., 1983).

Cardiac disorders not associated with myotonic dystrophy include coronary heart disease and hypertension. In fact *hypotension* is a consistent feature of the disorder (O'Brien et al., 1983), though this does not appear to result in symptoms. The extent to which cardiomyopathy is associated is debatable; it is certainly unusual at a clinical level, though postmortem evidence may be found (Nguyen et al., 1988). Anaesthetic hazards are outlined below under Management.

Smooth muscle

Smooth muscle of all organs may be affected in myotonic dystrophy (Table 27.4) and this causes considerable morbidity and sometimes mortality (Ronneblom et al., 1996;

Table 27.4. Smooth muscle involvement in myotonic dystrophy

Area affected	Effects
Pharynx and oesophagus	Delayed relaxation, loss of peristalsis; dysphagia, aspiration
Gall bladder	Delayed emptying, frequent calculi
Colon	Abdominal pain and other 'spastic colon' symptoms; rarely megacolon
Anal sphincter	Abnormal dilatation (especially childhood)
Uterus	Incoordinate contraction in labour
Ciliary body	Low intraocular pressure

Table 27.5. Myotonic dystrophy: extramuscular features

System	Effects
CNS	Lethargy, somnolence, mental retardation (children)
Peripheral nerves	Abnormalities in terminal arborization (usually insignificant clinically)
Ophthalmic	Cataract, retinopathy, blepharitis
Endocrine	Testicular atrophy, complications of pregnancy and labour, diabetes, early balding

Harper 2001). Swallowing problems are frequent and complex, with both voluntary and smooth muscle contributing, and with all stages of the swallowing mechanism involved, including jaw muscles, pharynx and oesophagus (Eckhardt et al., 1986). Oesophageal dysfunction may be incoordination or loss of peristalsis. If swallowing difficulties are a significant symptom, or if aspiration is suspected, full investigation is wise to establish where the defect lies.

Abdominal pain and variable bowel habits owing to large bowel dysfunction are extremely common and under-recognized complaints in both adults and children. Bowel motility is commonly abnormal (Goldberg and Sheft, 1972) but serious loss of function is rare. Confusion is possible between colonic and gall-bladder symptoms; while biliary calculi are increased in frequency in myotonic dystrophy, it is possible that unnecessary and hazardous gall-bladder surgery may at times be performed when the cause of pain is mainly colonic.

Other systems

Table 27.5 summarizes some of the important systemic problems that are not primary or secondary consequences of muscle dysfunction. Central nervous system (CNS) involvement is probably the most important of these and its extent is closely related to age at onset. It is normally absent in those with late-onset and minimal neuromuscular disease and most prominent in patients with congenital or childhood onset. As with most clinical aspects, it correlates with the degree of expansion in the trinucleotide repeat sequence (Tsilfidis et al., 1992).

The most striking feature of many (but by no means all) patients with myotonic dystrophy is a marked degree of apathy and inertia, resulting in many fewer symptoms than would seem reasonable for a given degree of weak-ness and myotonia, but also in a much less adequate level of function. This aspect is most commonly commented on by spouses and other relatives, and it may be the deciding factor in determining whether a patient can continue to work. Somnolence can be prominent, even in those with little involvement of respiratory muscles (Rubinsztein et al., 1998; Phillips et al., 1999). All these features, along with the occurrence of mental retardation in the congenital form, indicate a degree of CNS involvement in the disorder, though the objective radiological and neuropathological changes are not striking (Rosman and Kakulas, 1966). Thorough neuropsychiatric studies have been carried out (Woodward et al., 1982; Brumback and Wilson, 1984).

Other clinical features

Cataract has been recognized to be an integral part of myotonic dystrophy since the earliest description (Greenfield, 1911; Fleischer, 1918) and the disorder should be considered in any occurrence of cataract in early adult life. In older patients, cataract may be the only symptomatic clinical problem, with only minimal myotonia to indicate the diagnosis. Such patients commonly remain undiagnosed until more typical myotonic dystrophy is recognized in another relative, and their prognosis for retaining normal muscle function is excellent. The results of cataract surgery are good, but some patients have an associated retinopathy that must be considered if visual acuity remains poor. In its early stages, the cataract of myotonic dystrophy is characteristic, with multicoloured, refractile opacities visible in the anterior and posterior subcapsular regions when examined with a slit lamp. The use of lens opacities as a predictive test in those at risk has proved to be unreliable and has been superseded by molecular testing. Several studies have now shown that some individuals, predicted to be gene carriers on account of minor lens changes, show no evidence of the myotonic dystrophy mutation on molecular analysis (Brunner et al., 1991; Ashizawa et al., 1992; Reardon et al., 1992a,b).

Endocrine abnormalities are frequent but do not usually cause serious symptoms. Testicular atrophy is seen in most postpubertal males (Vazquez et al., 1990) but does not usually cause loss of secondary sexual function. Fertility is moderately reduced in both sexes, but there is a high fetal wastage in females (O'Brien and Harper, 1984). Alterations in the pituitary fossa and occasional pituitary tumours may result from persistently increased gonadotrophin secretion (Mahler and Parizel, 1982). Diabetes occurs occasionally but most patients show a consistent hyperinsulinism and insulin resistance, even at an early stage of their illness (Moxley et al., 1984). This seems likely to result from an RNA effect on insulin receptor function (Morrone et al., 1997).

Congenital myotonic dystrophy

Although the onset of typical myotonic dystrophy can frequently be traced back to childhood, the congenital form of the disorder is clinically distinctive and until recently has been underdiagnosed. It was originally described by Vanier (1960) and even now it is not fully recognized by many adult neurologists and general paediatricians, though with modern techniques of neonatal intensive care and ventilation it is becoming recognized as one of the major neuromuscular causes of respiratory insufficiency.

Some of the prominent features are listed in Table 27.6; many are quite unlike those seen in myotonic dystrophy of later life (Harper, 1975; Hageman et al., 1993); conversely, myotonia is not seen as a clinical feature in infancy. Most of the symptoms can be traced back into intrauterine life; indeed, in a pregnancy at risk the disorder can often be predicted by the poor fetal movements and polyhydramnios. The hypotonia and immobility of the affected newborn infant may be profound; the lungs are hypoplastic (Silver et al., 1984). Inadequate ventilation previously resulted in death for many without a specific diagnosis, but most now survive following resuscitation to allow recognition that a generalized neuromuscular disorder is present (Rutherford et al., 1989).

Unless a family history of myotonic dystrophy has been recognized, it may be difficult to distinguish congenital myotonic dystrophy from other congenital myopathies. The severe X-linked form of myotubular myopathy is particularly likely to be confused; molecular as well as pathological analysis is now of diagnostic help. Features suggesting myotonic dystrophy include a disproportionate weakness of face and jaw, the occurrence of a greatly raised and hypoplastic diaphragm on chest radiograph and at

Table 27.6. Congenital myotonic dystrophy – principal features

	Features
Intrauterine	Hydramnios
	Poor fetal movement
Neonatal	Facial diplegia
	Hypotonia (no significant myotonia)
	Respiratory failure
	Feeding problems
	Talipes (sometimes more general contractures)
	Disproportionate face and jaw weakness
	Thin ribs, elevated diaphragm on chest radiograph
Later	Marked facial and jaw muscle weakness
	Progressive general muscle weakness and wasting
	Mental retardation
	Myotonia
Investigations	Muscle histology: marked immaturity, abundant satellite cells
	Molecular analysis: very large ($>$1000 repeats) CTG expansion

postmortem (Bossen et al., 1974), and thin ribs on chest radiograph resulting from hypoplastic intercostal muscles. Talipes is frequent, but more general congenital contractures sometimes occur. Figure 27.2 illustrates the facial features at different ages. In most cases, confirmation is obtained by the recognition of features of myotonic dystrophy in the mother, which are often mild and relatively symptomless. EMG shows at most a few myotonic potentials (Swift et al., 1975); myotonia becomes conspicuous only after infancy. Muscle biopsy is helpful, not only in allowing other specific causes to be recognized but also in showing unusual features of immature fibres (Sarnat and Silbert, 1976; Silver et al., 1984) with central nuclei and abundant satellite cells in contrast to the appearance in myotubular myopathy. On histochemical examination, peripheral regions show deficiency of oxidative enzymes (Karpati et al., 1973).

The outlook for severely affected patients with congenital disease is poor with regard to both physical and mental function, and mental retardation is present in almost all survivors, even when anoxia has not been a major problem (Harper, 1975). A longitudinal study (Reardon et al., 1993) has shown that very few patients are able to live an independent adult life. Consequently, undertaking major measures of resuscitation in an infant recognized as being affected in the newborn period deserves careful

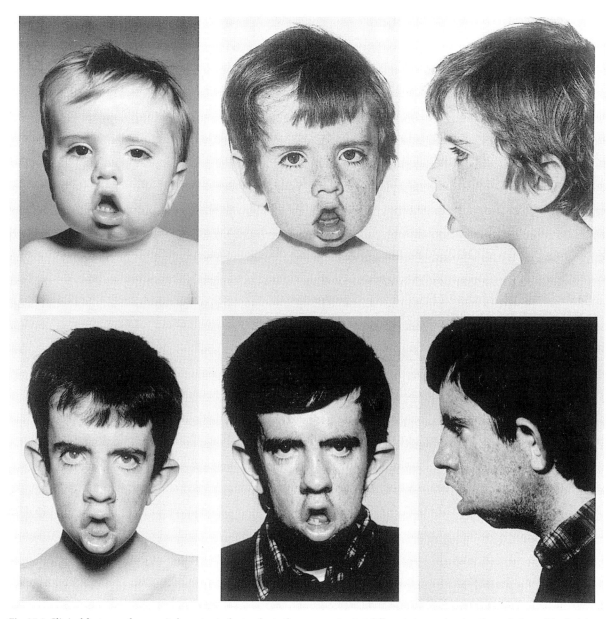

Fig. 27.2. Clinical features of congenital myotonic dystrophy in the same patient at different stages, showing the evolution of the facial characteristics.

consideration and discussion with the parents. Death is unusual once neonatal complications are overcome, and once an active course is embarked on it is not easy to abandon. The duration of any assisted ventilation that is required gives some guide to likely survival (Rutherford et al., 1989).

The almost universal maternal transmission of congenital myotonic dystrophy and its occurrence in the offspring of relatively mildly affected mothers are good examples of previously puzzling aspects of the disorder that have been largely resolved by the recognition of the instability of the myotonic dystrophy mutation. The topics of anticipation and parent of origin effects are discussed along with other genetic aspects below. Childhood-onset noncongenital disease is an intermediate group with important cognitive and behavioural problems (Steyaert et al., 1997).

Diagnostic investigations

Molecular analysis

Molecular analysis for the myotonic dystrophy mutation is the most important investigation in myotonic

Table 27.7. Diagnostic investigations in myotonic dystrophy

Molecular analysis for CTG repeat
  primary diagnosis or confirmation
  presymptomatic and carrier detection
  prenatal testing
Electromyography
Muscle biopsy (rarely needed)
Ophthalmological assessment (cataract, retinopathy)
Electrocardiogram (conduction defects)
Glucose and insulin studies (diabetes, insulin resistance)

dystrophy (MacMillan et al., 1992; Shelbourne et al., 1993), but it must be emphasized that clinical assessment, particularly an awareness of the disorder and a careful examination for its key features, remain essential if molecular analysis (or any other test) is to be used appropriately.

Table 27.7 summarizes the main uses of molecular analysis in myotonic dystrophy. Its value is enhanced by high specificity and sensitivity. The facts that a single mutation is responsible for virtually all cases worldwide, albeit variable in extent, and that the test can be performed on blood or any other tissue add to its power.

As a primary diagnostic test, mutation analysis is especially valuable in the absence of a clear family history, notably in suspected congenital cases (MacMillan et al., 1992) but also for atypical cases in adult life (Reardon et al., 1992b); it is always essential to explain clearly the genetic nature and implications of the test when it is being undertaken, not afterwards when an abnormal result has been obtained. In a known family, genetic testing is extremely helpful in deciding whether equivocal or atypical features are likely to be related to the family disorder. (It is always important first to confirm that the mutation is in fact present in at least one affected member of the family (Barnes et al., 1994).) When healthy relatives are being considered, it is extremely important to be aware that such predictive or presymptomatic testing for presence of the mutation is *not* diagnostic, and that it should be performed only following the general guidelines for such testing in late-onset genetic disorders generally (Advisory Committee on Genetic Testing, 1998). In particular, healthy young children should not be tested on grounds of parental concern alone, while older healthy children or adolescents should be involved in consent as far as they are able. Written consent for presymptomatic testing is essential.

A normal molecular result in a healthy relative will essentially exclude the later development or transmission of the disorder, and this is of considerable value in making the testing of offspring or prenatal diagnosis unnecessary. The main demand for prenatal diagnosis is from women who have had a congenitally affected child. Attitudes to prenatal testing vary considerably according to the experiences of the specific family. Early prenatal diagnosis by chorion villus sampling provides a highly accurate prenatal test (Myring et al., 1992; Smeets et al., 1992). New techniques of pre-implantation diagnosis are currently being evaluated (Sermon et al., 1997).

While molecular analysis is extremely accurate in terms of presence or absence of the mutation, a difficult issue arises in how far the size of the repeat expansion in an abnormal result can be correlated with likely outcome (Harley et al., 1992a; Gennarelli et al., 1996). As discussed later, it is wise to be cautious, but the fact that the ranges for congenital cases and for those with minimal disease do not overlap does allow an approximate guide that is useful in the context of prenatal and presymptomatic test results.

Other investigations

Specific molecular analysis has eliminated the need for many other forms of investigation.

EMG remains useful in confirming that clinical myotonia is indeed true myotonia; it is also useful in cases without a clear family history. It is no longer necessary when the diagnosis in the family is already clear and not needed for presymptomatic detection. A normal EMG can confirm that an individual carrying a 'minimal' mutation is free from overt neurological involvement (Reardon et al., 1992b).

Muscle biopsy is not needed if molecular testing is diagnostic. In fatal congenital disease, muscle may be a valuable source of DNA that can allow molecular analysis for congenital myotonic dystrophy (MacMillan et al., 1992).

The remaining investigations listed (in Table 27.7) are related to management. None should form part of presymptomatic testing, since all have a considerably greater frequency of false-positive and false-negative tests than molecular analysis. However, for those established as having the disorder or carrying the gene, it is clearly helpful to know whether there is any evidence of cardiac, ophthalmological or endocrine involvement, and such investigations may be needed on a regular basis.

Proximal myotonic myopathy (PROMM)

PROMM is a newly recognized disorder identified through a combination of careful clinical and electrophysiological documentation and the advent of specific molecular analysis. The extensive studies of Ricker and colleagues over

Table 27.8. Comparative clinical features of myotonic dystrophy and proximal myotonic myopathy (PROMM)

Abnormalities	Myotonic dystrophy	PROMM
Neuromuscular abnormalities		
Myotonia	+	+
Progressive muscle weakness and wasting	+	+
Facial weakness	+	–
Predominant distribution of weakness	Distal	Proximal
Muscle pain	–	+
Other symptoms		
Cardiac arrythmias	+	+
Cataract	+	+
CNS involvement	+	–
Genetic aspects		
Inheritance	Dominant	Dominant
Anticipation	+	+
Gene localization	19q	3q (some families)
Specific molecular basis	Trinucleotide repeat expansion	Unknown

Source: Based on Harper and Johnson (2000).

many years (Moxley and Ricker, 1995; Ricker et al., 1995) had established that a significant group of patients were not typical for myotonic dystrophy but yet had a progressive myotonic disorder. When these were considered alongside those patients thought to have myotonic dystrophy but showing no trinucleotide (CTG) expansion, it became clear that a specific entity existed; although PROMM has been generally adopted as a descriptor, the phenotype is not yet fully defined (Udd et al., 1997) and the muscle weakness is not always mainly proximal. An additional factor now needing to be considered is the large family described by Ranum et al. (1998) as 'type 2 myotonic dystrophy' with a mutation located on chromosome 3, which may be the same disorder as some families with PROMM (Day et al., 1999). It is probably wise to confine the terms 'type 1', 'type 2', etc. to the genetic nomenclature.

Table 27.8 summarizes some of the main features of PROMM by comparison with myotonic dystrophy; both share progressive muscle disease with myotonia, though the weakness is often milder and slowly progressive in PROMM, as well as more proximal in distribution. Cardiac involvement and cataract are also common to both, but patients with PROMM do not show clear CNS involvement, nor has any comparable condition to congenital myotonic

dystrophy been documented in PROMM families. In genetic terms, the loci are clearly distinct and PROMM may itself be heterogeneous. Both are autosomal but anticipation in PROMM is less marked and no trinucleotide repeat defect has been identified.

The genetics of myotonic dystrophy

Few disorders can have received so much attention or have raised so many puzzling genetic questions as has myotonic dystrophy. From the earliest studies it was recognized as following Mendelian autosomal dominant inheritance, a finding confirmed by systematic family studies (Bell, 1947), but a number of unexplained features were apparent. Notable among these was the remarkable clinical variation in severity and age at onset and the apparent worsening with successive generations. This 'anticipation' was first documented by Fleischer in 1918 when he showed that different families with established myotonic dystrophy could be linked through individuals with cataract alone or, on occasion, who were entirely healthy. The difficulty in providing a mechanism by which a genetic disorder might deteriorate led to a protracted debate as to whether it actually existed (Penrose, 1948; Höweler et al., 1989), which was only resolved when the molecular basis of the disorder was found to be an unstable trinucleotide repeat mutation (see Harper (1998) for a review).

A further puzzling feature was the maternal transmission of virtually all cases of congenital myotonic dystrophy (Harper and Dyken, 1972), again unexplained until it was recognized that not only do such cases have exceptionally large repeat expansions in the gene but that (for reasons still not fully understood) there is a size limit to transmission of such expansions by sperm that does not apply to the ovum (Ashizawa et al., 1994a). A comparable but opposite parent of origin effect exists for the smallest expansions, where paternally transmitted expansion is greater, accounting for the excess of cases at the 'top' of a pedigree transmitted by healthy or minimally affected males (Brunner et al., 1993; Lopez de Munain et al., 1995).

The main genetic features of myotonic dystrophy families are summarized in Table 27.9. They are of practical importance since it is general experience that every 'new' case of myotonic dystrophy diagnosed is likely to bring to light a series of secondary cases and gene carriers whose existence had not previously been suspected.

The myotonic dystrophy mutation

The isolation of the myotonic dystrophy gene and the identification of the responsible mutation both occurred

Table 27.9. Genetic aspects of myotonic dystrophy

Autosomal dominant inheritance: 50% risk to offspring of
affected parent

Extreme clinical variability within a kindred: partly correlated
with size of mutation expansion

Anticipation: earlier onset and greater severity likely in successive
generations

Parent of origin effects: maternal transmission of congenital
cases; mainly paternal ancestral origin

No true 'new' mutations: origin in families through healthy
transmitters of 'minimal' mutations

Single major genetic locus on chromosome 19

in rapid succession in the Spring of 1992, following a 10 year period of painstaking positional cloning research by a series of closely communicating groups internationally. Indeed, the mapping of the gene began before the advent of molecular techniques made actual isolation of the gene a possibility. This gene mapping and positional cloning effort, described in the previous edition of this book and elsewhere (Jansen et al., 1992; Shutler et al., 1992), will not be repeated here, but the key indication that the mutation had been identified was the discovery of an altered DNA sequence in patients with myotonic dystrophy in the small critical region where the gene was known to lie (Aslanidis et al., 1992; Buxton et al., 1992; Harley et al., 1992b).

Further study of this altered sequence in families with myotonic dystrophy showed a remarkable finding that explained many of the genetic problems of the disorder. Not only did the variable sequence differ between affected individuals (Fig. 27.3*a*) but a stepwise increase in fragment size was seen in successive generations (Fig. 27.3*b*); this finding was closely correlated with the clinical observation of anticipation. The interpretation of these observations was accelerated by the fact that, 6 months previously (Oberlé et al., 1991), a similar phenomenon had been encountered as the basis for fragile X mental retardation. In this disorder anticipation is also seen, a finding which had led to the suggestion that a comparable unstable DNA sequence might be found in myotonic dystrophy (Sutherland et al., 1991).

The initial observations of the unstable sequence showed that there was a correlation between size of the expanded repeat sequence and severity or earlier age at onset (Harley et al., 1992a; Reardon et al., 1992b; Tsilfidis et al., 1992). It can be seen from Fig. 27.4 that while there is a degree of overlap between the individual groups, the minimal and severe groups are distinct, a finding that has been confirmed by subsequent studies and which is of

considerable importance for genetic counselling and prenatal diagnosis. Since the expansion of the unstable sequence is seen in the offspring of both male and female patients, it cannot alone explain the exclusively maternal transmission of congenital myotonic dystrophy.

Study of the expanded sequence in families has thrown important light on the question of new mutations, mentioned above. Analysis of a series of families in which neither parent showed any identifiable neuromuscular abnormality has shown that in all cases one parent, most commonly the father, shows a minimal expansion (Reardon et al., 1992b; Lopez de Munain, 1995). Therefore, those rare cases that might have represented new mutations have proved not to be so, a finding of practical consequence for genetic counselling.

The properties of the gene itself are considered later, but two key findings relating to the mutation emerged from this initial research. First, it was located in the 3′ untranslated region and, therefore, was not expected to be reflected in the sequence of the protein produced. Second, it was a trinucleotide repeat (CTG), with variation in the number of repeats present. This discovery in myotonic dystrophy, along with the similar finding for fragile X mental retardation, confirmed the existence of a new type of mutational mechanism – that of trinucleotide repeat disorders – paving the way for later recognition of the same mutational mechanism in Huntington's disease and hereditary ataxias (Harper, 1996; Wells and Warren, 1998).

Table 27.10 summarizes the main properties of the myotonic dystrophy mutation that are clinically relevant. Almost all of these can be attributed to two distinctive general properties: first is the instability of the mutation, particularly the germline instability that underlies the variability of the disorder, the anticipation between generations and the parent of origin effects; second, the universal nature of the mutation, giving the practical application that virtually all individuals carrying the mutation can be detected by a single, relatively simple, molecular diagnostic test.

Germline instability

Germline instability (Table 27.11) is the key factor underlying the numerous unusual and previously puzzling aspects of the inheritance of myotonic dystrophy. The fact that mutation has to be looked at as a progressive process requires a considerable change of thought by comparison with more conventional genetic disorders. It is now clear that even minimally affected individuals or normal mutation carriers show significant genetic instability, and that expansion of the mutation into the clinically significant range is likely in the following generations. The instability

Table 27.10. The myotonic dystrophy mutation: clinically relevant aspects

CTG trinucleotide repeat expansion in the gene for the myotonic dystrophy protein kinase (DMPK) does not appear in protein

Normal individuals show <50 repeats; severest (congenital) disease shows >1500 repeats

There is an approximate correlation between repeat size and clinical severity

Virtually all cases worldwide result from the same mutational mechanism

Clinically normal mutation carriers are the source of all apparently new cases

A single molecular test can provide accurate detection or exclusion of mutation at any point in life

Table 27.11. Genetic instability of the myotonic dystrophy trinucleotide repeat sequence

Instability	Consequences
Germline instability	Size dependent: greater instability with increasing repeat number
	Sex dependent: greater expansion of small repeats with male transmission; preferential expansion of large female transmitted repeats
	Expansion more likely than contraction: hence anticipation
	Contraction of repeat occurs mainly in male transmission
Somatic instability	No obvious clinical consequences
	Range of sizes in larger expansions may 'blur' expanded sequence in affected adults
	Not sufficient to confuse prenatal or preimplantation diagnosis
	Repeat lengths in muscle larger and more variable than in blood

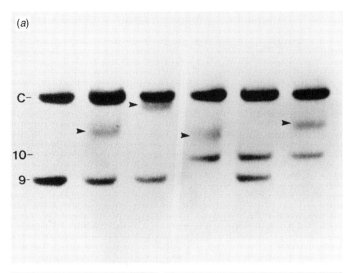

(a)

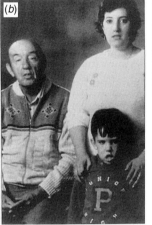

(b)

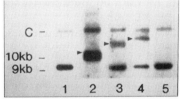

Fig. 27.3. The original studies of the myotonic dystrophy mutation. (*a*) The variable unstable sequence can be seen (arrowed) in affected individuals. Lanes 1 and 5 are unaffected individuals, showing the normal polymorphism with 9 and 10 kb fragments from the normal allele. C is a constant band. (*b*) DNA analysis of a three-generation family with myotonic dystrophy, demonstrating the molecular basis of anticipation. Lane 1 and 5 are unaffected individuals. Lanes 2, 3 and 4 are from the minimally affected grandfather, moderately affected mother and congenitally affected child, respectively, showing the corresponding small, moderate and large DNA expansions in the gene in successive generations. With permission (from (*a*) Harley et al., 1992a and (*b*) Harper, 1998.)

is directly related to the degree of expansion (Lavedan et al., 1993); as a result extinction of the mutation on account of severity and genetic lethality is usual within a few generations (de Die-Smulders et al., 1994), though some kindreds have been documented with relatively little change (Simmons et al., 1998).

This progressive instability is the basis of the striking anticipation that has always been the hallmark of myotonic dystrophy (Harper et al., 1992), but it is important to recognize that the repeat sequence may also diminish in size (Brunner et al., 1993; Ashizawa et al., 1994b), though

less frequently than an expansion. This is seen particularly for male transmissions in the larger size range (Ashizawa et al., 1994b) and may reflect an adverse effect on sperm, reducing the chance of fertilization by a sperm bearing a large expansion.

Such differences between male and female meiosis

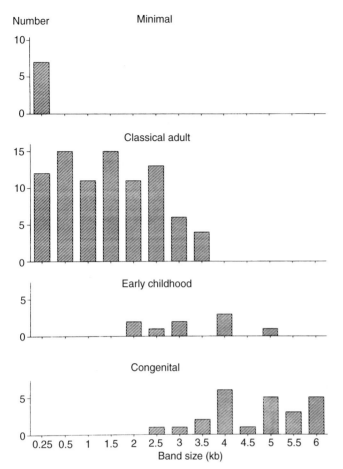

Fig. 27.4. Correlation of DNA expansion with phenotype in myotonic dystrophy. Note that while overlap exists between the different clinical categories, there is a clear distinction between the severe congenital and the minimally affected groups. (With permission from Harley et al., 1992b.)

explain, at least in part, the parent of origin effects already described; the limitations of male transmission of large expansions is likely to be the main reason why congenitally affected disease is so rarely transmitted through the male line; only six such cases have been documented among the thousands of known congenital cases (Bergoffen et al., 1994; Ohya et al., 1994). By contrast, for smaller expansions of under 100 repeats, there is a greater degree of increase during male transmission, in common with other trinucleotide repeat disorders such as Huntington's disease, in which the degree of expansion rarely exceeds this level. This explains the predominant origin of the disease from males in the grandparental generation (Lopez de Munain et al., 1995).

It needs to be recognized that the germline is essentially mosaic, at least in sperm where this can be documented; consequently, a wide range of expansion sizes is present in a single semen sample, offering an equally wide range of

outcomes in terms of any eventual pregnancy (Monckton et al., 1995). Such variability is also relevant to the practical development of pre-implantation diagnosis of the disorder (Sermon et al., 1997).

Somatic instability

Somatic instability is also a feature of the myotonic dystrophy mutation (Jansen et al., 1994; Worhle et al., 1995), especially for large expansions, which often appear on analysis of blood as a 'smear' rather than a sharp band. This somatic instability is also seen in fragile X mental retardation, which shares the occurrence of extremely large repeat expansions (Oberlé et al., 1991). By comparison, in the CAG polyglutamine expansion disorders of the CNS, where expansions are much smaller, somatic instability is inconspicuous (Telenius et al., 1994).

The widespread somatic instability of the repeat sequence in myotonic dystrophy has been documented by postmortem studies of a wide range of tissues (Kinoshita et al., 1996) and by studies on muscle biopsies, which have shown a more variable but generally increased range compared with blood from the same individual (Thornton et al., 1994). In view of the finding that somatic genetic instability underlies such serious neoplastic disorders as hereditary colon cancer, it is perhaps surprising that none of the clinical complications of myotonic dystrophy can at present be related to somatic cell instability.

Genetic instability is also seen during development and accounts for differences between identical twins (though clinically these are usually very similar in severity; Lopez de Munain et al., 1994) and tissue differences seen in embryonic development (Worhle et al., 1995). It is interesting, and of particular importance, that even the largest expansions have a clear-cut size when detected prenatally by chorion biopsy (Myring et al., 1992).

One final point deserving mention in relation to the myotonic dystrophy mutation is that a series of homozygotes for the mutation have now been documented (Cobo et al., 1993; Martorell et al., 1996), and that these appear not to be more severely affected than heterozygotes for the same repeat size. The same has proved to be the case for Huntington's disease (Wexler et al., 1987) and indicates that simple loss of gene function is unlikely to be the basis for the disease state.

Genetic heterogeneity

Throughout the prolonged period that the myotonic dystrophy gene was being mapped, the evidence pointed unequivocally to the existence of a single genetic locus on chromosome 19 (Wieringa et al., 1988) and no clearly unlinked families were documented. This homogeneity was reinforced when the specific trinucleotide repeat expansion was found to underlie almost all cases and, as discussed below, that their shared haplotype suggested a remote common origin.

This homogeneity still remains true to a remarkable extent, but two important exceptions need to be noted, the importance of which in understanding disease mechanisms may prove to be out of all proportion to their frequency The first, already described at a clinical level, is PROMM which is now clearly recognized as a distinct disorder, albeit with many affinities to myotonic dystrophy. It should be noted that its recognition as a specific entity only occurred when testing for the myotonic dystrophy mutation became feasible, allowing molecular study of atypical cases as well as causing a clinical re-assessment of the small number of cases diagnosed as having myotonic dystrophy but showing no repeat expansion.

The discovery of a single large kindred with apparent myotonic dystrophy but without the mutation and with the gene mapped to chromosome 3 (Ranum et al., 1998; Day et al., 1999) has now permitted a genetic assessment of PROMM families as well, making it clear that at least some of them (but not all) also map to chromosome 3. It is also widening the phenotype to make it clear that the clinical phenotypes may indeed be extremely comparable. The nature of these other genes and mutations is unknown at present, but at a practical level, it remains true that the overwhelming majority of patients with clinical myotonic dystrophy across the world will show the expected trinucleotide repeat expansion on chromosome 19.

Population origins of the myotonic dystrophy mutation

The population origins of the mutation has proved to be one of the most interesting and unexpected outcomes of identifying the myotonic dystrophy gene and mutation and illustrates well how research primarily focused on a genetic disease can illuminate important normal biological processes – in this case the course of human evolution. Long before the gene was isolated, two features were recognized that later became central to this field: the apparent lack of new mutations and ethnic differences in prevalence of the disorder. Each has proved to illustrate an important aspect of population genetics: the recent history and the remote origins of the disorder, respectively.

The lack of new mutations was a feature documented by all the early family studies (Harper, 1989); in almost all kindreds the origin of the disease could not be clearly established to arise de novo in a specific individual. Either one of the presumed healthy parents proved when examined to show minor features of the disease, or collateral branches of the family proved to be affected, showing that the origin

must be further back. The explanation for this is now clear; the clinical disorder indeed does not arise truly de novo, but from a parent carrying an expansion outside the normal range who may or may not show minor clinical features such as cataract (Reardon et al., 1992b). Unlike the mutations for most genetic disorders, which arise as a sudden change, in myotonic dystrophy there is a progressive increase in successive generations that will at some point cross the threshold required for clinical effects to occur.

That such a process can occur over many generations is illustrated by the occurrence of the disorder at high frequency in large isolated population groups such as those in Labrador (Pryse-Phillips et al., 1982), Northern Sweden (Rolander and Floderus, 1961) and, most notably, Northern Québec (Mathieu et al., 1990). Such populations have undergone rapid population growth. In the case of the Québec isolate, all cases of myotonic dystrophy can be traced to a common ancestor (presumably clinically normal) originating from France over 300 years ago (Bouchard et al., 1989).

The ethnic variation in prevalence of myotonic dystrophy has proved to be considerably more important than originally thought likely (Ashizawa and Epstein, 1991). While most differences in Caucasian populations can be explained on the basis of relatively recent factors, and while the disorder is also frequent in most Asian populations, there has always been a conspicuous absence of myotonic dystrophy in Black African populations. Originally attributed to underascertainment, it is now clear that it is of major biological significance (Goldman et al., 1994), reflecting a deficiency of the large 'normal range' repeats that are likely to be the source of subsequent unstable and eventually clinically significant alleles. Interestingly, the only well-documented African family, from Nigeria (Dada, 1973; Krahe et al., 1995), has arisen on a separate haplotype of surrounding markers, indicating an entirely different origin. All other cases worldwide share a common haplotype, suggesting a remote single origin in the progenitors of these other races that is not present in those of African origin (Goldman et al., 1996; Tishkoff et al., 1998).

These factors, along with analysis of the normal variation in repeat number at the myotonic dystrophy locus, are providing a powerful tool for evolutionary biologists to study the remote origins of different ethnic groups, and indeed of humans themselves.

Normal and abnormal gene function in myotonic dystrophy

Within a few months of the identification of the myotonic dystrophy mutation, the gene itself was isolated (Brook et

(a)

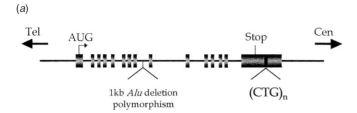

1kb *Alu* deletion
polymorphism

(CTG)$_n$

(b)

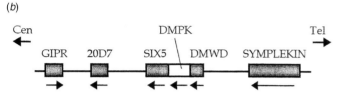

Fig. 27.5. The myotonic dystrophy genomic region of chromosome 19, showing (a) the structure of the molecular architecture of the region and the exon for the gene for myotonic dystrophy protein kinase (DMPK) and (b) the relationship of the gene for DMPK and neighbouring genes. (With permission from Newman and Brook, 2001.)

al., 1992; Fu et al., 1992; Mahadevan et al., 1992) and information became available on its DNA sequence, structural organization, homologies and the predicted properties of its protein product. Sequence data immediately made it clear that the protein had affinities with the protein kinase family, and the name myotonic dystrophy protein kinase (DMPK) has been generally adopted.

Despite this early promise, it soon became clear that, while our understanding of the genetic aspects and clinical variability was being rapidly illuminated by the nature of the mutation, the functional role of the gene in both normal individuals and in patients with myotonic dystrophy was going to be much more complex and difficult to determine. After eight years of research, we are still only beginning to see consistent results, and those outlined here remain provisional. Because of this, and because as yet they impinge little on the clinical interpretation and management of the condition, they are only summarized here; they are more fully covered in other reviews (Epstein and Jin, 1998; Monckton et al., 1998; Winchester and Johnson, 1998; Harper and Johnson, 2000; Harper, 2001).

The first factor requiring recognition is that DMPK is probably not the only gene product with its function disrupted by the trinucleotide expansion. It was already known from gene mapping and physical studies that this particular region of chromosome 19 is extremely gene rich (Alwassan et al., 1998). There are at least two other genes, lying immediately 5' and 3' to DMPK that require consideration, as shown in Fig. 27.5b.

The gene termed '59' (Shaw et al., 1993), and its mouse

counterpart *DMR-N9* (Jansen et al., 1995), was first identified by sequencing of the region and lies 1.1 kb from *DMPK*. It is a small gene (five exons) and widely expressed in many tissues including brain, but no clear disturbance of mRNA levels or of other properties has been identified in patients with myotonic dystrophy and so its role in the disorder remains uncertain.

Immediately 3' to *DMPK*, and hence very close to the CTG repeat, is another gene, giving rise to myotonic dystrophy-associated homeodomain protein (DMAHP) (Boucher et al., 1995; Heath et al., 1997) recently renamed *SIX5*, which, as the original name implies, encodes a homeodomain protein. This gene is also widely expressed in different tissues, including muscle, heart and lens; reduced mRNA synthesis has been shown in patients with myotonic dystrophy (Klesert et al., 1997). Since homeodomain proteins often act by regulating transcription of other genes (Englekamp and van Heyningen, 1996), DMAHP could act in myotonic dystrophy not only directly but also by effects on other key genes not necessarily in the immediate vicinity. It is attractive also to think that DMAHP might be particularly involved in the cataract of myotonic dystrophy (Winchester et al., 1999), since this gene is strongly expressed in lens (in contrast to DMPK), transgenic mice deficient in this gene show cataracts (Klesert et al., 2000) and since the closeness of the gene for DMAHP to the CTG repeat might allow its function to be disturbed preferentially by a small expansion.

Returning to the role of DMPK itself, this has now been intensively studied in terms of gene structure and sequence (Fig. 27.5b), RNA production, the nature and distribution of the protein and its functional properties (Epstein and Jin, 1998). There is general agreement on the expression of the gene in skeletal and heart muscle (Lam et al., 2000), but studies on RNA and protein levels in myotonic dystrophy have given conflicting results (Fu et al., 1993; Sabourin et al., 1993; Krahe et al., 1995), which may, in part, have resulted from differences in techniques used and tissues studied as well as reflecting possible differences between adult and congenital disease. More recently, it has been suggested that the effect of the mutation may be principally on DMPK RNA processing and maturation and that this may also affect the function of other RNAs by holding them within the nucleus as aggregates with CUG-binding proteins (Timchenko et al., 1996a). This mechanism could involve multiple genes that were not physically close.

Similar confusion has accompanied studies of the size of the DMPK protein as identified by different antibodies, with values found from 53 to 79 kDa (see Epstein and Jin, 1998; Harper and Johnson, 2000). It is not yet clear to what extent this signifies different isoforms in different tissues.

Localization to neuromuscular junctions and intercalated discs of striated muscle has been shown (van der Ven et al., 1993), but again it is possible that different isoforms may have different localizations (Dunne et al., 1996; Pham et al., 1998).

Functional studies have confirmed that DMPK does indeed show serine-threonine protein kinase activity (Dunne et al., 1996; Epstein and Jin, 1998), while comparison with allied structures shows it to be part of a large family of molecules involved in cell signalling (Leung et al., 1998).

A final area of potential complexity is that CTG repeat expansions have been shown to have direct effects on transcription, affecting the formation of nucleosomes and possibly through this affecting the function of genes in the region (Otten and Tapscott, 1995; Wang and Griffiths, 1995; Timchenko et al., 1996b). Altogether, it can be seen that the variety of mechanisms involved and their potential interactions mean that the unravelling of the factors involved in the cell biology of myotonic dystrophy is likely to be exceedingly complex.

Both knock-out and transgenic mouse models are now available (Monckton et al., 1998); knock-out mice for DMPK result only in mild myopathy, even in homozygous state (Jansen et al., 1996; Reddy et al., 1996), whereas transgenic mice produce more marked muscle changes, particularly when a large human repeat sequence is present (Gourdon et al., 1997). Recently, a large CTG expansion in transgenic mice was shown to affect the function of multiple RNAs and to reproduce the myotonia and myopathy, probably by interfering with CTG-binding proteins (Mankodi et al., 2000).

Management

The identification of the myotonic dystrophy mutation and the genes likely to be involved in the disease pathology have given a new impetus to therapeutic strategies, which has been enhanced by the possibility of assessing the effects of new agents on transgenic animal models. Results from preliminary trials of more conventional approaches have also emerged and have emphasized the value of having systematic assessment programmes in place that will allow detection of any change produced by therapy in this variable and slowly changing disorder. However, at present, no specific therapeutic agent exists that is of proven value. General aspects of management remain those of most benefit to patients.

Table 27.12 summarizes the main aspects of management. Most are relatively simple and obvious, yet it is surprising how many patients are left with no medical supervision and inadequate knowledge of the potential problems of the disease.

Table 27.12. Relevant factors in the management of myotonic dystrophy

Awareness of potential hazards and complications, by patients, family members and professionals

Regular medical surveillance
Support from lay groups
Avoidance of surgical and anaesthetic hazards
Early detection of swallowing problems
Regular electrocardiographic monitoring for cardiac conduction defects
Cataract surgery
Drug therapy for myotonia if severe and affecting function
Provision of appliances and mobility aids
Genetic counselling

Awareness is a key feature and should extend to relatives and to the family doctor as well as the patient. Only if those involved are full aware of the potential complications and hazards are serious avoidable problems likely to be prevented. Written information is useful and the internet an increasingly valuable source of details.

Regular medical surveillance is extremely helpful, especially on a multidisciplinary basis, with monitoring for cardiac conduction defects, and provision of appliances, physiotherapy and speech and swallowing therapy.

Surgery in myotonic dystrophy can carry high risks from a combination of cardiac arrhythmias, anaesthetic sensitivity and postoperative respiratory depression or aspiration, unless these hazards are clearly anticipated. It always needs to be asked whether the operation is actually necessary. Too often cholecystectomy or other abdominal surgery is performed for abdominal pain, which is likely to be colonic in origin and unlikely to be helped by surgical measures. If surgery is needed, it should only be undertaken where there are proper intensive care facilities available in case problems do arise. However, necessary surgery, such as cataract removal or correction of childhood orthopaedic deformities, should not be declined.

Drug therapy for myotonia plays only a small part in the management of myotonic dystrophy; in contrast to myotonia congenita, where the myotonia may be severe and disabling in some patients, most patients with myotonic dystrophy are troubled much more by their weakness than by myotonia, and they rarely require, or persist with, specific treatment for it.

Patients and relatives should be given the opportunity to have full and accurate information on the inheritance of myotonic dystrophy, both in general and in the specific context of their own situation.

References

Advisory Committee for genetic testing for Late Onset Disorders (1998). London: HMSO Department of Health.

Alwassan, M., Hamshere, M. G., Lennon, G. and Brook, J. D. (1998). Six transcripts map within 200 kilobases of the myotonic dystrophy expanded repeat. *Mammal. Genome* **9**, 485–487.

Ashizawa, T. and Epstein, H. F. (1991). Ethnic distribution of myotonic dystrophy gene. [Letter] *Lancet* **7**, 642–643.

Ashizawa, T., Hejtmanik, J. F., Liu, J., Perryman, M. B., Epstein, H. F. and Koch, D. D. (1992). Diagnostic value of ophthalmologic findings in myotonic dystrophy: comparison with risks calculated by haplotype analysis of closely linked restriction fragment length polymorphisms. *Am. J. Med. Genet.* **42**, 55.

Ashizawa, T., Dunne, P. W., Ward, P. A., Seltzer, W.K. and Richards, C. S. (1994a). Effects of the sex of myotonic dystrophy patients on the unstable triplet repeat in their affected offspring. *Neurology* **44**, 120–122.

Ashizawa, T., Anvret, M., Baiget, M. et al. (1994b). Characteristics of intergenerational contractions of the CTG repeat in myotonic dystrophy. *Am. J. Hum. Genet.* **54**, 414–423.

Aslanidis, C., Jansen, G., Amemiya, C. et al. (1992). Cloning of the essential myotonic dystrophy region and mapping of the putative defect. *Nature* **255**, 548–551.

Barnes, P. R., Hilton-Jones, D., Norbury, G., Roberts, A. and Huson, S. M. (1994). Incorrect diagnosis of myotonic dystrophy and its potential consequences revealed by subsequent direct genetic analysis. *J. Neurol. Neurosurg. Psychiatry* **57**, 662.

Batten, F. E. and Gibb, H. P. (1909). Myotonia atrophica. *Brain* **32**, 187–205.

Bell, J. (1947). Dystrophia myotonica and allied diseases. In: *Treasury of Human Inheritance*, Part V, ed. L. S. Penrose, pp. 343–410. Cambridge, UK: Cambridge University Press.

Bergoffen, J., Kant, J., Sladky, J., McDonald-McGinn, D., Zackai, E. H. and Fischbeck, K. H. (1994). Paternal transmission of congenital myotonic dystrophy. *J. Med. Genet.* **31**, 518–520.

Bossen, E. H., Selburne, J. D. and Verkauf, B. S. (1974). Respiratory muscle involvement in infantile myotonic dystrophy. *Arch. Pathol.* **97**, 250.

Bouchard, G., Roy, R., Declos, M., Mathieu, J. and Kouladjian, K. (1989). Origin and diffusion of the myotonic dystrophy gene in the Saguenay region (Québec). *Canad. J. Neurol. Sci.* **16**, 119–122.

Boucher, C. A., King, S. K., Carey, N. et al. (1995). A novel homeodomain encoding gene is associated with a large CpG island interrupted by the myotonic dystrophy unstable CTG repeat. *Hum. Mol. Genet.* **4**, 1919–1925.

Brewster, B., Groenen, P. and Wieringa, B. (1998). Myotonic dystrophy: clinical and molecular aspects. In: *Neuromuscular Disorders: Clinical and Molecular Genetics*, ed. A. E. H. Emery, pp. 323–364. Chichester: Wiley.

Brook, J. D., McCurrach, M. E., Harley, H. G. et al. (1992). Molecular basis of myotonic dystrophy: expansiohn of a trinucleotide (CTG) repeat at the 3′ end of a transcript encoding a protein kinase family member. *Cell* **68**, 799–808.

Brumback, R. A. and Wilson, H. (1984). Cognitive and personality function in myotonic dystrophy. *J. Neurol. Neurosurg. Psychiatry* **47**, 888–889.

Brunner, F. G., Smeets, H. J. M., Nillesen, et al. (1991). Myotonic dystrophy. *Brain* **114**, 2303.

Brunner, H. G., Nillesen, W., van Oost, B. A. et al. (1992). Presymptomatic diagnosis of myotonic dystrophy. *J. Med. Genet.* **29** 780–784.

Brunner, H. G., Bruggenwirth, H. T., Nillesen, W. et al (1993). Influence of sex of the transmitting parent as well as of parental allele size on the CTG expansion in myotonic dystrophy. *N. Engl. J. Med.* **328**, 476–480.

Bryant, S. H. (1977). The physiological basis of myotonia. In: *Pathogenesis of Human Muscular Dystrophies*, ed. L. P. Rowland, pp. 715–728. Amsterdam: Excerpta Medica.

Buxton, J., Shelbourne, P., Davies, J. et al. (1992). Detection of an unstable fragment of DNA specific to individuals with myotonic dystrophy. *Nat. Genet.* **6**, 355, 547–548.

Cobo, A., Martinez, J. M., Martorell, L. et al (1993). Molecular diagnosis of homozygous myotonic dystrophy in two asymptomatic sisters. *Hum. Mol. Genet.* **2**, 711–715.

Dada, T. O. (1973). Dystrophia myotonica in a Nigerian family. *E. Afr. Med.* **50**, 214–228.

Day, J. D., Roelofs, R., Leroy, B., Pech, I., Benzow, K. and Ranum, L. P. W. (1999). Clinical and genetic characteristics of a five generation family with a novel form of myotonic dystrophy (DM2) *Neuromusc. Disord.* **9**, 19–27.

de Die-Smulders, C. E., Höweler, C. J., Mirandolle, J. F. et al. (1994). Anticipation resulting in elimination of the myotonic dystrophy gene: a follow-up study of one extended family. *J. Med. Genet.* **31**, 595–601.

Dunne, P. W., Ma, L., Casey, D. L., Harati, Y. and Epstein, H. F. (1996). Localization of myotonic dystrophy protein kinase and its alteration with disease. *Cell. Motil. Cytoskel.* **33**, 52–63.

Eckhardt, V. F., Nix, W., Kraus, W. and Bohl, J. (1986). Esophageal motor function in patients with muscular dystrophy. *Gastroenterology* **90**, 628–635.

Engelkamp, D. and van Heyningen, V. T. (1996). Transcription factors in disease. *Curr. Opin. Genet. Dev.* **6**, 334–342.

Epstein, H. F. and Jin, S. (1998). Biochemical studies of DM protein kinase (DMPK). In: *Genetic Instabilities and Hereditary Neurological Diseases*, eds. R. D. Wells and S. T. Warren, pp. 147–167. New York: Academic Press.

Fleischer, B. (1918). Uber myotonische Dystrophie mit Katarakt. *Albrecht von Graefes Arch. Klin. Ophthalmol.* **96**, 91–133.

Fragola, P. V., Luzi, M., Calo, L. et al (1994). Cardiac involvement in myotonic dystrophy. *Am. J. Cardiol.* **74**, 1070–1072.

Fu, Y.-H., Pizzuti, A. M., Fenwick, R. G. et al. (1992). An unstable triplet repeat in a gene related to myotonic muscular dystrophy. *Science* **255**, 1256–1258.

Fu, Y.-H., Friedman, D. L., Richards, S. et al. (1993). Decreased expression of myotonin-protein kinase messenger RNA and protein in adult form of myotonic dystrophy. *Science* **260**, 235–238.

Gennarelli, M., Novelli, G., Andreasi Bassi, F. et al. (1996). Prediction of myotonic dystrophy clinical severity based on the number of intragenic (CTG) (n) trinucleotide repeats. *Am. J. Med. Genet.* **11**, 342–347.

Goldberg, J. I. and Sheft, D. J. (1972). Oesophageal and colon changes in myotonic dystrophica. *Gastroenterology* **63**, 134–189.

Goldman, A., Ramsay, M. and Jenkins, T. (1994). Absence of myotonic dystrophy in southern African Negroids is associated with a significantly lower number of CTG trinucleotide repeats. *J. Med. Genet.* **31**, 37–40.

Goldman, A., Ramsay, M. and Jenkins, T. (1996). Ethnicity and myotonic dystrophy: a possible explanation for its absence in sub-Saharan Africa. *Ann. Hum. Genet.* **60**, 57–65.

Gourdon, G., Radvanyi, F., Lia, A. S. et al. (1997). Moderate intergenerational and somatic instability of a 55 CTG repeat in transgenic mice. *Nat. Genet.* **15**, 190–192.

Greenfield, J. (1911). Notes on a family with myotonia atrophica and early cataract with report of an additional case of myotonia atrophica. *Rev. Neurol. Psychiatry* **9**, 169–181.

Hageman, A. T., Gabreels, F. J., Liem, K. D., Renkawek, K. and Boon, J. M. (1993). Congenital myotonic dystrophy; a report on thirteen cases and a review of the literature. [See comments] *J. Neurolog. Sci.* **115**, 95–101.

Harley, H. G., Brook, J. D., Rundle, S. A. et al. (1992a). Expansion of an unstable DNA region and phenotypic variation in myotonic dystrophy. *Nature* **6**, 545–546.

Harley, H. G., Rundle, S. A., Reardon, W. et al. (1992b). Unstable DNA sequence in myotonic dystrophy. *Lancet* **339**, 1125.

Harper, P. S. (1975). Congenital myotonic dystrophy in Britain. 1. Clinical aspects. *Arch. Dis. Child.* **50**, 505–513.

Harper, P. S. (1989). *Myotonic Dystrophy*, 2nd edn. Philadelphia, PA: Saunders.

Harper, P. S. (1996). *Huntington's Disease*. London: Saunders.

Harper, P. S. (1998). Myotonic dystrophy as a trinucleotide repeat disorder. In: *Genetic Instabilities and Hereditary Neurological Diseases*, eds. R. D. Wells and S. T. Warren, pp. 115–130. New York: Academic Press.

Harper, P. S. (2001). *Myotonic Dystrophy*, 3rd edn. London. PA: Saunders.

Harper, P. S. and Dyken, P. R. (1972). Early onset dystrophia myotonica – evidence supporting a maternal environmental factor. *Lancet* **ii**, 53–55.

Harper, P. S. and Johnson, K. J. (eds.) (2000). Myotonic dystrophy. In: *The Molecular and Metabolic Basis of Inherited Disease*. New York: McGraw-Hill, in press.

Harper, P. S. and Rüdel, R. (1993). Myotonic dystrophy. In: *Myology*, 2nd edn, ed. A. Engel, pp. 1192–1219. New York: McGraw Hill.

Harper, P. S., Harley, H. G., Reardon, W. and Shaw, D. J. (1992). Anticipation in myotonic dystrophy: new light on an old problem. *Am. J. Hum. Genet.* **51**, 10–16.

Hawley, R. J., Gottdiener, J. S., Day, J. A. and Engel, W. K. (1983). Families with myotrophic dystrophy with and without cardiac involvement. *Arch. Intern. Med.* **143**, 2134–2135.

Heath, S. K., Carne, S., Hoyle, C., Johnson, K. J. and Wells D. J. (1997). Characterisation of expression of mDMAHP, a homeodomain encoding gene at the murine DM locus. *Hum. Mol. Genet.* **6**, 651–657.

Höweler, C. J., Busch, H. F., Geraedts, J. P., Niermeijer, M. F. and Staal, A. (1989). Anticipation in myotonic dystrophy: fact or fiction? *Brain* **112**, 779–797.

Jansen, G., de Jong, P. J., Amemiya, C. et al. (1992). Physical and genetic characterization of the distal segment of the myotonic-dystrophy area on 19q. *Genomics* **13**, 509–517.

Jansen, G., Willems, P., Coerwinkel, M. et al. (1994). Gonosomal mosaicism in myotonic dystrophy patients: involvement of mitotic events in (CTG) (n) repeat variation and selection against extreme expansion in sperm. *Am. J. Hum. Genet.* **54**, 575–585.

Jansen, G., Bachner, D., Coerwinke, M., Wormskam, N. and Wieringa, B. (1995). Structural organisation and developmental expression pattern of the mourse WD-repeat gene DMR-N9 immediately upstream of the myotonic dystrophy locus. *Hum. Mol. Genet.* **4**, 843–852.

Jansen, G., Groenen, P. J. T. A., Bachner, D. et al. (1996). Abnormal myotonic dystrophy protein kinase levels produce only mild myopathy in mice. *Nat. Genet.* **13**, 316–324.

Karpati, G., Carpenter, S., Watters, G. V., Eisen, A. E. and Andermann, F. (1973). Infantile myotonic dystrophy. Histochemical and electron microscopic features in skeletal muscle. *Neurology* **23**, 1066–1077.

Kinoshita, M., Takahashi, R., Hasegawa, T. (1996). (CTG)n expansions in various tissues from a myotonic dystrophy patient. *Muscle Nerve* **19**, 240–242.

Klesert, T. R., Otten, A. D., Bird, T. D. and Tapscott, S. J. (1997). Trinucleotide repeat expansion at the myotonic dystrophy locus reduces expression of DMAHP. *Nat. Genet.* **16**, 402–406.

Krahe, R., Eckhart, M., Ogunniyi, A. O., Osuntokun, B. O., Siciliano, M. J. and Ashizawa, T. (1995). De novo myotonic dystrophy mutation in a Nigerian kindred. *Am. J. Hum. Genet.* **56**, 1067–1074.

Lam, L. T., Pham, Y. C. N., Man, N. and Morris, G. E. (2000). Characterization of a monoclonal antibody shows that the myotonic dystrophy protein kinase, DMPK, is expressed almost exclusively in muscle and heart. *Hum. Mol. Genet.* **9**, 2167–2174.

Lavedan, C., Hofmann-Radvanyi, H., Rabes, J. P., Roume, J. and Junien, C. (1993). Different sex-dependent constraints in CTG length variation as explanation for congenital myotonic dystrophy. *Lancet* **23**, 875–883.

Leung, T., Chen, X., Tan, I., Manser, E. and Lim, L. (1998). Myotonic dystrophy kinase-related Cdc42-binding kinase acts as a Cdc42 effector in promoting cytoskeletal reorganisation. *Mol. Cell Biol.* **18**, 130–140.

Lopez de Munain, A., Cobo, A. M., Huguet, E., Marti Masson, J. F., Johnson, K. and Baiget, M. (1994). CTG trinucleotide repeat variability in identical twins with myotonic dystrophy. *Ann. Neurol.* **35**, 374–375.

Lopez de Munain, A., Cobo, A. M., Poza, J. J. et al. (1995). Influence of the sex of the transmitting grandparent in congenital myotonic dystrophy. *J. Med. Genet.* **32**, 689–691.

MacMillan, J. C., Myring, J., Harley, H. G., Reardon, W., Harper, P. S. and Shaw, D. J. (1992). Molecular analysis for the myotonic dystrophy mutation in neuromuscular. *Neuromusc. Disord.* **2**, 405–411.

Mahadevan, M, Tsilfidis, C., Sabourin, L. et al. (1992). Myotonic dystrophy mutation: an unstable CTG repeat in the 3′ untranslated region of the gene. *Science* **255**, 1253–1255.

Mahler, C. and Parizel, G. (1982). Hypothalamic pituitary function in myotonic dystrophy. *J. Neurol.* **226**, 233–242.

Mankodi, A., Logigian, E., Callahan, L. et al. (2000). Myotonic dystrophy in transgenic mice expressing an expanded CUG repeat. *Science* **289** 1769–1773.

Martorell, L., Illa, I., Rosell, J., Benitez, J., Sedano, B. J. and Baiget, M. (1996). Homozygous myotonic dystrophy: clinical and molecular studies of three unrelated cases. *J. Med. Genet.* **33**, 783–785.

Mathieu, J., de Braekeleer, M. and Prevost, C. (1990). Genealogical reconstruction of myotonic dystrophy in the Saguenay-Lac-Saint-Jean area. *Neurology* **40**, 839–842.

Monckton, D. G., Wong, L. J., Ashizawa, T. and Caskey, C. T. (1995). Somatic mosaicism, germline expansion, germline reversions and intergenerational reductions in myotonic dystrophy males – small pool PCR analyses. *Hum. Mol. Genet.* **4**, 1–8.

Monckton, D. G., Ashizawa, T. and Siciliano, M. J. (1998). Murine models for myotonic dystrophy, In: *Genetic Instabilities and Hereditary Neurological Disease*, eds. R. Wells and S. Warren, pp. 181–193. San Diego, CA: Academic Press.

Morrone, A., Pegoraro, E., Angelini, C., Zammarchi, E., Marconi, G. and Hoffman, E. P. (1997). RNA metabolism in myotonic dystrophy; patient muscle shows decreased insulin receptor RNA and protein consistent with abnormal insulin resistance. *J. Clin. Invest.* **99**, 1691–1698.

Moxley, R. T. and Ricker, K. (1995). Proximal myotonic dystrophy. *Muscle Nerve* **18**, 557.

Moxley, R. T., Corbett, A. J., Minaker, M. L. and Rowe, J. W. (1984). Whole body insulin resistance in myotonic dystrophy. *Ann. Neurol.* **15**, 157–162.

Myring, J., Meredith, A. L., Harley, H. G. et al. (1992). Specific molecular prenatal diagnosis for the CTG mutation in myotonic dystrophy. *J. Med. Genet.* **29**, 785–788.

Newman, E. and Brook, J. D. (2001). Molecular and cell biology of myotonic dystrophy. In: *Myotonic Dystrophy*, 3rd edn, ed. P. S. Harper. London: Saunders.

Nguyen, H. H., Wolfe, J. T., Holmes, D. R. and Edwards, W. D. (1988). Pathology of the cardiac conduction system in myotonic dystrophy: a study of 12 cases. *J. Am. Coll. Cardiol.* **11**, 662–671.

Oberlé, I., Rousseau, F., Heitz, D. et al (1991). Amazing instability of a 550 bp DNA segment and abnormal methylation in fragile X syndrome. *Science* **252**, 1097.

O'Brien, T. and Harper, P. S. (1984). Reproductive problems and neonatal loss in women with myotonic dystrophy. *Brit. J. Obstet. Gynaecol.* **4**, 170–173.

O'Brien, T., Harper, P. S. and Newcombe, R. G. (1983). Blood pressure and myotonic dystrophy. *Clin. Genet.* **23**, 366–369.

Ohya, K., Tachi, N., Chiba, S. et al. (1994). Congenital myotonic dystrophy transmitted from an asymptomatic father. *Neurology* **44**, 1958–1960.

Olofsson, B.-O., Forsberg, H., Andersson, S., Bjerle, P., Henriksson, A. and Wedin, I. (1988). Electrocardiographic findings in myotonic dystrophy. *Brit. Heart J.* **59**, 47.

Otten, A. D. and Tapscott, S. J. (1995). Triplet repeat expansion in myotonic dystrophy alters the adjacent chromatin structure. *Proc. Natl. Acad. Sci. USA* **92**, 5465–5469.

Penrose, L. S. (1948). The problem of anticipation in pedigrees of dystrophia myotonica. *Ann. Eugen.* **14**, 125–132.

Pham, Y. C. N., thi Man, N., Lam, L. T. and Morris, G. E. (1998). Localization of myotonic dystrophy protein kinase in human and rabbit tissues using a new panel of monoclonal antibodies. *Hum. Mol. Genet.* **7**, 1957–1965.

Phillips, M. F. and Harper, P. S. (1997). Cardiac disease in myotonic dystrophy. *Cardiovasc. Res.* **33**, 13–22.

Phillips, M., Steer, H. M., Soldan, J. R., Wildes, C. M. and Harper, P. S. (1999). Daytime somnolence in myotonic dystrophy. *J. Neurol.* **246**, 275–282.

Pryse-Phillips, W., Johnson, G. J. and Larsen, B. (1982). Incomplete manifestations of myotonic dystrophy in a large kinship in Labrador. *Ann. Neurol.* **11**, 582–591.

Prystowsky, E. N., Prichett, E. L., Roses, A. D. and Gallagher, J. (1979). The natural history of conduction system disease in myotonic muscular dystrophy as determined by serial electrophysiologic studies. *Circulation* **60**, 1360–1364.

Ranum, L. P., Rasmussen, P. F., Benzow, K. A., Koob, M. D. and Day, J. W. (1998). Genetic mapping of a second myotonic dystrophy locus. *Nat. Genet.* **19**, 196–198.

Reardon, W., Harley, H. G., Brook, J. D. et al. (1992a). Minimal expression of myotonic dystrophy: a clinical and molecular analysis. *J. Med. Genet.* **29**, 770–773.

Reardon, W., Harley, H. G., Brook, J. D. et al. (1992b). Minimal expression of myotonic dystrophy: a clinical and molecular analysis. *J. Med. Genet.* **29**, 770.

Reardon, W., Newcombe, R., Fenton, I., Sibert, J. and Harper, P. S. (1993). The natural history of congenital myotonic dystrophy; mortality and long term clinical aspects. *Arch. Dis. Child.* **68**, 177–181.

Reddy, S., Sith, D. B. J., Rich, M. M. et al. (1996). Mice lacking the myotonic dystrophy protein kinase develop a late onset progressive myopathy. *Nat. Genet.* **13**, 325–335.

Ricker, K., Koch, M. C., Lehmann-Horn, F. et al. (1995). Proximal myotonic myopathy. Clinical features of a multisystem disorder similar to myotonic dystrophy. *Arch. Neurol.* **52**, 25–31.

Rolander, A. and Floderus, S. (1961). Dystrophia myotonica I Norbottens. *Svensk Lakartida* **58**, 648–652.

Ronnblom, A., Forsberg, H. and Danielsson, A. (1996). Gastrointestinal symptoms in myotonic dystrophy. *Scand. J. Gastroenterol.* **31**, 654–657.

Rosman, N. P. and Kakulas, B. A. (1966). Mental deficiency associated with muscular dystrophy. A neuropathological study. *Brain* **89**, 769–787.

Rubinsztein, J. S., Rubinsztein, D. C., Goodlum, S. and Holland, A. J. (1998). Apathy and hypersommia are common features of myotonic dystrophy. *J. Neurol. Neurosurg. Psychiatry* **64**, 510–515.

Rüdel, R. and Lehmann-Horn, F. (1996). Non-dystrophic myotonias and periodic paralyses. In: *Emery and Rimoin's Principles and Practice of Medical Genetics*, eds. D. L. Rimoin, J. M. Connor and R. E. Pyeritz, pp. 1006–1011. New York: Churchill Livingstone.

Rutherford, M. A., Heckmatt, J. Z. and Dubowitz, V. (1989). Congenital myotonic dystrophy: respiratory function at birth determines survival. *Arch. Dis. Child.* **64**, 191–195.

Sabourin, L. A., Mahadevan, M. S., Narang, M., Lee, D. S. C., Surh, L. C. and Korneluk, R. G. (1993). Effect of the myotonic dystrophy DM mutation on mRNA levels of the DM gene. *Nat. Genet.* **4**, 233–238.

Sarnat, H. B. and Silbert, S. W. (1976). Maturational arrest of fetal muscle in neonatal myotonic dystrophy. *Arch. Neurol.* **33**, 466–474.

Sermon, K., Lissens, W., Joris, H. et al. (1997). Clinical application of preimplantation diagnosis for myotonic dystrophy. *Prenat. Diagn.* **17**, 925–932.

Shaw, D. J., McCurrach, M., Rundle, S. A. et al. (1993). Genomic organisation and transcriptional units at the myotonic dystrophy locus. *Genomics* **18**, 673–679.

Shelbourne, P., Davies, J., Buxton, J. et al. (1993). Direct diagnosis of myotonic dystrophy with a disease-specific DNA marker. *N. Engl. J. Med.* **328**, 471–475.

Shutler, G., Korneluk, R. G., Tsilfidis, C. et al. (1992). Physical mapping and cloning of the proximal segment of the myotonic dystrophy gene region. *Genomics* **13**, 518–525.

Silver, M. M., Vilos, G. A., Silver, M. D., Shaheed, W. S. and Turner, K. L. (1984). Morphologic and morphometric analyses of muscle in the neonatal myotonic dystrophy syndrome. *Hum. Pathol.* **15**, 1171.

Simmons, Z., Thornton, C. A., Seltzer, W. K. and Richards, C. S. (1998). Relative stability of a minimal CTG repeat expansion in a large kindred with myotonic dystrophy. *Neurology* **50**, 1501–1504.

Smeets, H. J., Nillesen, W. M., Los, F. et al. (1992). Prenatal diagnosis of myotonic dystrophy by direct mutation analysis. *Lancet* **340**, 237–238.

Steinert, H. (1909). Uber das klinische und anatomische Bild des Muskelschwundes de Myotoniker. *Dtsch. Z. Nervenhlk.* **37**, 58–104.

Steyaert, J., Umans, S., Willekens, D. et al. (1997). A study of the cognitive and psychological profile in 16 children with congenital or juvenile myotonic dystrophy. *Clin. Genet.* **52**, 135–141.

Sutherland, G. R., Haan, E. A., Kremer, E. et al (1991). Hereditary unstable DNA: a new explanation for some old genetic questions? *Lancet* **338**, 289.

Swift, T. R., Ignacino, O. J. and Dyken, P. R. (1975). Neonatal dystrophia myotonica: electrophysiological studies. *Am. J. Dis. Child.* **129**, 734–737.

Telenius, H., Kremer, B., Goldberg, P., Theilmann, J. et al. (1994). Somatic and gonadal mosaicism of the Huntington disease gene CAG repeat in brain and sperm. *Nat. Genet.* **6**, 409–414.

Thomsen, J. (1876). Tonische krampfe in willkurlich beweglichen Muskeln infolge von ererbter psychischer Disposition (Ataxia muscularis). *Arch. Psychiatr. Nervenkr.* **6**, 702.

Thornton, C. A., Johnson, K. and Moxley, III, R. T. (1994). Myotonic dystrophy patients have larger CTG expansions in skeletal muscle than in leukocytes. *Ann. Neurol.* **35**, 104–107.

Timchenko, L. T., Miller, J. W., Timchenko, N. A. et al. (1996a). Identification of a (CUG)n triplet repeat RNA-binding protein and its expression in myotonic dystrophy. *Nucl. Acids Res.* **24**, 4407–4414.

Timchenko, L. T., Timchenko, N. A., Caskey, C. T. and Roberts, R. (1996b). Novel proteins with binding specificity for DNA CTG and RNA CUG repeats: implications for myotonic dystrophy. *Hum. Mol. Genet.* **5**, 115–121.

Tishkoff, S. A., Goldman, A., Calafell, F. et al. (1998). A global haplotype analysis of the myotonic dystrophy locus: Implications for the evolution of modern humans and for the origin of myotonic dystrophy mutations. *Am. J. Hum. Genet.* **62**, 1389–1402.

Tsilfidis, C., MacKenzie, A. E., Mellter, G., Barcelo, J. and Korneluk, R. G. (1992). Correlation between CTG trinucleotide repeat length and frequency of severe congenital myotonic dystrophy. *Nat. Genet.* **1**, 192–195.

Udd, B., Krahe, R., Wallgren-Pattersson, C. et al. (1997). Proximal myotonic myopathy – a family with proximal muscular dystrophy, myotonia, cataracts and hearing loss. *Neuromusc. Disord.* **7**, 217–228.

van der Ven, P. F. M., Jansen, G., van Kuppevelt, T. H. M. S. M. et al. (1993). Myotonic dystrophy kinase is a component of neuromuscular junctions. *Hum. Mol. Genet.* **2**, 1889–1894.

Vanier, T. M. (1960). Dystrophia myotonica in childhood. *Brit. Med. J.* **2**, 1284–1288.

Vazquez, J. A., Pinies, J. A., Martul, P., de Los, R., Gatzambide, S. and Busturia, M. A. (1990). Hypothalamic–pituitary–testicular function in 70 patients with myotonic dystrophy. *J. Endocrinol. Invest.* **13**, 375–379.

Wang, Y. H. and Griffiths, J. (1995). Expanded CTG triplet blocks from the myotonic dystrophy gene create the strongest known natural nucleosome positioning elements. *Genomics* **25**, 570–573.

Wells, R. D. and Warren, S. T. (eds). (1998). *Genetic Instabilities and Hereditary Neurological Diseases.* New York: Academic Press

Wexler, N. S., Young, A. B., Tanzi, R. E. et al. (1987). Homozygotes for Huntington's disease. *Nature* **326**, 194–197.

Wieringa, B., Brunner, H., Hulsebos, T., Schonk, D. and Ropers, H. H. (1988). Genetic and physical demarcation of the locus for dystrophia myotonica. In: *Advances in Neurology*, Vol. 48, *Molecular Genetics of Neurological and Neuromuscular Diseases*, eds. DiDonato et al., pp. 47–69. New York: Raven.

Winchester, C. L. and Johnson, K. J. (1998). Is myotonic dystrophy (DM) the result of a contiguous gene defect? In: *Genetic Instabilities and Hereditary Neurological Disease*, eds. R. Wells and S. Warren, pp. 169–179. San Diego, CA: Academic Press.

Winchester, C. L., Ferrier, R. K., Sermoni, A., Clark, B. J and Johnson, K. J. (1999). Characterization of expression of DMPK and SIX5 in the human eye and implications for pathogenesis in myotonic dystrophy, *Hum. Mol. Genet.* **8**, 481–492.

Wohrle, D., Kennerknecht, I., Wolf, M., Enders, H., Schwemmle, S. and Steinbach, P. (1995). Heterogeneity of DNA kinase repeat expansion in different fetal tissues. *Hum. Mol. Genet.* **4**, 1147–1153.

Woodward, J. B., Heaton, R. K., Simon, D. B. and Ringel, S. P. (1982). Neuropsychological findings in myotonic dystrophy. *J. Clin. Neuropsychol.* **4**, 335–342.

28

The metabolic myopathies

Richard T. Moxley III, Patrick Chinnery and Douglas Turnbull

Introduction

Inherited disorders of glycogen and fatty acid metabolism frequently cause skeletal muscle dysfunction as well as alterations in other organs, such as the heart and the liver (Tein, 1999). Patients typically present in one of three ways: (i) with progressive weakness and hypotonia (glycogenoses, such as the deficiencies of acid maltase, debrancher enzyme and brancher enzyme (GBE); and disorders of fatty acid oxidation, such as decreased uptake of carnitine and a deficiency of carnitine acylcarnitine translocase); (ii) with recurrent, reversible, muscle dysfunction associated with exercise intolerance and myoglobinuria with or without muscle cramps (glycogenoses, such as deficiencies of phosphorylase, phosphofructokinase (PFK) and phosphoglycerate kinase (PGK), and defects in fatty acid oxidation, such as a deficiency of carnitine palmitoyltransferase II (CPT II); or (iii) with a combination of (i) and (ii) (deficiencies in very-long-chain acyl coenzyme A dehydrogenase (VLCAD), short-chain L-3-hydroxyacyl-CoA dehydrogenase (SCAD) and trifunctional protein (MTP)). Episodes of lethargy, seizures and hypoglycaemia, or sudden unexpected death, are nonmuscle manifestations that occur in neonates and infants with these metabolic defects. Those manifestations may obscure detection of muscle weakness and deter arriving at the correct diagnosis. Chronic progressive weakness or episodic exercise-induced muscle pain and myoglobinuria occur as signs of metabolic myopathy later in childhood and in adult life.

Identification of the specific mutations responsible for many of the hereditary metabolic disorders of muscle is now possible as a result of breakthroughs in molecular biology. However, in vitro enzyme assays in cultured fibroblasts and muscle tissue still provide an important means to establish a specific diagnosis. Detection of metabolites in urine and plasma both at rest and during episodes of encephalopathy or weakness are usually necessary, and testing, such as forearm exercise with measurements of muscle release of lactate and ammonia, often points toward the likely alteration in muscle metabolism.

This chapter focuses on the hereditary disorders of glycogen and fatty acid metabolism that cause myopathy.

The glycogenoses

All the glycogenoses are autosomal recessive disorders except for PGK deficiency, which is an X-linked recessive, and some forms of phosphorylase b kinase (PbK) deficiency. Most of the defects involve cytoplasmic enzymes that act at different levels in glycogen breakdown and glycolysis (see Chapters 5 and 8). GBE involves the glycogen synthesis pathway and acid maltase deficiency the intralysosomal glycogen degradation pathway. Muscle weakness may occur in isolation or in association with other systemic complaints. If the inherited enzyme defect exists in a single molecular form identical for all tissues, it causes generalized disease, such as that occurring in the infantile form of acid maltase deficiency (AMD). However, most of the enzymes involved in glycogen metabolism and glycolysis exist in multiple isoforms and tissue-specific regulation during development occurs (DiMauro et al., 1997). The varying severity of organ involvement in specific diseases of glycogen metabolism and glycolysis may relate to the protective effects of uninvolved isoforms of a particular enzyme or from low residual concentrations of the enzyme in specific target tissues. However, many questions remain about the variability of the clinical phenotypes of the metabolic myopathies. In childhood and adult-onset AMD, there is a selective weakness of specific muscles although the enzyme defect is generalized.

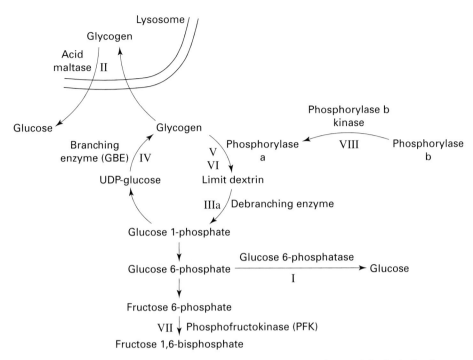

Fig. 28.1. Glycogen and early glucose metabolism to show the enzymes that are defective in the glycogenoses (I–VIII).

Recent reports have raised the hypothesis of 'double trouble'. For example, the autosomal recessive mutation that produces a deficiency of the main muscle isozyme of adenylate deaminase (myoadenylate deaminsae, AMPD) is common and occurs in approximately 2% of the population (Morisaki et al., 1992). Most individuals with this mutation are asymptomatic. Of interest are two children with AMPD deficiency who developed unusually early onset of myoglobinuria. Could these patients having very early onset of more severe symptoms of their glycogenosis represent an interactive 'double trouble' effect between the deficiencies of AMPD and myophosphorylase/PFK? These questions and many others require further study to investigate the relationship between phenotype and genotype(s).

At present disorders of glycogen metabolism cause two main clinical syndromes: one that involves progressive weakness of the limb and trunk musculature, sparing extraocular and facial muscles, and the other a syndrome of exercise intolerance, muscle cramps and intermittent muscle necrosis and myoglobinuria. The following section reviews the specific enzyme deficiencies that cause muscle symptoms. The first group are those involved in glycogen metabolism and glucose activation (Fig. 28.1). The second group can be described as the distal glycolytic pathway and are involved in breakdown of glucose to acetyl-CoA for other uses (Fig. 28.2).

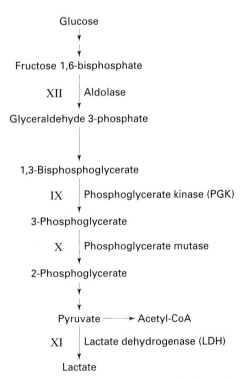

Fig. 28.2. Enzyme defects in the distal glycolytic pathway giving rise to glycogenoses (IX–XII).

Glycogen metabolism and glucose activation

Acid maltase deficiency

Acid maltase (lysosomal α-glucosidase) hydrolyses both (1–4)- and (1–6)-α-glycosidic linkages. In early life, degradation of lysosomal glycogen to glucose is essential to mobilize glycogen from the liver. Later in life the principal function of acid maltase is to prevent glycogen storage in lysosomes. The gene (GAA) for acid maltase maps to chromosome 17q21-q23, and contains 20 exons (D'Ancona et al., 1979; Hoefsloot et al., 1988, 1990; Martiniuk et al., 1985, 1986, 1990, 1991). The biosynthesis and processing of the enzyme includes multiple steps (Hoefsloot et al., 1988, 1990; Hermans et al., 1993; Wisselaar et al., 1993). Although AMD was the first lysosomal disorder to be identified (Hers, 1963), the precise metabolic role for the enzyme is still enigmatic. Massive amounts of glycogen, and at times mucopolysaccharides, accumulate in cells lacking the enzyme and attest to its biological significance, yet severe deficiency of the enzyme can exist in some cells and tissues without glycogen excess or functional impairment.

There are three forms of AMD: infantile, juvenile, and adult. Infants have hypotonia and weakness, enlargement of the heart, tongue and liver. Respiratory and feeding difficulties develop and death occurs before the age of two years. The childhood type presents later with weakness of proximal greater than distal limb muscles. Respiratory muscles have relatively selective severe damage (Rosenow and Engel, 1978; Martin et al., 1983; Trend et al., 1985; Margolis and Hill, 1986) and the heart is typically spared. Occasionally, calf enlargement develops, which simulates muscular dystrophy (Hers and Van Hoff, 1968; Swaiman et al., 1968, Engel et al., 1973). The adult form presents after 20 years of age with slowly progressive myopathy, typically affecting the proximal leg muscles first (Sander et al., 1998; de Jager et al., 1998; DiMauro et al., 1997). As many as one-third of the adult cases present with respiratory failure (Rosenow and Engel, 1978; Kurz et al., 1998), and eventually respiratory involvement occurs in all adults and is the usual cause of death (DiMauro et al., 1978a). Glycogen accumulation in skeletal muscle and other tissues varies in the various forms of AMD. Vacuoles appear in muscle tissue in all three forms but the amount is less marked in children and adults. A detailed review of the light microscopic and electron microscopic characteristics of the glycogen deposition is covered in a recent review (Engel and Hirschhorn, 1994).

The molecular defects associated with infantile AMD differ from those recently reported in some adult patients with AMD. AMD results from a heterogenous group of mutations affecting exons 2, 5, 10, 11, 14, 15, 18 and 19 as well as introns 1 and 10 (Raben et al., 1995a; Reuser et al., 1995; Huie et al., 1998). Mutations in exons 14 and 18 are common in infantile AMD while a splice out of exon 2 is common in adult AMD (Raben et al., 1995a; Reuser et al., 1995). Infantile AMD contrasts in its molecular biology from adult AMD. Over half the infantile patients have no detectable GAA mRNA (Martiniuk et al., 1986, 1990; van der Ploeg et al., 1988) while adult patients often have GAA mRNA of normal structure in skeletal muscle but deficient enzyme activity (Raben et al., 1995a; Hirschhorn, 1995). As a rule the clinical severity of AMD correlates with the level of enzyme activity assayed in leukocytes, fibroblasts or muscle tissue, with patients with the adult-onset disease having greater residual enzyme activity than those with the infantile-onset disease (Hirschhorn, 1995; Hers et al., 1989). However, some patients with adult-onset AMD have unusually low levels of enzyme activity that are more typical of those seen in infantile AMD (Raben et al., 1995a). The discordance between clinical severity and assays for residual enzyme activity may relate to the tissue selected for analysis. Recently, investigators described a close relationship between the degree of residual enzyme activity and clinical severity when using maltose as a substrate and carefully comparing activity with that in unaffected individuals (Huie et al., 1998).

Diagnostic clues of AMD consist of organomegaly in infants and children, the firm consistency of the weak muscle, selectively severe involvement of respiratory muscles and of hip adductor muscles in some of the adults, abnormal electrical irritability with myotonic-like discharges on electromyography (EMG), and vacuolar myopathy with high glycogen content and acid phosphatase activity of the vacuoles. However, none of the clinical or morphological findings is specific, and enzymatic analysis of muscle, cultured fibroblasts or leukocytes is necessary to reach a diagnosis. Prenatal diagnosis is possible by chorionic villus sampling (Reuser et al., 1995). An elevation in serum enzymes of muscle origin, especially creatine kinase, is common in all types of AMD. A diagnostic protocol for adult-onset AMD using an elevation of serum creatine kinase as the start point is available (Ausems et al., 1999) and recommends an initial assay for GAA in leukocytes in adults with elevated serum creatine kinase and clinical manifestations suggesting AMD. Adults without significant elevation of creatine kinase proceed to muscle biopsy and other diagnostic tests.

Treatment is supportive. Enzyme replacement remains a possibility for the future (DiMauro et al., 1997). A high-protein diet may help in certain patients (Slonim et al., 1983; Isaacs et al., 1986; Margolis and Hill, 1986; Umpleby et al., 1989). Recent gene transfer studies in fibroblasts and myoblasts from patients (Nicolino et al., 1998; Yang et al., 1998) and in animal models of AMD (including the Japanese Quail (Tsujino et al., 1998), mice (Raben et al., 1998) and neonatal rat (Pauly et al., 1998)) offer hope that some form of gene therapy will prove effective.

Debranching enzyme deficiency (glycogenosis IIIa; Cori–Forbes disease)

Debranching enzyme is bifunctional. It hydrolyses glycogen branch points (amylo-(1–6)-glucosidase activity) and transfers those three glucose residues adjacent to the branch points that resist cleavage by phosphorylase (oligo-(α1,4$\rightarrow$1–4)glucantransferase) activity (Brown and Illingworth, 1962). The enzyme is normally present in all tissues and can be assayed in leukocytes, erthyrocytes, cultured fibroblasts, muscle, liver and heart (Ding et al., 1990).

Three types of debrancher enzyme deficiency exist based upon a classification using the enzymatic and immunological assays. Transferase and glucosidase activities are deficient and cross-reacting material (CRM) is absent in both muscle and liver in type IIIa. In type IIIb both enzymatic activities are deficient but CRM is normal in muscle and heart with only the liver having a marked deficiency. In type IIIc there is a selective loss of transferase activity in liver and muscle with preservation of CRM in tissues typically affected. Specific mutations in the gene *AGL* occur in the different forms of debrancher deficiency. Mutations in exons 30 and 32 cause type IIIa in Ashkenazi Jews from North Africa (Parvari et al., 1997, 1998). Mutations in exon 3 cause type IIIb in some patients, but an insertion in intron 32 also can produce the type IIIb phenotype (Shen et al., 1996; Okubo et al., 1998).

Glycogenosis IIIa comprises a small subgroup with clinically significant myopathy (DiMauro et al., 1997). A protuberant abdomen in childhood, which decreases in adolescence, and muscle fatigue or aching on heavy exercise since an early age are common. Progressive weakness begins in early childhood or more commonly in adult life. Serum enzymes of muscle origin are increased from twice to more than ten times the upper limit of normal. EMG shows changes consistent with myopathy. Increased insertional activity, myotonic discharges and fibrillation potentials may occur (Brunberg et al., 1971; DiMauro et al., 1979). Muscle glycogen concentration varies between 3 and 6% and the iodine absorption spectrum of glycogen resembles that of limit dextrin. Histopathological studies show vacuolar myopathy.

Myopathic symptoms in debrancher enzyme deficiency typically start in the third or fourth decade at a time when hepatomegaly may be less prominent (DiMauro et al., 1984, 1997). Because the wasting is often in distal leg muscles and intrinsic hand muscles an erroneous diagnosis of motor neuron disease or peripheral neuropathy may occur. Sensory findings are rare. Confirmation of the diagnosis requires biochemical assay for debranching enzyme activity.

Frequent feedings and nocturnal gastric infusions of glucose and uncooked corn starches are used for hypoglycaemia, especially in childhood (Tein, 1999). No specific treatment is effective for the myopathy.

Branching enzyme deficiency

GBE (amylo-(1,4$\rightarrow$1,6)-transgylcosylase) introduces branch points into glycogen by transferring a terminal fragment from a 4-position on a branch terminus to a 6-position in the interior of the polymer. A deficiency of GBE results from mutation in *GBE* on chromosome 3 (Bao et al., 1996a,b; Lossos et al., 1998). The disease is an autosomal recessive disorder (Chen and Burchell, 1995) and has a variable clinical picture. Some patients even present in adulthood with central and peripheral nervous system dysfunction associated with the accumulation of polyglucosan bodies in the nervous system (so-called adult polyglucosan disease) (Lossos et al., 1991; Bruno et al., 1993; Bornemann et al., 1996; Lossos et al., 1998).

The precise molecular basis for the symptoms in GBE deficiency and for the variability in clinical patterns is not known. There are no tissue-specific isoforms and the variation in residual enzyme activity does not reliably predict the clinical severity (Brown and Brown, 1983; Tang et al., 1994; Bornemann et al., 1996; McConkie-Rosell et al., 1996; Lossos et al., 1998). The accumulation of basophilic, abnormally staining polysaccharide material that resists digestion with diastase is variable and can vary within different tissues in the same patient (Chen and Burchell, 1995).

Diagnosis of GBE deficiency is suggested by progressive hepatosplenomegaly and failure to thrive in infancy, muscle weakness (if present), and periodic acid–Schiff (PAS)-positive, diastase-fast deposits in affected tissues. Enzymatic assays and structural analysis of glycogen provide confirmatory evidence.

Treatment is supportive. Liver transplantation has proven beneficial in 10 children (Selby et al., 1991), but this therapy does not protect against the development of disease symptoms in other organs. Two years after liver transplantation, a child with GBE deficiency died of intractible cardiomyopathy (Sokal et al., 1992).

Myophosphorylase deficiency (type V glycogenosis; McArdle's disease)

Myophosphorylase deficiency is an autosomal recessive disease predicted by McArdle to occur from a deficiency of muscle phosphorylase (McArdle, 1951) and confirmed in 1959 (Mommaerts et al., 1959; Schmidt and Mahler, 1959). Phosphorylase deficiency results from mutations in chromosome 11q13 (Lebo et al., 1984; Burke et al., 1987; Tsujino et al., 1995a; Kubisch et al., 1998; Vorgerd et al., 1998; Andreu et al., 1999; Bruno et al., 1999a,b; Rubio et al., 1999). The nonsense point mutation at codon 9 is the most common, occurring in patients from the USA, UK, Germany, Italy and Spain. Japanese patients do not have this common mutation and myophosphorylase deficiency results in 72% of this population from mutations in codon 708/709 in exon 17 (Tsujino et al., 1995a). McArdle's disease is genetically heterogenous and occurs in patients with homozygous nonsense or missense mutations and in compound heterozygotes having a combination of alleles with missense and nonsense mutations (Vorgerd et al., 1998). Over 16 different mutations lead to McArdle's disease. Most mutations lead to no detectable myophosphorylase activity in muscle tissue; however, mRNA levels may be decreased, absent or show a truncated form (Beynon et al., 1995; Tsujino et al., 1995a). Variability in the level of expression of mRNA for myophosphorylase as well as variability in the level of residual activity may account for the different degrees of severity and spectrum of ages for the onset of clinical symptoms. These factors may contribute to the preponderance of males with phosphorylase deficiency.

Onset of symptoms in myophosphorylase deficiency typically occurs in late childhood or early teens with muscular pain, weakness and stiffness during slight-to-moderate exertion. Pain on exercise can occur in any muscle, even those of the jaw. Rest rapidly relieves the symptoms provoked by moderate exercise, but the more intense or prolonged the exercise, the longer the symptoms persist, sometimes for several days. Myoglobinuria occurs in approximately one-half of those affected and mild muscle weakness and atrophy in about one-third. A common symptom is an inability to extend the fingers fully after maintaining a sustained powerful grip. Repetitive, ischaemic type, forearm exercise results in rapid fatigue and a prolonged contracture of the muscle. Moderate whole-body exercise often provokes muscle stiffness in the limbs, tachycardia, dyspnoea, rapid exhaustion and, occasionally, nausea and vomiting. To avoid or lessen these symptoms, patients typically will 'warm up their muscles' for a few minutes, rest and after this warm up begin more prolonged exercise. This permits mobilization of fatty acids as a fuel and permits an improvement in overall exercise tolerance. This is referred to as 'second wind' phenomenon.

The precise cause for fatigue in myophosphorylase deficiency remains a mystery. Recent investigations suggest that the decrease in endurance and the abnormally hyperkinetic cardiorespiratory response to whole-body exercise result from a decreased density of Na^+/K^+ pumps on skeletal muscle fibres, which causes a failure of skeletal muscle fibre membrane excitability (Haller et al., 1998). The decreased number of Na^+/K^+ pumps may also lead to the hyperkalaemia that occurs during exercise. The decreased Na^+/K^+ pump density in muscle fibres may develop secondary to decreased physical activity and may also decrease the ease with which a contracture can occur. The mechanism of the electrically silent muscle contracture remains unclear, but it may result from a combination of increased sensitivity to calcium of the contractile proteins and an associated elevation in intracellular calcium (Ruff, 1996).

Serum levels of muscle enzymes are usually elevated at rest. Even clinically asymptomatic patients with myophosphorylase deficiency have elevated levels of serum creatine kinase (Gospe et al., 1998). Following exercise, the level of muscle enzymes can increase markedly. EMG studies occasionally show alterations consistent with myopathy. There is electrical silence of muscle fibres during contracture. Repetitive stimulation of motor nerves produces a decline in amplitude of the evoked compound muscle potential and a decline in the force (Haller et al., 1998). Absence of phosphorylase is apparent histochemically in fresh frozen muscle. Enzyme activity is absent from skeletal muscle fibres but present in smooth muscle cells of blood vessels. Detection of phosphorylase in muscle depends upon the presence of a glycogen primer; the enzyme is not demonstrable even in normal muscle that is depleted of glycogen, which can occur following prolonged storage of a specimen at room temperature or after death. Mature muscle fibres in patients lack phosphorylase activity; however, the fetal isozyme can reappear in immature-regenerating muscle fibres (Sato et al., 1977; DiMauro et al., 1978b; Martinuzzi et al., 1999). Assay of skeletal muscle for myophosphorylase activity establishes the diagnosis (<5% of normal). Analysis of muscle recovering following a bout of rhabdomyolysis can hamper diagnosis because of the appearance of the fetal isozyme.

Forearm exercise testing is helpful. One protocol involves collecting forearm venous blood at rest and after ischaemic exercise. This protocol has risk. A blood pressure cuff is placed around the arm, inflated to 80–100 mmHg above resting systolic blood pressure. Repetitive maximum hand grip exercise occurs for 1 minute (approximately

30 grips) using a hand dynamometer to record grip force. At the conclusion of the 1 minute of ischaemic exercise the blood pressure cuff is released and venous forearm blood is obtained 1, 2, 5 and 10 minutes after exercise for measurement of lactate and ammonia. This test introduces a risk of provoking a forearm muscle contracture and rhabdomyolysis. Ischaemic forearm exercise testing may lead to a compartment syndrome with ulnar nerve damage or to myoglobinuria with renal failure in some patients (Meinck et al., 1982).

The preferred protocol for forearm exercise is a nonischaemic forearm exercise test without a blood pressure cuff. Repetitive maximum isometric contractions using a hand dynamometer occur, each maintained for 1.5 seconds followed by 0.5 second of rest, performed for 1 minute. Forearm venous blood samples are collected prior to exercise and 1, 2, 4, 6 and 10 minutes following cessation of exercise and analysed for venous lactate and ammonia. A threefold elevation in lactate indicates a normal response. Lactate levels rise immediately after exercise, while ammonia rises gradually, beginning 3–4 minutes after completion of exercise. Patients with a defect in muscle glycogenolysis will fail to have a normal rise in lactate and will have an exaggerated increase in ammonia.

Treatment remains a challenge. Moderate low intensity aerobic exercise is safe and an important part of the treatment in myophosphorylase deficiency. Monitoring serum creatine kinase levels between exercise sessions is useful to assure that the appropriate intensity of exercise is being used. Excessive intensity of exercise provokes an abnormally marked increase in creatine kinase and reflects associated muscle injury. Patients should avoid maximal exercise, but they should also avoid a highly sedentary lifestyle. Such deconditioning makes patients more dependent on glycolysis. Past attempts to treat patients with frequent ingestion of glucose or fructose, injections of glucagon and the administration of branch-chain amino acids have proven ineffective (MacLean, et al., 1958; Tein, 1999).

Aggressive treatment of rhabdomyolysis and myoglobinuria is essential for the acute management of pigmenturia in patients with myophosphorylase deficiency and other metabolic myopathies that cause rhabdomyolysis. A marked elevation in serum creatine kinase should prompt urine testing with haemastix to check for myoglobin. Increased fluid intake, urgent medical evaluation, admission and careful monitoring for renal failure may be indicated. Decreasing the pH of the urine with bicarbonate treatment is often necessary. Some patients require intravenous mannitol and furosemide (frusemide) to maintain urine output. Occasionally haemodialysis is required.

Phosphorylase b kinase deficiency (glycogenosis VIII)

PbK deficiency causes a variety of clinical syndromes; two involve skeletal muscle. The kinase is a multimeric enzyme composed of four different subunits: α, β, γ and δ. The α- and β-subunits are regulatory. The γ-subunit is catalytic, and the δ-subunit confers calcium sensitivity through its calmodulin-like activity (Wehner and Kilimann, 1995; Bruno et al., 1998a). Wehner et al. (1994) have proposed three sites for mutations that may cause PbK deficiency. These are the muscle-specific α-subunit gene on the X chromosome, the muscle-specific exon of the β-subunit on chromosome 16 and the muscle-specific γ-subunit gene on chromosome 7. At present there are two mutations in the α_M-subunit on the X chromosome (Xq12-q13) that cause the myopathic form of PbK deficiency (Wehner et al., 1994; Bruno et al., 1998a). Another form of PbK deficiency presents in early childhood with hepatomegaly and nonprogressive myopathy (Madlom et al., 1989; van den Bergl and Berger, 1990). Still another form, which is mainly myopathic, presents in childhood or adolescence with exercise intolerance, stiffness and weakness of the exercising muscles (Clemens et al., 1990; Shin, 1990; Wilkinson et al., 1994). Less commonly, patients present with respiratory failure, hypotonia and cardiomyopathy (Mizuta et al., 1984; Servidei et al., 1988; Sahin et al., 1998; Regalado et al., 1999). The hepatic form of PbK deficiency begins in infancy or childhood and causes hepatomegaly, motor delay, failure to thrive and hypoglycaemia (van den Bergl and Berger, 1990). Inheritance in these cases is X-linked recessive or occasionally autosomal recessive.

Patients with myopathy have a variable elevation of serum creatine kinase. Forearm exercise may produce a normal, impaired or a flat curve for venous lactate after exercise (Abarbanel et al., 1986; Wilkinson et al., 1994). There is often an abnormal elevation of venous ammonia after exercise (Laforet et al., 1996). Muscle biopsy shows subsarcolemmal accumulations of glycogen, typically in type IIB fibres (Wilkinson et al., 1994). No glycogen storage is present in satellite cells, fibroblasts, endothelial cells, pericytes, smooth muscle of intramuscular blood vessels, in axons or Schwann cells of intramuscular nerves (Clemens et al., 1990). Histochemical staining for phosphorylase is normal. Assay of muscle for PbK shows no activity or a severe deficiency (Wehner and Kilimann, 1995; Laforet et al., 1996; Bruno et al., 1998b; Sahin et al., 1998).

There is no specific treatment. A high-protein diet is a consideration. A trial of prednisone 30mg per day for 3 months failed to improve patients (Clemens et al., 1990). Supportive care and moderate exercise remain the mainstay of therapy.

Phosphofructokinase deficiency (glycogenosis VII; Tarui's disease)

PFK deficiency is an autosomal recessive disorder and results from point mutations in chromosome 1q32 involving both introns and exons (Nakagawa et al., 1995; Nakajima et al., 1995; Raben et al., 1995a). Fewer than 40 cases of PFK deficiency have been reported. Mutations affecting exon 5 account for 60% of the mutations that cause PFK deficiency in Ashkenazi Jewish patients (Raben et al., 1995b). Clinical findings resemble those associated with myophosphorylase deficiency. The onset of exercise intolerance, myalgias and cramps without definite weakness usually occurs in early childhood. Occasionally patients will have prominent gouty arthritis, haemolysis and gastric ulcer in association with exercise intolerance (Nakagawa et al., 1995). Jaundice occurs in some patients as does myoglobinuria.

Forearm exercise testing in PFK deficiency is abnormal. There is decreased production of lactate and an increased production of ammonia. Both PFK and myophosphorylase deficiencies show this pattern (Mineo and Tarui, 1995; Tarui, 1995). However, glucose infusion leads to a different effect on muscle purine degradation in myophosphorylase deficiency compared with PFK deficiency. In myophosphorylase deficiency, intravenous infusion of 5% dextrose during forearm exercise prevents the rise in venous ammonia and hypoxanthine. Intravenous glucose accompanying forearm exercise in patients with PFK deficiency leads to an even more abnormal rise in plasma ammonia and hypoxanthine levels than with exercise alone (Mineo and Tarui, 1995). Glucose infusion actually lowers exercise performance in patients with PFK deficiency and impairs muscle oxidative phosphorylation (Haller and Lewis, 1991). Increased glucose entry into exercising muscle provides an energy substrate in patients with myophosphorylase deficiency. In contrast, in PFK deficiency, the antilipolytic effect of glucose deprives exercising muscle of free fatty acids, which are the critical fuel for skeletal muscle in this disorder. Of interest is the presence of insulin resistance in patients with PFK deficiency (Ristow et al., 1997). Insulin resistance may have developed to exert a protective effect since insulin normally inhibits lipolysis.

Studies of isometric plantar flexion exercise performed both aerobically and anaerobically indicate that a reduced turnover of the tricarboxylic acid cycle accounts for the fatigue and muscle cramps in PFK deficiency (Grehl et al., 1998). Heterozygotes showed moderate alterations from normal while homozygotes showed a markedly elevated ATP demand during exercise. There was a dramatic increase in the concentration of phosphomonoesters (Grehl et al., 1998). Animal studies using the PFK-deficient dog model indicate impaired oxidative metabolism and impaired extraction of oxygen by skeletal muscle during electrically stimulated muscle exercise (McCully et al., 1999).

The subsarcolemmal glycogen deposits in muscle resemble those seen in myophosphorylase deficiency. Structurally abnormal glycogen, resembling the amylopectin that accumulates in GBE deficiency, has been observed in muscle fibres in a few patients (Agamanolis et al., 1980; Hays et al., 1981). Diagnosis depends on assay of skeletal muscle for the specific muscle isoform of PFK (Nakagawa et al., 1995; Nikajima et al., 1995; Raben et al., 1995a).

Treatment differs somewhat from that for myophosphorylase deficiency in view of the worsening of muscle metabolism that occurs with the administration of glucose. Acutely ill infants benefit from a ketogenic diet (Swoboda et al., 1997). A diet relatively high in protein may also help older patients, although no controlled studies are available. Moderate aerobic exercise is desirable. However, excessive exercise may increase haemolysis (Toyoda et al., 1996), and monitoring of exercise intensity is required as noted previously for myophosphorylase deficiency.

Defects in the distal glycolytic pathway

Deficiencies of PGK, phosphoglycerate mutase, lactate dehydrogenase (LDH) and aldolase are 'distal pathway' glycogenoses (Fig. 28.2) and share certain common features:

- severe exercise provokes attacks of myoglobinuria (this is similar to myophosphorylase and PFK deficiencies)
- there is mild or no glycogen accumulation in the muscle fibres
- forearm ischaemic exercise testing is either positive, or there is only a modest (less than twofold) elevation of venous lactate in blood collected from the exercised muscles
- muscle fibres have some detectable residual enzyme activity.

Phosphoglycerate kinase deficiency (glycogenosis IX)

PGK deficiency is the only glycogenosis transmitted by X-linked recessive inheritance. At present three clinical phenotypes of PGK deficiency are known: a myopathic form, a haemolytic form and a mixed form. The myopathic form develops in childhood or adult life with exertional intolerance, muscle cramps, myoglobinuria and central nervous system (CNS) symptoms, such as mental retardation and seizures (Rosa et al., 1982; DiMauro et al., 1983; Tonin et al., 1989; Schroder et al., 1996; Sugie et al., 1998).

A variety of missense mutations cause PGK deficiency (Tsujino et al., 1995b; Sugie et al., 1998). There is no clear correlation between the specific mutation or the biochemical features of PGK activity assayed in muscle and the phenotypic manifestations (Tsujino et al., 1995b; Schroder et al., 1996; Sugie et al., 1998). Serum creatine kinase is occasionally elevated. Diagnosis depends upon assay of muscle for PGK activity. Treatment is symptomatic. The haemolytic anaemia may respond to spleenectomy.

Phosphoglycerate mutase deficiency (glycogenosis X)

Phosphoglycerate mutase deficiency is an autosomal recessive disorder characterized by muscle cramps and pain provoked by sudden vigorous exercise (DiMauro et al., 1981, 1982; Bresolin et al., 1983; Kissel et al., 1985; Vita et al., 1990; Toscano et al., 1996; Vissing et al., 1999). Only 11 cases have been reported. Recurrent myoglobinuria occurs in some patients. The enzyme is dimeric with muscle isoform MH dominating in adult muscle and brain isoform BB in developing muscle.

Mutations in the gene on chromosome 7p12–7p13 cause the disorder. There is genetic heterogeneity. The disorder occurs more frequently in African-Americans in whom codons 78 and 89 are involved (Tsujino et al., 1995c) while Caucasians develop symptoms through mutation at codon 90 in exon 1 (Toscano et al., 1996). All three gene lesions cause similar phenotypes (Tsujino et al., 1995c).

Somewhat greater exercise tolerance occurs in patients with phosphoglycerate mutase deficiency compared with patients with deficiencies of myophosphorylase or PFK. Forearm ischaemic exercise typically produces low rather than no elevation in venous lactate (1.5–2-fold increase above resting values) (DiMauro et al., 1997; Vissing et al., 1999). Plasma ammonia rises abnormally, increasing sevenfold compared with the normal fourfold elevation (Vissing et al., 1999). Phosphoglycerate mutase activity is markedly decreased in muscle, to 2–6% of the values seen in normal individuals (Tsujino et al., 1995c; Toscano et al., 1996; Vissing et al., 1999).

Ischaemic exercise provokes muscle contracture, similar to that in other glycogenoses. Muscle contractures may result from an increased release of calcium from the sarcoplasmic reticulum (Vissing et al., 1999). One patient treated with dantrolene sodium at a maintenance dose of 200 mg daily had significant amelioration of his muscle cramping (Vissing et al., 1999). In selected patients, dantrolene sodium may be a useful treatment.

Lactate dehydrogenase deficiency (glycogenosis XI)

LDH deficiency presents with exercise intolerance, myalgias, myoglobinuria and skin rash (erythematous, non-itchy patches on extensor surfaces and soles and ankles) (Kanno et al., 1980; Bryan et al., 1990; Kanno and Maekawa, 1995). LDH is a tetrameric enzyme composed of various combinations of muscle (M) and heart (H) subunits. As in the case of phosphoglycerate mutase, the expression of various isozymes in different tissues is developmentally regulated. The M_4 form predominates in mature muscle and in skin (Kanno and Maekawa, 1995). This may account for the prominent alterations in the skin that accompany the muscle symptoms. The M subunit is abundant in the liver, skeletal muscles, skin and the uterus. Symptoms related to hepatic dysfunction are not present. However, in females uterine stiffness can develop in the early stages of labour and delivery. Three women have required Caesarean section, and frequent monitoring during pregnancy is necessary (Kanno and Maekawa, 1995).

There is genetic heterogeneity in the mutations causing LDH deficiency (Kanno and Maekawa, 1995). Total LDH activity in muscle is less than 5% of normal. LDH deficiency accounts for the remarkable increase in venous pyruvate and the impaired increase in lactate following ischaemic forearm exercise. The marked elevation of pyruvate accompanied by an impaired release of lactate during exercising is characteristic for LDH deficiency. In contrast with myophosphorylase deficiency, patients with LDH deficiency demonstrate an increase in venous pyruvate and alanine following forearm exercise (Wahren et al., 1973; Kanno and Maekawa, 1995). Specific diagnosis requires assay of skeletal muscle for LDH activity. The diagnosis can be suspected if plasma levels of muscle enzymes are elevated after a bout of muscle pain or rhabdomyolysis. In this circumstance, the plasma creatine kinase levels show a marked elevation while there is only a modest rise in plasma LDH. This suggests a decreased content of LDH in muscle.

There is no specific treatment. Patients are at risk for rhabdomyolysis and subsequent renal failure. Women require close monitoring during pregnancy.

Aldolase deficiency (glycogenosis XII)

Aldolase A is one of three isozymes of aldolase (other two are B and C) responsible for the conversion of fructose 1,6-bisphosphate into glyceraldehyde 3-phosphate and dihydroxyacetone phosphate in the glycolytic pathway (Gamblin et al., 1991). Deficiency of aldolase A can cause haemolytic anaemia (Beutler et al., 1973; Miwa et al., 1981). A recent report describes the occurrence of rhabdomyolysis and myopathy in a child with a deficiency of aldolase A resulting from a mutation involving a single base transversion from guanine to adenine at position 619 (Kreuder et al., 1996). This 4½-year-old boy presented with muscle weakness, exercise intolerance and a fever. His inability to walk for more than 10 minutes or climb more than two flights of steps at a time occurred in the setting of an upper respiratory tract infection. Following recovery from his infection, his serum creatine kinase level declined from being markedly elevated (over 40 times normal) to a level approximately three times above normal two weeks after resolution of his febrile illness. He subsequently had less severe elevations of creatine kinase, which occurred after whole-body exercise and after general anaesthesia for a tonsillectomy. Muscle biopsy showed well-preserved architecture but an increased variability in the diameters of both type I and type II fibres. Electron microscopy revealed dilated intermyofibrillar spaces containing fine, electron-dense accumulations of lipid-myelin figures, and an increased variation in the shape and size of mitochondria. There was a profound decrease in assayable aldolase activity. Residual aldolase activity in red blood cells was 4% of normal. The aggravation of his symptoms and the provocation of rhabdomyolysis by his infection and associated fever is unusual as a precipitating circumstance in a metabolic myopathy. It is possible that the mutation in this patient had affected a portion of the enzyme that controls its thermolability (Kreuder et al., 1996). Further studies of this rare enzyme deficiency are necessary. However, in the work-up of patients with exercise intolerance and myoglobinuria, analysis of aldolase activity in skeletal muscle specimens needs to be included.

Myoadenylate deaminase deficiency (AMPD-1 deficiency)

AMPD converts AMP to inosine monophosphate (IMP) with liberation of ammonia. The biological role of this enzyme remains uncertain.

In 1978 Fishbein, Armbrustmacher and Griffin described five men with muscle weakness or cramping after exercise beginning in childhood. All five men had a severe deficiency of AMPD activity in their muscle. Their symptoms appeared to correlate with the loss of enzyme activity. Subsequent genetic studies have shown that AMPD-1 deficiency results from autosomal recessive inheritance of mutations involving the gene on chromosome 1p13–p21 (Sabina et al., 1990, 1992; Gross, 1997; Verzijl et al., 1998).

A nonsense mutation involving exon 2 of *AMPD-1* accounts for the disorder in the vast majority of patients. Approximately 2% of the general Dutch population (Verzijl et al., 1998) and 1.5% of randomly selected individuals in Germany (Gross, 1997) are homozygous for the mutation. It is interesting to note that the frequency of this mutation

and presence of deficient enzyme activity on muscle biopsy is much higher than the prevalence of muscle complaints attributed to this metabolic myopathy. This lack of correlation remains unexplained. Gross (1997) suggests that there is alternative splicing of exon 2, which harbours the mutation, that occurs frequently and protects the majority of individuals carrying the mutation from manifesting symptoms. This hypothesis requires confirmation.

Two types of AMPD-1 deficiency have been proposed: one transmitted as autosomal recessive manifesting in adult life with muscle cramping and exercise intolerance; the second type having higher residual enzyme activity in skeletal muscle (1–10%) occurring in association with a variety of neurogenic and myopathic disorders. This classification of AMPD-1 deficiency has received careful examination in a recent study (Verzijl et al., 1998). The results have raised serious questions about the existence of the second type of AMPD-1 deficiency and further questions about the significance of the primary deficiency and its clinical symptoms. Thirty three individuals with severe deficiency of AMPD-1 on muscle biopsy underwent detailed clinical and molecular genetic investigation. In 23 of these, a primary AMPD-1 deficiency was seen without signs of other neuromuscular pathology on muscle biopsy. The remaining 10 patients had other diseases in addition to a deficiency of AMPD-1, including myotonic dystrophy, facioscapulohumeral muscular dystrophy, AMD and hereditary motor sensory neuropathy type I. Of 100 normal volunteers, two had homozygous mutations for the AMPD-1 gene and 18 had heterozygous mutations. All 33 patients with a deficiency of AMPD-1 had mutations at the typical site (codon 12 in exon 2 of chromosome 1 in *AMPD-1*). There was no significant correlation between clinical symptoms or the lack of symptoms and AMPD-1 deficiency in the groups studies. The investigators have proposed that AMPD-1 deficiency in the Dutch population is only a harmless polymorphism and is not a disease in itself. This interpretation has prompted disagreement (Fishbein, 1999). Further investigation is necessary to clarify the pathophysiological significance of AMPD-1 deficiency.

There is no clearly established therapy. Most patients receive symptomatic treatment and adjust the intensity and duration of exercise to control symptoms. A few patients have improved with 10–20g/h ribose during prolonged exercise.

Malignant hyperthermia

Since its recognition (Denborough and Lovell, 1960), malignant hyperthermia (MH) has aroused the special interest of anesthesiologists (see Chapters 10 and 30). The clinical syndrome has the following elements. Exposure to both halothane and suxamethonium (succinylcholine) (or similar agents) leads to: (i) a sharp rise in body temperature; (ii) stiffness of masseter and limb muscles (probably owing to contracture); (iii) lactic acidosis; (iv) cardiac arrhythmia; (v) muscle necrosis; and (vi) marked elevation of serum creatine kinase with myoglobinuria. There is excellent agreement comparing the European and the North American protocols for detection of MH susceptibility (Allen et al., 1998; Hopkins, et al., 1998; Fletcher et al., 1999; Islander and Twetman, 1999). Contracture testing is now widely used to identify individuals having a susceptibility to MH, specifically for individuals who have had a reaction to inhaled halogenated anaesthetics and/or suxamethonium suggestive of MH. The European protocol uses incremental doses of halothane up to 2% and incremental doses of caffeine to test muscle tissue in vitro for a contracture. In North America, a single dose of 3% halothane and incremental doses of caffeine are used. Individuals who have a contracture to 3% halothane of 0.5 g or more and a contracture to 2 mmol/l caffeine of 0.2 g or more are considered to be susceptible to MH (Denborough, 1998). Occasionally there is a discrepancy between the halothane and the caffeine contractures. The Europeans refer to such results as 'equivocal' while workers in North America classify the results as 'susceptible'.

MH susceptibility in humans has genetic heterogeneity. Approximately 10% of patients have mutations in the region of chromosome 19q13.1 involving the ryanodine receptor (Denborough, 1998) that predispose patients to MH (Richter et al., 1997; Tong et al., 1997; Manning et al., 1998; Barone et al., 1999; Fortunato et al., 1999). Mutations in other loci can also cause MH, for example affecting the α_1-subunit of the human dihydropyridine-sensitive calcium channel (Monnier et al., 1997) and the adult skeletal muscle sodium channel (Moslehi et al., 1998). The diagnosis at present relies on the use of either the European or North American protocols for in vitro contracture testing. Treatment is outlined in Table 28.1 and described in detail in recent reviews (Bertorini, 1997; Abraham et al., 1998; Denborough, 1998). Screening for MH susceptibility needs consideration in any individuals having a persistent unexplained elevation in serum creatine kinase levels (Weglinski et al., 1997).

Several detailed reviews of MH have recently been published (Abraham et al., 1998; Denborough, 1998; Loke and MacLennan, 1998), and they offer a thorough discussion of current management and diagnosis. Other recent reviews (Bertorini, 1997; Chan et al., 1997; Naguib and Magboul, 1998) discuss drug-induced syndromes, including MH and

Table 28.1. Treatment for malignant hyperthermia

Malignant hyperthermia crisis
  Stop volatile anesthetics/suxamethonium (succinylcholine)
  Hyperventilate: 100% oxygen
  Intravenous dantrolene sodium in boluses 2–3 mg/kg up to 10 mg/kg total
  Sodium bicarbonate 1–2 mEq/kg (1–2 mmol/kg)
  Administer ice saline intravenously, and lavage stomach, bladder and rectum
  Monitor end-tidal CO_2, blood gases, serum potassium, clotting studies, and urine output
  Treat hyperkalaemia and acidosis
  Monitor electrocardiograph for arrhythmias and treat with antiarrhythmic agents but avoid calcium channel blockers
Postacute-crisis care
  Intensive care monitoring for at least 48 hours
  Renal protective therapy
  Continue dantrolene sodium 1–2 mg/kg intravenously every 4 hours for at least 36 hours

the neuroleptic malignant syndrome, which appear to have a different pathogenesis to MH (Keck, et al., 1995; Bertorini 1997).

Defects of mitochondrial fatty acid oxidation

Mitochondrial fatty acid oxidation is discussed in detail in Chapter 8. Figure 28.3 shows main areas affected by defects.

Pathophysiology of the disease

A defect in β-oxidation can cause both accumulation of intermediates proximal to the defect in the mitochondria, and a shortage of end-products, particularly of acetyl-CoA, and reduced nicotinamide and flavine adenine dinucleotides (NADH and $FADH_2$, respectively). As a result, the muscle disease seen in patients can result from a variety of consequences of the metabolic disorder. First, there is a shortage of energy under specific physiological conditions: fasting and prolonged exercise. During short-term exercise, energy can be derived from muscle glycogen and blood glucose. The shortage of energy is complicated by impaired fatty acid oxidation in the liver, which results in low ketone body concentrations – important metabolic fuels both in skeletal and cardiac muscle. Second, accumulation of intermediates of fatty acid oxidation may inhibit the breakdown of fat and result in the accumulation of fat

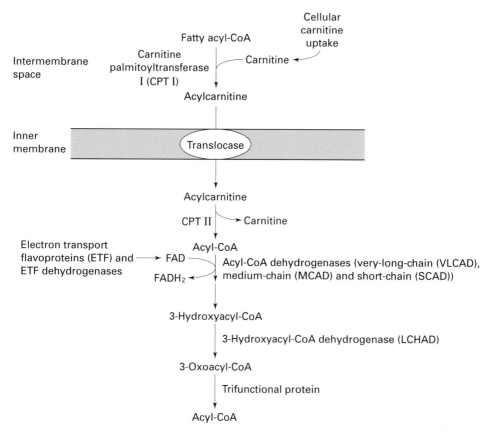

Fig. 28.3. Mitochondrial oxidation of long-chain fatty acids showing the position of enzyme defects.

as lipid droplets in skeletal muscle of some patients with defects of mitochondrial fatty acid oxidation. It is important to be aware that in many patients, however, lipid accumulation in muscle is not a feature. Third, rhabdomyolysis can occur; the mechanism of this is not known but some of the accumulating intermediates (acyl-CoA and acylcarnitine esters) have detergent properties and may have an effect on membrane permeability.

Clinical features

Since the defects of fatty acid oxidation have similar effects on metabolism, the clinical features may be very similar, or identical, for different enzyme defects. Patients, especially adults, with abnormalities of fatty acid oxidation often present with muscle symptoms, although it is essential to be aware that involvement of other organs is common. The muscle-related symptoms are predominantly of exercise-induced muscle pain and rhabdomyolysis and/or weakness. The muscle pain is usually induced by prolonged exercise and may be severe enough to stop the patient continuing with the exercise. More characteristically, the patient will develop muscle pain some time after the exercise. This is associated with stiffness of the muscles and the patient may at this stage notice myoglobinuria. Patients are also at risk at times of infection, especially when food intake is limited or if there is persistent vomiting. If severe, the rhabdomyolysis and muscle necrosis can lead to severe muscle weakness, resulting in respiratory failure and renal failure owing to myoglobinuria. In the majority of patients, this muscle weakness and rhabdomyolysis is self-limiting.

Another presentation of patients with disorders of fatty acid oxidation is proximal muscle weakness without pain or rhabdomyolysis. This weakness can be profound and may occur over a period of several days. Again illness and the associated fasting may precipitate the episodes. In some patients, there is a more slowly progressive weakness, although in our experience this is uncommon.

Involvement of other organs may result in other, and life-threatening, symptoms. In children the most common presentation of an β-oxidation disorder is a metabolic crisis with hypoketotic hypoglycaemia. Metabolic decompensation is often provoked by prolonged fasting or intercurrent infections. These fulminating symptoms may be associated with cardiomyopathy and myopathy. The mortality in these acute episodes is high, especially if the condition is not recognized.

Cardiomyopathy is a prominent feature in some patients and its identification is very important. These patients are at risk of cardiac arrest owing to arrhythmias (intraventricular tachycardia, third-degree heart block) and from progressive cardiac failure.

Neurological clinical features may result from the hypoglycaemia seen in some patients. In addition, neurological features may be a prominent feature of MTP and LCHAD deficiency. These patients may develop severe and progressive pigmentary retinopathy. In other patients peripheral neuropathy is a prominent feature (Dionisi-Vici et al. 1991).

Special features of individual β-oxidation defects

Primary carnitine deficiency

Primary carnitine deficiency is a rare disorder and presents in childhood with progressive proximal muscle weakness, cardiomyopathy and in some cases hypoglycaemia (Stanley et al. 1991). It is caused by impaired cellular carnitine uptake, and mutations have been detected in a gene encoding a sodium dependent carnitine transporter (Nezu et al., 1999; Seth et al., 1999; Tang et al., 1999). This disorder has to be separated from secondary carnitine deficiency, which is common in many patients with metabolic disorders.

Carnitine palmitoyltransferase (CPT) deficiency

CPT deficiency was the first β-oxidation defect to be described and clinically and biochemically, can be classified under three subtypes.

- A muscle form presents in adolescence or adulthood with recurrent episodes of myalgia; rhabdomyolysis is typically induced by fasting and/or prolonged exercise. In these patients, the biochemical abnormality involves CPT II. Between episodes, most patients are symptom free but in approximately 20% a mild muscle weakness can be found. In the muscle there is often minimal or no lipid storage. The defect is inherited in an autosomal recessive manner and the molecular defect has been identified in many patients (Taroni et al., 1992, 1993; Kaufmann et al., 1997).
- A hepatomuscular form of CPT II deficiency has been described with severe disease in infancy associated with hypoglycaemic cardiomyopathy, hypotonia and renal cysts (Demaugre et al., 1988).
- A rarer infantile hepatic form associated with hypoglycaemia, hyperketonaemia in the relative absence of

muscle symptoms. In these patients CPT I is low in liver and fibroblasts but not in muscle (Demaugre et al., 1988).

Carnitine-acylcarnitine translocase deficiency

Deficiency of carnitine-acylcarnitine translocase is a rare β-oxidation defect that is inherited in an autosomal recessive manner. When the deficiency is near total, it results in a very severe phenotype with severe hypoglycaemia, cardiac involvement and myopathy (Stanley et al., 1992; Pande et al. 1993; Pande 1999). The condition in its severe form is usually fatal although there have been reports of partial deficiency with a milder phenotype (Dionisi-Vici et al., 1995; Morris et al. 1998). The genetic defect has been identified in some patients (Huizing et al., 1997).

Very-long-chain acyl-CoA dehydrogenase deficiency

Patients with deficiency of VLCAD may present with fairly severe episodes of hypoglycaemia, vomiting and coma brought on by fasting. This illness has a high mortality and is often associated with a lipid storage myopathy and cardiomyopathy (Vianey-Saban et al., 1997). A second group of patients is characterized by a much later onset often without metabolic disturbance but with prominent muscle symptoms (Oglivie et al., 1994; Straussberg et al., 1997; Smelt et al., 1998). In these patients, the muscle symptoms may resemble CPT deficiency with prominent exercise-induced myalgia and rhabdomyolysis. These patients often do not have cardiac abnormalities and the lipid storage in muscle may be mild.

Medium-chain acyl-CoA dehydrogenase deficiency

Whilst medium-chain acyl-CoA dehydrogenase (MCAD) deficiency is probably the most common fatty acid oxidation disorder, with a proposed incidence of 1 in 6000 births in the UK (Blakemore et al., 1991), the symptoms rarely involve muscle. These patients usually present with metabolic crises associated with a Reye-like syndrome with stupor, encephalopathy, hypoketotic hypoglycaemic and sudden death in some children. Rarely patients present in adult life with muscle pain, lipid-storage myopathy and rhabdomyolysis (Ruitenbeck et al., 1995). Cardiomyopathy has not been reported in patients with MCAD deficiency.

Short-chain acyl-CoA dehydrogenase deficiency

SCAD deficiency appears to be very rare, having been identified in only a few patients. Clinically two forms can be distinguished.

- A severe infantile form has hypoglycaemic episodes, vomiting, lethargy, muscle weakness, microcephaly and psychomotor retardation (Amendt et al., 1987; Coates et al., 1988). These children all have systemic SCAD deficiency.

- A mild late-onset form occurs with slowly progressive proximal lipid storage myopathy and secondary carnitine deficiency. The enzyme defect is limited to muscle. Some cases of this myopathic form of SCAD deficiency may represent a riboflavin-responsive multiple acyl-CoA dehydrogenase deficiency.

Electron transfer flavoprotein (EFT) or EFT dehydrogenase deficiency (glutaric aciduria type II)

Deficiency of electron transfer flavoproteins (ETF) or ETF dehydrogenases give rise to glutaric aciduria type II. The defect involves not only fatty acid oxidation but also amino acid metabolism. The dehydrogenases involved in amino acid metabolism also feed electrons into the respiratory chain via ETF and ETF dehydrogenase. For this reason many of the symptoms observed are more likely to be related to the disturbance of amino acid rather than fatty acid oxidation.

The clinical features are variable (Loehr et al., 1990), but a number of patients present with a very severe form that is present at birth with congenital abnormalities, hyperketotic hypoglycaemia and results in early death (Amendt et al., 1986). These patients excrete glutaric acid derived from amino acid metabolism in high concentration, hence the name of the disorder. Other patients may present with a milder form of the illness but usually presenting in childhood. Lipid-storage myopathy may be a prominent clinical feature.

Riboflavin-responsive multiple acyl-CoA-dehydrogenase deficiency

Multiple deficiency of acyl-CoA dehydrogenase is an important disorder to recognize because of its remarkable response to riboflavin treatment. These patients often present with muscle pain and proximal muscle weakness, often precipitated by fasting or illness (Antozzi et al., 1994).

Long-chain 3-hydroxyacyl-CoA dehydrogenase and mitochondrial trifunctional protein deficiency

Patients with long-chain 3-hydroxyacyl-CoA dehydrogenase (LCHAD) and MTP deficiency may present in a similar manner to other patients with defects of mitochondrial fatty acid oxidation with either profound hypoketotic hypoglycaemia in early childhood (Jackson et al., 1991, 1992, Morris et al., 1997) or a proximal myopathy and rhabdomyolysis later in life (Schaefer et al., 1996; Miyajima et al., 1997). What is particularly unusual about this condition is that patients may present with other neurological features such as a sensory motor peripheral neuropathy and pigmentary retinopathy (Ibdah et al., 1998). In addition, female carriers of an LCHAD-deficient fetus have increased frequency of pre-eclampsia associated with complications of pregnancy and this may lead to acute fatty liver of pregnancy.

Investigation of fatty acid oxidation defect

Metabolic studies

Most abnormalities caused by a β-oxidation defect can be detected in routine laboratory tests only during acute symptoms or after prolonged fasting. Characteristic features, which are detectable during acute hypoglycaemia, are a hypoketotic response and an increased concentration of nonesterified fatty acids. During the stable phase of the disease, excretion of organic acids may also be normal, but following fasting this often generates a characteristic pattern of urinary organic acids.

Carnitine and acylcarnitine analysis

Serum carnitine analysis was originally a mainstay in the investigation of patients. However, it is now recognized that the changes in carnitine concentration may be primary or secondary. Very low concentrations are seen in carnitine transporter defects, but carnitine concentration can be entirely normal in some patients with defects of the carnitine shuttle. Acylcarnitine analysis in blood has transformed the investigation of fatty acid oxidation disorders. In the majority of patients, acylcarnitines are abnormal even when the patient is metabolically stable (Millington et al., 1992; Rashed et al., 1995; Vianey-Saban et al., 1997). In addition, the pattern of acylcarnitines in blood may also give information about the level of the enzyme defect. In vitro stress tests looking at the generation of intermediates of β-oxidation in skin fibroblasts and muscle may also have a role in identifying the presence and site of a defect (Schaefer et al., 1997).

Molecular diagnosis

The definitive diagnosis can be verified by detecting reduced enzyme activity in cultured cells or detecting prevalent disease-causing mutations in blood or tissue specimens. In MCAD and LCHAD deficiencies, molecular genetic diagnosis is particularly useful because about 90% of these patients have a common disease-causing mutation (Ijlst et al., 1997; Matern et al., 1999). In some defects, such as VLCAD deficiency, there is a clear correlation of the genotype with the disease phenotype (Andresen et al., 1996, 1997).

Prenatal or neonatal screening

Prenatal diagnosis or routine neonatal screening by acylcarnitine analysis may be warranted in disorders with severe clinical course or in populations with high-frquency of the disorder, respectively (Nada et al., 1996; Clayton et al., 1998).

Management of patients with fatty acid oxidation defects

Avoidance of exacerbating factors

In many patients avoidance of exacerbating factors is an important part of the management. In children, fasting and infection are the major causes of metabolic decompensation and rhabdomyolysis (Dionisi-Vici et al., 1991; Straussberg et al., 1997). Both fasting and endocrine stress responses will promote lipolysis and decrease availability of carbohydrates. These patients, therefore, need to avoid fasting and maintain a regular carbohydrate intake during infections to try to reduce lipolysis. In adults, whilst exercise is a major precipitant of rhabdomyolysis, fasting often raises serum creatine kinase and reduces exercise tolerance (Miyajima et al., 1997).

Dietary intervention

In all β-oxidation defects, the main purpose of therapeutic intervention is to ensure that there is sufficient provision of calories by carbohydrates during periods of metabolic stress and fasting. The other purpose is to prevent the accumulation of β-oxidation intermediates and lipid by providing only the amount of fats required to meet the need for essential fatty acids. A low-fat, high-carbohydrate diet with less than 10–15% of total energy delivered from triacylglycerols and replacing part of the dietary fat by medium-chain fatty acids are regarded useful in disorders of long-chain fatty acid oxidation. Medium-chain triacylglycerols (MCT) are absorbed from the gut into the portal vein. Within hepatocytes, the medium-chain fatty acids are converted into ketone bodies. Ketone bodies are oxidized by cardiac and skeletal muscle in preference to fatty acids and may be protective by suppressing the production of intermediates of long-chain fatty acid oxidation. Anecdotal evidence is strongly suggestive that MCT is beneficial in MTP or VLCAD deficiency presenting with cardiomyopathy (Jackson et al., 1991; Morris et al., 1997). In these infants, cardiac function deteriorated relentlessly until the introduction of MCT. The evidence in favour of MCT is less convincing in patients whose problem is recurrent rhabdomyolysis; in some patients dietary modification appeared to reduce the frequency of rhabdomyolysis (Oglivie et al., 1994; Schaefer et al., 1996) but it was not effective in others (Smelt et al., 1998).

Carnitine supplementation

Carnitine is unequivocally beneficial in those with primary carnitine deficiency, but the role of carnitine supplementation in other fatty acid oxidation disorders remains controversial. While secondary carnitine deficiency is common, the levels are probably not low enough to limit β-oxidation. Controlled trials of carnitine have still not been undertaken, despite years of debate.

Riboflavin

In some patients with MAD deficiency presenting with a myopathy, there is an excellent response to riboflavin treatment.

References

Abarbanel, J. M., Bashan, N., Potashnik, R., Osimani, A., Moses, S. W. and Herishanu, Y. (1986). Adult muscle phosphorylase 'b' kinase deficiency. *Neurology* **36**, 560–562.

Abraham, R. B., Adnet, P., Glauber, V. and Perel, A. (1998). Malignant hyperthermia. [Review] [48 refs]. *Postgrad. Med. J.* **74**, 11–17.

Agamanolis, D. P., Askari, A. D., Di Mauro, S. et al. (1980). Muscle phosphofructokinase deficiency: two cases with unusual polysaccharide accumulation and immunologically active enzyme protein. *Muscle Nerve* **3**, 456–467.

Allen, G. C., Larach, M. G. and Kunselman, A. R. (1998). The sensitivity and specificity of the caffeine–halothane contracture test: a report from the North American Malignant Hyperthermia Registry. The North American Malignant Hyperthermia Registry of MHAUS. *Anesthesiology* **88**, 579–588.

Amendt, B. A. and Rhead, W. J. (1986). The multiple acyl-coenzyme A dehydrogenation disorders, glutaric aciduria type II and ethylmalonic-adipic aciduria. Mitochondrial fatty acid oxidation, acyl-coenzyme A dehydrogenase and electron transfer flavoprotein activities in fibroblasts. *J. Clin. Invest.* **78**, 205–213.

Amendt, B. A., Greene, C., Sweetman, L. et al. (1987). Short-chain acyl-coenzyme A dehydrogenase deficiency. Clinical and biochemical studies in two patients. *J. Clin. Invest.* **79**, 1303–1309.

Andresen, B. S., Bross, P., Vianey-Saban, C. et al. (1996). Cloning and characterization of human very-long-chain acyl-CoA dehydrogenase cDNA, chromosomal assignment of the gene and identification in four patients of nine different mutations within the VLCAD gene. [Published erratum appears in *Hum. Mol. Genet.* (1996), 5, *Hum. Mol.Genet.* **5**, 461–472.

Andresen, B. S., Bross, P., Udvari, S. et al. (1997). The molecular basis of medium-chain acyl-CoA dehydrogenase (MCAD) deficiency in compound heterozygous patients: is there correlation between genotype and phenotype? *Hum. Mol. Genet.* **6**, 695–707.

Andreu, A. L., Bruno, C., Tamburino, L. et al. (1999). A new mutation in the myophosphorylase gene (Asn684Tyr) in a Spanish patient with McArdle's disease. *Neuromusc. Disord.* **9**, 171–173.

Antozzi, C., Garavaglia, B., Mora, M. et al. (1994). Late-onset riboflavin-responsive myopathy with combined multiple acyl coenzyme A dehydrogenase and respiratory chain deficiency. *Neurology* **44**, 2153–2158.

Ausems, M. G., Lochman, P., van Diggelen, D. P., van Arnstel, K., Reuser, A. J. and Wokke, J. H. (1999). A diagnostic protocol for adult-onset glycogen storage disease type II. *Neurology* **52**, 851–853.

Bao, Y., Kishnani, P., Wu, J.Y. and Chen, Y.T. (1996a). Hepatic and neuromuscular forms of glycogen storage disease type IV caused by mutations in the same glycogen-branching enzyme gene. *J. Clin. Invest.* **97**, 941–948.

Bao, Y., Dawson, T. J. and Chen, Y. T. (1996b). Human glycogen debranching enzyme gene (AGL): complete structural organization and characterization of the 5′ flanking region. *Genomics* **38**, 155–165.

Barone, V., Massa, O., Intravaia, E. et al. (1999). Mutation screening of the RYR1 gene and identification of two novel mutations in Italian malignant hyperthermia families. *J. Med. Genet.* **36**, 115–118.

Bertorini, T. E. (1997). Myoglobinuria, malignant hyperthermia, neuroleptic malignant syndrome and serotonin syndrome. [Review] *Neurol. Clin.* **15**, 649–671.

Beutler, E., Scott, S., Bishop, A., Margolis, N., Matsumoto, F. and Kuhl, W. (1973). Red cell aldolase deficiency and hemolytic anaemia: a new syndrome. *Trans. Assoc. Am. Physic.* **86**, 154–166.

Beynon, R. J., Bartram, C., Hopkins, P. et al. (1995). McArdle's disease: molecular genetics and metabolic consequences of the phenotype. *Muscle Nerve* **3**, S18–S22.

Blakemore, A. I., Singleton, H., Pollitt, R. J. et al. (1991). Frequency of the G985 MCAD mutation in the general population. [Letter] *Lancet* **337**, 298–299.

Bornemann, A., Besser, R., Shin, Y. S. and Goebel, H. H. (1996). A mild adult myopathic variant of type IV glycogenosis. *Neuromusc. Disord.* **6**, 95–99.

Bresolin, N., Ro, Y. I., Reyes, M., Miranda, A. F. and DiMauro, S. (1983). Muscle phosphoglycerate mutase (PGAM) deficiency: a second case. *Neurology* **33**, 1049–1053.

Brown, D. H. and Brown, B. I. (1983). Studies of the residual glycogen branching enzyme activity present in human skin fibroblasts from patients with type IV glycogen storage disease. *Biochem. Biophys. Res. Commun.* **111**, 636–643.

Brown, D. H. and Illingworth, B. (1962). The properties of an oligo-(1,4→1,4)-glucantransferase from animal tissue. *Proc. Natl. Acad. Sci. USA* **48**, 1783

Brunberg, J. A., McCormick, W. F. and Schochet, S. S. (1971). Type 3 glycogenosis. An adult with diffuse weakness and muscle wasting. *Arch. Neurol.* **25**, 171–178.

Bruno, C., Servidei, S., Shanske, S. et al. (1993). Glycogen branching enzyme deficiency in adult polyglucosan body disease. *Ann. Neurol.* **33**, 88–93.

Bruno, C., Manfredi, G. Andreu, A. L., Shanske, S., Krishna, S., Ilse, W. K. and DiMauro, S. (1998a). A splice junction mutation in the alpha(M) gene of phosphorylase kinase in a patient with myopathy. *Biochem. Biophys. Res. Commun.*, **249**, 648–651.

Bruno, C., Minetti, C., Shanske, S. et al. (1998b). Combined defects of muscle phosphofructokinase and AMP deaminase in a child with myoglobinuria. *Neurology* **50**, 296–298.

Bruno, C., Lofberg, M., Tamburino, L. et al. (1999a). Molecular characterization of McArdle's disease in two large Finnish families. *J. Neurol. Sci.* **165**, 121–125.

Bruno, C., Tamburino, L., Kawashima, N. et al. (1999b). A nonsense mutation in the myophosphorylase gene in a Japanese family with McArdle's disease. *Neuromusc. Disord.* **9**, 34–37.

Bryan, W., Lewis, S. F., Bertocci, L. et al. (1990). Muscle lactate dehydrogenase deficiency: a disorder of anaerobic glycogenolysis associated with exertional myoglobinuria. *Neurology* **40**, 203–203.

Burke, J., Hwang, P., Anderson, L., Lebo, R., Gorin, F. and Fletterick, R. (1987). Intron/exon structure of the human gene for the muscle isozyme of glycogen phosphorylase. *Proteins* **2**, 177–187.

Chan, T. C., Evans, S. D. and Clark, R. F. (1997). Drug-induced hyperthermia. [Review] *Crit. Care Clin.* **13**, 785–808.

Chen, Y. T. and Burchell, A. (1995). Glycogen storage diseases. In: *The Metabolic and Molecular Basis of Inherited Diseases*, eds. C. R. Scriver, W. S. Beaudet, W. S. Sly and D. Valle, pp. 935–965. New York: McGraw-Hill.

Clayton, P. T., Doig, M., Ghafari, S. et al. (1998). Screening for medium chain acyl-CoA dehydrogenase deficiency using electrospray ionisation tandem mass spectrometry. *Arch. Dis. Child.* **79**, 109–115.

Clemens, P. R., Yamamoto, M. and Engel, A. G. (1990). Adult phosphorylase b kinase deficiency. [Review] *Ann. Neurol.* **28**, 529–538.

Coates, P. M., Hale, D. E., Finocchiaro, G., Tanaka, K. and Winter, S. C. (1988). Genetic deficiency of short-chain acyl-coenzyme A dehydrogenase in cultured fibroblasts from a patient with muscle carnitine deficiency and severe skeletal muscle weakness. *J. Clin. Invest.* **81**, 171–175.

D'Ancona, G. G., Wurm, J. and Croce, C. M. (1979). Genetics of type II glycogenosis: assignment of the human gene for acid alpha-glucosidase to chromosome 17. *Proc. Natl. Acad. Sci. USA* **76**, 4526–4529.

de Jager, A. E., van der Vliet, T. M., van der Ree, T. C., Oosterink, B. J. and Loonen, M. C. (1998). Muscle computed tomography in adult-onset acid maltase deficiency. *Muscle Nerve* **21**, 398–400.

Demaugre, F., Bonnefont, J. P., Mitchell, G. et al. (1988). Hepatic and muscular presentations of carnitine palmitoyl transferase deficiency: two distinct entities. *Ped. Res.* **24**, 308–311.

Denborough, M. (1998). Malignant hyperthermia. [Review] *Lancet* **352**, 1131–1136.

Denborough, M. A. and Lovell, R. R. H. (1960). Anaesthetic deaths in a family. *Lancet* **ii**, 45.

DiMauro, S., Stern, L. Z., Mehler, M., Nagle, R. B. and Payne, C. (1978a). Adult-onset acid maltase deficiency: a postmortem study. *Muscle Nerve* **1**, 27–36.

DiMauro, S., Arnold, S., Miranda, A. and Rowland, L. P. (1978b). McArdle disease: the mystery of reappearing phosphorylase activity in muscle culture – a fetal isoenzyme. *Ann. Neurol.* **3**, 60–66.

DiMauro, S., Hartwig, G. B., Hays, A. et al. (1979). Debrancher enzyme deficiency: neuromuscular disorder in 5 adults. *Ann. Neurol.* **5**, 422–436.

DiMauro, S., Miranda, A.F., Khan, S., Gitlin, K. and Friedman, R. (1981). Human muscle phosphoglycerate mutase deficiency: newly discovered metabolic myopathy. *Science* **212**, 1277–1279.

DiMauro, S., Miranda, A. F., Olarte, M., Friedman, R. and Hays, A. P. (1982). Muscle phosphoglycerate mutase deficiency. *Neurology* **32**, 584–591.

DiMauro, S., Dalakas, M. and Miranda, A. F. (1983). Phosphoglycerate kinase deficiency: another cause of recurrent myoglobinuria. *Ann. Neurol.* **13**, 11–19.

DiMauro, S., Bresolin, N. and Hays, A. P. (1984). Disorders of glycogen metabolism. In: *Critical Reviews in Clinical Neurobiogy*, ed. A. D. Roses, pp. 83. Boca Raton, FL: CRC Press.

DiMauro, S., Servidei, S. and Tsujino, S. (1997). Disorders of carbohydrate metabolism: Glycogen storage diseases. In: *The Molecular and Genetic Basis of Neurological Disease*, 2nd edn, eds. R. N. Rosenberg, S. B. Prusiner, S. DiMauro and R. J. Barohn, pp. 1067–1097. Boston, MA: Butterworth-Heinemann.

Ding, J. H., de Barsy, B. T., Brown, B. I., Coleman, R. A. and Chen, Y. T. (1990). Immunoblot analyses of glycogen debranching enzyme in different subtypes of glycogen storage disease type III. *J. Ped.* **116**, 95–100.

Dionisi-Vici, C., Burlina, A. B., Bertini, E. et al. (1991). Progressive neuropathy and recurrent myoglobinuria in a child with long-chain 3-hydroxyacyl-coenzyme A dehydrogenase deficiency. *J. Ped.* **118**, 744–746

Engel, A. G. and Hirschhorn, R. (1994). Acid maltase deficiency. In: *Myology*, eds. A. Engel and C. Franzini-Armstrong, pp. 1533–1553. New York: McGraw-Hill.

Engel, A. G., Gomez, M. R., Seybold, M. E. and Lambert, E. H. (1973). The spectrum and diagnosis of acid maltase deficiency. *Neurology* **23**, 95–106.

Fishbein, W. N. (1999). Primary, secondary and coincidental types of myoadenylate deaminase deficiency. [Letter; comment] *Ann. Neurol.* **45**, 547–548.

Fishbein, W. N., Armbrustmacher, V. W. and Griffin, J. L. (1978). Myoadenylate deaminase deficiency: a new disease of muscle. *Science* **200**, 545–548.

Fletcher, J. E., Rosenberg, H. and Aggarwal, M. (1999). Comparison of European and North American malignant hyperthermia diagnostic protocol outcomes for use in genetic studies. [See comments] *Anesthesiology* **90**, 654–661.

Fortunato, G., Carsana, A., Tinto, N., Brancadoro, V., Canfora, G. and Salvatore, F. (1999). A case of discordance between genotype and phenotype in a malignant hyperthermia family. *Eur. J. Hum. Genet.* **7**, 415–420.

Gamblin, S. J., Davies, G. J., Grimes, J. M., Jackson, R. M., Littlechild, J. A. and Watson, H. C. (1991). Activity and specificity of human aldolases. *J. Mol. Biol.* **219**, 573–576.

Gospe, S. J., El-Schahawi, M., Shanske, S. et al. (1998). Asymptomatic McArdle's disease associated with hyper-creatine kinase-emia and absence of myophosphorylase. *Neurology* **51**, 1228–1229.

Grehl, T., Muller, K., Vorgerd, M., Tegenthoff, M., Malin, J. P. and Zange, J. (1998). Impaired aerobic glycolysis in muscle phosphofructokinase deficiency results in biphasic post-exercise phosphocreatine recovery in 31P magnetic resonance spectroscopy. *Neuromusc. Disord.* **8**, 480–488.

Gross, M. (1997). Clinical heterogeneity and molecular mechanisms in inborn muscle AMP deaminase deficiency. [Review] *J. Inher. Metabolic Dis.* **20**, 186–192.

Haller, R. G. and Lewis, S. F. (1991). Glucose-induced exertional fatigue in muscle phosphofructokinase deficiency [see comments]. *N. Engl. J. Med.* **324**, 364–369.

Haller, R. G., Clausen, T. and Vissing, J. (1998). Reduced levels of skeletal muscle Na$^+$K$^+$-ATPase in McArdle disease. [See comments] *Neurology* **50**, 37–40.

Hays, A. P., Hallett, M., Delfs, J. et al. (1981). Muscle phosphofructokinase deficiency: abnormal polysaccharide in a case of late-onset myopathy. *Neurology* **31**, 1077–1086.

Hermans, M. M., Wisselaar, H. A., Kroos, M. A., Oostra, B. A. and Reuser, A. J. (1993). Human lysosomal alpha-glucosidase: functional characterization of the glycosylation sites. *Biochem. J.* **289**, 681–686.

Hers, H. G. (1963). a-Glucosidase deficiency in generalized glycogen storage disease (Pompe's disease). *Biochem. J.* 11

Hers, H. G. and Van Hoff, F. (1968). Glycogen storage diseases: type II and type VI glycogenosis. In: *Carbohydrate Metabolism and its Disorders*, eds. F. Dickens, P. J. Randle and W. J. Whelan, pp. 151–160. New York: Academic Press.

Hers, H. G., Van Hoff, F. and DeBarsy, T. (1989). Glycogen storage diseases. In: *The Metabolic Basis of Inherited Disease*, eds. C. R. Scriver, W. S. Sly and E. Balle, pp. 425–452. New York: McGraw-Hill.

Hirschhorn, K. (1995). Glycogen Storage Disease. In: *The Metabolic and Molecular Basis of Inherited Diseases*, eds. C. R. Scriver, A. L. Beaudeat, W. S. Sly and D. Valle, pp. 2443–2465. New York: McGraw-Hill.

Hoefsloot, L. H., Hoogeveen-Westerveld, M., Kroos, M.A. et al. (1988). Primary structure and processing of lysosomal alpha-glucosidase; homology with the intestinal sucrase–isomaltase complex. *EMBO J.* **7**, 1697–1704.

Hoefsloot, L. H., Hoogeveen-Westerveld, M., Reuser, A. J. and Oostra, B. A. (1990). Characterization of the human lysosomal alpha-glucosidase gene. *Biochem. J.* **272**, 493–497.

Hopkins, P. M., Hartung, E. and Wappler, F. (1998). Multicentre evaluation of ryanodine contracture testing in malignant hyperthermia. The European Malignant Hyperthermia Group. *Br. J. Anaesth.* **80**, 389–394.

Huie, M. L., Tsujino, S., Sklower, B. S. et al. (1998). Glycogen storage disease type II: identification of four novel missense mutations (D645N, G648S, R672W, R672Q) and two insertions/deletions in the acid alpha-glucosidase locus of patients of differing phenotype. *Biochem. Biophys. Res. Commun.* **244**, 921–927.

Huizing, M., Iacobazzi, V., Ijlst, L. et al. (1997). Cloning of the human carnitine-acylcarnitine carrier cDNA and identification of the molecular defect in a patient. *Am. J. Hum. Genet.* **61**, 1239–1245.

Ibdah, J. A., Tein, I., Dionisi-Vici, C., et al. (1998). Mild trifunctional protein deficiency is associated with progressive neuropathy and myopathy and suggests a novel genotype-phenotype correlation. *J. Clin. Invest.* **102**, 1193–1199.

Ijlst, L., Oostheim, W., Ruiter, J. P. and Wanders, R. J. (1997). Molecular basis of long-chain 3-hydroxyacyl-CoA dehydrogenase deficiency: identification of two new mutations. *J. Inher. Metab. Dis.* **20**, 420–422.

Isaacs, H., Savage, N., Badenhorst, M. and Whistler, T. (1986). Acid maltase deficiency: a case study and review of the pathophysiological changes and proposed therapeutic measures. *J. Neurol. Neurosurg. Psychiatry* **49**, 1011–1018.

Islander, G. and Twetman, E. R. (1999). Comparison between the European and North American protocols for diagnosis of malignant hyperthermia susceptibility in humans. *Anesth. Analg.* **88**, 1155–1160.

Jackson, S., Bartlett, K., Land, J. et al. (1991). Long-chain 3-hydroxyacyl-CoA dehydrogenase deficiency. *Ped. Res.* **29**, 406–411.

Jackson, S., Kler, R. S., Bartlett, K. et al. (1992). Combined enzyme defect of mitochondrial fatty acid oxidation. *J. Clin. Invest.* **90**, 1219–1225.

Kanno, T. and Maekawa, M. (1995). Lactate dehydrogenase M-subunit deficiencies: clinical features, metabolic background and genetic heterogeneities. *Muscle Nerve* **3**, S54–S60

Kanno, T., Sudo, K., Takeuchi, I. et al. (1980). Hereditary deficiency of lactate dehydrogenase M-subunit. *Clin. Chim. Acta* **108**, 267–276.

Kaufmann, P., El-Schahawi, M. and DiMauro, S. (1997) Carnitine palmitoyltransferase II deficiency: diagnosis by molecular analysis of blood. *Mol. Cell. Biochem.* **174**, 237–239.

Keck, P. E., Caroff, S. N. and McElroy, S. L. (1995). Neuroleptic malignant syndrome and malignant hyperthermia: end of controversy? *J. Neuropyschol. Clin. Neurosci.* **7**, 135–144.

Kissel, J. T., Beam, W., Bresolin, N., Gibbons, G., DiMauro, S. and Mendell, J. R. (1985). Physiologic assessment of phosphoglycerate mutase deficiency: incremental exercise test. *Neurology* **35**, 828–833.

Kreuder, J., Borkhardt, A., Repp, R. et al. (1996). Brief report: inherited metabolic myopathy and hemolysis due to a mutation in aldolase A. [See comments] *N. Engl. J. Med.* **334**, 1100–1104.

Kubisch, C., Wicklein, E. M. and Jentsch, T. J. (1998). Molecular diagnosis of McArdle disease: revised genomic structure of the myophosphorylase gene and identification of a novel mutation. *Hum. Mut.* **12**, 27–32.

Kurz, D., Aguzzi, A. and Scherer, T. A. (1998). Decompensated cor pulmonale as the first manifestation of adult-onset myopathy. *Respiration* **65**, 317–319.

Laforet, P., Eymard, B., Lombes, A. et al. (1996). Exercise intolerance caused by muscular phosphorylase kinase deficiency. Contribution of in vivo metabolic studies. [Review] *Rev. Neurol.* **152**, 458–464.

Lebo, R. V., Gorin, F., Fletterick, R. J. et al. (1984). High-resolution chromosome sorting and DNA spot-blot analysis assign McArdle's syndrome to chromosome 11. *Science* **225**, 57–59.

Loehr, J. P., Goodman, S. I. and Frerman, F. E. (1990). Glutaric acidemia type II: heterogeneity of clinical and biochemical phenotypes. *Ped. Res.* **27**, 311–315.

Loke, J. and MacLennan, D. H. (1998). Malignant hyperthermia and central core disease: disorders of Ca2+ release channels. [Review] *Am. J. Med.* **104**, 470–486.

Lossos, A., Barash, V., Soffer, D. et al. (1991). Hereditary branching enzyme dysfunction in adult polyglucosan body disease: a possible metabolic cause in two patients. *Ann. Neurol.* **30**, 655–662.

Lossos, A., Meiner, Z., Barash, V. et al. (1998). Adult polyglucosan body disease in Ashkenazi Jewish patients carrying the Tyr329Ser mutation in the glycogen-branching enzyme gene. *Ann. Neurol.* **44**, 867–872.

Maclean, D., Vissing, J., Vissing, S. F. and Haller, R. J. (1958). Oral branch chain amino acids do not improve exercise capacity in McArdle's disease. *Neurology* **51**, 1456–1459.

Madlom, M., Besley, G. T., Cohen, P. T. and Marrian, V. J. (1989). Phosphorylase b kinase deficiency in a boy with glycogenosis affecting both liver and muscle. *Eur. J. Ped.* **149**, 52–53.

Manning, B. M., Quane, K. A., Ording, H. et al. (1998). Identification of novel mutations in the ryanodine-receptor gene (RYR1) in malignant hyperthermia: genotype–phenotype correlation. *Am. J. Hum. Genet.* **62**, 599–609.

Margolis, M. L. and Hill, A. R. (1986). Acid maltase deficiency in an adult. Evidence for improvement in respiratory function with high-protein dietary therapy. *Am. Rev. Resp. Dis.* **134**, 328–331.

Martin, R. J., Sufit, R. L., Ringel, S. P., Hudgel, D. W. and Hill, P. L. (1983). Respiratory improvement by muscle training in adult-onset acid maltase deficiency. *Muscle Nerve* **6**, 201–203.

Martiniuk, F., Ellenbogen, A., Hirschhorn, K. and Hirschhorn, R. (1985). Further regional localization of the genes for human acid alpha glucosidase (GAA), peptidase D (PEPD) and alpha mannosidase B (MANB) by somatic cell hybridization. *Hum. Genet.* **69**, 109–111.

Martiniuk, F., Mehler, M., Pellicer, A., et al. (1986). Isolation of a cDNA for human acid alpha-glucosidase and detection of genetic heterogeneity for mRNA in three alpha-glucosidase-deficient patients. *Proc. Natl. Acad. Sci. USA* **83**, 9641–9644.

Martiniuk, F., Mehler, M., Tzall, S., Meredith, G. and Hirschhorn, R. (1990). Sequence of the cDNA and 5′-flanking region for human acid alpha-glucosidase, detection of an intron in the 5′ untranslated leader sequence, definition of 18-bp polymorphisms and differences with previous cDNA and amino acid sequences. *DNA Cell Biol.* **9**, 85–94.

Martiniuk, F., Bodkin, M., Tzall, S. and Hirschhorn, R. (1991). Isolation and partial characterization of the structural gene for human acid alpha glucosidase. *DNA Cell Biol.* **10**, 283–292.

Martinuzzi, A., Schievano, G., Nascimbeni, A. and Fanin, M. (1999). McArdle's disease. The unsolved mystery of the reappearing enzyme. *Am. J. Pathol.* **154**, 1893–1897.

Matern, D., Strauss, A. W., Hillman, S. L., Mayatepek, E., Millington, D. S. and Trefz, F. K. (1999). Diagnosis of mitochondrial trifunctional protein deficiency in a blood spot from the newborn screening card by tandem mass spectrometry and DNA analysis. *Ped. Res.* **46**, 45–49.

McArdle, B. (1951). Myopathy due to a defect in muscle glycogen breakdown. *Clin. Sci.* **24**, 13–33.

McConkie-Rosell, A., Wilson, C., Piccoli, D. A. et al. (1996). Clinical and laboratory findings in four patients with the non-progressive hepatic form of type IV glycogen storage disease. *J. Inher. Metab. Dis.* **19**, 51–58.

McCully, K., Chance, B. and Giger, U. (1999). In vivo determination of altered hemoglobin saturation in dogs with M-type phosphofructokinase deficiency. *Muscle Nerve* 22, 621–627.

Meinck, H. M., Goebel, H. H., Rumpf, K. W., Kaiser, H. and Neumann, P. (1982). The forearm ischaemic work test – hazardous to McArdle patients? *J. Neurol. Neurosurg. Psychiatry* 45, 1144–1146.

Millington, D. S., Terada, N., Chace, D. H. et al. (1992). The role of tandem mass spectrometry in the diagnosis of fatty acid oxidation disorders. *Prog. Clin. Biol. Res.* 375, 339–354.

Mineo, I. and Tarui, S. (1995). Myogenic hyperuricemia: what can we learn from metabolic myopathies? [Review] *Muscle Nerve* 3, S75–S81

Miwa, S., Fujii, H., Tani, K. et al. (1981). Two cases of red cell aldolase deficiency associated with hereditary hemolytic anemia in a Japanese family. *Am. J. Hematol.* 11, 425–437.

Miyajima, H., Orii, K. E., Shindo, Y. et al. (1997). Mitochondrial trifunctional protein deficiency associated with recurrent myoglobinuria in adolescence. *Neurology* 49, 833–837.

Mizuta, K., Hashimoto, E., Tsutou, A. et al. (1984). A new type of glycogen storage disease caused by deficiency of cardiac phosphorylase kinase. *Biochem. Biophys. Res. Commun.* 119, 582–587.

Mommaerts, W. F., Illingworth, B., Pearson, C. M., Guillory, R. J. and Seraydarian, K. (1959). A functional disorder of muscle associated with the absence of phosphorylase. *Proc. Natl. Acad. Sci. USA* 45, 791

Monnier, N., Procaccio, V., Stieglitz, P. and Lunardi, J. (1997). Malignant-hyperthermia susceptibility is associated with a mutation of the alpha 1-subunit of the human dihydropyridine-sensitive L-type voltage-dependent calcium-channel receptor in skeletal muscle [see comments]. *Am. J. Hum. Genet.* 60, 1316–1325.

Morisaki, T., Gross, M., Morisaki, H., Pongratz, D., Zollner, N. and Holmes, E. W. (1992). Molecular basis of AMP deaminase deficiency in skeletal muscle. *Proc. Natl. Acad. Sci. USA* 89, 6457–6461.

Morris, A. A., Clayton, P. T., Surtees, R. A. and Leonard, J. V. (1997). Clinical outcomes in long-chain 3-hydroxyacyl-coenzyme A dehydrogenase deficiency. [Letter; comment] *J. Ped.* 131, 938.

Morris, A. A., Olpin, S. E., Brivet, M., Turnbull, D. M., Jones, R.A. and Leonard, J. V. (1998). A patient with carnitine-acylcarnitine-translocase deficiency with a mild phenotype. [See comments] *J. Ped.* 132, 514–516.

Moslehi, R., Langlois, S., Yam, I. and Friedman, J. M. (1998). Linkage of malignant hyperthermia and hyperkalemic periodic paralysis to the adult skeletal muscle sodium channel (*SCN4A*) gene in a large pedigree. *Am. J. Med. Genet.* 76, 21–27.

Nada, M. A., Vianey-Saban, C., Roe, C. R. et al. (1996). Prenatal diagnosis of mitochondrial fatty acid oxidation defects. *Prenat. Diagn.* 16, 117–124.

Naguib, M. and Magboul, M. M. (1998). Adverse effects of neuromuscular blockers and their antagonists. [Review] *Drug Safety* 18, 99–116.

Nakagawa, C., Mineo, I., Kaido, M. et al. (1995). A new variant case of muscle phosphofructokinase deficiency, coexisting with

gastric ulcer, gouty arthritis and increased hemolysis. *Muscle Nerve* 3, S39–S44

Nakajima, H., Hamaguchi, T., Yamasaki, T. and Tarui, S. (1995). Phosphofructokinase deficiency: recent advances in molecular biology. [Review] *Muscle Nerve* 3, S28–S34

Nezu, J., Tamai, I., Oku, A. et al. (1999). Primary systemic carnitine deficiency is caused by mutations in a gene encoding sodium ion-dependent carnitine transporter. *Nat. Genet.* 21, 91–94.

Nicolino, M. P., Puech, J. P., Kremer, E. J. et al. (1998). Adenovirus-mediated transfer of the acid alpha-glucosidase gene into fibroblasts, myoblasts and myotubes from patients with glycogen storage disease type II leads to high level expression of enzyme and corrects glycogen accumulation. *Hum. Mol. Genet.*, 7, 1695–1702.

Ogilvie, I., Pourfarzam, M., Jackson, S., Stockdale, C., Bartlett, K. and Turnbull, D. M. (1994). Very long-chain acyl coenzyme A dehydrogenase deficiency presenting with exercise-induced myoglobinuria. *Neurology* 44, 467–473.

Okubo, M., Horinishi, A., Nakamura, N. et al. (1998). A novel point mutation in an acceptor splice site of intron 32 (IVS32 A-12→G) but no exon 3 mutations in the glycogen debranching enzyme gene in a homozygous patient with glycogen storage disease type IIIb. [See comments] *Hum. Genet.* 102, 1–5.

Pande, S. V. (1999). Carnitine-acylcarnitine translocase deficiency. [Review] *Am. J. Med. Sci.* 318, 22–27.

Pande, S. V., Brivet, M., Slama, A., Demaugre, F., Aufrant, C. and Saudubray, J. M. (1993). Carnitine-acylcarnitine translocase deficiency with severe hypoglycemia and auriculo ventricular block. Translocase assay in permeabilized fibroblasts. *J. Clin. Invest.* 91, 1247–1252.

Parvari, R., Moses, S., Shen, J., Hershkovitz, E., Lerner, A. and Chen, Y. T. (1997). A single-base deletion in the 3′-coding region of glycogen-debranching enzyme is prevalent in glycogen storage disease type IIIA in a population of North African Jewish patients. *Eur. J. Hum. Genet.* 5, 266–270.

Parvari, R., Shen, J., Hershkovitz, E., Chen, Y. T. and Moses, S. W. (1998). Two new mutations in the 3′ coding region of the glycogen debranching enzyme in a glycogen storage disease type IIIa Ashkenazi Jewish patient. *J. Inher. Metab. Dis.* 21, 141–148.

Pauly, D. F., Johns, D. C., Matelis, L. A., Lawrence, J. H., Byrne, B. J. and Kessler, P. D. (1998). Complete correction of acid alpha-glucosidase deficiency in Pompe disease fibroblasts in vitro and lysosomally targeted expression in neonatal rat cardiac and skeletal muscle. *Gene Ther.* 5, 473–480.

Raben, N., Nichols, R. C., Boerkoel, C. and Plotz, P. (1995a). Genetic defects in patients with glycogenosis type II (acid maltase deficiency). [Review] *Muscle Nerve* 3, S70–S74

Raben, N., Sherman, J. B., Adams, E., Nakajima, H., Argov, Z. and Plotz, P. (1995b). Various classes of mutations in patients with phosphofructokinase deficiency (Tarui's disease). *Muscle Nerve* 3, S35–S38

Raben, N., Nagaraju, K., Lee, E. et al. (1998). Targeted disruption of the acid alpha-glucosidase gene in mice causes an illness with critical features of both infantile and adult human glycogen storage disease type II. *J. Biol. Chem.* 273, 19086–19092.

Rashed, M. S., Ozand, P. T., Bucknall, M. P. and Little, D. (1995). Diagnosis of inborn errors of metabolism from blood spots by acylcarnitines and amino acids profiling using automated electrospray tandem mass spectrometry. *Ped. Res.* **38**, 324–331.

Regalado, J. J., Rodriguez, M. M. and Ferrer, P. L. (1999). Infantile hypertrophic cardiomyopathy of glycogenosis type IX: isolated cardiac phosphorylase kinase deficiency. *Ped. Cardiol.* **20**, 304–307.

Reuser, A. J., Kroos, M. A., Hermans, M. M. et al. (1995). Glycogenosis type II (acid maltase deficiency). [Review] *Muscle Nerve* **3**, S61–S69

Richter, M., Schleithoff, L., Deufel, T., Lehmann-Horn, F. and Herrmann-Frank, A. (1997). Functional characterization of a distinct ryanodine receptor mutation in human malignant hyperthermia-susceptible muscle. *J. Biol. Chem.* **272**, 5256–5260.

Ristow, M., Vorgerd, M., Mohlig, M., Schatz, H. and Pfeiffer, A. (1997). Deficiency of phosphofructo-1-kinase/muscle subtype in humans impairs insulin secretion and causes insulin resistance. *J. Clin. Invest.* **100**, 2833–2841.

Rosa, R., George, C., Fardeau, M., Calvin, M. C., Rapin, M. and Rosa, J. (1982). A new case of phosphoglycerate kinase deficiency: PGK creteil associated with rhabdomyolysis and lacking hemolytic anemia. *Blood* **60**, 84–91.

Rosenow, E. C. and Engel, A. G. (1978). Acid maltase deficiency in adults presenting as respiratory failure. *Am. J. Med.* **64**, 485–491.

Rubio, J. C., Martin, M. A., Garcia, A. et al. (1999). McArdle's disease associated with homozygosity for the missense mutation Gly204Ser of the myophosphorylase gene in a Spanish patient. *Neuromusc. Disord.* **9**, 174–175.

Ruff, R. L. (1996). Elevated intracellular Ca^{2+} and myofibrillar Ca^{2+} sensitivity cause iodoacetate-induced muscle contractures. *J. Appl. Physiolol.* **81**, 1230–1239.

Ruitenbeek, W., Poels, P. J., Turnbull, D. M. et al. (1995). Rhabdomyolysis and acute encephalopathy in late onset medium chain acyl-CoA dehydrogenase deficiency. *J. Neurol. Neurosurg. Psychiatry* **58**, 209–214.

Sabina, R. L., Morisaki, T., Clarke, P. et al. (1990). Characterization of the human and rat myoadenylate deaminase genes. *J. Biol. Chem.* **265**, 9423–9433.

Sabina, R. L., Fishbein, W. N., Pezeshkpour, G., Clarke, P. R. and Holmes, E. W. (1992). Molecular analysis of the myoadenylate deaminase deficiencies. *Neurology* **42**, 170–179.

Sahin, G., Gungor, T., Rettwitz-Volk, W. et al. (1998). Infantile muscle phosphorylase-b-kinase deficiency. A case report. *Neuropediatrics* **29**, 48–50.

Sander, H. W., Menkes, D. L., Hood, D. C. and Williams, D. A. (1998). A 60-year-old woman with weakness, fatigue and acute respiratory failure: case report and discussion of the differential diagnosis. *Military Med.* **163**, 715–718.

Sato, K., Imai, F., Hatayama, I. and Roelofs, R. I. (1977). Characterization of glycogen phosphorylase isoenzymes present in cultured skeletal muscle from patients with McArdle's disease. *Biochem. Biophys. Res. Commun.* **78**, 663–668.

Schaefer, J., Jackson, S., Dick, D. J. and Turnbull, D. M. (1996). Trifunctional enzyme deficiency: adult presentation of a usually fatal beta-oxidation defect. *Ann. Neurol.* **40**, 597–602.

Schaefer, J., Jackson, S., Taroni, F., Swift, P. and Turnbull, D. M. (1997). Characterization of carnitine palmitoyltransferases in patients with a carnitine palmitoyltransferase deficiency: implications for diagnosis and therapy. *J. Neurol. Neurosurg. Psychiatry* **62**, 169–176.

Schmidt, R. and Mahler, R. (1959). Chronic progressive myopathy with myoglobinuria: demonstration of a glycogenolytic defect in the muscle. *J. Clin. Invest.*, **38**, 2044

Schroder, J. M., Dodel, R., Weis, J., Stefanidis, I. and Reichmann, H. (1996). Mitochondrial changes in muscle phosphoglycerate kinase deficiency. *Clin. Neuropathol.* **15**, 34–40.

Selby, R., Starzl, T. E., Yunis, E., Brown, B. I., Kendall, R. S. and Tzakis, A. (1991). Liver transplantation for type IV glycogen storage disease. *N. Engl. J. Med.* **324**, 39–42.

Servidei, S., Metlay, L. A., Chodosh, J. and DiMauro, S. (1988). Fatal infantile cardiopathy caused by phosphorylase b kinase deficiency. *J. Ped.*, **113**, 82–85.

Seth, P., Wu, X., Huang, W., Leibach, F. H. and Ganapathy, V. (1999). Mutations in novel organic cation transporter (OCTN2), an organic cation/carnitine transporter, with differential effects of the organic cation transport function and the carnitine transport function. *J. Biol. Chem.* **274**, 33388–33392.

Shen, J., Bao, Y., Liu, H. M., Lee, P., Leonard, J. V. and Chen, Y. T. (1996). Mutations in exon 3 of the glycogen debranching enzyme gene are associated with glycogen storage disease type III that is differentially expressed in liver and muscle. *J. Clin. Invest.* **98**, 352–357.

Shin, Y. S. (1990). Diagnosis of glycogen storage disease. *J. Inher. Metab. Dis.* **13**, 419–434.

Slonim, A. E., Coleman, R. A., McElligot, M. A. et al. (1983). Improvement of muscle function in acid maltase deficiency by high-protein therapy. *Neurology* **33**, 34–38.

Smelt, A. H., Poorthuis, B. J., Onkenhout, W. et al. (1998). Very long chain acyl-coenzyme A dehydrogenase deficiency with adult onset. *Ann. Neurol.* **43**, 540–544.

Sokal, E. M., van Hoof, H. F., Alberti, D. et al. (1992). Progressive cardiac failure following orthotopic liver transplantation for type IV glycogenosis. *Eur. J. Ped.* **151**, 200–203.

Stanley, C. A., DeLeeuw, S., Coates, P. M. et al. (1991). Chronic cardiomyopathy and weakness or acute coma in children with a defect in carnitine uptake. [Review] *Ann. Neurol.* **30**, 709–716.

Stanley, C. A., Hale, D. E., Berry, G. T., de Leeuw, S., Boxer, J. and Bonnefont, J. P. (1992). Brief report: a deficiency of carnitine-acylcarnitine translocase in the inner mitochondrial membrane. *N. Engl. J. Med.* **327**, 19–23.

Straussberg, R., Harel, L., Varsano, I., Elpeleg, O. N., Shamir, R. and Amir, J. (1997). Recurrent myoglobinuria as a presenting manifestation of very long chain acyl coenzyme A dehydrogenase deficiency. *Pediatrics* **99**, 894–896.

Sugie, H., Sugie, Y., Ito, M. and Fukuda, T. (1998). A novel missense mutation (837T→C) in the phosphoglycerate kinase gene of a patient with a myopathic form of phosphoglycerate kinase deficiency. *J. Child Neurol.* **13**, 95–97.

Swaiman, K. F., Kennedy, W. R. and Sauls, H. S. (1968). Late infantile acid maltase deficiency. *Arch. Neurol.* **18**, 642–648.

Swoboda, K. J., Specht, L., Jones, H. R., Shapiro, F., DiMauro, S. and Korson, M. (1997). Infantile phosphofructokinase deficiency with arthrogryposis: clinical benefit of a ketogenic diet. [Review] *J. Ped.* **131**, 932–934.

Tang, N. L., Ganapathy, V., Wu, X. et al. (1999). Mutations of OCTN2, an organic cation/carnitine transporter, lead to deficient cellular carnitine uptake in primary carnitine deficiency. [Published erratum appears in *Hum. Mol. Genet.* (1999) 8, 943.] *Hum. Mol. Genet.* **8**, 655–660.

Tang, T. T., Segura, A. D., Chen, Y. T. et al. (1994). Neonatal hypotonia and cardiomyopathy secondary to type IV glycogenosis. *Acta Neuropathol.* **87**, 531–536.

Taroni, F., Verderio, E., Fiorucci, S. et al. (1992). Molecular characterization of inherited carnitine palmitoyltransferase II deficiency. *Proc. Natl. Acad. Sci. USA* **89**, 8429–8433.

Taroni, F., Verderio, E., Dworzak, F., Willems, P. J., Cavadini, P. and DiDonato, S. (1993). Identification of a common mutation in the carnitine palmitoyltransferase II gene in familial recurrent myoglobinuria patients. *Nat. Genet.* **4**, 314–320.

Tarui, S. (1995). Glycolytic defects in muscle: aspects of collaboration between basic science and clinical medicine. [Review] *Muscle Nerve* **3**, S2–S9

Tein, I. (1999). Neonatal metabolic myopathies. [Review] *Sem. Perinatol.* 125–151.

Tong, J., Oyamada, H., Demaurex, N., Grinstein, S., McCarthy, T. V. and MacLennan, D. H. (1997). Caffeine and halothane sensitivity of intracellular Ca2$^+$ release is altered by 15 calcium release channel (ryanodine receptor) mutations associated with malignant hyperthermia and/or central core disease. *J. Biol. Chem.* **272**, 26332–26339.

Tonin, P., Shanske, S. and Brownell, A. K. (1989). Phosphoglycerate kinase (PGK) deficiency: a third case with recurrent myoglobinuria. *Neurology* **39**, S359

Toscano, A., Tsujino, S., Vita, G., Shanske, S., Messina, C. and DiMauro, S. (1996). Molecular basis of muscle phosphoglycerate mutase (PGAM-M) deficiency in the Italian kindred. *Muscle Nerve* **19**, 1134–1137.

Toyoda, H., Nakase, T., Toméoku, M. et al. (1996). Improvement of hemolysis in muscle phosphofructokinase deficiency by restriction of exercise. *Inter. Med.* **35**, 222–226.

Trend, P. S., Wiles, C. M., Spencer, G. T., Morgan-Hughes, J. A., Lake, B. D. and Patrick, A. D. (1985). Acid maltase deficiency in adults. Diagnosis and management in five cases. *Brain* **108**, 845–860.

Tsujino, S., Shanske, S., Nonaka, I. and DiMauro, S. (1995a). The molecular genetic basis of myophosphorylase deficiency (McArdle's disease). *Muscle Nerve* **3**, S23–S27

Tsujino, S., Shanske, S. and DiMauro, S. (1995b). Molecular genetic heterogeneity of phosphoglycerate kinase (PGK) deficiency. *Muscle Nerve* **3**, S45–S49

Tsujino, S., Shanske, S., Sakoda, S., Toscano, A. and DiMauro, S. (1995c). Molecular genetic studies in muscle phosphoglycerate mutase (PGAM-M) deficiency. *Muscle Nerve* **3**, S50–S53

Tsujino, S., Kinoshita, N., Tashiro, T. et al. (1998). Adenovirus-mediated transfer of human acid maltase gene reduces glycogen

accumulation in skeletal muscle of Japanese quail with acid maltase deficiency. *Hum. Gene Ther.* **9**, 1609–1616.

Umpleby, A. M., Trend, P. S., Chubb, D. et al. (1989). The effect of a high protein diet on leucine and alanine turnover in acid maltase deficiency. *J. Neurol. Neurosurg. Psychiatry* **52**, 954–961.

van den Bergl, E. and Berger, R. (1990). Phosphorylase b kinase deficiency in man: a review. [Review] *J. Inher. Metab. Dis.* **13**, 442–451.

van der Ploeg, A. T., Bolhuis, P. A., Wolterman, R. A. et al. (1988). Prospect for enzyme therapy in glycogenosis II variants: a study on cultured muscle cells. *J. Neurol.* **235**, 392–396.

Verzijl, H. T., van Engelen, G., Luyten, J. A. et al. (1998). Genetic characteristics of myoadenylate deaminase deficiency. [See comments] *Ann. Neurol.* **44**, 140–143.

Vianey-Saban, C., Guffon, N., Delolne, F., Guibaud, P., Mathieu, M. and Divry, P. (1997). Diagnosis of inborn errors of metabolism by acylcarnitine profiling in blood using tandem mass spectrometry. *J. Inher. Metab. Dis.* **20**, 411–414.

Vissing, J., Lewis, S. F., Galbo, H. and Haller, R. G. (1992). Effect of deficient muscular glycogenolysis on extramuscular fuel production in exercise. *J. Appl. Physiol.* **72**, 1773–1779.

Vissing, J., Schmalbruch, H., Haller, R. G. and Clausen, T. (1999). Muscle phosphoglycerate mutase deficiency with tubular aggregates: effect of dantrolene. *Ann. Neurol.* **46**, 274–277.

Vita, G., Toscano, A., Bresolin, N. et al. (1990). Muscle phosphoglycerate mutase (PGAM) deficiency in the first caucasian patient. *Neurology* **40**, 297

Vorgerd, M., Kubisch, C., Burwinkel, B. et al. (1998). Mutation analysis in myophosphorylase deficiency (McArdle's disease). *Ann. Neurol.* **43**, 326–331.

Wahren, J., Felig, P., Havel, R. J., Jorfeldt, L., Pernow, B. and Saltin, B. (1973). Amino acid metabolism in McArdle's syndrome. *N. Engl. J. Med.* **288**, 774–777.

Weglinski, M. R., Wedel, D. J. and Engel, A. G. (1997). Malignant hyperthermia testing in patients with persistently increased serum creatine kinase levels. *Anesth. Analg.* **84**, 1038–1041.

Wehner, M. and Kilimann, M. W. (1995). Human cDNA encoding the muscle isoform of the phosphorylase kinase gamma subunit (PHKG1). *Hum. Genet.* **96**, 616–618.

Wehner, M., Clemens, P. R., Engel, A. G. and Kilimann, M. W. (1994). Human muscle glycogenosis due to phosphorylase kinase deficiency associated with a nonsense mutation in the muscle isoform of the alpha subunit. *Hum. Mol. Genet.*, **3**, 1983–1987.

Wilkinson, D. A., Tonin, P., Shanske, S., Lombes, A., Carlson, G. M. and DiMauro, S. (1994). Clinical and biochemical features of 10 adult patients with muscle phosphorylase kinase deficiency. *Neurology* **44**, 461–466.

Wisselaar, H. A., Kroos, M. A., Hermans, M. M., van Beeumen, J. and Reuser, A. J. (1993). Structural and functional changes of lysosomal acid alpha-glucosidase during intracellular transport and maturation. *J. Biol. Chem.* **268**, 2223–2231.

Yang, B. Z., Ding, J. H., Roe, D., Dewese, T., Day, D. W. and Roe, C. R. (1998). A novel mutation identified in carnitine palmitoyltransferase II deficiency. *Mol. Genet. Metab.* **63**, 110–115.

29

Oxidative phosphorylation diseases of muscle

John M. Shoffner and Eric A. Shoubridge

Introduction

Contemporary concepts of oxidative phosphorylation (OXPHOS) diseases originated with the description of a multisystem disorder called Kearns–Sayre syndrome and a rare hypermetabolic disorder called Luft's disease (Ernster et al., 1959; Luft et al., 1962). Kearns–Sayre syndrome is characterized by chronic progressive external ophthalmoplegia, retinitis pigmentosa and mitochondrial myopathy. Luft's disease is characterized by increased body temperature, structural abnormalities in mitochondria and abnormal OXPHOS function. Early descriptions of the neuromuscular manifestations of OXPHOS diseases played an important role in formulating the criteria used by clinicians to diagnose OXPHOS diseases for over three decades. Patient diagnosis depended on the recognition of characteristic phenotypes, the identification of histological and ultrastructural abnormalities in skeletal muscle mitochondria and the identification of abnormalities in OXPHOS enzyme activities. Although the mitochondrial DNA (mtDNA) encodes only 13 polypeptide subunits of the OXPHOS enzymes, there are more than 70 nuclear-encoded subunits and a much larger number of factors necessary for the assembly and maintenance of a functional respiratory chain. This degree of complexity makes the diagnosis of OXPHOS diseases a challenging process. The term 'mitochondrial medicine' emerged to encompass the complex synthesis of clinical, biochemical, pathological and genetic information required for patient diagnosis. The phenotypic spectrum of OXPHOS diseases is very broad; this chapter focuses on selected examples of OXPHOS diseases that have some neuromuscular involvement and it presents an algorithm to facilitate patient diagnosis.

Oxidative phosphorylation biochemistry and genetics

Mitochondria are generally about $0.1–0.5\,\mu$m in diameter and in adult human muscle account for about 4% of the total fibre volume (Jerusalem et al., 1975). They are cytoplasmic structures with an inner and outer membrane separated by an intermembrane space. The outer membrane is permeable to most small molecules and ions and it contains a variety of proteins such as monoamine oxidase, long-chain acyl-CoA synthetase, carnitine palmitoyltransferase I (CPTI) and mitochondrial protein import proteins. The inner mitochondrial mebrane is impermeable to most metabolites. It has a convoluted structure with multiple folds called cristae. The inner membrane has a high content of protein and cardiolipin. It contains the enzymes of OXPHOS as well as multiple classes of translocases. The space surrounded by the inner mitochondrial membrane, called the mitochondrial matrix, contains an array of enzymes including those for the tricarboxylic acid cycle (Krebs cycle), the pyruvate dehydrogenase complex, β-oxidation of fatty acids, urea cycle, ketone metabolism, amino acid metabolism, haem metabolism, nucleotide metabolism and the peptidases plus chaperonins necessary for mitochondrial protein import and OXPHOS enzyme assembly and maintenance.

The matrix also contains mtDNA, a 16 569 nucleotide pair, double-stranded, circular molecule that codes for two ribosomal RNAs (rRNA), 22 transfer RNAs (tRNA), and 13 polypeptides that are integral components of the enzyme complexes that constitute the mitochondrial respiratory chain (see Figs. 5.1 and 5.2, pp. 81 and 82).

OXPHOS uses about 95% of the oxygen delivered to tissues, producing most of the ATP that is required by cells. The expression of the genes involved in the OXPHOS pathway and the assembly of the five OXPHOS enzyme complexes (complex I to V) into the inner mitochondrial membrane is a highly ordered and coordinated process that depends on gene expression from the mtDNA as well as the nuclear DNA. MtDNA encodes 13 polypeptide subunits of the OXPHOS enzymes; however, a much larger number of proteins (perhaps hundreds) are estimated to be necessary for proper OXPHOS function. OXPHOS enzymes are located in the mitochondrial inner membrane and are designated as complex I (NADH:ubiquinone oxidoreductase, EC 1.6.5.3), complex II (succinate:ubiquinone oxidoreductase, EC 1.3.5.1), complex III (ubiquinol:ferrocytochrome c oxidoreductase, EC 1.10.2.2), complex IV (ferrocytochrome c:oxygen oxidoreductase or cytochrome c oxidase (COX), EC 1.9.3.1), and complex V (adenine trisphosphate (ATP) synthase, EC 3.6.1.34). Complex I transfers electrons to ubiquinone (coenzyme Q_{10} (CoQ)) through a long series of redox groups which include flavin mononucleotide (FMN) and six iron-sulphur clusters. This large and fragile enzyme is composed of approximately 43 subunits, seven encoded by mtDNA and the remainder by nuclear DNA. Complex II performs a key step in the tricarboxylic acid cycle in which succinate is dehydrogenated to fumarate and the electrons are donated to ubiquinone in the mitochondrial inner membrane. It is localized to the matrix side of the mitochondrial inner membrane and is the only OXPHOS enzyme in which all subunits are coded by nuclear DNA. Complex III catalyses electron transfer between two mobile electron carriers, ubiquinol and cytochrome c, and also translocates protons across the mitochondrial inner membrane. This enzyme is composed of 11 polypeptides, only one of which is encoded by mtDNA. Complex IV or COX is the terminal enzyme complex of the electron transport chain. It collects electrons transferred from reduced cytochrome c and donates them to oxygen, which is then reduced to water. In conjunction with this process, protons are pumped across the mitochondrial inner membrane into the intermembrane space. Mammalian complex IV is composed of 13 polypeptide subunits, three of which are encoded by mtDNA. Complex V uses the electrochemical gradient created by complexes I, III and IV as a source of energy for synthesizing ATP from adenine diphosphate (ADP) and inorganic phosphate (P_i). This enzyme is composed of two parts, the F_1 segment, which catalyses ATP synthesis, and the F_0 segment, which translocates protons into the mitochondrial matrix. It is composed of 12–13 subunits, two encoded by mtDNA (ATPase six and eight genes) and 11–12 subunits encoded by nuclear DNA. The synthesis of ATP by complex V is functionally coupled to electron transport through complexes I, III, IV and the reduction of oxygen. In coupled mitochondria, electron transport and oxygen consumption increase when ADP is available and decline to a minimum constant level when ADP is limiting.

The transmission of mtDNA in mammals is, as far as is known, strictly maternal. Although paternal mtDNA enters the oocyte at fertilization (in the mitochondria of the sperm midpiece), paternal mitochondria are eliminated in the early embryo by still ill-defined mechanisms. The only known exception to this rule was reported in interspecific mouse crosses in which leakage of paternal mtDNA was observed (Gyllensten et al., 1991; Kaneda et al., 1995). Therefore, in humans, transmission of mtDNA mutations is expected to occur exclusively along maternal lineages. When a pathogenic mtDNA mutation is present, the consequences of maternal transmission are influenced by whether the mtDNA is homoplasmic (all mtDNAs share the same sequence) or heteroplasmic (different sequence variants coexist). As the majority of pathogenic mutations are heteroplasmic, it is important to understand the transmission genetics of mtDNA sequence variants. Although oocytes contain about 100 000 copies of mtDNA, rapid shifts in the proportion of mutant mtDNAs have been observed between generations. This is the result of a genetic bottleneck for mtDNA in early oogenesis (Hauswirth and Laipis, 1982; Jenuth et al., 1996). The practical consequence of this phenomenon is that the risk of having affected offspring is not trivial at any degree of heteroplasmy.

When heteroplasmy exists in somatic cells, the normal and mutant mtDNAs segregate randomly during cytokinesis to the daughter cells. The rate of replicative segregation is faster than expected because the replication of mtDNA is not tied to the cell cycle (Clayton, 1982). Consequently, mtDNA templates can replicate more than once or not at all during the cell cycle. Once the mutant mtDNAs reach a critical level, the cellular phenotype changes rapidly from normal to abnormal. The relationship between genotype and phenotype is more complex for pathogenic mtDNA mutations that are homoplasmic. Disease expression appears to be influenced by poorly understood genetic and environmental interactions.

Algorithm for patient diagnosis

OXPHOS defects can result from mutations in any of the mitochondrial genes or in any of the nuclear OXPHOS genes. Since the genes for OXPHOS are located in two distinct genomes, the inheritance of OXPHOS diseases can be maternal, Mendelian (autosomal dominant, autosomal recessive, X-linked) or sporadic. The basic elements of the

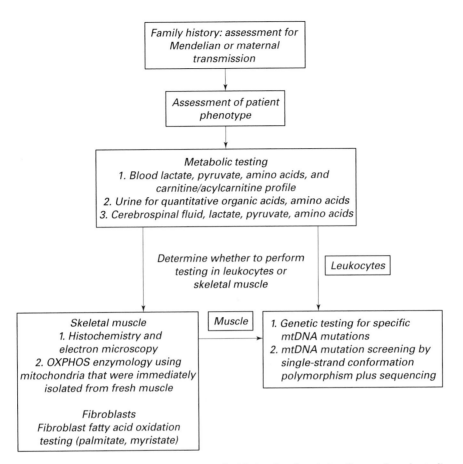

Fig. 29.1. Diagnostic algorithm for assessment of oxidative phosphorylation diseases. In order to diagnose most patients, clinical and laboratory data are collected and assessed.

algorithm are (i) phenotype recognition, (ii) metabolic testing, (iii) assessment for skeletal muscle pathology, (iv) OXPHOS biochemistry and (v) genetic testing (Fig. 29.1).

Phenotype recognition

Because of the large number of phenotypes that are described, phenotype recognition can be difficult. Table 29.1 outlines major classes of phenotype–genotype association in patients with OXPHOS diseases.

Metabolic testing in OXPHOS diseases

Abnormalities in oxidative phosphorylation can produce identifiable defects in related metabolic pathways such as glycolysis, pyruvate metabolism, the tricarboxylic acid cycle, protein catabolism, and fatty acid oxidation. Although the quantification of organic acids and amino acids in blood, urine and cerebrospinal fluid can provide useful diagnostic information, normal values for metabolic

tests do not exclude the diagnosis. Metabolic acidosis as well as elevations of lactate, pyruvate, lactate/pyruvate ratio (>20), alanine, tricarboxylic acid cycle intermediates, dicarboxylic acids and/or a generalized amino aciduria can be important diagnostic clues to the presence of an OXPHOS disease. Other metabolites that may also be increased include triglcylglycine, ethylmalonic acid, 3-methylglutaconic acid, 2-ethylhydracrylic acid, 2-methyl-succinate, butyrylglycine, isovalerylglycine and ammonia. Excretion of carnitine esters may be associated with reduced blood and tissue carnitine levels. A 24-hour urine collection is useful since it can provide an integrated evaluation of organic and amino acids as well as insight into the function of the highly OXPHOS-dependent proximal renal tubules. Although this is easily accomplished in adults, a 24-hour urine collection is difficult in paediatric patients and spot urine collection is used. Analysis of organic and amino acids in venous blood can be complicated by technical factors such as duration of tourniquet application, activity such as recent seizures or vigorous crying and

Table 29.1. Oxidative phosphorylation disease phenotype and genotype associations for the most frequently encountered mtDNA mutations: mutations in mtDNA can occur spontaneously, exhibit maternal inheritance or exhibit Mendelian inheritance patterns

Phenotypes	References
Deletions/duplications (sporadic, clonal)	
Kearns–Sayre and chronic progressive external ophthalmoplegia syndromes	Holt et al., 1988; Moraes et al., 1989; Shoubridge et al., 1990
Kearns–Sayre syndrome, mitochondrial encephalomyopathy, lactic acidosis, stroke-like episodes (MELAS), hypoparathyroidism, diabetes mellitus	Zupanc et al., 1991
Kearns–Sayre syndrome (delivery of healthy children)	Kokot et al., 1996; Larsson et al., 1992
Kearns–Sayre syndrome, hypoparathyroidism	Tengan et al., 1998; Wilichowski et al., 1997
Kearns–Sayre syndrome, hypoparathyroidism, diabetes mellitus	Isotani et al., 1996
Kearns–Sayre syndrome, pernicious anaemia, hypoparathyroidism	Abramowicz et al., 1996
Kearns–Sayre syndrome, pituitary hypothyroidism, periventricular white matter abnormalities	Yasui et al., 1993
Kearns–Sayre syndrome, corneal decompensation	Chang et al., 1994
Kearns–Sayre syndrome, choroideraemia-like fundus	Herzberg et al., 1993
Kearns–Sayre syndrome, dilated cardiomyopathy with successful cardiac transplantation	Tranchant et al., 1993
Kearns–Sayre syndrome, oculocerebrorenal syndrome (Lowe syndrome)	Moraes et al., 1991b
Kearns–Sayre syndrome, anhidrosis, de Toni–Fanconi–Debre syndrome	Mori et al., 1991
Kearns–Sayre syndrome, Bartter syndrome	Goto et al., 1990a
Chronic progressive external ophthalmoplegia presenting with unilateral ptosis	Rossier and Hatt, 1996
Chronic progressive external ophthalmoplegia, pregnancy complicated by preterm labour, hypertension	Ewart and Burrows, 1997
Chronic progressive external ophthalmoplegia plus stroke, epilepsy	Furuya et al., 1997
Chronic progressive external ophthalmoplegia, periventricular white matter lesions, pituitary hypothyroidism	Yasui et al., 1993
Ptosis, pigmentary retinopathy, normal ocular motility, no ragged-red fibres	Ota et al., 1994
Chronic progressive external ophthalmoplegia, deafness, cardiomyopathy with successful cardiac transplantation	Tranchant et al., 1993
Chronic progressive external ophthalmoplegia, familial hypercholesterolaemia	Orimo et al., 1992
Chronic progressive external ophthalmoplegia, abnormal markers of oxidative stress	Andreetta et al., 1991
Chronic progressive external ophthalmoplegia, marfanoid appearance, cytoplasmic bodies in muscle	Sahashi et al., 1990
Adult-onset mitochondrial myopathy	Manfredi et al., 1997
Pearson syndrome	Rotig et al., 1988, 1989
Pearson syndrome, Kearns–Sayre syndrome	Simonsz et al., 1992
Pearson syndrome with neonatal death	Muraki et al., 1997
Pearson syndrome, multiple renal cysts	Gurgey et al., 1996
Pearson syndrome, Leigh disease	Santorelli et al., 1996a; Yamadori et al., 1992
Pearson syndrome, de Toni–Debre–Fanconi syndrome	Niaudet et al., 1994
Pearson syndrome variant: sideroblastic anaemia with vacuolization of haematopoietic precursors	Mielot et al., 1997
Pearson's syndrome, zonular cataract, secondary strabismus	Cursiefen et al., 1998
Pearson syndrome variant: exocrine pancreas dysfunction, mitochondrial myopathy	Morris et al., 1997
Pearson syndrome variant: congenital hypoplastic anaemia, diabetes mellitus, exocrine pancreas insufficiency, renal tubule dysfunction, cerebral atrophy	Majander et al., 1991
Pearson syndrome variant: altered tricarboxylic acid and urea cycle metabolites, adrenal insufficiency, corneal opacities	Ribes et al., 1993
Pearson syndrome, 3-methylglutaconicaciduria	Gibson et al., 1992
Cerebellar ataxia, hypogonadotrophic hypogonadism, chorioretinal dystrophy	Barrientos et al., 1997
Cerebral palsy and growth hormone deficiency	Gucuyener et al., 1998
Developmental delay, regression, brainstem dysfunction, lactic acidosis, pancytopenia, failure to thrive, absence of ragged-red and cytochrome-oxidase-negative fibres	Blok et al., 1995

Table 29.1. (*cont.*)

Phenotypes	References
Adrenal insufficiency	Bruno et al., 1998
Adrenal insufficiency, growth retardation, deafness, leukodystrophy	Nicolino et al., 1997
Diabetes mellitus, optic atrophy, deafness (diabetes inspidus, diabetes mellitus, optic atrophy, deafness (DIDMOAD) Wolfram phenotype)	Rotig et al., 1993
Diabetes mellitus, cataracts, deafness, macular dystrophy	Souied et al., 1998
Diabetes mellitus, mitochondrial myopathy, leukodystrophy	Nicolino et al., 1997
Diabetes mellitus, diabetic amyotrophy, diabetic myoatrophy, diabetic fatty liver	Hinokio et al., 1995
Diabetes mellitus, Fanconi syndrome	Luder and Barash, 1994
Mitochondrial myopathy, axonal neuropathy	Molnar et al., 1996
Mitochondrial myopathy, multiple symmetric lipomatosis	Campos et al., 1996b
MELAS, Fanconi sydnrome	Campos et al., 1995b
Leigh disease	Rahman et al., 1996
Infantile cardio-encephalomyopathy with decreased carnitine acetyltransferase	Melegh et al., 1995
Cluster headache	Montagna et al., 1998; Odawara et al., 1997
Migrainous strokes (complicated migraines); ragged-red fibres	Bresolin et al., 1991
Leukodystrophy, chronic renal failure, tubulointerstitial nephritis	Rotig et al., 1995
Hypoparathyroidism, ataxia, spastic paraparesis, myopathy, deafness, short stature, vitiligo, hirsuitism, anaemia, diabetes, exocrine pancreas dysfunction	Tulinius et al., 1995
Renal tubule dysfunction (polydipsia, polyuria), fatigue, ataxia, deafness	Tulinius et al., 1995
Leukodystrophy ataxia, bulbar palsy, ragged-red fibre myopathy	Nakai et al., 1994
Chronic tubulointerstitial nephropathy, megaloblastic anaemia, growth retardation, partial renal Fanconi syndrome	Szabolcs et al., 1994b
Recurrent myoglobinuria	Ohno et al., 1991a,b
Chronic diarrhoea, villous atrophy	Cormier-Daire et al., 1994
Inclusion body myositis	Oldfors et al., 1993
Affective disorder	Stine et al., 1993

Deletion (sporadic, clonal) plus maternally transmitted point mutation in tRNA$^{Leu(UUR)}$ (A3243G)

Kearns–Sayre syndrome, autoimmune polyglandular syndrome (Addison's disease, autoimmune insulin-dependent diabetes mellitus, Hashimoto thyroiditis, primary ovarian failure)	Ohno et al., 1996

Deletion/duplication (maternally transmitted)

Kearns–Sayre syndrome	Akaike et al., 1995
Diabetes, deafness	Ballinger et al., 1992, 1994; Dunbar et al., 1993; Gebhart et al., 1996
Wolfram syndrome (optic atrophy, diabetes mellitus, diabetes insipidus, deafness, urinary tract abnormalities, neurological dysfunction)	Rotig et al., 1993; Barrientos et al., 1996a
Chronic progressive external ophthalmoplegia	Ozawa et al., 1988; Tanaka et al., 1989
Chronic progressive external ophthalmoplegia in mother and Pearson syndrome in son	Bernes et al., 1993
Chronic progressive external ophthalmoplegia in mother and daughters with proximal tubulopathy, diabetes mellitus, cerebellar ataxia	Rotig et al., 1992
Chronic progressive external ophthalmoplegia, diabetes mellitus	Dunbar et al., 1993

Point mutations in tRNA$^{Leu(UUR)}$ (A3243G)

MELAS (maternally inherited, sporadic)	Goto et al., 1990b
MELAS, cataracts	Terauchi et al., 1996
MELAS, laminar cortical necrosis, severe cortical atrophy	Valanne et al., 1996
MELAS, cardiomyopathy	Cristofari et al., 1995
MELAS, diabetes mellitus, hyperthyroidism	Yang et al., 1995; Li et al., 1996
MELAS, chronic renal failure	Ihara et al., 1996

Table 29.1. (*cont.*)

Phenotypes	References
MELAS with ophthalmoplegia, developmental delay, pigmentary retinopathy, or intestinal pseudo-obstruction	Morgan-Hughes et al., 1995
MELAS, ophthalmoplegia, pigmentary retinopathy	Rummelt et al., 1993
MELAS without ragged-red fibre myopathy, normal lactate level (rest and post-exercise)	Ujike et al., 1993
Late-onset MELAS (> 50 years)	Kimata et al., 1998; Minamoto et al., 1996
Myopathy, seizures	Degoul et al., 1994
Myopathy, leukoencephalopathy	Degoul et al., 1994
Myopathy, cardiomyopathy	Zeviani et al., 1991
Variable combinations of deafness, mitochondrial myopathy, diabetes mellitus, mental retardation	Damian et al., 1995
Variable intrafamilial combinations of deafness, retinal pigmentary degeneration, migraine headaches, hypothalamic hypogonadism, mitochondrial myopathy	Mosewich et al., 1993
Encephalopathy, deafness, ataxia, dementia	Morgan-Hughes et al., 1995
Chronic mild encephalopathy, short stature, hearing loss	Damian et al., 1994
Myoclonus epilepsy with ragged red fibres (MERRF)	Chang et al., 1993; Crimmins et al., 1993; Folgero et al., 1995; Hammans et al., 1995; Lee et al., 1997
MERRF, basal ganglia calcifications	Fabrizi et al., 1996
MERRF/MELAS overlap	Chen et al., 1993
Hypertrophic cardiomyopathy	Matthews et al. 1994; Cristofari et al., 1995; Hiruta et al., 1995
Kearns–Sayre syndrome	Crimmins et al., 1993
Chronic progressive external ophthalmoplegia syndromes (variable expression of deafness, diabetes mellitus, pigmentary retinopathy)	Chang et al., 1993; Martinuzzi et al., 1992; Moraes et al., 1993
Chronic progressive external ophthalmoplegia, MELAS	Fang et al., 1993; Jean-Francois et al., 1994
Chronic progressive external ophthalmoplegia, MELAS, MERRF features	Chang et al., 1993
Chronic progressive external ophthalmoplegia, MELAS, carnitine deficiency	Hsu et al., 1995
Juvenile cataract + retinal pigmentary degeneration	Isashiki et al., 1998
Renal failure	Damian et al., 1998
Cardiomyopathy	Silvestri et al., 1997; Vilarinho et al., 1997; Damian et al., 1998
Mitochondrial myopathy	Kawakami et al., 1994; Campos et al., 1995a; Hammans et al., 1995; Morgan-Hughes et al., 1995; Smith et al., 1997
Deafness	Crimmins et al., 1993; Jean-Francois et al., 1994
Diabetes mellitus ± deafness, ± islet cell antibodies	Reardon et al., 1992; van den Ouweland et al., 1992; Onishi et al., 1993
Diabetes mellitus, pancreatic exocrine dysfunction	Onishi et al., 1998
Diabetes mellitus, cardiomyopathy, sick sinus syndrome (first-degree atrioventricular block, incomplete right bundle branch block) progressing to sinus arrest	Inamori et al., 1997
Diabetes mellitus, hearing loss, cardiomyopathy	Gerbitz et al., 1993; Shinomiya et al., 1998
Diabetes mellitus, pregnancy, spontaneous abortion	Yanagisawa et al., 1995
Diabetes mellitus, hypertrophic cardiomyopathy	Kitaoka et al., 1995; Takeda, 1995, 1997; Yoshida et al., 1995
Diabetes mellitus, hyperechogenic cardiomyopathy	Kuzuya et al., 1994
Diabetes mellitus, decreased cerebral blood perfusion	Odawara et al., 1995
Diabetes mellitus, pigmentary retinopathy	Vialettes et al., 1995
Diabetes mellitus, deafness, cerebellar ataxia	Arai and Ohshima, 1997

Table 29.1. (*cont.*)

Phenotypes	References
Diabetes mellitus, deafness, Leigh disease variant with asymptomatic basal ganglia and subcortical increase of T_2 MRI signal (adult)	Bowen et al., 1998
Diabetes mellitus, mental retardation, growth hormone deficiency, nephropathy	Yorifuji et al., 1996
Diabetes mellitus, psychiatric symptoms	Inagaki et al., 1997
Diabetes mellitus, deafness, macular dystrophy, retinal branch vein occlusion	Souied et al., 1998
Diabetes mellitus, deafness, macular pattern retinal dystrophy	Massin et al., 1995; Bonte et al., 1996
Diabetes mellitus, deafness, progressive non-diabetic kidney disease (Alport-like phenotype)	Jansen et al., 1997
Diabetic embryopathy (anal atresia, caudal dysgenesis, multicystic dysplastic kidneys	Feigenbaum et al., 1996
Diabetes mellitus, retinitis pigmentosa, hypothalamic hypogonadism, mitochondrial myopathy (variable manifestations within a pedigree)	Mosewich et al., 1993
Gestational diabetes	Chuang et al., 1995
MERRF, chronic progressive external ophthalmoplegia overlap	Verma et al., 1996
MERRF/MELAS overlap	Chen et al., 1993; Campos et al., 1996a
Leigh disease	Nakase, 1993
Psychosis, mitochondrial myopathy, Alzheimer-like neuropathology	Kaido et al., 1996
Infantile intractable seizures, developmental delay	Feigenbaum et al., 1996
Cardiac and gastrointestinal abnormalities	Dougherty et al., 1994
Recurrent respiratory failure	Kamakura et al., 1995
Depressive disorder	Onishi et al., 1997
Cluster headache	Seibel et al., 1996
No association with larger populations of cluster headache patients	Cortelli et al., 1995
VACTERL (vertebral, anal, cardiovascular, tracheo-oesophageal, renal, limb defects)	Damian et al., 1996
Failure to thrive, developmental delay	Koo et al., 1993
Failure to thrive, developmental delay, microcephaly, seizures, lactic acidosis, pancreatitis	Kishnani et al., 1996
Demyelinating polyneuropathy	Rusanen et al., 1995; King et al., 1996
Peripheral neuropathy, rhabdomyolysis, severe lactic acidosis	Hara et al., 1994a
Subacute dementia, cerebral atrophy, myoclonus, periodic synchronous discharge (EEG) (Creutzfeldt–Jakob-like presentation)	Isozumi et al., 1994
Parkinsonism, dementia, vertical supranuclear ophthalmoplegia, deafness	Hara et al., 1994a
Ataxia, vertical supranuclear ophthalmoplegia, deafness	Hara et al., 1994b
Chronic asthma, depression	Shanske et al., 1993
Analysis of fetus	Matthews et al., 1994
Point mutation in tRNA$^{Leu(UUR)}$ (A3243T)	
Mitochondrial encephalomyopathy	Shaag et al., 1997
Point mutation in tRNA$^{Leu(UUR)}$ (A3271C)	
MELAS	Goto et al., 1991
Diabetes mellitus	Tsukuda et al., 1997
Point mutation in tRNA$^{Leu (UUR)}$ (3271 deletion)	
Mitochondrial encephalomyopathy with severe intracerebral calcifications (Fahr disease variant)	Shoffner et al., 1995
Point mutation in tRNA^{Lys} (A8344G)	
MERRF	Seibel et al., 1990; Shoffner et al., 1990; Yoneda et al., 1990
MERRF, pigmentary retinal degeneration	Isashiki et al., 1998
MERRF, bilateral optic atrophy	Isashiki et al., 1994
MERRF, overwhelming lactic acidosis	Sanger and Jain, 1996
MERRF, multiple symmetrical lipomatosis with clonal chromosome 6 deletion in lipomas	Larsson et al., 1995
MERRF, dizygotic twins	Penisson-Besnier et al., 1992

Table 29.1. (*cont.*)

Phenotypes	References
Late-onset MERRF (63 years)	Nomura et al., 1993
Mitochondrial myopathy	Graf et al., 1993; Silvestri et al., 1993
Mitochondrial myopathy, sensory neuropathy	Graf et al., 1993
Cardiomyopathy	Ozawa et al., 1995
Rapid-onset dementia	Ozawa et al., 1995
Ekbom syndrome (photomyoclonus, cerebellar ataxia, cervical lipoma)	Calabresi et al., 1994; Traff et al., 1995
Multiple symmetric lipomatosis	Holme et al., 1993; Klopstock et al., 1997; Naumann et al., 1997
Truncal lipomas, myopathy	Silvestri et al., 1993
Leigh disease, dystonia	Huang et al., 1995
Leigh disease	Hammans et al., 1993; Nakase, 1993; Silvestri et al., 1993; Sweeney et al., 1994
MELAS	Hammans et al., 1993
Chronic progressive external ophthalmoplegia	Hammans et al., 1993
Chronic progressive external ophthalmoplegia, lipoma, mitochondrial myopathy	Suomalainen et al., 1992
Spinocerebellar degeneration	Howell et al., 1996
Atypical Charcot–Marie–Tooth disease	Howell et al., 1996
Diabetes mellitus	Suzuki, 1994; Suzuki et al., 1994
Late-onset dementia, seizures, myopathy	Nomura et al., 1993
Point mutation in tRNA^{Lys} (T8356G)	
MERRF/MELAS overlap	Silvestri et al., 1992; Zeviani et al., 1993
MERRF	Masucci et al., 1995
Point mutation in ATP6 (T8993G)	
Leigh disease (sporadic or maternally transmitted)	Sakuta et al., 1992; Shoffner et al., 1992; Tatuch et al., 1992
Leigh disease, hypertrophic cardiomyopathy	Pastores et al., 1994
Leigh disease, ragged-red fibres	Mak et al., 1996
Neuropathy, ataxia, retinitis pigmentosa (NARP)	Holt et al., 1990; Tatuch and Robinson, 1993
NARP, prenatal diagnosis	Harding et al., 1992
Retinitis pigmentosa, ataxia, mental retardation	Puddu et al., 1993
Severe infantile lactic acidosis, encephalopathy	Houstek et al., 1995
Kearns–Sayre syndrome	Santorelli et al., 1997
Mental retardation, ataxia	de Coo et al., 1996
Mental retardation, ataxia, retinitis pigmentosa	Puddu et al., 1993
Nonspecific developmental delay	Fryer et al., 1994
Cerebral palsy	Fryer et al., 1994
Lactic acidosis	Klement et al., 1994
Point mutation in ATP6 (T8993C)	
Leigh disease	de Vries et al., 1993; Santorelli et al., 1994

struggling that occurs in some children during venipuncture and delays in sample processing. In order to enhance the accuracy of lactate, pyruvate and amino acid analysis as well as our ability to compare serial determinations reliably, the blood is collected as a morning sample after an overnight fast.

Skeletal muscle pathology in OXPHOS diseases

Most patients who are suspected of having an OXPHOS disease will require a muscle biopsy. The primary goals of the muscle biopsy are (i) to assess the muscle for other diseases; (ii) to isolate mitochondria for biochemical testing; (iii) to isolate DNA for testing; (iv) to look for pathological

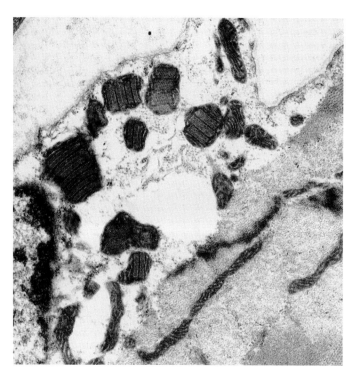

Fig. 29.3. Electron microscopy of mitochondrial paracrystalline inclusions. These condensations of the mitochondrial isoform of creatine kinase between the inner and outer mitochondrial membranes are present in skeletal muscle and are important clues to the presence of a mitochondrial disease. Paracrystalline inclusions often indicate that a mitochondrial DNA mutation is present in the patient, particularly one that impairs mitochondrial protein synthesis.

changes in the muscle, such as fibrosis and inflammation that would produce secondary abnormalities in the muscle biochemistry; and (v) to search for histochemical and ultrastructural changes that support the presence of an OXPHOS disease.

There are only a few histochemical changes that are predictive of the presence of an OXPHOS disease: ragged-red fibres, abnormal succinate dehydrogenase reactions and COX-deficient fibres (Fig. 29.2, colour plate). Ragged-red fibres are characterized by large proliferations of subsarcolemmal mitochondria and replacement of some of the contractile elements with intermyofibrillar accumulations of mitochondria. These appear red as detected by Gomori–Trichrome staining (Engel and Cunningham, 1963) and have a moth-eaten appearance because of the loss of some of the contracile elements. The percentage of ragged-red fibres shows large interindividual variability, ranging from approximately 2% to 70% of the total fibres. Ragged-red

fibres also have mild accumulations of glycogen and neutral lipid. Pathological alterations are segmental and do not extend the length of the myofibre, thus emphasizing the heterogeneous nature of the skeletal muscle manifestations (Yamamoto and Nonaka, 1988; Shoubridge et al., 1990). The abnormal myofibre segments can have sharp boundaries as in Kearns–Sayre and chronic progressive external ophthalmoplegia (CPEO) syndromes or be somewhat diffuse. Ragged-red fibres usually show increased reactivity for succinate dehydrogenase (which is a more sensitive indicator of mitochondrial proliferation than the Gomori–trichrome stain) and a decreased activity for COX reaction (COX-negative or COX-deficient fibres). Frequently, the number of COX-negative or COX-deficient fibres is larger than the number of ragged-red fibres, suggesting that the biochemical abnormality is a prerequisite for the morphological abnormality. These changes are observed in a wide variety of OXPHOS diseases including mtDNA depletion, mtDNA deletions and mitochondrial tRNA mutations. The mutation in the mitochondrial gene for tRNA[Leucine(UUR)] (A3243G substitution) is an important exception to this pattern of histopathology. This mutation is the most common cause for mitochondrial encephalomyopathy, lactic acidosis, and stroke-like episodes (MELAS). In many patients, the ragged-red fibres may be COX deficient or show a positive COX reaction (Yamazaki et al., 1991; Hasegawa et al., 1992, 1993; Chikama et al., 1994; Mita et al., 1995). In addition, the blood vessels characteristically show an increased succinate dehydrogenase reaction (Yamazaki et al., 1991; Hasegawa et al., 1992, 1993; Chikama et al., 1994; Mita et al., 1995). It is important to note that COX-deficient fibres, increased succinate dehydrogenase reaction and ragged-red fibres may be observed in a variety of conditions including normal ageing, zidovudine myopathy, myotonic dystrophy, limb girdle dystrophy, inclusion body myositis, inflammatory myopathies and nemaline myopathy (Muller-Hocker, 1989, 1990; Yamamoto et al., 1989; Oldfors et al., 1993, 1995; Santorelli et al., 1996b; Moslemi et al., 1997; Schroder and Molnar, 1997; Horvath et al., 1998).

Ultrastructural analysis of the muscle may reveal structurally abnormal mitochondria with paracrystalline inclusions, which are intermembranous condensations of mitochondrial creatine kinase and possibly other mitochondrial proteins (Stadhouders et al., 1990) (Fig. 29.3). When this ultrastructural abnormality is found in conjunction with ragged-red fibres, increases in succinate dehydrogenase reactivity, and COX-deficient fibres, the presence of a mtDNA mutation that impairs mitochondrial protein synthesis, such as a mtDNA deletion, mtDNA depletion, or a mitochondrial tRNA point mutation, is suggested. This can be important in focusing the genetic testing.

Unfortunately, most patients with OXPHOS diseases do not show any of the above characteristic muscle changes. The muscle pathology may show neurogenic changes, internal nuclei, fibre splitting, myofibre hypertrophy or hypotrophy involving either type I or type II fibres, accumulations of lipid or mild increases in glycogen (Koo et al., 1993; Reichmann et al., 1993). In some individuals, the muscle histology may even be normal. Patients with OXPHOS defects (mtDNA or nuclear DNA) do not usually display dystrophic changes in muscle such as increased connective tissue or significant myonecrosis. This observation can be important in distinguishing patients with OXPHOS diseases from other classes of neuromuscular disease.

OXPHOS biochemistry

The presence of an OXPHOS disease can be confirmed by biochemical and genetic testing. When specific gene mutations are not suggested by the clinical examination, OXPHOS enzyme analysis in skeletal muscle mitochondria can be used to classify a disorder as an OXPHOS disease. In order to perform accurate assessments of this delicate enzyme system, immediate isolation of mitochondria from fresh muscle biopsies can be helpful. This approach avoids artifacts in OXPHOS enzyme analysis that can be associated with freezing the biopsy prior to mitochondrial isolation (Zheng et al., 1990). Although it is now possible to achieve a precise diagnosis of certain OXPHOS diseases by DNA analysis alone, OXPHOS enzymology is necessary in the majority of patients. To determine the specific activities of OXPHOS enzymes, complex I, complex III and complex IV assays are used to assess electron flow across single OXPHOS complexes and the complex I+III and complex II+III assays assess the movement of electrons between complexes (see Fig. 5.2, p. 82). The specificity of these assays is demonstrated by using specific respiratory inhibitors. The proper functioning of the reagents used in these assays can be ensured by performing each enzyme assay in mitochondria isolated from mouse or rat skeletal muscle in parallel with the patient assays.

Complex I deficiencies are commonly observed in patient samples; however, distinguishing between pathogenic defects and those produced by technical factors can be difficult. In order to assess complex I function, three different assays can be used. These employ different electron acceptors: (i) n-decyl coenzyme Q (CoQ) as the electron acceptor, (ii) CoQ_1 as the electron acceptor and (iii) the traditional complex I+III assay. The first two assays are the most specific for mitochondrial complex I activity, but CoQ reduction probably occurs at different sites owing to the more hydrophilic nature of CoQ_1 and the more lipophilic nature of n-decylCoQ. The complex I+III assays measures the rate of electron flow between complexes I and III. However, approximately 50% of the observed activity is nonmitochondrial and must be accounted for in the interpretation.

Because of the complexities associated with the measurement of respiratory chain enzyme activities, corroborative data can be sought by testing for abnormalities in skin fibroblast β-oxidation: β-oxidation of substrates like palmitate ($C_{16:0}$) and myristate ($C_{14:0}$) is often reduced in patients with OXPHOS defects. In patients evaluated at Children's Healthcare of Atlanta, β-oxidation was observed in about 24% of fibroblast cultures from patients who had skeletal muscle OXPHOS defects, most commonly complex I defects (unpublished observation). During the first step of β-oxidation, a double bond is added to the fatty acid, electrons are transferred to the electron transfer flavoprotein via reduced flavin adenine dinucleotide ($FADH_2$) and electrons are transferred to complex I via reduced nicotinamide adenine dinucleotide (NADH) (see Fig. 5.2, p. 82). OXPHOS defects, particularly those involving complex I, reduce the oxidation of palmitate and myristate to levels that are approximately 40–60% of the control mean. This contrasts with diseases like CPT deficiency and medium-chain acyldehydrogenase deficiency, which reduce the oxidation of these fatty acids to <10% and <20% of the control means, respectively. Long-chain fatty acid oxidation by the trifunctional protein is normal in patients who harbour OXPHOS defects.

Genetic testing of OXPHOS diseases

At the time of muscle biopsy, a small portion of the biopsy is frozen in liquid nitrogen for DNA isolation. The integrated clinical–genetic, metabolic and biochemical–genetic protocol increases the probability of reaching the correct biochemical and genetic diagnosis, which is necessary for accurate genetic counselling and effective patient management. Table 29.1 is designed to assist physicians in recognizing genotype and phenotype associations. It is important to remember that, although a large number of mtDNA mutations are known, most mutations are private or semi-private (i.e. occurring in relatively few families). If one of the known mtDNA mutations is not found in a proband then it can be useful to exclude a mtDNA mutation. This can be done with a comprehensive analysis of mtDNA by single-strand conformational polymorphism and DNA sequencing. If a cell line is available, cytoplasts derived from patient cells, can be fused to rho⁰ cells to test for rescue of the biochemical phenotype. Transfer of the biochemical defect would suggest a mtDNA mutation, while rescue of the phenotype would suggest a nuclear gene defect.

Mitochondrial DNA mutations: frequently encountered OXPHOS diseases

Three classes of pathogenic mtDNA mutation exist: (i) mtDNA rearrangements in which mtDNA genes are deleted or duplicated, (ii) mtDNA point mutations in genes for tRNA or rRNA resulting in defects in mitochondrial protein synthesis, and (iii) missense mutations that change an amino acid, thus altering a critical function of an OXPHOS polypeptide. A comprehensive review of OXPHOS diseases and mtDNA mutations is presented by Shoffner and Wallace (1995). The OXPHOS diseases known to be caused by nuclear DNA mutations are inherited in an autosomal dominant or autosomal recessive pattern. A brief synopsis of the most important OXPHOS diseases with neuromuscular involvement is given below.

Kearns–Sayre and chronic progressive external ophthalmoplegia syndromes

Ptosis, ophthalmoplegia and a ragged-red fibre myopathy represent a clinical triad that is highly predictive for the presence of a mtDNA mutation. Patients with these manifestations can be classified into one of three groups according to their age of onset and the severity of their clinical symptoms. The most severe variant is the Kearns–Sayre syndrome, which is characterized by infantile, childhood or adolescent onset of disease manifestations and significant multisystem involvement, which can include cardiac abnormalities (cardiomyopathies and cardiac conduction defects), diabetes mellitus, cerebellar ataxia, deafness and evidence of multifocal neurodegeneration. Some patients will present in infancy with an atypical variant called Pearson syndrome. These individuals manifest anaemia, leukopenia and thrombocytopenia, resulting in a need for frequent transfusions. Exocrine pancreas dysfunction is an important manifestation of this disease. Patients with Pearson syndrome may have severe systemic manifestations or may be oligosymptomatic. However, if patients survive infancy and early childhood, Kearns–Sayre syndrome develops.

CPEO plus refers to a disorder of intermediate severity that has an adolescent or adult onset and variable involvement of tissues other than the eyelids and eye muscles. The mildest variant is isolated CPEO, in which clinical signs and symptoms develop during adulthood and are limited to the eyelids and eye muscles. In each of these classification groups, patients worsen with age. Individuals who are initially classified as isolated CPEO can progress to CPEO plus, and patients with Kearns–Sayre syndrome often develop more severe multisystem involvement.

The most common cause for Kearns–Sayre and CPEO syndromes is a rearrangement of mtDNA, either a large-scale deletion or a partial duplication (Holt et al., 1988a; Poulton et al., 1989a,b, 1993). The mtDNA deletion mutation has the simplest structure, consisting of a mtDNA molecule that is missing contiguous tRNA and protein-coding genes, thus yielding a mtDNA molecule that is smaller than the normal 16.6 kb mtDNA. The structurally more complex mtDNA duplication mutation produces a mtDNA molecule that is larger than the normal mtDNA and contains two tandemly arranged mtDNA molecules consisting of a full length 16.6 kb mtDNA coupled to a mtDNA deletion (Poulton et al., 1989a,b, 1993). Leukocytes and platelets containing mtDNA rearrangements tend to be lost from the circulation. By contrast, there is evidence for an accumulation of mtDNA deletions in skeletal muscle (Larsson et al., 1990). Assessment for mtDNA deletions in blood samples is probably the most common mistake made by physicians when requesting mtDNA genetic testing. In most cases, the analysis is uninformative. Skeletal muscle is nearly always necessary for detection of large-scale mtDNA rearrangements.

Approximately 80% of patients with Kearns–Sayre syndrome, 70% with CPEO plus, and 40% with CPEO harbour mtDNA rearrangements (Holt et al., 1989; Moraes et al., 1989). In most patients with mtDNA rearrangements, the mutation was not inherited but appears to be a spontaneous event that occurred during oogenesis or very early embryogenesis. Because of replicative segregation of mutant and wild-type mtDNAs, the identification of maternal inheritance of a mtDNA rearrangement by clinical criteria can be difficult and often requires analysis of skeletal muscle mtDNA from maternal lineage relatives of the proband. Of the two classes of mtDNA rearrangement, the mtDNA duplication mutation has the greatest probability of being maternally transmitted. Point mutations in mitochondrial genes for tRNA, which are usually maternally inherited, are also an important cause for Kearns–Sayre and CPEO syndromes. Characterization of the mtDNA mutation in a patient with either Kearns–Sayre or CPEO syndrome is important for genetic counselling of the patient and family members.

Myoclonic epilepsy and ragged-red fibre disease

Myoclonic epilepsy and ragged-red fibre disease (MERRF) can begin at any age, ranging from late childhood to adulthood. The clinical features that are most predictive for a diagnosis of MERRF are epilepsy (myoclonic epilepsy, generalized seizures or focal seizures), cerebellar ataxia and a ragged-red fibre myopathy. Other manifestations include dementia, corticospinal tract degeneration, peripheral neuropathy, optic atrophy, deafness, proximal renal tubule dysfunction, cardiomyopathy and lactic acidaemia plus hyperalaninaemia. Myoclonic jerks occur at rest and increase in frequency and amplitude with movement. The myoclonus in patients with MERRF is best categorized as cortical reflex myoclonus and can be associated with epileptiform discharges and photic sensitivity, with large amplitude occipital wave forms detected by electroencephalography as well as giant cortical somatosensory evoked responses (Rosing et al., 1985; Wallace et al., 1988; Thompson et al., 1994). As many as 80–90% of patients with MERRF have an A-to-G substitution resulting from a change in a conserved nucleotide affecting the TψC loop of the tRNA^{Lysine} at position 8344 of the mtDNA (A8344G) (Shoffner et al., 1990). A small percentage of patients with MERRF harbour a T-to-C mutation at position 8356 of the mtDNA (Silvestri et al., 1992; Zeviani et al., 1993).

Mitochondrial encephalomyopathy, lactic acidosis, and stroke-like episodes

Disease manifestations in patients with MELAS can appear at essentially any age. Patients are generally below 45 years of age and are characterized as 'stroke in the young'. They present with a large or small vessel stroke that can be associated with a migraine headache and/or seizures. Delineating this presentation from the long list of other causes of stroke in the young can be difficult and is assisted by recognizing myopathy, ataxia, cardiomyopathy, diabetes mellitus, retinitis pigmentosa, proximal renal tubule defects, or lactic acidaemia and hyperalaninaemia. Since these systemic manifestations are not present in all patients, biochemical and genetic studies are essential in establishing the diagnosis. Cerebellar ataxia is often observed in patients with MELAS and may precede the development of stroke by many years. However, careful patient evaluation usually reveals manifestations in other organs, thus distinguishing these patients from those with other classes of cerebellar ataxia.

An A-to-G mutation in the gene for tRNA$^{Leucine(UUR)}$ (A3243G) accounts for approximately 80% of the MELAS cases. A mutation at position 8356 of the gene for tRNA^{Lysine} has been associated with features of both MERRF and MELAS (Zeviani et al., 1993). An important feature of the A3243G mutation (van den Ouweland et al., 1994) as well as some mtDNA rearrangements (Ballinger et al., 1994a) is that they significantly increase the risk of developing diabetes mellitus. As many as 1% of randomly selected patients with adult-onset diabetes mellitus may harbour the A3243G mutation (Otabe et al., 1994). OXPHOS diseases are important considerations in the differential diagnosis of patients with diabetes mellitus and stroke. The A3243G mutation is an important cause for Kearns–Sayre and CPEO syndromes and should be considered in the differential diagnosis of these disorders. The identification of this mutation is important in these patients since it is maternally inherited and is associated with a greater risk of stroke than the mtDNA rearrangements.

Leigh syndrome and cerebellar ataxia plus pigmentary retinopathy syndromes

Leigh syndrome or subacute necrotizing encephalopathy is suspected when cranial nerve abnormalities, respiratory dysfunction and ataxia are observed in conjunction with bilateral hyperintense signals on T$_2$-weighted magnetic resonance images in the basal ganglia, cerebellum or brainstem. The age of onset for disease manifestations is usually during infancy or early childhood. Two mtDNA mutations, a T-to-G (Shoffner et al., 1992; Tatuch et al., 1992) (T8993G) or a T-to-C (Santorelli et al., 1994) substitution in the ATPase 6 gene at position 8993 (T8993C) are important causes for Leigh disease. The T8993G mutation is the most frequently encountered of the two and changes an evolutionarily conserved leucine to an arginine in the proton channel of the ATPase 6 polypeptide, impairing ATP synthesis (Tatuch et al., 1994; Trounce et al., 1994). The T8993G mutation is the most frequently encountered of these two mutations and was originally identified in patients with retinitis pigmentosa plus cerebellar ataxia syndromes (Holt et al., 1990).

The T8993G mutation acts in a recessive manner. Patients generally have no manifestations when the levels of the mutation in tissues is less than approximately 60–70% of the total mtDNA. Patients that harbour approximately 70–90% mutant mtDNAs in their tissues have highly variable disease manifestations. In mildly affected individuals, a pigmentary retinopathy can be the only clinical manifestation. In more severely affected individuals, cerebellar ataxia and retinitis pigmentosa are commonly observed together. Brain imaging of these patients can show isolated cerebellar atrophy or more extensive cerebellar and brainstem involvement with olivopontocerebellar atrophy. Additional manifestations that can be observed are hypertrophic cardiomyopathy, sensory and motor neuropathies, muscle weakness and elevated lactate or alanine levels in blood or urine. Aproximately 7% to 20% of patients with Leigh disease harbour the T8993G mutation (Shoffner et al., 1992; Santorelli et al., 1993; Tatuch et al., 1994; Trounce et al., 1994).

Nuclear DNA mutations and OXPHOS disease

Mitochondrial DNA depletion diseases

MtDNA depletion diseases are an important group of disorders affecting infants and neonates in which a quantitative reduction in mtDNA copy number exists within various tissues (Boustany et al., 1983; Moraes et al., 1991a; Figarella-Branger et al., 1992; Telerman-Toppet et al., 1992; Tritschler et al., 1992). Patients have variable combinations of mitochondrial myopathy with COX-negative fibres, hypotonia, hepatopathy, progressive external ophthalmoplegia and severe lactic acidosis. The diagnosis is made using quantitative Southern blot analysis, which demonstrates that the copy number of the mtDNA is greatly reduced in affected tissues. Interestingly, the unaffected tissues of some patients may show normal levels of mtDNA. The disorder appears to be transmitted in an autosomal recessive fashion in most cases.

Kearns–Sayre and chronic progressive external ophthalmoplegia syndromes

Kearns–Sayre and CPEO syndromes can be transmitted in an autosomal dominant or recessive fashion (McAuley, 1956; Berenberg et al., 1977; Barron et al., 1979; Bastiaensen et al., 1979; Zeviani et al., 1989). mtDNA analysis of affected individuals in these families revealed that each harbours an array of deleted mtDNAs (Zeviani et al., 1989). Clinical manifestations include ophthalmoplegia, proximal muscle weakness, sensorineural hearing loss and abnormal vestibular responses, tremor, ataxia and sensorimotor neuropathy (Zeviani, 1992). Although multiple mtDNA deletions accumulate in various tissues of some patients, clinical manifestations within the same pedigree are often highly variable, ranging from individuals with severe manifestations to individuals who are asymptomatic. In one family with this disorder, the male proband exhibited the manifestations of Kearns–Sayre syndrome

and Leigh disease (Cormier et al., 1991). Elevations in blood lactate, a ragged-red fibre myopathy and OXPHOS defects primarily affecting complexes I and IV occur. The biochemical abnormalities are typical of mutations that cause defects in mitochondrial protein synthesis. The mtDNA deletions are best detected in skeletal muscle biopsies (Zeviani et al., 1989). These mutations are generally absent in populations of rapidly dividing cells such as cultured fibroblasts, peripheral blood cells, cultured myoblasts (Servidei et al., 1991), myotubes, or in vitro innervated muscle cells (Zeviani, 1992). Autosomal dominant forms of the disease map to chromosome 10q23.3–24.3 (Suomalainen et al., 1995) and chromosome 3p14.1–21.2 (Kaukonen et al., 1996).

Myoneurogastrointestinal disorder and encephalopathy

Myoneurogastrointestinal disorder and encephalopathy (MNGIE) is an autosomal recessive disorder characterized by a progressive external ophthalmoplegia, dementia with a progressive leukodystrophy, mitochondrial myopathy, peripheral neuropathy, and prominent involvement of the gastrointestinal tract (Ionasescu, 1983; Ionasescu et al., 1983, 1984; Bardosi et al., 1987; Blake et al., 1990; Simon et al., 1990; Rowland, 1992). The gastrointestinal manifestations are heralded by significant diarrhoea, malabsorption and weight loss with normal pancreatic function. Radiological investigations may show marked thickening of the small intestines, which reflects the pathological findings of extensive mural thickening and fibrosis of the submucosa and subserosa. Lactate may be elevated along with other tricarboxylic acid cycle intermediates. This disorder is linked to chromosome 22q13.32-qter (Hirano et al., 1998). Recent investigations demonstrated that this disorder is caused by loss-of-function mutations in the gene for thymidine phosphorylase (Nishino et al., 1999). Thymidine phosphorylase converts thymidine to 2-deoxy-D-ribose 1-phosphate and may function to regulate thymidine availability for DNA synthesis. Thymidine phosphorylase is widely expressed in human tissues. Interestingly, this enzyme is apparently not expressed in skeletal muscle, even though disease manifestations are identifiable in this tissue. At this time, the mechanism for disease expression in skeletal muscle is unknown.

Wolfram syndrome

Wolfram syndrome is characterized by diabetes insipidus, insulin-dependent diabetes mellitus, optic atrophy and deafness. In a small percentage of patients, multiple mtDNA deletions are observed in tissues of these individuals. Muscle biopsy may reveal COX-deficient fibres and ragged-red fibres. This autosomal recessive disorder is linked to chromosome 4p16 (Barrientos et al., 1996a,b; Barrientos et al., 1996).

Leigh syndrome

Leigh syndrome can be caused by defects in aerobic energy metabolism including pyruvate dehydrogenase (Stansbie et al., 1986), however, OXPHOS defects (complex I and IV) are the most commonly identified biochemical abnormality in this group of patients (DiMauro et al., 1987; Robinson et al., 1987; Morris et al., 1996; Rahman et al., 1996). All nuclear OXPHOS gene mutations reported are transmitted in an autosomal recessive fashion.

Four mutations in genes encoding nuclear-encoded respiratory chain subunits have been identified in patients with Leigh syndrome. One is in the gene coding for the flavoprotein subunit of complex II (Bourgeron et al., 1995). The other three mutations groups involve complex I subunits. One is a mutation affecting the 18 kDa (AQDQ) complex I subunit, which maps to chromosome 5 (van den Heuvel et al., 1998), the second affects the NDUSF9 (TYKY) subunit (Loeffen et al., 1998) and the third the 51 kDa subunit (NDUFV1) (Schuelke, et al., 1999). A patient with the complex I mutated 18 kDa subunit showed normal organic and amino acids, skeletal muscle light microscopy and electron microscopy. The complex I defect was present in both skeletal muscle and in fibroblasts. This patient provides genetic confirmation for the common observation that complex I defects generally do not produce detectable metabolic abnormalities. Additional phenotypic heterogeneity was observed with the mutations affecting the 51 kDa subunit. One individual was diagnosed as having Alexander disease, which is characterized by megalencephaly with progressive spasticity and dementia (Schuelke et al., 1999).

Although complex IV defects are frequently observed, mutations affecting the nuclear-encoded subunits of complex IV were not found in patients with Leigh syndrome (Adams et al., 1997). Three complementation groups appear to encompass the majority of these patients (Brown and Brown, 1996). In one complementation group, mutations in a highly evolutionarily conserved gene, *SURF1* (chromosome 9q34) were found to be the cause of systemic COX (complex IV) deficiency (Tiranti et al., 1998; Zhu et al., 1998). All of these patients had Leigh syndrome with early-onset hypotonia, ataxia, brainstem abnormalities, regression and the characteristic bilateral basal ganglia lesions. *SURF1* appears to be essential for complex IV assembly. Mutations in *SURF1* are heterogeneous consisting of small deletions and insertions, nonsense mutations and donor-splice site mutants; most patients are compound heterozygotes. All reported mutations are loss-of-function and predict a truncated protein product. Functional complementation, which was used to discover this gene defect in these patients, promises to be a powerful tool in uncovering novel mechanisms for OXPHOS disease pathogenesis.

A group of patients with Leigh syndrome, referred to as the Saguenay Lac-Saint-Jean type, shows complex IV deficiency (Merante et al., 1993; Morin et al., 1993; Heyer, 1995; Lee et al., 1998). Although phenotypically similar to the patients harbouring mutations in *SURF1*, this recessively transmitted disorder maps to chromosome 2. Whereas, the complex IV defect in the group with *SURF1* mutations is systemic, the Saguenay Lac-Saint-Jean group has 50% activity in muscle, fibroblasts and amniocytes; less than 10% activity in brain and liver; and normal activity in kidney and heart.

Hereditary spastic paraplegia with ragged-red fibre myopathy

An autosomal recessive form of spastic paraparesis was identified at chromosome 16q24.3 (de Michele et al., 1998). Patients experience progressive weakness, spasticity mild decreases in vibratory sensation as their major manifestations, and they have ragged-red, COX-deficient fibres in their skeletal muscle. Dysphagia, scoliosis and optic nerve atrophy have also occurred. This unique form of hereditary spastic paraplegia is caused by mutations in the gene called *paraplegin*, which is localized to the mitochondria (Casari et al., 1998). Paraplegin has a high degree of homology with a subclass of ATPases belonging to the AAA family. These ATPases are metalloproteases with both proteolytic and chaperonin functions, suggesting that paraplegin plays a role in the assembly and maintenance of the respiratory chain enzyme complexes.

Friedreich ataxia

Friedreich ataxia was recently discovered to be a mitochondrial disease. Clinical manifestations are systemic and include hypoactive or absent deep tendon reflexes, ataxia, corticospinal tract dysfunction, impaired vibratory and proprioceptive function, hypertrophic cardiomyopathy and diabetes mellitus. This autosomal recessive disorder was mapped to chromosome 9q13. This disease is caused by a GAA trinucleotide repeat expansion in the first intron of the gene frataxin (Campuzano et al., 1996).

Frataxin is a mitochondrial protein (Koutnikova, Campuzano, et al., 1997) that is involved in iron homeostasis. Mutations in *frataxin* result in impaired activity of the iron–sulphur containing enzymes within the mitochondria: complex I, complex II, complex III and aconitase (Rotig et al., 1997).

Summary

Physicians in all specialties are becoming increasingly aware of OXPHOS diseases. Although the prevalence of OXPHOS diseases in the general population is unknown, the number of requests for paedriatic and adult evaluations are increasing rapidly. A basic awareness of OXPHOS disease phenotypes as well as of the essential elements of patient evaluation are important for appropriate patient management and referrals. Centres that specialize in OXPHOS disease evaluations can be instrumental in working with referring physicians to develop a diagnostic plan that suits each individual patient's needs. After a complete evaluation, genetic counselling based on Mendelian or mtDNA principles of inheritance can be applied. Although approaches that assess patients for mtDNA mutations are evolving rapidly, significant ambiguity in diagnosis often remains even after detailed testing is complete. Advances in our understanding of mutations in nuclear genes for OXPHOS functions will provide a powerful addition to our ability to diagnose, manage and counsel patients with these disorders.

Acknowledgements

This work was supported by an NIH grant NS33999 and a grant from the United Mitochondrial Disease Association awarded to J. M. S.

References

Abramowicz, M. J., Cochaux, P., Cohen, L. H.and Vamos, E. (1996). Pernicious anaemia and hypoparathyroidism in a patient with Kearns–Sayre syndrome with mitochondrial DNA duplication. *J. Inher. Metab. Dis.* **19** (2), 109–111.

Adams, P. L., Lightowlers, R. N. and Turnbull, D. M. (1997). Molecular analysis of cytochrome c oxidase deficiency in Leigh's syndrome. *Ann. Neurol.* **41**, 268–270.

Akaike, M., Kawai, H., Kashiwagi, S., Kunishige, M. and Saito, S. (1995). A case of Kearns–Sayre syndrome whose asymptomatic mother had abnormal mitochondria in skeletal muscle. *Rinsho Shinkeigaku* **35**, 190–194.

Andreetta, F., Tritschler, H. J., Schon, E. A., DiMauro, S.and Bonilla, E. (1991). Localization of mitochondrial DNA in normal and pathological muscle using immunological probes: a new approach to the study of mitochondrial myopathies. *J. Neurol. Sci.* **105**, 88–92.

Arai, M. and Ohshima, S. (1997). Maternally inherited diabetes and deafness with cerebellar ataxia: a new clinical phenotype associated with the mitochondrial DNA 3243 mutation. [Letter] *J. Neurol.* **244**, 468–469.

Ballinger, S. W., Shoffner, J. M., Hedaya, E. V. et al. (1992). Maternally transmitted diabetes and deafness associated with a 10.4kb. *Nat. Genet.* **1**, 11–15.

Ballinger, S. W., Shoffner, J. M., Gebhart, S., Koontz, D. A. and Wallace, D. C. (1994). Mitochondrial diabetes revisited. *Nat. Genet.* **7**, 458–459.

Bardosi, A., Creutzfeldt, W., DiMauro, S. et al. (1987). Myo-, neuro-, gastrointestinal encephalomyopathy (MNGIE syndrome) due to partial deficiency of cytochrome c oxidase. A new mitochondrial multisystem disorder. *Acta Neuropathol.* **74**, 248–258.

Barrientos, A., Casademont, J., Saiz, A. et al. (1996a). Autosomal recessive Wolfram syndrome associated with an 8.5-kb mtDNA single deletion. *Am. J. Hum. Genet.* **58**, 963–970.

Barrientos, A., Volpini, V., Casademont, J. et al. (1996b). A nuclear defect in the 4p16 region predisposes to multiple mitochondrial DNA deletions in families with Wolfram syndrome. *J. Clin. Invest.* **97**, 1570–1576.

Barrientos, A., Casademont, J., Genis, D. et al. (1997). Sporadic heteroplasmic single 5.5kb mitochondrial DNA deletion associated with cerebellar ataxia, hypogonadotropic hypogonadism, choroidal dystrophy and mitochondrial respiratory chain complex I deficiency. *Hum. Mutat.* **10**, 212–216.

Barron, S. A., Heffner, R. R. J. and Zwirecki, R. (1979). A familial mitochondrial myopathy with central defect in neural transmission. *Arch. Neurol.* **36**, 553–556.

Bastiaensen, L. A., Jaspar, H. H. J. and Stadhouders, A. M. (1979). Ophthalmoplegia-plus. *Doc. Ophthalmol.* **46**, 365–380.

Berenberg, R. A., Pellock, J. M., DiMauro, S. et al. (1977). Lumping or splitting? 'Ophthalmoplegia-plus' or 'Kearns–Sayre syndrome'. *Ann. Neurol.* **1**, 37–54.

Bernes, S. M., Bacino, C., Prezant, T. R. et al. (1993). Identical mitochondrial DNA deletion in mother with progressive external ophthalmoplegia and son with Pearson marrow-pancreas syndrome. *J. Pediatr.* **123**, 598–602.

Blake, D., Lombes, A. and Minetti, C. (1990). MNGIE syndrome: report of 2 new patients. *Neurology*, **40**(Suppl. 1), 294.

Blok, R. B., Thorburn, D. R., Danks, D. M. and Dahl, H. H. (1995). mtDNA deletion in a patient with symptoms of mitochondrial cytopathy but without ragged red fibers. *Biochem. Mol. Med.* **56**, 26–30.

Bonte, C., Leys, A., Matthijs, G. and Missotten, L. (1996). Fundus changes in patients with the mitochondrial DNA point mutation at position 3243. *Bull. Soc. Belge Ophtalmol.* **261**, 9–12.

Bourgeron, T., Rustin, P., Chretien, D. et al. (1995). Mutation of a nuclear succinate dehydrogenase gene results in mitochondrial respiratory chain deficiency. *Nat. Genet.* **11**, 144–149.

Boustany, R. N., Aprille, J. R., Halperin, J., Levy, H.and DeLong, G. R. (1983). Mitochondrial cytochrome deficiency presenting as a myopathy with hypotonia, external ophthalmoplegia and lactic acidosis in an infant and as fatal hepatopathy in a second cousin. *Ann. Neurol.* **14**, 462–470.

Bowen, J., Richards, T. and Maravilla, K. (1998). MR imaging and proton MR spectroscopy in A-to-G substitution at nucleotide position 3243 of leucine transfer RNA. *Am. J. Neuroradiol.* **19**, 231–234.

Bresolin, N., Martinelli, P., Barbiroli, B. et al. (1991). Muscle mitochondrial DNA deletion and 31P-NMR spectroscopy alterations in a migraine patient. *J. Neurol. Sci.* **104**, 182–189.

Brown, R. M.and Brown, G. K. (1996). Complementation analysis of systemic cytochrome oxidase deficiency presenting as Leigh syndrome. *J. Inherit. Metab. Dis.* **19**, 752–760.

Bruno, C., Minetti, C., Tang, Y. et al. (1998). Primary adrenal insufficiency in a child with a mitochondrial DNA deletion. *J. Inherit. Metab. Dis.* **21**, 155–161.

Calabresi, P. A., Silvestri, G., DiMauro, S. and Griggs, R. C. (1994). Ekbom's syndrome: lipomas, ataxia and neuropathy with MERRF. *Muscle Nerve* **17**, 943–945.

Campos, Y., Bautista, J., Gutierrez-Rivas, E. et al. (1995a). Clinical heterogeneity in two pedigrees with the 3243 bp tRNA(Leu(UUR)) mutation of mitochondrial DNA. *Acta Neurol. Scand.* **91**, 62–65.

Campos, Y., Garcia-Silva, T., Barrionuevo, C. R., Cabello, A., Muley, R. and Arenas, J. (1995b). Mitochondrial DNA deletion in a patient with mitochondrial myopathy, lactic acidosis and stroke-like episodes (MELAS) and Fanconi's syndrome. *Pediatr. Neurol.* **13** (1), 69–72.

Campos, Y., Martin, M. A., Lorenzo, G., Aparicio, M., Cabello, A. and Arenas, J. (1996a). Sporadic MERRF/MELAS overlap syndrome associated with the 3243 tRNA(Leu(UUR)) mutation of mitochondrial DNA. *Muscle Nerve* **19**, 187–190.

Campos, Y., Martin, M. A., Navarro, C., Gordo, P. and Arenas, J. (1996b). Single large-scale mitochondrial DNA deletion in a patient with mitochondrial myopathy associated with multiple symmetric lipomatosis. *Neurology* **47**, 1012–1014.

Campuzano, V., Montermini, L., Molto, M. D. et al. (1996). Friedreich's ataxia: autosomal recessive disease caused by an intronic GAA triplet repeat expansion. *Science* **271**, 1423–1427.

Casari, G., De Fusco, M., Ciarmatori, S. et al. (1998). Spastic paraplegia and OXPHOS impairment caused by mutations in paraplegin, a nuclear encoded mitochondrial metalloprotease. *Cell* **93**, 973–983.

Chang, T. S., Johns, D. R., Walker, D., de la Cruz, Z., Maumence, I. H. and Green, W. R. (1993). Ocular clinicopathologic study of the mitochondrial encephalomyopathy overlap syndromes. *Arch. Ophthalmol.* **111**, 1254–1262.

Chang, T. S., Johns, D. R., Stark, W. J., Drachman, D. B. and Green, W. R. (1994). Corneal decompensation in mitochondrial ophthalmoplegia plus (Kearns–Sayre) syndrome. A clinicopathologic case report. *Cornea* **13**, 269–273.

Chen, R. S., Huang, C. C., Lee, C. C. et al. (1993). Overlapping syndrome of MERRF and MELAS: molecular and neuroradiological studies. *Acta Neurol. Scand.* **87**, 494–498.

Chikama, M., Himoto, Y. and Nonaka, I. (1994). Mitochondrial myopathy, encephalopathy, lactic acidosis and stroke-like episodes with delayed and decreased cerebral blood flow on cerebral angiography – a case report. *Rinsho Shinkeigaku* **34**, 167–169.

Chuang, L. M., Wu, H. P., Chiu, K. C., Lai, C. S., Tai, T. Y. and Lin, B. J. (1995). Mitochondrial gene mutations in familial non-insulin-dependent diabetes mellitus in Taiwan. *Clin. Genet.* **48**, 251–254.

Clayton, D. A. (1982). Replication of animal mitochondrial DNA. *Cell* **28**, 693–705.

Cormier, V., Rotig, A., Tardieu, M., Colonna, M., Saudubray, J. M. and Munnich, A. (1991). Autosomal dominant deletions of the mitochondrial genome in a case of progressive encephalomyopathy. *Am. J. Hum. Genet.* **48**, 643–648.

Cormier-Daire, V., Bonnefont, J. P., Rustin, P. et al. (1994). Mitochondrial DNA rearrangements with onset as chronic diarrhea with villous atrophy. *J. Pediatr.* **124**, 63–70.

Cortelli, P., Zacchini, A., Barboni, P., Malpassi, P., Carelli, V. and Montagna, P. (1995). Lack of association between mitochondrial tRNA(Leu(UUR)) point mutation and cluster headache. [Letter; comment] *Lancet* **345**, 1120–1121.

Crimmins, D., Morris, J. G., Walker, G. L. et al. (1993). Mitochondrial encephalomyopathy: variable clinical expression within a single kindred. *J. Neurol. Neurosurg. Psychiatry* **56**, 900–905.

Cristofari, M., Bertocchi, P. and Vigano, M. (1995). The MELAS syndrome and dilated-hypertrophic cardiomyopathy: a case report. [Not in English.] *G. Ital. Cardiol.* **25**, 69–76.

Cursiefen, C., Kuchle, M., Scheurlen, W. and Naumann, G. O. (1998). Bilateral zonular cataract associated with the mitochondrial cytopathy of Pearson syndrome. *Am. J. Ophthalmol.* **125**, 260–261.

Damian, M. S., Reichmann, H., Seibel, P., Bachmann, G., Schachenmayr, W. and Dorndorf, W. (1994). MELAS syndrome. Clinical aspects, MRI, biochemistry and molecular genetics. *Nervenarzt* **65**, 258–263.

Damian, M. S., Seibel, P., Reichmann, H. et al. (1995). Clinical spectrum of the MELAS mutation in a large pedigree. *Acta Neurol. Scand.* **92**, 409–415.

Damian, M. S., Seibel, P., Schachenmayr, W., Reichmann, H. and Dorndorf, W. (1996). VACTERL with the mitochondrial np 3243 point mutation. *Am. J. Med. Genet.* **62**, 398–403.

Damian, M. S., Hertel, A., Seibel, P. et al. (1998). Follow-up in carriers of the 'MELAS' mutation without strokes. *Eur. Neurol.* **39**, 9–15.

de Coo, I. F., Smeets, H. J., Gabreels, F. J., Arts, N. and van Oost, B. A. (1996). Isolated case of mental retardation and ataxia due to a de novo mitochondrial T8993G mutation. [Letter] *Am. J. Hum. Genet.* **58**, 636–638.

Degoul, F., Diry, M., Pou-Serradell, A., Lloreta, J.and Marsac, C. (1994). Myo-leukoencephalopathy in twins: study of 3243-myopathy, encephalopathy, lactic acidosis and strokelike episodes mitochondrial DNA mutation. *Ann. Neurol.* **35**, 365–370.

de Michele, G., de Fusco, M., Cavalcanti, F. et al. (1998). A new locus for autosomal recessive hereditary spastic paraplegia maps to chromosome 16q24.3. *Am. J. Hum. Genet.* **63**, 135–139.

de Vries, D. D., van Engelen, B. G., Gabreels, F. J., Ruitenbeek, W. and van Oost, B. A. (1993). A second missense mutation in the mitochondrial ATPase 6 gene in Leigh's syndrome. *Ann. Neurol.* **34**, 410–412.

DiMauro, S., Servidei, S., Zeviani, M. et al. (1987). Cytochrome c oxidase deficiency in Leigh syndrome. *Ann. Neurol.* **22**, 498–506.

Dougherty, F. E., Ernst, S. G. and Aprille, J. R. (1994). Familial recurrence of atypical symptoms in an extended pedigree with the syndrome of mitochondrial encephalomyopathy, lactic acidosis and stroke-like episodes (MELAS). *J. Pediatr.* **125**, 758–761.

Dunbar, D. R., Moonie, P. A., Swingler, R. J., Davidson, D., Roberts, R. and Holt, I. J. (1993). Maternally transmitted partial direct tandem duplication of mitochondrial DNA associated with diabetes mellitus. *Hum. Mol. Genet.* **2**, 1619–1624.

Engel, W. K. and Cunningham, G. G. (1963). Rapid examination of muscle tissue. An improved method for fresh-frozen biopsy sections. *Neurology* **13**, 919–923.

Ernster, L., Ikkos, D. and Luft, R. (1959). Enzyme activities of human skeletal muscle mitochondria: A tool in clinical metabolic research. *Nature* **184**, 1851.

Ewart, R. M. and Burrows, R. F. (1997). Pregnancy in chronic progressive external ophthalmoplegia: a case report. *Am. J. Perinatol.* **14**, 293–295.

Fabrizi, G. M., Cardaioli, E., Grieco, G. S. et al. (1996). The A to G transition at nt 3243 of the mitochondrial tRNALeu(UUR) may cause an MERRF syndrome. *J. Neurol. Neurosurg. Psychiatry* **61**, 47–51.

Fang, W., Huang, C. C., Lee, C. C., Cheng, S. Y., Pang, C. Y. and Wei, Y. H. (1993). Ophthalmologic manifestations in MELAS syndrome. *Arch. Neurol.* **50**, 977–980.

Feigenbaum, A., Chitayat, D., Robinson, B. et al. (1996). The expanding clinical phenotype of the tRNA(Leu(UUR)) A→G mutation at np 3243 of mitochondrial DNA: diabetic embryopathy associated with mitochondrial cytopathy. *Am. J. Med. Genet.* **62**, 404–409.

Figarella-Branger, D., Pellissier, J. F., Scheiner, C., Wernert, F. and Desnuelle, C. (1992). Defects of the mitochondrial respiratory chain complexes in three paediatric cases with hypotonia and cardiac involvement. *J. Neurol. Sci.* **108**, 105–113.

Folgero, T., Torbergsen, T. and Oian, P. (1995). The 3243 MELAS mutation in a pedigree with MERRF. *Eur. Neurol.* **35**, 168–171.

Fryer, A., Appleton, R., Sweeney, M. G., Rosenbloom, L. and Harding, A. E. (1994). Mitochondrial DNA 8993 (NARP) mutation presenting with a heterogeneous phenotype including 'cerebral palsy'. *Arch. Dis. Child.* **71**, 419–422.

Furuya, H., Sugimura, T., Yamada, T., Hayashi, K. and Kobayashi, T. (1997). A case of incomplete Kearns–Sayre syndrome with a stroke like episode. *Rinsho Shinkeigaku* **37**, 680–684.

Gebhart, S. S., Shoffner, J. M., Koontz, D., Kaufman, A. and Wallace, D. (1996). Insulin resistance associated with maternally inherited diabetes and deafness. *Metabolism* **45**, 526–531.

Gerbitz, K. D., Paprotta, A., Jaksch, M., Zierz, S. and Drechsel, J. (1993). Diabetes mellitus is one of the heterogeneous phenotypic features of a mitochondrial DNA point mutation within the tRNALeu(UUR) gene. *FEBS Lett.* **321**, 194–196.

Gibson, K. M., Bennett, M. J., Mize, C. E. et al. (1992). 3-Methylglutaconic aciduria associated with Pearson syndrome. *J. Pediatr.* **121**, 940–942.

Goto, Y., Itami, N., Kajii, N., Tochimaru, H., Endo, M. and Horai, S. (1990a). Renal tubular involvement mimicking Bartter syndrome in a patient with Kearns–Sayre syndrome. *J. Pediatr.* **116**, 904–910.

Goto, Y., Nonaka, I. and Horai, S. (1990b). A mutation in the tRNA(Leu)(UUR) gene associated with the MELAS subgroup of mitochondrial encephalomyopathies. *Nature* **348**, 651–653.

Goto, Y., Nonaka, I. and Horai, S. (1991). A new mutation in the tRNA-Leu(UUR) gene associated with mitochondrial myopathy, lactic acidosis and stroke-like episodes. *Biochem. Biophys. Acta*, **1097**, 238–240.

Graf, W. D., Sumi, S. M., Copass, M. K. et al. (1993). Phenotypic heterogeneity in families with the myoclonic epilepsy and ragged-red fiber disease point mutation in mitochondrial DNA. *Ann. Neurol.* **33**, 640–645.

Gucuyener, K., Seyrantepe, V., Topaloglu, H. and Ozguc (1998). Mitochondrial deletion in a boy with growth hormone deficiency mimicking cerebral palsy. *J. Inherit. Metab. Dis.* **21**, 173–174.

Gurgey, A., Ozalp, I., Rotig, A. et al. (1996). A case of Pearson syndrome associated with multiple renal cysts. *Pediatr. Nephrol.* **10**, 637–638.

Gyllensten, U., Wharton, D., Josefsson, A. and Wilson, A. C. (1991). Paternal inheritance of mitochondrial DNA in mice. *Nature* **352**, 255–257.

Hammans, S. R., Sweeney, M. G., Brockington, M. et al. (1993). The mitochondrial DNA transfer RNA(Lys)A→G(8344) mutation and the syndrome of myoclonic epilepsy with ragged red fibres (MERRF). Relationship of clinical phenotype to proportion of mutant mitochondrial DNA. *Brain* **116**, 617–632.

Hammans, S. R., Sweeney, M. G., Hanna, M. G., Brockington, M., Morgan-Hughes, J. A. and Harding, A. E. (1995). The mitochondrial DNA transfer RNALeu(UUR) A→G(3243) mutation. A clinical and genetic study. *Brain* **118**, 721–734.

Hara, H., Wakayama, Y., Kouno, Y., Yamada, H., Tanaka, M. and Ozawa, T. (1994a). Acute peripheral neuropathy, rhabdomyolysis and severe lactic acidosis associated with 3243 A to G mitochondrial DNA mutation [letter]. *J. Neurol. Neurosurg. Psychiatry* **57**, 1545–1546.

Hara, K., Yamamoto, M., Anegawa, T., Sakuta, R. and Nakamura, M. (1994b). Mitochondrial encephalomyopathy associated with parkinsonism and a point mutation in the mitochondrial tRNA(Leu)(UUR)) gene. *Rinsho Shinkeigaku* **34** (4), 361–365.

Harding, A. E., Holt, I. J., Sweeney, M. G., Brockington, M. and Davis, M. B. (1992). Prenatal diagnosis of mitochondrial DNA8993 T→G disease. *Am. J. Hum. Genet.* **50**, 629–633.

Hasegawa, H., Matsuoka, T., Goto, Y. and Nonaka, I. (1992). Vascular pathology in chronic progressive external ophthalmoplegia with ragged-red fibers. *Rinsho Shinkeigaku* **32**, 155–160.

Hasegawa, H., Matsuoka, T., Goto, Y.and Nonaka, I. (1993). Cytochrome c oxidase activity is deficient in blood vessels of patients with myoclonus epilepsy with ragged-red fibers. *Acta Neuropathol. (Berlin)* **85**, 280–284.

Hauswirth, W. W. and Laipis, P. J. (1982). Mitochondrial DNA polymorphism in a maternal lineage of Holstein cows. *Proc. Natl. Acad. Sci. USA* **79**, 4686–4690.

Herzberg, N. H., van Schooneveld, M. J., Bleeker-Wagemakers, E. M. et al. (1993). Kearns–Sayre syndrome with a phenocopy of choroideremia instead of pigmentary retinopathy. *Neurology* **43**, 218–221.

Heyer, E. (1995). Mitochondrial and nuclear genetic contribution of female founders to a contemporary population in northeast Quebec. *Am. J. Hum. Genet.* **56**, 1450–1455.

Hinokio, Y., Suzuki, S., Komatu, K. et al. (1995). A new mitochondrial DNA deletion associated with diabetic amyotrophy, diabetic myoatrophy and diabetic fatty liver. *Muscle Nerve* **3**, S142–149.

Hirano, M., Garcia-de-Yebenes, J., Jones, A. C. et al. (1998). Mitochondrial neurogastrointestinal encephalomyopathy syndrome maps to chromosome 22q13.32-qter. *Am. J. Hum. Genet.* **63**, 526–533.

Hiruta, Y., Chin, K., Shitomi, K. et al. (1995). Mitochondrial encephalomyopathy with A to G transition of mitochondrial transfer RNA(Leu(UUR)) 3243 presenting hypertrophic cardiomyopathy. *Intern. Med.* **34**, 670–673.

Holme, E., Larsson, N. G., Oldfors, A., Tulinius, M., Sahlin, P. and Stenman, G. (1993). Multiple symmetric lipomas with high levels of mtDNA with the tRNA(Lys) A→G(8344) mutation as the only manifestation of disease in a carrier of myoclonus epilepsy and ragged-red fibers (MERRF) syndrome. *Am. J. Hum. Genet.* **52**, 551–556.

Holt, I. J., Harding, A. E. and Morgan, H. J. A. (1988). Deletions of muscle mitochondrial DNA in patients with mitochondrial myopathies. *Nature* **331**, 717–719.

Holt, I. J., Harding, A. E., Cooper, J. M. et al. (1989). Mitochondrial myopathies: clinical and biochemical features of 30 patients with major deletions of muscle mitochondrial DNA. *Ann. Neurol.* **26**, 699–708.

Holt, I. J., Harding, A. E., Petty, R. K. and Morgan-Hughes, J. A. (1990). A new mitochondrial disease associated with mitochondrial DNA heteroplasmy. *Am. J. Hum. Genet.* **46**, 428–433.

Horvath, R., Fu, K., Johns, T., Genge, A., Karpati, G. and Shoubridge, E. A. (1998). Characterization of the mitochondrial DNA abnormalities in the skeletal muscle of patients with inclusion body myositis. *J. Neuropathol. Exp. Neurol.* **57**, 396–403.

Houstek, J., Klement, P., Hermanska, J. et al. (1995). Altered properties of mitochondrial ATP-synthase in patients with a T→G mutation in the ATPase 6 (subunit a) gene at position 8993 of mtDNA. *Biochem. Biophys. Acta*, **1271**, 349–357.

Howell, N., Kubacka, I., Smith, R., Frerman, F., Parks, J. K. and Parker, W. D., Jr. (1996). Association of the mitochondrial 8344 MERRF mutation with maternally inherited spinocerebellar degeneration and Leigh disease. *Neurology* **46**, 219–222.

Hsu, C. C., Chuang, Y. H., Tsai, J. L. et al. (1995). CPEO and carnitine deficiency overlapping in MELAS syndrome. *Acta Neurol. Scand.* **92**, 252–255.

Huang, W. Y., Chi, C. S., Mak, S. C., Wu, H. M. and Yang, M. T. (1995). Leigh syndrome presenting with dystonia: report of one case. *Chung Hua Min Kuo Hsiao Erh Ko I Hsueh Hui Tsa Chih* **36**, 378–381.

Ihara, M., Tanaka, H., Yashiro, M. and Nishimura, Y. (1996). Mitochondrial myopathy, encephalopathy, lactic acidosis and stroke-like episodes (MELAS) with chronic renal failure: report of mother-child cases. *Rinsho Shinkeigaku*, **36**, 1069–1073.

Inagaki, T., Ishino, H., Seno, H., Ohguni, S., Tanaka, J. and Kato, Y. (1997). Psychiatric symptoms in a patient with diabetes mellitus associated with point mutation in mitochondrial DNA. *Biol. Psychiatry* **42**, 1067–1069.

Inamori, M., Ishigami, T., Takahashi, N. et al. (1997). A case of mitochondrial cardiomyopathy with heart failure, sick sinus syndrome and diabetes mellitus: mitochondrial DNA adenine-to-guanine transition at 3243 of mitochondrial tRNA(LEU)(UUR) gene. *J. Cardiol.* **30**, 341–347.

Ionasescu, V. (1983). Oculogastrointestinal musclular dystrophy. *Am. J. Med. Genet.* **15**, 103–112.

Ionasescu, V., Thompson, S. H., Ionasescu, R. et al. (1983). Inherited ophthalmoplegia with intestinal pseudo-obstruction. *J. Neurol. Sci.* **59**, 215–228.

Ionasescu, V., Thompson, H. S., Aschenbrener, C., Anuras, S. and Risk, W. S. (1984). Late-onset oculogastrointestinal muscular dystrophy. *Am. J. Med. Genet.* **18**, 781–788.

Isashiki, Y., Nakagawa, M., Yamada, H. and Miyata, M. (1994). Ocular manifestations in mitochondrial DNA abnormalities. *Nippon Ganka Gakkai Zasshi*, **98**, 3–12.

Isashiki, Y., Nakagawa, M., Ohba, N. et al. (1998). Retinal manifestations in mitochondrial diseases associated with mitochondrial DNA mutation. *Acta Ophthalmol. Scand.* **76**, 6–13.

Isotani, H., Fukumoto, Y., Kawamura, H. et al. (1996). Hypoparathyroidism and insulin-dependent diabetes mellitus in a patient with Kearns–Sayre syndrome harbouring a mitochondrial DNA deletion. *Clin. Endocrinol.* **45**, 637–641.

Isozumi, K., Fukuuchi, Y., Tanaka, K., Nogawa, S., Ishihara, T. and Sakuta, R. (1994). A MELAS (mitochondrial myopathy, encephalopathy, lactic acidosis and stroke-like episodes) mtDNA mutation that induces subacute dementia which mimicks Creutzfeldt–Jakob disease. *Intern. Med.* **33**, 543–546.

Jansen, J. J., Maassen, J. A., van der Woude, F. J. et al. (1997). Mutation in mitochondrial tRNA(Leu(UUR)) gene associated with progressive kidney disease. *J. Am. Soc. Nephrol.* **8**, 1118–1124.

Jean-Francois, M. J., Lertrit, P., Berkovic, S. F. et al. (1994). Heterogeneity in the phenotypic expression of the mutation in the mitochondrial tRNA(Leu) (UUR) gene generally associated with the MELAS subset of mitochondrial encephalomyopathies. *Aust. N. Z. J. Med.* **24**, 188–193.

Jenuth, J. P., Peterson, A. C., Fu, K. and Shoubridge, E. A. (1996). Random genetic drift in the female germline explains the rapid segregation of mammalian mitochondrial DNA. *Nat. Genet.* **14**, 146–151.

Jerusalem, F., Engel, A. G. and Peterson, H. A. (1975). Human muscle fiber fine ultrastructure: morphometric data on controls. *Neurology* **25**, 127.

Kaido, M., Fujimura, H., Soga, F. et al. (1996). Alzheimer-type pathology in a patient with mitochondrial myopathy, encephalopathy, lactic acidosis and stroke-like episodes (MELAS). *Acta Neuropathol. (Berlin)* **92**, 312–318.

Kamakura, K., Abe, H., Tadano, Y. et al. (1995). Recurrent respiratory failure in a patient with 3243 mutation in mitochondrial DNA. [letter] *J. Neurol.* **242**, 253–255.

Kaneda, H., Hayashi, J., Takahama, S., Taya, C., Lindahl, K. F. and Yonekawa, H. (1995). Elimination of paternal mitochondrial DNA in intraspecific crosses during early mouse embryogenesis. *Proc. Natl. Acad. Sci. USA* **92**, 4542–4546.

Kaukonen, J. A., Amati, P., Suomalainen, A. et al. (1996). An autosomal locus predisposing to multiple deletions of mtDNA on chromosome 3p. *Am. J. Hum. Genet.* **58**, 763–769.

Kawakami, Y., Sakuta, R., Hashimoto, K. et al. (1994). Mitochondrial myopathy with progressive decrease in mitochondrial tRNA(Leu)(UUR) mutant genomes. *Ann. Neurol.* **35**, 370–373.

Kimata, K. G., Gordan, L., Ajax, E. T., Davis, P. H. and Grabowski, T. (1998). A case of late-onset MELAS. *Arch. Neurol.* **55**, 722–725.

King, M. D., O'Neill, G., Poulton, J. et al. (1996). Polyneuropathy in the mtDNA base pain 3243 point mutation. [Letter; comment] *Neurology* **46**, 1495–1496.

Kishnani, P. S., Van Hove, J. L., Shoffner, J. S., Kaufman, A., Bossen, E. H. and Kahler, S. G. (1996). Acute pancreatitis in an infant with lactic acidosis and a mutation at nucleotide 3243 in the mitochondrial DNA tRNALeu(UUR) gene. *Eur. J. Pediatr.* **155**, 898–903.

Kitaoka, H., Kameoka, K., Suzuki, Y. et al. (1995). A patient with diabetes mellitus, cardiomyopathy and a mitochondrial gene mutation: confirmation of a gene mutation in cardiac muscle. *Diabetes Res. Clin. Pract.* **28**, 207–212.

Klement, P., Zeman, J., Hansikova, H., Houstkova, H., Baudysova, M. and Houstek, J. (1994). Different restriction fragment pattern of mtDNA indicative of generalized 8993 point mutations in a boy with lactic acidosis. *J. Inherit. Metab. Dis.* **17**, 249–250.

Klopstock, T., Naumann, M., Seibel, P., Shalke, B., Reiners, K. and Reichmann, H. (1997). Mitochondrial DNA mutations in multiple symmetric lipomatosis. *Mol. Cell. Biochem.* **174**, 271–275.

Kokot, W., Iwaszkiewicz-Bilikiewiczowa, B., Lewczuk, A. and Sworczak, K. (1996). A case of Kearns–Sayre syndrome. *Klin. Oczna* **98**, 327–330.

Koo, B., Becker, L. E., Chuang, S. et al. (1993). Mitochondrial encephalomyopathy, lactic acidosis, stroke-like episodes (MELAS): clinical, radiological, pathological and genetic observations. *Ann. Neurol.* **34**, 25–32.

Koutnikova, H., Campuzano, V., Foury, F., Dolle, P., Cazzalini, O. and Koenig, M. (1997). Studies of human, mouse and yeast homologues indicate a mitochondrial function for frataxin. *Nat. Genet.* **16**, 345–351.

Kuzuya, N., Noda, M., Fujii, M. and Kanazawa, Y. (1994). A pedigree with maternally transmitted diabetes mellitus, deafness and cardiomyopathy. *Nippon Rinsho* **52**, 2611–2615.

Larsson, N. G., Holme, E., Kristiansson, B., Oldfors, A. and Tulinius, M. (1990). Progressive increase in the mutated mitochondrial DNA fraction in Kearns–Sayre syndrome. *Pediatr. Res.* **28**, 131–136.

Larsson, N. G., Eiken, H. G., Boman, H., Holme, E., Oldfors, A. and Tulinius, M. H. (1992). Lack of transmission of deleted mtDNA from a woman with Kearns–Sayre syndrome to her child. *Am. J. Hum. Genet.* **50**, 360–363.

Larsson, N. G., Tulinius, M. H., Holme, E. and Oldfors, A. (1995). Pathogenetic aspects of the A8344G mutation of mitochondrial DNA associated with MERRF syndrome and multiple symmetric lipomas. *Muscle Nerve* **3**, S102–S106.

Lee, H. C., Song, Y. D., Li, H. R. et al. (1997). Mitochondrial gene transfer ribonucleic acid (tRNA)Leu(UUR) 3243 and tRNA(Lys) 8344 mutations and diabetes mellitus in Korea. *J. Clin. Endocrinol. Metab.* **82**, 372–374.

Lee, N., Morin, C., Mitchell, G. and Robinson, B. (1998). Saguenay Lac Saint Jean cytochrome oxidase deficiency: sequence analysis of nuclear encoded COX subunits, chromosomal localization and a sequence anomaly in subunit VIc. *Biochem. Biophys. Acta* **27**, 1–4.

Li, J. Y., Kong, K. W., Chang, M. H. et al. (1996). MELAS syndrome associated with a tandem duplication in the D-loop of mitochondrial DNA. *Acta Neurol. Scand.* **93**, 450–455.

Loeffen, J., Smeitink, J., Triepels, R. et al. (1998). The first nuclear-encoded complex I mutation in a patient with Leigh syndrome. *Am. J. Hum. Genet.* **63**, 1598–1608.

Luder, A. and Barash, V. (1994). Complex I deficiency with diabetes, Fanconi syndrome and mtDNA deletion. *J. Inherit. Metab. Dis.* **17**, 298–300.

Luft, R., Ikkos, D., Palmieri, G., Ernster, L. and Afzelius, B. (1962). A case of severe hypermetabolism of nonthyroid origin with a defect in the maintenance of mitochondrial respiratory control: a correlated clinical, biochemical and morphological study. *J. Clin. Invest.* **41**, 1776–1804.

Majander, A., Suomalainen, A., Vettenranta, K. et al. (1991). Congenital hypoplastic anemia, diabetes and severe renal tubular dysfunction associated with a mitochondrial DNA deletion. *Ped. Res.* **30**, 327–330.

Mak, S. C., Chi, C. S., Liu, C. Y., Pang, C. Y. and Wei, Y. H. (1996). Leigh syndrome associated with mitochondrial DNA 8993 T→G mutation and ragged-red fibers. *Ped. Neurol.* **15**, 72–75.

Manfredi, G., Vu, T., Bonilla, E. et al. (1997). Association of myopathy with large-scale mitochondrial DNA duplications and deletions: which is pathogenic? *Ann. Neurol.* **42**, 180–188.

Martinuzzi, A., Bartolomei, L., Carrozzo, R. et al. (1992). Correlation between clinical and molecular features in two MELAS. *J. Neurol. Sci.* **113**, 222–229.

Massin, P., Guillausseau, P. J., Vialettes, B. et al. (1995). Macular pattern dystrophy associated with a mutation of mitochondrial DNA. *Am. J. Ophthalmol.* **120**, 247–248.

Masucci, J. P., Davidson, M., Koga, Y., Schon, E. A. and King, M. P. (1995). In vitro analysis of mutations causing myoclonus epilepsy with ragged-red fibers in the mitochondrial tRNA(Lys)gene: two genotypes produce similar phenotypes. *Mol. Cell. Biol.* **15**, 2872–2881.

Matthews, P. M., Hopkin, J., Brown, R. M., Stephenson, J. B., Hilton-Jones, D. and Brown, G. K. (1994). Comparison of the relative levels of the 3243 (A→G) mtDNA mutation in heteroplasmic adult and fetal tissues. *J. Med. Genet.* **31**, 41–44.

McAuley, F. D. (1956). Progressive external ophthalmoplegia. *Br. J. Ophthalmol.* **40**, 686–690.

Melegh, B., Seress, L., Sumegi, B. et al. (1995). Mitochondrial DNA deletion in hereditary cardio-encephalo-myopathy. *Orv. Hetil.* **136**, 1275–1279.

Merante, F., Petrova-Benedict, R., MacKay, N. et al. (1993). A biochemically distinct form of cytochrome oxidase (COX) deficiency in the Saguenay-Lac-Saint-Jean region of Quebec. *Am. J. Hum. Genet.* **53**, 481–487.

Mielot, F., Bader-Meunier, B., Tchernia, G. and Dommergues, J. P. (1997). Myelodysplasia in children and mitochondrial cytopathies. *Pathol. Biol. (Paris)* **45**, 594–599.

Minamoto, H., Kawabata, K., Okuda, B. et al. (1996). Mitochondrial encephalomyopathy with elderly onset of stroke-like episodes. *Intern. Med.* **35**, 991–995.

Mita, S., Tokunaga, M., Kumamoto, T., Uchino, M., Nonaka, I. and Ando, M. (1995). Mitochondrial DNA mutation and muscle pathology in mitochondrial myopathy, encephalopathy, lactic acidosis and strokelike episodes. *Muscle Nerve* **3**, S113–S118.

Molnar, M., Zanssen, S., Buse, G. and Schroder, J. M. (1996). A large-scale deletion of mitochondrial DNA in a case with pure mitochondrial myopathy and neuropathy. *Acta Neuropathol. (Berlin)* **91**, 654–658.

Montagna, P., Cortelli, P. and Barbiroli, B. (1998). A case of cluster headache associated with mitochondrial DNA deletions. [Letter; comment] *Muscle Nerve* **21**, 127–129.

Moraes, C. T., DiMauro, S., Zeviani, M. et al. (1989). Mitochondrial DNA deletions in progressive external ophthalmoplegia and Kearns–Sayre syndrome. *N. Eng. J. Med.* **320**, 1293–1299.

Moraes, C. T., Shanske, S., Tritschler, H. J. et al. (1991a). mtDNA depletion with variable tissue expression: a novel genetic abnormality in mitochondrial diseases. *Am. J. Hum. Genet.* **48**, 492–501.

Moraes, C. T., Zeviani, M., Schon, E. A. et al. (1991b). Mitochondrial DNA deletion in a girl with manifestations of Kearns–Sayre and Lowe syndromes: an example of phenotypic mimicry? *Am. J. Hum. Genet.* **41**, 301–305.

Moraes, C. T., Ciacci, F., Silvestri, G. et al. (1993). Atypical clinical presentations associated with the MELAS mutation at position 3243 of human mitochondrial DNA. *Neuromusc. Disord.* **3**, 43–50.

Morgan-Hughes, J. A., Sweeney, M. G., Cooper, J. M. et al. (1995). Mitochondrial DNA (mtDNA) diseases: correlation of genotype to phenotype. *Biochrm. Biophys. Acta* **1271**, 135–140.

Mori, K., Narahara, K., Ninomiya, S., Goto, Y. and Nonaka, I. (1991). Renal and skin involvement in a patient with complete Kearns–Sayre syndrome. *Am. J. Med. Genet.* **38**, 583–587.

Morin, C., Mitchell, G., Larochelle, J. et al. (1993). Clinical, metabolic and genetic aspects of cytochrome c oxidase deficiency in Saguenay-Lac-Saint-Jean. *Am. J. Hum. Genet.* **53**, 488–496.

Morris, A. A., Leonard, J. V., Brown, G. K. et al. (1996). Deficiency of respiratory chain complex I is a common cause of Leigh disease. *Ann. Neurol.* **40**, 25–30.

Morris, A. A., Lamont, P. J. and Clayton, P. T. (1997). Pearson's syndrome without marrow involvement. *Arch. Dis. Child.* **77**, 56–57.

Mosewich, R. K., Donat, J. R., DiMauro, S. et al. (1993). The syndrome of mitochondrial encephalomyopathy, lactic acidosis and strokelike episodes presenting without stroke. *Arch. Neurol.* **50**, 275–278.

Moslemi, A. R., Lindberg, C. and Oldfors, A. (1997). Analysis of multiple mitochondrial DNA deletions in inclusion body myositis. *Hum. Mutat.* **10**, 381–386.

Muller-Hocker, J. (1989). Cytochrome *c* oxidase deficient cardiomyocytes in the human heart. An age-related phenomenon. *Am. J. Pathol.* **134**, 1167–1171.

Muller-Hocker, J. (1990). Cytochrome *c* oxidase deficient fibers in the limb muscle and diaphragm of man without muscular disease: an age-related alteration. *J. Neurol. Sci.* **100**, 14–21.

Muraki, K., Goto, Y., Nishino, I. et al. (1997). Severe lactic acidosis and neonatal death in Pearson syndrome. *J. Inherit. Metab. Dis.* **20**, 43–48.

Nakai, A., Goto, Y., Fujisawa, K. et al. (1994). Diffuse leukodystrophy with a large-scale mitochondrial DNA deletion. *Lancet* **343**, 1397–1398.

Nakase, H. (1993). Leigh's syndrome and mitochondrial myopathy. *Nippon Rinsho* **51**, 2403–2408.

Naumann, M., Kiefer, R., Toyka, K. V., Sommer, C., Seibel, P. and Reichmann, H. (1997). Mitochondrial dysfunction with myoclonus epilepsy and ragged-red fibers point mutation in nerve, muscle and adipose tissue of a patient with multiple symmetric lipomatosis. *Muscle Nerve* **20**, 833–839.

Niaudet, P., Heidet, L., Munnich, A. et al. (1994). Deletion of the mitochondrial DNA in a case of de Toni-Debre-Fanconi syndrome and Pearson syndrome. *Pediatr. Nephrol* **8**, 164–168.

Nicolino, M., Ferlin, T., Forest, M. et al. (1997). Identification of a large-scale mitochondrial deoxyribonucleic acid deletion in endocrinopathies and deafness: report of two unrelated cases with diabetes mellitus and adrenal insufficiency, respectively. *J. Clin. Endocrinol. Metab.* **82**, 3063–3067.

Nishino, I., Spinazzola, A. and Hirano, M. (1999). Thymidine phosphorylase gene mutations in MNGIE, a human mitochondrial disorder. *Science* **283**, 689–692.

Nomura, T., Ota, M., Kotake, N. and Tanaka, K. (1993). Two cases of MERRF (myoclonus epilepsy associated with ragged red fibers) showing different clinical features in the same family. *Rinsho Shinkeigaku* **33**, 1198–1200.

Odawara, M., Tada, K. and Yamashita, K. (1995). Decreased cerebral blood perfusion in an NIDDM patient with an A-to-G mutation in the mitochondrial gene; a possible contribution to cognition deficits in diabetes. *Diabetologia* **38**, 1004–1005.

Odawara, M., Tamaoka, A., Mizusawa, H. and Yamashita, K. (1997). A case of cluster headache associated with mitochondrial DNA deletions. [Letter] *Muscle Nerve* **20**, 394–395.

Ohno, K., Tanaka, M., Ino, H. et al. (1991a). Direct DNA sequencing from colony: analysis of multiple deletions of the mitochondrial genome. *Biochem. Biophys. Acta* **1090**, 9–16.

Ohno, K., Tanaka, M., Sahashi, K. et al. (1991b). Mitochondrial DNA deletions in inherited recurrent myoglobinuria. *Ann. Neurol.* **29**, 364–369.

Ohno, K., Yamamoto, M., Engel, A. G. et al. (1996). MELAS- and Kearns–Sayre-type co-mutation with myopathy and autoimmune polyendocrinopathy. [Published erratum appears in *Ann. Neurol.* (1996) **40**, 480.] *Ann. Neurol.* **39**, 761–766.

Oldfors, A., Larsson, N. G., Lindberg, C. and Holme, E. (1993). Mitochondrial DNA deletions in inclusion body myositis. *Brain* **116**, 325–336.

Oldfors, A., Moslemi, A. R., Fyhr, I. M., Holme, E., Larsson, N. G. and Lindberg, C. (1995). Mitochondrial DNA deletions in muscle fibers in inclusion body myositis. *J. Neuropathol. Exp. Neurol.* **54**, 581–587.

Onishi, H., Inoue, K., Osaka, H. et al. (1993). Mitochondrial myopathy, encephalopathy, lactic acidosis and stroke-like episodes (MELAS) and diabetes mellitus: molecular genetic analysis and family study. *J. Neurol. Sci.* **114**, 205–208.

Onishi, H., Kawanishi, C., Iwasawa, T. et al. (1997). Depressive disorder due to mitochondrial transfer RNALeu(UUR) mutation. *Biol. Psychiatry.* **41**, 1137–1139.

Onishi, H., Hanihara, T., Sugiyama, N. et al. (1998). Pancreatic exocrine dysfunction associated with mitochondrial tRNA(Leu)(UUR) mutation. *J. Med. Genet.* **35**, 255–257.

Orimo, S., Arai, M., Hiyamuta, E. and Goto, Y. (1992). A case of chronic progressive external ophthalmoplegia associated with familial hypercholesterolemia. *Rinsho Shinkeigaku* **32**, 37–41.

Ota, Y., Miyake, Y., Awaya, S., Kumagai, T., Tanaka, M. and Ozawa, T. (1994). Early retinal involvement in mitochondrial myopathy with mitochondrial DNA deletion. *Retina* **14**, 270–276.

Otabe, S., Sakura, H., Shimokawa, K. et al. (1994). The high prevalence of the diabetic patients with a mutation in the mitochondrial gene in Japan. *J. Clin. Endocrinol. Metab.* **79**, 768–771.

Ozawa, M., Goto, Y., Sakuta, R., Tanno, Y., Tsuji, S. and Nonaka, I. (1995). The 8344 mutation in mitochondrial DNA: a comparison between the proportion of mutant DNA and clinico-pathologic findings. *Neuromusc. Disord.* **5**, 483–488.

Ozawa, T., Yoneda, M., Tanaka, M. et al. (1988). Maternal inheritance of deleted mitochondrial DNA in a family with mitochondrial myopathy. *Biochem. Biophys. Res. Commun.* **154**, 1240–1247.

Pastores, G. M., Santorelli, F. M., Shanske, S. et al. (1994). Leigh syndrome and hypertrophic cardiomyopathy in an infant with a mitochondrial DNA point mutation (T8993G). *Am. J. Med. Genet.* **50**, 265–271.

Penisson-Besnier, I., Degoul, F., Desnuelle, C. et al. (1992). Uneven distribution of mitochondrial DNA mutation in MERRF dizygotic. *J. Neurol. Sci.* **110**, 144–148.

Poulton, J., Deadman, M. E. and Gardiner, R. M. (1989a). Duplications of mitochondrial DNA in mitochondrial myopathy. *Lancet* **i**, 236–240.

Poulton, J., Deadman, M. E. and Gardiner, R. M. (1989b). Tandem direct duplications of mitochondrial DNA in mitochondrial myopathy: analysis of nucleotide sequence and tissue distribution. *Nucl. Acids Res.* **17**, 10223–10229.

Poulton, J., Deadman, M. E., Bindoff, L., Morten, K., Land, J. and Brown, G. (1993). Families of mtDNA re-arrangements can be detected in patients with mtDNA deletions: duplications may be a transient intermediate form. *Hum. Mol. Genet.* **2**, 23–30.

Puddu, P., Barboni, P., Mantovani, V. et al. (1993). Retinitis pigmentosa, ataxia and mental retardation associated with mitochondrial DNA mutation in an Italian family. *Br. J. Ophthalmol.* **77**, 84–88.

Rahman, S., Blok, R. B., Dahl, H. H. et al. (1996). Leigh syndrome: clinical features and biochemical and DNA abnormalities. *Ann. Neurol.* **39**, 343–351.

Reardon, W., Ross, R. J. M., Sweeney, M. G. et al. (1992). Diabetes mellitus associated with a pathogenic point mutation in mitochondrial DNA. *Lancet* **340**, 1376–1379.

Reichmann, H., Gold, R., Meurers, B. et al. (1993). Progression of myopathology in Kearns–Sayre syndrome: a morphological follow-up study. *Acta Neuropathol. (Berlin)* **85**, 679–681.

Ribes, A., Riudor, E., Valcarel, R. et al. (1993). Pearson syndrome: altered tricarboxylic acid and urea-cycle metabolites, adrenal insufficiency and corneal opacities. *J. Inherit. Metab. Dis.* **16**, 537–540.

Robinson, B. H., De Meirlei, R. L., Glerum, M., Sherwood, G. and Becker, L. (1987). Clinical presentation of mitochondrial respiratory chain defects in NADH-coenzyme Q reductase and cytochrome oxidase: clues to pathogenesis of Leigh disease. *J. Pediatr.* **110**, 216–222.

Rosing, H. S., Hopkins, L. C., Wallace, D. C., Epstein, C. M. and Weidenheim, K. (1985). Maternally inherited mitochondrial myopathy and myoclonic epilepsy. *Ann. Neurol.* **17**, 228–237.

Rossier, J. and Hatt, M. (1996). Atypical manifestation of progressive external ophthalmoplegia. *Klin. Monatsbl. Augenheilkd.* **208**, 366–367.

Rotig, A., Colonna, M., Blanche, S. et al. (1988). Deletion of blood mitochondrial DNA in pancytopenia. [Letter] *Lancet* **2**, 567–568.

Rotig, A., Colonna, M., Bonnefont, J. P. et al. (1989). Mitochondrial DNA deletion in Pearson's marrow/pancreas syndrome. *Lancet* **i**, 902–903.

Rotig, A., Bessis, J. L., Romero, N. et al. (1992). Maternally inherited duplication of the mitochondrial genome in a syndrome of proximal tubulopathy, diabetes mellitus and cerebellar ataxia. *Am. J. Hum. Genet.* **50**, 364–370.

Rotig, A., Cormier, V., Chatelain, P. et al. (1993). Deletion of mitochondrial DNA in a case of early-onset diabetes mellitus, optic atrophy and deafness (DIDMOAD, Wolfram syndrome). *J. Inherit. Metab. Dis.* **16**, 527–530.

Rotig, A., Goutieres, F., Niaudet, P. et al. (1995). Deletion of mitochondrial DNA in patient with chronic tubulointerstitial nephritis. *J. Pediatr.* **126**, 597–601.

Rotig, A., de Lonlay, P., Chretien, D. et al. (1997). Aconitase and mitochondrial iron–sulphur protein deficiency in Friedreich ataxia. *Nat. Genet.* **17**, 215–217.

Rowland, L. P. (1992). Progressive external ophthalmoplegia and ocular myopathies. In: *Handbook of Clinical Neurology*, Vol. 18, eds. L. P. Rowland and S. DiMauro, pp. 287–329. North Holland: Elsevier Science.

Rummelt, V., Folberg, R., Ionasescu, V., Yi, H. and Moore, K. C. (1993). Ocular pathology of MELAS syndrome with mitochondrial DNA nucleotide 3243 point mutation. *Ophthalmology* **100**, 1757–1766.

Rusanen, H., Majamaa, K., Tolonen, U., Remes, A. M., Myllyla, R. and Hassinen, I. E. (1995). Demyelinating polyneuropathy in a patient with the tRNA(Leu)(UUR) mutation at base pair 3243 of the mitochondrial DNA. *Neurology* **45**, 1188–1192.

Sahashi, K., Ohno, K., Tanaka, M. et al. (1990). Cytoplasmic body and mitochondrial DNA deletion. *J. Neurol. Sci.* **99**, 291–300.

Sakuta, R., Goto, Y., Horai, S. et al. (1992). Mitochondrial DNA mutation and Leigh's syndrome. [Letter] *Ann. Neurol.* **32**, 597–598.

Sanger, T. D. and Jain, K. D. (1996). MERRF syndrome with overwhelming lactic acidosis. *Pediatr. Neurol.* **14**, 57–61.

Santorelli, F. M., Shanske, S., Macaya, A., DeVivo, D. C. and DiMauro, S. (1993). The mutation at nt 8993 of mitochondrial DNA is a common cause of Leigh's syndrome. *Ann. Neurol.* **34**, 827–834.

Santorelli, F. M., Shanske, S., Jain, K. D., Tick, D., Schon, E. A. and DiMauro, S. (1994). A T→C mutation at nt 8993 of mitochondrial DNA in a child with Leigh syndrome. *Neurology* **44**, 972–974.

Santorelli, F. M., Barmada, M. A., Pons, R., Zhang, L. L. and DiMauro, S. (1996a). Leigh-type neuropathology in Pearson syndrome associated with impaired ATP production and a novel mtDNA deletion. *Neurology* **47**, 1320–1323.

Santorelli, F. M., Sciacco, M., Tanji, K. et al. (1996b). Multiple mitochondrial DNA deletions in sporadic inclusion body myositis: a study of 56 patients. *Ann. Neurol.* **39**, 789–795.

Santorelli, F. M., Tanji, K., Shanske, S. and DiMauro, S. (1997). Heterogeneous clinical presentation of the mtDNA NARP/T8993G mutation. *Neurology* **49**, 270–273.

Schroder, J. M. and Molnar, M. (1997). Mitochondrial abnormalities and peripheral neuropathy in inflammatory myopathy, especially inclusion body myositis. *Mol. Cell. Biochem.* **174**, 277–281.

Schuelke, M., Smeitink, J., Mariman, E. et al. (1999). Mutant NDUFV1 subunit of mitochondrial complex I causes leukodystrophy and myoclonic epilepsy. *Nat. Genet.* **21**, 260–261.

Seibel, P., Degoul, F., Romero, N., Marsac, C. and Kadenbach, B. (1990). Identification of point mutations by mispairing PCR as exemplified in MERRF disease. *Biochem. Biophys. Res. Commun.* **173**, 561–565.

Seibel, P., Grunewald, T., Gundolla, A., Diener, H. C. and Reichmann, H. (1996). Investigation on the mitochondrial transfer RNA(Leu)(UUR) in blood cells from patients with cluster headache. *J. Neurol.* **243**, 305–307.

Servidei, S., Zeviani, M., Manfredi, G. et al. (1991). Dominantly inherited mitochondrial myopathy with multiple deletions of mitochondrial DNA: clinical, morphologic and biochemical studies. *Neurology* **41**, 1053–1059.

Shaag, A., Saada, A., Steinberg, A., Navon, P. and Elpeleg, O. N. (1997). Mitochondrial encephalomyopathy associated with a novel mutation in the mitochondrial tRNA(leu)(UUR) gene (A3243T). *Biochem. Biophys. Res. Commun.* **233**, 637–639.

Shanske, A. L., Shanske, S., Silvestri, G., Tanji, K., Wertheim, D. and Lipper, S. (1993). MELAS point mutation with unusual clinical presentation. *Neuromusc. Disord.* **3**, 191–193.

Shinomiya, H., Fukuda, N., Takeichi, N. et al. (1998). Evaluation of cardiac function by various cardiac imaging techniques in mitochondrial cardiomyopathy: a case report. *J. Cardiol.* **31**, 109–114.

Shoffner, J. M. and Wallace, D. C. (1995). Oxidative phosphorylation diseases. In: *The Metabolic and Molecular Bases of Inherited Disease*, eds. C. R. Scriver, A. L. Beaudet, W. S. Sly et al., pp. 1535–1610. New York: McGraw-Hill.

Shoffner, J. M., Lott, M. T., Lezza, A. M., Seibel, P., Ballinger, S. W. and Wallace, D. C. (1990). Myoclonic epilepsy and ragged-red fiber disease (MERRF) is associated with a mitochondrial DNA tRNA(Lys) mutation. *Cell* **61**, 931–937.

Shoffner, J. M., Fernhoff, P. M., Krawiecki, N. S. et al. (1992). Subacute necrotizing encephalopathy: oxidative phosphorylation defects. *Neurology* **42**, 2168–2174.

Shoffner, J. M., Bialer, M. G., Pavlakis, S. G. et al. (1995). Mitochondrial encephalomyopathy caused by a single nucleotide deletion in the mitochondrial tRNA-leucine(UUR) gene. *Neurology* **45**, 286–292.

Shoubridge, E. A., Karpati, G. and Hastings, K. E. (1990). Deletion mutants are functionally dominant over wild type mitochondrial genomes in skeletal muscle fiber segments in mitochondrial disease. *Cell* **62**, 43–49.

Silvestri, G., Moraes, C. T., Shanske, S., Oh, S. J. and DiMauro, S. (1992). A new mutation in the tRNA-Lys gene associated with myoclonic epilepsy and ragged-red fibers (MERRF). *Am. J. Hum. Genet.* **51**, 1213–1217.

Silvestri, G., Ciafaloni, E., Santorelli, F. M. et al. (1993). Clinical features associated with the A→G transition at nucleotide 8344 of mtDNA ('MERRF mutation'). *Neurology* **43**, 1200–1206.

Silvestri, G., Bertini, E., Servidei, S. et al. (1997). Maternally inherited cardiomyopathy: a new phenotype associated with the A to G AT nt.3243 of mitochondrial DNA (MELAS mutation). *Muscle Nerve* **20**, 221–225.

Simon, L. T., Horoupian, D. S., Dorfman, L. J. et al. (1990). Polyneuropathy, ophthalmoplegia, leukoencephalopathy and intestinal pseudo-obstruction: POLIP syndrome. *Ann. Neurol.* **28**, 349–360.

Simonsz, H. J., Barlocher, K. and Rotig, A. (1992). Kearns–Sayre's syndrome developing in a boy who survived pearson's syndrome caused by mitochondrial DNA deletion. *Doc. Ophthalmol.* **82**, 73–79.

Smith, M. L., Hua, X. Y., Marsden, D. L. et al. (1997). Diabetes and mitochondrial encephalomyopathy with lactic acidosis and stroke-like episodes (MELAS): radiolabelled polymerase chain reaction is necessary for accurate detection of low percentages of mutation. *J. Clin. Endocrinol. Metab.* **82**, 2826–2831.

Souied, E. H., Sales, M. J., Soubrane, G. et al. (1998). Macular dystrophy, diabetes and deafness associated with a large mitochondrial DNA deletion. *Am. J. Ophthalmol.* **125**, 100–103.

Stadhouders, A., Jap, P. and Walliman, T. H. (1990). Biochemical nature of mitochondrial crystals. *J. Neurol. Sci.* **98**(Suppl.), 304–305.

Stansbie, D., Wallace, S. J. and Marsac, C. (1986). Disorders of the pyruvate dehydrogenase complex. *J. Inher. Metab. Dis.* **9**, 105–109.

Stine, O. C., Luu, S. U., Zito, M. and Casanova, M. (1993). The possible association between affective disorder and partially deleted mitochondrial DNA. *Biol. Psychiatry* **33**, 141–142.

Suomalainen, A., Ciafaloni, E., Koga, Y., Peltonen, L., DiMauro, S. and Schon, E. A. (1992). Use of single strand conformation polymorphism analysis to detect. *J. Neurol. Sci.* **111**, 222–226.

Suomalainen, A., Kaukonen, J., Amati, P. et al. (1995). An autosomal locus predisposing to deletions of mitochondrial DNA. *Nat. Genet.* **9**, 146–151.

Suzuki, S. (1994). Clinical characterization of diabetes mellitus in the families with mitochondrial encephalomyopathies. *Nippon Rinsho* **52**, 2606–2610.

Suzuki, S., Hinokio, Y., Hirai, S. et al. (1994). Diabetes with mitochondrial gene tRNALYS mutation. *Diabetes Care* **17**, 1428–1432.

Sweeney, M. G., Hammans, S. R., Duchen, L. W. et al. (1994). Mitochondrial DNA mutation underlying Leigh's syndrome: clinical, pathological, biochemical and genetic studies of a patient presenting with progressive myoclonic epilepsy. *J. Neurol. Sci.* **121**, 57–65.

Szabolcs, M. J., Seigle, R., Shanske, S., Bonilla, E., DiMauro, S. and D'Agati, V. (1994). Mitochondrial DNA deletion: a cause of chronic tubulointerstitial nephropathy. *Kidney Int.* **45**, 1388–1396.

Takeda, N. (1995). Mitochondrial DNA mutations in diabetes mellitus and heart disease. [Editorial; comment] *Intern. Med.* **34**, 931–932.

Takeda, N. (1997). Cardiomyopathies and mitochondrial DNA mutations. *Mol. Cell. Biochem.* **176**, 287–290.

Tanaka, M., Yoneda, M., Ohno, K. et al. (1989). Differently deleted mitochondrial genomes in maternally inherited chronic progressive external ophthalmoplegia. *J. Inherit. Metab. Dis.* **12**, 359–362.

Tatuch, Y. and Robinson, B. H. (1993). The mitochondrial DNA mutation at 8993 associated with NARP slows the rate of ATP synthesis in isolated lymphoblast mitochondria. *Biochem. Biophys. Res. Commun.* **192**, 124–128.

Tatuch, Y., Christodoulou, J., Feigenbaum, A. et al. (1992). Heteroplasmic mitochondrial DNA mutation (T to G) at 8993 can cause Leigh disease when the percentage of abnormal mtDNA is high. *Am. J. Hum. Genet.* **50**, 852–858.

Tatuch, Y., Pagon, R. A., Vlcek, B., Roberts, R., Korson, M. and Robinson, B. H. (1994). The 8993 mtDNA mutation: heteroplasmy and clinical presentation in three families. *Eur. J. Hum. Genet.* **2**, 35–43.

Telerman-Toppet, N., Biarent, D., Bouton, J. M. et al. (1992). Fatal cytochrome *c* oxidase-deficient myopathy of infancy associated with mtDNA depletion. Differential involvement of skeletal muscle and cultured fibroblasts. *J. Inherit. Metab. Dis.* **15**, 323–326.

Tengan, C. H., Kiyomoto, B. H., Rocha, M. S. et al. (1998). Mitochondrial encephalomyopathy and hypoparathyroidism associated with a duplication and a deletion of mitochondrial deoxyribonucleic acid. *J. Clin. Endocrinol. Metab.* **83**, 125–129.

Terauchi, A., Tamagawa, K., Morimatsu, Y., Kobayashi, M., Sano, T. and Yoda, S. (1996). An autopsy case of mitochondrial encephalomyopathy, lactic acidosis and stroke-like episodes (MELAS) with a point mutation of mitochondrial DNA. *Brain Dev.* **18**, 224–229.

Thompson, P. D., Hammans, S. R. and Harding, A. E. (1994). Cortical reflex myoclonus in patients with the mitochondrial DNA transfer RNA-Lys(8344) (MERRF) mutation. *J. Neurol.* **241**, 335–340.

Tiranti, V., Hoertnagel, K., Carrozzo, R. et al. (1998). Mutations of SURF-1 in Leigh disease associated with cytochrome c oxidase deficiency. *Am. J. Hum. Genet.* **63**, 1609–1621.

Traff, J., Holme, E., Ekbom, K. and Nilsson, B. Y. (1995). Ekbom's syndrome of photomyoclonus, cerebellar ataxia and cervical lipoma is associated with the tRNA(Lys) A8344G mutation in mitochondrial DNA. *Acta Neurol. Scand.* **92**, 394–397.

Tranchant, C., Mousson, B., Mohr, M. et al. (1993). Cardiac transplantation in an incomplete Kearns–Sayre syndrome with. *Neuromusc. Disord.* **3**, 561–566.

Tritschler, H. J., Andreetta, F., Moraes, C. T. et al. (1992). Mitochondrial myopathy of childhood associated with depletion of mitochondrial DNA. *Neurology* **42**, 209–217.

Trounce, I., Neill, S. and Wallace, D. C. (1994). Cytoplasmic transfer of the mtDNA nt 8993 T→G (ATP6) point mutation associated with Leigh syndrome into mtDNA-less cells demonstrates cosegregation with a decrease in state III respiration and ADP/O ratio. *Proc. Natl. Acad. Sci. USA* **91**, 8334–8338.

Tsukuda, K., Suzuki, Y., Kameoka, K. et al. (1997). Screening of patients with maternally transmitted diabetes for mitochondrial gene mutations in the tRNA[Leu(UUR)] region. *Diabet. Med.* **14**, 1032–1037.

Tulinius, M. H., Oldfors, A., Holme, E. et al. (1995). Atypical presentation of multisystem disorders in two girls with mitochondrial DNA deletions. *Eur. J. Pediatr.* **154**, 35–42.

Ujike, H., Wakagi, T., Kohira, I., Kuroda, S., Otsuki, S. and Sato, T. (1993). MELAS without ragged red fibers or lactic acidosis diagnosed by. *Jpn. J. Psychiatry Neurol.* **47**, 637–641.

Valanne, L., Paetau, A., Suomalainen, A., Ketonen, L. and Pihko, H. (1996). Laminar cortical necrosis in MELAS syndrome: MR and neuropathological observations. *Neuropediatrics* **27**, 154–160.

van den Heuvel, L., Ruitenbeek, W., Smeets, R. et al. (1998). Demonstration of a new pathogenic mutation in human complex I deficiency: A 5 bp duplication in the nuclear gene encoding the 18 kD (AQDQ) subunit. *Am. J. Hum. Genet.* **62**, 262–268.

van den Ouweland, J. M., Lemkes, H. H., Ruitenbeek, W. et al. (1992). Mutation in mitochondrial tRNA(Leu)(UUR) gene in a large pedigree with. *Nat. Genet.* **1**, 368–371.

van den Ouweland, J. M., Lemkes, H. H., Trembath, R. C. et al. (1994). Maternally inherited diabetes and deafness is a distinct subtype of diabetes and associates with a single point mutation in the mitochondrial tRNA(Leu(UUR)) gene. *Diabetes* **43**, 746–751.

Verma, A., Moraes, C. T., Shebert, R. T. and Bradley, W. G. (1996). A MERRF/PEO overlap syndrome associated with the mitochondrial DNA 3243 mutation. *Neurology* **46** , 1334–1336.

Vialettes, B., Paquis-Fluckinger, V., Silvestre-Aillaud, P. et al. (1995). Extra-pancreatic manifestations in diabetes secondary to mitochondrial DNA point mutation within the tRNALeu(UUR) gene. *Diabetes Care* **18**, 1023–1028.

Vilarinho, L., Santorelli, F. M., Rosas, M. J., Tavares, C., Melo-Pires, M. and DiMauro, S. (1997). The mitochondrial A3243G mutation presenting as severe cardiomyopathy. *J. Med. Genet.* **34**, 607–609.

Wallace, D. C., Zheng, X. X., Lott, M. T. et al. (1988). Familial mitochondrial encephalomyopathy (MERRF): genetic, pathophysiological and biochemical characterization of a mitochondrial DNA disease. *Cell* **55**, 601–610.

Wilichowski, E., Gruters, A., Kruse, K. et al. (1997). Hypoparathyroidism and deafness associated with pleioplasmic large scale rearrangements of the mitochondrial DNA: a clinical and molecular genetic study of four children with Kearns–Sayre syndrome. *Pediatr. Res.* **41**, 193–200.

Yamadori, I., Kurose, A., Kobayashi, S., Ohmori, M. and Imai, T. (1992). Brain lesions of the Leigh-type distribution associated with a mitochondriopathy of Pearson's syndrome: light and electron microscopic study. *Acta Neuropathol. (Berlin)* **84**, 337–341.

Yamamoto, M. and Nonaka, I. (1988). Skeletal muscle pathology in chronic progressive external ophthalmoplegia with ragged-red fibers. *Acta Neuropathol.* **76**, 558.

Yamamoto, M., Koga, Y., Ohtaki, E. and Nonaka, I. (1989). Focal cytochrome *c* oxidase deficiency in various neuromuscular diseases. *J. Neurol. Sci.* **91**, 207.

Yamazaki, M., Igarashi, H., Hamamoto, M., Miyazaki, T. and Nonaka, I. (1991). A case of mitochondrial encephalomyopathy with schizophrenic psychosis, dementia and neuroleptic malignant syndrome. *Rinsho Shinkeigaku.* **31**, 1219–1223.

Yanagisawa, K., Uchigata, Y., Sanaka, M. et al. (1995). Mutation in the mitochondrial tRNA(leu) at position 3243 and spontaneous abortions in Japanese women attending a clinic for diabetic pregnancies. *Diabetologia* **38**, 809–815.

Yang, C. Y., Lam, H. C., Lee, H. C. et al. (1995). MELAS syndrome associated with diabetes mellitus and hyperthyroidism: a case report from Taiwan. *Clin. Endocrinol.* **43**, 235–239.

Yasui, M., Kihira, T., Ota, K. et al. (1993). A case of chronic progressive external ophthalmoplegia with pituitary hypothyroidism. *No To Shinkei* **45**, 741–745.

Yoneda, M., Tanno, Y., Horai, S., Ozawa, T., Miyatake, T. and Tsuji, S. (1990). A common mitochondrial DNA mutation in the t-RNA(Lys) of patients with myoclonus epilepsy associated with ragged-red fibers. *Biochem. Int.* **21**, 789–796.

Yorifuji, T., Kawai, M., Momoi, T. et al. (1996). Nephropathy and growth hormone deficiency in a patient with mitochondrial tRNA(Leu(UUR)) mutation. *J. Med. Genet.* **33**, 621–622.

Yoshida, R., Ishida, Y., Abo, K. et al. (1995). Hypertrophic cardiomyopathy in patients with diabetes mellitus associated with mitochondrial tRNA(Leu)(UUR) gene mutation. *Intern. Med.* **34**, 953–958.

Zeviani, M. (1992). Nucleus-driven mutations of human mitochondrial DNA. *J. Inherit. Metab. Dis.* **15**, 456–471.

Zeviani, M., Servidei, S., Gellera, C., Bertini, E., DiMauro, S. and DiDonato, S. (1989). An autosomal dominant disorder with multiple deletions of mitochondrial DNA starting at the D-loop region. *Nature* **339**, 309–311.

Zeviani, M., Gellera, C., Antozzi, C. et al. (1991). Maternally inherited myopathy and cardiomyopathy: association with mutation in mitochondrial DNA tRNA(Leu)(UUR). *Lancet* **338**, 143–147.

Zeviani, M., Muntoni, F., Savarese, N. et al. (1993). A MERRF/MELAS overlap syndrome associated with a new point mutation in the mitochondrial DNA tRNA(Lys) gene. [Published erratum appears in *Eur. J. Hum. Genet.* (1993) **1**, 124.] *Eur. J. Hum. Genet.* **1**, 80–87.

Zheng, X. X., Shoffner, J. M., Voljavec, A. S. and Wallace, D. C. (1990). Evaluation of procedures for assaying oxidative phosphorylation enzyme activities in mitochondrial myopathy muscle biopsies. *Biochem. Biophys. Acta* **1019** , 1–10.

Zhu, Z., Yao, J., Johns, T. et al. (1998). SURF1, encoding a factor involved in the biogenesis of cytochrome c oxidase. *Nat. Genet.* **20**, 337–343.

Zupanc, M. L., Moraes, C. T., Shanske, S., Langman, C. B., Ciafaloni, E. and DiMauro, S. (1991). Deletion of mitochondrial DNA in patients with combined features of Kearns–Sayre and MELAS syndromes. *Ann. Neurol.* **29**, 680–683.

30

Ion channel disorders of muscle

Louis J. Ptáček and Saïd Bendahhou

Introduction

Electrical excitability of skeletal muscle cells results from a balance of inhibitory and excitatory influences. Ionic concentration gradients established by ATP-dependent pumps can be maintained because the lipid bilayer is an extremely good insulator. Once ionic concentrations are established, movement of one or more ions down their respective concentration gradients can establish voltage differences across a membrane. Movement of Cl^- down their concentration gradient through passive, voltage-gated ion channels results in polarization of the resting membrane. At rest, membrane conductance results from movement of Cl^-. Similar movement of sodium ions through voltage-gated ion channels is responsible for generating action potentials in human skeletal muscle. Movement of potassium and Cl^- through channels opened by membrane depolarization is the basis of repolarization. The depolarization of the plasma membrane caused by sodium ion flux is transmitted along the T-tubule membrane thereby propagating the depolarization throughout the cell. This electrical depolarization initiates a conformational change of voltage-sensitive L-type calcium channels that physically interact with the ryanodine receptor in the sarcoplasmic reticulum (SR), in turn leading to opening of the calcium slow-release channel of the ryanodine receptor. It is the Ca^{2+} released from the SR that results in mechanical activation of the contractile myofibrils within the muscle cells. Disruption of any of these cellular functions would be expected to result in abnormal excitability of cells. The myotonic disorders have long been recognized as disorders of muscle membrane excitability, since neither nerve block nor neuromuscular junction blockade with curare alters the myotonia in these patients. They are, therefore, logical candidates as the site of defect in the periodic paralyses/nondystrophic myotonias (Ptáček et al., 1991a,b, 1993a).

It is not surprising that the disruption of the balance of excitability of muscle cells might lead to neurological phenotypes. However, large changes in excitability of muscle or nerve may well be lethal. Therefore, nature selects against such major changes. A growing body of evidence suggests that subtle changes in some ion channels can lead to a slight increase in membrane excitability that results in a neurological phenotype. Interestingly, these phenotypes are frequently episodic. That is, under many circumstances, muscle (or nerve) may be functioning properly; however, a precipitating event can lead to abnormal excitability resulting in one of any number of phenotypes of periodic paralysis, an episodic movement disorder or epilepsy (depending on the tissue involved). In this chapter, discussion will be focused on a number of muscle disease phenotypes that are known to result from specific mutations of ion channels.

Proteins involved with muscle membrane excitability and excitation–contraction coupling

Acetylcholine receptor

Electrical signals from motor neurons are transduced to biochemical signals at the presynaptic nerve terminal. Acetylcholine (ACh) is released into the synaptic cleft and binds to the ACh receptor (AChR) thereby leading to Na^+ conductance at the motor endplate through AChR-associated sodium channels. The ACh receptor is a complex of proteins that can lead to myasthenic syndromes when mutated (Chapter 32).

Voltage-gated cation channel structure

A family of genes encoding voltage-gated cation channel α-subunits has been cloned from various species. These cDNAs represent genes that share significant DNA homology with one another. The functional subunits of sodium, calcium and potassium channels are all homologous. Voltage-dependent sodium and calcium channels are membrane proteins that consist of a single large polypeptide containing 1800 to 2000 amino acid residues. The proteins show a high degree of evolutionary conservation in regions presumed to be critical for channel function. The conserved regions include areas thought to function in voltage-sensitive gating, inactivation and ion selectivity. There are four regions of internal homology in voltage-gated sodium and calcium channels (domains I to IV) each encompassing 225 to 325 amino acid residues (Ptáček et al., 1991b). In potassium channels, there is only a single domain, and four of these molecules must come together to form a functional channel. Analysis of these repeat domains has revealed at least six hydrophobic segments within each domain (Fig. 30.1). These segments (S1 to S6) are putative transmembrane helices and are located at conserved regions in each domain (Ptáček et al., 1991b). The S4 helix contains a repeating motif with a positively charged amino acid at every third position and serves as a 'voltage sensor' for the channel.

Potassium channel

Potassium channels are formed by an α-subunit with a single domain with six membrane-spanning segments (Fig. 30.1). Four α-subunits must associate as a multimer in order to form a functional channel. This multimer is thought to associate with a single β-subunit. As noted above, the positively charged S4 segment is known to act as the voltage sensor for these channels. Since the potassium channel α-subunit has only one domain, there is no cytoplasmic loop between domains (as in sodium channels where interdomain III–IV is the inactivation particle, see below). A series of very elegant studies has shown that the N-terminal portion of the potassium channel α-subunit protein functions as the inactivation gate (Hoshi et al., 1990). Since there are no skeletal muscle disorders yet recognized resulting from potassium channel mutations, these channels will not be discussed further here. However, it is quite likely that one or more hyperexcitability disorders of skeletal muscle will eventually be shown to result from mutant potassium channels.

Sodium channel

A family of genes encoding voltage-gated sodium channel α-subunits has been cloned from *Drosophila*, electric eel, rat and human. These cDNAs represent genes that share significant DNA homology with one another. The functional subunits of these sodium channels are homologous to potassium and calcium channels (Fig. 30.1); together they form a large family of ion channel proteins. Voltage-dependent sodium channels are membrane proteins that consist of a single large polypeptide of approximately 260000 molecular weight containing 1800 to 2000 amino acid residues and are 25 to 30% carbohydrate by weight. There are four regions of internal homology in sodium channels (domains I to IV). Interestingly, these domains are each homologous to the potassium channels above. Sodium channels have presumably arisen from gene duplication and reduplication events such that four homologous domains are now in tandem. A single sodium channel peptide is thought to form a functional channel (in contrast to potassium channels where the functional channel is a tetramer of single-domain subunits). In addition to the α-subunit, mammalian sodium channels may contain one or more smaller β-subunits. They serve, in part, to modulate channel kinetics in vivo (Isom et al., 1994).

Calcium channel

The skeletal muscle dihydropyridine (DHP) receptor is a complex of five subunits (α_1, α_2, β, γ, δ,). The α_1-subunit forms the structural channel and is homologous to voltage-gated sodium channels (Fig. 30.1). DHP receptors serve two functions, excitation–contraction (EC) coupling and voltage-gated calcium conductance. When expressed in vitro, this protein induces calcium currents that are voltage sensitive and can be blocked by DHPs (Tanabe et al., 1988). In addition, this protein is critical for EC coupling in skeletal muscle. However, calcium conductance through this channel is not necessary for EC coupling. In vitro study of muscle cells in a calcium-free bath shows preservation of EC coupling. The calcium ions that ultimately lead to activation of the contractile apparatus of muscle cells are released from slow-release channels (ryanodine receptor 1 (RYR1), see below) in the SR. Muscular dysgenesis is an autosomal recessive disease in mice caused by a single base pair deletion in the DHP receptor, which prevents its expression (Powell and Fambrough, 1973; Chaudhari, 1992). Muscular dysgenesis is caused by a lethal mutation, resulting in complete absence of skeletal muscle contraction owing to the failure of depolarization of the T-tubular membrane to trigger calcium release from the SR. EC coupling can be restored to muscular dysgenesis myotubes growing in culture when they are transfected with a vector containing cDNA for the wild-type DHP receptor (Tanabe et al., 1988).

The S4 segments of this voltage-gated calcium channel also function as voltage sensors for both EC coupling and calcium conductance. Movements of these charged parts

(a) **Potassium channels**

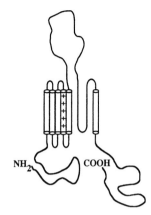

(b) **Sodium and calcium channels**

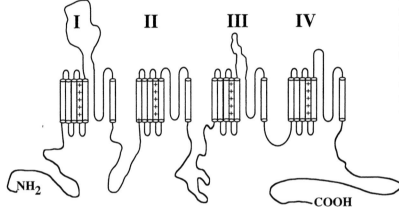

(c) **Chloride channels**

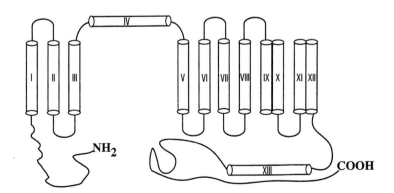

Fig. 30.1. Voltage-gated ion channels. (*a*) Potassium channels are single-domain proteins with six membrane-spanning segments. Four of these proteins must coassemble in a tetramer to form a functional channel. The S4 segment has a high charge density, with arginine and lysine residues (+) at every third position. This part of the channel serves as a voltage sensor by responding to changes in membrane potential. The N-terminus of the protein is an inactivation particle, which falls into the conducting pore to inactivate the channels after they have opened. (*b*) Sodium and calcium channels share homology with potassium channels but have four domains in tandem that are thought to have resulted from a gene duplication and reduplication of a progenitor potassium channel-like gene. A single protein subunit is thought to form a functional channel. Each of the four domains in the sodium and calcium channel proteins share homology with the one domain of potassium channels. (*c*) A model of the voltage-gated chloride channel from skeletal muscle is shown; much less is known about this protein. It has 13 hydrophobic segments but not all of these apparently cross the membrane. Details regarding orientation of the different segments are not entirely clear, particularly for domains IX through XII. These channels share no homology with the voltage-gated cation channels.

of the proteins could, for example, occur in response to depolarization and lead to alterations of the protein conformation. This, in turn, could lead to interaction of the cytoplasmic loop between domains II and III with the RYR1 in such a way as to lead to opening of a calcium channel in the SR (Tanabe et al., 1990). Opening of this RYR1 channel allows calcium from the SR to move into the cytoplasm where it interacts with the contractile proteins to effect muscle contraction (Fig. 30.2).

Voltage-gated chloride channel structure

The skeletal muscle chloride channel (ClC-1) is a member of an extended gene family expressed in a wide range of organisms. Genes for voltage-gated chloride channel have been cloned more recently than those for the other ion channels (Jentsch et al., 1990; Steinmeyer et al., 1991; Thiemann et al., 1992) and much less is known about their structure and molecular properties. The chloride channel protein is about 1000 amino acid residues in length and 90–100 kDa. Hydropathy plots predict 12 (or 13) membrane-spanning segments (Fig. 30.1). More recent models suggest that only 10 of these segments actually traverse the membrane. Biophysical data led to a kinetic model in which chloride channels were thought to form homodimers, the so-called double-barrelled channel (Hanke and Miller, 1983; Bauer et al., 1991).

Ryanodine receptor

The skeletal muscle calcium release channel RYR1 is a large ligand-gated ion channel localized in specialized areas of the SR. The channel protein consists of four subunits (560 kDa) and four small 12 kDa binding proteins. The RYR1 acts as a calcium-release channel and as a foot structure bridging the gap between the SR and the T-tubules. The gene for RYR1 is a complex structure that consists of 106 exons of a total 160 kb (Phillips et al., 1996). In skeletal muscle, calcium release is triggered by direct activation of RYR1 by the voltage-gated calcium channel (DHP receptor) located at the cell membrane (Fig. 30.2) (Rios and Pizarro, 1991).

Definitions

Myotonia

The myotonic muscle disorders represent a heterogeneous group of clinically similar diseases sharing the common feature of myotonia: delayed relaxation of muscle after voluntary contraction (action myotonia, Fig. 30.3) or mechanical stimulation (percussion myotonia). Electrophysiologically, myotonia is characterized by highly orga-

nized repetitive electrical activity of muscle fibres (Fig. 30.4). The repetitive discharges wax and wane in amplitude and frequency, which results in the classic 'dive-bomber' quality to this phenomenon when heard on an audio monitor.

Warm-up phenomenon

Myotonia represents abnormal relaxation of muscle. Not surprisingly, it was noted early on that patients with myotonia congenita were very stiff. They complain that they are particularly stiff after sitting or resting for a period of time and that they have difficulty getting up out of chairs. Their initial movements are stiff and robot-like but muscles become more fluid as they warm up. For this reason, this clinical symptom was termed the 'warm-up phenomenon'. This finding can be seen in patients with myotonia of different causes but is particularly noted in patients with myotonia congenita.

Paradoxical myotonia

In contrast to the warm-up phenomenon, some patients with myotonia have worsening of their symptoms with repeated muscle activity. This is termed paradoxical myotonia. It is particularly noted in patients with paramyotonia congenita but also in patients with hyperkalaemic periodic paralysis (hyperKPP). For example, in paramyotonia congenita, patients closing their eyes tightly and repeatedly develop increasing difficulty opening their eyes owing to worsening myotonia of the orbicularis oculi muscles. This can be a particularly helpful sign in making the diagnosis of paramyotonia congenita.

Potassium sensitivity

The periodic paralyses have been classified into both hypo- and hyperkalaemic forms. This has created a significant amount of misunderstanding among clinicians, however, since many patients with hyperKPP have normal potassium levels during their attacks. Potassium sensitivity, especially in hyperKPP, refers to the ability to precipitate attacks by manipulation of the serum potassium. For example, in hyperKPP, patients may have normal potassium levels during spontaneous attacks but, invariably, it is possible to induce attacks by administration of adequate doses of potassium. In contrast, patients with hypokalaemic periodic paralysis (hypoKPP) always have low serum potassium levels during their spontaneous clinical attacks. This can also be confusing as patients with paramyotonia congenita can also have low potassium levels during attacks. As noted below, these observations can be

Dihydropyridine receptor

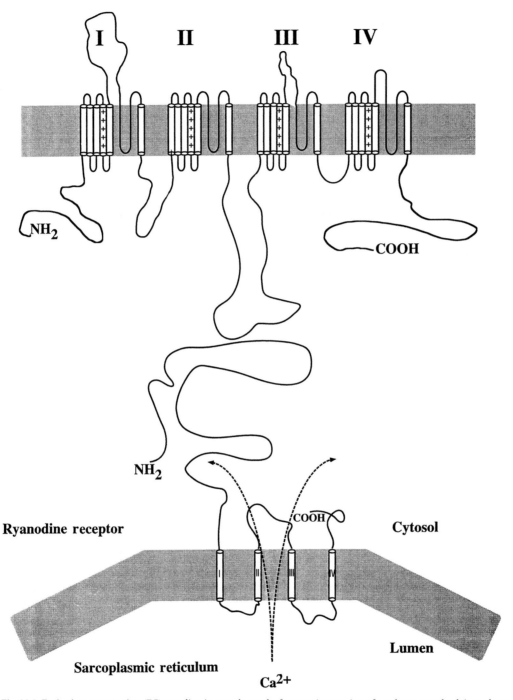

Fig. 30.2. Excitation–contraction (EC) coupling in muscle results from an interaction of a voltage-gated calcium channel (dihydropyridine receptor) skeletal muscle. This voltage-gated calcium channel serves as a voltage sensor for changes in membrane potential. An interaction of the cytoplasmic loops between domains II and III with the 'foot region' of the ryanodine receptor leads to opening of a slow-release calcium channel in the sarcoplasmic reticulum. Depolarization of the membrane as sensed by the voltage-gated calcium channel leads to a conformational change in the ryanodine receptor and opening of the slow-release channel with subsequent movement of Ca^{2+} out of the sarcoplasmic reticulum into the cytosol.

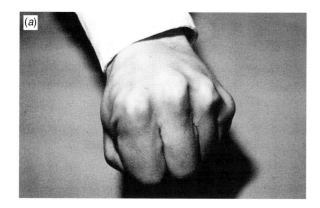

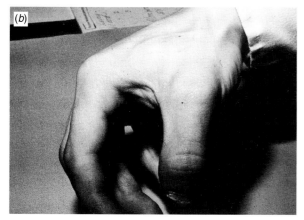

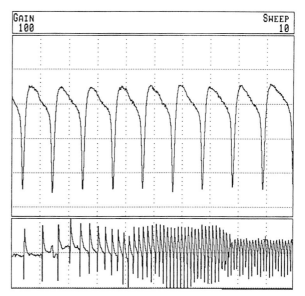

Fig. 30.4. Electrical myotonia can be examined by electromyography. The placement of a needle in the abductor pollicus brevis shows prominent myotonia in the patient shown in Fig. 30.3. A portion of the myotonic run shown at the bottom of the figure is ended in the upper part of the figure to show the prominent myotonic discharges. Of note, in this figure, is the waxing and waning amplitude and frequency that is characteristic of myotonia.

Fig. 30.3. In action myotonia, patients have difficulty in muscle relaxation. A patient with myotonia is asked to clench his fists (*a*) and then to open it as quickly as he can. When the patient attempts to release his grip, he has difficulty since the muscle is not relaxing normally. This results in a slow opening of the hands (*b*). The patients are able to open the fingers somewhat by flexing the wrist and making use of the extensor tendons of the fingers to counteract the muscles of flexion that were activated and not relaxing.

very helpful in making a diagnosis in a patient but great care must be taken as they can also lead to misdiagnosis.

Temperature sensitivity

Temperature-sensitive mutants are well recognized in organisms such as *Drosophila melanogaster*; temperature-sensitive mutants in humans are uncommon. A notable exception however, are those involved in paramyotonia congenita. In these patients, muscle cooling leads to worsening of myotonia initially, which may transition into paralysis. Therefore, in these patients, lowered muscle temperature can elicit both myotonia and episodic weakness. All patients with myotonia, and many patients without muscle diseases, complain of stiffness with muscle

cooling. Therefore, to make a diagnosis of temperature-sensitive myotonia or periodic paralysis, it is critical that objective measures of temperature sensitivity be obtained. These have been well described in the literature (Jackson et al., 1994) and primarily refer to the ability to elicit compound motor action potential decrement with muscle cooling. Attempts to cool the muscle by placing the forearm, for example, in ice water are often unsuccessful since this is uncomfortable for patients. In fact, because of the discomfort, it is difficult to get the muscle core temperature down significantly when cooling the forearm in this way. It is much more effective to place the patient's forearm in a 15 °C waterbath for 30 to 45 minutes. This is generally well tolerated by patients and also is much more successful in reducing the core muscle temperature. It is possible to use a needle thermistor to measure the core temperature if such documentation is desired.

Clinical phenotypes

Periodic paralyses and nondystrophic myotonias

The periodic paralyses have traditionally been divided into hypokalaemic, hyperkalaemic, normokalaemic and paramyotonic forms (Ptáček et al., 1993a). During the 1990s, a combination of electrophysiological and molecular biological studies have clarified the classification of the disease. It has become apparent that there are two broad categories of disease: hypoKPP and hyperKPP. All forms of periodic paralysis are either autosomal dominantly inherited or occur as sporadic cases that are probably the result of new mutations. HyperKPP usually results from a disorder of the skeletal muscle voltage-gated sodium channel. The molecular alterations have been defined for many patients (Ptáček et al., 1991b; Rojas et al., 1991). It is becoming clear that a number of disorders once considered separate entities are in fact allelic to hyperKPP including paramyotonia congenita (Ptáček et al., 1992a; McClatchey et al., 1992a), and a form of myotonia without periodic paralysis that is potassium sensitive (Ptáček et al., 1994a). There are, however, a small proportion of patients with hyperKPP that is not allelic (Wang et al., 1993). The gene causing hypoKPP has also been identified (Ptáček et al., 1994a; Fouad et al., 1997). Three mutations have been identified to date and lead to phenotypically similar disorders. Remarkably, transient weakness also characterizes a disorder of the chloride channel (Ptáček et al., 1993a). This chapter describes the clinical and historical features of the periodic paralyses, delineates the laboratory abnormalities that have been identified in patients, reviews genetic and molecular studies in the disorders, relates molecular abnormalities to phenotypic variation and summarizes current treatment for symptoms of the disorders.

Hyperkalaemic periodic paralysis

Patients who had normo- or hyperkalaemia rather than hypokalaemia during attacks of weakness were first recognized in 1951 (Tyler et al., 1951). Patients with hyperKPP have the onset of symptoms in infancy or early childhood; frequently, myotonia is clinically evident in infancy and episodic weakness develops subsequently. Attacks are frequent, last much shorter periods of time than those of hypoKPP (often 30 minutes to 2 to 3 hours) but are similarly precipitated by rest after exercise and by emotional stress. In these patients, hyperkalaemia is not present during many attacks of weakness. Potassium levels tend to rise at the onset of weakness but are often normal and occasionally fall to hypokalaemic levels. The disease is defined by the patient's response to potassium rather than by the absolute potassium level during attacks. Patients are initially of normal strength during attack-free intervals but develop persistent interattack weakness after years of attacks (Ptáček et al., 1993b). Myotonia is often but not invariably evident during attack-free intervals.

Laboratory evaluation frequently discloses slightly elevated serum potassium at times when patients are not reporting attacks and the serum creatine kinase level is often elevated. Other serum parameters are normal. Electromyography often discloses myotonia; muscle histology is usually abnormal and may show vacuoles, degenerating or atrophic fibres. Most patients described as having 'normokalaemic periodic paralysis' have been potassium sensitive and, therefore, cannot be distinguished from those with hyperKPP (Ptáček et al., 1993a). Rare kindreds have been reported where neither elevating nor lowering the serum potassium level provoked attacks. Controversy exists concerning the relationship of this disorder to hyperKPP. It is not clear whether these patients are distinct from the population of typical patients with hyperKPP.

Paramyotonia congenita

Eulenburg originally described paramyotonia congenita, noting paradoxical myotonia (myotonia that worsens with activity), cold exacerbation of myotonia and attacks of weakness that are provoked by cold or can occur without cold exposure (Eulenburg, 1886). Paradoxical myotonia contrasts with the expected improvement with exercise seen in most forms of classical myotonia. Interattack weakness commonly develops after years of attacks much as in other forms of periodic paralyses.

Laboratory studies are normal in many patients with paramyotonia congenita. Electromyography usually demonstrates myotonia. Muscle histology may show degenerating fibres, vacuoles or atrophic fibres. The cold sensitivity that is seen in paramyotonia congenita can be quantified using electromyography with standard protocols (Jackson et al., 1994).

Patients with paramyotonia congenita are often sensitive to potassium. As with hyperKPP, weakness can sometimes also be provoked by *hypo*kalaemic challenge (Ptáček et al., 1993a).

Phenotype of mixed potassium and temperature sensitivity

A phenotype that is an interesting hybrid between the potassium- and temperature-sensitive forms of periodic paralysis has been well documented in patients (de Silva et al., 1990). To make this diagnosis, it is necessary to demonstrate weakness induced by potassium loading and to obtain objective measures of temperature sensitivity (Jackson et al., 1994). This disorder may have variable degrees of potassium or temperature sensitivity, one or the other being more prominent in different patients. This diagnosis does not have any bearing on therapy separate from that of either the potassium- or the temperature-sensitive disorders themselves (see below).

Potassium aggravated myotonia

Potassium-aggravated myotonia (PAM) is a sodium channel disorder of particular interest because of the potassium-sensitive myotonia that these individuals demonstrate (Trudell et al., 1987). Their symptoms are, therefore, episodic although they do not have periodic paralysis. The myotonia of these patients is markedly improved by lowering potassium levels. It is not temperature sensitive.

Hypokalaemic periodic paralysis

The clinical syndrome of hypoKPP was first described in 1885 (Westphal, 1885). It was not until 1934, however, that the association of hypokalaemia with the syndrome of periodic paralysis was first identified (Biemond and Daniels, 1934). In the typical patient, an apparently normal person suddenly awakens with severe weakness of the limbs. There is no alteration of consciousness and the limbs are painless. Patients are often unable to walk and at times may be totally quadriplegic. Attacks of weakness typically resolve over 3 to 4 hours but may occasionally persist for as long as 24 hours (Ptáček et al., 1993a). Once the attack has resolved, patients are again completely normal. The weakness that occurs during attacks of paralysis is usually confined to the limbs; facial and respiratory muscle weakness can occasionally occur. Extraocular muscle weakness is rarely, if ever, observed. During attacks of severe weakness, patients lose their muscle stretch reflexes. Patients may have subjective sensory symptoms but tests of sensation are invariably normal. Myotonia cannot be detected by electromyographic examination but eyelid myotonia is frequently present even during attack-free intervals.

Attacks of weakness in hypoKPP typically have their onset in the second decade but can begin as early as three or four years of age. Almost invariably, attacks of familial hypoKPP begin before 30 years of age. The appearance of typical attacks of hypokalaemic weakness in patients after 30 years of age is usually indicative of either thyrotoxic hypoKPP, a secondary cause of hypokalaemia leading to periodic paralysis, or perhaps a similar (but distinct) genetic disorder (Fouad et al., 1997).

Within families, the severity of periodic attacks is greater in males than females. Attacks usually occur either while the patient is sleeping at night or at other times when the patient has rested following exercise. Attacks are precipitated by manoeuvres that lower serum potassium levels, such as high-carbohydrate and high-sodium meals and by emotional stress. Gentle exercise of an affected limb will restore strength to that limb more rapidly than occurs in an unexercised limb.

After years of attacks of paralysis, interattack weakness will appear in many patients and progress in severity, particularly in patients who are untreated. Attack frequency is often reported to diminish with age, but it is frequently replaced by disabling weakness, which ultimately may progress to the point of wheelchair confinement. Patients are often unaware of this weakness early in the course of their illness. They are, moreover, equally unaware of the fact that they are having major fluctuations in strength during times when they consider that their strength is normal. During attack-free intervals, and early in the course of the illness, physical examination is usually normal. The one exception is the presence of eyelid myotonia (Ptáček and Griggs, 1996).

Episodes of weakness occurring in patients with hypoKPP are characteristically associated with low serum potassium levels. In a small proportion of patients, the serum potassium declines but remains within normal limits (Torres et al., 1981). Blood studies in patients with periodic paralysis are unrevealing during attack-free intervals. Muscle biopsy is invariably abnormal during attacks when vacuoles are numerous. It is usual for the biopsy to remain abnormal during attack-free intervals, showing either vacuoles or atrophic changes. Vacuoles have been shown by electron microscopy to be dilated SR, possibly as a result of water movement across the membrane in response to ion fluxes across the sarcolemma.

Approximately two-thirds of patients with hypoKPP have a family history of a disorder, in which case it is invariably autosomal dominant. Approximately one-third of patients occur as sporadic cases; these can then transmit the disease to subsequent generations. Some result from new mutations. Another example of sporadic disease may arise in an affected child of a gene carrier who is nonpenetrant for the mutation (Fouad et al., 1997).

Thyrotoxic hypokalaemic periodic paralysis

Thyrotoxic periodic paralysis usually appears as an acquired, sporadic disorder that resolves with treatment of the underlying thyrotoxicosis; it will recur if thyrotoxicosis recurs. Attacks of thyrotoxic periodic paralysis are invariably associated with hypokalaemia and resemble those of familial hypoKPP. Thyrotoxic periodic paralysis occurs most frequently in oriental adults, although it can occur in all races. Despite the higher incidence of thyrotoxicosis in women, less than 5% of cases of thyrotoxic periodic paralysis occur in women. As many as 10% of thyrotoxic oriental males may develop thyrotoxic periodic paralysis; the proclivity to develop periodic paralysis when thyrotoxic has been transmitted as an autosomal dominant disorder (Ptáček et al., 1993a).

Thyrotoxicosis is often clinically inapparent but is suspected when a patient over the age of 30 years first develops typical periodic paralysis. Examination during attack-free intervals often demonstrates proximal weakness from the thyrotoxicosis. Other signs of thyrotoxicosis may be completely lacking. The usual laboratory indicator of thyrotoxicosis, an elevation of thyroxine, is often lacking. Elevations in triiodothyronine are sometimes present but normal thyroid hormone levels may be found. In such instances a depression of thyroid-stimulating hormone and increased radioactive iodine uptake by the thyroid gland are the sole evidence for thyrotoxicosis (Ptáček et al., 1993a).

Myotonia congenita

Autosomal recessive myotonia (Becker's myotonia)
Becker's myotonia is an autosomal recessive disorder (Becker, 1979) that is associated not only with myotonia but also with transient weakness that can eventually be 'warmed up' to normal strength (Ptáček et al., 1993a). This weakness is, therefore, analogous to typical myotonia, which lessens with repeated muscle contraction. The transient weakness often results in major disability and suggests a diagnosis of either a periodic paralysis or muscular dystrophy. The diagnosis is evident clinically by careful evaluation of patients, because strength is characteristically normal on the initial voluntary contraction and then diminishes rapidly. Repeated muscle contraction then results in a return to normal strength. Muscles are generally large or normal in size, in contrast to the atrophy seen in muscular dystrophy.

Autosomal dominant myotonia (Thomsen's disease)
Thomsen's disease is a disorder characterized by autosomal dominant inheritance and painless myotonia (Ptáček et al., 1993a). Patients do not experience weakness nor can weakness be detected on examination. In fact, these patients often appear Herculean with large, well-developed musculature. The myotonia does, however, 'warm up' with repeated activity such that it may be totally abolished. This warm-up contrasts with the worsening of myotonia (paradoxical myotonia) seen with sodium channel myotonia. Electromyography invariably shows myotonia in all forms of myotonia congenita.

Andersen syndrome

Patients with Andersen syndrome have a potassium-sensitive periodic paralysis and frequent ectopic ventricular premature beats, most commonly bigeminy or bidirectional tachycardia. The recognition of a form of periodic paralysis associated with dysmorphic features, including short stature, hypertelorism, low-set ears, mandibular hypoplasia and clinodactyly, is credited to Andersen (Andersen et al., 1971). Only subsequently, however, was the nature of the periodic paralysis recognized (Tawil et al., 1994; Sansone et al., 1997). Cardiac arrhythmia detected by physical examination is often the presenting manifestation of the disorder. In some patients, the cardiac arrhythmia and periodic paralysis are mirror images of each other in terms of provocative and therapeutic tests: raising serum potassium levels precipitates weakness but normalizes the electrocardiogram, whereas lowering serum potassium improves strength but worsens the electrocardiographic abnormalities. However, there is an increasing awareness that some of these patients are actually hypokalaemic during their attacks (Tawil et al., 1994; Sansone et al., 1997).

Other periodic paralyses

Studies of large populations of patients with periodic paralysis and myotonia with the disorders discussed above have identified a large number of mutations in a number of different genes for muscle membrane ion channel (Ptáček et al., 1993a,b, 1994a,b; Zhang et al., 1996; Fouad et al., 1997). However, there remains a large group of patients in whom no mutations have been identified (L. J. Ptáček and S. Bendahhou, unpublished data). Among these patients with molecularly unexplained disease, some of them are likely to have mutations in other genes (perhaps ion channels?) that are as yet unrecognized. Energies are being directed at identifying such genes which may be predicted from the genetic and physiological studies described below. Another part of this patient population is likely to result from phenocopies and misdiagnosis. For example, some of these patients, though diagnosed as having nondystrophic myotonia or periodic paralysis, may in fact have some other metabolic disorder, or other unusual disorders such as episodic ataxia. In episodic ataxia, the intermittent discoordination is perceived by many patients as weakness and so, based on clinical history, a diagnosis of periodic paralysis will sometimes be made. In fact, it was through serendipity that acetazolamide came to be recognized as a good treatment for patients with episodic ataxia (Griggs et al., 1978). Furthermore, these patients can also be sensitive to potassium levels, which further complicates this differentiation. There are also likely to be other nongenetic causes of episodic weakness, and of a differential diagnosis of hypo- and hyperkalaemia must be examined carefully as sufficiently high or low potassium levels can lead to weakness of a nongenetic type (Table 30.1).

Table 30.1. Differential diagnosis of secondary hypokalaemic periodic paralysis

Thyrotoxic periodic paralysis
Paralysis secondary to urinary K^+ wasting
Hypertension, alkaline urine, metabolic alkalosis
    Primary hyperaldosteronism
    Liquorice intoxication
    Excessive thiazide therapy for hypertension
    Excessive mineralocorticoid therapy for Addison's disease
Normotension, alkaline urine, metabolic acidosis
    Hyperplasia of juxtaglomerular apparatus with
    hyperaldosteronism
Alkaline urine, metabolic acidosis
    Primary renal tubular acidosis
    Fanconi's syndrome
Acid urine, metabolic acidosis
    Chronic ammonium chloride ingestion
    Recovery phase of diabetic coma
    Bilateral ureterocolostomy
    Recovery phase of acute renal tubular necrosis
Antibiotic therapy: Amphotericin β, gentamicin, carbenicillin and
    ticarcillin
Paralysis secondary to gastrointestinal K^+ wastage
    Nontropical sprue
    Laxative abuse
    Pancreatic gastrin-secreting adenoma with severe diarrhoea
    Villous adenoma of the rectum
    Severe or chronic diarrhoea
    Draining of gastrointestinal fistula
    Prolonged gastrointestinal intubation or vomiting
    Clay ingestion
Pharmacotherapy: β-adrenergic agonists, insulin
Athletic training and profuse sweating
Barium-induced periodic paralysis: insecticides and rat poison

Malignant hyperthermia

Malignant hyperthermia (MH) was first identified in 1960 (Denborough and Lovell, 1960). A history of anaesthesia-related deaths was present in 10 of 24 relatives who had received anaesthetics and this suggested that the syndrome was an inherited disorder. A similar syndrome occurs in various strains of pigs and is referred to as either MH or porcine stress syndrome. The syndrome is associated with exposure to halogenated volatile anaesthetics or depolarizing neuromuscular blocking agents in otherwise normal patients (Gronert, 1994). Because of the variability of clinical signs of MH and the similarity of these signs to those of other perioperative complications, a commonly agreed upon set of signs that estimates the likelihood of a MH episode has, until recently, not been firmly established. A MH clinical grading scale has now been developed by agreement among a panel of experts (Larach et al., 1994).

Susceptibility to MH (MHS) cannot be predicted in the absence of a challenge with triggering agents, or a positive family history. In the latter, transmission is as an autosomal dominant trait. The syndrome usually includes several or all of the following signs: temperature elevation, muscle rigidity, systemic acidosis, rhabdomyolysis (elevated serum potassium and creatine kinase values, myoglobinuria) and arrhythmias (Rosenberg, 1988; Gronert, 1994). The earliest signs include masseter muscle rigidity, tachycardia, increased end-tidal carbon dioxide levels, and diffuse muscle rigidity. Hyperthermia usually occurs later in the syndrome and may not occur at all. The most sensitive and specific indicator of MHS is an increased end-tidal carbon dioxide level. Whole-body rigidity after treatment with suxamethonium (succinylcholine), while less sensitive, is very specific for MH provided that a myotonic disorder has been excluded for the patient. The syndrome has a wide range of presentations, from a prolonged onset (hours) and extremely mild signs to rapid onset (seconds to minutes) and death. The syndrome can be fatal if not aborted early in its course. Complete recovery is the most usual course if the appropriate treatment (see below) is promptly administered. In this case, most (or all) of the muscle damage is reversible. While mortality of MH was at one time as high as 80%, it has decreased to about 10% since the widespread availability of dantrolene (Harrison, 1988) (see below).

MH has been identified in both genders, with a male-to-female predominance of about 3 to 1. The disorder also occurs in people of all ethnic backgrounds. In the absence of coexisting neuromuscular disease, 1 in 50000 patients anaesthetized with depolarizing muscle relaxants (e.g. suxamethonium) or volatile inhalational agents (e.g. halothane, isoflurane) suffer fulminant rigidity, rhabdomyolysis, hypercarbia and acidosis (Hogan, 1998). It is critical to distinguish MHS from perioperative conditions with overlapping clinical presentations, such as thyrotoxicosis, sepsis, phaeochromocytoma, transfusion reaction, etc. The syndrome triggered by certain antipsychotic agents, termed the neuroleptic malignant syndrome, while similar to MH in some ways, appears to be a distinctly different entity (Brownell, 1988). Exertional heat stroke may be associated with, but is not identical to, MH (Hopkins et al., 1991).

The prevalence of triggered crises rises to 1 in 5000 patients when surveys are confined to anaesthesia in childhood (O'Flynn et al., 1994) and may be even higher in specific ethnic groups. History of an analogous complication in a close relative is a strong predictor of MHS (Hogan, 1998). Elevated serum creatine kinase values in a relative of someone known to have MHS significantly increase the likelihood of MHS. Also, the presence of coexisting neuromuscular diseases, such as various muscular dystrophies, carnitine palmitoyltransferase II deficiency or Brody myopathy, may elevate the risk of a myopathic episode resembling MH to 50–100%. A complicating feature of MH is that even patients who have undergone an uneventful general anaesthetic may have an episode during a future anaesthesia exposure (Halsall et al., 1979).

The observation that a contracture of peripheral muscle occurred in vitro in response to low doses of caffeine (Kalow et al., 1970) and halothane (Ellis et al., 1971; Ellis and Harriman, 1973) in individuals susceptible to MH formed the basis for a diagnostic test and suggested that skeletal muscle was the primary tissue involved (in vitro contracture test; IVCT). The halothane and caffeine contracture test is the only diagnostic test for MHS. The patient must be referred to a testing centre for the diagnosis of MH, since it requires muscle biopsy and the tissue is not viable for a sufficient length of time for shipment. Furthermore, it is crucial that the surgeon performing the biopsy be very familiar with the procedure, and it is advisable to remove additional small specimens to examine for histochemical evidence of muscle disorder. The primary muscle used is the vastus lateralis. The muscle is usually removed under local anaesthetic, but nontriggering general anaesthesia can be used. There are two protocols used for the in vitro contracture test. There is a European MH Group protocol and a North American MH Group (1984) protocol. Both tests employ halothane or caffeine addition to tissue baths containing fibre bundles and determine the resulting contracture response (increase in resting tension). The sensitivity and specificity of this test is far from perfect. It is common that a patient suffering a MH reaction may have had uneventful anaesthesia exposures in the past. One multicentre trial reported that of 105 individuals surviving fulminant MH events 15 had equivocal IVCT and one had a normal IVCT (Ording et al., 1997).

Hotlines are available for assistance. In the USA this is the MH Association of the United States (1-800-MH-HYPER). The same hotline can be reached from outside the USA, at 1-315-428-7924. In Canada, the contact is the MH Association of Canada (1-416-447-0052). In the UK, the contact is on 01345-333-1111 and in Germany it is 07131-48-20-50. The North American MH Registry was formed as a repository for patient information. The registry has recently merged with the MH Association of the United States and information can be reached by calling 1-800-98-MHAUS.

The genetics of periodic paralysis/non-dystrophic myotonias

The gene for the sodium channel on chromosome 17q (SCN4A)

Physiological abnormalities characterized in vitro in muscle from patients with hyperKPP first suggested a gene coding for a skeletal muscle sodium channel as the site of defect in these patients (Lehmann Horn et al., 1987a). Linkage analysis with genetic probes for sodium channels supported this hypothesis even before the genomic localization of this gene was known (Ptáček et al., 1991a; Fontaine et al., 1990). These data proved that hyperKPP must be caused by mutations in the gene for the sodium channel or in some other gene that resides very close to this. The disease allele in one hyperKPP family is not linked to the sodium channel locus (Wang et al., 1993), suggesting that a second hyperKPP gene is present. However, a large majority of hyperKPP disease alleles are linked to the gene for the sodium channel. Genetic linkage analysis subsequently showed that the nonmyotonic form of hyperKPP is also linked to the sodium channel on chromosome 17 (Ebers et al., 1991). These data suggested that the myotonic and nonmyotonic forms of hyperKPP are allelic disorders.

Hyperkalaemic periodic paralysis with myotonia

Two distinct mutations have been identified in patients with hyperKPP and established the gene for the sodium channel as the disease gene in these families (Ptáček et al., 1991b; Rojas et al., 1991). These two mutations account for a large majority of the hyperKPP families (Feero et al., 1993; Ptáček et al., 1993b, 1994b). The two mutations give rise to amino acid changes (T704M and M1592V) in putative membrane-spanning segments of the sodium channel and are predicted to reside very close to the cytoplasmic side of the membrane (Fig. 30.5). HyperKPP is recognized as a pathological condition in American quarter horses and a mutation in the horse homologue of the skeletal muscle voltage-gated sodium channel has been characterized (Rudolph et al., 1992). It corresponds to F1419L, which results from the homologous mutation in the human gene (Fig. 30.5). This mutation has not yet been seen in human patients with this disease.

Hyperkalaemic periodic paralysis myotonia

Interestingly, though hyperKPP without myotonia breeds true in families and is distinct from the myotonic form of hyperKPP, mutation analysis demonstrated that these patients have one of the mutations described above (Ptáček et al., 1991b). The reason for the phenotypic

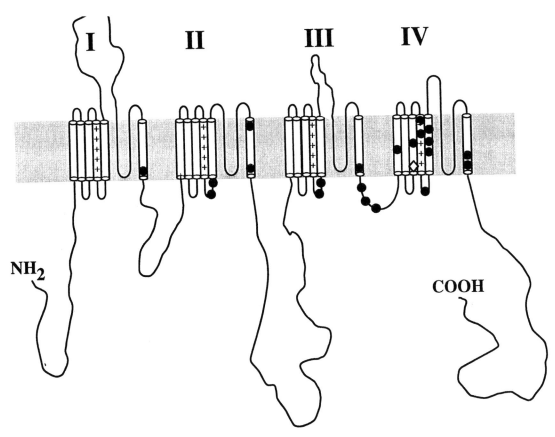

Fig. 30.5. Mutations affecting the sodium channel in the periodic paralyses/nondystrophic myotonias. Twenty-five mutations have been described thus far in the α-subunit of the skeletal muscle sodium channel. The approximate locations of these mutations are shown by black dots. The white diamond in the S3 segment of domain IV represents the homologous location of a mutation that was identified in a horse model of periodic paralysis.

difference between families with and without myotonia is not understood.

The fact that both phenotypes breed true in families with the disease suggests that the modulating factor must be co-segregating with the disease allele. Two possibilities exist. First, there may be a distinct gene closely linked to the gene for the sodium channel that somehow modulates sodium channel function. Second, there may be a normal alteration within the sodium channel itself (polymorphism) that does not cause abnormal sodium channel function but does interact with the mutation causing T704M in such a way as to modulate its abnormal function. Several poly-morphisms are known to exist in the gene for the sodium channel (Rojas et al., 1991; McClatchey et al., 1992b). In either case, the modulating factor would be tightly linked (genetically) to the mutation causing T704M. Then the mutation and the modulating factor would co-segregate and the resulting phenotype would be consistent within any one family. Clinical and electrophysiological charac-terization of additional families with various phenotypes and molecular alterations may reveal other examples where one mutation yields different family-specific phe-notypes. Exploration of the electrophysiological pheno-type and its association with the clinical phenotypes may shed light on sodium channel structure–function relation-ships that are not currently understood.

Paramyotonia congenita

In vitro study of muscle from patients with paramyotonia congenita showed sodium conductance abnormalities that were similar to those seen in hyperKPP (Lehmann-Horn et al., 1987b). These electrophysiological similarities, along with clinical similarities, led to the hypothesis that paramyotonia congenita and hyperKPP are allelic disor-ders. The first genetic support of this hypothesis was the demonstration of genetic linkage of this disease locus to the gene for the sodium channel on chromosome 17 (Ptáček et al., 1991a).

Seven recognized sodium channel mutations are associated with a pure temperature-sensitive phenotype of myotonia and periodic paralysis (giving rise to substitutions S804F, T1313M, L1433R, R1448H, R1448C, R1448P, R1448S; Fig. 30.5) (McClatchey et al., 1992a,b; Ptáček et al., 1993b; Wang et al., 1995; Bendahhou et al., 1999a). Four of these mutations affect the same amino acid residue (1448) in the S4 segment. These mutations replace this arginine residue with cysteine, histidine, proline or serine and therefore neutralize this highly conserved S4 positive charge (the charge on histidine (pK_a6) will be dependent on its local environment but it is not likely to have a strong positive charge). Although the exact functional consequences of neutralizing arginine 1448 in hSkM1 can only be revealed by a detailed electrophysiological study of the mutant channel itself, some insight can be gained from studies of the effects of S4 segment mutants in other voltage-dependent sodium and potassium channels. Site-directed mutagenesis experiments involving the S4 segment of the rat brain II sodium channel and the *Shaker B* potassium channel support the hypothesis that this segment does act as the voltage sensor in the biophysical mechanism of activation (Stuhmer et al., 1989; Papazian et al., 1991). Substitution of a neutral amino acid for individual positively charged residues in S4 of domains I and II of the rat brain II channel decreases the steepness of the voltage dependence of activation and shifts the midpoint of the activation curve along the voltage axis (Stuhmer et al., 1989). Mutations neutralizing charges in the *Shaker* potassium channel S4 have a less predictable effect but also shift both the slope of the activation curve and the location of the curve on the voltage axis. In addition, mutations affecting S4 in the *Shaker* potassium channel indicate coupling between channel activation and inactivation.

A characteristic of the paramyotonia congenita phenotype is the presence of both cold-induced myotonia and intermittent weakness, suggesting that these mutations can, under different physiological circumstances, lead to either repetitive sodium channel activation or failure of activation and onset of paralysis. Although repetitive activity could result from either a shift in the voltage dependence of activation to more negative potentials or a shift of inactivation to more positive potentials, the persistent sodium currents reported in electrophysiological recordings from paramyotonia congenita muscle (Lehmann-Horn et al., 1987b) suggest that channel inactivation may be the process that is primarily affected. It has been shown that failure of sodium channel inactivation, even in a small percentage of the channel population, can lead to membrane depolarization, inactivation of the other normal sodium channels and muscle paralysis (Cannon et al.,

1991). Given the effects of mutations in *Shaker* affecting S4, it is also possible that the mutations described here could affect both inactivation and activation. However, since these mutations insert different amino acids than the substitution studied at the comparable location in *Shaker*, this point can only be resolved through the study of the mutated paramyotonia congenita channel expressed in vitro.

A third mutation affects the adjacent S3 segment and introduces a positively charged arginine for the normal leucine. The mutation giving rise to T1313M occurs in the sodium channel 'inactivation gate', the cytoplasmic loop connecting domains III and IV. This mutation probably interferes, through some stearic alteration, with the ability of this gate to interact normally with its docking site. The mutation giving rise to S804F occurs neither in the 'voltage sensor' or 'inactivation gate' of the sodium channel. Rather, this mutation resides in the S6 segment of domain II in a region predicted to be near the cytoplasmic surface of the membrane (McClatchey et al., 1992b). Unfortunately, results of potassium provocation in these patients are not reported and, therefore, it is possible that patients with this mutation will eventually be reclassified as a mixed hyperKPP/paramyotonia congenita phenotype. McClatchey and her colleagues suggested that the substitution of this polar serine with the larger, nonpolar phenylalanine at the cytoplasmic face of segment S6 of domain II opposite the III–IV interdomain might indicate a role for this part of the channel in receiving the inactivation gate as it pivots to block the channel pore. This is an analogous situation to that suggested for the two human hyperKPP mutations that are also predicted to affect postions located on the cytoplasmic face of the membrane (Ptáček et al., 1993a). The location of these five paramyotonia congenita sodium channel mutations is distinct from the two reported hyperKPP mutations, and this molecular heterogeneity is likely to be responsible for differences in the clinical presentation of these two syndromes.

The temperature sensitivity of symptoms is an interesting aspect of the paramyotonia congenita phenotype and we can speculate as to how this relates to sodium channel defects. Structural changes caused by the mutations reported here might alter the relative energy levels of various conformations associated with different sodium channel gating modes. If the factors stabilizing such states differ in their entropic contributions between mutant and wild-type channels, changes in temperature may differentially affect the preferred channel conformation in each case, and lower temperatures might serve to stabilize the mutant channel in a state associated with an abnormal gating mode. This might be anticipated if, for example, hydrophobic interactions play a prominent role in stabilizing a particular conformation. Alternatively, the mutations may render the channel abnormally sensitive to other cellular processes that are themselves temperature sensitive, such as phosphorylation or G-protein interaction. Ultimately, the correlation between the mutations described here and the pathophysiology of excitation in paramyotonia congenita will require the expression and analysis of human skeletal muscle sodium channels in which this mutation has been introduced.

Mutants with both temperature and potassium sensitivity

Two mutations resulting in changes in the sodium channel (A1156T, G1306V) have been identified in patients with both potassium- and cold-sensitive myotonia and episodic weakness (Fig. 30.5) (de Silva et al., 1990; McClatchey et al., 1992a,b). The relationship of both temperature- and potassium-sensitive phenotype in the same patients remains a mystery. Electrophysiological study of these mutants may lead to understanding of this relationship. Because patients harbouring these two mutations are rare among patients with periodic paralysis, only a few patients have been subjected to rigorous electrophysiological study. It will be important to study additional families with these mutations to determine whether they consistently produce this phenotype. As noted above, the patients with the mutation giving rise to S804F have not been subjected to potassium challenge and may, ultimately, be reclassified as having the hyperKPP/paramyotonia congenita phenotype once that has been clarified. Alternatively, these distinctions may simply represent discreet points on a continuous spectrum of potassium and temperature sensitivity.

Sodium channel myotonia without associated weakness

Despite the lack of episodic weakness in patients with myotonia without associated weakness, the potassium-sensitive and acetazolamide-responsive myotonia suggested that this disorder was also allelic to hyperKPP and paramyotonia congenita (Trudell et al., 1987). This hypothesis was also supported by genetic linkage to the chromosome 17 sodium channel locus (Ptáček et al., 1992a). Muscle from these patients has not yet been studied in vitro.

Patients with one of these mutations (Fig. 30.5) never have episodic weakness. The myotonia caused by I1160V and V1589M is worsened by potassium administration (Heine et al., 1993; Ptáček et al., 1994b). Potassium sensitivity has not yet been assessed in patients with G1306A

and G1306E (Lerche et al., 1993). The reason for muscle membrane hyperexcitability in all of these patients in the absence of any weakness is not known. One possibility is that these mutations result in physiological abnormalities that are more minor than the myotonia in other families. An attenuated physiological abnormality might be sufficiently severe to cause myotonia but not dramatic enough to result in inactivation of most or all of the skeletal muscle sodium channels. Alternatively, if these mutations result in altered activation of sodium channels without affecting channel inactivation and without causing persistent sodium conductance, then muscle cells might be hyperexcitable while retaining their ability to inactivate and reactivate completely. This might yield regenerative action potentials (myotonia) without inactivating all of the voltage-gated sodium channels in muscle (periodic paralysis). The explanation for the behaviour of these mutants may be much clearer once the mutations are expressed in vitro and physiological data are available.

The gene for the calcium channel on chromosome 1q (CACNA1S)

The shared clinical features of periodic paralysis seen in both hypo- and hyperKPP suggested the possibility that these disorders might be allelic. This hypothesis was tested in several large hypoKPP pedigrees using linkage analysis. Recombinants were noted between the disease allele in several hypoKPP families and the gene for the sodium channel locus on chromosome 17 (Fontaine et al., 1991; Casley et al., 1992). This demonstrated that a distinct gene causes hypoKPP in these families. The homogeneity seen in the clinical presentation of hypoKPP families suggests that a single gene may be responsible for this disorder. However, it does not rule out the possibility that more than one gene can lead to the hypoKPP phenotype. Recently, a hypoKPP was reported to be genetically linked to a locus on chromosome 1q (Fontaine et al., 1994; Ptáček et al., 1994a) near a gene encoding a DHP-sensitive, voltage-gated calcium channel. No recombinants were noted between the disease allele in the reported families and an intragenic marker for the gene for the calcium channel. While it is possible that another hypoKPP gene exists, there is, to date, no genetic evidence supporting that hypothesis.

Genetic linkage of the hypoKPP disease allele to the CACNA1S locus led to a search for mutations to prove that this DHP receptor/calcium channel was indeed the affected site in hypoKPP. Two mutations were identified and occurred in adjacent nucleotide positions in the region of the gene encoding the S4 segment of domain IV (Fig. 30.6) (Ptáček et al., 1994a). One of these mutations

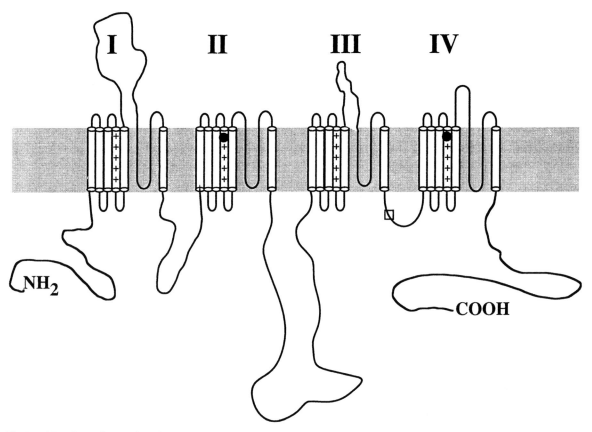

Fig. 30.6. Mutations affecting the calcium channel in hypokalaemic periodic paralysis and malignant hyperthermia susceptibility. Three mutations giving rise to hypokalaemic periodic paralysis have been identified at two sites in the skeletal muscle calcium channel. Both regions involve an arginine residue in the S4 segment of either domain II or IV. R528H occurs in approximatly one-third of hypokalemic periodic paralysis mutants and R1239H occurs in about two-thirds of these patients. A third mutation, resulting in R1239G, at the same location as the R1239H, has only been recognized in a single family. The empty square in the cytoplasmic loop between domains III and IV represents the location of the R1086H mutation recognized in a patient with a malignant hyperthermia-like reaction.

accounted for a large proportion of the disease (about two-thirds of more than 30 hypoKPP families) and arose as a de novo mutation in one patient with sporadic disease. The second mutation was found in only one family (Ptáček et al., 1994a; Fouad et al., 1997). Identification of these mutations, therefore, established the DHP-sensitive calcium channel as the site affected in hypoKPP. Subsequently, a third mutation, resuting in a change in the S4 segment of domain II has been reported (Jurkat Rott et al., 1994; Fouad et al., 1997).

The gene for the chloride channel on chromosome 7q (*CLCN1*)

In vitro physiological studies of patient muscle implicated abnormal chloride conductance in Thomsen disease (Lipicky and Bryant, 1973) and led to genetic linkage

experiments using markers near the human skeletal muscle voltage-gated chloride channel locus. Tight linkage supported the hypothesis that this chloride channel is the site of defect in this disease (Abdalla et al., 1992).

Because of the implication of chloride channels in the mouse model of this disorder (Mehrke et al., 1988) and the known chloride channel mutation in the mouse model of autosomal recessive myotonia (Steinmeyer et al., 1991), mutational analysis of the chloride channel gene *CLCN1* was performed directly. This led to identification of chloride channel mutations in some of these patients (Koch et al., 1992).

A mouse with an autosomal recessive myotonic phenotype was known to have altered chloride conductance (Mehrke et al., 1988). This led Steinmeyer and colleagues to show genetic linkage of *ClC-1* to *adr* and then to identify a transposon insertion in mouse *ClC-1* (Steinmeyer et al.,

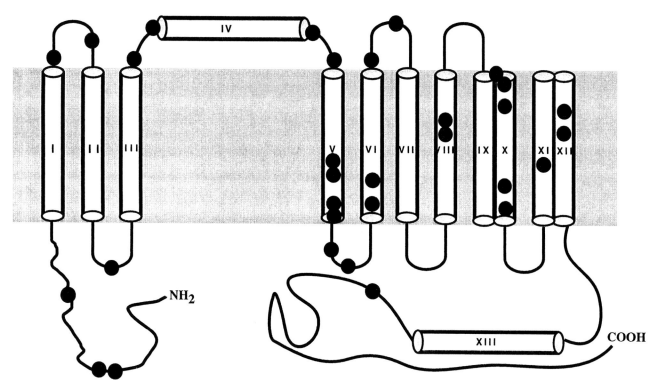

Fig. 30.7. Mutations affecting the chloride channel in myotonia congenita. Thirty-six mutations in the voltage-gated chloride channel have been recognized now in patients with Thompsen's or Becker's myotonia congenita, dispersed throughout the channel and at the locations shown by black dots in the chloride channel protein.

1991). Subsequently, a mutation was noted affecting the chloride channel of humans with the same autosomal recessive myotonia phenotype. This mutation resulted in a phenylalanine to cysteine change in the eighth putative transmembrane domain of the chloride channel (Koch et al., 1992). Subsequently, over 25 mutations resulting in Becker's myotonia congenita have been identified (Fig. 30.7). To date, several mutations have been identified to cause the autosomal dominant myotonia congenita phenotype. The mutation resulting in G230E was noted in three of four families studied by George and colleagues (1993) and affects a part of the chloride channel protein thought to be an extracellular loop between putative membrane-spanning segments D3 and D4. They postulated that the negatively charged glutamic acid residue introduces an electrostatic force that affects conductance of chloride through the channel and/or ion selectivity. A second mutation, results in a proline to leucine substitution at position 480 in the loop connecting the ninth and tenth putative membrane-spanning segments (Steinmeyer et al., 1994). This mutation was noted in descendants of Julius Thomsen, who was afflicted with the disease and was the first to characterize the typical autosomal dominant

form of myotonia congenita that has come to bear his name. Additional mutations giving rise to Thomsen's myotonia congenita mutations have now been identified.

Genetics of malignant hyperthermia

MHS1: the gene for the ryanodine receptor on chromosome 19q (*RYR1*)

Because the gene for malignant hyperpyrexia in the pig is linked to glucose phosphate isomerase and since this enzyme belongs to a linkage group conserved in vertebrates, one group investigated the possibility that susceptibility to MH might be located on human chromosome 19, which carries the gene for glucose phosphate isomerase (McCarthy et al., 1990). They found evidence for linkage to this region of chromosome 19. Another group of investigators found co-segregation of MHS with markers for the gene for RYR1 (MacLennan et al., 1990). They argued from this evidence, as well as from the fact that the function of the product of *RYR1* is the calcium release channel of the SR, that the basic defect in MH resides in this gene.

Subsequently, a growing list of *RYR1* mutations are now known to cause MH, MH with central core disease or central core disease alone (Fujii et al., 1991; Gillard et al., 1991, 1992; Quane et al., 1993, 1994a; Zhang et al., 1993; Keating et al., 1994; Tong et al., 1997, 1999; Manning et al., 1998; Monsieurs et al., 1998; Lynch et al., 1999). Of note, the *RYR1* mutation giving rise to R614C seen in the porcine MHS (Fujii et al., 1991) is also found in human MHS (Gillard et al., 1991).

MHS2: the gene for the sodium channel on chromosome 17q (*SCN4A*)

In some families, it became clear that the MHS phenotype was not linked to the locus on 19q13.1, thus indicating genetic heterogeneity. Linkage in such families led to identification of a second locus on chromosome 17 (Levitt et al., 1992). Support for the location of a gene affecting MHS on 17q and the basis of the disorder caused by mutation in *SCN4A* was strengthened by the report of a family in which both hyperKPP and MH were inherited as autosomal dominant traits and both showed linkage to polymorphic markers within *SCN4A* (Moslehi et al., 1998). Subsequently, we have identified an unusual double mutant (on a single allele) in *SCN4A* (Fig. 30.5), (Bendahhou et al., 2000).

MHS3: the gene for the calcium channel α_2- and δ-subunits on chromosome 7q

Families with MHS were then identified in whom the disease locus was neither on chromosome 19 nor on 17. In some of these, linkage was noted with no recombination to markers flanking *CACNL2A* on chromosome 7 (Iles et al., 1994). Since this gene encodes a subunit of the L-type voltage-dependent calcium channel that is intimately associated at the skeletal muscle triadic junctions with RYR1, it is possible that the mutation is located in this gene.

MHS4: unknown gene on chromosome 3q

In a single German pedigree with classic MH, a fourth MHS locus was mapped (Sudbrak et al., 1995). These investigators found a maximum multipoint LOD score of 3.22 for linkage to markers defining a 1 cM interval on chromosome 3q13.1. The MH phenotype in this family was determined by the IVCT performed on a sample of freshly obtained muscle.

MHS5: gene for the calcium channel on chromosome 1q (*CACN1AS*);

In a collaborative study in three pedigrees in Europe in which disease status was classified according to the European IVCT, a genomewide linkage screen detected two further MHS loci (Robinson et al., 1997). One of these loci is located on 1q32, where an interesting candidate gene (*CACNA1S*) resides. This gene had already been shown to cause another muscle disease, hypoKPP (Ptáček et al., 1994a; Fouad et al., 1997). Subsequently, a mutation in *CACNA1S* (R1086H, Fig. 30.6), distinct from the hypoKPP mutations, was identified in members of a large French family affected by MHS (Monnier et al., 1997).

MHS6: unidentified gene on chromosome 5p

A second locus identified in the above mentioned linkage study was located on chromosome 5p in a Belgian MHS kindred (Robinson et al., 1997). Disease status in this family was also classified according to the European IVCT protocol. Multipoint linkage analysis showed linkage to the region on 5p that coded for an area on chromosome 5 between D5S419 and D5S398. However, no gene or mutation giving rise to MHS has yet been identified at this locus.

Chromosome 1 CPT2 gene

Mitochondrial oxidation of long-chain fatty acids is initiated by the sequential action of carnitine palmitoyltransferase I, which is located in the outer membrane and is detergent labile, carnitine palmitoyltransferase II, which is located in the inner membrane and is detergent stable, and a carnitine-acylcarnitine translocase. In one report, three individuals were identified as heterozygotes for a missense mutation giving rise to R503C in a highly conserved region of carnitine palmitoyl transferase II (Vladutiu et al., 1998). Sequence analysis showed no other change in this gene in these patients. One individual with R503C survived an episode of MH during surgery at four years of age, during which creatine phosphokinase levels were elevated to over 5 000 mU/ml. The patient remained negative for myopathic symptoms at the age of 21 years. The second patient experienced progressive weakness over a 20-year period and myopathic symptoms worsened transiently after surgery. Lymphoblasts and biopsied muscle showed carnitine palmitoyltransferase II activities of 47% and 13% of normal, respectively, in the two patients. Muscle enzymes of oxidative phosphorylation were decreased in activity to values ranging from 22 to 49% of normal (Taggart et al., 1999). The 24-year-old son of the second patient was also

Table 30.2. Mutations affecting the sodium channel

Amino acid change[a]	Disease	Location		Activation shift	Inactivation		Deactivation	Recovery from inactivation
		Domain	Segment		Fast	Slow		
V445M	PAM	I	S6	R	s	E	—	s
I693T	PC	II	S4–S5	L	NC	I	—	NC
T704M	HyperKPP	II	S5	L	s	I	s	s
S804F	PAM	II	S6	NC	s	NC	—	f
A1156T	HyperKPP	III	S4–S5	R	s	NC	—	f
I1160V	PAM	III	S4–S5	NC	NC	NC	s	f
V1293I	PAM	III	S6	L	NC	NC	—	f
G1306A	PAM	III–IV		NC	s	—	—	—
G1306E	PAM			NC	s	NC	s	NC
G1306V	PAM			NC	s	—	—	—
T1313M	PC	III–IV		NC	s	NC	s	f
M1360V	HyperKPP	IV	S1	NC	s	NC	—	f
F1419L	HyperKPP	IV	S3		s			
L1433R	PC	IV	S3	NC	s	—	NC	f
R1448C	PC	IV	S4	NC	s	NC	s	f
R1448H	PC			NC	s	—	—	f
R1448P	PC			NC	s	NC	s	f
R1448S	PC			NC	s	NC	s	f
G1456E	PC	IV	S4	—	—	—	—	—
V1458F	PC	IV	S4	—	—	—	—	—
F1473S	PC	IV	S4–S5	NC	s	—	—	f
F1490L–M1493I	HyperKPP	IV	S5	—	—	—	—	—
I1495F	HyperKPP	IV	S5	L	s	E	NC	s
V1589M	PAM	IV	S6	NC	NC	NC	—	—
M1592V	HyperKPP	IV	S6	L	NC	I	—	f

Notes:

PAM, potassium-aggravated myotonia; PC, paramyotonia congenita; HyperKPP and HypoKPP, hyper- and hypokalaemic periodic paralyses, respectively; NC, no change; s, slow; f, fast; L, left; R, right; E, enhanced; I, impaired

[a] Single code symbols for amino acids.

heterozygous for the R503C substitution and had myopathic symptoms.

Pathophysiology

Sodium channel

Twenty-five missense mutations have been described up to date occurring in *SCN4A*, encoding the human skeletal muscle voltage-gated sodium channel (hSkM1) and causing hyperKPP, paramyotonic congenita, or PAM (Table 30.2). Despite the fact that these mutations have effects scattered throughout the channel, there are three locations considered as 'hotspots': S4 segment of domain IV, interdomain III–IV, and cytoplasmic membrane interface (Fig.

30.5). All of these mutations (except two) have been studied in either *Xenopus* oocytes or in a mammalian cell line to characterize the functional consequences of mutations. This has led to a better understanding of the disease and of normal structure–function relationships.

It is possible to postulate that the amino acids facing the intracellular milieu are implicated in pathophysiology since it was shown that protease treatment of the intracellular face of the membrane resulted in a disruption of sodium channel inactivation (Armstrong et al., 1973). Furthermore, mutagenesis studies showed a critical role in channel fast activation of amino acid residues located in the III–IV cyoplasmic linker, in domain IV at the S4–S5 intracellular loop and the S6 transmembrane segment (West et al., 1992; Tang et al., 1996; Lerche et al., 1997; McPhee et al., 1998). The alteration of channel inactivation by naturally occurring mutations on the extracellular face of the membrane remains 'puzzling' but indicates the functional complexity of the voltage-gated ion channels. Other defects were also reported with these mutations and include shifts of activation and inactivation curves, slowed deactivation, slowed recovery from fast inactivation and either an impairment or an enhancement of slow inactivation. The functional consequences of these mutations are diverse.

Mutations linked to hyperkalaemic periodic paralysis

Seven point mutations are known to cause hyperKPP, resulting in T704M (Cannon and Strittmatter, 1993; Cummins et al., 1993; Yang et al., 1994; Cummins and Sigworth, 1996; Hayward et al., 1997; Bendahhou et al., 1999b), A1156T (Yang et al., 1994), M1360V (Wagner et al., 1997), I1495F (Bendahhou et al., 1999b), M1592V (Hayward et al., 1997) and the F1490L/M1493I double mutant (Bendahhou et al. 2000). These are all localized at the intracellular interface except I1495F, which is located in the transmembrane segment S5 of domain IV. A noninactivating (termed also 'sustained' or 'persistent') sodium current was first thought to underlay the manifestations of either hyperexcitability or inexcitability of the muscle during attacks (Cannon et al., 1991). Many mutants indeed, but not all of them, exhibited a sustained current as a result of a late first opening, reopening or long-lasting opening of the aberrant channels (Table 30.2). Expression studies in the human embryonic kidney cell line (HEK 293) of rT698M (rat homologue of the human T704M) and rM1585V (rat homologue of the human M1592V) revealed the presence of a sustained current that ranged from 3 to 16% of the peak current at the end of 40 millisecond test pulse (Cannon and Strittmatter, 1993). Interestingly, these studies failed to show the sensitivity of the expressed channels to elevated extracellular potassium. This remains puzzling since in vitro studies of myoballs from patients with the M1592V substitution showed that these channels were sensitive to high extracellular potassium concentrations (Lehmann-Horn et al., 1987a). Using the same mutations and the same expression system, other groups have shown that other defects occurred. They proposed that a hyperpolarizing shift of the activation curve causes an increased overlap between the activation and the steady-state inactivation curve that results in a persistent or window current between -70 and -35 mV (Cummins et al., 1993; Rojas et al., 1999). These window currents would activate at negative voltages where the wild-type channels would not yet be activated and can account for enhanced depolarization recorded in muscle fibres of patients with hyperKPP. The voltage dependence of the window current is also consistent with the non-inactivating currents that Lehmann-Horn et al. (1987a) observed in biopsied muscle fibres at membrane potentials between the resting potential (-80 mV) and the normal threshold for the fast sodium current (-65 mV). More recently, studies have revealed that not only fast inactivation could be affected with these mutations but also slow inactivation. An impairment of slow inactivation was first reported with rT698M (Cummins and Sigworth, 1996; Hayward et al., 1997) and confirmed on the human homologue T704M (Bendahhou et al., 1999b; Hayward et al., 1999). This was postulated to explain the manifestation of myotonia in hyperKPP patients. However, our group observed an enhancement of slow inactivation with the I1495F change, which may account for the manifestation of paralysis (Bendahhou et al., 1999b).

Mutations linked to paramyotonic congenita

Ten point mutations have been associated with paramyotonic congenita, which occur in one gene copy: I693T (Plassart-Schiess et al., 1998), T1313M (Hayward et al., 1996), L1433L (Ji et al., 1996), R1448C-H-P-S (Chahine et al., 1994; Yang et al., 1994; Ji et al., 1996; Lerche et al., 1996a; Richmond et al., 1997a; Featherstone et al., 1998; Bendahhou et al., 1999a) G1456E (Sasaki et al., 1999), V1458F and F1473S (Mitrovic et al., 1996) (Table 30.2). These mutations are located in domain II in the linker S5–S6, in the interdomain III–IV and in domain IV, in the S3 transmembrane segment, near the intracellular face of the membrane in the domain IV S4–S5 linker and in the S4 transmembrane segment thought to be the voltage sensor (Fig. 30.5). The last represents the most common mutations in paramyotonic congenita and occurs at arginine 1448. The four mutations found at this location (arginine changed to cysteine, histidine, proline or serine) caused no significant shift in activation despite the location of these mutations in one of the putative voltage-sensing segments. The principal effect of these mutations is that the time constants for fast inactivation are longer. All of these mutations also showed an enhanced recovery from fast inactivation and slower deactivation time constant, which was postulated to account, in part, for the onset of the paramyotonic congenita in these patients. Surprisingly, the most dramatic defect was observed in channel inactivation. Indeed, these mutations resulted in a slower rate of inactivation and a shift in the inactivation curve to hyperpolarizing potentials. Temperature had a slightly greater effect on the fast inactivation kinetics of channels changed at R1448C than it did on either the normal wild-type channels or those carrying substitution R1448H (Chahine et al., 1994). Alkaline extracellular pH, however, slowed the inactivation kinetics of R1448H channels but had no effect on either wild-type or R1448C channels. No mutant showed a sensitivity to extracellular potassium. Slow inactivation was not affected in any of the mutants studied except the I693T substitution, which showed an impairment of slow inactivation (Hayward et al., 1999). Interestingly, this amino acid is located in the domain II linker S5–S6, ten residues away from another mutation that causes hyperKPP (T704M substitution) and that was also shown to impair slow inactivation.

The slower rate of inactivation and the more rapid recovery from inactivation seen in mutant channels paramyotonic congenita may lead to the hyperexcitability and episodes of myotonia observed in these patients. Other groups hypothesized that a combination of slower rate of inactivation and a defect in channel deactivation may account for the onset of the myotonia (Richmond et al., 1997b; Featherstone et al., 1998; Bendahhou et al., 1999a). This was shown using mutant channels with the changes R1448C, R1448P, R1448S and I1160V. The process by which these mutations might lead to the development of paralysis is not clear.

Mutations linked to potassium-aggravated myotonia

Eight missense mutations have been associated with PAM. These result in V445M (Takahashi and Cannon, 1999), S804F (Green et al., 1998), I1160V (Ptáček et al., 1994b), V1293I (Green et al., 1998), G1306A, G1306E and G1306V (Lerche et al., 1993; Hayward et al., 1996) and V1589M. The affected amino acids are located in regions that are shown to be specifically involved in channel fast inactivation (domain I S6, domain II S6, domain III S4–S5, and S6, interdomain III–IV, and domain IV S6). However, expression studies showed mixed results for mutant fast inactivation kinetics. While some of these mutants exhibited a slowed rate of inactivation (V445M and G1306A, G1306E, and G1306V) (Lerche et al., 1993; Takahashi and Cannon, 1999), others did not exhibit any change in channel kinetics (Table 30.2). The V1589M substitution is another example of an amino acid change causing PAM studied in a mammalian cell background (Mitrovic et al., 1994). The principal effect of this change was to destabilize channel inactivation. While the rate of fast inactivation was not altered, steady-state fast inactivation was slightly shifted in the depolarizing direction and recovery from fast inactivation was enhanced. Slow inactivation was not affected in any of the mutant channels causing PAM except in the V445M substitution, where slow inactivation was particularly enhanced (Takahashi and Cannon, 1999). This residue is located in the S6 segment that was shown to be involved in sodium channel slow inactivation. The peculiarity of the

patients with these PAM mutations is their high sensitivity to elevated potassium concentration. Several groups have tested the effect of elevated extracellular potassium concentration on biopsied muscle cells (Cannon et al., 1991), on mutant channels expressed in heterologous systems (Cannon and Strittmatter, 1993) or in theoretical models (Cannon et al., 1993). Despite the sensitivity of the mutant sodium channels in biopsied muscle to high potassium concentration, the same mutant channels expressed in HEK293 cells were not sensitive to elevated extracellular potassium. In a computer-simulated model of an excitable muscle membrane, it was shown that high-extracellular potassium concentrations, only in conjunction with defects in both channel deactivation and recovery from inactivation, can produce an action potential train that may underlay myotonia in patients with the I1160V substitution (Richmond et al., 1997a). The heterologous expression systems may be lacking endogenous factors that are necessary for the manifestations of myotonia and paralysis after potassium ingestion. The role of potassium levels in the manifestation of PAM remains unclear.

Calcium channel

Unlike sodium, chloride and calcium release channels, few mutations have been identified on the L-type calcium channels (DHP receptor). Three mutations were found in patients suffering from hypoKPP and one mutation in patients with MH (Monnier et al., 1997). Interestingly, the hypoKPP substitutions are located in two segments that presumably contribute to the calcium channel voltage sensor (Fig. 30.6): R528H, R1239H, and R1239G (Jurkat Rott et al., 1994; Ptáček et al., 1994a; Fouad et al., 1997).

The location of the three substitutions within the putative voltage sensor are expected to affect calcium channel voltage dependence of activation. Studies were conducted both on myotubes from patients with hypoKPP and on mutant channels overexpressed in heterologous expression systems. When studied in biopsied myotubes, R528H mutant channels exhibited a dramatic hyperpolarizing shift in the inactivation curve (Sipos et al., 1995). This was not confirmed by other groups since either a modest hyperpolarizing shift or even no change in the voltage dependence of steady-state inactivation were reported (Lapie et al., 1996; Lerche et al., 1996b). An erratum was published later to show that in biopsied muscle, no significant shift in the steady-state inactivation was recorded (Sipos et al., 1995). The same mutation was introduced into the cardiac L-type calcium channel and functionally expressed in HEK293 cells (Lerche et al., 1996b). No significant change in the inactivation curve was observed.

Despite the location of R528 within the putative voltage sensor, the expression studies revealed no change in the voltage dependence of activation. However, in the mutant R528H, a slower rate in channel activation combined with a significant reduction in current density of the mutant channels was widely observed (Sipos et al., 1995; Lapie et al., 1996; Morrill et al., 1998). It is conceivable that a mutation that causes such an aberrant expression level could underlay the manifestations of paralysis in patients with hypoKPP.

Patients with hypoKPP typically have low serum potassium levels associated with the attacks of weakness. Electrophysiological characterization of calcium current in muscle fibres showed that a reduction in the extracellular concentration of potassium caused a paralytic depolarization in biopsied muscle fibres, whereas normal fibres were hyperpolarized (Rüdel et al., 1984). A depolarization of muscle fibres to –50 mV may be sufficient to inactivate voltage-gated sodium channels, rendering the muscle fibres inexcitable and leading to paralysis.

Chloride channel

Thirty-six mutations in *CLCN1* encoding the skeltal muscle voltage-gated chloride channel have been identified (Table 30.3) in patients with myotonia congenita. These mutations are associated with either Thomsen's (dominant) or Becker's (recessive) myotonia congenita. In some cases, the same mutations may have different modes of transmission in different families (Zhang et al., 1996; Plassart-Schiess et al., 1998b). Unlike mutations affecting sodium and calcium channel mutations that are exclusively missense, various mutations (missense, nonsense, deletion and insertion) have been found in the chloride channel gene. Another major difference with other voltage-gated channels is the absence of a clear picture about the topology of the chloride channel. No well-defined transmembrane segment with positive or negative charges has been identified as a putative voltage sensor and no pore-forming region has been clearly defined. In the absence of any information about such functional domains, studying these mutations in expression systems may be valuable in identifying such molecular structures and may help to define the topology of these channels.

Expression of these mutations in *Xenopus* oocytes or in a mammalian cell background confirmed what was already established from in vitro data studying patient muscle. There is a reduction in chloride conductance that is sufficient to cause myotonia (Lipicky et al., 1971). Indeed, the dominant mutations were shown to reduce chloride channel conductance greatly (Table 30.3).

Most of the mutations have been studied in *Xenopus* oocytes, in HEK293 cells or in the tsA201 cell line. These studies, summarized in Table 30.3, show a simplistic way by which these altered channels cause myotonia. A reduction in current density is a common defect in these mutations. The open channel probability is often dramatically shifted to the depolarizing potential range where the chloride channel does not contribute to maintaining rest potential close to −90 mV, increasing the hyperexcitability of the cell membrane thereby leading to myotonia. In some substitutions (G230E and P480L), the single channel conductance is reduced. The selectivity is altered in G230E when studied in tsA201 cells, suggesting the involvement of this residue in the pore structure (Fahlke et al., 1997a). In order to assess the dominant negative effect of these mutations, increasing ratios of mutant to wild-type cRNA was injected into oocytes. The channel conductance was decreased as the amount of mutant cRNA increased.

It is not clear what makes a mutation dominant or recessive. The location of the amino acid residue, where the disease-causing change occurs, does not necessarily determine the nature of the trait. I290M, which results from a dominant mutation, is adjacent to E291K, which is the result of a recessive change. Another example of this confusion is the two adjacent residues G285 and V286. Substitutions at these positions to E and A, respectively, cause myotonia congenita with dominant and recessive traits. Furthermore, co-expression of the wild-type channels and the dominant mutations resulted in a partial reversion of the positive shift in the voltage dependence compared with the mutant alone (Pusch et al., 1995).

Single-channel characterization of two *ClC-1* carrying either a dominant (I290M) or a recessive (I556N) mutation suggested that ClC-1 channels may have the same double-barrelled structure as the *Torpedo* channels ClC-0 (Saviane et al., 1999). The conductance of the ClC-1 channel would occur through a dimeric protein with two independent pores controlled by a common gate, as proposed for ClC-0 (Miller, 1982). The pattern of inheritance may arise from differential modifications on the double pore caused by these mutations.

Ryanodine receptor

Eighteen point mutations have been identified in the human *RYR1* at 16 different locations: these give rise to C35R, G248R, G341R, R552W, R614C/L, R2163C, V2168M, T2206M, G2435R and R2458C/H causing MH, and to R163C, I403M, Y522S, R2163H, R2436H, and I4898T linked to both central core disease and MH (Gillard et al., 1991; Quane et al., 1993, 1994a,b; 1997; Zhang et al., 1993; Keating

Table 30.3. Chloride channel mutations

Mutation	Inheritance	Current density	Open probability shift	Conductance	References
G200R	Dominant	NC	Right		Wollnik et al., 1997; Wagner et al., 1998
G230R	Dominant	Reduced	Left	Reduced	Steinmeyer et al., 1994; Fahlke et al., 1997a
V286A	Dominant		Right	Reduced	Kubisch et al., 1998
I290M	Dominant		Right/WT		Pusch et al., 1995
F307S	Dominant		Right	Reduced	Kubisch et al., 1998
R317Q	Dominant		Right		Pusch et al., 1995
P480L	Dominant	Reduced	Right/WT	Reduced/WT	Pusch et al., 1995
Q552R	Dominant	Abolished	Right/WT		Pusch et al., 1995
R105C	Recessive				Meyer Kleine et al., 1995
D136G	Recessive				Fahlke et al., 1995, 1997b
Y150C	Recessive		NC	NC	Wollnik et al., 1997
V165G	Recessive				Meyer Kleine et al., 1995
F167L	Recessive				George et al., 1994
V236L	Recessive		Right	Reduced	Kubisch et al., 1998
Y261C	Recessive		NC	NC	Wollnik et al., 1997
V269A	Recessive				Our unpublished data
G285E	Recessive	Abolished	NC/WT	Reduced	Kubisch et al., 1998
E291K	Recessive	Abolished	NC/WT	Reduced/WT	Pusch et al., 1995
A313T	Recessive		Right	Increased	Kubisch et al., 1998
I329T	Recessive				Meyer Kleine et al., 1995
R338Q	Recessive				George et al., 1994
F413C	Recessive				Koch et al., 1992
A415V	Recessive				Mailander et al., 1996
G482R	Recessive				Meyer Kleine et al., 1995
G485V	Recessive		Left?	Reduced	Wollnik et al., 1997
R496S	Recessive	Abolished			Lorenz et al., 1994
G499R	Recessive				Our unpublished data
A531V	Recessive				Papponen et al., 1999
I556N	Recessive		Right	Reduced	Kubisch et al., 1998
Q68X	Recessive				Zhang et al., 1996
Q74X	Recessive				Mailander et al., 1996
R300X	Recessive				George et al., 1994
R894X	Recessive	Reduced			Meyer Kleine et al., 1995
del. 1095–1096	—				Meyer Kleine et al., 1995
del. 1278–1281	—				Heine et al., 1994
del. 1437–1450	—				Meyer Kleine et al., 1995
ins. +1962	—				Meyer Kleine et al., 1995

Notes:
NC, no change; WT, wild type; del., deletion; ins., insertion.

et al., 1994, 1997; Phillips et al., 1994; Lynch et al., 1997, 1999; Manning et al., 1998). All these mutations are clustered in the MH-linked domains I and II except the recent reported mutation I4898T, which is located in the C-terminal transmembrane/luminal region of the RYR1 (Fig. 30.2).

Functional studies were carried out on biopsied muscle from patients with MH using the in vitro tests for MH discussed above (p. 614). Using the IVCT, these muscles were found to have increase sensitivity to caffeine and halothane (Fletcher et al., 1990, 1991, 1993; Fill et al., 1991; Valdivia et al., 1991; Nelson 1992). When this test was conducted on muscle from patients with identified mutations, there was a good correlation between caffeine threshold and tension values (Manning et al., 1998). Other groups have conducted binding assay studies on membrane preparations from patients with known mutations in the RYR1.

These studies showed that these mutations enhance the sensitivity of the RYR1 to activating concentrations of calcium, in response to exogenous ligands such as caffeine (Richter et al., 1997). Functional studies have also been carried out by introducing mutations identified as linked to MH into rabbit RYR1 cDNA and expressing the wild-type and mutant channels in HEK293 cells. A large study of 15 such mutations showed that intracellular calcium release from the SR is more sensitive to extracellular applications of caffeine and halothane for the mutant than for wild-type RYR1 (Tong et al., 1997).

The I4898T substitution is unique for several reasons. First, it occurs in a region where no mutation was previously described and far from the two known MH mutation hotspots. Second, all affected family members suffer from a clinically severe and highly penetrant form of central core disease. Third, the response of the mutant channels to caffeine and halothane was not enhanced as reported for the other mutant channels. It was abolished in the I4898T alone mutant and was normal in the I4898T/wild-type heterozygous mutant cells when expressed in HEK293 cells. Binding of [^{3}H]-ryanodine was reduced. The authors speculate that the abnormal channel behaviour result from a disruption of the interactions of RYR1 with associated luminal proteins such as calsequestrin and triadin. Other mechanisms are proposed, for example, the I4898T substitution may alter the regulation of the RYR1 by luminal calcium, or this residue may be part of the pore region of the RYR1 (Balshaw et al., 1999).

Studying mutations causing MH and central core disease offered a possibility of defining the mechanism for the pathophysiology of these disorders. An enhanced sensitivity of the RYR1 to activating concentrations of calcium ions may favour a depletion of the internal calcium store, which may lead to muscle weakness (MacLennan et al., 1996).

Mutations in RYR account for only a portion of the cases of MHS. It is interesting that MHS is seen with higher frequency in populations of patients with different muscle diseases. Furthermore, mutations in a number of other genes have been implicated in MHS. These include genes encoding the skeletal muscle calcium and sodium channels (CACNA1S and SCN4A) and carnitine palmitoyltransferase II (Monnier et al., 1997; Taggart et al., 1999; Bendahhou et al., 2000). A unifying model has been proposes in which MH results from loss of calcium homeostasis in skeletal muscle cells (Hogan, 1998). While this can clearly occur as a result of RYR1 mutations, massive depolarization of muscle cell membranes from mutations affecting sodium channels is another way in which intracellular calcium levels may be elevated. Mutations in

CACNA1S may lead to altered calcium conductance through the encoded L-type calcium channel or to altered regulation of RYR1 channel opening. It is known that activation of the RYR1 calcium release channel in SR can be effected by palmitoylcarnitine (el-Hayek et al., 1993). A mutation in carnitine palmitoyltransferase II that increases the level of this endogenous RYR1 modulator provides a physiological rationale for the linkage of mutations affecting this enzyme with MHS.

It is important to recall that an individual's risk for a MH reaction is related to age and that previous uncomplicated anaesthesia does not rule out MHS. These observations suggest that other endogenous factors and environmental influences affect MHS (Fig. 30.8).

Diagnosis and treatment

The periodic paralyses and nondystrophic myotonias

The attacks of all forms of periodic paralysis respond to treatment. Myotonia seen with the sodium and chloride channel disorders requires different therapies (Table 30.4) than those used for episodic weakness (Table 30.5). Acute paralyses can be treated and once the diagnosis is established, prophylactic treatment can usually be devised to prevent attacks. The best regimen(s) has not been established nor is it clear that prevention of attacks will forestall the development of the disabling interattack weakness that patients develop. A multicentre, randomized controlled trial has recently been completed and established daranide, a carbonic anhydrase inhibitor as being very effective in preventing attacks of both hypo- and hyperKPP (Tawil et al., 2000).

Acute attacks of hypoKPP can be aborted by the administration of oral potassium preparations (Ptáček et al., 1993a). Intravenous potassium treatment should be avoided if possible since the solutions used to dilute the potassium salts often worsen hypokalaemia. Attack prevention strategies include dietary modification with a low-carbohydrate, low-sodium diet. Attack prevention usually requires the administration of a carbonic anhydrase inhibitor such as acetazolamide or dichlorphenamide. A small proportion of patients are dramatically worsened by carbonic anhydrase inhibitors (Torres et al., 1981) and may have a genetically distinct disorder. Triamterene has proved effective for attack prevention in such patients (Torres et al., 1981). Both acetazolamide and dichlorphenamide can produce some improvement in persistent interattack weakness; it is not known whether such weakness

Table 30.4. Treatment strategy for periodic paralyses:

	Response to acetazolamide	Other medication	Diet
Sodium channel disorders			
Hyperkalaemic periodic paralysis	Yes	Thiazides	Low potassium
Paramyotonia congenita	Yes	Mexiletine	
Calcium channel disorder			
Hypokalaemic periodic paralysis	Yes	Spironolactone Triameterene	Low carbohydrate, low sodium
Chloride channel disorder			
Transient weakness in Beckers's myotonic congenita	Yes	Mexiletine	
Disorders of uncertain aetiology			
Thyrotoxic periodic paralysis	No	β-blockade	

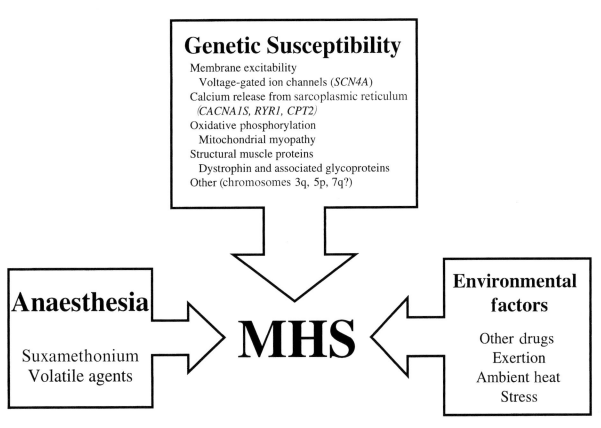

Fig. 30.8. A scheme to explain susceptibility to malignant hyperthermia (MHS). This appears to arise as a result of both genetic and environmental factors. Here, MHS is shown to be modulated by any one of a number of recognized genetic factors as well as by exposure to volatile or polarizing anaesthetics or other environmental factors.

Table 30.5. Treatment for myotonia

	Response to acetazolamide	Other medications
Sodium channel disorder	Yes	Mexiletine
Chloride channel disorder		
Thomsen's disease	No	Quinine, procainamide, phenytoin
Becker's disease	Yes	Mexiletine, tocainide

can be totally prevented. No agent has returned strength to normal once severe weakness has developed.

Thyrotoxic periodic paralysis responds to correction of thyrotoxicosis. Carbonic anhydrase inhibitors worsen the symptoms of these patients. Beta-blockade treatment of thyrotoxicosis usually eliminates periodic paralysis providing time for specific antithyroid treatment to become effective. In patients with no other signs of thyrotoxicosis, β-blockade may be the only treatment necessary (Griggs et al., 1996).

The mechanism of action of carbonic anhydrase inhibitors for hypoKPP has not yet been established. Since there is no sulphonamide-inhibited carbonic anhydrase in muscle (Riggs and Griggs, 1979), it is probable that a systemic metabolic effect is responsible for attack prevention. The metabolic acidosis produced may underlie the salutatory effects since the ingress of potassium to muscle is lessened in subjects treated with acetazolamide (Riggs et al., 1984).

In hyperKPP, acute individual attacks are mild and seldom require treatment. Patients themselves often discover that carbohydrate-containing food promptly improves weakness. An alternative strategy includes the administration of beta-adrenergic agonists such as salbutamol (albuterol). When used as an inhalant salbutamol is convenient and relatively safe. Patients with cardiac arrhythmia must be carefully excluded before such treatment is considered. Prophylactic treatment of hyperKPP includes kaliopenic diuretics such as thiazides or carbonic anhydrase inhibitors. Whether the regular use of these agents will prevent the development of interattack weakness is not known. Since patients often decline long-term treatment that will prevent attacks, it is important to determine whether such prophylactic treatment is of value in improving or preventing the persistent weakness that often develops after many years.

Most patients with paramyotonia congenita have

sufficiently symptomatic myotonia that it overshadows their infrequent attacks of episodic weakness. Patients seldom require medication for prevention of attacks of weakness; acetazolamide is occasionally useful for prevention of weakness or treatment of myotonia but has also precipitated acute weakness in certain patients (Ptáček and Griggs, 1996).

Paramyotonia congenita and acetazolamide-responsive myotonia congenita are both responsive to carbonic anhydrase inhibitors in terms of their effect on myotonia. Since potassium administration dramatically worsens myotonia in many of these patients, the kaliopenic effect of carbonic anhydrase inhibitors probably underlies their therapeutic effect in myotonia as well as in periodic paralysis (Ptáček and Griggs, 1996). Paramyotonia congenita and acetazolamide-responsive myotonia congenita both respond well to mexiletine and tocainide (Ptáček and Griggs, 1996).

The weakness of autosomal recessive myotonia congenita is markedly improved by the orally absorbed, methylated lignocaine (lidocaine) derivative mexiletine (Ptáček et al., 1993a). Some patients derive benefit from acetazolamide but the response is variable (Ptáček et al., 1993a).

Malignant hyperthermia

In general, preoperative screening by the anaesthetist for family history of MH or for signs of the syndrome in previous surgeries is important. However, the lack of an eventful anaesthesia even with triggering anaesthetics is no guarantee that the patient is not susceptible. An immediate response of the anaesthesiologist to the earliest signs of MHS and the availability of dantrolene in the operating room are the two most important means of preventing the syndrome from becoming fatal.

Since the disorder is inherited in an autosomal dominant pattern in humans, members of families in which MH has been identified are at high risk. Signs of MHS during a previous anaesthetic, including masseter muscle and whole body rigidity, elevated creatine kinase values and myoglobinuria, are also indicative of high risk (O'Flynn et al., 1994). Patients with central core disease, King–Denborough syndrome and Duchenne muscular dystrophy are also at higher than normal risk (Brownell, 1988). The response of patients with Duchenne muscular dystrophy may be different from prototypic MH and is marked by dramatic hyperkalaemia and cardiac arrest, especially after suxamethonium administration. For the patient known or suspected to have MHS, nontriggering anaesthesia is recommended, including nitrous oxide, barbiturates, opioids, local anaesthetics and any nondepolarizing neuromuscular blocking agents (the use of curare is controversial). Since anaesthesia may be required in an emergency, patients who have had a previous MH episode or who are at high risk are advised to wear a medic alert bracelet.

When considering anaesthesia for individuals with known or suspected MH, safe alternatives do exist. The main triggering agents that should be avoided are the halogenated volatile anaesthetics (halothane, enflurane, isoflurane, methoxyflurane, desflurane) and the depolarizing neuromuscular blocking agent suxamethonium. For tracing family histories of anaesthetic problems, cyclopropane and ether are also regarded as triggering agents. Controversy surrounds the use of curare and the phenothiazines, and they are probably best avoided. Drugs that appear safe for use in patients with MHS include antibiotics, antihistamines, antipyretics, atracurium, barbiturates, benzodiazepines, droperidol, ketamine, local anaesthetics, mivacurium, opioids, nitrous oxide, pancuronium, propofol, propranolol, vasoactive drugs and vecuronium.

A full-blown MH episode can be avoided by immediate discontinuation of triggering anaesthesia upon the first signs (O'Flynn et al., 1994). The patient should be hyperventilated (two to four times minute ventilation) with 100% oxygen at high flow rates.

Dantrolene, an antagonist of calcium release from intracellular stores, was found to be an effective therapeutic and prophylactic agent (Kolb et al., 1982). With increased awareness among physicians, the availability of dantrolene, and the development of the IVCT, the mortality from MH has decreased from about 80% to about 10% (Harrison, 1988). With a rapid and proper response, the prognosis is good. The syndrome usually resolves rapidly. However, both acute (hours) and delayed (days) recrudescences have been reported. Complications during and for several hours after the episode include disseminated intravascular coagulation and myoglobinuric renal failure. Since dantrolene is not readily soluble, assistance should be obtained to mix each ampoule of 20 mg with 50 ml bacteriostatic Water for Injection. The initial intravenous dose should be at least 2.5 mg/kg and this should be repeated as needed. Although a maximum of 10 mg/kg is recommended, higher doses may be deemed necessary in extreme cases. Dantrolene and bicarbonate are titrated while monitoring heart rate, body temperature, and arterial partial pressure of carbon dioxide. If significant acidosis occurs, 2 to 4 mEq/kg bicarbonate (2–4 nmo/kg) should be given. Monitoring carbon dioxide excretion with a capnometer is highly advised. Calcium channel blockers should be avoided as they can induce hyperkalaemia in the presence of dantrolene. To reduce body temperature, use external ice packs and gastric (fastest, most practical), wound and rectal lavage. Stop cooling at 38°C to avoid hypothermia. Central mixed venous blood gas determinations are highly recommended to assess acidosis. Femoral venous blood gases are less desirable alternatives. Hyperkalaemia is managed in the usual fashion (including treatment with bicarbonate, glucose, insulin and calcium), being aware that hypokalaemia frequently results. Since potassium may retrigger the syndrome, potassium replacement is not advised. The patient is monitored in the intensive care unit for 36 to 72 hours and is given dantrolene for 2 to 4 days, converting to the oral form when convenient. Because of the possibility of disseminated intravascular coagulation, coagulation studies should be carried out during and following an episode. The presence of *myoglobinuria* dictates therapy with diuretics, fluid loading and bicarbonate.

The use of reassuring counselling, nontriggering anaesthaesia and careful monitoring of heart rate, end-tidal carbon dioxide, muscle tone and temperature should result in an uneventful anaesthetic. Dantrolene is the drug of choice for an episode of MH and the prophylactic use of 2.5 mg/kg is recommended by some for those who have previously experienced an episode of MH. Ordinarily, dantrolene pretreatment is not needed.

References

Abdalla, J. A., Casley, W. L., Cousin, H. K. et al. (1992). Linkage of Thomsen disease to the T-cell-receptor beta (TCRB) locus on chromosome 7q35. *Am. J. Hum. Genet.* **51**, 579–584.

Andersen, E. D., Krasilnikoff, P. A. and Overvad, H. (1971). Intermittent muscular weakness, extrasystoles, and multiple developmental anomalies. *Acta. Paediatr. Scand.* **60**, 559–564.

Armstrong, C. M., Bezanilla, F. and Rojas, E. (1973). Destruction of sodium conductance inactivation in squid axons perfused with pronase. *J. Gen. Physiol.* **62**, 375–391.

Balshaw, D., Gao, L. and Meissner, G. (1999). Luminal loop of the ryanodine receptor: a pore-forming segment? *Proc. Natl. Acad. Sci.* USA **96**, 3345–3347.

Bauer, C. K., Steinmeyer, K., Schwarz, J. R. and Jentsch, T. J. (1991). Completely functional double-barreled chloride channel expressed from a single Torpedo cDNA. *Proc. Natl. Acad. Sci. USA* **88**, 11052–11056.

Becker, P. E. (1979). Heterozygote manifestation in recessive generalized myotonia. *Hum. Genet.* **46**, 325–329.

Bendahhou, S., Cummins, T. R., Kwiecinski, H., Waxman, S. G., and Ptáček, L. J. (1999a). Characterization of a new sodium channel mutation at arginine 1448 associated with moderate paramyotonia congenita in humans. *J. Physiol. (Lond.)* **518**, 337–344.

Bendahhou, S., Cummins, T. R., Tawil, R., Waxman, S. G. and Ptáček, L. J. (1999b). Activation and inactivation of the voltage-gated sodium channel: role of segment S5 revealed by a novel hyperkalaemic periodic paralysis mutation. *J. Neurosci.* **19**, 4762–4771.

Bendahhou, S., Cummins, T., Hahn, A., Langlois, S., Waxman, S. G. and Ptáček, L. J. (2000). Enhancement of slow inactivation in a double-mutation in the human skeletal muscle sodium channel causing hyperkalaemic periodic paralysis. *J. Clin. Invest.* **106**, 431–438.

Biemond, A. and Daniels, A. P. (1934). Familial periodic paralysis and its transition into spinal muscular atrophy. *Brain* **57**, 90–108.

Brownell, A. K. (1988). Malignant hyperthermia: relationship to other diseases. *Br. J. Anaesth.* **60**, 303–308.

Cannon, S. C. and Strittmatter, S. M. (1993). Functional expression of sodium channel mutations identified in families with periodic paralysis. *Neuron* **10**, 317–326.

Cannon, S. C., Brown, R. H., Jr and Corey, D. P. (1991). A sodium channel defect in hyperkalemic periodic paralysis: potassium-induced failure of inactivation. *Neuron* **6**, 619–626.

Cannon, S. C., Brown, R. J. and Corey, D. P. (1993). Theoretical reconstruction of myotonia and paralysis caused by incomplete inactivation of sodium channels. *Biophys. J.* **65**, 270–288.

Casley, W. L., Allon, M., Cousin, H. K. et al. (1992). Exclusion of linkage between hypokalemic periodic paralysis (HOKPP) and three candidate loci. *Genomics* **14**, 493–494.

Chahine, M., George, A. L., Jr, Zhou, M., Ji S., Sun, W., Barchi, R. L. and Horn, R. (1994). Sodium channel mutations in paramyotonia congenita uncouple inactivation from activation. *Neuron* **12**, 281–294.

Chaudhari, N. (1992). A single nucleotide deletion in the skeletal muscle-specific calcium channel transcript of muscular dysgenesis (*mdg*) mice. *J. Biol. Chem.* **267**, 25636–25639.

Cummins, T. R. Sigworth, F. J. (1996). Impaired slow inactivation in mutant sodium channels. *Biophys. J.* **71**, 227–236.

Cummins, T. R., Zhou, J., Sigworth, F. J. et al. (1993). Functional consequences of a Na$^+$ channel mutation causing hyperkalemic periodic paralysis. *Neuron* **10**, 667–678.

de Silva, S. M., Kuncl, R. W., Griffin, J. W., Cornblath, D. R. and Chavoustie, S. (1990). Paramyotonia congenita or hyperkalemic periodic paralysis? Clinical and electrophysiological features of each entity in one family. *Muscle Nerve* **13**, 21–26.

Denborough, M. A. and Lovell, R. R. H. (1960). Anaesthetic deaths in a family. *Lancet* **ii**, 45.

Ebers, G. C., George, A. L., Barchi, R. L. et al. (1991). Paramyotonia congenita and hyperkalemic periodic paralysis are linked to the adult muscle sodium channel gene. *Ann. Neurol.* **30**, 810–816.

el-Hayek, R., Valdivia, C., Valdivia, H. H., Hogan, K. and Coronado R. (1993). Activation of the Ca^{2+} release channel of skeletal muscle sarcoplasmic reticulum by palmitoyl carnitine. *Biophys. J.* **65**, 779–789.

Ellis, F. R. and Harriman, D. G. (1973). A new screening test for susceptibility to malignant hyperpyrexia. *Br. J. Anaesth.* **45**, 638.

Ellis, F. R., Harriman, D. G., Keaney, N. P., Kyei-Mensah, K. and Tyrrell, J. H. (1971). Halothane-induced muscle contracture as a cause of hyperpyrexia. *Br. J. Anaesth.* **43**, 721–722.

European Malignant Hyperthermia (1984). A protocol for the investigation of malignant hyperpyrexia susceptibility. *Br. J. Anaesth.* **56**, 1267–1271.

Eulenburg, A. (1886). Über eine familiäre, durch 6 Generationen verfolgbare Form Congenitaler Paramyonie. *Z. Neurol.* **5**, 265–272.

Fahlke, C., Rudel, R., Mitrovic, N., Zhou, M. and George, A. L., Jr (1995). An aspartic acid residue important for voltage-dependent gating of human muscle chloride channels. *Neuron* **15**, 463–472.

Fahlke, C., Beck, C. L., George, A. L., Jr. (1997a). A mutation in autosomal dominant myotonia congenita affects pore properties of the muscle chloride channel. *Proc. Natl. Acad. Sci. USA* **94**, 2729–2734.

Fahlke, C., Knittle, T., Gurnett, C . A., Campbell, K.P. and George, A. L., Jr (1997b). Subunit stoichiometry of human muscle chloride channels. *J. Gen. Physiol.* **109**, 93–104.

Featherstone, D. E., Fujimoto, E. and Ruben, P. C. (1998). A defect in skeletal muscle sodium channel deactivation exacerbates hyperexcitability in human paramyotonia congenita. *J. Physiol.* (*Lond.*) **506**, 627–638.

Feero, W. G., Wang, J., Barany, F. et al. (1993). Hyperkalemic periodic paralysis: rapid molecular diagnosis and relationship of genotype to phenotype in 12 families. *Neurology* **43**, 668–673.

Fill, M., Mejia-Alvarez, R., Zorzato, F., Volpe, P. and Stefani, E. (1991). Antibodies as probes for ligand gating of single sarcoplasmic reticulum Ca^{2+}-release channels. *Biochem. J.* **273**, 449–457.

Fletcher, J. E., Tripolitis, L., Erwin, K. et al. (1990). Fatty acids modulate calcium-induced calcium release from skeletal muscle heavy sarcoplasmic reticulum fractions: implications for malignant hyperthermia. *Biochem. Cell. Biol.* **68**, 1195–1201.

Fletcher, J. E., Mayerberger, S., Tripolitis, L., Yudkowsky, M. and Rosenberg, H. (1991). Fatty acids markedly lower the threshold for halothane-induced calcium release from the terminal cisternae in human and porcine normal and malignant hyperthermia susceptible skeletal muscle. *Life Sci.* **49**, 1651–1657.

Fletcher, J. E., Calvo, P.A. and Rosenberg, H. (1993). Phenotypes associated with malignant hyperthermia susceptibility in swine genotyped as homozygous or heterozygous for the ryanodine receptor mutation. *Br. J. Anaesth.* **71**, 410–417.

Fontaine, B., Khurana, T. S., Hoffman, E. P. et al. (1990). Hyperkalemic periodic paralysis and the adult muscle sodium channel alpha-subunit gene. *Science* **250**, 1000–1002.

Fontaine, B., Trofatter, J., Rouleau, G. A. et al. (1991). Different gene loci for hyperkalemic and hypokalemic periodic paralysis. *Neuromusc. Disord.* **1**, 235–238.

Fontaine, B., Vale, Santos, J., Jurkat Rott K. et al. (1994). Mapping of the hypokalaemic periodic paralysis (HypoPP) locus to chromosome 1q31–32 in three European families. *Nat. Genet.* **6**, 267–272.

Fouad, G., Dalakas, M., Servedei, S. et al. (1997). Genotype-phenotype correlations of DHP receptor alpha-1 gene mutations causing hypokalemic periodic paralysis. *Neuromusc. Disord.* **7**, 33–38.

Fujii, J., Otsu, K., Zorzato, F. et al. (1991). Identification of a mutation in porcine ryanodine receptor associated with malignant hyperthermia. *Science* **253**, 448–451.

George, A. L., Jr, Crackower, M. A., Abdalla, J. A. and Hudson, A. J., Ebers, G.C. (1993). Molecular basis of Thomsen's disease (autosomal dominant myotonia congenita). *Nat. Genet.* **3**, 305–310.

George, A. L., Jr, Sloan Brown, K., Fenichel, G. M., Mitchell, G. A., Spiegel, R. and Pascuzzi, R. M. (1994). Nonsense and missense mutations of the muscle chloride channel gene in patients with myotonia congenita. *Hum. Mol. Genet.* **3**, 2071–2072.

Gillard, E. F., Otsu, K., Fujii, J. et al. (1991). A substitution of cysteine for arginine 614 in the ryanodine receptor is potentially causative of human malignant hyperthermia. *Genomics* **11**, 751–755.

Gillard, E. F., Otsu, K., Fujii, J. et al. (1992). Polymorphisms and deduced amino acid substitutions in the coding sequence of the ryanodine receptor (RYR1) gene in individuals with malignant hyperthermia. *Genomics* **13**, 1247–1254.

Griggs, R. C., Moxley, R. T., Lafrance, R. A. and McQuillen, J. (1978). Hereditary paroxysmal ataxia: response to acetazolamide. *Neurology* **28**, 1259–1264.

Green, D. S., George, A. L. Jr and Cannon, S. C. (1998). Human sodium channel gating defects caused by missense mutations in S6 segments associated with myotonia: S804F and V1293I. *J. Physiol. (Lond.)* **510**, 685–694.

Griggs, R. C., Bender, A. N. and Tawil, R. (1996). A puzzling case of periodic paralysis. *Muscle Nerve* **19**, 362–364.

Gronert, G. A. (1994). Malignant hyperthermia. In *Myology*, eds. A. G. Engel and C. Franzini-Armstrong, pp. 1661–1678. New York: McGraw-Hill.

Halsall, P. J., Cain, P. A. and Ellis, F. R. (1979). Retrospective analysis of anaesthetics received by patients before susceptibility to malignant hyperpyrexia was recognized. *Br. J. Anaesth.* **51**, 949–954.

Hanke, W. and Miller, C. (1983). Single chloride channels from *Torpedo electroplax*. Activation by protons. *J. Gen. Physiol.* **82**, 25–45.

Harrison, G. G. (1988). Malignant hyperthermia. Dantrolene – dynamics and kinetics. *Br. J. Anaesth.* **60**, 279–286.

Hayward, L. J., Brown, R. H., Jr and Cannon, S. C. (1996). Inactivation defects caused by myotonia-associated mutations in the sodium channel III–IV linker. *J. Gen. Physiol.* **107**, 559–576.

Hayward, L. J., Brown, R. H., Jr and Cannon, S. C. (1997). Slow inactivation differs among mutant Na$^+$ channels associated with myotonia and periodic paralysis. *Biophys. J.* **72**, 1204–1219.

Hayward, L. J., Sandoval, G. M., Cannon, S. C. (1999). Defective slow inactivation of sodium channels contributes to familial periodic paralysis. *Neurology* **52**, 1447–1453.

Heine, R., Pika, U. and Lehmann Horn, F. (1993). A novel SCN4A mutation causing myotonia aggravated by cold and potassium. *Hum. Mol. Genet.* **2**, 1349–1353.

Heine, R., George, A. L., Jr, Pika, U., Deymeer, F., Rudel, R. and Lehmann Horn, F. (1994). Proof of a non-functional muscle chloride channel in recessive myotonia congenita (Becker) by detection of a 4 base pair deletion. *Hum. Mol. Genet.* **3**, 1123–1128.

Hogan, K. (1998). The anesthetic myopathies and malignant hyperthermias. *Curr. Opin. Neurol.* **11**, 469–476.

Hopkins, P. M., Ellis, F. R. and Halsall, P. J. (1991). Evidence for related myopathies in exertional heat stroke and malignant hyperthermia. *Lancet* **338**, 1491–1492.

Hoshi, T., Zagotta, W. N. and Aldrich, R. W. (1990). Biophysical and molecular mechanisms of Shaker potassium channel inactivation. *Science* **250**, 533–538.

Iles, D. E., Lehmann-Horn, F., Scherer, S. W. et al. (1994). Localization of the gene encoding the alpha 2/delta-subunits of the L-type voltage-dependent calcium channel to chromosome 7q and analysis of the segregation of flanking markers in malignant hyperthermia susceptible families. *Hum. Mol. Genet.* **3**, 969–975.

Isom, L. L., de Jongh, K. S. and Catterall and W. A. (1994). Auxiliary subunits of voltage-gated ion channels. *Neuron* **12**, 1183–1194.

Jackson, C. E., Barohn, R. J. and Pták, L. J. (1994). Paramyotonia congenita: abnormal short exercise test, and improvement after mexiletine therapy. *Muscle Nerve* **17**, 763–768.

Jentsch, T. J., Steinmeyer, K. and Schwarz, G. (1990). Primary structure of *Torpedo marmorata* chloride channel isolated by expression cloning in *Xenopus* oocytes. *Nature* **348**, 510–514.

Ji, S., George, A. L., Jr, Horn, R. and Barchi, R. L. (1996). Paramyotonia congenita mutations reveal different roles for segments S3 and S4 of domain D4 in hSkM1 sodium channel gating. *J. Gen. Physiol.* **107**, 183–194.

Jurkat Rott, K., Lehmann, Horn, F., Elbaz, A., Heine, R. et al. (1994). A calcium channel mutation causing hypokalemic periodic paralysis. *Hum. Mol. Genet.* **3**, 1415–1419.

Kalow, W., Britt, B. A., Terreau, M. E. and Haist, C. (1970). Metabolic error of muscle metabolism after recovery from malignant hyperthermia. *Lancet* **ii**, 895–898.

Keating, K. E., Quane, K. A., Manning, B. M. et al. (1994). Detection of a novel RYR1 mutation in four malignant hyperthermia pedigrees. *Hum. Mol. Genet.* **3**, 1855–1858.

Keating, K. E., Giblin, L., Lynch, P. J. et al. (1997). Detection of a novel mutation in the ryanodine receptor gene in an Irish malignant hyperthermia pedigree: correlation of the IVCT response with the affected and unaffected haplotypes. *J. Med. Genet.* **34**, 291–296.

Koch, M. C., Steinmeyer, K., Lorenz, C. et al. (1992). The skeletal muscle chloride channel in dominant and recessive human myotonia. *Science* **257**, 797–800.

Kolb, M. E., Horne, M. L. and Martz, R. (1982). Dantrolene in human malignant hyperthermia. *Anesthesiology* **56**, 254–262.

Kubisch, C., Schmidt-Rose, T., Fontaine, B., Bretag, A. H. and Jentsch, T. J. (1998). ClC-1 chloride channel mutations in myotonia congenita: variable penetrance of mutations shifting the voltage dependence. *Hum. Mol. Genet.* **7**, 1753–1760.

Lapie, P., Goudet, C., Nargeot, J., Fontaine, B. and Lory, P. (1996). Electrophysiological properties of the hypokalaemic periodic paralysis mutation (R528H) of the skeletal muscle alpha 1s subunit as expressed in mouse L cells. *FEBS Lett.* **382**, 244–248.

Larach, M. G., Localio, A. R., Allen, G. C. et al. (1994). A clinical grading scale to predict malignant hyperthermia susceptibility. *Anesthesiology* **80**, 771–779.

Lehmann-Horn, F., Kuther G., Ricker, K., Grafe, P., Ballanyi, K. and Rüdel, R. (1987a). Adynamia episodica hereditaria with myotonia: a non-inactivating sodium current and the effect of extracellular pH. *Muscle Nerve* **10**, 363–374.

Lehmann-Horn, F., Rüdel, R. and Ricker, K. (1987b). Membrane defects in paramyotonia congenita (Eulenburg). *Muscle Nerve* **10**, 633–641.

Lerche, H., Heine, R., Pika, U. et al. (1993). Human sodium channel myotonia: slowed channel inactivation due to substitutions for a glycine within the III–IV linker. *J. Physiol. (Lond.)* **470**, 13–22.

Lerche, H., Mitrovic, N., Dubowitz, V. and Lehmann-Horn, F. (1996a). Paramyotonia congenita: the R1448P Na⁺ channel mutation in adult human skeletal muscle. *Ann. Neurol.* **39**, 599–608.

Lerche, H., Klugbauer, N., Lehmann-Horn, F., Hofmann, F. and Melzer, W. (1996b). Expression and functional characterization of the cardiac L-type calcium channel carrying a skeletal muscle DHP-receptor mutation causing hypokalaemic periodic paralysis. *Pflügers Arch.* **431**, 461–463.

Lerche, H., Peter, W., Fleischhauer, R. et al. (1997). Role in fast inactivation of the IV/S4–S5 loop of the human muscle Na⁺ channel probed by cysteine mutagenesis. *J. Physiol. (Lond.)* **505**, 345–352.

Levitt, R. C., Olckers, A., Meyers, S. et al. (1992). Evidence for the localization of a malignant hyperthermia susceptibility locus (*MHS2*) to human chromosome 17q. *Genomics* **14**, 562–566.

Lipicky, R. J. and Bryant, S. H. (1973). A biophysical study of the human myotonias. In *New Developments in Electromyography and Clinical Neurophysiology*, ed. J. E. Desmedt, pp. 451–463. Basel: Karger. .

Lipicky, R. J., Bryant, S. H. and Salmon, J. H. (1971). Cable parameters, sodium, potassium, chloride, and water content, and potassium efflux in isolated external intercostal muscle of normal volunteers and patients with myotonia congenita. *J. Clin. Invest.* **50**, 2091–2103.

Lorenz, C., Meyer Kleine, C., Steinmeyer, K., Koch, M. C. and Jentsch, T. J. (1994). Genomic organization of the human muscle chloride channel CIC-1 and analysis of novel mutations leading to Becker-type myotonia. *Hum. Mol. Genet.* **3**, 941–946.

Lynch, P. J., Krivosic-Horber, R., Reyford, H. et al. (1997). Identification of heterozygous and homozygous individuals with the novel RYR1 mutation Cys35Arg in a large kindred. *Anesthesiology* **86**, 620–626.

Lynch, P. J., Tong, J., Lehane, M. et al. (1999). A mutation in the transmembrane/luminal domain of the ryanodine receptor is associated with abnormal Ca²⁺ release channel function and severe central core disease. *Proc. Natl. Acad. Sci. USA* **96**, 4164–4169.

MacLennan, D. H., Duff, C., Zorzato, F. et al. (1990). Ryanodine receptor gene is a candidate for predisposition to malignant hyperthermia. *Nature* **343**, 559–561.

MacLennan, D. H., H. P. M. and Zhang, Y. (1996). Molecular biology of membrane transport disorders. In: *Molecular Biology of Membrane Transport Disorders*, ed. S. G. Schultz, pp. 181–200. New York: Plenum.

Mailander, V., Heine, R., Deymeer, F. and Lehmann-Horn, F. (1996). Novel muscle chloride channel mutations and their effects on heterozygous carriers. *Am. J. Hum. Genet.* **58**, 317–324.

Manning, B. M., Quane, K. A., Ording, H. et al. (1998). Identification of novel mutations in the ryanodine-receptor gene (RYR1) in malignant hyperthermia: genotype-phenotype correlation. *Am. J. Hum. Genet.* **62**, 599–609.

McCarthy, T. V., Healy, J. M., Heffron, J. J. et al. (1990). Localization of the malignant hyperthermia susceptibility locus to human chromosome 19q12–13.2. *Nature* **343**, 562–564.

McClatchey, A. I., van den Bergh, P., Pericak Vance, M. A. et al. (1992a). Temperature-sensitive mutations in the III–IV cytoplasmic loop region of the skeletal muscle sodium channel gene in paramyotonia congenita. *Cell* **68**, 769–774.

McClatchey, A. I., McKenna Yasek, D. Cros, D. et al. (1992b). Novel mutations in families with unusual and variable disorders of the skeletal muscle sodium channel. *Nat. Genet.* **2**, 148–152.

McPhee, J. C., Ragsdale, D. S., Scheuer, T. and Catterall, W. A. (1998). A critical role for the S4–S5 intracellular loop in domain IV of the sodium channel alpha-subunit in fast inactivation. *J. Biol. Chem.* **273**, 1121–1129.

Mehrke, G., Brinkmeier, H. and Jockusch, H. (1988). The myotonic mouse mutant ADR: electrophysiology of the muscle fiber. *Muscle Nerve* **11**, 440–446.

Meyer Kleine, C., Steinmeyer, K., Ricker, K., Jentsch, T. J. and Koch, M. C. (1995). Spectrum of mutations in the major human skeletal muscle chloride channel gene (CLCN1) leading to myotonia. *Am. J. Hum. Genet.* **57**, 1325–1334.

Miller, C. (1982). Open-state substructure of single chloride channels from *Torpedo electroplax*. *Philos. Trans. R. Soc. Lond. B. Biol. Sci.* **299**, 401–411.

Mitrovic, N., George, A. L., Jr, Heine, R. et al. (1994). K(+)-aggravated myotonia: destabilization of the inactivated state of the human muscle Na⁺ channel by the V1589M mutation. *J. Physiol. (Lond.)* **478**, 395–402.

Mitrovic, N., Lerche, H., Heine, R. et al. (1996). Role in fast inactivation of conserved amino acids in the IV/S4–S5 loop of the human muscle Na⁺ channel. *Neurosci. Lett.* **214**, 9–12.

Monnier, N., Procaccio, V., Stieglitz, P. and Lunardi, J. (1997). Malignant-hyperthermia susceptibility is associated with a mutation of the alpha 1-subunit of the human dihydropyridine-sensitive L-type voltage-dependent calcium-channel receptor in skeletal muscle. *Am. J. Hum. Genet.* **60**, 1316–1325.

Monsieurs, K. G., Van Broeckhoven, C., Martin, J. J., van Hoof, V. O., and Heytens, L. (1998). Gly341Arg mutation indicating malignant hyperthermia susceptibility: specific cause of chronically elevated serum creatine kinase activity. *J. Neurol. Sci.* **154**, 62–65.

Morrill, J. A., Brown, R. H., Jr, Cannon, S. C. (1998). Gating of the L-type Ca channel in human skeletal myotubes: an activation defect caused by the hypokalemic periodic paralysis mutation R528H. *J. Neurosci.* **18**, 10320–10334.

Moslehi, R., Langlois, S., Yam, I. and Friedman, J. M. (1998). Linkage of malignant hyperthermia and hyperkalemic periodic paralysis to the adult skeletal muscle sodium channel (SCN4A) gene in a large pedigree. *Am. J. Med. Genet.* **76**, 21–27.

Nelson, T. E. (1992). Halothane effects on human malignant hyperthermia skeletal muscle single calcium-release channels in planar lipid bilayers. *Anesthesiology* **76**, 588–595.

O'Flynn, R. P., Shutack, J. G., Rosenberg, H. and Fletcher, J. E. (1994). Masseter muscle rigidity and malignant hyperthermia susceptibility in paediatric patients. An update on management and diagnosis. *Anesthesiology* **80**, 1228–1233.

Ording, H., Brancadoro, V., Cozzolino, S. et al. (1997). In vitro contracture test for diagnosis of malignant hyperthermia following the protocol of the European MH Group: results of testing patients surviving fulminant MH and unrelated low-risk subjects. The European Malignant Hyperthermia Group. *Acta Anaesthesiol. Scand.* **41**, 955–966.

Papazian, D. M., Timpe, L. C., Jan, Y. N. and Jan, L. Y. (1991). Alteration of voltage-dependence of Shaker potassium channel by mutations in the S4 sequence. *Nature* **349**, 305–310.

Papponen, H., Toppinen, T., Baumann, P. et al. (1999). Founder mutations and the high prevalence of myotonia congenita in northern Finland. *Neurology* **53**, 297–302.

Phillips, M. S., Khanna, V. K., de Leon, S., Frodis, W., Britt, B. A. and MacLennan, D. H. (1994). The substitution of Arg for Gly2433 in the human skeletal muscle ryanodine receptor is associated with malignant hyperthermia. *Hum. Mol. Genet.* **3**, 2181–2186.

Phillips, M. S., Fujii, J., Khanna, V. K. et al. (1996). The structural organization of the human skeletal muscle ryanodine receptor (RYR1) gene. *Genomics* **34**, 24–41.

Plassart-Schiess, E., Lhuillier, L., George, A. L., Jr, Fontaine, B. and Tabti, N. (1998a). Functional expression of the Ile693Thr Na+ channel mutation associated with paramyotonia congenita in a human cell line. *J. Physiol. (Lond.)* **507**, 721–727.

Plassart-Schiess, E., Gervais, A., Eymard, B. et al. (1998b). Novel muscle chloride channel (CLCN1) mutations in myotonia congenita with various modes of inheritance including incomplete dominance and penetrance. *Neurology* **50**, 1176–1179.

Powell, J. A. and Fambrough, D. M. (1973). Electrical properties of normal and dysgenic mouse skeletal muscle in culture. *J. Cell. Physiol.* **82**, 21–38.

Pták, L. J. and Griggs, R.C. (1996). Familial periodic paralyses. In *The Molecular Biology of Membrane Transport Disorders*, ed T. Andreoli, pp. 625–642. New York: Plenum.

Pták, L. J., Tyler, F., Trimmer, J. S., Agnew, W. S. and Leppert, M. (1991a). Analysis in a large hyperkalemic periodic paralysis pedigree supports tight linkage to a sodium channel locus. *Am. J. Hum. Genet.* **49**, 378–382.

Pták, L. J., George, A. L., Jr, Griggs, R. C. et al. (1991b). Identification of a mutation in the gene causing hyperkalemic periodic paralysis. *Cell* **67**, 1021–1027.

Pták, L. J., Tawil, R., Griggs, R. C., Storvick, D. and Leppert, M. (1992a). Linkage of atypical myotonia congenita to a sodium channel locus. *Neurology* **42**, 431–433.

Pták, L. J., George, A. L., Jr, Barchi, R. L. et al. (1992b). Mutations in an S4 segment of the adult skeletal muscle sodium channel cause paramyotonia congenita. *Neuron* **8**, 891–897.

Pták, L. J., Johnson, K. J. and Griggs, R. C. (1993a). Genetics and physiology of the myotonic muscle disorders. *N. Engl. J. Med.* **328**, 482–489.

Pták, L. J., Gouw, L., Kwiecinski, H. et al. (1993b). Sodium channel mutations in paramyotonia congenita and hyperkalemic periodic paralysis. *Ann. Neurol.* **33**, 300–307.

Pták, L. J., Tawil, R., Griggs, R. C. et al. (1994a). Dihydropyridine receptor mutations cause hypokalemic periodic paralysis. *Cell* **77**, 863–868.

Ptáček, L. J., Tawil, R., Griggs, R. C. et al. (1994b). Sodium channel mutations in acetazolamide-responsive myotonia congenita, paramyotonia congenita, and hyperkalemic periodic paralysis. *Neurology* **44**, 1500–1503.

Pusch, M., Steinmeyer, K., Koch, M. C. and Jentsch, T. J. (1995). Mutations in dominant human myotonia congenita drastically alter the voltage dependence of the ClC-1 chloride channel. *Neuron* **15**, 1455–1463.

Quane, K. A., Healy, J. M., Keating, K. E. et al. (1993). Mutations in the ryanodine receptor gene in central core disease and malignant hyperthermia. *Nat. Genet.* **5**, 51–55.

Quane, K. A., Keating, K. E., Manning, B. M. et al. (1994a). Detection of a novel common mutation in the ryanodine receptor gene in malignant hyperthermia: implications for diagnosis and heterogeneity studies. *Hum. Mol. Genet.* **3**, 471–476.

Quane, K. A., Keating, K. E., Healy, J. M. et al. (1994b). Mutation screening of the RYR1 gene in malignant hyperthermia: detection of a novel Tyr to Ser mutation in a pedigree with associated central cores. *Genomics* **23**, 236–239.

Quane, K. A., Ording, H., Keating, K. E. et al. (1997). Detection of a novel mutation at amino acid position 614 in the ryanodine receptor in malignant hyperthermia. *Br. J. Anaesth.* **79**, 332–337.

Richmond, J. E., Featherstone, D. E. and Ruben, P. C. (1997a). Human Na+ channel fast and slow inactivation in paramyotonia congenita mutants expressed in *Xenopus laevis* oocytes. *J. Physiol. (Lond.)* **499**, 589–600.

Richmond, J. E., van de Carr, D., Featherstone, D. E., George, A. L., Jr, and Ruben, P. C. (1997b). Defective fast inactivation recovery and deactivation account for sodium channel myotonia in the I1160V mutant. *Biophys. J.* **73**, 1896–1903.

Richter, M., Schleithoff, L., Deufel, T., Lehmann-Horn, F. and Herrmann-Frank, A. (1997). Functional characterization of a distinct ryanodine receptor mutation in human malignant hyperthermia-susceptible muscle. *J. Biol. Chem.* **272**, 5256–5260.

Riggs, J. E. and Griggs, R. C. (1979). Diagnosis and treatment of the periodic paralyses. *Neuropharmacology* **4**, 123–128.

Riggs, J. E., Griggs, R. C. and Moxley, R. T. D. (1984). Dissociation of glucose and potassium arterial-venous differences across the forearm by acetazolamide. A possible relationship to acetazolamide's beneficial effect in hypokalemic periodic paralysis. *Arch. Neurol.* **41**, 35–38.

Rios, E. and Pizarro, G. (1991). Voltage sensor of excitation-contraction coupling in skeletal muscle. *Physiol. Rev.* **71**, 849–908.

Robinson, R. L., Monnier, N., Wolz, W. et al. (1997). A genome wide search for susceptibility loci in three European malignant hyperthermia pedigrees. *Hum. Mol. Genet.* **6**, 953–961.

Rojas, C. V., Wang, J. Z., Schwartz, L. S., Hoffman, E. P., Powell, B. R. and Brown, R. H., Jr. (1991). A Met-to-Val mutation in the skeletal muscle Na+ channel alpha-subunit in hyperkalaemic periodic paralysis. *Nature* **354**, 387–389.

Rojas, C. V., Neely, A., Velasco-Loyden, G., Palma, V. and Kukuljan, M. (1999). Hyperkalemic periodic paralysis M1592V mutation modifies activation in human skeletal muscle Na+ channel. *Am. J. Physiol.* **276**, C259–C266.

Rosenberg, H. (1988). Clinical presentation of malignant hyperthermia. *Br. J. Anaesth.* **60**, 268–273.

Rüdel, R., Lehmann-Horn, F., Ricker, K. and Kuther, G. (1984). Hypokalemic periodic paralysis: in vitro investigation of muscle fiber membrane parameters. *Muscle Nerve* 7, 110–120.

Rudolph, J. A., Spier, S. J., Byrns, G., Rojas, C. V., Bernoco, D. and Hoffman, E. P. (1992). Periodic paralysis in quarter horses: a sodium channel mutation disseminated by selective breeding. *Nat. Genet.* **2**, 144–147.

Sansone, V., Griggs, R. C., Meola, G. et al. (1997). Andersen's syndrome: a distinct periodic paralysis. *Ann. Neurol.* **42**, 305–312.

Sasaki, R., Takano, H., Kamakura, K. et al. (1999). A novel mutation in the gene for the adult skeletal muscle sodium channel alpha-subunit (SCN4A) that causes paramyotonia congenita of von Eulenburg. *Arch. Neurol.* **56**, 692–696.

Saviane, C., Conti, F. and Pusch, M. (1999). The muscle chloride channel ClC-1 has a double-barreled appearance that is differentially affected in dominant and recessive myotonia. *J. Gen. Physiol.* **113**, 457–468.

Sipos, I., Jurkat-Rott, K., Harasztosi, C., Fontaine, B., Kovacs, L., Melzer, W. and Lehmann-Horn, F. (1995). Skeletal muscle DHP receptor mutations alter calcium currents in human hypokalaemic periodic paralysis myotubes. [Published erratum appears in *J. Physiol.* (*Lond.*) 1998 **508**, 955.] *J. Physiol.* (*Lond.*) **483**, 299–306.

Steinmeyer, K., Klocke, R., Ortland, C. et al. (1991). Inactivation of muscle chloride channel by transposon insertion in myotonic mice. *Nature* **354**, 304–308.

Steinmeyer, K., Lorenz, C., Pusch, M., Koch, M. C. and Jentsch, T. J. (1994). Multimeric structure of ClC-1 chloride channel revealed by mutations in dominant myotonia congenita (Thomsen). *EMBO J.* **13**, 737–743.

Stuhmer, W., Conti, F., Suzuki, H. et al. (1989). Structural parts involved in activation and inactivation of the sodium channel. *Nature* **339**, 597–603.

Sudbrak, R., Procaccio, V., Klausnitzer, M. et al. (1995). Mapping of a further malignant hyperthermia susceptibility locus to chromosome 3q13.1. *Am. J. Hum. Genet.* **56**, 684–691.

Taggart, R. T., Smail, D., Apolito, C. and Vladutiu, G. D. (1999). Novel mutations associated with carnitine palmitoyltransferase II deficiency. *Hum. Mutat.* **13**, 210–220.

Takahashi, M. P. and Cannon, S. C. (1999). Enhanced slow inactivation by V445M: a sodium channel mutation associated with myotonia. *Biophys. J.* **76**, 861–868.

Tanabe, T., Beam, K. G., Powell, J. A. and Numa, S. (1988). Restoration of excitation–contraction coupling and slow calcium current in dysgenic muscle by dihydropyridine receptor complementary DNA. *Nature* **336**, 134–139.

Tanabe, T., Beam, K. G., Adams, B. A, Niidome, T. and Numa, S. (1990). Regions of the skeletal muscle dihydropyridine receptor critical for excitation-contraction coupling. *Nature* **346**, 567–569.

Tang, L., Kallen, R. G. and Horn, R. (1996). Role of an S4–S5 linker in sodium channel inactivation probed by mutagenesis and a peptide blocker. *J. Gen. Physiol.* **108**, 89–104.

Tawil, R., Ptáček, L. J., Pavlakis, S. G. et al. (1994). Andersen's syndrome: potassium-sensitive periodic paralysis, ventricular ectopy, and dysmorphic features. *Ann. Neurol.* **35**, 326–330.

Tawil, R., McDermott, M. P., Brown, R. B. S. et al. (2000). Randomized trials of dichlorphenamide in the periodic paralyses. *Ann. Neurol.* **47**, 46–53. .

Thiemann, A., Grunder, S., Pusch, M. and Jentsch, T. J. (1992). A chloride channel widely expressed in epithelial and non-epithelial cells. *Nature* **356**, 57–60.

Tong, J., Oyamada, H., Demaurex, N., Grinstein, S., McCarthy, T. V. and MacLennan, D. H. (1997). Caffeine and halothane sensitivity of intracellular Ca^{2+} release is altered by 15 calcium release channel (ryanodine receptor) mutations associated with malignant hyperthermia and/or central core disease. *J. Biol. Chem.* **272**, 26332–26339.

Tong, J., McCarthy, T. V. and MacLennan, D. H. (1999). Measurement of resting cytosolic Ca^{2+} concentrations and Ca^{2+} store size in HEK-293 cells transfected with malignant hyperthermia or central core disease mutant Ca^{2+} release channels. *J. Biol. Chem.* **274**, 693–702.

Torres, C. F., Griggs, R. C., Moxley, R. T. and Bender, A. N. (1981). Hypokalemic periodic paralysis exacerbated by acetazolamide. *Neurology* **31**, 1423–1428.

Trudell, R. G., Kaiser, K. K. and Griggs, R. C. (1987). Acetazolamide-responsive myotonia congenita. *Neurology* **37**, 488–491.

Tyler, F. H., Stephens, F. E., Gunn, F. D. and Perkoff, G. T. (1951). Studies in disorders of muscle VII. Clinical manifestations and inheritance of a type of periodic paralysis without hypopotassimia. *J. Clin. Invest.* **30**, 492–502.

Valdivia, H. H., Hogan, K. and Coronado, R. (1991). Altered binding site for Ca^{2+} in the ryanodine receptor of human malignant hyperthermia. *Am. J. Physiol.* **261**, C237–C245.

Vladutiu, G. D., Taggart, R. T., Smail, D., Lindsley, H. B. and Hogan, K. (1998). A carnitine palmitoyl transferase II (CPT2) Arg503635 ys mutation confers malignant hyperthermia and variable myopathy. *Am. J. Hum. Genet.* **63**, A5.

Wagner, S., Lerche, H., Mitrovic, N., Heine, R., George, A. L. and Lehmann-Horn, F. (1997). A novel sodium channel mutation causing a hyperkalemic paralytic and paramyotonic syndrome with variable clinical expressivity. *Neurology* **49**, 1018–1025.

Wagner, S., Deymeer, F., Kurz, L. L., Benz, S. et al. (1998). The dominant chloride channel mutant G200R causing fluctuating myotonia: clinical findings, electrophysiology, and channel pathology. *Muscle Nerve* **21**, 1122–1128.

Wang, J., Zhou, J., Todorovic, S. M. et al. (1993). Molecular genetic and genetic correlations in sodium channelopathies: lack of founder effect and evidence for a second gene. *Am. J. Hum. Genet.* **52**, 1074–1084.

Wang, J., Dubowitz, V., Lehmann-Horn, F., Ricker, K., Ptáček, L. and Hoffman, E. P. (1995). In vivo sodium channel structure/function studies: consecutive Arg1448 changes to Cys, His, and Pro at the extracellular surface of IVS4. *Soc. Gen. Physiol. Ser.* **50**, 77–88.

West, J. W., Patton, D. E., Scheuer, T., Wang, Y., Goldin, A. L and Catterall, W. A. (1992). A cluster of hydrophobic amino acid residues required for fast Na$^+$-channel inactivation. *Proc. Natl. Acad. Sci. USA* **89**, 10910–10914.

Westphal, C. (1885). Über einen merkqurdigen fall von periodischer lahmung aller vier extremitaten mit gleichzeitigem erloschen der elektrischen erregbarkeit wahrend der lahmung. *Klin. Wochenschr.* **22**, 489–491.

Wollnik, B., Kubisch, C., Steinmeyer, K. and Pusch, M. (1997). Identification of functionally important regions of the muscular chloride channel CIC-1 by analysis of recessive and dominant myotonic mutations. *Hum. Mol. Genet.* **6**, 805–811.

Yang, N., Ji, S., Zhou, M., Ptáček, L. J. et al. (1994). Sodium channel mutations in paramyotonia congenita exhibit similar biophysical phenotypes in vitro. *Proc. Natl. Acad. Sci. USA* **91**, 12785–12789.

Zhang, Y., Chen, H. S., Khanna, V. K. et al. (1993). A mutation in the human ryanodine receptor gene associated with central core disease. *Nat. Genet.* **5**, 46–50.

Zhang, J., George, A. L., Jr., Griggs, R. C. et al. (1996). Mutations in the human skeletal muscle chloride channel gene (CLCN1) associated with dominant and recessive myotonia congenita. *Neurology* **47**, 993–998.

31

Inflammatory myopathies

Marinos C. Dalakas and George Karpati

Introduction

Inflammatory myopathies (IM) constitute a heterogeneous group of subacute, chronic and, rarely, acute acquired diseases of skeletal muscle which have in common the presence of moderate to severe muscle weakness and inflammation on muscle biopsy. The diseases are clinically important because they represent the largest group of acquired and potentially treatable myopathies both in children and adults.

A practical classification of all the IM, based on aetiology and pathogenesis has four groups: (i) idiopathic IM (IIM), which comprise the largest group and will be the main focus of this chapter; (ii) secondary IM, occurring in association with other systemic or connective tissue diseases, or with bacterial, viral or parasitic infections; (iii) infantile, childhood or congenital forms; and (iv) miscellaneous forms.

Idiopathic inflammatory myopathies

Based on distinct clinical, immunopathological, histological and prognostic criteria, as well as different responses to therapies, IIM can be separated into three major and distinct subsets: polymyositis (PM), dermatomyositis (DM) and inclusion body myositis (IBM). PM and DM would appear to have primarily an autoimmune pathogenesis, based on their association with other putative or definite autoimmune diseases or viral infections, the evidence for a T-cell-mediated myocytotoxicity or complement-mediated microangiopathy (DM) and their varying response to immunotherapies (Dalakas, 1988, 1991; Hohlfeld et al., 1993; Karpati and Carpenter 1993a; Engel et al., 1994; Karpati and Currie, 1994). In IBM, the autoimmune features coexist with 'degenerative' features including myo-

nuclear abnormalities, vacuolization, amyloid deposition and mitochondrial proliferation. This chapter will review the main clinical and histological features, the underlying immunopathology and the response to immunotherapeutic interventions.

Overall clinical features

The incidence of PM, DM and IBM is approximately 1 in 100 000. DM affects both children and adults, and females more often than males, whereas PM is seen after the second decade of life and very rarely in childhood. IBM is three times more frequent in men than in women, is more common in whites than in blacks, and is most likely to affect persons over the age of 50 years.

All three forms have in common a myopathy characterized by proximal and often symmetric muscle weakness, which usually develops subacutely or chronically (weeks to months) or very insidiously, as in IBM. Patients usually report increasing difficulty with everyday tasks predominantly requiring the use of proximal muscles, such as getting up from a chair, climbing steps, stepping onto a curb, lifting objects or combing their hair. Fine motor movements that depend on the strength of distal muscles, such as buttoning a shirt, sewing, knitting or writing, are affected only late in the course of DM and PM but earlier in IBM, where distal weakness is common and may even predominate. Falling is common among patients with IBM because of early involvement of the quadriceps muscle and buckling of the knees. Ocular muscles remain normal, even in advanced, untreated disease, and if these muscles were affected, the diagnosis of inflammatory myopathy would be in doubt. Facial muscles also remain normal except, rarely, in advanced disease. Mild facial muscle weakness, however, is seen in up to 60% of patients with sporadic IBM (s-IBM). The pharyngeal and neck flexor muscles are often involved, causing dysphagia or fatigue and difficulty in holding up the head. In advanced disease, and rarely in acute DM, respiratory muscles may also be affected. Severe weakness is almost always associated with muscular wasting. Sensation remains normal. The tendon reflexes are preserved but may be absent in severely weakened or atrophied muscles, especially in s-IBM, where atrophy of the quadriceps and the distal muscle is common. Exercise-induced myalgia and muscle tenderness may occur in some patients, usually early in the disease, particularly in DM but not in PM or s-IBM. Weakness in PM and DM progresses over a period of weeks or months, in contrast with the much slower progression of limb girdle dystrophies, from which they sometimes need to be differentiated. However, IBM may progress very slowly for years, and its clinical features may simulate those of limb girdle muscular dystrophy or peroneal muscular atrophy.

Specific features

Dermatomyositis

DM occurs in both children and adults. It is a distinct clinical entity identified by a characteristic rash accompanying or, more often, preceding the muscle weakness. The skin manifestations include a heliotrope rash (blue-purple discoloration) on the upper eyelids with oedema (Fig. 31.1, p. 00), a flat red rash on the face and upper trunk, and erythema of the knuckles with a raised violaceous scaly eruption (Gottron's rash) that later results in scaling of the skin. The erythematous rash can also occur on other body surfaces, including the knees, elbows, malleoli, neck and anterior chest (often in a V sign), or back and shoulders (shawl sign), and it may be exacerbated by exposure to the sun. In some patients, the rash is pruritic especially in the scalp, chest and back. Dilated capillary loops at the base of the fingernails are also characteristic of DM. The cuticles may be irregular, thickened and distorted, and the lateral and palmar areas of the fingers may become rough and cracked, with irregular, 'dirty' horizontal lines, resembling mechanics' hands. The degree of weakness can be mild, moderate or severe leading to quadriparesis. At times, the muscle strength appears normal, hence the term 'dermatomyositis sine myositis' (Otero et al., 1992). When muscle biopsy is performed in such cases, however, significant perivascular and perimysial inflammation is often seen. DM in children resembles the adult disease except for more frequent extramuscular manifestations, as discussed below. A common early abnormality in children is 'misery', defined as an irritable child that feels uncomfortable, has a red flush on the face, is fatigued, does not feel like socializing and has a varying degree of proximal muscle weakness. A tiptoe gait caused by flexion contracture of the ankles is also common.

DM usually occurs alone but may overlap with systemic sclerosis and mixed connective tissue disease (Dalakas, 1991, 1992). Fasciitis and skin changes similar to those found in DM have occurred in patients with the eosinophilia–myalgia syndrome associated with the ingestion of contaminated L-tryptophan (Hertzmann et al., 1990; Illa et al., 1993).

Polymyositis

Patients with PM do not present with any distinctive clinical feature that would confirm the diagnosis. Unlike DM, in which the rash secures early recognition, the actual onset of PM is difficult to pinpoint. The patients present with subacute onset of proximal muscle weakness and very rarely myalgia, which may exist for several months before they seek medical advice. The diagnosis of PM is based on finding subacute inflammatory myopathy, which progresses steadily and occurs in adults who do not have a rash, involvement of the extraocular and facial muscles (mild facial weakness is seen in IBM but not in PM), family history of a neuromuscular disease, history of exposure to myotoxic drugs or toxins, endocrinopathy, neurogenic disease, dystrophy, biochemical muscle disorder or IBM, as determined by muscle pathology and histochemistry.

PM can be viewed as a syndrome from diverse causes that may occur separately or in association with systemic autoimmune or connective tissue diseases and certain known viral or bacterial infections. With the exception of D-penicillamine and zidovudine (AZT), in which there may be endomysial inflammatory infiltrates similar to those seen in PM, myotoxic drugs, such as emetine, chloroquine, steroids, cimetidine, ipecac and lovastatin, do not cause PM. Instead, they elicit a toxic noninflammatory myopathy that is histologically different from PM and does not require immunosuppressive therapy (Dalakas, 1991, 1992; and Chapter 33).

Inclusion body myositis

IBM is the most common of the inflammatory myopathies. It affects men more often than women and is more frequent above the age of 50 years. It is the most commonly acquired myopathy in men above 50 years of age. Although IBM may only be suspected when a patient with presumed polymyositis does not respond to therapy, involvement of distal muscles, especially foot extensors and deep finger flexors in almost all cases, should be a clue to an early clinical diagnosis (Dalakas, 1991, 1992; Hohlfeld et al., 1993; Karpati and Carpenter, 1993a,b; Sekul

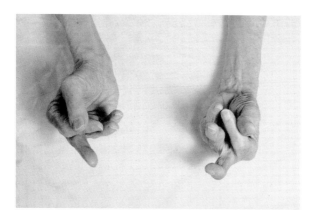

Fig. 31.2. Severe preferential weakness in finger flexors in a patient with sporadic inclusion body myositis.

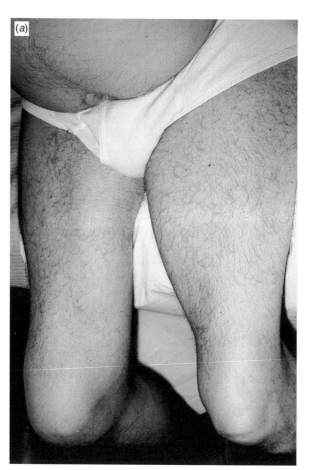

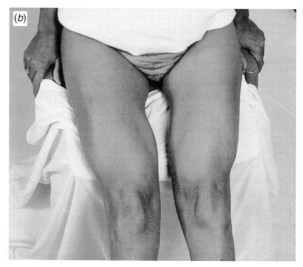

Fig. 31.3. Quadricep changes in patients with inclusion body myositis (IBM). (*a*) Prominent muscle weakness and wasting in the quadriceps muscles of a patient with sporadic IBM. (*b*) A patient with hereditary sparing IBM, linked to chromosome 9p, showing the quadriceps-sparing phenotype in contrast to that seen in (*a*).

and Dalakas, 1993; Engel et al., 1994; Griggs et al., 1995; Carpenter, 1996; Karpati, 1997) to be confirmed by muscle biopsy. Some patients present with falls because their knees collapse owing to early weakness of the quadriceps muscles. Others present with weakness in the small muscles of the hands, especially finger flexors, and complain of inability to hold certain objects such as golf clubs, play the guitar, turn a key or tie a knot (Fig. 31.2). The weakness and the accompanying atrophy can be asymmetric with, preferential involvement of the quadriceps (Fig. 31.3*a*), iliopsoas, triceps, biceps and finger flexors in the forearm. This is in contrast to the hereditary quadriceps-sparing IBM (Sivarkumar and Dalakas, 1996, 1997) in which the quadriceps remains strong in spite of the weakness in the other muscles (Fig. 31.3*b*). The selective involvement of the flexor digitorum profundus has been confirmed with MRI imaging (Sekul et al., 1997). Some dysphagia is common, occurring in up to 60% of the patients, especially late in the disease, but it rarely requires gastrostomy. Because of the distal and at times asymmetric weakness and atrophy and the early loss of the patellar reflex, a lower motor neuron disease is often suspected, especially since serum creatine kinase (CK) activity is either not elevated or only moderately increased (Dalakas, 1991). Sensory examination is generally normal except for a mildly diminished vibratory sensation at the ankles, presumably related to the patient's age. Contrary to early suggestions, the distal weakness does not represent neurogenic involvement but is part of the distal myopathic process, as confirmed with macro electromyography (EMG) (Luciano and Dalakas, 1997). However, an axonal neuropathy seems to occur in IBM patients more frequently than would be expected by chance alone (Schroder and Molnar, 1997). In contrast to PM and DM in which facial muscles are spared, mild facial muscle weakness has been noted in 60% of IBM patients (Sekul and Dalakas, 1993).

Sporadic IBM can be associated with systemic autoimmune or connective tissue diseases in at least 20% of affected patients (Koffman et al., 1998a). An increased frequency of $DR\beta_1 0301$ and $DQ\beta_1 0201$ alleles associated with DR and DQ phenotypes has been documented in up to 75% of patients (Koffman et al., 1998b). Hereditary IBM is usually recessive but can, less frequently, be dominant, some with an associated leukoencephalopathy (Cole et al., 1988) and others with sparing of the quadriceps (Griggs et al., 1995; Sivakumar and Dalakas, 1996; Argov et al., 1997). At present, hereditary IBM includes various ill-defined vacuolar, myopathies affecting distal more than proximal muscles and with clinical profiles that differ from the one described above for s-IBM (Griggs et al., 1995; Argov et al., 1997). Hereditary IBM (inclusion body myopathy) with sparing of the quadriceps occurs not only in Iranian Jews, as initially described (Argov and Yarom, 1984; Massa et al., 1991), but also in other ethnic groups (Sivakumar and Dalakas, 1996; Argov et al., 1997). Further description and genetic data on hereditary IBM are not provided in this review because these diseases lack muscle inflammation and, therefore, do not represent a true inflammatory myopathy. There is, however, a subset of patients with familial IBM, that have the typical phenotype of s-IBM, with histological and immunopathological features identical to the sporadic form (Sivakumar et al., 1997).

Progression of s-IBM is slow but steady. The degree of disability in relation to the duration of the disease has not been systematically studied. Review of the course of 14 randomly chosen patients with symptoms for more than five years revealed that 10 of them required a cane or other support for ambulation by the fifth year after onset of disease while three of five patients with symptoms for 10 years or more were using wheelchairs. Using quantitative muscle strength testing, we have found a 10% drop in muscle strength over a one- and two-year period (Sekul and Dalakas, 1993). Recent data from our 86 consecutively studied patients indicate that progression is faster when the disease begins later in life. The patients whose disease begins in their sixties may require an assistive device many years later compared with those patients whose disease begins in their seventies, presumably because of lesser reserves (Peng et al., 2000).

Extramuscular manifestations

In addition to the primary disturbance of the skeletal muscles, extramuscular manifestations may be prominent in patients with IIM. Dysphagia is most prominent in IBM

and DM because of involvement of the oropharyngeal striated muscles and distal oesophagus. Cardiac abnormalities consist of atrioventricular conduction defects, tachyarrythmias, low ejection fraction and dilated cardiomyopathy, either from the disease itself or from hypertension associated with long-term steroid use. Pulmonary involvement results from primary weakness of the thoracic muscles, drug-induced pneumonitis, (e.g. from methotrexate) or interstitial lung disease. Interstitial lung disease may precede the myopathy or occur early in the disease and develops in up to 10% of patients with PM or DM, the majority of whom have anti-Jo-1 antibodies (directed against histidyl-transfer RNA synthetase). Fatality related to adult respiratory distress syndrome has been noted in PM patients with anti-Jo-1 antibodies (Clawson and Oddis, 1995), emphasizing the diagnostic importance of these antibodies. Pulmonary capillary angiitis with varying degrees of diffuse alveolar haemorrhage has also been described (Schwarz et al., 1995). Subcutaneous calcifications, sometimes extruding to the surface and causing ulcerations and infections (Fig. 31.4, colour plate), are found in patients with DM, mostly in children but also in some adults (Dalakas, 1995c). Intestinal infarcts are seen more often in childhood DM and result from vasculitis and infarction. Contractures of the joints are seen particularly in childhood DM. General systemic disturbances, such as fever, malaise, weight loss, arthralgia and Raynaud's phenomenon can occur, particularly when the inflammatory myopathy is associated with a connective tissue disorder. Finally, there is an increased incidence of malignancies in patients with DM (particularly over 50 years of age), but not in PM or IBM. Because tumours are usually uncovered by abnormal findings in the medical history and physical examination rather than by a radiological blind search, it is our practice to recommend a complete physical examination, with focus on breast, pelvic and rectal examinations, urinalysis, complete blood cell count, relevant blood chemistry tests (i.e. prostate-specific antigen (PSA) and carcinoembryonic antigen (CEA)) and a chest X-ray film, to be repeated at six-monthly intervals for several years.

Diagnosis

The clinically suspected diagnosis of PM, DM or IBM is established or confirmed by elevated activity of the muscle-derived serum enzymes, electromyographic findings and the muscle biopsy.

Muscle-derived serum enzyme levels

The most sensitive indicator enzyme is CK, which, in the presence of active disease, can be elevated in serum by as much as 50 times above the normal level. Although serum CK usually parallels the disease activity, it can be normal in active DM and even, rarely, in active PM. In IBM, serum CK is not usually elevated more than tenfold, and in some patients may be normal even from the beginning of the illness. Serum CK may also be normal in patients with untreated, even active, childhood DM and in some patients with PM or DM associated with a connective tissue disease, reflecting the restriction of the pathological process to the intramuscular vessels and perimysium. Along with the serum CK, glutamate oxaloacetate transaminase (GOT), glutamate pyruvate transaminase (GPT) and lactate dehydrogenase (LDH) may be elevated, which sometimes is erroneously interpreted as a sign of liver disease. Serum aldolase activity may also be elevated.

Electromyography
Needle EMG shows myopathic motor unit potentials characterized by short-duration, low-amplitude polyphasic units on voluntary activation, and increased spontaneous activity with fibrillations, complex repetitive discharges and positive sharp waves. This EMG pattern also occurs in a variety of acute, toxic and active myopathic processes and should not be considered diagnostic for the inflammatory myopathies. Mixed myopathic and neurogenic potentials (polyphasic units of short and long duration) are more often seen in IBM, but they can be seen in both PM and DM as a consequence of muscle fibre regeneration and chronicity of the disease or presence of an associated peripheral neuropathy. Contrary to previous reports, our findings using macro-EMG have failed to show a neurogenic pattern of involvement in patients with IBM (Luciano and Dalakas, 1997) even though histological evidence of an axonal neuropathy may be present in some patients especially of older age. EMG studies, therefore, are generally useful for excluding primary neurogenic disorders in such patients (Schroder and Molnar, 1997).

Muscle biopsy
For definite diagnosis of an inflammatory myopathy, microscopic examination of a muscle biopsy is essential (Carpenter and Karpati, 1981; Karpati and Carpenter 1993a; Engel and Banker, 1986; Mastaglia and Walton, 1992). For maximum diagnostic information, three major prerequisites are essential.
1. Proper choice of muscle. As a rule of thumb, a clinically moderately weak muscle offers the best chance for a positive biopsy. Imaging techniques such as computed tomography or magnetic resonance imaging are rarely required to select an involved region of a muscle. Simultaneous biopsies from more than one site are to

be discouraged, although a repeat biopsy from a different site occasionally becomes necessary. Open biopsy done by an expert is strongly recommended in preference to needle biopsy, since open biopsy offers a larger sample and is far better suited for ultrastructural study.
2. The biopsy specimens should be used for the preparation of cryostat sections, semithin plastic-embedded sections and, for selected patients, ultrathin sections for ultrastructural scrutiny. Each of these preparations should be stained by appropriate techniques. Cryostat sections are to be used mainly for routine histological and histochemical stains and reactions and for class I major histocompatibility complex (MHC) immunocytochemistry. However, in selected patients, they are also used for immunocytochemical localization of various lymphocytic subsets, cytokines, adhesion molecules and expression of 'alien' molecules in muscle fibres in IBM, as well as immunoglobulins and complement components. Semithin plastic-embedded sections or laminin cytochemistry also offer reliable means for the determination of capillary density of muscle, which is essential information in the differential diagnosis of DM from PM and IBM (Carpenter and Karpati, 1992; Karpati and Carpenter, 1993a). Electron microscopic examination is required for the detection of tubuloreticular inclusions in endothelial cells of blood vessels in DM (Jerusalem et al., 1974) or for the identification of the tubular filamentous inclusions in IBM (Carpenter, 1996; Karpati, 1997).
3. Interpretation of the biopsy requires special expertise in myopathology to avoid the several pitfalls that can lead to erroneous diagnosis (vide infra). The principal pathological features in the muscle biopsy are: changes affecting muscle fibres, alterations in blood vessels and the inflammatory cell profile plus any special immunopathological features.

A constellation of these abnormalities is usually characteristic of DM, PM, IBM, or certain other forms of inflammatory myopathy. In some instances, the number of typical changes falls short of being pathognomonic for a given form of IM. In such cases, only a 'probable' diagnosis is made. Table 31.1 summarizes these changes in adult DM, as well as in PM and IBM and Figs. 31.5–31.10, 31.12–31.16 and 31.11 (colour plate) illustrate many of these changes.

A number of comments must be made about these changes. Several of these abnormalities are pathognomonic even in isolation. Muscle infarcts (Fig. 31.6), perifascicular atrophy, A-band or focal myofibrillar loss (Fig. 31.8), capillary necrosis (Fig. 31.13a) (de Visser et al., 1989; Emslie-Smith and Engel, 1990), membrane attack complex

Table 31.1. Pathological features in idiopathic inflammatory myopathies (IIM)

	Dermatomyositis	Polymyositis	Inclusion body myositis
Muscle fibres			
Necrosis of muscle fibres			
Scattered necrosis (Fig. 31.5)	±	+	+
Infarcts (Fig. 31.6)	+	−	−
Sluggish phagocytosis (Fig. 31.6)	**+**	−	−
Regeneration	±	+	+
Atrophy			
Grouped	−	−	−
Scattered	+	+	+
Perifascicular (Fig. 31.7)	**+**	−	−
Hypertrophy	−	−	+
Z-disc streaming	+	+	+
Zonal myofibrillar loss (Fig. 31.8)	+	−	−
A band loss	+	−	−
Intrinsic lysosomal activation with exocytosis	−	+	−
Rimmed vacuoles and eosinophilic masses (Fig. 31.9)	−	−	**+**
Nuclear abnormalities (15 nm filaments) (Fig. 31.10)	−	±	**+**
Ragged-red fibres	−	−[a]	+
Amyloid-staining inclusions (Fig. 31.11, p. 00)	−	−	**+**
Ubiquitin-positive inclusions	−	−	+
'Alien' molecules[b] (Fig. 31.12)	−	−	+
Adhesion molecules (ICAM-1)	+	−	−
Blood vessels			
Increased capillarity	−	−	+
Capillary necrosis ± loss (Fig. 31.13a)	**+**	± (secondary)	−
Undulating tubules and other endothelial abnormalities	**+**	−	−
Arterial necrosis or thrombosis	+	−	−
Immunoglobulin deposition	**+**	−	−
Complement (5b-9) deposition (membrane attack complex) (Fig. 31.13b)	+	−	−
Adhesion molecules (VCAM-1)	+	−	−
Inflammatory and immunopathology			
Lymphocytes			
Endomysial ($CD4^+/CD8^+$T cells) (Fig. 31.14)	+	+	+
Septal (B cells + $CD4^+$ T cells)	+	−	−
Partial invasion (T cytotoxic $CD8^+$ cells and activated macrophages) (Fig. 31.15)	−	**+**	+
Plasma cells	−	±	−
Expression of sarcolemmal class I major histocompatibility complex protein products (Fig. 31.16)	+	+	+
Other			
Marked regional variability of pathology in clinically affected muscles	+	−	−
Interstitial fibrosis	+ (in severe cases)	+ (variable)	+ (focal)

Notes:

+, Present; −, absent. Since microscopic scrutinies should be directed to muscle fibres, blood vessels and inflammatory cells changed in these domains are shown separately. Certain highly characteristic pathological changes are marked **+** and the presence of at least two of these changes in a given biopsy would provide a practically pathognomonic diagnosis for a given entity.

[a] Ragged-red fibres occur in rare cases of polymyositis that seem to constitute a treatment-resistant subgroup.

[b] 'Alien' molecules include α_1-chymotrypsin, apolipoprotein E, prion protein, β-amyloid precursor, etc.

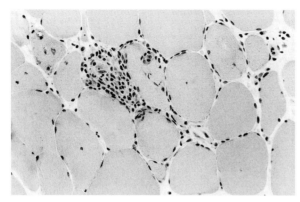

Fig. 31.5. Adult polymyositis. A single necrotic fibre is undergoing phagocytosis by macrophages. (Haematoxylin and eosin, ×350.)

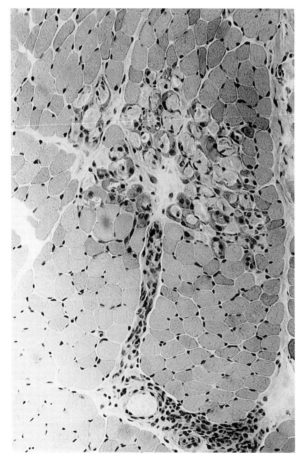

Fig. 31.6. Childhood dermatomyositis. A triangular area contains necrotic fibres in which phagocytosis is sparse despite some activation of satellite cells, which appear as peripheral myoblasts. The entire area represents an infarct. An interfascicular septum leading downwards from the infarct is infiltrated with mononuclear cells. (Haematoxylin and eosin, ×350.)

(MAC) deposition in vessel walls (Fig. 31.13*b*) (Kissel et al., 1986; 1991b), arterial thrombosis or undulating tubules in endothelial cells are characteristic for DM. Partial invasion of non-necrotic muscle fibres by CD8+ cytotoxic lymphocytes and activated macrophages (Fig. 31.15) is typical for either PM or IBM but does not occur in DM (Arahata and Engel, 1984, 1986). The presence of 15–18 nm tubular filamentous masses in nuclei or cytoplasm of muscle fibres (Fig. 31.10) is essential for the diagnosis of IBM but its demonstration may require extensive ultrastructural scrutiny (Lotz et al., 1989). However, it has become clear that these filamentous masses are not disease-specific for sporadic IBM nor are rimmed vacuoles (Fig. 31.9) (Massa et al., 1991). The presence of multinucleated giant cells among elongated inflammatory ('epitheloid') cells, macrophages or lymphocytes is characteristic of granulomatous myopathy. The presence of encysted trichinellal larvae in muscle fibres in the midst of a florid inflammatory reaction with abundant polymorphonuclear leucocytes is typical for *Trichinella* myositis.

Uniform expression of class I MHC products at the surface of all muscle fibres is characteristic of PM (Fig. 31.16), whereas in DM this phenomenon may be evident only in the perifascicular or other random regions and in IBM it occurs mainly in fibres that show partial invasion by CD8+ lymphocytes (Karpati et al., 1988; Emslie-Smith et al., 1989). MHC class I expression does not occur in limb girdle dystrophy, denervating diseases or metabolic myopathies (except in regenerating fibres), which makes MHC immunostaining a very helpful diagnostic tool.

The most common cause of a clinical misdiagnosis of inflammatory myopathies is an erroneous pathological interpretation of the biopsy (Karpati and Carpenter, 1988).

A relatively common erroneous practice is to combine PM and DM as the 'DM–PM complex'. Another source of confusion is the failure to distinguish IBM from PM. In the vast majority of patients, clear distinctions between these entities can be made reliably, which is important for investigative, therapeutic and prognostic reasons.

There are a number of pitfalls that could lead to erroneous interpretation of the muscle biopsy. Failure to assess blood vessel pathology may occur through lack of awareness of its importance or lack of appropriate preparations or stains to assess it. The failure to find IBM filaments is usually related to inadequate electron microscopic samples and insufficient search. The failure to distinguish between muscle fibre necrosis and partial invasion of muscle fibres by cytotoxic lymphocytes and macrophages is usually related to the lack of awareness of this phenomenon. In DM, the pathological involvement may be spotty and a given biopsy may not contain convincing pathological changes. In other instances, even if the biopsy contains changes typical of DM, the lack of inflammatory cell infiltrates in the biopsy could lead to the conclusion of 'non-specific abnormalities'. In some diseases other than inflammatory myopathies (i.e. Duchenne muscular dystrophy, myasthenia gravis), endomysial infiltration by lymphocytes may also occur (Kissel et al., 1991a; Maselli et al., 1991).

In addition to muscle biopsy, skin biopsy may be indicated in DM, preferably from a clinically involved area; however, pathological alteration is often present in clinically uninvolved skin. The changes include a thinning of the epithelial cell layer with attenuation or absence of rete pegs, perivascular mononuclear inflammatory cell infiltrates and oedema of the superficial dermis.

Aetiology and pathogenesis

Immune-mediated mechanisms

Serum autoantibodies
Various autoantibodies against nuclear (antinuclear antibodies) and cytoplasmic antigens are found in up to 20% of patients with inflammatory myopathies (Dalakas, 1991, 1992; Plotz et al., 1989; Targoff, 1990; Ge et al., 1995). The antibodies to cytoplasmic antigens are directed against cytoplasmic ribonucleoproteins, which are involved in translation and protein synthesis. They include antibodies against various synthetases, translation factors, and proteins of the signal-recognition particles. The antibody anti-Jo-1 accounts for 75% of all the antisynthetases; it is clinically useful because up to 80% of patients with anti-Jo-1 antibodies have interstitial lung disease. In general, these antibodies may be nonmuscle-specific because they are directed against ubiquitous targets; and they are almost always associated with interstitial lung disease even in patients who do not have active myositis. In addition, they are seen in all three subtypes (PM, DM and IBM), in spite of their clinical and immunopathological differences. Therefore, their pathogenic role in producing muscle damage is doubtful.

Immunopathology of dermatomyositis
The primary antigenic target in DM consists of components of the vascular endothelium of the larger endomysial blood vessels and capillaries (Banker, 1975; Carpenter et al., 1976). The earliest pathological alterations are changes in the endothelial cells, consisting of pale and swollen cytoplasm with microvacuoles and undulating tubules in the smooth endoplasmic reticulum followed by obliteration, vascular necrosis or thrombi formation (Carpenter et

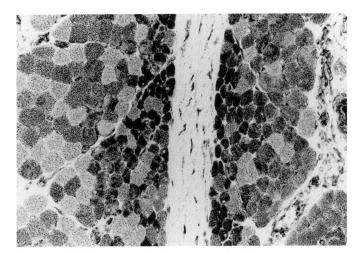

Fig. 31.7. Adult dermatomyositis. A narrow mantle of the periphery of two adjacent fascicles separated by an interfascicular septum contains markedly atrophic fibres with excessive oxidative enzyme activity. The interior of the fascicle appears normal. (NADH-tetrazolium reductase stain, ×140.)

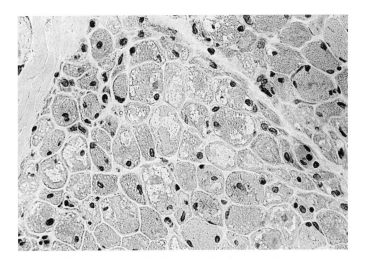

Fig. 31.8. Adult dermatomyositis. Many muscles fibres contain irregular, optically empty areas, from where the myofibrils have been lost ('punched out' zones). Myonuclei are conspicuous by their large size and sometimes internal location. (Haematoxylin and eosin, ×350.)

al., 1976). Such alterations in the microvasculature occur early in the disease through deposition of the C5b-9 MAC, the lytic component of the complement pathway, on the endothelium of capillaries. This occurs before the onset of inflammatory or structural changes in the muscle fibres (Whitaker and Engel, 1972; Emslie-Smith and Engel, 1990). Utilizing an in vitro assay system that uses radiolabelled anti-C9 antibodies to measure C3 consumption by sensitized erythrocytes (Basta and Dalakas, 1994), it was further

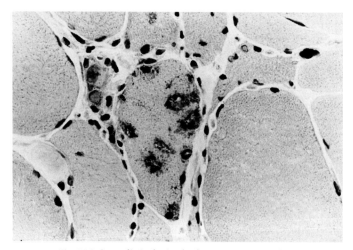

Fig. 31.9. Sporadic inclusion body myositis. A muscle fibre contains several 'rimmed' vacuoles. Most of these are at the periphery of the fibre. (Modified trichrome, ×520.)

found that patients with active, but not chronic DM, have very high C3 uptake in their serum. MAC and the active fragments of the early complement components C3b and C4b were also found to be increased in the patients' serum using a radioimmunoassay (Basta and Dalakas, 1994).

Sequentially, the disease begins when putative antibodies directed against endothelial cells of the endomysium (Cervera et al., 1991) activate complement C3, which forms C3b and C4b fragments and leads to formation and deposition of MAC on the endomysial microvasculature. The deposition of MAC leads, through somatic lysis of the endothelial cells, to necrosis of the capillaries and perivascular inflammation. The effects of ischaemia on muscle

fibres are microinfarcts, various sublethal cellular changes or fibre atrophy, especially at the perifascicular regions (Fig. 31.7). The perifascicular atrophy often seen in more chronic stages is a reflection of the endofascicular hypoperfusion, which is prominent at the periphery of fascicles where capillarity normally is less than elsewhere. There is marked reduction in the number of capillaries per muscle fibre (Carpenter and Karpati, 1992), with dilatation of the remaining capillaries occurring in an effort to compensate for the impaired perfusion. The mechanism is shown in Fig. 31.17.

The putative complement fixing anti-endothelial cell antibodies can be detected by enzyme-linked immunosorbant assay (ELISA) using human umbilical vein endothelial cells as antigen (Stein et al., 1993). However, characterization of the pathogenicity of these antibodies has not yet been performed. The activation of complement by the putative anti-endothelial cell antibodies is believed to be responsible for the induction of cytokines (Lundberg et al., 1995) which, in turn, upregulate the expression of vascular cell adhesion molecule 1 (VCAM-1) and intercellular adhesion molecule 1 (ICAM-1) on the endothelial cells (Stein and Dalakas, 1993) and facilitate the exit of activated lymphoid cells to the perimysial and endomysial spaces. The main immune factors that play a role in the pathogenesis of DM are shown in Fig. 31.17.

Immunophenotypic analysis of the lymphocytic infiltrates in the muscle biopsies of patients with DM demonstrates that B cells and CD4+ cells are the predominant cells in the perimysial and perivascular regions, supporting the view of a humoral-mediated process, as described

(a)

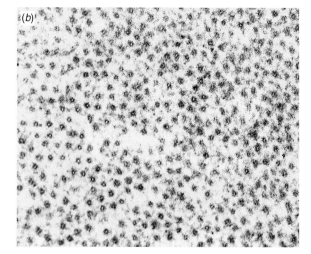

Fig. 31.10. Nuclear abnormalities. (a) A large collection of abnormal filaments is present on the surface of a muscle fibre. The filamentous mass is surrounded by whorls of cytomembrane, which on light microscope would appear as a rimmed vacuole. The shape and size of the filamentous mass suggests that it used to fill a myonucleus, but the nuclear membrane had been fully dissolved. (b) High power shows the 18 nm diameter filaments, typical of inclusion body myositis, to be tubular.

above (Arahata and Engel, 1986; Engel et al., 1994; Dalakas, 1995b).

Immunopathology of polymyositis and inclusion body myositis

Cytotoxic T cells

In PM and IBM, there is evidence not of microangiopathy and muscle ischaemia, as in DM, but of an antigen-directed cytotoxicity mediated by cytotoxic T cells targeting muscle fibres (Engel and Arahata, 1984, 1986; Arahata and Engel, 1986; Hohlfeld et al., 1993; Engel et al., 1994; Dalakas 1995b). This conclusion is supported by the presence of CD8$^+$ cells, which, along with macrophages, initially surround the healthy but MHC class I-expressing non-necrotic muscle fibres that they eventually invade and destroy. These T cells are activated, as evidenced by their expression of ICAM-1 and MHC class I and II antigens on their surface, and exert, through deleterious cytokines (Tews and Goebel, 1996; Lundberg et al., 1995) a cytotoxic effect against muscle fibres. This process is supported by several lines of evidence.

- Cell lines established from muscle biopsies of patients with PM exert cytotoxicity to the autologous myotubes in vitro (Hohlfeld and Engel, 1991).
- By immunoelectron microscopy, CD8$^+$ cells and macrophages send spike-like processes into non-necrotic muscle fibres that traverse the basal lamina and focally displace or compress the muscle fibres ('partial invasion') (Arahata and Engel, 1986).
- The cytotoxic autoinvasive CD8$^+$ T cells contain perforin and granzyme granules (Goebel et al., 1996), which are directed towards the surface of the fibres and on release induce pores in the cell membrane and cell destruction.

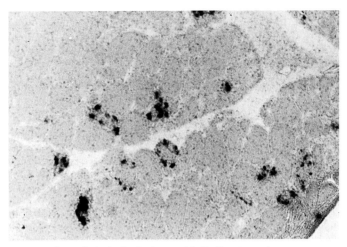

Fig. 31.12. Sporadic inclusion body myositis. Radioautograph using a radiolabelled single-stranded M13 phage DNA shows discrete binding sites in scattered muscle fibres. The binding sites are in or near rimmed vacuoles or in myonuclei. (×140.)

Efforts to document apoptotic cell death in these myofibres have repeatedly failed (Schneider et al., 1996). The prevailing view at the moment is that damage to the myofibre in PM results from atrophy and/or necrosis.

- On the basis of T cell receptor (TCR) analysis, there is clonal expansion of T cells with restricted usage of the TCR variable region of certain TCR gene families, notable Vα1, Vβ15 and Vβ6, indicating that the T cell response is driven by a muscle-specific antigen (Mantegazza et al., 1993; Bender et al., 1995; O'Hanlon et al., 1994a,b). This is true not only for PM but also for s-IBM (Bender et al., 1995; Fyhr et al., 1996, 1997). In the latter, the TCR of the autoinvasive CD8$^+$ T cells showed predominance of Vβ3, Vβ6, and Vβ5 gene families. When these families were

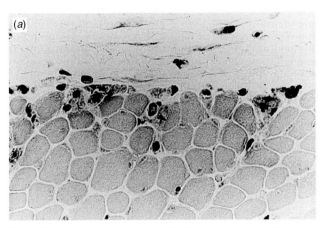

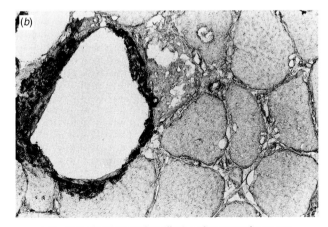

Fig. 31.13. Adult dermatomyositis. (a) Acid phosphatase-positive macrophages mark the sites of endomysial capillaries. The macrophages are presumably engaged in phagocytosis of necrotic endothelial cells (×350). (b) A large vein shows immunoreactive membrane attack complex deposited in its wall. (×520.)

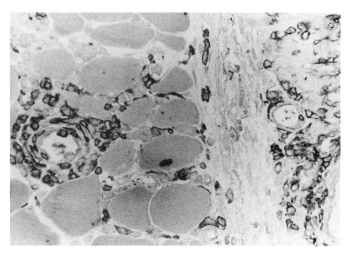

Fig. 31.14. Adult dermatomyositis. Helper T cells surround an endomysial arteriole on the right. On the left, an interfascicular septum contains mainly B lymphocytes. (Immunoperoxidase with antibodies for CD4 and CD20 antigens, respectively; ×350.)

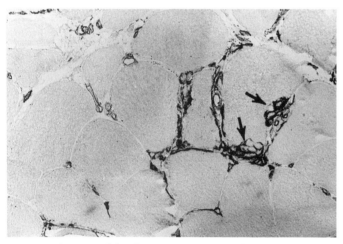

Fig. 31.15. Adult polymyositis. CD8 antigen-bearing (cytotoxic) lymphocytes partially invade a non-necrotic muscle fibre (arrows). (×320.)

cloned and sequenced, restriction in the amino acid sequence of the joining CDR3 region was noted (Bender et al., 1995). In s-IBM, the restricted expression of the TCR gene families among the autoinvasive T lymphocytes and the homologies in the CDR3 region persist over time, suggesting a continuous antigen-driven T cell response (Amemiya et al., 2000).

- The cytotoxicity mediated by the CD8$^+$ cells appears to be antigen-specific because, in addition to clonal expansion of certain TCR gene families described above, the T cells invade muscle fibres expressing MHC class 1 antigen, a prerequisite for antigen recognition by the

CD8$^+$ cells. MHC class 1 antigen is not present on normal muscle fibres but it is ubiquitously expressed on the sarcolemma of the muscle fibres in patients with PM and IBM (Karpati and Carpenter, 1993a). MHC class I expression is probably upregulated by cytokines secreted by activated T cells, macrophages or viruses (in a setting of a viral infection), as discussed below. Recent data indicate that the muscle fibres in PM and s-IBM express the BB1 marker of the antigen-presenting cells and their autoinvasive T cells express the CTLA-4 and CD28 receptor (Murata and Dalakas, 1999). It appears, therefore, that the muscle fibres are not only targets of cytotoxicity but also have the potential to behave as professional antigen-presenting cells (Bender et al., 1998). The nature of the antigenic peptides bound by the MHC class I for presentation to the CD8$^+$ cells is not known. It is believed that such antigens are probably endogenous sarcolemmal or cytoplasmic self-proteins originating from within the muscle fibre. The possibility of antigens being viral peptides appears unlikely because several laboratories have failed to amplify viruses within the muscle fibres not only in patients with PM triggered by a putative viral infection (Leff et al., 1992; Leon-Monzon and Dalakas, 1992), but also in patients with classic PM associated with infection with human immunodeficiency virus 1 (HIV-1) or human T cell leukaemia/lymphoma virus (HTLV-1) (Illa et al., 1991; Leon-Monzon et al., 1993, 1994).

- In three rare cases, γ/δ cells or natural killer cells were the main participating cells in the myocytotoxicity of PM and IBM (Hohlfeld et al., 1991; Puschke et al., 1992; Dalakas and Illa, 1995).
- Expression of metalloproteinases MMP-2 and MMP-9, zinc-dependent endopeptidases, is upregulated on the fibres expressing MHC class I and some CD8$^+$ autoinvasive T cells. Because the muscle membrane contains extracellular matrix proteins such as collagen IV and fibronectin, which are substrates for MMP-2 and MMP-9, these metalloproteinases may facilitate adhesion of T cells to the muscle and enhance cytotoxicity (Choi and Dalakas, 2000).

Cytokines and adhesion molecules

The T cell-derived cytokines (interleukins 2, 4 and 5 and interferon-γ), the macrophage-derived cytokines (interleukins 1 and 2 and tumour necrosis factor α), and cytokines that are derived from either T cells or macrophages (such as macrophage colony stimulating factor or transforming growth factor β) have been variably amplified with the reverse transcriptase polymerase chain reaction (PCR) in the muscles of patients with PM, DM and IBM. Among the adhesion molecules and their receptors, ICAM-1,

VCAM and endothelial leukocyte adhesion molecule (ELAM), and their respective ligands integrins β_1 and β_2, are also upregulated on the endothelial cells or the infiltrating T cells in patients with PM, DM and IBM. These may facilitate the adhesion, penetration and exit of activated T cells through the endothelial cell wall (de Bleecker and Engel, 1994; Dalakas, 1995a,b, 1998; Lundberg et al., 1995; Tews and Goebel, 1995). Figure 31.18 illustrates the immunopathology of PM and s-IBM.

Non-immune features in muscles in inclusion body myositis

The muscle biopsy is the key investigative tool for confirming the diagnosis of IBM. For the most informative sample, it is essential to avoid biopsy of a severely weak or of normal strength muscle.

Key microscopic findings of the muscle biopsy are summarized in Table 31.1 and illustrated in the figures cited therein (Dalakas, 1990; Dalakas and Sivakumar, 1996; Karpati, 1997).

Rimmed vacuoles are not specific for IBM, but when they occur in great abundance, they are highly characteristic (Fig. 31.9), particularly in association with the other features listed in Table 31.1. The blue granules that are located in or along the wall of the vacuoles correspond to whorls of cytomembranes or myelin figures, detectable by electron microscopy. On epon-embedded sections, the actual vacuolar space is much less conspicuous than on cryostat sections. The round or oval masses (2–4 μm by 6–8 μm) correspond to masses of irregularly stacked 14–18 μm thick filaments, which, on suitable orientation, can be shown to be tubular. The contention of a group of investigators that these filaments are identical to the paired helical filaments found in neurons in Alzheimer's disease (Askanas et al., 1994) has not been confirmed. The nature of the tubular filaments is still obscure. They do not represent viral particles. They possibly consist of altered myonuclear matrix material (vide infra).

Electron microscopy is necessary to show precisely the myonuclear abnormalities. These include abnormal heterochromatin distribution indicative of either a shut-off or activation of genomic activity, masses of the typical IBM tubular filaments and actual nuclear disintegration. In rare instances, the nuclear IBM filaments can be caught in the process of being discharged to the cytoplasm as a result of myonuclear breakdown.

Congophilic material, best visualized by Texas-red fluorescent optics (Fig. 31.11, colour plate), can be found in a variable number of fibres usually in or near rimmed vacuoles (Askanas et al., 1992a,b, 1993). However, this is by no means specific for IBM, as it has been found in other myo-

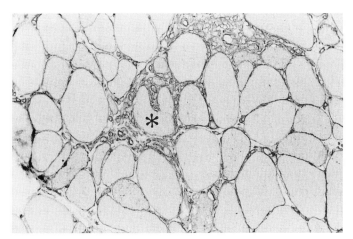

Fig. 31.16. Adult polymyositis. Immunoreactive class 1 major histocompatability complex protein is present at the surface of all muscle fibres as well as the surface of endomysial mononuclear inflammatory cells. The star indicates a fibre that is partially invaded by inflammatory cells. (×350.)

pathies (de Bleecker et al., 1996). or even in chronic neurogenic conditions such as the postpolio syndrome (Semino-Mora and Dalakas, 1998). The same applies to a variety of 'alien' molecules (Figs. 31.11 (colour plate) and 3.12), such as β-amyloid and its precursor protein, α-chymotrypsin, tau, apolipoprotein E, prion protein, etc. (Mendell et al., 1991; Askanas and Engel, 1995), which are found in a small percentage of fibres. Ubiquitin-positive masses are relatively frequent but are also nonspecific (Askanas and Engel, 1995).

A single-stranded DNA-binding protein accumulates in up to 5% of muscle fibres. This is demonstrated by in situ hybridization using a variety of DNA probes (Nalbantoglu et al., 1994). The sites of these accumulations correspond to existing or disintegrated myonuclei (Fig. 31.12). The identity of this protein is undetermined. Ragged-red, cytochrome oxidase-negative muscle fibres with mitochondrial excess are common. Multiple mitochondrial DNA deletions have been demonstrated in most examined cases (Horvath et al., 1998).

Viral infections

Several viruses, including coxsackievirus, influenza, parymyxoviruses, cytomegalovirus and Epstein–Barr virus, have been directly associated with chronic and acute myositis (Chou, 1986; Dalakas et al., 1986b; Nishino et al., 1989; Hays and Gamboa, 1994; Dalakas, 1995a). A possible molecular mimicry phenomenon has been proposed with the coxsackieviruses because of structural homology between Jo-1 antibody and the genomic RNA of an animal

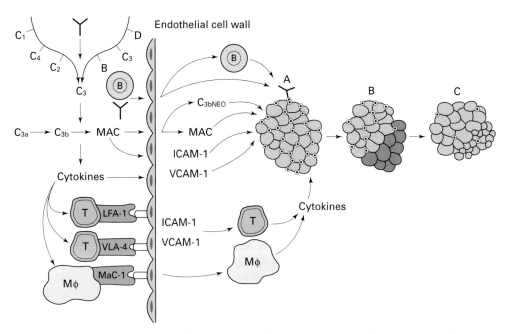

Fig. 31.17. Diagrammatic illustration of the main immune factors connected with the pathogenesis of dermatomyositis from the initiation of the disease. MAC, membrane attack complex; ICAM-1, intercellular adhesion molecule 1, VCAM-1, vascular cell adhesion molecule 1; LFA-1, leukocyte function associated antigen; VLA-4, very late antigen 4; C, complement components, Mϕ, macrophages. (See text for details.)

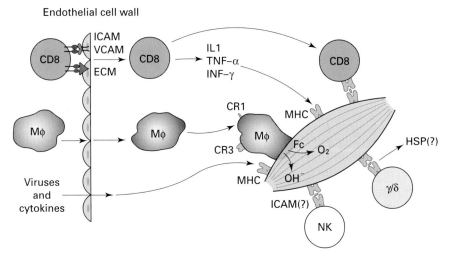

Fig. 31.18. Diagrammatic illustration of the main immune factors associated with the immunopathogenesis of polymyositis and sporadic inclusion body myositis. ICAM, intercellular adhesion molecule; VCAM, vascular cell adhesion molecule, CD8, CD8+ T cells; IL1, interleukin 1, TNF-α, tumour necrosis factor α; INF-γ, interferon-γ; CR, cellular receptor; MHC, major histocompatibility complex; HSP, heat shock protein, NK, natural killer; Mϕ, macrophages. (See text for details.)

picornavirus and the encephalomyocarditis virus (Plotz et al., 1989; Leff et al., 1992). Our very sensitive PCR studies, however, have repeatedly failed to confirm the presence of such viruses in these patients' muscle biopsies, suggesting that it is unlikely, although not impossible, for these viruses to replicate in the muscles of patients with PM, DM and IBM (Dalakas et al., 1986a,b, 1987; Dalakas and Pezeshkpour, 1988; Morgan et al., 1989; Dalakas, 1994b).

The best evidence of viral connection in PM and IBM is with retroviruses, which have been associated with inflammatory myopathy in monkeys infected with the simian immunodeficiency virus (Dalakas et al., 1986a, 1987), and in humans infected with HIV and HTLV-I (Dalakas et al., 1986b; Leon-Monzon et al., 1994; Cupler et al., 1996). In HIV-positive patients, an inflammatory myopathy (HIV-PM) can occur either as an isolated clinical phenomenon, being the first clinical indication of HIV infection, or concurrently with other manifestations of the acquired immunodeficiency syndrome (AIDS) (Dalakas and Pezeshkpour, 1988; Dalakas, 1994b). HIV seroconversion can also coincide with myoglobulinuria and acute myalgia, suggesting that myotropism for HIV may be symptomatic early in the infection. In addition, HTLV-1 causes not only a myeloneuropathy – referred to as tropical spastic paraparesis (TSP) – but also PM, which may coexist with TSP or may be the only clinical manifestation of HTLV-1 infection (Dalakas and Pezeshkpour, 1988; Dalakas, 1994b; Karpati and Currie, 1994). Of interest, IBM can also occur in a setting of HIV or HTLV-I infection (Cupler et al., 1996). Using in situ hybridization, PCR immunocytochemistry and electron microscopy, we could detect viral antigens within the muscle fibres of biopsies from patients with HIV and HTLV-1 but only in occasional endomysial macrophages (Illa et al., 1991; Leon-Monzon et al., 1993, 1994; Dalakas, 1994b; Cupler et al., 1996). We have interpreted these observations to suggest that in PM and IBM associated with HIV-1 and HTLV-1 there is no evidence of persistent infection of the muscle fibre with the virus or viral replication within the muscle. The predominant endomysial cells in HIV-1 and HTLV-1 PM and IBM are the CD8[+], nonviral-specific, cytotoxic T cells, which along with macrophages invade or surround non-necrotic muscle fibres expressing MHC class I. Because this immunopathological pattern is identical to the one described earlier for retroviral-negative PM and IBM, we have proposed that a T-cell-mediated and MHC class I-restricted cytotoxic process is a common pathogenetic mechanism in both retroviral-negative and retroviral-positive PM and IBM, but in the latter, viral-induced cytokines trigger the process.

Nonviral microbial myositis

Several animal parasites, such as protozoa (*Toxoplasma, Trypansoma* spp.), cestodes (cysticerci), and nematodes (trichinae), may produce a focal of diffuse IM known as parasitic PM. *Staphylococcus aureus, Yersinia* spp., *Streptococcus* spp. and anaerobes may produce a suppurative myositis, known as tropical PM or pyomyositis. Pyomyositis, a previous rarity in western countries, can now be seen in rare patients with AIDS. Certain bacteria, such as *Borrelia burgdorferi* of Lyme disease and *Legionella pneumophila* of Legionnaire's disease, may infrequently be the cause of polymyositis.

Inflammatory myopathies in collagen vascular diseases

Neuromuscular impairment may occur in any of the collagen vascular diseases from a variety of causes, such as muscle ischaemia, cachexia, peripheral nerve involvement, musculoskeletal deformities, therapeutic steroid-related side effect, etc. True IM is another possibility but occurs relatively infrequently (Rosenberg et al., 1988). In a large series of patients with systemic sclerosis, a DM-like picture was found in about 12% of the patients, particularly in those having anti-PM-Scl antibodies (Mimori, 1987). Among the inflammatory myopathies, DM is the only form that truly overlaps with systemic sclerosis. In systemic lupus, the true incidence in the form of PM has been estimated at 5–8% (Foote et al., 1982). In our experience, prominent class I MHC expression at the surface of muscle fibres appears to be a constant feature in these patients. In Sjögren's syndrome, both a DM and IBM picture has been observed; however, the overall incidence is low (Ringel et al., 1982). In rheumatoid arthritis and periarteritis nodosa, a clinically evident inflammatory muscle disease is very rare, although muscle biopsies may show focal interstitial or perivascular mononuclear inflammatory cell infiltrates or necrotic arteritis (Fig. 31.13*a*) respectively, without major muscle fibre damage.

In practical terms, if a patient with any of the above collagenoses, as defined by rigorous diagnostic criteria, shows undue muscle weakness that cannot otherwise be explained, and particularly if serum CK activity is significantly elevated and if there is an EMG abnormality consistent with an IM, a muscle biopsy from a carefully selected site is justified.

It appears that DM or PM in association with collagen vascular diseases shows the same pathological features as the ones found in idiopathic DM and PM.

Miscellaneous forms of inflammatory myopathies

Granulomatous myopathy

Granulomatous myopathy can occur in a number of conditions (Carpenter and Karpati, 1984; Mastaglia and Walton, 1992). While many patients with systemic sarcoidosis have asymptomatic microscopic granulomata in muscle, which can be helpful in the diagnosis, a clinically manifest myopathy is rare. These patients present with an insidious limb girdle syndrome and muscle biopsy shows noncaseating granulomas with giant cells. Muscle fibre damage is usually limited. In some patients, intranuclear filaments can be seen in myonuclei that are indistinguishable from those observed in IBM. In a special group of patients, usually postmenopausal women, a similar clinical and pathological picture in muscle is present without evidence of systemic sarcoidosis. In some of these patients myasthenia gravis may also develop. The relationship of this granulomatous myopathy to classical sarcoidosis is unclear.

A granulomatous myopathy may rarely develop into Crohn's disease (Ménard et al., 1976) and in association with thymoma.

Myopathy in hypersensitivity vasculitis

Vasculitis in muscle may be present in the many forms of IM including DM and the collagenoses. In addition, there are patients who present with a nonspecific vasculitis, which either involves skeletal muscles alone or their tissues as well. In many instances, the aetiological factor remains obscure. In these patients, the pathology consists of mononuclear infiltration of vessel walls and their vicinity without necrosis or thrombosis of the vessels themselves. The clinical picture is variable but severe muscle weakness rarely develops.

Eosinophilic syndromes

Three types of inflammatory disease are associated with either prominent presence of eosinophilic polymorphonuclear leukocytes in muscle (or fascia) or systemic eosinophilia, or both.

In *eosinophilic polymyositis* (Layzer et al., 1977), muscle involvement is part of a systemic hypereosinophilic syndrome. A marked systemic eosinophilia is present. Myocardium is often involved in the inflammatory process. Proximal limb muscles show stiffness, pain and variable weakness. Serum CK activity is moderately elevated. The pathological picture is similar to that of idiopathic PM, except that there is a conspicuous presence of eosinophilic polymorphonuclear leukocytes in the inflammatory infiltrates.

In *eosinophilic fasciitis*, the inflammatory reaction is restricted to the fascia and is best shown by a biopsy of the fascia lata (Simon et al., 1982). *Necrotizing fasciitis* is a misnomer because the basic process is a hyperacute necrotizing myopathy caused usually by β-haemolytic streptococci, presumably acting as a superantigen (File et al., 1998; Gardam et al., 1998). It may follow a variety of wounds and surgical interventions. If early treatment with high-dose intravenous immunoglobulins and antistreptococcal antibiotics is missed, amputation of the affected limb may be necessary to avoid a fatal outcome.

The *eosinophilia–myalgia syndrome* was caused by prolonged oral intake of large doses of a contaminated L-tryptophan preparation as a therapeutic agent, mainly for insomnia (Hertzmann et al., 1990). There was marked systemic eosinophilia with generalized myalgia and moderate muscle weakness (Martin et al., 1990). Another important feature is thickening of the skin, mimicking scleroderma. In severe disease, myocarditis and other visceral involvements can supervene. The lymphocytic inflammatory infiltrates (CD8[+] cytotoxic cells) also include either abundant or few eosinophilic polymorphonuclear leukocytes, mainly in the perimysial region, but less often also in the interstitial space of muscle (Emslie-Smith et al., 1991; Illa et al., 1993). Muscle fibre necrosis was rare and serum CK activity did not rise significantly. Coexisting peripheral neuropathy may cause denervation atrophy. In some cases, the muscle biopsy shows no abnormality, despite clinical symptoms.

The pathogenic factor appears to be a contamination of L-tryptophan with an acetaldehyde ditryptophan derivative, which seems to induce an autosensitization. The disease usually subsides after cessation of exposure but resolution may be slow. Corticosteroid therapy may help to accelerate recovery.

Macrophagic myofasciitis

A distinctive inflammatory muscle disorder was recently identified in up to 80 French patients who presented with myalgias, fatigue and mild muscle weakness (Cherin et al., 1999). Muscle biopsy revealed pronounced infiltration of the connective tissue around the muscle (epimysium, perimysium and perifascicular endomysium) by sheets of periodic acid–Schiff base-positive macrophages and occasional CD8[+] T cells. Serum CK or erythrocyte sedimentation may at times be elevated. Most patients respond to glucocorticoid therapy, and the overall prognosis is favourable. The pathology is almost always seen at the sites of previous vaccinations, even several months later, and has been linked to a type of aluminium component used as a substrate for preparation of the vaccines. Macrophagic myofasciitis has been reported exclusively from France.

Localized forms

IM, usually of the PM type, may be restricted to one muscle or to one group of muscles (Heffner et al., 1977; Bharucha and Morgan-Hughes, 1981). These localized forms of IM may involve forearm muscles, quadriceps, sternomastoids, masseter or shoulder-girdle muscles. The last is probably the best known variety, since it mimics facioscapulohumeral dystrophy (Munsat et al., 1972). It may be sporadic or familial (autosomal dominant). The response to corticosteroid therapy is poor.

Another form of localized muscle inflammation can occur in any large muscle presenting as a muscle mass (Heffner et al., 1977). Necrosis and regeneration of muscle fibres and focal inflammatory infiltrates are present. The aetiology of this peculiar muscle reaction is unknown. It has to be differentiated from neoplasms or abscesses.

Inflammatory myopathy with 'pipe-stem' capillaries

In three patients, a peculiar form of necrotizing and to a lesser extent IM with a microangiopathy has been described (Emslie-Smith and Engel, 1991). The hallmark of the pathology is so-called 'pipe stem' capillaries, which stand out by their thickened wall. MAC was demonstrated in the walls of some of these vessels. The capillarization of the muscle is usually reduced. While there are similarities between this vascular pathology and that occurring in DM, the two entities are different. It should be noted that capillaries with thickened walls, presumably caused by a widening of the basal lamina, can occur in a variety of diseases including diabetes, collagen vascular disorders (such as systemic lupus erythematosus) as well as unspecified myopathies and neuropathies.

Drug-induced inflammatory myopathy

Reduced intramuscular injection of pentazocine in habitual users of the analgesic drug produces a necrotic IM with massive increase of endomysial and perimysial connective tissue, resulting in joint contractures. A peculiar effect of this process is the inability of arms to be fully lowered next to the trunk ('arm levitation phenomenon'). It is not known what chemical feature of pentazocine is responsible for this peculiar pathological reaction in muscle.

Systemic use of D-penicillamine (Doyle et al., 1983), procainamide and phenytoin may cause vasculitis involving skeletal muscles. Reduced muscle strength, however, is usually mild. D-Penicillamine, in fact, more often causes a myasthenia-like picture than vasculitis. (See also Chapter 33). Zidovudine, used in the treatment of AIDS, causes a mitochondrial myopathy that may coexist with endomysial inflammatory infiltrants related to HIV (Dalakas et al., 1995).

Graft-versus-host reaction

In the graft-versus-host reaction, interstitial infiltration of muscle with lymphocytes may occur, but clinical muscle weakness is mild or not discernable.

Combined inflammatory and mitochondrial myopathy

Combined inflammatory and mitochondrial myopathy occurs in middle-aged patients with a chronic limb girdle syndrome and prominent quadriceps weakness (Carpenter et al., 1992; Blume et al., 1997). They have markedly elevated serum CK activity with typical muscle pathological features of PM and mitochondrial myopathy. The response to corticosteroids is poor. This entity appears distinct from IBM.

Special forms of myopathies in children

Benign acute childhood myositis

Benign acute childhood myositis (BACM) is also called myalgia cruris epidemica since the cardinal manifestations include acute pain and swelling of the muscles in the calves and anterior tibial compartment. The disease runs a self-limiting course of a few days up to two weeks (Anthony et al., 1979). Cases tend to cluster, which would be consistent with an infectious aetiology. Influenza A and B virus have been found in patients with BACM (Ruff and Secrist, 1982). Muscle biopsy may be normal or it may show intense lymphocytic infiltration and oedema.

Childhood dermatomyositis

Childhood DM is the most common form of acquired muscle disease in childhood (Carpenter et al., 1976; Banker and Engel, 1986). Onset of symptoms may occur as early as two years. The peak incidence is 14–16 years of age. The female-to-male ratio of occurrence is about 3:2. In approximately 25% of children, an acute viral-like disease precedes the onset.

The course of the disease is usually subacute, but acute cases are not too infrequent. Symptoms include weakness of the shoulder and hip girdle muscles, as well as proximal limb muscles. Muscles are often tender to touch and may be swollen. Muscle pain and arthralgia are exaggerated by exercise. The skin rash is similar to that described in adult DM. Raynaud's phenomenon does not occur and carcinoma is not associated with childhood DM.

Extramuscular manifestations, which are nowadays rare, may include ischaemic necrosis of the intestinal wall with perforation. Subcutaneous calcinosis is not uncommon and causes skin ulceration and limb deformities. Interstitial pulmonary fibrosis is very rare. Childhood DM is self-limiting after a course of two to four years; however, if it is left untreated, severe residual muscle wasting and weakness may occur.

The serum CK activity is elevated and the EMG shows a characteristic pattern that is similar to that of adult DM.

The light and electron microscopic histological features on muscle biopsy are very similar to those of adult DM, but perifascicular atrophy and muscle infarcts are more common in childhood DM. The vascular changes include capillary necrosis, reduced capillary density of muscle, endothelial cell abnormalities and thrombosis of medium-sized arteries and veins.

Polymyositis in children

Chronic IM of the adult PM type is exceedingly rare in children (Thompson, 1982). Two peculiar types of chronic IM deserve comment. Although these entities are rare they are still important because they are potentially treatable and require differentiation from congenital muscular dystrophy and other congenital myopathies.

Infantile polymyositis with sick myonuclei

Infantile PM with sick myonuclei (Sripathi et al., 1996) develops during the first year. Early signs include an inability to stand, falling, weak arm elevation and poor head control owing to weakness of neck muscles. The atrophy of arm muscles with relatively normal bulk of forearm musculature confers a 'Popeye' type of arm contour. Craniobulbar deficits are lacking and there are no extramuscular manifestations. Tendon reflexes are usually lost early in the disease.

The EMG findings are similar to those described for adult idiopathic PM. Muscle biopsy abnormalities include interstitial infiltrates of lymphocytes but without partial invasion of muscle fibres of the type described in PM, marked smallness of most muscle fibres, scattered muscle fibre necrosis and regeneration. Failed regeneration, however, is common and as a result numerous scattered

foci of muscle fibre loss and fibrosis are common features. Sarcolemmal class I MHC expression in muscle fibres occurs, which tends to confirm the inflammatory nature of the disease.

A distinctive feature of the pathology consists of prominent myonuclear abnormalities (Figs 31.10) including abnormally large size, irregular or even bizarre shapes with cytoplasmic invaginations and various inclusions. Inclusions may take the form of 4 nm filaments resembling actin filaments, hexagonal arrays of 22 nm filaments and microtubules. Excess heterochromatin is present in many nuclei.

This disease appears to be self-limiting but even with corticosteroid therapy (which is somewhat helpful) major permanent muscle wasting and weakness remain.

Congenital inflammatory myopathy

In cogenital IM (Roddy et al., 1986; Shevell et al., 1990), fetal movements are reduced and muscular hypotonia is noted at birth. Motor milestones are considerably delayed. Muscle weakness involves the neck, limb, face and respiratory territories. Contractures are common in the limbs. Stretch reflexes are depressed or absent. Most patients have microencephaly and mental subnormality. The muscle biopsy reveals necrosis and regeneration, extensive muscle fibre loss and fibrosis, focal interstitial lymphocytic infiltration and sarcolemmal class I MHC expression in large groups of nonregenerating muscle fibres. Dystrophin immunostaining of muscle fibres is normal.

Steroid responsiveness of this disease is variable but never dramatic and CNS features are not affected.

This syndrome must be differentiated from Fukuyama congenital dystrophy (Olney and Miller, 1983), as well as the Walker Walburg syndrome and merosin-negative congenital dystrophy (see Chapter 25). In the last, the muscle biopsy may show prominent endomysial inflammatory infiltrates.

Treatment

Because the specific target antigens in DM, PM and IBM are unknown, the presently employed immunosuppressive therapies are not selectively targeting either the autoreactive T cells or the complement-mediated process affecting intramuscular blood vessels. Instead, they are inducing a nonselective and largely nonspecific immunosuppression or immunomodulation. Furthermore, many of these therapies are empirical and are based mostly on uncontrolled experience.

The practical goal of therapy in IM is to improve the function in the activities of daily living and improving muscle strength. In essence, the therapy is also designed to induce a remission of the dysimmune state or to minimize muscle fibre loss before a spontaneous remission occurs. Although when the muscle strength improves, the serum CK tends to fall concurrently, the reverse is not always true because most of the immunosuppressive therapies can result in decrease of serum muscle enzymes without necessarily improving muscle strength. Unfortunately, this has been interpreted as 'chemical improvement' and led to the erroneous practice of 'chasing' or 'treating' the serum CK level instead of the muscle weakness. This practice may lead to prolonged use of unnecessary immunosuppressive drugs and erroneous assessment of their efficacy (Dalakas, 1988, 1989, 1991, 1992, 1994a, 1995a).

Drugs of use in treating inflammatory myopathies

Corticosteroids

Prednisone is the first-line drug for treatment for DM or PM. Its action is unclear but it may exert a beneficial effect by inhibiting recruitment and migration of lymphocytes to the areas of muscle inflammation and interfering with the production of lymphokines. Its effect on interleukin 1 may be important because this lymphokine is myotoxic (Leon-Monzon and Dalakas, 1994) and is secreted by the activated macrophages that invade the muscle fibres. Steroid-induced suppression of ICAM-1 may also be relevant because downregulation of ICAM-1 can prevent the passage of lymphocytes across the endothelial cell wall towards the muscle fibres.

Because the effectiveness and relative safety of prednisone therapy will determine the future need for stronger immunosuppressive drugs, our preference has been to start with a high-dose prednisone, 80–100 mg per day, early in the disease. After an initial period of three to four weeks, prednisone is tapered over a 10-week period to 80–100 mg in a single daily dose, alternate days by gradually reducing the alternate 'off day' dose by 10 mg per week, or faster if necessitated by side effects, though this carries a greater risk of breakthrough of disease. If there is evidence of efficacy, and no serious side effects, the dosage is reduced gradually by 5–10 mg every three to four weeks until the lowest possible dose that controls the disease is reached. If by the time the dosage has been reduced to 80–100 mg every other day (approximately 14 weeks after initiating therapy), there has been no objective benefit (defined as unimproved muscle strength) the patient may be considered unresponsive to prednisone and an accelerated tapering regimen is introduced while the next-in-line immunosuppressive drug is started (Dalakas, 1988, 1989, 1992, 1995a). An important alternative to high-dose oral steroids is high-dose intermittent intravenous methylprednisolone, at 500–1000 mg two to three times weekly, depending on disease severity and tolerance. In fact, this is the highly preferred first-line treatment of one of the authors (G.K.). This route of administration minimizes muscular (and extramuscular) side effects, which are particularly prone to occur in the aged and those with malnutrition and major disease atrophy. In such cases, it is our preferred initial treatment. When the dose can be reduced, a switch to a much lower oral therapy can be made.

Although almost all the patients with bona fide PM or DM respond to steroids to some degree at least for some period of time, a number of them fail to respond or become steroid resistant. Many authorities recommend immunosuppressive drugs, such as azathioprine along with corticosteroids at the outset, while others base the decision to start an immunosuppressive drug in patients with PM or DM on the following factors: (i) need for its 'steroid-sparing' effect, when in spite of steroid responsiveness the patient has developed significant complications; (ii) attempts to lower a high-steroid dosage have repeatedly resulted in a new relapse; (iii) adequate dose of prednisone for at least a two to three month period has been ineffective; and (iv) rapidly progressive disease with evolving severe weakness and respiratory failure. One author of this chapter (G.K.) prefers to use immunosuppressants at the outset, while the other author (M.D.) delays it for the above-cited special circumstances. The preference for selecting immunosuppressive therapy is, however, empirical. The choice is usually based on our own prejudices, our personal experience with each drug and our own assessment of the relative efficacy and safety ratio. A number of immunosuppressive agents have been used.

Azathioprine

Azathioprine is a derivative of 6-mercatopurine; it is given orally. Although lower doses (1.5–2 mg/kg) are commonly used, we prefer higher doses, up to 3 mg/kg for effective immunosuppression. This drug is well tolerated, has fewer side effects and, empirically, it appears to be as effective for long-term therapy as the other drugs. If liver function tests become impaired, the drug should be stopped. Some degree of anaemia however is tolerated.

Methotrexate

Methotrexate is an antagonist of folate metabolism. Although its superiority to azathioprine has not been established, it does have a faster action. It can be given intravenously over 20–60 minutes at weekly doses of 0.4 up to 0.8 mg/kg with sufficient fluids, or orally starting at 7.5 mg weekly for the first 3 weeks (given in a total of three doses, 2.5 mg every 12 hours), increasing it gradually by 2.5 mg per week up to a total of 25 mg weekly. A relevant side effect is methotrexate pneumonitis, which can be difficult to distinguish from the interstitial lung disease of the primary inflammatory myopathy, the latter often associated with Jo-1 antibodies.

Cyclophosphamide

Cyclophosphamide is an alkylating agent that is given intravenously or orally, at doses of 2–2.5 mg/kg, usually 50 mg orally three times a day. Cyclophosphamide has not been effective in our hands (Cronin et al., 1989) in spite of occasional promising results reported by others (Bombardieri et al., 1989).

Chlorambucil

Chlorambucil is an antimetabolite that has been tried in some patients with variable results (Sinoway and Callen, 1993).

Cyclosporin

Although the toxicity of cyclosporin (cyclosporine) can now be monitored by measuring optimal trough serum levels (optimal levels are 100–250 mg/ml), its effectiveness in PM and DM needs confirmation (Heckmatt et al., 1989). The advantage of cyclosporin is that it acts faster than azathioprine or methotrexate and the results (positive or negative) may therefore become apparent early (Grau et al., 1994).

Plasmapheresis

A double-blind, placebo-controlled study did not show any advantage from plasmapheresis (Miller et al., 1992).

Total lymphoid irradiation

Total lymphoid irradiation has been helpful in rare patients and may have long-lasting benefit. The long-term side effects of this treatment, however, should be seriously considered before deciding on this experimental and rather extreme approach. Total lymphoid irradiation has been ineffective in IBM (Kelly et al., 1986).

Intravenous immunoglobulin

The use of intravenous immunoglobulin (IVIg) is a promising, but expensive therapy. It has been reported to be effective in uncontrolled studies (Cherin et al., 1991; Lang et al., 1991; Jan et al., 1992). In the first double-blind study conducted for DM, IVIg was effective in patients with refractory DM; not only did strength improve but also the underlying immunopathology may resolve (Dalakas et al.,

1993). The improvements begin after the first IVIg infusion and are clearly evident by the second monthly infusion. The benefit is short lived (not more than eight weeks), requiring repeated infusions every six to eight weeks for an indefinite period to maintain improvement.

IVIg may act in DM by inhibiting the deposition of activated complement fragment on the capillaries (Basta and Dalakas, 1994), by suppressing cytokines especially ICAM-1, or by saturating Fc receptors and interfering with the action of macrophages (Dalakas et al., 1997a,b; Dalakas, 1997).

A controlled double-blind study for PM is still underway although the drug has been effective in our hands in up to 80% of the patients in uncontrolled studies.

IVIg has also exerted some benefit in IBM in uncontrolled studies (Soueidan and Dalakas 1993). Others, however, have not confirmed it (Amato et al., 1994). Benefit was seen in up to 30% of patients, although not statistically significant, in our controlled double-blind study (Dalakas et al., 1997a). Although the improvement was not dramatic, it made a difference to the lifestyle of these patients. In a further study that examined treatment with IVIg in combination with prednisone, no benefit of IVIg could be shown (Dalakas et al., 1997a); similar results were seen in an uncontrolled study (Barohn et al., 1995).

A treatment regimen

Until further control drug trials are completed, the following step-by-step empirical approach for the treatment of PM and DM is suggested:

Step 1: high-dose corticosteroid (oral or intermittent intravenous)

Step 2: initial and/or subsequent optional immunosuppressants, i.e. azathioprine or methotrexate

Step 3: if step 2 fails, try high-dose IVIg

Step 4: if step 3 fails, consider a trial, with guarded optimism, of one of the following agents, chosen according to the patient's age, degree of disability, tolerance, experience with the drug and the patient's general health: cyclosporin or chlorambucil, cyclophosphamide or mycophenolate.

The ultimate aim of treatment is the elimination of the aetiological factor. That is rarely attainable at present. Short of that, the development of specific immunotherapies aimed at targeting precise pathogenic events operating in the particular inflammatory myopathy is the goal. This may include inhibition of antigen presentation, curtailment of inflammatory cell activiation and mobility or inhibition of the production or action of specific pathogenic antibodies.

References

Amato, A. A., Barohn, R. J., Jackson, C. E., Pappert, E. J., Sahenk, Z. and Kissel, J. T. (1994). Inclusion body myositis: treatment with intravenous immunoglobulin. *Neurology* **44**, 1516–1518.

Amemiya, K., Granger, R. P. and Dalakas, M. C. (2000). Clonal restriction of T-cell receptor expression by infiltrating lymphocytes in inclusion body myositis persists over time. Studies in repeated muscle biopsies. *Brain* **123**, 2030–2039.

Anthony, J. H., Procopis, P. G. and Ourvrier, R. A. (1979). Benign acute childhood myositis. *Neurology* **29**, 1068–1071.

Arahata, K. and Engel, A. G. (1984). Monoclonal antibody analysis of mononuclear cells in myopathies. I: Quantitation of subsets according to diagnosis and sites of accumulation and demonstration and counts of muscle fibres invaded by T cells. *Ann. Neurol.* **16**, 193–208.

Arahata, K. and Engel, A. G. (1986). Monoclonal antibody analysis of mononuclear cells in myopathies III. Immunoelectron microscopy aspects of cell-mediated muscle fibre injury. *Ann. Neurol.* **19**, 112–125.

Argov, Z. and Yarom, R. (1984). 'Rimmed vacuole myopathy' sparing the quadriceps: a unique disorder in Iranian Jews. *J. Neurol. Sci.* **64**, 33–43.

Argov, Z., Tiram, E., Eisenberg, I. et al. (1997). Various types of hereditary inclusion body myopathies map to chromosome 9p1-q1. *Ann. Neurol.* **41**, 548–551.

Askanas, V. and Engel, W. K. (1995). New advances in the understanding of sporadic inclusion body myopathies. *Curr. Opin. Rheum.* **7**, 486–496.

Askanas, V., Serdaroglu, P., Engel, W. K. and Alvarez, R. B. (1992a). Immunocytochemical localization of ubiquitin in inclusion body myositis allows its light-microscopic distinction from polymyositis. *Neurology* **42**, 460–461.

Askanas, V., Engel, W. K., Alvarez, R. B. and Glenner, G. G. (1992b). β-Amyloid protein immunoreactivity in muscle of patients with inclusion-body myositis. *Lancet* **339**, 560–561.

Askanas, V., Engel, W. K. and Alvarez, R. B. (1993). Enhanced detection of Congo-red-positive amyloid deposits in muscle fibers of inclusion body myositis and brain of Alzheimer disease using fluorescence technique. *Neurology* **43**, 1265–1267.

Askanas, V., Engel, W. K., Bilak, M., Alvarez, R. B. and Selkoe, D. J. (1994). Twisted tubulofilaments of inclusion body myositis muscle resemble paired helical filaments of Alzheimer brain containing hyperphosphorylated tau. *Am. J. Pathol.* **144**, 177–187.

Banker, B. Q. (1975). Dermatomyositis of childhood. Ultrastructural alterations of muscle and intramuscular blood vessels. *J. Neuropathol. Exp. Neurol.* **35**, 46–75.

Banker, B. Q. and Engel, A. G. (1986). The polymyositis and dermatomyositis syndromes In: *Myology*, eds. A. G. Engel, and B. Q. Banker, pp. 1385–1422. New York: McGraw Hill.

Barohn, R. J., Amato, A. A., Sahenk, Z., Kissel, J. T., Mendell, J. R. (1995). Inclusion body myositis: explanation for poor response to immunosuppressive therapy. *Neurology* **45**, 1302–1304.

Basta, M. and Dalakas, M. C. (1994). High-dose intravenous immunoglobulin exerts its beneficial effect in patients with derma-tomyositis by blocking endomysial deposition of activated complement fragments. *J. Clin. Invest.* **94**, 1729–1735.

Bender, A., Ernst, N., Iglesias, A., Dornmair, K., Wekerle, H. and Hohlfeld, R. (1995). T cell receptor in polymyositis: clonal expansion of autoaggressive CD8⁺ T cells. *J. Exp. Med.* **181**, 1863–1868.

Bender, A., Behrens, L., Engel, A. G. and Hohlfeld, R. (1998). T-cell heterogeneity in muscle lesions of inclusion body myositis. *J. Neuroimmunol* **84**, 86–91.

Bharucha, N. E. and Morgan-Hughes, J. A. (1981). Chronic focal polymyositis in the adult. *J. Neurol. Neurosurg. Psychiatr.* **44**, 419–425.

Blume, G., Pestronk, A., Frank, B. and Johns, D. R. (1997). Polymyositis with cytochrome oxidase negative muscle fibres. Early quadriceps weakness and poor response to immunosuppressive therapy. *Brain* **120**, 39–45.

Bombardieri, S., Hughes, G. R. V., Neri, R., Del Bravo, P. and Del Bono, L. (1989). Cyclophosphamide in severe polymyositis. *Lancet* **i**, 1138–1139.

Carpenter, S. (1996). Inclusion body myositis, a review. *J. Neuropath. Exp. Neurol.* **55**, 1105–1114.

Carpenter, S. and Karpati, G. (1981). The major inflammatory myopathies of unknown cause. *Pathol. Ann.* **16**, 205–237.

Carpenter, S. and Karpati, G. (1984). Granulomatous myopathies. In: *Pathology of Skeletal Muscle*, eds. S. Carpenter, and G. Karpati, pp. 557–558. New York: Churchill-Livingstone.

Carpenter, S. and Karpati, G. (1992). The pathological diagnosis of specific inflammatory myopathies. *Brain Pathol.* **2**, 13–19.

Carpenter, S., Karpati, G., Rothman, S. and Walters, G. (1976). The childhood type of dermatomyositis. *Neurology* **26**, 952–962.

Carpenter, S., Karpati, G., Johnston, W., Shoubridge, E. and Gavel, M. (1992). Coexistence of polymyositis (PM) with mitochondrial myopathy (MM). *Neurology* **42** (Suppl. 3), 388.

Cervera, R., Ramires, G., Fernandez-Sola, J. et al. (1991). Antibodies to endothelial cells in dermatomyositis: association with interstitial lung disease. *Br. Med. J.* **302**, 880–881.

Cherin, P., Herson, S., Wechsler, B. et al. (1991). Efficacy of intravenous immunoglobulin therapy in chronic refractory polymyositis and dermatomyositis. An open study with 20 adult patients. *Am. J. Med.* **91**, 162–168.

Cherin, P., Laforet, P., Gherardi, R. K. et al. (1999). Macrophagic myofasciitis: description and etiopathogenic hypothesis. Study and Research Group on Acquired and Dysimmunity-related Muscular Diseases (GERMMAD) of the French Association against Myopathies (AFM). *Rev. Med. Int.* **206**, 483–499.

Choi, Y. C. and Dalakas, M. C. (2000). Expression of matrix metalloproteinases in the muscle of patients with inflammatory myopathies. *Neurology* **54**, 65–71.

Chou, S. M. (1986). Inclusion body myositis: a possible chronic persistent mumps myositis? *Hum. Pathol.* **17**, 765–776.

Clawson, K. and Oddis, C. V. (1995). Adult respiratory distress syndrome in polymyositis patients with the anti-Jo-I antibody. *Arthritis Rheum.* **38**, 1519–1523.

Cole, A. J., Kuzniecky, R., Karpati, G., Carpenter, S., Andermann, E. and Andermann, F. (1988). Familial myopathy with changes resembling inclusion body myositis and periventricular leucoencephalopathy. *Brain* **111**, 1025–1037.

Cronin, M. E., Miller, F. W., Hicks, J. E., Dalakas, M. and Plotz, P. H. (1989). The failure of intravenous cyclophosphamide therapy in refractory idiopathic inflammatory myopathy. *J. Rheumatol.* **16**, 1225–1228.

Cupler, E. J., Leon-Monzon, M., Miller, J., Semino-Mora, C., Anderson, T. L. and Dalakas, M. C. (1996). Inclusion body myositis in HIV-I and HTLV-I infected patients. *Brain* **19**, 1887–1893.

Dalakas, M. C. (ed.) (1988). *Polymyositis and Dermatomyositis.* Boston, MA: Butterworths.

Dalakas, M. C. (1989). Treatment of polymyositis and dermatomyositis. *Curr. Opin. Rheumatol.* **1**, 443–449.

Dalakas, M. C. (1990). Inflammatory myopathies. *Curr. Opin. Neurol. Neurosurg.* **3**, 689–696.

Dalakas, M. C. (1991). Polymyositis, dermatomyositis, and inclusion-body myositis. *N. Engl. J. Med.* **325**, 1487–1498.

Dalakas, M. C. (1992). Inflammatory myopathies: pathogenesis and treatment. *Clin. Neuropharmacol.* **5**, 327–351.

Dalakas, M. C. (1994a). Current treatment of the inflammatory myopathies. *Curr. Opin. Rheumatol.* **6**, 595–601.

Dalakas, M. C. (1994b). Retroviral myopathies. In: *Myology*, vol. II, eds. A. G. Engel and C. Franzini-Armstrong, pp. 1419–1437. New York: McGraw-Hill.

Dalakas, M. C. (1995a). How to diagnose and treat the inflammatory myopathies. *Semin. Neurol.* **14**, 137–145.

Dalakas, M. C. (1995b). Immunopathogenesis of inflammatory myopathies. *Ann. Neurol.* **37**, 74–86.

Dalakas, M. C. (1995c). Calcifications in dermatomyositis. *N. Engl. J. Med.* **333**, 978.

Dalakas, M. C. (1997). Intravenous immunoglobulin therapy for neurological diseases. *Ann. Intern. Med.* **126**, 721–730.

Dalakas, M. C. (1998). Molecular immunology and genetics of inflammatory muscle diseases. *Arch. Neurol.* **55**, 1509–1512.

Dalakas, M. C. and Illa, I. (1995). Common variable immunodeficiency and inclusion body myositis: a distinct myopathy mediated by natural killer cells. *Ann. Neurol.* **37**, 806–810.

Dalakas, M. C. and Pezeshkpour, G. H. (1988). Neuromuscular diseases associated with human immunodeficiency virus infection. *Ann. Neurol.* **23**(Suppl.), 38–48.

Dalakas, M. C. and Sivakumar, K. (1996). The immunopathologic and inflammatory differences between dermatomyositis, polymyositis and inclusion body myositis. *Curr. Opin. Neurol. Neurosurg.* **9**, 235–239.

Dalakas, M. C., London, W. T., Gravell, M. and Sever, J. L. (1986a). Polymyositis in an immunodeficiency disease in monkeys induced by a type D retrovirus. *Neurology* **36**, 569–572

Dalakas, M. C., Pezeshkpour, G. H., Gravell, M. and Sever, J. L. (1986b). Polymyositis in patients with AIDS. *JAMA* **256**, 2381–2383.

Dalakas, M. C., Gravell, M., London, W. T., Cunningham, G. and Sever, J. L. (1987). Morphological changes of an inflammatory myopathy in rhesus monkeys with simian acquired immunodeficiency syndrome (SAIDS). *Proc. Soc. Exp. Biol. Med.* **185**, 368–376.

Dalakas, M. C., Illa, I., Dambrosia, J. M. et al. (1993). A controlled trial of high-dose intravenous immunoglobulin infusions as treatment for dermatomyositis. *N. Engl. J. Med.* **329**, 1993–2000.

Dalakas, M. C., Illa, I., Pezeshkpour, G. H. et al. (1995). Mitochondrial myopathy caused by long-term zidovudine therapy. *N. Engl. J. Med.* **332**, 1098–1105.

Dalakas, M. C., Sonies, B., Koffman, B. et al. (1997a). High-dose intravenous immunoglobulin (IVIg) combined with prednisone in the treatment of patients with inclusion-body myositis (IBM): a double blind, randomized controlled trial. *Neurology* **48**, 332S.

Dalakas, M. C., Sekul, E. A., Cupler, E. J. and Sivakumar, K. (1997b). The efficacy of high dose intravenous immunoglobulin (IVIg) in patients with inclusion-body myositis (IBM). *Neurology* **48**, 712–716.

de Bleecker, J. L. and Engel, A. G. (1994). Expression of cell adhesion molecules in inflammatory myopathies and Duchenne dystrophy. *J. Neuropathol. Exp. Neurol.* **53**, 369–376.

de Bleecker, J. L., Ertl, B. B. and Engel, A. G. (1996). Patterns of abnormal parotein expression in target formations and unstructured cores. *Neuromusc. Disord.* **6**, 339–349.

de Visser, M., Emslie-Smith, A. M. and Engel, A. G. (1989). Early ultrastructural alterations in adult dermatomyositis. Capillary abnormalities precede other structural changes in muscle. *J. Neurol. Sci.* **94**, 181–192.

Doyle, D. R., McCurley, T. L. and Sergent, J. S. (1983). Fatal polymyositis in D-penicillamine-treated rheumatoid arthritis. *Ann. Intern. Med.* **98**, 327–330.

Emslie-Smith, A. M. and Engel, A. G. (1990). Microvascular changes in early and advanced dermatomyositis: a quantitative study. *Ann. Neurol.* **27**, 343–356.

Emslie-Smith, A. M. and Engel, A. G. (1991). Necrotizing myopathy with pipestem capillaries, microvascular deposition of the complement membrane attack complex (MAC), and minimal cellular infiltration. *Neurology* **41**, 936–939.

Emslie-Smith, A. M., Arahata, K. and Engel, A. G. (1989). Major histocompatibility complex class I antigen expression, immunolocalization of interferon subtypes, and T cell-mediated cytotoxicity in myopathies. *Hum. Pathol.* **20**, 224–231.

Emslie-Smith, A. M., Engel, A. G., Duffy, J. and Bowles, C. A. (1991). Eosinophilia myalgia syndrome: I. Immunocytochemical evidence for a T-cell-mediated immune effector response. *Ann. Neurol.* **29**, 524–528.

Engel, A. G. and Arahata, K. (1984). Monoclonal antibody analysis of mononuclear cells in myopathies. II: phenotypes of autoinvasive cells in polymyositis and inclusion body myositis. *Ann. Neurol.* **16**, 209–215.

Engel, A. G. and Arahata, K. (1986). Mononuclear cells in myopathies: quantitation of functionally distinct subsets, recognition of antigen-specific cell-mediated cytotoxicity in some diseases, and implications for the pathogenesis of the different inflammatory myopathies. *Hum. Pathol.* **17**, 702–721.

Engel, A. G., and Banker, B. Q. (1986). *Myology.* New York: McGraw-Hill.

Engel, A. G., Hohlfeld, R. and Banker, B. Q. (1994). The polymyositis and dermatomyositis syndrome. In: *Myology*, eds. A. G. Engel and C. Franzini-Armstrong, pp. 1335–1383. New York: McGraw-Hill.

File, T. M. Jr, Tan, S.J. and DiPersio, J. R. (1998). Group A streptococcal necrotizing fasciitis. Diagnosing and treating the 'flesh-eating bacteria syndrome'. *Cleveland Clinic. J. Med.* **65**, 241–249.

Foote, R. A., Kimbrough, S. M. and Stevens, J. C. (1982). Lupus myositis. *Muscle and Nerve* **5**, 65.

Fyhr, I. M., Moslemi, A. R., Tarkowski, A., Lindberg, C. and Oldfors, A. (1996). Limited T-cell receptor V gene usage in inclusion body myositis. *Scand. J. Immunol.* **43**, 109–114.

Fyhr, I. M., Moslemi, A. R., Mosavi, A. A., Lindberg, C., Tarkowski, A. and Oldfors, A. (1997). Oligoclonal expansion of muscle infiltrating T cells in inclusion body myositis. *J. Neuroimmunol.* **79**, 185–189.

Gardam, M. A., Low, D. E., Saginur, R., Miller, M. A. (1998). Group B streptococcal necrotizing fasciitis and streptococcal toxic shock-like syndrome in adults. *Arch. Int. Med.* **158**, 1704–1708.

Ge, Q., Nilasena, D. S., O'Brien, C. A., Frank, M. B. and Targoff, I. N. (1995). Molecular analysis of a major antigenic region of the 240-kD protein of Mi-2 autoantigen. *J. Clin. Invest.* **96**, 1730–1737.

Goebel, N., Michaelis, D., Engelhardt, M. et al. (1996). Differential expression of perforin in muscle-inflammatory T cells in polymyositis and dermatomyositis. *J. Clin. Invest.* **97**, 2905–2910.

Grau, J. M., Herrero, C., Casademont, J., Fernandez-Sola, J. and Urbano-Marquez, A. (1994). Cyclosporine A as first choice for dermatomyositis. *J. Rheumatol.* **21**, 381–382.

Griggs, R. C., Askanas, V., DiMauro, S. et al. (1995). Inclusion body myositis and myopathies. *Ann. Neurol.* **38**, 705–713.

Hays, A. P. and Gamboa, E. T. (1994). Acute viral myositis. In: *Myology*, eds. A. G. Engel, and C. Franzini-Armstrong, pp. 1399–1418. New York: McGraw-Hill.

Heckmatt, J., Hasson, N., Saunders, C. et al. (1989). Cyclosporin in juvenile dermatomyositis. *Lancet* **i**, 1063–1066.

Heffner, R. R., Armbrustmacher, V. W. and Earle, K. M. (1977). Focal myositis. *Cancer* **40**, 301–306.

Hertzmann, P. A., Blevins, W. L., Mayer, J., Greenfield, B., Ting, M. and Gleich, G. J. (1990). Association of the eosinophilia-myalgia syndrome with the ingestion of tryptophan. *N. Engl. J. Med.* **322**, 869–873.

Hohlfeld, R. and Engel, A. G. (1991). Coculture with autologous myotubes of cytotoxic T cells isolated from muscle in inflammatory myopathies. *Ann. Neurol.* **29**, 498–507.

Hohlfeld, R., Engel, A. G., Kunio, L. I. and Harper, M. C. (1991). Polymyositis mediated by T lymphocytes that express the gamma/delta receptor. *N. Engl. J. Med.* **324**, 877–881.

Hohlfeld, R., Goebels, N. and Engel, A. G. (1993). Cellular mechanisms in inflammatory myopathies. *Baillière's Clin. Neurol.* **2**, 617–636.

Horvath, R., Fu, K., Genge, A., Karpati, G. and Shoubridge, E. A. (1998). Characterization of the mitochondiral DNA abnormalities in the skeletal muscle of patients with inclusion body myositis. *J. Neuropath. Exp. Neurol.* **57**, 396–403.

Illa, I., Nath, A. and Dalakas, M. C. (1991). Immunocytochemical and virological characteristics of HIV-associated inflammatory myopathies: similarities with seronegative polymyositis. *Ann. Neurol.* **29**, 474–481.

Illa, I., Dinsmore, S. and Dalakas, M. C. (1993). Immune-mediated mechanisms and immune activation of fibroblasts in the pathogenesis of eosinophilia-myalgia syndrome induced by L-tryptophan. *Hum. Pathology* **24**, 702–709.

Jan, S., Beretta, S., Moggio, M., Alobbati, L., Pellegrini, G. (1992). High-dose intravenous human immunoglobulin in polymyositis resistant to treatment. *J. Neurol. Neurosurg. Psychiatry* **55**, 60–64.

Jerusalem, F., Rakusa, M., Engel, A. G. and Macdonald, R. D. (1974). Morphometric analysis of skeletal muscle capillary ultrastructure in inflammatory myopathies. *J. Neurol. Sci.* **23**, 391–401.

Karpati, G. (1997). Inclusion body myositis – Status 1997. *Neurologist* **3**, 201–208.

Karpati, G. and Carpenter, S. (1988). Idiopathic inflammatory myopathies. *Curr. Opin. Neurol. Neurosurg.* **1**, 804–814,

Karpati, G. and Carpenter, S. (1993a). Pathology of the inflammatory myopathies. *Baillière's Clin. Neurol.* **2**, 527–556.

Karpati, G. and Carpenter, S. (1993b). Evolving concepts about inclusion body myositis. In: *Actualités Neuromusculaires: Acquisition Récentes*. eds. G. Serratrice, J. F., Pellesier, J. Pouget et al., pp. 93–98. Paris: *Exp. Scient. Française*.

Karpati, G. and Currie, G. S. (1994). The inflammatory myopathies. In: *Disorders of Voluntary Muscle*, eds. J. Walton, G. Karpati, D. Hilton-Jones, pp. 619–646. Edinburgh: Churchill-Livingston.

Karpati, G., Pouliot, Y., Carpenter, S. (1988). Expression of immunoreactive major histocompatability complex products in human skeletal muscles. *Ann. Neurol.* **23**, 64–72.

Kelly, J. J. Jr, Madoc-Jones, H., Adelman, L. S., Andres, P. L. and Munsat, T. L. (1986). Total body irradiation is not effective in inclusion body myositis. *Neurology* **36**, 1264–1266.

Kissel, J. T., Mendell, J. R. and Rammohan, K. W. (1986). Microvascular deposition of complement membrane attack complex in dermatomyositis, *N. Engl. J. Med.* **314**, 329.

Kissel, J. T., Burrow, K. L., Rammohan, K. W. for the CIDD Group (1991a). Mononuclear cell analysis of muscle biopsies in prednisone-treated and untreated Duchenne muscular dystrophy. *Neurology* **41**, 667–672.

Kissel, J. T., Halterman, R. K., Rammohan, K. W. and Mendell, J. R. (1991b). The relationship of complement-mediated microvasculopathy to the histologic features and clinical duration of disease in dermatomyositis. *Arch. Neurol.* **48**, 26–30.

Koffman, B. M., Rugiero, M. and Dalakas, M. C. (1998a). Autoimmune diseases and autoantibodies associated with sporadic inclusion body myositis. *Muscle and Nerve* **21**, 115–117.

Koffman, B. M., Sivakumar, K., Simonis, T., Stroncek, D. and Dalakas, M. C. (1998b). HLA allele distribution distinguishes sporadic inclusion body myositis from hereditary inclusion body myopathies. *J. Neuroimmunol.* **84**, 139–142.

Lang, B., Laxer, R. M., Murphy, G., Silverman, E. D. and Roifman, C. M. (1991). Treatment of dermatomyositis with intravenous immunoglobulin. *Am. J. Med.* **91**, 169–172.

Layzer, R. B., Shearn, M. A. and Satya-Murti, S. (1977). Eosinophilic polymyositis. *Ann. Neurol.* **1**, 65–71.

Leff, R. L., Love, L. A., Miller, F. W. et al. (1992). Viruses in the idiopathic inflammatory myopathies: absence of candidate viral genomes in muscle. *Lancet* **339**, 1192–1195.

Leon-Monzon, M. and Dalakas, M. C. (1992). Absence of persistent infection with enteroviruses in muscles of patients with inflammatory myopathies. *Ann. Neurol.* **32**, 219–222.

Leon-Monzon, M. and Dalakas, M. C. (1994). Interleukin-1 (IL-1) is toxic to human muscle. *Neurology* **44**(Suppl.) A132.

Leon-Monzon, M., Lamperth, L. and Dalakas, M. C. (1993). Search for HIV proviral DNA and amplified sequences in the muscle biopsies of patients with HIV-polymyositis. *Muscle and Nerve* **16**, 408–413.

Leon-Monzon, M., Illa., I., Dalakas, M. C. (1994). Polymyositis in patients infected with HTLV-1: the role of the virus in the cause of the disease. *Ann. Neurol.* **36**, 643–649.

Lotz, B. P., Engel, A. G., Nishino, H., Stevens, J. C. and Litchy, W. J. (1989). Inclusion body myositis. Observations in 40 patients. *Brain* **112**, 727–747.

Luciano, C. A. and Dalakas, M. C. (1997). A macro-EMG study in inclusion-body myositis: no evidence for a neurogenic component. *Neurology* **48**, 29–33.

Lundberg, I., Brengman, J. M. and Engel, A. G. (1995). Analysis of cytokine expression in muscle in inflammatory myopathies, Duchenne's dystrophy and non-weak controls. *J. Neuroimmunol.* **63**, 9–16.

Mantegazza, R., Andreette, F., Bernasconi, P. et al. (1993). Analysis of T cell receptor repertoire of muscle infiltrating T lymphocytes in polymyositis. *J. Clin. Invest.* **91**, 2880–2886.

Martin, R. W., Duffy, J., Engel, A. G. et al. (1990). The clinical spectrum of eosinophilia–myalgia syndrome associated with L-tryptophan ingestion. *Ann. Int. Med.* **113**, 124.

Maselli, R. A., Richman, D. P. and Wollmann, R. L. (1991). Inflammation at the neuromuscular junction in myasthenia gravis. *Neurology* **41**, 1497–1504.

Massa, R., Weller, B., Karpati, G., Shoubridge, E. and Carpenter, S. (1991). Familial inclusion body myositis among Kurdish-Iranian Jews. *Arch. Neurol.* **48**, 519–522.

Mastaglia, F. L. and Walton, J. N. (1992). Inflammatory myopathies. In: *Skeletal Muscle Pathology*, 2nd edn, eds. F. L. Mastaglia and J. N. Walton, p. 360. Edinburgh: Churchill Livingstone.

Ménard, D. B., Haddad, H., Blain, J. G., Beaudry, R., Devroede, G. and Masse, S. (1976). Granulomatous myositis and myopathy associated with Crohn's disease. *N. Engl. J. Med.* **295**, 818–819.

Mendell, J. R., Sahenk, Z., Gales, T. and Paul, L. (1991). Amyloid filaments in inclusion body myositis. *Arch. Neurol.* **48**, 1229–1234.

Miller, F. W., Leitman, S. F., Cronin, M. E. et al. (1992). Controlled trial of plasma exchange and leukopheresis in patients with polymyositis and dermatomyositis. *N. Engl. J. Med.* **326**, 1380–1384.

Mimori, T. (1987). Scleroderma–polymyositis overlap syndrome: clinical and seriologic aspects. *Int. J. Dermatol.* **26**, 419–425.

Morgan, O. St C., Rodgers-Johnson, P., Mora, C. and Char, G. (1989). HTLV-1 and polymyositis in Jamaica. *Lancet* **ii**, 1184–1187.

Munsat, T. L., Piper, D., Cancilla, P. and Mednick, J. (1972). Inflammatory myopathy with facioscapulohumeral distribution. *Neurology* **22**, 335–347.

Murata, K. and Dalakas, M. C. (1999). Expression of the costimulatory molecule BB-1, the ligands CTLA-4 and CD28 and their mRNA in inflammatory myopathies. *Am. J. Pathol.* **155**, 453–460.

Nalbantoglu, J., Karpati, G. and Carpenter, S. (1994). Conspicuous accumulation of a single- stranded DNA binding protein in skeletal muscle fibres in inclusion body myositis. *Am. J. Pathol.* **144**, 874–882.

Nishino, H., Engel, A. G., Rima, B. K. (1989). Inclusion body myositis: the mumps virus hypothesis. *Ann. Neurol.* **25**, 260–264.

O'Hanlon, T. P., Dalakas, M. C., Plotz, P. H. and Miller, F. W. (1994a). Predominant TCR-alpha-beta variable and joining gene expression by muscle-infiltrating lymphocytes in the idiopathic inflammatory myopathies. *J. Immunol.* **152**, 2569–2576.

O'Hanlon, T. P., Dalakas, M. C., Plotz, P. H. and Miller, F. W. (1994b). The IJ T cell receptor repertoire in inclusion body myositis: diverse patterns of gene expression by muscle infiltrating lymphocytes. *J. Autoimmunity* **7**, 321–333.

Olney, R. K. and Miller, R. K. (1983). Inflammatory infiltration in Fukuyama type congenital muscular dystrophy. *Muscle and Nerve* **6**, 75.

Otero, C., Illa, I. and Dalakas, M. C. (1992). Is there dermatomyositis (DM) without myositis? *Neurology* **42**, 388S.

Peng, A., Koffman, B. M., Malley, J. D. and Dalakas, M. C. (2000). Disease progression in sporadic inclusion body myositis (s-IBM): observations in 78 patients. *Neurology* **55**, 296–298.

Plotz, P. H., Dalakas, M., Leff, R. L., Love, L. A., Miller, F. W. and Cronin, M. E. (1989). Current concepts in the idiopathic inflammatory myopathies: polymyositis, dermatomyositis and related disorders. *Ann. Intern. Med.* **111**, 143–157.

Puschke, G., Ruegg, D., Hohlfeld, R. and Engel, A.G. (1992). Autoaggressive myocytotoxic T-lymphocytes expressing an unusual gamma delta T cell receptor. *J. Exp. Med.* **176**, 1785–1789.

Ringel, S. P., Forstot, J. Z., Tan, E. M., Wehling, C., Griggs, R. C. and Butcher, D. (1982). Sjögren's syndrome and polymyositis or dermatomyositis. *Arch. Neurol.* **39**, 157.

Roddy, S. M., Ashwal, S., Peckham, N. and Mortensen, S. (1986). Infantile myositis: a case diagnosed in the neonatal period. *Ped. Neurol.* **2**, 241.

Rosenberg, N. L., Carry M. R. and Ringel, S.P. (1988). Association of inflammatory myopathies with other connective tissue disorders and malignancies. In: *Polymyositis and Dermatomyositis*, ed. M. C. Dalakas, p. 37. Boston MA: Butterworth.

Ruff, R. L. and Secrist, D. (1982). Viral studies in benign acute childhood myositis. *Arch. Neurol.* **39**, 261.

Schneider, C., Gold, R., Dalakas, M. C. et al. (1996). MHC class I-mediated cytotoxicity does not induce apoptosis in muscle fibres nor in inflammatory T cells: studies in patients with polymyositis, dermatomyositis and inclusion body myositis. *J. Neuropathol. Exp. Neurol.* **55**, 1205–1209.

Schroder, J. M. and Molnar, M. (1997). Mitochondrial abnormalities and peripheral neuropathy in inflammatory myopathy, especially inclusion body myositis. *Mol. Cell. Biochem.* **174**, 277–282.

Schwarz, M. I., Sutarik, J. M., Nick, J. A., Leff, R. L., Emlen, J. W. and Tuder, R. M. (1995). Pulmonary capillaritis and diffuse alveolar hemmorrhage: a primary manifestation of polymyositis. *Am. J. Respir. Crit. Care Med.* **151**, 2037–2040.

Sekul, E. A. and Dalakas, M. C. (1993). Inclusion body myositis: new concepts. *Semin. Neurol.* **13**, 256–263.

Sekul, E. A,. Chow, C. and Dalakas, M. C. (1997). Magnetic resonance imaging of the forearm as a diagnostic aid in patients with inclusion body myositis. *Neurology* **48**, 863–866.

Semino-Mora, C. and Dalakas, M. C. (1998). Rimmed vacuoles with β-amyloid and ubiquitinated filamentous deposits in the muscles of patients with long-standing denervation (post-poliomyelitis muscular atrophy): similarities with inclusion body myositis. *Hum. Pathol.* **29**, 1128–1133.

Shevell, M., Rosenblatt, B., Silver, C. M., Carpenter, S. and Karpati, G. (1990). Congenital inflammatory myopathy. *Neurology* **40**, 1111–1114.

Simon, D. B., Ringel, S. F. and Sufit, R. I. (1982). Clinical spectrum of fascial inflammation. *Muscle Nerve* **5**, 525.

Sinoway, T. A. and Callen, J. P. (1993). Chlorambucil: an effective corticosteroid-sparing agent for patients with recalcitrant dermatomyositis. *Arthritis. Rheum.* **36**, 319–324.

Sivakumar, K. and Dalakas, M. C. (1996). The spectrum of familial inclusion body myopathies in 13 families and description of a quadriceps sparing phenotype in non-Iranian Jews. *Neurology* **47**, 977–984.

Sivakumar, K. and Dalakas, M. C. (1997). Inclusion body myositis and myopathies. *Curr. Opin. Neurol.* **10**, 413–420.

Sivakumar, K., Semino-Mora, C. and Dalakas, M. C. (1997). An inflammatory, familial, inclusion body myositis with autoimmune features and a phenotype identical to sporadic inclusion body myositis: studies in 3 families. *Brain* **120**, 653–661.

Soueidan, S. A. and Dalakas, M. C. (1993). Treatment of inclusion-body myositis with high-dose intravenous immunoglobulin. *Neurology* **43**, 876–879.

Sripathi, N., Karpati, G. and Carpenter, S. (1996). A distinctive type of infantile inflammatory myopathy with abnormal myonuclei. *J. Neurol. Sci.* **136**, 1–2.

Stein, D. P. and Dalakas, M. C. (1993). Intercellular adhesion molecule-1 expression is upregulated in patients with dermatomyositis (DM). *Ann. Neurol.* **34**, 268.

Stein, D. P., Jordan, S. C., Toyoda, M., Gallera, O. and Dalakas, M. C. (1993). Anti-endothelial cell antibodies (AECA) in dermatomyositis (DM). *Neurology* **43** (Suppl.), 356.

Targoff, I. N. (1990). Immune mechanisms of myositis. *Curr. Opin. Rheumatol.* **2**, 882–888.

Tews, D. S. and Goebel, H. H. (1995). Expression of cell adhesion molecules in inflammatory myopathies. *J. Neuroimmunol.* **59**, 185–194.

Tews, D. S. and Goebel, H. H. (1996). Cytokine expression profiles in idiopathic inflammatory myopathies. *J. Neuropathol. Exp. Neurol.* **55**, 342–347.

Thompson, C. E. (1982). Infantile myositis. *Dev. Med. Child Neurol.* **24**, 307–313.

Whitaker, J. N. and Engel, W. K. (1972). Vascular deposits of immunoglobulin and complement in idiopathic inflammatory myopathy. *N. Engl. J. Med.* **286**, 333–338.

32

Myasthenia gravis and myasthenic syndromes: autoimmune and genetic disorders

John Newsom-Davis and David Beeson

Introduction

The principal disease process affecting neuromuscular transmission is autoimmunity, and this underlies three disorders: myasthenia gravis (MG), the Lambert–Eaton myasthenic syndrome (LEMS) and acquired neuromyotonia (NMT). In these disorders ion channels are targets, and they are particularly vulnerable to antibody-mediated attack at the neuromuscular junction for two reasons: they lie outside the blood–nerve barrier and, therefore, lack the protection this offers to the remainder of the nervous system, and they have extracellular domains that are accessible to circulating antibodies.

But the last few years have seen the characterization of a further important group of disorders, namely the congenital myasthenic syndromes (CMS). These genetic disorders arise from mutations affecting the muscle acetylcholine receptor (AChR) and, in a few patients, the anchor protein (ColQ) for acetylcholinesterase (AChE). Additionally, the neuromuscular junction is the target for neurotoxins such as botulinum toxin (Shapiro et al., 1998), and those contained in certain snake venoms; these will not be considered further in this chapter. The neuromuscular junction and the role of toxins is discussed in greater detail in Chapter 9.

The neuromuscular junction

Figure 32.1 illustrates the key features of the neuromuscular junction. The nerve terminal is separated from the postsynaptic muscle fibre membrane by a narrow synaptic cleft that contains the basement membrane, to which AChE is attached by the ColQ protein (not shown). The muscle membrane has a series of folds in the postsynaptic region, the AChRs being concentrated on the peaks of the folds, which are aligned with the active zones of the nerve termi-nal from which vesicle exocytosis occurs. The AChRs comprise five subunits ($\alpha_2, \beta \ \gamma/\varepsilon, \delta$) arranged around a central ion channel (Fig. 32.2). (The two α-subunits are of the α_1 type, see Chapter 9.) The γ-subunit in fetal muscle AChR (α_2, γ, δ) is replaced by an ε-subunit by 34 weeks of gestation in humans to form the adult type ($\alpha_2, \beta, \delta, \varepsilon$). In denervated muscle, AChRs revert to the fetal type.

The depolarizing phase of the nerve action potential is generated by the opening of voltage-gated sodium channels (VGSCs); their inactivation and the opening of voltage-gated potassium channels (VGKCs) repolarizes the nerve membrane. Invasion of the nerve terminal by the action potential leads to the opening of P/Q-type voltage-gated calcium channels (VGCCs) and the local influx of calcium, which triggers the release of about 30 vesicles (quanta) of acetylcholine (ACh), each containing about 10 000 molecules. Transient binding of an ACh molecule to each of the two α-subunits of the AChR leads to brief opening of the central ion pore, the influx of small cations (mainly sodium), and the production of a potential change. The spontaneous release of a single quantum (vesicle) gives rise to a miniature endplate potential (MEPP). The endplate potential (EPP) is generated by the nerve-evoked synchronous release of 30 or so quanta (the 'quantal content' of the EPP). The EPP activates VGSCs in the clefts of the synaptic folds, which then generate the muscle action potential that propagates along the muscle fibre membrane and activates contraction.

Autoimmune disorders

Myasthenia gravis

Clinical features

Ocular symptoms (diplopia and/or ptosis) are the most common presenting symptoms, but any striated muscle

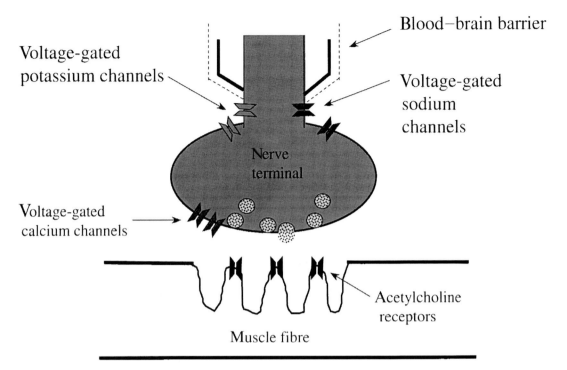

Fig. 32.1. Schematic diagram of the neuromuscular junction.

can be involved, including respiratory muscles. The characteristic features of the weakness in MG are its variability, its increase with muscle usage and improvement with rest, and its exacerbation by emotional stress and by infection.

Signs include progressive weakness during sustained effort (e.g. fatiguable ptosis), variable diplopia, occasionally 'pseudo'-nystagmus, nasal speech, nasal regurgitation, difficulty with swallowing and weakness of jaw closure and of neck extension, leading to jaw propping and head droop. The smile may have a snarling quality. Proximal and distal weakness of the upper limbs and proximal weakness of the lower limbs is usual in patients moderately affected. Ankle dorsiflexion, however, is typically preserved except in those most severely affected. Paralysis of the diaphragm is life threatening and associated with profound orthopnoea. Tendon reflexes are almost always brisk. Sphincter control is usually unaffected.

The balance of the evidence from neuropsychological testing argues against central nervous system (CNS) involvement (Glennerster et al., 1996). Psychiatric studies also fail to reveal any specifically associated disorders when appropriate controls are studied.

Heart disease was reported to be present in 16% of 108 patients with MG studied (Mygland et al., 1991), but this incidence was no higher than in a control group of patients with spinal muscular atrophy. Significantly, however, these

abnormalities were much commoner in those with thymoma (50%), which is likely to relate to the anticardiac antibodies that have been detected in these patients.

Clinical subtypes
The clinical expression of MG is heterogeneous, comprising several subgroups that need to be distinguished because of the implications for therapy and for pathogenesis.

The principal subdivision is between the 85% of patients who are seropositive for anti-AChR antibodies (seropositive MG) and those who are not (seronegative MG). In terms of pathogenesis, as discussed further below, these can be considered as different disorders. But even

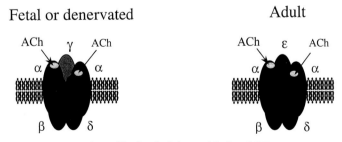

Fig. 32.2. A comparison of fetal and adult acetylcholine (ACh) receptors.

among the seropositive patients there are important differences in thymic pathology and immune response gene associations. About 10% of patients have a thymoma. Among the remainder, patients with early-onset disease (<45 years) are more often female and typically have thymic hyperplasia. Late-onset cases are more likely to be male and the thymus is usually atrophic (i.e. normal for age).

Juvenile myasthenia, a term infrequently used now, is not a distinct subgroup and should be considered with the early-onset group.

Seronegative myasthenia is misleadingly named because these patients too have pathogenetic antibodies although to targets other than AChRs, as discussed in the next section. Seronegative patients are not distinguishable clinically from those who are seropositive. Ocular symptoms are more common (about 50% of such patients are seronegative). Thymoma is extremely rare.

Neonatal myasthenia arises from placental transfer of maternal antibodies and is, therefore, the result of 'passive immunization' rather than active disease. These infants usually have only a transient myasthenic disorder. In rare instances, neonatal MG associates with arthrogryposis multiplex congenita, principally because some or all of the maternal antibodies are targeting the fetal form of AChR. In the latter, the mother herself can be unaffected (Vincent et al., 1997). Neonatal myasthenia needs to be distinguished from the genetic group of CMS, described in a later section.

Penicillamine-induced MG has been most frequently observed in patients with rheumatoid arthritis, but has also been reported in Wilson's disease and primary biliary cirrhosis treated with penicillamine. Serum anti-AChR antbodies are detectable, and the clinical characteristics do not differ from those found in recent-onset idiopathic MG. The pathophysiological features are also similar. There is an association with HLA-Bw35 and with HLA-DR1. Symptoms usually decline over several months following drug withdrawal.

Natural history

MG can present at any age from about one year onwards. The progress of the disease is variable. In some, the disorder stays confined to the eye muscles (ocular myasthenia) and if this lasts for two years or more, particularly if the anti-AChR antibody is undetectable or at very low titre, the chance of the disorder becoming generalized is greatly diminished. Oosterhuis (1989) found a remission rate of about 1% per year in over 180 patients with generalized MG treated with anticholinesterase medication alone, followed for a mean period of 17 years. The remission rate in simi-

larly treated patients with ocular myasthenia was about twice this.

Epidemiology

MG can affect all races, although the clinical expression can differ. Chinese patients have a greater proportion of early-onset and ocular myasthenia and less late-onset severe disease than do Caucasians (Chiu et al., 1987). Immunogenetic associations also differ (see below). A survey by Somnier et al. (1991) in Denmark gave a point prevalence (in 1988) of 9.6 per 100 000 for women and 5.7 per 100 000 for men. The annual incidence in this population was 0.44 per million. But a recent study by Robertson et al. (1998) indicates a prevalence (at least in the East Anglian population of the UK he studied) of 15 per 100 000, and an annual incidence of 1 per 100 000. Moreover, there is evidence that the incidence may be increasing in the elderly, particularly in men (Schon et al., 1996). A study of mortality and survival in a Danish myasthenic population indicated a prognosis only a little less good than that of the corresponding control group. Old age, severe disease and the presence of a thymoma were, as might be expected, associated with a less favourable prognosis (Christensen et al., 1998).

Immunological associations

One of the earliest clues to the immunological nature of MG was its association with other autoimmune disorders. In a personal series of 600 cases, a history of hyperthyroidism was present in 3%, rheumatoid arthritis in 2% systemic lupus erythematosus in 1% and polymyositis in 0.5%. MG can also associate with LEMS and with NMT.

In early-onset caucasoid patients with MG, there is a strong association with the HLA-A1–B8–DR3–DQ2 extended haplotype (Janer et al., 1999). The association is consistently stronger in females than in males in this early-onset group, and with HLA-B8 rather than with HLA-DR3. In patients with late-onset disease, there is a much weaker association with HLA-B7 and HLA-DR2, and HLA-DR2 is also often present in patients with early-onset disease who lack HLA-DR3. These associations are influenced by race. In Chinese patients with early-onset MG, the association is with HLA-B46 and HLA-DR9, the latter being stronger. In Japanese patients, there are strong associations not only with HLA-DR9 but also with HLA-DRw13 and HLA-DQw3. No strong associations have been identified in patients with thymoma, in ocular myasthenia or in those who are seronegative for anti-AChR antibodies. There is, however, an association in late-onset disease with particular immunoglobulin heavy chain genes, emphasizing the immunogenetic heterogeneity of the disorder.

Pathophysiology

The primary defect in MG is a reduction in the number of functional AChRs at the postsynaptic membrane, causing a decreased amplitude of the EPP, which may fail to reach the critical firing threshold for the muscle cell and lead to conduction block. MEPP amplitudes are also reduced.

The mechanism of loss of functional AChRs differs between seropositive and seronegative MG, but in both forms its antibody-mediated nature has been shown by passive transfer studies to mice.

Antibodies to the acetylcholine receptor

Anti-AChR antibodies are of IgG class and are heterogeneous, i.e. they differ in their sites of binding to the AChR. Many of them bind to sites within the main immunogenic region of the α-subunit, which includes residues 60–75 on the extracellular domain. The antibodies are usually assayed using human muscle that contains both adult and fetal-type AChRs that are labelled with [^{125}I] labelled α-bungarotoxin.

Several mechanisms can underlie loss of functional AChRs in seropositive MG: complement-mediated lysis, modulation and pharmacological block. The first of these lead to widening and simplification of the postsynaptic folds. There may also be loss of endplate VGSCs (Ruff and Lennon, 1998).

Antibodies in seronegative myasthenia gravis

Several lines of evidence point to the presence of pathogenetic antibodies in patients with MG in whom anti-AChR antibodies are undetectable. First, babies born to seronegative mothers may exhibit neonatal myasthenia (nature's experiment). Second, mice injected with seronegative immunoglobulins show reduced MEPPs, and a reduced number of functional AChRs but without evidence of antibodies bound to AChRs. Third, seronegative plasmas and the non-IgG fractions can inhibit AChR function in a human muscle cell line (TE671) expressing the fetal form of the receptor, without evidence of AChR binding. One proposed explanation for the effects of seronegative plasma is the presence of antibodies, some of which may be of IgM class, that target muscle membrane determinant(s) other than AChRs and inactivate AChRs through an intracellular second messenger system, perhaps involving AChR phosphorylation.

Thymus pathology

The thymus in patients with early-onset disease typically shows the changes of hyperplasia, comprising lymphoid follicles with germinal centres that together with their surrounding T cell areas appear to be invading the thymic medulla. In well-advanced disease, there appears to be breakdown of the laminin layer that normally separates the T cell areas from the medullary bands. Thymic cells cultured from such thymuses spontaneously synthesize anti-AChR antibodies, the rates of production in culture correlating positively with the serum titre. No anti-AChR antibody production can be detected in thymuses from seronegative patients. The hyperplastic thymus is enriched for AChR-reactive T cells. This observation, together with the spontaneous production of anti-AChR antibodies, points to the presence of antigen within the thymus. Thymic myoid cells have been shown to contain AChRs and may be the targets for AChR-reactive T cells.

In late-onset MG, the thymus is usually 'normal' or atrophic (Willcox et al., 1991). In a comparison with an age-matched control group, no differences could be detected (Myking et al., 1998). For instance, germinal centres were found in 7 of 22 of the MG group and in 6 of 20 of the controls.

In seronegative patients, the thymus is usually normal (Verma and Oger, 1992).

Thymomas appear to arise from rare cortical epithelial cells that are positive for cortical and for medullary epithelial cell markers (Willcox et al., 1987). They are characterized by the presence of very large numbers of immature thymic cells, giving them their lymphoepithelial cell appearance. Thymic epithelial cells have been shown to express mRNA for α- and ε-subunits (MacLennon et al., 1998; Zheng et al., 1999), and their epithelial cells may select and immunize T cells specifically for AChR and for other muscle proteins (e.g. titin, ryanodine receptor) to which antibodies are also made.

Acetylcholine receptor-reactive T cells

Anti-AChR antibody production in MG is believed to be T cell dependent as it is in experimental autoimmune MG. It has proved extraordinarily difficult to raise AChR-reactive T cell lines to the α-subunit, despite the fact that antibodies in MG appear to be directed principally to the main immunogenic region on the N-terminal extracellular domain of this subunit. Recent studies suggest that epitopes to the ε-subunit may be more important (Hill et al., 1999).

Diagnosis

The presence of anti-AChR antibodies unequivocally establishes the diagnosis of seropositive MG, although the actual antibody titre is not an index of disease severity between individuals. Confirmatory evidence would be the presence of an increased decrement in the compound muscle action potential (>10%) at 3 Hz stimulation,

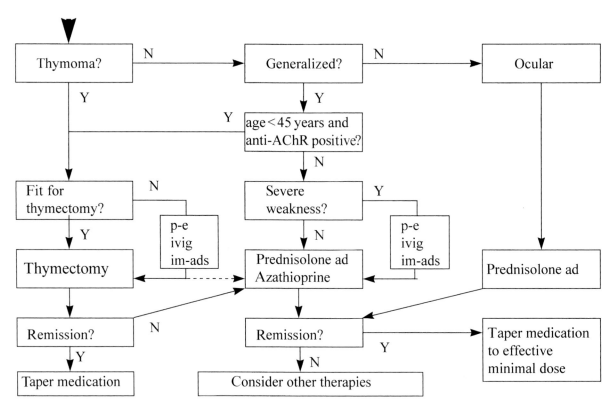

Fig. 32.3. A flow diagram for the immunological treatment of myasthenia gravis. p-e, plasma exchange; ivig, intravenous immunoglobulin; im-ads, immunoadsorption; ad, alternate day; N, no; Y, yes; AChR, acetylcholine receptor.

increased jitter or blocking on single-fibre electromyography, and response to anticholinesterase medication. In practice, these tests are not necessary when the antibody test is positive.

In seronegative MG, electromyography becomes particularly important, especially single-fibre studies, although it needs to be remembered that increased jitter can occur in other conditions besides myasthenia (e.g. mitochondrial myopathy). Where such studies are not possible, a neostigmine or edrophonium test may need to be done. For the latter, premedication with atropine is advisable, as well as a test dose (2 mg). Some patients with ocular MG may show a positive response to this alone, making it unnecessary to give the full dose (8 mg). In occasional cases of seronegative MG, the diagnosis can be established by a clear-cut response to plasma exchange. An assay for the antibodies in this form of MG is not yet available for clinical use.

In seropositive patients, thymus imaging (computed tomography or magnetic resonance) is essential to exclude the presence of a thymoma. Thymic hyperplasia cannot be diagnosed with certainty from the scanning appearances.

Management

Pyridostigmine, an anticholinesterase compound, will produce symptomatic improvement and is given initially at a dosage (for adults) of 30 mg four or five times daily, increasing to 60 mg if required. Higher dosage is associated with greater adverse effects, particularly gastrointestinal, which can be partially controlled by propantheline or loperamide. Neostigmine (15 mg) can be used as an alternative to pyridostigmine but is shorter acting. The need to use higher anticholinesterase doses indicates that immunological treatment may be required. Moreover, high anticholinesterase dosage runs the risk of inducing cholinergic toxicity and of downregulating the number of AChRs, as has been shown in animal experiments.

Figure 32.3 provides a framework for the immunological treatment of patients with MG. The first question focuses on thymoma. If imaging reveals the presence of a tumour, thymectomy is indicated to reduce the risk of local infiltration. However, removal of the tumour does not usually result in any improvement in muscle strength, and further immunological treatment will usually be needed. As the figure illustrates, treatment with prednisolone either alone or combined with azathioprine is then indicated. If the thymoma was invasive and incompletely removed, local radiotherapy or chemotherapy should be considered, although no randomized clinical trial data seem to be available (Hejna et al., 1999).

If a thymoma has been excluded, and the patient's symptoms are purely ocular and poorly controlled by pyridostigmine, treatment with alternate day prednisolone is recommended (Fig. 32.3). This can be undertaken in outpatients, the dose being increased weekly by 5 mg either until symptoms resolve or until a provisional ceiling dose is reached (e.g. 1 mg/kg body weight). Pyridostigmine should be tapered and withdrawn, and the initial prednisolone maintenance dose held until the patient has been symptom free for two to three months before being slowly reduced to define the effective minimal dose. When symptoms return, the dose can be adjusted upwards as required to regain control. At a later stage, further attempts to reduce the dose can be made, but it is unusual to be able to withdraw prednisolone fully without symptoms returning. If symptoms are not adequately controlled at the dosage suggested above, a higher dose of steroids can be used, or an additional immunosuppressive agent such as azathioprine can be introduced. Complete failure to respond to steroids should raise the question of whether the diagnosis is correct. The adverse effects of prednisolone are well known, but the use of the alternate day regimen seems to reduce the risk of steroid myopathy (the author has never encountered this in patients treated with the alternate day regimen). The bisphosphanates (e.g. etidronate) have also greatly reduced the morbidity from steroid-induced bone disease.

Thymectomy has never been subjected to a prospective trial but retrospective studies by neurologists from several different countries indicate an expected remission rate of 25–30%, most of the improvement occurring in the first year. Evaluation of the contribution of thymectomy to outcome is complicated in many published series by the coincident use of immunosuppressive drugs. The group that is most likely to be helped comprises patients with early-onset disease (<45 years) who are seropositive for anti-AChR antibodies. In the author's experience, seronegative patients do not appear to benefit and, as pointed out in an earlier section, the thymus in these patients does not show the changes of medullary hyperplasia that characterize the seropositive patients. Similarly, patients with late-onset disease often have an atrophic thymus and are less likely to benefit from surgery. Consequently, until a randomized trial is undertaken, thymectomy is best restricted to those with imaging evidence of a thymoma or to seropositive patients who are under the age of 45 years at disease onset. As to the type of thymectomy, most centres appear still to adopt the trans-sternal approach, although a few are beginning to use a video-assisted endoscopic approach (Mantegazza et al., 1998). Transcervical thymectomy runs the risk of incomplete thymus removal.

In children thymectomy seems of greatest value in those with a history of less than two years who are seropositive for anti-AChR antibodies (Seybold, 1998).

As Figure 32.3 indicates, patients who are seronegative for anti-AChR antibodies, or who are over the age of 45 years at disease onset, or who have failed to respond to thymectomy should be considered for immunosuppressive drug therapy.

Many retrospective uncontrolled trials have argued quite convincingly for the benefits of corticosteroid treatment. A recent randomized trial comparing intravenous methylprednisolone with placebo infusion has shown objectively a significant short-term improvement in those receiving the active preparation (Lindberg et al., 1998), although in the author's view the intravenous route has no advantages over oral treatment.

A recent randomized double-blind trial comparing prednisolone (alternate day) plus azathioprine versus prednisolone (alternate day) plus placebo clearly demonstrated the advantages of the former (Palace et al., 1998). Azathioprine was given at a dose of 2.5 mg/kg body weight. Prednisolone in both groups was increased (in hospital) in steps of 10 mg to the peak dose (1.5 mg/kg body weight or 100 mg alternate days, whichever was the lower). This dose was maintained until anticholinesterase-free remission had developed, when it was slowly reduced (10 mg/month until a dose of 60 mg alternate day was reached, and by 5 mg/month thereafter). The dose of prednisolone required to maintain remission was significantly lower in those receiving the combined regimen, treatment failures were less common, remissions lasted longer and the medications were better tolerated. At three years, it was possible to withdraw prednisolone fully in over 60% of those in the group receiving combined treatment whereas the median dose in the groups receiving prednisolone alone was over 40 mg on alternate days. One interesting feature of the trial was the time lag of over one year before azathioprine appeared to become effective. In patients who are intolerant of azathioprine, cyclosporin (up to 5 mg/kg) or methotrexate (up to 25 mg weekly) are alternatives.

Plasma exchange, intravenous immunoglobulin and immunoadsorption are useful in the short-term control of severe myasthenic symptoms. They can be used to overcome a myasthenic crisis, to prepare patients for thymectomy, to cover postoperative deterioration of muscle strength or to control severe myasthenic weakness in the longer term while awaiting the response to immunosuppressive treatment. A consecutive daily course of plasma exchange appears more effective than an alternate day regimen (Yeh and Chiu, 1999). A recent prospective trial comparing plasma exchange with intravenous immunoglobulin showed the procedures to be of equal benefit (Gajdos et al., 1997). In the presence of sepsis (a cause of myasthenic crisis), intravenous immunoglobulin is the preferred treatment.

Pregnancy does not worsen the long-term outcome in MG (Batocchi et al., 1999). As indicated above, babies born to myasthenic mothers may develop neonatal myasthenia and, in extreme cases, this may lead to arthrogryposis multiplex congenita and to fetal death. There are, therefore, rational grounds for continuing immunotherapy during pregnancy, particularly since there are no compelling reasons for regarding azathioprine and prednisolone as teratogenic. For example, a mother who had experienced three consecutive fetal deaths associated with arthrogryposis underwent thymectomy followed by prednisolone and azathioprine; she conceived again while receiving these medications, which were continued through the pregnancy, and gave birth to a healthy boy. Plasma exchange and intravenous immunoglobulins also appear to be safe (Batocchi et al., 1999).

Drugs that can interfere with neuromuscular transmission

Drugs that should be used with caution in patients with poorly controlled MG include quinine, quinidine, procainamide, aminoglycoside antibiotics and β-blockers. Neuromuscular blocking agents used in anaesthesia and botulinum toxin injections for the treatment of movement disorders may reveal clinically silent MG.

Lambert–Eaton myasthenic syndrome

Clinical features

Difficulty in walking is usually the first complaint in patients with LEMS, followed by weakness of the arms (O'Neill et al., 1988). Double vision is unusual. Autonomic symptoms are common (dry mouth, constipation, erectile failure) and are sometimes the first to occur, but they are often not volunteered by the patient. Rarely patients present in respiratory failure.

Gait in LEMS has a characteristic rolling quality. Proximal weakness, unless it is very severe, is easy to overlook because of the augmentation in strength that occurs during the first few seconds of a voluntary effort, and which is caused by post-tetanic potentiation. Reflexes are depressed or absent and can also show post-tetanic potentiation. A mild degree of ptosis and diplopia may be present, but eye movements are not grossly restricted.

Clinical subtypes and natural history

About 60% of patients are smokers and have an associated small cell lung cancer. In this group (C-LEMS), the peak incidence is in the fourth to sixth decades, and in many patients survival is limited by the tumour. Importantly, the neurological disorder may precede radiological or other evidence of the tumour by up to five years. The incidence of C-LEMS in patients with small cell lung cancer was estimated at about 3% in a prospective trial (Elrington et al., 1991), giving an annual incidence of about 250 cases in the UK. Patients sometimes have an associated cerebellar syndrome (Mason et al., 1997). There is also a weak association of LEMS with lymphoma.

There is no cancer association in the remaining patients (NC-LEMS), and in this group disease onset can be in childhood or adulthood, up to extreme old age. The disorder is at least 10-fold less common than MG. Onset may follow influenza, and be subacute. Subsequently, the disability can be stable or slowly increase. Spontaneous remissions are rare. Apart from the presence of the tumour and its implications for prognosis, there appears to be no difference in the clinical features of NC- and C-LEMS.

Immunological associations

As in MG, other autoimmune diseases associate with LEMS, principally in those with NC-LEMS. Vitiligo is particularly common. There is also a strong association with HLA-B8 and HLA-DR3 in patients with NC-LEMS.

Pathophysiology

The primary defect in both forms of LEMS is a reduction in the number of quanta released by each nerve impulse. The quantal content of the EPP may thus be 10 or less, compared with more than 30 at healthy endplates, the number increasing during the first few impulses of a high-frequency train (e.g. 40 Hz) of nerve stimuli (post-tetanic potentiation). MEPPs are of normal amplitude. The pathophysiological changes are consistent with the loss of nerve terminal VGCCs. Freeze-fracture electron microscopy of the nerve terminal P face showed paucity and disorganization of the active zone particles that represent VGCCs. The antibody-dependent nature of these changes (Fig. 32.4) was shown by the passive transfer to mice of the pathophysiological and morphological changes by injection of patients' immunoglobulins.

Antibodies to P/Q-type voltage-gated calcium channels

Anti-P/Q-type VGCC antibodies are of the IgG class and are detected in over 90% of patients with LEMS (whether of the C-LEMS or NC-LEMS, type) but not in healthy controls or

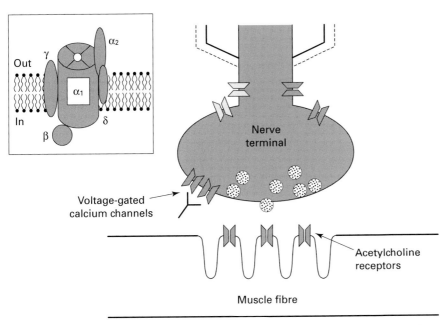

Fig. 32.4. The neuromuscular junction in the Lambert–Eaton myasthenic syndrome. A model of the voltage-gated calcium channel is shown (inset); the α_1-subunit contains the ion pore and is the primary target for the autoantibodies.

in those with other neurological disorders (Motomura et al., 1995). The specificities of the antibodies in C-LEMS and NC-LEMS do not appear to differ. The antibodies reduce the number of functional presynaptic P/Q-type VGCCs by cross-linking and modulation, thereby decreasing the calcium influx on which quantal release depends. They appear to target specifically the α_1-subunit (Fig. 32.4) of these channels (Pinto et al., 1998). The antibodies also underlie the cholinergic and adrenergic autonomic defects in LEMS (Waterman et al., 1997), as has been show by passive transfer to mice. Additionally, the antibodies block P-type and both P- and Q-type VGCCs in cerebellar Purkinje cells and granule cells, respectively (Pinto et al., 1998), suggesting that they may be implicated in the ataxia present in some patients. However, although these antibodies underlie the neurological deficits in LEMS, they may also play a role in controlling tumour growth in C-LEMS, since survival of these patients was found to be significantly longer than that of patients with small cell lung cancer without LEMS in a matched study (Maddison et al., 1999), although lead-time bias may have contributed to this outcome.

The antibodies are assayed using human cerebellar P/Q-type VGCCs radiolabelled with MVIIC conotoxin (Motomura et al., 1995). In some patients, serum antibodies to N-type VGCCs can be detected, but current evidence argues against these having a substantial pathogenetic role in the majority of patients (Motomura et al., 1997). There appears also to be a rare seronegative form of LEMS.

Role of small cell lung cancer
Small cell cancers are believed to be neuroectodermal in origin. They express antigenic determinants including P/Q-type VGCCs that are shared with the CNS. C-LEMS and NC-LEMS IgG blocks potassium-stimulated (voltage-dependent) calcium influx into cultured small cell lung cancer cells, suggesting that in C-LEMS the autoantibodies are provoked by tumour VGCCs. In strong support of this is the improvement in the neurological syndrome that often occurs following specific tumour therapy (Chalk et al., 1990). The immune response is presumably initiated early in the life of the tumour, in view of the sometimes long interval between LEMS onset and the tumour declaring itself. The autoimmune stimulus in NC-LEMS is unknown.

Diagnosis
Electromyography will show a reduced amplitude of the compound muscle action potential, which increases by more than 50% (Maddison et al., 1998) following 15 seconds maximal voluntary contraction. In some patients,

the increase can exceed 1000%. Other nonspecific features of a defect of neuromuscular transmission may also be present: an increased decrement at low rates of stimulation and increased jitter in single-fibre studies. The diagnosis is established by the detection of a raised titre of anti-P/Q-type VGCC antibodies, found in patients with both C-LEMS and NC-LEMS (Motomura et al., 1995).

Management

Most patients will experience symptomatic improvement with 3,4-diaminopyridine (which is only available from specialist pharmacies), at an initial dose in adults of 10 mg four times daily increasing to 20 mg if necessary (McEvoy et al., 1989). A total daily dose of 100 mg should probably not be exceeded; an overdose leads to CNS excitation and seizures. The compound acts by blocking nerve VGKC, thereby prolonging the action potential at motor nerve terminals and increasing quantal release. Patients usually experience perioral and sometimes peripheral paraesthesias about an hour after ingestion. Guanidine offers an alternative therapy, but bone marrow depression and kidney damage are serious drawbacks. Pyridostigmine is only of modest benefit.

Specific tumour therapy will, of course, be necessary in those with an overt lung cancer, and as discussed earlier this may result in an improvement or even full recovery in muscle strength. More commonly, the tumour will not be detectable initially, but continued vigilance will be required (e.g. thoracic imaging) because of the long latent interval. In C-LEMS, prednisolone can be used as an immunosuppressive agent in those failing to respond to tumour therapy and pharmacological treatment. Azathioprine is probably better avoided in this group in view of its very slow action.

In NC-LEMS, patients will often respond to combined prednisolone and azathioprine. Cyclosporin can be considered in those intolerant of azathioprine, or who fail to respond. The treatment protocol can be similar to that described in the section on MG.

In severe disease, plasma exchange can be followed by useful improvement, although this can only be expected to last for a few weeks. Intravenous immunoglobulin treatment offers an alternative approach. A recent randomized blinded crossover study showed significant improvement in those receiving the active preparation (a total of 2 g/kg body weight given over two days), which reached its peak at two to four weeks and thereafter slowly declined (Bain et al., 1996). This improvement was associated with a decline in the anti-VGCC antibody titre, which took over a week to develop, arguing against anti-idiotypic neutralization of the antibody by intravenous immunoglobulin.

Autoimmune neuromyotonia

Clinical features

Muscle twitching ('myokymia') is the cardinal feature of autoimmune neuromyotonia, which is usually associated with muscle cramps (Newsom-Davis and Mills, 1993). The myokymia may be generalized or confined to a few muscle groups. Patients may complain of muscle stiffness or weakness, and pseudomyotonia may be present, for example in slowness of release of hand grip or of withdrawal of the protruded tongue. Patients are sometimes aware of muscle hypertrophy, although this is usually first recognized by the examiner. Sweating may be increased. Some patients experience paraesthesias, poor sleep and, rarely, hallucinations.

The myokymia has an undulating quality. It may be enhanced by previous voluntary muscle activation, which sometimes evokes cramp. Superficially it may resemble the fasciculation of denervation (with which it is sometimes confused), but the muscles are likely to be hypertrophied rather than wasted. It can affect limb muscles, trunk muscles (e.g. buttocks, pectoralis, neck) and bulbar muscles (face and tongue). Sometimes the myokymia only becomes evident after the patient has contracted the muscle. Reflexes can be difficult to elicit in some muscles.

Clinical subtypes

As in MG and LEMS, autoimmune neuromyotonia can occur as a paraneoplastic disorder. A literature survey and a review of our own series of patients indicates that thymoma occurs in 15–20%. There also appears to be an association with small cell lung cancer (Newsom-Davis and Mills, 1993). A number of patients have evidence of a mild neuropathy.

Immunological associations

Neuromyotonia can associate with MG, with thymoma (see above) and with other autoimmune diseases (Newsom-Davis, 1997). It can also occur in the Guillain–Barré syndrome. As in MG, it can be provoked by penicillamine.

Pathophysiology

Neuromyotonia arises because of an increased excitability of peripheral motor nerves, leading to the characteristic 'myokynic' discharges. These consist of spontaneous doublet, triplet or multiplet motor unit discharges that have high intraburst frequencies (40–300 Hz) and that occur irregularly (Newsom-Davis and Mills, 1993). Fasciculation and fibrillation potentials may also be observed. Prolonged discharges may follow voluntary

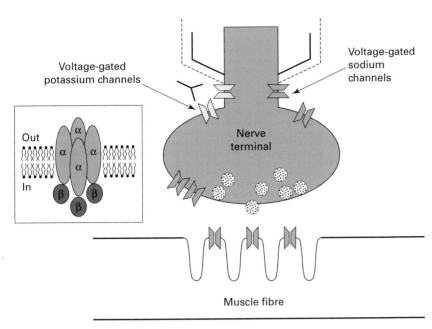

Fig. 32.5. The neuromuscular junction in autoimmune neuromyotonia. A model of the voltage-gated potassium channel is shown (inset). The α-subunits are the primary targets for the autoantibodies; the β-subunits are intracellular.

activation. Isaacs (1961) showed that many of these discharges were arising in the distal arborization of motor nerves since they were unaffected by distal motor block by local anaesthetic, although in some they may occur more proximally (Newsom-Davis and Mills, 1993). The discharges continue during sleep or general anaesthesia, distinguishing them from the discharges of the stiff man syndrome.

The humoral nature of the disorder was shown by the striking reduction in neuromyotonic discharges following plasma exchange (Sinha et al., 1991). These findings suggested the possible presence of antibodies that downregulated VGKC (Fig. 32.5). Their effect would be to increase the quantal content of the EPP (by lengthening the action potential) and to lead to repetitive firing. This was confirmed by a highly significant increase in the quantal content of the EPP in mice injected with neuromyotonic IgG (Shillito et al., 1995). Moreover, neuromyotonic IgG applied to cultured rat dorsal root ganglion cells led to repetitive firing, as did 3,4-diaminopyridine, which also blocks VGKC.

Antibodies to voltage-gated potassium channel

Anti-VGKC antibodies are of IgG class and appear to target members of the *shaker*-related family of VGKCs. They can be detected using radiolabelled α-dendrotoxin (which is a ligand for some members of this family) in about 50% of patients. A molecular-immunohistochemical assay using *Xenopus* oocytes expressing the relevant human gene for the VGKC enabled antibodies to be detected to one or more of the VGKC subtypes in all 20 patients studied (Hart et al., 1997).

Diagnosis

Myokymia and associated neuromyotonic discharges on electromyography should establish the diagnosis. The antibody assay is a useful confirmation if positive, but the absence of a detectable antibody does not exclude the diagnosis. Imaging of the thorax is important because of the risk of associated thymoma or lung cancer.

Management

The neuromyotonia often responds to anticonvulsant medications that downregulate sodium channels (e.g. carbamazepine, phenytoin, lamotrigine). In those failing to respond adequately, treatment with prednisolone alone or combined with azathioprine should be considered. In the authors' experience, some patients will respond, but not all will do so. No prospective trials have yet been undertaken in this disorder. As in myasthenia, removal of a thymoma does not appear greatly to influence the underlying disorder.

In severe disease, or to help in establishing an antibody-mediated disease process, plasma exchange can be undertaken. Improvement will only last for a few weeks. Some patients may also respond to intravenous immunoglobulin therapy.

Congenital myasthenic syndromes

The CMS are inherited disorders of neuromuscular transmission that do not have an underlying autoimmune mechanism. They are a heterogeneous group of disorders caused by a variety of genetic defects and are rare compared with autoimmune forms of myasthenia. They have in common the symptom of fatigable muscle weakness. The phenotypes of the various CMS are often similar, but clinical, electrophysiological, cytochemical and morphological analysis has helped to delineate those associated with defects in postsynaptic, synaptic or presynaptic functions (reviewed in Engel, 1993; Beeson et al., 1997). More recently, mutations responsible for a number of the CMS have been identified, and it is likely that in the future CMS will be classified according to their underlying molecular basis.

Postsynaptic abnormalities

Mutations within the genes that encode muscle AChR are the primary cause of abnormalities in neuromuscular postsynaptic function. Its subunits are encoded by separate genes of between 10 and 12 exons, with the *CHRNA* (α), *CHRNG* (γ) and *CHRND* (δ) loci located on chromosome 2 and the *CHRNB* (β) and *CHRNE* (ε) loci on chromosome 17 (Beeson et al., 1990, 1993). Various mutations within these genes can give rise to very different clinical syndromes.

Acetylcholine receptor deficiency
Clinical features
AChR deficiency is the most common form of CMS seen in the UK. It is a recessive disorder, and there is often consanguinity within the family. Weakness is usually evident at birth or within the first few years of life and is characterized by feeding difficulties, ptosis, impaired eye movements and delayed motor milestones. The weakness is generalized and muscle wasting does not occur. Muscle biopsies show a markedly reduced number of AChRs, as measured by binding of [^{125}I]-labelled α-bungarotoxin and very small MEPPs. Staining, for AChE is typically patchy and the endplates are elongated. Concurrent with the reduced α-bun-

garotoxin binding, there may also be loss of postsynaptic membrane folding. There is usually a good response to anticholinesterase treatment; on occasions, 3,4-diaminopyridine, which increases transmitter release from the nerve terminal, may be a useful alternative treatment in older children (Palace et al., 1991).

Molecular basis
Mutations underlying AChR deficiency are concentrated at the AChR ε-subunit gene locus (Fig. 32.6). Patients may have a homozygous mutation or be heterozygous for two different defective ε-subunit alleles. The mutations are located along the length of the gene, and the lack of any founder effect suggests a constant low level of mutation of this gene within human populations. The mutations may be missense mutations affecting amino acid residues essential for AChR function, such as $\varepsilon C128S$, which alters one of the cysteine residues that is present in all members of the 'cys-loop' gene superfamily and is essential for correct subunit folding, or $\varepsilon S143L$, which disrupts the N-glycosylation site conserved in all the AChR subunits. The mutations may also be insertions, deletions, splice site and nonsense mutations that lead to truncation of the ε-subunit; or mutations in the promoter region of the ε-subunit gene that result in the loss of transcription.

Some missense mutations and some truncations affecting areas near to the C-terminus of the ε-subunit may result in low expression of the adult AChR ($\alpha_2\beta\delta\varepsilon$), whereas mutations of residues essential for AChR function or that truncate the ε-subunit prior to the M3–M4 cytoplasmic loop will almost certainly be null alleles. In these cases, neuromuscular transmission is likely to be mediated through the fetal form of the AChR ($\alpha_2\beta\gamma\delta$-subunits). Immunocytochemical evidence has been obtained showing the presence of fetal AChR at the endplates of patients with CMS caused by ε-subunit null alleles. In both normal and ε-subunit-deficient human muscle biopsies, mRNA encoding the AChR γ-subunit can be readily detected by both reverse transcriptase polymerase chain reaction and RNase protection assays. Consequently, in human muscle, there will probably be a low level of the γ-subunit available for recruitment into AChR pentamers and this would rescue the phenotype from the potentially fatal consequence of the ε-subunit null alleles. Recent identification of mutations in control elements within the ε-subunit gene promoter that disrupt transcription of the ε-subunit mRNA gives support to the hypothesis that the synaptic transmission is mediated through fetal AChR and suggests that mutations in proteins which control AChR synthesis could also be responsible for AChR-deficiency syndromes (Nichols et al., 1999).

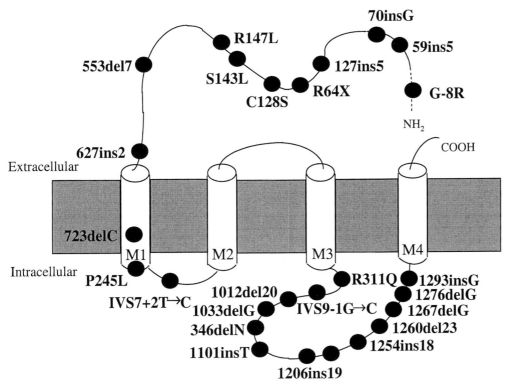

Fig. 32.6. Schematic diagram of the acetylcholine receptor ε-subunit illustrating the position affected by 25 mutations responsible for AChR deficiency (reviewed in Engel et al., 1999).

Low-affinity, fast-channel syndrome
Clinical features
The phenotypes of the low-affinity, fast-channel syndrome and AChR deficiency are similar. Both have a recessive pattern of inheritance and a reduced response to ACh. Whereas in AChR deficiency, this results from a loss of AChR number, in the fast-channel syndrome it results from kinetic abnormalities of AChR function. Therefore, muscle biopsies from these patients do not show the ultrastructural changes of the neuromuscular junction often found in patients with AChR deficiency, although they may show reduced α-bungarotoxin binding (Wang et al., 1999).

Molecular basis
The combination of a null allele (εS143L) or a low-expression allele (εG-8R) with εP121L unmasks the phenotypic effects of this mutation, which are not seen in the heterozygous state. εP121L causes AChR activations to be fewer and shorter than normal and thus a reduced response to ACh. A similar effect is seen for αV285I in combination with the null allele αF233V, indicating that these fast-channel syndrome mutations might occur in any of the genes for AChR subunit.

Slow-channel syndrome
Clinical features
The slow-channel syndrome was first described by Engel et al. (1982). The disorder shows dominant inheritance. Age of onset and severity are variable and in some individuals the phenotypic effects of a mutant allele may remain subclinical. Limb and girdle muscles are most affected, and weakness of scapular and finger extensor muscles is characteristic. Frequently, though not always, on electromyography there is a repetitive response to a single nerve stimulus, and electrophysiological studies on biopsied muscle show a prolonged decay of the MEPPs or endplate currents. Ultrastructural studies often show an endplate myopathy, particularly in affected muscles, which is thought to be caused by 'calcium overload' in the endplate region. Unlike AChR deficiency and the fast-channel syndrome, the disorder is slowly progressive and patients do not respond to anticholinesterase treatments. However, recent studies show that quinidine sulphate at doses to give serum levels of 0.7 to 2.5 μg/ml are beneficial, although dose-related side effects may occur (Harper and Engel, 1998).

Molecular basis
To date, 14 different mutations underlying the slow-channel syndrome have been reported (Fig. 32.7). The

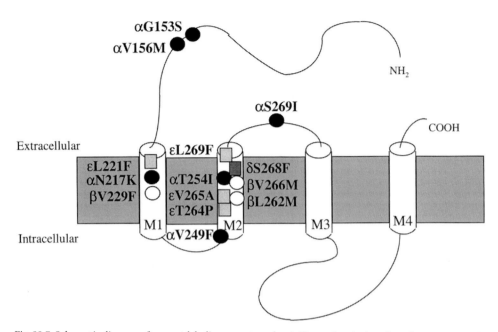

Fig. 32.7. Schematic diagram of an acetylcholine receptor subunit illustrating the location of 14 mutations that underlie slow-channel syndromes (reviewed in Engel et al., 1999).

mutations occur in different subunits and in different functional domains within the subunits. Each results in a single amino acid change and in vitro expression demonstrates that each prolongs ion-channel activations and thus is responsible for a pathogenic gain of function for the AChR. An animal model in which transgenic mice with slow-channel mutations were generated confirmed the pathogenicity of these mutations (Gomez et al., 1997). The majority affect the M2 transmembrane domain and are thought to act predominantly by slowing channel closure, resulting in long individual channel openings. The primary effect of other mutations is to enhance the affinity of the AChR for ACh, which causes repeated reopenings of the channel during the extended period of ACh occupancy. The mechanism through which prolonged channel activations cause endplate myopathy is not yet clear, but it is thought that excess calcium entry leads to 'calcium overload', inhibition of mitochondrial respiration and activation of degenerative enzymes. In addition to this excitotoxic effect, muscle dysfunction may occur because at physiological rates of stimulation the prolonged EPPs summate, leading to persistent depolarization of the endplate and inactivation of the VGSC involved in the generation of the muscle action potential.

Synaptic abnormalities

Within the synaptic cleft the action of ACh is terminated via hydrolysis by AChE. The asymmetric form of AChE is con-centrated and anchored to the basal lamina at the endplate by the collagen-like tail molecule ColQ.

Endplate acetylcholinesterase deficiency
Clinical features
Inheritance of AChE deficiency is autosomal recessive. There is generalized weakness, exacerbated by exercise, that is usually apparent at birth or in early childhood. Symptoms may progress during early life. On electromyography, there is often, but not always, a repetitive response to a single-nerve stimulus. On muscle biopsy, staining of endplates show loss or marked reduction of AChE and, as a result, the MEPPs have an extended decay phase. Morphological changes may include a reduced nerve terminal area and degeneration of the junctional folds. Patients do not respond to acetylcholinesterase inhibitors.

Molecular basis
Eleven mutations underlying this disorder have been described (Fig. 32.8). Each is within the gene encoding ColQ, located on chromosome 3p24.2 (Donger et al., 1998; Ohno et al., 1998). The ColQ polypeptide contains a proline-rich attachment domain (PRAD) that binds the AChE tetramers, a central collagen domain and a C-terminal domain responsible for anchoring in the basal lamina and initiating assembly of the triple helix collagen structure. The mutations may be homozygous or heteroallelic,

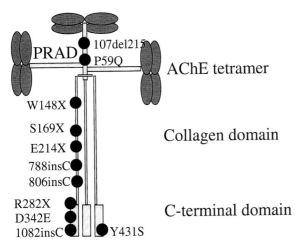

PRAD ● 107del21S
      ● P59Q   AChE tetramer

W148X ●
S169X ●   Collagen domain
E214X ●
788insC●
806insC●
R282X ●   C-terminal domain
D342E ●
1082insC● ● Y431S

Fig. 32.8. Schematic diagram of the asymmetric form of acetylcholinesterase illustrating the positions of 11 mutations that have been identified in *COLQ*.

are present in each of the functional domains and illustrate genetic heterogeneity for this disorder.

The physiological consequences show similarities to the slow-channel syndrome. Prolonged exposure to ACh will cause desensitization of AChRs; persistent depolarization of the endplate will inactivate the VGSCs in the postsynaptic membrane, and persistent stimulation will cause an endplate myopathy. This condition illustrates a pathology mediated through AChRs although caused by defects in an associated functional molecule.

Presynaptic abnormalities

A number of reports describe disorders in which presynaptic dysfunction resulting in reduced ACh release is implicated; however, their molecular basis has yet to be determined. These include inherited disorders with features similar to LEMS, a syndrome attributed to a paucity of synaptic vesicles and familial infantile myasthenia.

Familial infantile myasthenia
Clinical features
Inheritance of familial infantile myasthenia is autosomal recessive. Onset is usually in the neonatal period and is characterized by severe episodic respiratory and bulbar difficulties. Facial weakness and fluctuating ptosis may be evident but there is little or no extraocular involvement. Episodic crises become less frequent with age. Electromyographic findings may be normal in rested muscle but, characteristically, abnormal decrement of the compound muscle action potential amplitudes and

reduced MEPP are induced following stimulation at 10 Hz for several minutes. It is thought that the defect of reduced quantal size may involve the process of uptake/resynthesis or packaging of ACh. Patients respond well to anti-acetylcholinesterase preparations.

References

Bain, P. G., Motomura, M., Newsom-Davis, J. et al. (1996). Effects of intravenous immunoglobulin on muscle weakness and calcium channel antibodies in the Lambert–Eaton myasthenic syndrome. *Neurology* **47**, 678–683.

Batocchi, A. P., Majolini, L., Evoli, A., Lino, M. M., Minisci, C. and Tonali, P. (1999). Course and treatment of myasthenia gravis during pregnancy. *Neurology* **52**, 447–452.

Beeson, D., Jeremiah, S., West, L. et al. (1990). Assignment of the human nicotinic acetylcholine receptor genes: the α- and δ-subunit genes to chromosome 2 and the β-subunit gene to chromosome 17. *Ann. Hum. Genet.* **54**, 199–208.

Beeson, D., Brydson, M., Betty, M. et al. (1993). Primary structure of the human muscle acetylcholine receptor: cDNA cloning of the gamma and epsilon subunits. *Eur. J. Biochem.* **215**, 229–238.

Beeson, D., Palace, J. and Vincent, A. (1997). Congenital myasthenic syndromes. *Curr. Opin. Neurol.* **10**, 402–407.

Chalk, C. H., Murray, N. M., Newsom-Davis, J., O'Neill, J. H. and Spiro, S. G. (1990). Response of the Lambert–Eaton myasthenic syndrome to treatment of associated small-cell lung carcinoma. *Neurology* **40**, 1552–1556.

Chiu, H. C., Vincent, A., Newsom-Davis, J., Hsieh, K. H. and Hung, T. (1987). Myasthenia gravis: population differences in disease expression and acetylcholine receptor antibody titers between Chinese and Caucasians. *Neurology* **37**, 1854–1857.

Christensen, P. B., Jensen, T. S., Tsiropoulos, I. et al. (1998). Mortality and survival in myasthenia gravis: a Danish population based study. *J. Neurol. Neurosurg. Psychiatry* **64**, 78–83.

Donger, C., Krejci, E., Serradell, A. et al. (1998). Mutation in the human acetylcholinesterase-associated collagen gene, ColQ, is responsible for congenital myasthenic syndrome with end-plate acetylcholine esterase deficiency (type 1c). *Am. J. Hum. Genet.*, **63**, 967–975.

Elrington, G. M., Murray, N. M. F., Spiro, S. G. and Newsom-Davis, J. (1991). Neurological paraneoplastic syndromes in patients with small cell lung cancer: a prospective survey of 150 patients. *J. Neurol., Neurosurg. Psychiatry* **54**, 764–767.

Engel, A. G. (1993). The investigation of congenital myasthenic syndromes. *Ann. N. Y. Acad. Sci.* **681**, 425–434.

Engel, A. G., Lambert, E. H., Mulder, D. M. et al. (1982). A newly recognised congenital myasthenic syndrome attributed to prolonged open time of the acetylcholine-induced ion channel. *Ann. Neurol.* **11**, 553–569.

Engel, A. G., Ohno, K. and Sine, S. (1999). Congenital myasthenic syndromes. *Arch. Neurol.* **56**, 163–167.

Gajdos, P., Chevret, S., Clair, B., Tranchant, C., Chastang, C. and the Myasthenia Gravis Clinical Study Group. (1997). Clinical trial of plasma exchange and high-dose intravenous immunoglobulin in myasthenia gravis. *Ann. Neurol.* **41**, 789–796.

Glennerster, A., Palace, J., Warburton, D., Oxbury, S., and Newsom-Davis, J. (1996). Memory in myasthenia gravis: neuropsychological tests of central cholinergic function before and after effective immunologic treatment. *Neurology* **46**, 1138–1142.

Gomez, C., Maselli, R., Gundeck, J. et al. (1997). Slow-channel transgenic mice: a model of postsynaptic organelle degeneration at the neuromuscular junction. *J. Neurosci.* **17**, 4170–4179.

Hart, I. K., Waters, C., Vincent, A., et al. (1997). Autoantibodies detected to expressed K^+ channels are implicated in neuromyotonia. *Ann. Neurol.* **41**, 238–246.

Harper, C. M. and Engel, A. (1998). Safety and efficacy of quinidine sulphate in slow-channel congenital myasthenic syndrome. *Ann. N. Y. Acad. Sci.* **841**, 203–206.

Hejna, M., Haberl, I. and Raderer, M. (1999). Nonsurgical management of malignant thymoma. *Cancer* **85**, 1871–1884.

Hill, M., Beeson, D., Moss, P. et al. (1999). Early-onset myasthenia gravis: a recurring T-cell epitope in the adult-specific acetylcholine receptor epsilon subunit presented by the susceptibility allele HLA-DR52a. *Ann. Neurol.* **45**, 224–231.

Isaacs, H. (1961). A syndrome of continuous muscle fibre activity. *J. Neurol., Neurosurg. Psychiatry* **30**, 126–133.

Janer, M., Cowland, A., Picard, J. et al. (1999). A susceptibility region for myasthenia gravis extending into the HLA-class I sector telomeric to HLA-C. *Hum. Immunol.* **60**, 909–917.

Lindberg, C., Andersen, O. and Lefvert, A. K. (1998). Treatment of myasthenia gravis with methylprednisolone: a double blind study. *Acta Neurol. Scand.* **97**, 370–373.

MacLennan, C. A., Beeson, D., Willcox, N., Vincent, A. and Newsom-Davis, J. (1998). *Ann. N. Y. Acad. Sci.* **841**, 407–410.

Maddison, P., Newsom-Davis, J. and Mills, K. R. (1998). Distribution of electrophysiological abnormality in Lambert-Eaton myasthenic syndrome. *J. Neurol., Neurosurg. Psychiatry* **65**, 213–217.

Maddison, P., Newsom-Davis, J., Mills, K. R. and Souhami, R. L. (1999). Favourable prognosis in Lambert-Eaton myasthenic syndrome and small-cell lung carcinoma. *Lancet* **353**, 117–118.

Mantegazza, R., Confalonieri, P., Antozzi, C. et al. (1998). Video-assisted thoracoscopic extended thymectomy (VATET) in myasthenia gravis. *Ann. N. Y. Acad. Sci.* **841**, 749–752.

Mason, W. P., Graus, F., Lang, B. et al. (1997). Small-cell lung cancer, paraneoplastic cerebellar degeneration and the Lambert–Eaton myasthenic syndrome. *Brain* **120**, 1279–1300.

McEvoy, K. M., Windebank, A. J., Daube, J. R. and Low, P. A. (1989). 3,4-Diaminopyridine in the treatment of the Lambert–Eaton myasthenic syndrome. *N. Engl. J. Med.* **321**, 1567–1571.

Motomura, M., Johnston, I., Lang, B., Vincent, A. and Newsom-Davis, J. (1995). An improved diagnostic assay for Lambert–Eaton myasthenic syndrome. *J. Neurol. Neurosurg. Psychiatry* **58**, 85–87.

Motomura, M., Lang, B., Johnston, I., Palace, J., Vincent, A., and Newsom-Davis, J. (1997). Incidence of serum anti-P/Q-type and

anti-N-type calcium channel autoantibodies in the Lambert–Eaton myasthenic syndrome. *J. Neurol. Sci.* **47**, 35–42.

Mygland, A., Aarli, J., Hofstad, H. and Gilhus, N. E. (1991). Heart muscle antibodies in myasthenia gravis. *Autoimmunity* **10**, 263–267.

Myking, A. O., Skeie, G. O., Varhaug, J. E., Andersen, K. S., Gilhus, N. E. and Aarli, J. A. (1998). The histomorphology of the thymus in late onset, non-thymoma myasthenia gravis. *Eur. J. Neurol.* **5**, 401–405.

Newsom-Davis, J. (1997). Autoimmune neuromyotonia (Isaacs' syndrome): an antibody-mediated potassium channelopathy. *Ann. N. Y. Acad. Sci.* **835**, 111–119.

Newsom-Davis, J. and Mills, K. R. (1993). Immunological associations of acquired neuromyotonia (Isaacs' syndrome): report of 5 cases and literature review. *Brain* **116**, 453–469.

Nichols, P., Croxen, R., Vincent, A. et al. (1999). Mutation of the acetylcholine receptor ε-subunit promoter in congenital myasthenic syndrome. *Ann. Neurol.* **45**, 439–443.

Ohno, K., Brengman, J., Tsujino, A. et al. (1998). Human endplate acetylcholinesterase deficiency caused by mutations in the collagen-like tail subunit (ColQ) of the asymmetric enzyme. *Proc. Natl. Acad. Sci. USA* **95**, 9654–9659.

O'Neill, J. H., Murray, N. M. and Newsom-Davis, J. (1988). The Lambert–Eaton myasthenic syndrome: a review of 50 patients. *Brain* **111**, 577–596.

Oosterhuis, H. J. G. H. (1989). The natural course of myasthenia gravis: a long term follow up study. *J. Neurol. Neurosurg. Psychiatry* **52**, 1121–1127.

Palace, J., Wiles, C. M. and Newsom-Davis, J. (1991). 3,4-Diaminopyridine in the treatment of congenital (hereditary) myasthenia. *J. Neurol. Neurosurg. Psychiatry* **54**, 1069–1072.

Palace, J., Newsom-Davis, J., Lecky, B. and the Myasthenia Study Group (1998). A randomized double-blind trial of prednisolone alone or with azathioprine in myasthenia gravis. *Neurology* **50**, 1778–1783.

Pinto, A., Gillard, S., Moss, F. et al. (1998). Human autoantibodies specific for the α1A calcium currents in cerebellar neurons. *Proc. Natl. Acad. Sci. USA* **95**, 8328–8333.

Robertson, N. P., Deans, J. and Compston, D. A. (1998). Myasthenia gravis: a population based epidemiological study in Cambridgeshire, England. *J. Neurol. Neurosurg. Psychiatry* **65**, 492–496.

Ruff, R. L. and Lennon, V. A. (1998). End-plate voltage-gated sodium channels are lost in clinical and experimental myasthenia gravis. *Ann. Neurol.* **43**, 370–379.

Schon, F., Drayson, M. and Thompson, R. A. (1996). Myasthenia gravis and elderly people. *Age Ageing* **25**, 56–58.

Seybold, M. E. (1998). Thymectomy in childhood myasthenia gravis. *Ann. N. Y. Acad. Sci.* **841**, 731–741.

Shapiro, R. L., Hatheway, C. and Swerdlow, D. L. (1998). Botulism in the United States: a clinical and epidemiological review. *Ann. Int. Med.* **129**, 221–228.

Shillito, P., Molenaar, P. C., Vincent, A. et al. (1995). Acquired neuromyotonia: evidence for autoantibodies directed against K^+ channels of peripheral nerves. *Ann. Neurol.* **38**, 714–722.

Sinha, S., Newsom-Davis, J., Mills, K. R., Byrne, N., Lang, B. and Vincent, A. (1991). Autoimmune aetiology for acquired neuromyotonia (Isaacs' syndrome). *Lancet* **338**, 75–77.

Somnier, F. E., Keiding, N. and Paulson, O. B. (1991). Epidemiology of myasthenia in Denmark: a longitudinal and comprehensive population survey. *Arch. Neurol.* **48**, 733–739.

Verma, P. K. and Oger, J. J. (1992). Seronegative generalized myasthenia gravis: low frequency of thymic pathology. *Neurology* **42**, 586–589.

Vincent, A., Newland, C., Brueton, L., Riemersma, S., Huson S. M. and Newsom-Davis, J. (1997). Arthrogryposis multiplex congenita with maternal antibodies specific for a fetal antigen. *Lancet* **346**, 24–25.

Wang, H.-L., Milone, M., Ohno, K. et al. (1999). Acetylcholine receptor M3 domain, stereochemical and volume contributions to channel gating. *Nat. Neurosci.* **2**, 226–233.

Waterman, S. A., Lang, B. and Newsom-Davis, J. (1997). Effect of Lambert–Eaton myasthenic syndrome antibodies on autonomic neurons in the mouse. *Ann. Neurol.* **42**, 147–156.

Willcox, N., Schluep, M., Ritter, M. A., Schuurman, H. A., Newsom-Davis, J. and Christensson, B. (1987). Myasthenic and non-myasthenic thymoma: an expansion of a minor cortical subset? *Am. J Pathol.* **127**, 447–460.

Willcox, N., Schluep, M., Ritter, M. and Newsom-Davis, J. (1991). The thymus in seronegative patients. *J. Neurol.*, **238**, 256–261.

Yeh, J. H. and Chiu, H. C. (1999). Plasmapheresis in myasthenia gravis: a comparative study of daily versus alternately daily schedule. *Acta. Neurol. Scand.* **99**, 147–151.

Zheng, Y., Wheatley, L. M., Liu, T. and Levinson, A. I. (1999). Acetylcholine receptor alpha subunit mRNA expression in human thymus: augmented expression in myasthenia gravis and upregulation by interferon-gamma. *Clin. Immunol.* **91**, 170–177.

33

Toxic and iatrogenic myopathies and neuromuscular transmission disorders

Zohar Argov, Henry J. Kaminski, Ali Al-Mudallal and Robert L. Ruff

Introduction

Numerous drugs are myotoxic and injure muscle through a wide array of mechanisms, including inflammatory reactions, mitochondrial injury, electrolyte disturbance and compromise of lysosomal metabolism. With the ever increasing introduction of new therapeutic agents, the frequency of drug-related muscle injury is likely to increase. Of further importance is that muscle injury may resolve by simple withdrawal of the agent, while persistent injury may lead to widespread injury with rhabdomyolysis, leading to renal failure, irreversible disability and death. The pattern of muscle involvement is equally diverse, and this review attempts to classify drug-induced muscle disorders based on general clinical features to simplify their recognition (Argov and Mastaglia, 1994; Victor and Sieb, 1994; George and Pourmand, 1997). Table 33.1 summarizes major clinical characteristics and the major medications that are associated with these syndromes.

Myopathies

Focal myopathy

Localized muscle injury occurs with repeated intramuscular injections and is related to direct effects of needle insertion or the injected agent, but it may be further complicated by local haemorrhage or infection. Such focal myopathy is most commonly seen among drug addicts and can occur in several muscle groups. Previously, when intramuscular administration of antibiotics and therapeutic narcotics was more common, the quadriceps and deltoids were the most common sites of 'needle myopathy' (Argov and Mastaglia, 1994; Zaidat et al., 1999). Injection can produce local induration and fibrous contracture; in

addition focal necrosis may develop with serum creatine kinase (CK) elevation (George and Pourmand, 1997). The severity and mechanism of injury varies among agents. Digoxin, benzodiazepines, and lidocaine (lignocaine) may produce extensive necrosis, while chloroquine has a local toxic effect. The pH and osmolarity of the agent may be of particular importance in the extent of CK elevation and muscle necrosis. The damage produced by opiates and chlorpromazine is thought to be a consequence of histamine release. The appreciation of a focal myopathy is clinically important in order to avoid confusing CK elevations with those from other muscle disorders or myocardial infarction.

Acute or subacute painful myopathy

Numerous agents may produce muscle weakness of rapid onset, usually with proximal musculature most prominently effected. Muscle damage may be extensive and produce marked elevations of muscle enzymes in serum and myoglobinuria. Electromyography (EMG) will identify typical signs of muscle disease, and prominent spontaneous activity may be present. The pathogenesis of muscle damage varies among agents and the following presentation attempts to group drugs that produce muscle damage by similar mechanisms of action.

Toxic myopathy

Clofibrate and related agents, bezafibrate, etofibrate, beclofibrate, lovastatin and gemfibrozil, used for their cholesterol-lowering activity, induce a myopathy characterized by the acute onset of cramps, myalgias and weakness with an elevation of serum transaminases and CK. Myotonia develops in some patients in response to these agents, especially clofibrate. Accumulation of the active metabolite of clofibrate, chlorophenoxyisobutyric acid,

Table 33.1. Drug-induced myopathies

Major toxin-related syndromes	Drug
Necrotizing myopathy	Lovastatin, clofibrate, bezafibrate, etofibrate, gemfibrozil, epsilon-aminocaproic acid, organophosphates, ethanol
Lysosomal-related myopathy	Chloroquine, mepacrine (quinacrine), amiodarone, perhexiline
Inflammatory myopathy	Penicillamine, procainamide, phenytoin, levodopa, leuprolide, propylthiouracil, cimetidine
Antimicrotubular myopathy	Colchicine, vincristine
Mitochondrial myopathy	Zidovudine, germanium
Vitamin/amino acid-related myopathy	Vitamin E (excess and deficiency), etretinate, isotretinoin, tryptophan (eosinophilia-myalgia syndrome)
Hypokalaemia-related myopathy	Glycyrrhizic acid (liquorice), glycyrrhetic acid (enoxolone, carbenoxolone), amphotericin (amphotericin B), diuretics, laxatives, ethanol
Drugs of abuse	Phencyclidine (PCP, angel dust), cocaine, diamorphine (heroin), toluene
Critical illness myopathy	Combination high-dose steroids, nondepolarizing neuromuscular blockade, sepsis

appears to be particularly toxic, and the presence of renal failure, nephrotic syndrome or hypothyroidism appears to place patients at greater risk for development of myopathy. Some patients also have an associated peripheral neuropathy. Discontinuation or reduction in dose of the drug will lead to gradual recovery (Mastaglia, 1992). Nicotinic acid, which is also used for its lipid-lowering properties, may induce a painful myopathy with increased serum CK. In some patients, isolated serum CK elevations have been described. With all these agents, their withdrawal leads to resolution of the myopathy. Simvastatin, pravastatin, lovastatin and 3-hydroxy-3-methylglutaryl-coenzyme A reductase inhibitors rarely cause myopathy when used alone; however, in combination with gemfibrozil, mibefradil or cyclosporin (cyclosporine), they are more likely to cause muscle injury (Giordano et al., 1997; Nakahara et al., 1998; Schmassmann-Suhijar et al., 1998). Thirty per cent of cardiac transplant recipients receiving cyclosporin and reductase inhibitors will develop myopathy (Tobert, 1988). Cyclosporin alone may cause myopathy manifesting with myalgia or rhabdomyolysis. Serum CK levels may be normal or elevated 10–20 times. Muscle biopsy typically shows type II fibre atrophy, segmental necrosis and ragged-red fibres. Myopathy is believed to be dose dependent and subsides with reducing the dose.

Epsilon-aminocaproic acid inhibits fibrinolysis. The drug has been frequently used after subarachnoid haemorrhage in an attempt to limit rebleeding and has been used in various coagulation disorders. A myopathy affecting axial musculature, with symptoms beginning four or more weeks after initiation of treatment may occur. Its induction may be related to alterations in muscle membrane function or to muscle ischaemia (Mastaglia, 1992).

Some agents produce a myopathy by compromise of mitochondrial function. Zidovudine (AZT) causes a progressive, painful myopathy, thought to be dose related. Weakness is proximal muscle weakness, and myalgias occur in the thighs and calves, which are often exacerbated by exercise. Symptoms may start as late as 9 months after commencing the medication. Serum CK is normal or minimally increased. EMG may show fibrillations and positive waves in the proximal muscles. A clear distinction between zidovudine myopathy and HIV myositis is sometimes difficult to make. HIV myositis can resemble polymyositis with inflammatory infiltrates (see Chapter 31). Ragged-red fibres are found, but inflammatory infiltrates are usually absent in zidovudine myopathy. Germanium is an antineoplastic agent that affects mitochondria in many organ systems, leading often to renal failure and anaemia. Muscle demonstrates ragged-red fibres and vacuolization. Mitochondria show dense granules on electron microscopy.

Excess ingestion of vitamin E may result in proximal muscle weakness and elevated serum CK (Mastaglia, 1992). Vitamin E deficiency may also produce generalized muscle weakness, including the ocular muscles (Mastaglia, 1992). Etretinate is a vitamin A derivative that is used in treating psoriasis. Skeletal muscle damage is an uncommon side effect of its use and is manifested as proximal muscle weakness and tenderness (Mastaglia, 1992). Isotretinoin is used for treatment of severe acne. Mild and transient arthralgias and myalgias can occasionally be seen (Mastaglia, 1992).

Emetine is an amoebicide, an emetic and is used in alcoholic aversion therapy. Proximal limb and trunk muscles are primarily affected but a reversible, generalized myopathy may also occur. The degree of muscle damage depends on the dose and duration of exposure (Mastaglia, 1992). *Radix ipecacuanhae* contains the alkaloids cephaeline, psychotrine and the toxic emetine. Its primary indication is as an emetic in treatment of toxin or drug ingestion. Ingestion of emetine for more than 10 days in high doses results in a severe myopathy and cardiomyopathy. Coincident eating disorders, such as anorexia nervosa and bulimia nervosa, are common (Victor and Sieb, 1994; George and Pourmand, 1997). Occasionally, sensory symptoms may be observed. Serum enzymes associated with muscle damage are mildly to moderately elevated and the biopsy reveals predominance of type I fibres, a slight decrease in the average diameter of muscle fibre, isolated necrotic granular basophilic fibres and intracytoplasmic eosinophilic rod-like inclusions in the type I fibres. Treatment is supportive. Cessation of emetine ingestion leads to gradual recovery within several months in most cases.

Hypokalaemia-related myopathy

Agents that produce hypokalaemia with potassium serum levels below 2 mmol/l may induce muscle damage (Victor and Sieb, 1994; George and Pourmand, 1997). The most common agents to induce hypokalaemic myopathy are diuretics and laxatives when used therapeutically or abused. The antifungal agent amphotericin (amphotericin B) is nephrotoxic and may produce potassium depletion leading to the development of myopathy. Liquorice (licorice), which contains glycyrrhizic acid, and carbenoxolone, a drug for peptic ulcer disease that contains the related compound glycyrrhetic acid (enoxolone), have an aldosterone-like effect that induces potassium loss. Toluene may also induce potassium depletion and myopathy. A vacuolar myopathy that may show necrosis and regenerative fibres is seen histologically. Occasionally, the muscle injury may be so severe as to produce rhabdomyolysis.

Chronic alcoholism may also induce hypokalaemic myopathy (Finsterer et al., 1998). Hypokalaemia can also develop from alcohol-induced hypomagnesaemia. Weakness, hypotonia and depressed deep tendon reflexes occur and this can develop quickly to flaccid paralysis. The acute onset of painless weakness in the proximal limb muscles and limb girdle muscles without muscle cramps, tenderness or swelling is characteristic. Serum CK and aldolase are elevated. When the patient is hypokalaemic and hypomagnesaemic, the myopathy is often painful. Strength improves with potassium and magnesium replacement (Mastaglia, 1992).

Myositis

Several agents cause muscle disease by inducing an immune attack. D-Penicillamine may cause an inflamma-

tory myopathy indistinguishable from polymyositis. Myocardial involvement may be fatal. Halting the drug results in recovery (Mastaglia, 1992). Procainamide may cause interstitial myositis as part of a lupus-like vasculitic reaction (Mastaglia, 1992). Phenytoin, levodopa, leuprolide, propylthiouracil and cimetidine have been associated with an inflammatory myopathy but the relation is not as clearly established.

Tryptophan is an essential amino acid and is marketed as a nonprescription, nutritional supplement. In 1989 an epidemic of myalgia and eosinophilia occurred in association with tryptophan use. Proposed diagnostic criteria for the so-called eosinophilia-myalgia syndrome are (i) eosinophil count over 1000×10^6 cells, (ii) severe myalgia, and (iii) an absence of alternative explanations for eosinophilia. Manifestations may develop acutely with a severe respiratory illness followed by myalgia, fatigue and painful moderate to severe proximal or distal weakness. Patients may develop respiratory failure. Other manifestations include fever, rash, urticaria, livedo reticularis, alopecia, lymphadenopathy, scleroderma-like syndrome and paraesthesias. In addition to marked eosinophilia, patients may have increased serum CK in the acute phase. The onset of the syndrome may be delayed months or years after tryptophan ingestion (Clauw et al., 1990). Some patients develop severe axonal sensory–motor neuropathy (Emslie-Smith et al., 1994). Muscle biopsy reveals fibre atrophy and perimysial inflammation with T cell and eosinophilic infiltrate (Clauw et al., 1990). The pathogenesis remains obscure. Speculations emphasize the role of impurities and abnormalities of tryptophan metabolism with the development of this syndrome. Treatment is limited to stopping the offending agent plus commencing corticosteroid treatment. Some individuals develop a chronic scleroderma-like-syndrome, sensory motor polyneuropathy, a persistent proximal myopathy or episodic myalgias (Kaufman et al., 1991).

Acute rhabdomyolysis

Several of the commonly abused drugs may produce muscle weakness. Cocaine results in myoglobinuria. This is either a direct toxic effect from cocaine or secondary to cocaine-induced ischaemia. Excessive amounts of sympathomimetic drugs may produce acute rhabdomyalysis, myoglobinuria and renal failure (Mastaglia, 1992). Diamorphine (heroin) ingestion may produce acute rhabdomyolysis and commonly results in alteration in consciousness and subsequent pressure-induced damage to skeletal muscle (Mastaglia, 1992). Phencyclidine (PCP, angel dust) use may cause myoglobinuria and acute renal failure. Excessive isometric motor activity may be the cause of PCP myopathy as PCP does not have a direct toxic effect on muscle (Mastaglia, 1992). Chronic toluene abuse will often produce symmetric weakness with many associated peripheral and central nervous system (CNS) dysfunctions. Associated hypokalaemia, hypophosphataemia and acidosis may lead to myoglobinuria.

Severe myonecrosis can occur as a consequence of general anaesthesia, status epilepticus or prolonged unconsciousness; the last probably has its effect through pressure necrosis. In addition, a large number of agents, including the venoms of several snakes and spiders, have been implicated in acute myonecrosis with myoglobinuria. This condition is associated with extreme elevation in serum levels of muscle-associated enzymes and myoglobinuria. Extreme muscle swelling may produce compartment syndromes, leading to nerve entrapments and limb ischaemia. Numerous snake venoms are myotoxic at the bite site; others have more widespread effects, causing muscle necrosis and myoglobinuria. Snakes with venoms that are associated with diffuse rhabdomyolysis are the Tiger snake, Tiapan, Mulga and Seasnake. The venom of the Arkansas and Honduran tarantulas causes irreversible injury to the muscle fibre plasma membranes, leading to diffuse myonecrosis (Mastaglia, 1992).

Subacute or chronic painless proximal myopathy

Corticosteroids

Muscle weakness and wasting are also common complications of glucocorticoid administration (Kaminski and Ruff, 1994; Anagnos et al., 1997). Patients with steroid myopathy usually have other stigmata of glucocorticoid excess (i.e. 'moon facies', 'buffalo hump', fragile skin, osteoporosis, cataracts). The weakness is insidious in onset and primarily proximal, with the legs more severely involved than the arms. Myalgias frequently accompany the weakness (Kaminski and Ruff, 1994). Glucocorticoids may also produce muscle weakness by altering serum electrolytes, in particular through their mineralocorticoid activity in producing hypokalaemia (Kaminski and Ruff, 1994). Biopsies show a vacuolar degeneration pattern, which is characteristic of potassium depletion not steroid myopathy. Glucocorticoids may produce transient hypophosphataemia as a result of increased renal clearance of phosphate; if this is severe, muscle necrosis may result. However, potassium and phosphate depletion are not the usual causes of myopathy associated with glucorticoid use.

Serum concentrations of CK and aldolase are usually normal. The EMG findings are variable. Typically, insertional activity is normal and the motor unit potentials are of low amplitude and short duration. Despite isolated reports of fibrillation potentials accompanying the brief duration motor unit potentials, spontaneous electrical activity is typically absent. Histological studies show nonspecific changes or selective atrophy of type II muscle fibres, in particular type IIB fibres. Increased muscle glycogen is found in type IIA fibres. Prominent subsarcolemmal lipid deposits may be seen, but lipid excess is not characteristic of iatrogenic steroid myopathy. Electron microscopic studies reveal mitochondrial aggregation and vacuolization. These changes are not severe and correlate poorly with weakness (Kaminski and Ruff, 1994).

Estimates of the incidence of steroid myopathy associated with daily treatment lasting more than 90 days vary from 2 to 21%; however, these figures indicate only those patients who developed severe weakness. The steroid myopathy may be missed in patients using steroids for disorders that produce weakness, such as the inflammatory myopathies or CNS (Batchelor et al., 1997). Distinguishing between worsening of the condition, in particular inflammatory myopathy and steroid myopathy may be difficult. However, clinical clues do exist. Steroid myopathy takes time to develop; therefore, weakness developing at the onset of steroid treatment is probably caused by a flare in the inflammatory process. Weakness should be treated by continuing or increasing the dose of steroid. Steroid myopathy usually occurs with stigmata of steroid usage in their absence weakness is probably not steroid induced. Elevation in serum CK also would suggest that the weakness is partially caused by the inflammatory myopathy, but normal enzyme levels do not rule out a flare in inflammatory myopathy.

The dose and duration of steroid treatment associated with the onset of weakness varies widely, but patients who receive steroids for less than a month rarely develop severe steroid myopathy. The incidence of steroid myopathy varies with the glucocorticoid preparation. Although any glucocorticoid can produce steroid myopathy, the fluorinated steroids (triamcinolone, betamethasone and dexamethasone) are more likely to produce weakness. Patients develop weakness when switched from other steroids to equivalent anti-inflammatory doses of triamcinolone or dexamethasone and recover from dexamethasone- or triamcinolone-induced weakness when converted to an equivalent anti-inflammatory dose of another preparation (Kaminski and Ruff, 1994).

The prime method of treating steroid myopathy is to decrease the steroid dosage to the lowest possible level, but recovery may take many weeks. Conversion to a non-fluorinated steroid and to alternate-day dosing may limit side effects. Starvation or protein deprivation accelerates steroid myopathy, and steroid treatment slows or prevents recovery of muscle mass in the malnourished. Inactivity also worsens steroid myopathy, and exercise may prevent weakness and accelerate recovery. Physical therapy also may be useful in prevention and treatment of weakness and wasting (Kaminski and Ruff, 1994).

Colchicine
Colchicine induces a proximal myopathy especially in patients with renal insufficiency. Distal sensory involvement secondary to axonal neuropathy is common. Serum CK is usually elevated. Coincident administration of cyclosporin is suggested to potentiate colchicine myopathy, but the observation has not been confirmed. Discontinuation of colchicine improves strength and the sensory neuropathy (Mastaglia, 1992).

Vincristine
Although vincristine commonly causes an axonal peripheral neuropathy, some patients develop a proximal myopathy, manifesting with proximal muscle pain and weakness with muscle wasting; the EMG shows positive sharp waves with fibrillation potentials. These side effects are dose related and usually disappear six weeks after finishing treatment. Some patients, however, continue to have symptoms for prolonged periods of time.

Perhexiline
Perhexiline is a calcium channel blocker that with chronic use leads to peripheral neuropathy and less commonly to painless proximal myopathy. Systemic side effects includes hypoglycaemia, weight loss and hepatic disturbances. Characteristic intracytoplasmic inclusions, frequently associated with calcium deposits, are found either at the periphery of the muscle fibres or between the central myofibrils. These inclusions may also be found in endothelial cells, pericytes, Schwann cells and fibroblasts and vary in morphology depending on cell type. Discontinuation of the drug and supportive treatment leads to reversal of the myopathy (Zaidat et al., 1999).

Amiodarone
Amiodarone, an antiarrhythmic agent, frequently causes neurologic side effects including peripheral neuropathy, ataxia, tremor and, less commonly, a proximal and distal myopathy that may be painful or painless. Manifestations may begin as early as one month or up to three years after initiation of treatment. Marked distal motor weakness and stocking and gloves sensory impairment occur, usually associated with distal muscular atrophy. Enlargement of extraocular muscles that resembles endocrine ophthalmopathy may occur (Sundelin and Norrsell, 1997). Muscle biopsy reveals a vacuolar myopathy with lysosomal inclusions. High levels of amiodarone and its metabolite desethylamiodarone may be found in the muscle despite normal serum levels. Experimentally, prolonged dosing of mice with amiodarone produced myopathy characterized by autophagic vacuolation, phospholipid inclusions and necrosis mainly affecting type II fibres. Therefore, amiodarone or its metabolites may have a direct toxic effect on oxidative enzyme activity (Zaidat et al., 1999).

Antimalarial agents
Several antimalarial agents cause a myopathy that appears to affect the lysosomes. Chloroquine and hydroxychloroquine may cause progressive painless proximal muscle wasting and weakness. A neuropathy and cardiomyopathy may occur. Type I muscle fibres are affected and show vacuolar degeneration. EMG shows fibrillations with myopathic motor unit potentials. The myopathy slowly reverses after discontinuation of the medication. Plasmocid induces a proximal and painless myopathy with histological evidence of muscle necrosis and phagocytosis. Animal studies suggest that autodigestion by intramyofibral lysosomal proteases, followed by digestion of the necrotic fibres by macrophage proteases, occurs. Mepacrine (quinacrine, a drug no longer distributed in the USA) is an acridine dye also used to treat malaria and giardiasis. General side effects includes headache, dizziness, vomiting, diarrhoea, yellowish discoloration of urine, sclera and skin, and less commonly psychosis. Prolonged treatment produces a painless proximal myopathy.

Clozapine
Clozapine is a dibenzodiazepine derivative used as an antipsychotic that commonly causes mild elevations of serum CK. In a study of 37 patients, three had elevations to over 20 000 U/l but without myoglobinuria, and five had myopathic changes by EMG but muscle biopsy showed minimal alterations (Scelsa et al., 1996). An individual exposed to clozapine has been described who developed rhabdomyolysis; an inborn defect of the potassium channels was hypothesized to account for the muscle injury in this patient with clozapine therapy (Koren et al., 1998).

Myopathies associated with ethanol abuse
Acute and possibly chronic forms of alcoholic myopathy exist. Acute necrotizing myopathy commonly occurs against a background of chronic alcohol abuse. Excessive ingestion of alcohol results in noninflammatory muscle

necrosis characterized as an acute onset of severe muscle pain, cramps, weakness, swelling and tenderness, which may be generalized or focal. Recovery depends on the severity of muscle destruction and may take several months. Significant rhabdomyolosis may lead to acute renal failure (Mastaglia, 1992).

Definitive evidence of a chronic alcoholic myopathy does not exist. Some think that chronic alcohol use results in the insidious onset of painless proximal muscle weakness and wasting, but others consider this secondary to peripheral neuropathy (Mastaglia, 1992). Chronic drinkers who acutely increase their alcohol intake elevate their serum CK and myoglobin without a clinically evident myopathy. This may be an asymptomatic form of chronic alcoholic myopathy that could progress to persistent proximal weakness (Mastaglia, 1992).

Critical illness myopathy

Acute weakness of myopathic origin may develop in the intensive care setting (Gutmann et al., 1996; Rich et al., 1996; Ruff, 1996, 1998). Several factors appear to contribute to the rapid onset of weakness and wasting: immobility, use of nondepolarizing neuromuscular-blocking agents, concurrent sepsis and glucocorticoid use (Ruff, 1996). After liver transplantation, 8% of patients develop an acute necrotizing myopathy that is most closely associated with high doses of corticosteroid administration (Campellone et al., 1998). Asymmetric weakness may occur, which may misdirect diagnostic evaluation to a lesion of the brain or spinal cord (Sun et al., 1997). Muscle histopathology reveals myopathy with loss of thick filaments in almost 80%, mild myopathic changes in 14% and atrophy of type I and II fibres in a small number (Lacomis et al., 1996). Selective loss of thick filaments is particularly associated with use of intravenous corticosteroids. Rich et al. (1996) identified three patients with severe weakness whose muscle was inexcitable with direct electrical stimulation. Loss of muscle of membrane excitability can produce a response pattern on EMG testing that resembles axonal neuropathy (Rich et al., 1996, 1998; Ruff, 1996, 1998). From these observations, one can conclude that critical illness myopathy may have several pathogenic mechanisms. Despite the severity of weakness, patients may improve significantly with supportive care.

Diffuse muscle weakness may be a significant contributing factor to difficulty in weaning patients from ventilatory assistance. Many factors may contribute to muscle weakness. Muscle relaxants, aminoglycosides, β-agonists, theophylline, metabolic disturbances, sepsis, hypoxia, corticosteroids, neuromuscular-blocking agents and seda-

tives are commonly used in the critically ill patient and may contribute to weakness.

Drug-induced myasthenic syndromes

A substantial number of drugs and therapeutic agents interfere with neuromuscular junction transmission (NMT) producing various clinical disorders. These agents may either augment an already existing transmission defect in patients with neuromuscular junction disorders or interact with other drugs to produce a NMT block and even produce de novo a disorder of the junction. This section will only deal with drugs that caused NMT defects in humans.

Clinical presentations

Recognition of clinical patterns in which drug-induced disorders of NMT are manifested is important for patient management and for identifying previously undescribed side effects of known or new drugs. There are five major clinical pictures of drug-induced impairment of NMT:
- rapid-onset drug-induced myasthenia
- slow drug-induced myasthenia
- unmasked myasthenia gravis (MG)
- aggravated MG
- postoperative respiratory depression.

Rapid-onset drug-induced myasthenia
The development, within days, of myasthenic features in an apparently normal person should always be suspected as drug related. When the symptoms and signs develop shortly after starting a new medication, correct diagnosis is relatively easy. Most commonly affected are respiratory muscles, with a dramatic presentation, or extraocular muscles, with the appearance of double vision. Rapid disappearance of signs after drug withdrawal is considered a proof that the myasthenia was drug induced. In many of these apparently normal persons, the drug unmasks an underlying subclinical disorder of NMT. This was illustrated in the case of a patient with chloroquine-induced acute myasthenic syndrome, who continued to have abnormal electrophysiological findings in repetitive nerve stimulation and in single-fibre EMG several months after the drug-induced clinical disorder had completely resolved (Robberecht et al., 1989). A number of drugs have been implicated in causing such a complication (Table 33.2), probably through their strong blocking effects on NMT. Still, many of these drugs are commonly used and this side effect is rare, strengthening the notion that a

Table 33.2. Drug-induced myasthenia in humans: clinical presentations and mechanisms

Drug	Rapid myasthenia	Slow myasthenia	Unmasking of myasthenia	Aggravation of myasthenia	Postoperative respiratory depression	Mechanism[a]
Antibiotics and antimicrobials						
Neomycin	+				+	Combined
Kanamycin	+			+?	+	Presynaptic
Streptomycin	+	+		+	+	Combined
Gentamicin	+			+		Presynaptic
Tobramycin					+	Presynaptic
Amikacin					+	Presynaptic?
Polymyxin B (polymixin B)	+				+	Combined
Colistin	+			+	+	Combined
Tetracyclines				+		Postsynaptic
Lincomycin					+	Combined
Clindamycin					+	Combined
Erythromycin				+		Presynaptic?
Ampicillin			+			Unknown
Imipenem				+		Unknown
Clarithromycin	+?					Unknown
Bretylium	+					Postsynaptic
Emetine	+					Unknown
Ciprofloxacin			+	+		Unknown
Cardiovascular drugs						
Beta-blockers	+		+			Combined
Quinidine			+	+	+	Presynaptic
Procainamide	+	+		+		Combined
Verapamil	+			+		Combined
Trimetaphan	+				+	Unknown
Central nervous system drugs						
Phenytoin (diphenylhydantoin)		+	+	+		Combined
Trimethadione		+				Immune?
Lithium			+		+	Presynaptic?
Chlorpromazine				+		Combined
Benzhexol (trihexyphenidyl)	+					Unknown
Antirheumatic agents						
D-Penicillamine	+	+			+	Immune
Chloroquine	+	+			+	Combined
Prednisone				+		Postsynaptic
Other drugs						
Procaine/lignocaine (lidocaine)	+?					Presynaptic
D, L-Carnitine		+				Unknown
Lactate				+		Presynaptic
Methoxyflurane	+					Unknown
Magnesium	+			+		Presynaptic
Contrast agents				+		Unknown
Citrate anticoagulation				+		Presynaptic?
Aprotinin				+		Unknown
Ritonavir			+?			Unknown

Table 33.2. (*cont.*)

Drug	Clinical presentations					Mechanism[a]
	Rapid myasthenia	Slow myasthenia	Unmasking of myasthenia	Aggravation of myasthenia	Postoperative respiratory depression	
Levonorgestrel			+			Unknown
Desferoxamine (desferrioxamine)			+?			Unknown
Interferon-α	+			+		
Pyrantal pamoate			+	+		Unknown

Note:

[a] Neuromuscular junction affected pre- or postsynaptic or as a combination of both. ? indicates a clear understanding has not been established.

subclinical impairment of NMT already exists in the affected patients.

Slow drug-induced myasthenia

The gradual evolution of myasthenia (within weeks to many months) has been linked to a number of drugs, especially D-penicillamine (Table 33.2). The clinical syndrome is very similar to idiopathic MG and may be accompanied by a similar immune response: serum antibodies against the acetylcholine receptor can be detected. The major difference between 'classical' MG and the drug-induced disorder is that upon withdrawal of the offending medication gradual recovery is common. Full recovery after drug withdrawal, however, does not occur in all patients and MG may persist, with a need for immunosuppressive therapy. In such cases, it may be argued that the drug unmasked a pre-existing immune-mediated disorder of the neuromuscular junction. The causal role of the drug in the myasthenic disorder can only be identified retrospectively in this clinical presentation. This is because recovery, which is the hallmark of drug-induced disorders, depends on correct diagnosis and must be followed for a prolonged period. Consequently, recording drug usage history is essential in the evaluation of any myasthenic patient, and therapy withdrawal is an important diagnostic tool.

Unmasking myasthenia gravis

A previously undeclared MG that first manifests after exposure to a drug and remains clinically active even after the medication is withdrawn is the major feature of this group. Typically, a drug with NMT-blocking properties is given to a 'healthy' subject and a myasthenic syndrome appears within a short time (usually days but sometime a few weeks). Withdrawal of the drug does not affect the overall clinical course, although transient improvement can be observed. The drug may be regarded as the 'last straw' that led to the clinical appearance of MG. In many of these patients, immunological features of typical MG are already present at diagnosis. When antibodies to the acetylcholine receptor cannot be detected, the differentiation between this presentation and the first one depends on the response to drug cessation.

Aggravated myasthenia gravis

Aggravated MG is by now probably the most common presentation of drug-induced NMT impairment, and many drugs have been implicated (Table 33.2). When a patient with a relatively mild or well controlled MG is given a drug and this results in worsening of the muscle weakness or fatiguability, the recognition of the drug's contribution is easy and may be made by the patient himself. However, when the drug is given for a disease that in itself is deleterious to MG (e.g. antibiotics for infection), the additional harmful effects of the administered agent may be overlooked. As a result, several instances of possible antibiotic-induced aggravation of MG have not been clearly identified for a long time (e.g. with ampicillin). Knowledge of the possible harmful effects of a drug is essential for the management of patients with MG, but the use of such a drug is not necessarily an absolute contraindication (see Management).

Postoperative respiratory depression

Delayed recovery of muscle function, especially that of the respiratory muscles, after anaesthesia can have many causes, such as erroneous overdosage, pseudocholin esterase deficiency with depolarizing muscle relaxant usage drug-induced impairment of NMT in previously undetected MG. In many instances, the offending drug augments the function of NMT blockers traditionally used for muscle relaxation. In other cases, the patients may be unduly susceptible to the neuromuscular-blocking activity of a drug and this may be regarded as very-rapid-onset drug-induced myasthenia, similar to the first presentation. Patients with other diseases that reduce the safety factor for NMT, such as poliomyelitis, rapidly progressive amyotrophic lateral sclerosis, polymyositis and hypocalcaemia (Kaeser, 1984), should also be closely monitored for similar postanaesthetic complications. The surrounding circumstances of anaesthesia and the acute development of the complication make this a distinct presentation. Better recognition and monitoring of neuromuscular function during anaesthesia by electrophysiological methods of repetitive stimulation ('train of four' test) may prevent many of these complications as the state of NMT can be determined and extubation be delayed.

Identification

Recognition of one of the above-mentioned clinical syndromes is the first and essential part in identifying a possible hazardous drug for myasthenic patients. In drugs with strong neuromuscular-blocking activity (e.g. the aminoglycoside antibiotics) and relatively frequent use in MG, the deleterious effects become easily apparent. Drugs with weaker effects or infrequent use in MG are identified through rare single case reports (Table 33.2). This poses a problem because it is not always clear from such reports that the drug is the sole causative factor. The patient's condition may be unstable, and additional factors, such as infection, may contribute. A possible method for determining that a certain drug, especially one rarely used in MG, is dangerous in this disorder is rechallenge (Kaeser, 1984; Argov et al., 1986; Robberecht et al., 1989). This procedure necessitates the cooperation and consent of the subject and entails ethical problems. At times, however, it is an essential step.

The next step in identifying a hazardous drug was traditionally in vitro testing on a conventional preparation of the neuromuscular junction. Such experiments are important in elucidating the mechanisms of neuromuscular blockade by a drug but cannot always be used as a proof for the drug-induced myasthenic disorder. The validity of the in vitro models to the in vivo situation is questionable for the following reasons. First, higher concentrations of the tested drug are frequently required for in vitro experiments, because normal synapses are less sensitive to drug-blocking effects. This raises the question of whether the observed effect occurs in the lower therapeutic concentration range.

Second, several drugs have been shown to change some characteristics of NMT in these preparations, but this effect does not indicate that they are dangerous in MG (e.g. barbiturates; Proctor and Weakly, 1976). Third, drug effects on the junction in vivo may be mediated via mechanisms that are not operative in the isolated preparation. For instance, citrate anticoagulants used in plasmapheresis impair neuromuscular function by reducing free ionized calcium levels in the serum (and probably the synaptic cleft as well) (Wirguin et al., 1990). Such an effect cannot be identified in an isolated NMJ preparation where low calcium level in the medium is part of the basic technique.

Because of the above considerations, it is our belief that the experimental autoimmune MG (EAMG) animal model should be used to identify possible hazardous drugs clearly when only single clinical observations are available. The neuromuscular synapse of EAMG has a low safety factor, as in human MG, and generalized or indirect effects can be mimicked in the whole animal with in vivo testing. Also, doses can be adjusted to the human range (Argov et al., 1986; Eliashiv et al., 1990; Wirguin et al., 1990). The major disadvantage of EAMG for drug testing is that it is available in only few laboratories.

Mechanisms

Drug-induced myasthenia results from a direct pharmacological NMT-blocking property of the medication. The site of block may be presynaptic, postsynaptic or combined. NMT block may occur only when the safety factor of the neuromuscular junction is lowered either by another disorder or by the medication itself (e.g. hypocalcaemia induced by citrate anticoagulants) or when serum level of the drug is unduly high (e.g. in renal insufficiency) (Lindesmith et al., 1968; Pittinger et al., 1970). A completely different mechanism occurs in immune-mediated drug-induced myasthenia, when drugs impair the immunological system causing a disorder of the neuromuscular junction similar to idiopathic MG (Table 33.2) (Mastaglia and Argov, 1982; Penn et al., 1998).

Presynaptic block
The motor nerve action potential opens calcium channels and increases calcium entry into the presynaptic nerve terminal, resulting in higher probability of acetylcholine vesicle discharge. The amplitude and duration of this action potential determine the magnitude of transmitter release. Several drugs may reduce evoked transmitter release by interfering with these presynaptic processes (Table 33.2). This may be the result of a local anaesthetic-like action of a drug, which reduces the amplitude of the

invading nerve action potential (Argov and Yaari, 1979). Another possible presynaptic action is blocking of calcium channels directly. This is probably the mechanism of aggravation of MG (Howard, 1990) and for the occurrence of the Lambert–Eaton myasthenic syndrome with verapamil (Krendel and Hopkins, 1986). Both the interference with calcium entry and the local anaesthetic action lead to reduction in the quantal content of the evoked transmitter release, which can be demonstrated in an isolated neuromuscular preparation.

Postsynaptic action

A number of drugs block NMT postsynaptically (Table 33.2). This may occur by direct interference with acetylcholine binding to its receptor (a 'curariform' block) or by blocking ionic conductance across the muscle endplate membrane. A good clinical response to acetylcholinesterase inhibitors (edrophonium or neostigmine) strongly indicates a postsynaptic action in the offending medication (Sokoll and Gergis, 1981). However, this is not sufficient proof of mechanism and additional studies in an isolated neuromuscular synapse preparation are necessary.

Combined pre- and postsynaptic action

Many agents implicated in drug-induced myasthenia posses both pre- and postsynaptic inhibitory effects (Table 33.2). This combined action is typical to a group of drugs with 'membrane stabilizing' action (Argov and Mastaglia, 1979). In several of these drugs, the presynaptic block was shown to be calcium related (most probably interfering with calcium entry into nerve terminals) and the postsynaptic action was curariform.

Immune-mediated block

Immune-mediated block is typical of D-penicillamine but was also suggested in a few cases of other drug-induced disorders of the neuromuscular junction (Table 33.2). The clinical syndrome and the laboratory data D-penicillamine, are very similar to idiopathic MG with the presence of antibodies to the acetylcholine receptor. Induction of myasthenia by DPA occurs only after prolonged treatment (Bucknall, 1977), supporting the notion that this is not a pharmacological block. The fact that D-penicillamine-related myasthenia is drug induced is primarily supported by the observation of spontaneous recovery within few months after drug withdrawal and disappearance of the antibodies to the acetylcholine receptor. Spontaneous recovery without immunosuppressive therapy is rare in idiopathic MG but occurs in approximately two-thirds of these myasthenic patients after stoppage of D-penicillamine (Bucknall, 1977; Kuncl et al., 1986). The

remainder of these patients requires steroid therapy, usually for a brief period only. Attempts to produce the myasthenia in animals given only DPA have failed. However, chronic treatment with DPA made mice more susceptible to the induction of EAMG (Penn et al., 1998). The fact that this side effect is much more common when DPA is given in disorders with presumed autoimmune pathogenesis, like rheumatoid arthritis (Bucknall, 1977), biliary cirrhosis (Marcus et al., 1984), and systemic sclerosis (Steen et al., 1986), but was seen in only two patients with Wilson disease (Czlonskowska, 1975) suggests a basic immunological susceptibility. Supporting this is the finding of increased frequency of specific histocompatability antigen types related to idiopathic MG in patients with DPA-induced MG (Penn et al., 1998). Other studies, however, did not find the increased presence of DR3 (typical to idiopathic MG; Pirskanen, 1976) in DPA-related myasthenia. In DPA-induced MG in patients with rheumatoid arthritis, DR1 frequency was increased (Garlepp et al., 1983); in those with systemic sclerosis, DR5 rate was higher than controls (Steen et al., 1986).

DPA administration triggers immune responses to itself in addition to triggering response to the acetylcholine receptor (Penn et al., 1998). It was shown that DPA binds to the receptor and possibly changes its antigenic characteristics (Bever et al., 1982; Penn et al., 1998), suggesting a basis for the autoimmune reaction. It is also possible that D-penicillamine activates a B cell line to produce antibodies to the acetylcholine receptor (Fawcett et al., 1982). Another possible mechanism is impairment of the equilibrium between helper and suppressor T cells. This may explain the co-occurrence of other iatrogenic autoimmune disorders in DPA-treated patients, namely pemphigus, myositis, lupus erythematosus, Goodpasture syndrome and thyroiditis (Mastaglia and Argov, 1982; Howard, 1990; Penn et al., 1998).

A further immune mechanism for drug-induced MG is indicated by reports of a group of eight patients who were treated with interferon-α; seven developed MG de novo and one showed aggravation of pre-existing MG (Batocchi et al., 1995; Bora et al., 1996; Rohde et al., 1996; Uyama et al., 1996). This immunomudulator affects probably both major histocompatibility complex (MHC) class II and class I antigens and this may be related to the emergence of MG in the above patients, through disturbance of the normal cytokine network balance (Batocchi et al., 1995). In all patients, prolonged (months) exposure to interferon-α was reported and full recovery occurred after withdrawal of the agent. Although interferon-α was effective treatment for EAMG (Shenoy et al., 1995), it may be hazardous in humans, as is any other immunomudulator that can change the immune regulation status in vivo.

Management

As in any drug-induced disease, recognition and withdrawal of the suspected agent is the most important step in the patient's management. In mild disease, this approach suffices and the drug-related signs will rapidly resolve. In penicillamine-induced myasthenia, where recovery may take a few months, addition of pyridostigmine is necessary in many patients. A few patients may develop a severe disease that will require immunosuppressive therapy. Since in many of these patients the myasthenia is short-lasting, plasmapheresis theoretically has potential value.

In acute severe myasthenia, maintenance of respiratory function is essential. Although the pharmacological block resolves within hours to days, shortening the respirator time is a goal. This can be achieved by agents that counteract the neuromuscular block induced by the offending drug. Positive response to edrophonium should be followed by neostigmine (1.0–2.5 mg intramuscular). It should be repeated every 4 hours if the edrophonium test remains positive. As combined block is common in drug-induced myasthenia, calcium infusions (1 ampoule of calcium 10% given slowly) should be administered with the acetylcholinesterase inhibitors, especially if the offending drug is clearly identified and known to have a presynaptic action. The aminopyridines can also be considered if the edrophonium test shows no improvement or if there is worsening of signs in a patient with prolonged drug-induced myasthenic syndrome. Once myasthenia resolves or improves to baseline these additional drugs can be discontinued. However, the patient should be further monitored to avoid 'recurarization'.

Avoidance of a possible drug complication in myasthenics requires special consideration in two clinical situations: infection and elective operations. Myasthenic patients are prone to infection, mainly respiratory, for two major reasons: reduced respiratory muscles function and immunosuppressive treatment. It is essential to achieve early control of infection as it can aggravate the myasthenic condition and lead to myasthenic crisis. However, numerous antibiotics are known to impair NMT. If an ambulatory myasthenic patient needs antibiotics, it is mandatory to choose a 'safe' drug. To date, there are no reports of deterioration in myasthenia with combined sulphamethoxazole (sulfametoxazole)–trimethoprim (co-trimoxazole) preparations or with chloramphenicol and we consider these 'safe' for treatment of infection in ambulatory myasthenics. Penicillins should not be regarded as safe in all patients, although they are probably safe in most. Newer antibiotics that have not passed the time trial in myasthenia should not be regarded as safe even if no reports of drug-induced MG exist. When in doubt or in need of use of an antibiotic that is listed as hazardous, close monitoring is essential. We prefer to hospitalize such patients, as deterioration may be acute with rapid respiratory decompensation. In-hospital infection, especially in patients with a severe disorder, should be treated by the most suitable antibiotic according to bacterial sensitivity tests. However, avoidance of aminoglycosides should be attempted as these are the drugs with the strongest neuromuscular-blocking properties.

Myasthenic patients may require surgery, and a safe choice of anaesthetics is needed. Several anaesthetic agents have been shown to impair NMT in vitro (Howard, 1990) or aggravate the electrical decrement in patients (Nilsson et al., 1989). Pretreatment of myasthenic patients with plasmapheresis, especially before thymectomy, has reduced the rate of postoperative respiratory complications, but the risk remains. In one review, isoflurane and nitrous oxide were recommended (Howard, 1990); however, it has been shown that isoflurane has twice the blocking properties compared with halothane (Nilsson and Muller, 1990). Consequently, halothane may still be the best choice. HLA-B8 was reported to be associated with increased risk of anaesthetic-induced neuromuscular blockade in patients with antibodies to the acetylcholine receptor (Howard, 1990). Monitoring of the state of the neuromuscular junction by the 'train of four' method has long been practised by anaesthesiologists and is recommended for every patient with MG during surgery and in the early postoperative period. Whenever possible, muscle relaxants should be avoided in myasthenia, especially the curariform agents. There is a clear need for a controlled study on the best anaesthetic approach in myasthenia, as many of the above recommendations are based on studies of a single agent without comparisons with other drugs.

Specific Drugs

All drugs implicated in humans as causing or aggravating MG and Lambert–Eaton myasthenic syndrome or impairing NMT are reviewed in Table 33.2. The mechanisms are mentioned, when known although for many a clear understanding of the drug's mechanism has not been established.

Acknowledgements

This work was supported by the Office of Research and Development, Medical Research Service of the Department of Veterans Affairs (R. L. R., H. J. K.). Dr Kaminski is also supported by National Institutes of Health grant EY-11998.

References

Anagnos, A., Ruff, R. L. and Kaminski, H. J. (1997). Endocrine neuromyopathies. *Neurol. Clin.* **15**, 673–696.

Argov, Z. and Mastaglia, F. L. (1979). Disorders of neuromuscular transmission caused by drugs. *N. Eng. J. Med.* **301**, 409–413.

Argov, Z. and Mastaglia, F. L. (1994). Drug-induced neuromuscular disorders. In: *Disorders of Voluntary Muscle*, ed. J. Walton, G. Karpati, and D. Hilton-Jones, pp. 989–1029. Edinburgh: Churchill Livingstone.

Argov, Z. and Yaari, Y. (1979). The action of chlorpromazine at an isolated cholinergic synapse. *Brain Res.* **164**, 227–236.

Argov, Z., Brenner, T. and Abramsky, O. (1986). Ampicillin may aggravate clinical and experimental myasthenia gravis. *Arch. Neurol.* **43**, 255–227.

Batchelor, T. T., Taylor, L. P., Thaler, H. T., Posner, J. B. and DeAngelis, L. M. (1997). Steroid myopathy in cancer patients. *Neurology* **48**, 1234–1238.

Batocchi, A. P., Evoli, A., Servidei, S., Palmisani, M. T., Apollo, F. and Tonali, P. (1995). Myasthenia gravis during interferon alpha therapy. *Neurology* **45**, 382–383.

Bever, C. T., Chang, H. W., Penn, A. S., Jaffe, I. A. and Bock, E. (1982). Penicillamine-induced myasthenia gravis: Effects of penicillamine on acetylcholine receptor. *Neurology* **32**, 1077–1082.

Bora, I., Karli, N., Bakar, M., Zarifoglu, M., Turan, F. and Ogul, E. (1996). Myasthenia gravis following IFN-alpha-2a treatment. *Eur. Neurol.* **38**, 68.

Bucknall, R. C. (1977). Myasthenia associated with D-penicillamine therapy in rheumatoid arthritis. *Proc. Roy. Soc. Med.* **70**, 114–117.

Campellone, J. V., Lacomis, D., Kramer, D. J., van Cott, A. C. and Giuliani, M. J. (1998). Acute myopathy after liver transplantation. *Neurology* **50**, 46–53.

Clauw, D., Nashel, D., Umhau, A. and Katz, P. (1990). Tryptophan-associated eosinophilic connective-tissue disease. *J. Am. Med. Ass.* **263**, 1502–1506.

Czlonskowska, A. (1975). Myasthenia syndrome during penicillamine treatment. *Brit. Med. J.* **2**, 600–602.

Eliashiv, S., Wirguin, I., Brenner, T. and Argov Z. (1990). Aggravation of human and experimental myasthenia gravis by contrast media. *Neurology* **40**, 1623–1625.

Emslie-Smith, A., Mayeno, A., Nakano, S., Gleich, G. and Engel, A. G. (1994). 1,1′-Ethylidenebis[tryptophan] induces pathologic alterations in muscle similar to those observed in the eosinophilia-myalgia syndrome. *Neurology* **44**, 2390–2392.

Fawcett, P. R. W., McLachlan, S. M., Nicolson, L., Argov, Z. and Mastaglia, F. L. (1982). D-Penicillamine associated myasthenia gravis: immunological and electrophysiological studies. *Muscle Nerve* **5**, 328–334.

Finsterer, J., Hess, B., Jarius, C., Stöllberger, C., Budka, H. and Mamoli, B. (1998). Malnutrition-induced hypokalemic myopathy in chronic alcoholism. *Clin. Toxicol.* **36**, 369–373.

Garlepp, M. J., Dawkins, R. L. and Christiansen, F. T. (1983). HLA antigens and acetylcholine receptor antibodies in penicillamine induced myasthenia gravis. *Br. Med. J.* **286**, 338–340.

George, K. K. and Pourmand, R. (1997). Toxic myopathies. *Neurol. Clin.* **15**, 711–730.

Giordano, N., Sensi, M., Mattii, G., Battisti, E., Villanova, M. and Gennari, C. (1997). Polymyositis associated with simvastatin. *Lancet* **349**, 1600–1601.

Gutmann, L., Blumenthal, D., Gutmann, L. and Schochet, S. S. (1996). Acute type II myofiber atrophy in critical illness. *Neurology* **46**, 819–821.

Howard, J. F. Jr (1990). Adverse drug effects on neuromuscular transmission. *Semin. Neurol.* **10**, 89–102.

Kaeser, H. E. (1984). Drug-induced myasthenic syndromes. *Acta Neurolog. Scand.* **70**, 39–47.

Kaminski, H. J. and Ruff, R. L. (1994). Endocrine myopathies (hyper- and hypofunction of adrenal, thyroid, pituitary, and parathyroid glands) and iatrogenic corticosteroid myopathy. In *Myology*, eds. A. Engel and C. Franzini-Armstrong, pp. 1726–1753. New York: McGraw-Hill.

Kaufman, L., Gruber, B. and Gregersen, P. (1991). Clinical follow-up and immunogenetic studies of 32 patients with eosinophilia-myalgia syndrome. *Lancet* **337**, 1071–1074.

Koren, W., Koren, E., Nacasch, N., Ehrenfeld, M. and Gur, H. (1998). Rhabdomyolysis associated with clozapine treatment in a patient with decreased calcium-dependent potassium permeability of cell membranes. *Clin. Neuropharmacol.* **21**, 262–264.

Krendel, D. A. and Hopkins, L. G. (1986). Adverse effect of verapamil in a patient with the Lambert–Eaton Syndrome. *Muscle Nerve* **9**, 519–522.

Kuncl, R. W., Pestronk, A., Drachman, D. and Rechthland, E. (1986). The pathophysiology of penicillamine-induced myasthenia gravis. *Ann. Neurology* **20**, 740–744.

Lacomis, D., Giuliani, M. J., van Cott, A. and Kramer, D. J. (1996). Acute myopathy of intensive care: clinical, electromyographic, and pathological aspects. *Ann. Neurol.* **40**, 645–654.

Lindesmith, L. A., Banes, R. D., Bigelow, D. B. and Petty, T. L. (1968). Reversible respiratory paralysis associated with polymyxin therapy. *Ann. Intern. Med.* **68**, 318–327.

Marcus, S. N., Chadwick, D. and Walker, R. J. (1984). D-penicillamine-induced myasthenia gravis in primary biliary cirrhosis. *Gastroenterol.* **86**, 166–168.

Mastaglia, F. L. (1992). Toxic myopathies. In: *Myopathies*, eds. L. P. Rowland and S. DiMauro, pp. 595–622. New York: Elsevier.

Mastaglia, F. L. and Argov, Z. (1982). Immunologically-mediated drug-induced neuromuscular disorders. In: *Pseudo Allergic Reactions: Involvement of Drugs and Chemicals*, vol. 3, ed. H. D. Schlumerger, Basel: Karger.

Nakahara, K., Kuriyama, M., Sonoda, Y. et al. (1998). Myopathy induced by HMG-CoA reductase inhibitors in rabbits: A pathological, electrophysiological, and biochemical study. *Toxicol. Appl. Pharmacol.* **152**, 99–106.

Nilsson, E. and Muller, K. (1990). Neuromuscular effects of isoflurane in patients with myasthenia gravis. *Acta Anaesthesiol. Scand.* **34**, 126–131.

Nilsson, E., Paloheimo, M., Muller, K. and Heinonen, J. (1989). Halothane-induced variability in the neuromuscular transmission of patients with myasthenia gravis. *Acta Anaesthesiol. Scand.* **33**, 395–401.

Penn, A. S., Low, B. W., Jaffe, I., Luo, L. and Jacques, J. J. (1998). Drug-induced autoimmune myasthenia gravis. *Ann. N.Y. Acad. Sci.* **841**, 433–449.

Pirskanen, R. (1976). On the significance of HL-A and LD antigens in myasthenia gravis. *Ann. N.Y. Acad. Sci.* **274**, 451–460.

Pittinger, C. B., Eryasa, Y. and Adamson, R. (1970). Antibiotic-induced paralysis. *Anesthes. Analges.* **49**, 487–501.

Proctor, W. R. and Weakly, J. N. (1976). A comparison of the presynaptic and post-synaptic actions of pentobarbitone and phenobarbitone in the neuromuscular junction of the frog. *J. Physiol.* **258**, 257–268.

Rich, M., Teener, J., Raps, E., Schotland, D. and Bird, S. (1996). Muscle is electrically inexcitable in acute quadraplegic myopathy. *Neurology* **46**, 731–736.

Rich, M. M., Pinter, M. J., Kraner, S. D. and Barchi, R. L. (1998). Loss of electrical excitability in an animal model of acute quadriplegic myopathy. *Ann. Neurol.* **43**, 171–180.

Robberecht, W., Bednarik, J., Bourgeois, P., van Hess, H. and Carton, H. (1989). Myasthenic syndrome caused by direct effect of chloroquine on neuromuscular junction. *Arch. Neurol.* **46**, 464–468.

Rohde, D., Sliwka, U., Schweizer, K. and Jaske, G. (1996). Oculobulbar myasthenia gravis induced by cytokine treatment of a patient with metastasized renal cell carcinoma. *Eur. J. Clin. Pharmacol.* **50**, 471–473.

Ruff, R. L. (1996). Acute illness myopathy. *Neurology* **46**, 600–601.

Ruff, R. L. (1998). Why do ICU patients become paralyzed? *Ann. Neurol.* **43**, 154–155.

Scelsa, S. N., Simpson, D. M., McQuistion, H. L., Fineman, A., Ault, K. and Reichler, B. (1996). Clozapine-induced myotoxicity in patients with chronic psychotic disorders. *Neurology* **47**, 1518–1532.

Schmassmann-Suhijar, D., Bullingham, R., Gasser, R., Schmutz, J., and Haefeli, W. E. (1998). Rhabdomyolysis due to interaction of simvastatin with mibefradil. *Lancet* **351**, 1929–1930.

Shenoy, M., Baron, S., Wu, B., Goluszko, E. and Christadoss, P. (1995). IFN-a treatment suppresses the development of experimental autoimmune myasthenia gravis. *J. Immunol.* **154**, 6203–6208.

Sokoll, M. D. and Gergis, S. D. (1981). Antibiotics and neuromuscular function. *Anesthiology* **55**, 148–155.

Steen, V. D., Blair, S. and Medsger, T. A. Jr (1986). The toxicity of D-penicillamine in systemic sclerosis. *Ann. Intern. Med.* **104**, 699–705.

Sun, D. Y., Edgar, M. and Rubin, M. (1997). Hemiparetic acute myopathy of intensive care progressing to triplegia. *Arch. Neurol.* **54**, 1420–1422.

Sundelin, K. and Norrsell, K. (1997). Enlargement of extraocular muscles during treatment. *Acta Ophthalmol. Scand.* **75**, 333–334.

Tobert, J. A. (1988). Efficacy and long-term adverse effect pattern of lovastatin. *Am. J. Cardiol.* **62**, 28–34.

Uyama, E., Fujiki, N. and Uchino, M. (1996). Exacerbation of myasthenia gravis during interferon-a treatment. *J. Neurol. Sci.* **144**, 221–222.

Victor, M. and Sieb, J. P. (1994). Myopathies due to drugs, toxins, and nutritional deficiency. In: *Myology*, eds. A. G. Engel and C. Franzini-Armstrong, pp. 1697–1725. New York: McGraw-Hill.

Wirguin, I., Brenner, T., Shinar E., Argov, Z. (1990). Citrate-induced impairment of neuromuscular transmission in human and experimental autoimmune myasthenia gravis. *Ann. Neurol.* **27**, 328–330.

Zaidat, O., Ruff, R. L. and Kaminski, H. J. (1999). Endocrine and toxic myopathies. In *Muscle Diseases*, eds. A. Schapira and R. Griggs, M. A., p. 363. Woburn, Butterworth Heinemann.

34

Painful muscle syndromes

Russell Lane

Introduction

Muscle pain is one of the most common neuromuscular symptoms. It may result from disease or altered physiology in muscle (*primary* muscle pain) but it can also result from disease or dysfunction of peripheral nerves or nerve roots in which nerve fibres serving muscle nocioceptors are involved or from central nervous system (CNS) disorders that cause increase in muscle tone, such as spasticity, dystonia, parkinsonian rigidity, tetanus or stiff-man syndrome. In addition, pain resulting from disease of bones, joints and other connective tissues, and the viscera, may be referred to muscle. The quality of muscle pain and the factors that tend to aggravate and relieve it may help to determine its origin.

Primary muscle pain that is fairly persistent may be described as a deep aching or a feeling of tenseness, pressure or soreness and may be associated with tenderness on palpation, while myalgia associated with or following exertion is often described as a stiffness and may indeed be accompanied by a restriction in range of movement. Intermittent or paroxysmal muscle pain is usually described as a spasm, cramp or 'charley horse'. In any case, muscle pain may be focal or diffuse. By contrast, joint pain tends to be focal or multifocal and is exacerbated by joint movement, although it may be referred to a site remote from the pathology, such as the thigh muscles in hip disease. Joint disease may also be associated with painful reflex muscle spasm, as in cervical whiplash injuries. Bone pain tends to have a deep, boring, continuous quality, usually unaffected by joint movement, and it is often worse at night.

Pathogenesis of primary muscle pain

Muscle nocioceptors

Primary muscle pain can occur in normal individuals under predictable circumstances and in many disease states. The precise factors that determine the quality and magnitude of primary muscle pain are not fully understood. Nocioception in muscle appears to be mediated by thinly myelinated Aδ fibres and unmyelinated C fibres, the unencapsulated, multiple branched endings of which are distributed through the endomysium and other connective tissues, particularly in the regions of tendon insertions, fasciae and aponeuroses. By contrast, fibres subserving encapsulated Golgi tendon organs and muscle spindles do not transmit pain. Nocioceptors respond to mechanical and chemical stimuli; some appear to be unimodal, others polymodal. The most significant responses are induced by bradykinin, serotonin, histamine, potassium and hydrogen ions. Chemical stimuli result in slow-onset, chronic responses while mechanical stimuli tend to produce brief, rapid-onset pain (Mills et al., 1985).

Processes causing muscle pain

General processes involved in the pathogenesis of muscle pain are shown in Table 34.1.

Mechanical and chemical factors
Predictably, muscle pain results from processes that generate noxious chemical mediators, for example inflammatory myopathies and disorders of muscle metabolism, or that cause an increase in intramuscular pressure and stretching of connective tissues, such as muscle haematoma or infarction, cramp and contracture. By contrast, necrotic and degenerative processes affecting the myofibres per se, such

Table 34.1. Pathogenesis of muscle pain: General mechanisms and examples

Mechanisms	Examples
Mechanical factors	Excessive tension (e.g. cramps, contractures, reflex muscle spasm, hypertonia)
	Eccentric contraction
	Muscle haematoma
Muscle inflammation	Acute polymyositis
	Interstitial inflammation (e.g. myofasciitis)
Metabolic disorders	Disorders of intermediary muscle metabolism
Muscle ischaemia	Claudication, compartment syndromes, exercise-induced muscle ischaemia
	Muscle infarction

as dystrophies, are rarely associated with myalgia, even when the pathology is severe (Mills et al., 1985; Marchettini, 1993). Although there are some notable exceptions to this. It is well known that exertional myalgia may be the only notable symptom in dystrophinopathy and muscle pain may be a presenting feature in Becker dystrophy. Myalgia can also be a significant problem in some patients with facioscapulohumeral muscular dystrophy, but there is no relationship between myalgia and the extent of muscle pathology (Bushby et al., 1999)

Muscle pain may also result from sarcomeric disruption produced by *eccentric* muscle contraction. This type of muscle contraction is metabolically more efficient than concentric contraction but causes much more postexercise myalgia (Newham et al., 1983a). Myalgia from eccentric muscle contraction differs from mechanical pain resulting from muscle swelling or stretching, in that pain and tenderness develop progressively over the 24–72 hours after exercise and are associated with an increase in serum creatine kinase (CK) levels, which can reach tens of thousands of units if responses are followed for up to 5 days (Newham et al., 1983a). This is associated with a reduction in strength, which recovers over several days (Friden, 1984). Both Newham et al. (1983b) and Friden (1984) reported significant ultrastructural changes, including marked Z line disruption and streaming and disruption of myofibrillary architecture, in muscles that had contracted eccentrically during exercise, but not in muscles which had contracted concentrically. Friden (1984) reported that these changes could be seen immediately after exercise, indicating that they are a direct result of traumatic distrac-

tion. However, secondary changes including intracellular oedema, mitochondrial swelling and lysosomal activation with the generation of excess lipofuscin granules often followed (Friden, 1984). Leakage of muscle proteins such as CK presumably occurs through submicroscopic lesions in the sarcolemma; no surface membrane disruption could be seen on electron microscopy (Newham et al., 1983b; Friden, 1984). Support for the concept of early traumatic muscle lesions induced by eccentric exercise followed by a reactive inflammatory response comes from changes observed in acute-phase reactants that accompany the increases in serum CK and the development of muscle pain. Gleeson et al. (1995) reported that muscle pain was maximal two days after eccentric contraction; serum CK levels peaked one to seven days after exercise and C-reactive protein peaked 1–11 days after exercise. Total leukocyte count, neutrophils, monocytes and basophils fell to 15–20% below preexercise levels, with falls in iron, zinc, albumin and immunoglobulins G and M; lymphocytes, eosinophils and platelets were unchanged. These observations were interpreted as evidence of a rapid, acute-phase inflammatory response initiated within one day of exercise but without further marked changes despite muscle fibre necrosis. In keeping with this, another study showed that prostaglandin E_2 levels, which might have been expected to rise as a result of muscle membrane damage, did not change following eccentric or concentric contraction exercise (Croisier et al., 1996).

The myalgia caused by eccentric contraction damage does not seem to respond to treatment with anti-inflammatory analgesics, such as salicylates, but Giamberardino et al. (1996) showed that prior administration of L-carnitine significantly reduced pain, tenderness and CK release compared with placebo, possibly through its vasodilator properties, which might promote wash-out of allogenic metabolites.

Ischaemia

In addition to myalgia resulting from disease processes affecting muscle connective tissues, skeletal and cardiac muscle pain can also be induced by ischaemia. Familiar examples include angina and the intermittent claudication of the leg muscles owing to occlusive vascular disease, and jaw claudication in cranial arteritis. Ischaemic muscle pain is also a common experience in normal subjects as a result of high intensity work, such as forearm pain while carrying a heavy suitcase. The pathogenesis of ischaemic muscle pain is also unclear. It does not seem to result from ischaemic hypoxia, since postexercise pain is not worsened if ischaemia is maintained by occlusion of blood supply to a muscle, and it is not augmented by ischaemia prior to exercise (Mills et al., 1985). However, the pain is rapidly relieved by restoration of the blood supply, suggesting that effector molecules of low molecular weight might mediate the pain. For example, adenosine is produced in abundance in ischaemic muscle and can induce ischaemia-like pain after intra-arterial injection (Sylven et al., 1988). In a controlled clinical trial, caffeine, a nonselective adenosine receptor antagonist, was shown to exhibit considerable analgesic effects in ischaemic myalgia (Myers et al., 1997).

Experimental studies of muscle pain in humans

The investigation of the origins of muscle pain in humans began with the observations of Lewis (1932). He noted that pain reminiscent of ischaemic myalgia could be induced by injection of a variety of substances into muscle. These observations were extended by Kellgren (1937/38, 1939), who injected saline solutions into muscle or fascia while cutaneous receptors were blocked by local anaesthetic. He noted that localization of pain was less accurate when saline was injected into muscle compared with into fascia, and that pain became progressively more diffuse as the intensity increased: the greater the pain intensity, the less accurate the localization. He also noted that the radiation of pain did not follow dermatomes or radicular territories. Hockaday and Whitty (1967) showed that the referred pain could be abolished by blocking either the site of injection or the site of referral. Later studies compared the characteristics of cutaneous and muscle pain (Torebjork et al., 1984). Cutaneous nerve stimulation caused tingling, pins and needles and burning, while stimulation of muscle–nerve fascicles caused deep pain with cramp-like qualities. As the stimulus was increased, muscle pain was experienced in areas beyond the distribution of the stimulated nerve. As a generalization, cutaneous pain remains confined to the distribution of the stimulated nerve while muscle pain is referred more widely as intensity increases. These observations have clinical significance. For example, carpal tunnel syndrome can present with proximal deep pain in the upper limb (Golding, 1968; Kummel and Zazanis, 1973) and ulnar nerve compression at the elbow can cause deep pain in the ipsilateral scapular region (Marchettini, 1993). Deep pain characteristic of myalgia can also result from nerve root compression and in the thoracic region can simulate angina (Lindahl and Hamberg, 1981). Finally, any polyneuropathy that affects small myelinated or unmyelinated fibres subserving muscle nociception can produce deep muscle pain in addition to any typical superficial cutaneous pain symptoms.

Study of the saline infusion model of muscle pain has continued. In a series of reports, Graven-Nielsen and colleagues compared infusions of isotonic and hypertonic saline into tibialis anterior. They noted that pain was significantly greater with hypertonic saline than isotonic saline. The size of the saline pool produced at the infusion site in the muscle, and the resulting increase in intramuscular pressure, did not differ, but microdialysis probes demonstrated that increases in intramuscular sodium and potassium, and to some extent magnesium, were significantly greater with the hypertonic saline, suggesting that ionic mediators might be important in pain genesis in this model (Graven-Nielsen et al., 1997a). They also demonstrated temporal and spatial summation of nociceptive inputs from injured muscle, which facilitate pain responses in areas of referred pain (Arendt-Nielsen et al., 1997; Graven-Nielsen et al., 1997b). Myalgia caused by hypertonic saline infusion into tibialis anterior was shown to be associated with an increase in stretch reflexes but without an increase in H-reflex amplitude. It was suggested that this might be a result of an increase in muscle spindle sensitivity caused by a centrally mediated increase in gamma motor neuron efferent activity (Matre et al., 1998). A comparison of the intensity of pain from muscle produced by intramuscular electrical stimulation with cutaneous pain induced by a carbon dioxide laser demonstrated that, while both skin and muscle pain showed increasing but decelerating stimulus–response curves, muscle pain was consistently rated as more unpleasant (Svensson et al., 1997). This indicates that the central nociceptive processing determining sensitivity is similar for skin and muscle but muscle pain is relatively more intense as it is mediated by a greater activation of afferent inputs.

The sensitivity of nociceptors in skeletal muscle can be increased by substances released by pathological processes, including exercise-induced trauma. This may have relevance to the understanding of fibromyalgia (see below). Dorsal horn neurons that process inputs may develop wider or more numerous receptive fields, resulting in the spread and wider referral of deep muscle pain (Mense, 1991).

In summary, observations to date confirm Lewis's original conclusions. Muscle pain is a single discrete sensory entity in which spatial and/or temporal summation progressively modifies the intensity and location of the perception. The perceived change in quality of myalgia, from 'soreness' to 'tension' to 'cramp', reflecting increasing pain severity, simply relates to the intensity of nociceptive stimulation.

Chemical allogens

Much research has focused on attempting to define the principal chemical mediators of muscle pain. The determination of such factors would clearly have therapeutic implications. However, it seems likely that many substances generated during muscle metabolism and disease processes have the potential to stimulate muscle nociceptors and, as Lewis stated so long ago, the quality of pain evoked from somatic stuctures depends more on the structures stimulated than the nature of the stimulus. Some allogens, such as bradykinin, serotonin, histamine, potassium and hydrogen ions and adenosine have already been mentioned. The importance of hydrogen ions in the production of muscle pain was demonstrated in an experiment in which myalgia caused by ischaemia was compared with that induced by an infusion of acid phosphate buffer (pH 5.2) (Issberner et al., 1996). During ischaemic muscle contraction, muscle pain increased linearly as the pH in the region of the working muscles fell. Qualitatively similar deep muscle pain was induced with acid phosphate buffer infusion, with a similar linear correlation following a lag phase. However, on restoring circulation, pH rose more slowly than the decrease in muscle pain. This suggests that proton accumulation is an important mediator of muscle pain but the mechanisms involved are not simple. Furthermore, muscle pain is a feature of McArdle's disease and phosphofructokinase (PFK) deficiency, in which lactate and hydrogen ion production is minimal (Mills et al., 1985).

Exertional myalgia in normal subjects

Muscle pain related to exercise is a subject of particular interest in sports medicine, and studies of normal subjects have taught us much about muscle pain mechanisms in disease states. Two important processes in this regard, ischaemia and muscle fibre trauma from eccentric contraction, have already been discussed.

Muscle pain during exercise can be reliably assessed using a simple pain scale (Cook et al., 1997). Studies on normal volunteers using a cycle ergometer showed that pain threshold for the legs was reached at about 50% of maximal exercise capacity; pain perception then accelerated, becoming maximal at exhaustion. Hamilton et al. (1996) examined the relationship between work output and exercise-related sensations (leg effort, muscle tension, muscle discomfort, muscle pain and breathing discomfort, as assessed using a Borg category-ratio scale) in a bicycle ergometer test. Normal subjects exercised at between 20 and 120% of the 'maximal' work capacity achieved in a prior incremental exercise test to exhaustion. A hierarchy of perception thresholds was observed. Leg effort and muscle tension were first noticed at about one-third of maximal capacity, muscle and breathing discomfort at about 50% capacity, and muscle pain at about 60%. However, the intensity of other sensations then exceeded muscle pain and breathing discomfort at higher work rates. This suggests that muscle pain perception during muscular work is distinct and has possibly different origins from sensations of effort, muscle tension and muscular 'discomfort'.

Muscle pain as a symptom: muscle pain syndromes

Primary myalgia can be diffuse or focal, relatively persistent or paroxysmal, and exclusively exertional or exacerbated (or rarely alleviated) by exercise (Table 34.2). Paroxysmal muscle pain, usually described as 'cramp', is classified separately and must be distinguished from muscle contracture. Muscle pain is also a feature of certain defined neuromuscular disorders and syndromes. These conditions will be considered only in relation to their muscle pain component and the reader is referred to appropriate chapters in this volume for more detailed descriptions of the respective diseases.

Focal muscle pain

The causes of focal muscle pain can be classified in relation to whether muscle swelling is present or not. Swelling or induration associated with focal muscle pain can result from infections such as 'tropical' and 'nontropical' pyomyositis, haematoma formation, muscle infarction (e.g. in compartment syndromes) and idiopathic inflammatory and granulomatous disorders such as focal nodular myositis and sarcoidosis. Focal muscle pain with swelling can also result from toxic muscle injury, as in certain drug-induced myopathies and acute alcoholic myopathy.

Focal myalgia without swelling is most commonly the result of disease in other systems and tissues, such as nerve root irritation in disc prolapse, vascular disease resulting in intermittent claudication, and peripheral nerve diseases, for example restless legs syndrome or Spillane's syndrome of 'painful legs and moving toes' (Spillane et al., 1971).

Bacterial infections: tropical and nontropical pyomyositis
Bacterial infection of muscle produces a focal abscess or multiple abscesses but is usually preceded by a prodrome of fever, nonspecific malaise and more generalized

Table 34.2. Classification of muscle pain

Type of muscle pain	Causes
Focal muscle pain	
With swelling or induration	Haematoma, infarction, pyomyositis, nodular myositis, sarcoidosis, drugs, alcohol
Without swelling	Claudication, neurogenic disorders (e.g. brachial plexus neuritis), 'painful legs and moving toes syndrome'
Diffuse muscle pain	
With weakness	Inflammatory myopathies, infections (e.g. viruses, *Toxoplasma*), metabolic bone disease
Without weakness	Polymyalgia rheumatica, myofasciitis, fibromyalgia, chronic fatigue syndrome, drugs, alcohol, electrolyte disorders, steroid withdrawal
Paroxysmal muscle pain	
Cramps in normal subjects	Effort cramps (e.g. 'stitch', calf cramps in athletes), rest cramps (especially in the elderly), fluid and electrolyte disorders (e.g. hyponatraemia, hypomagnesaemia), pregnancy, hyperventilation (tetany)
Cramps in neuromuscular diseases	Neurogenic disorders (e.g. motor neuron disease), cramp-fasciculation syndromes, neuromyotonia, Flier's disease, Satoyoshi syndrome, secondary to systemic metabolic disorders (e.g. uraemia, cirrhosis, endocrine disorders)
Contractures	Glycogenolytic and glycolytic disorders, Brody's disease (sarcoplasmic Ca^{2+}-ATPase deficiency), rippling muscle disease
Myotonia	Sodium channelopathies, chloride channelopathies, proximal myotonic myopathy (PROMM)
Exertional myalgia	Glycogenolytic and glycolytic disorders, lipid storage myopathies (carnitine palmityltransferase deficiency), mitochondrial myopathies, myoadenylate deaminase deficiency, exertional muscle pain syndrome (EMPS), dystrophinopathies

myalgia, which may obscure the diagnosis, particularly if predisposing conditions that can themselves be associated with muscle pain are active. Patel et al. (1997) reviewed available literature on the subject and reported a series of 13 patients with nontropical pyomyositis. In 11, preceding or co-morbid conditions, including human immunodeficiency virus infection and trauma, may have predisposed to the condition. *Staphylococcus aureus* was the causative organism in seven patients; two had multiple organisms and no organism could be found in the remaining two. Computed tomographic scanning of muscle proved helpful in guiding muscle biopsy and drainage procedures and 11 patients recovered with intravenous antibiotics.

Muscle infarction

Muscle infarction can result in severe pain, sometimes associated with swelling and rhabdomyolysis. Occlusion of major nutrient arteries, for example as a result of sudden arteriosclerotic occlusion or embolism, can cause haemorrhagic infarction, fibre necrosis and vacuolation (Harriman, 1977). However, arteriosclerosis more often results in chronic ischaemia with neurogenic muscular atrophy, most marked distally (Farinon et al., 1984). Muscle infarction can also complicate arterial disease in diabetes, and several examples of this have been reported (Banker and Chester, 1973; Bjornskov et al., 1995). Haemorrhagic muscle infarcts were demonstrated on magnetic resonance imaging and biopsy in one study and it was suggested that this was the result of a hypercoagulable state together with endothelial damage. Long-term anticoagulation therapy was recommended to prevent recurrences (Bjornskov et al., 1995).

Patients with insulin-dependent diabetes will also sometimes develop severe diffuse muscle pain and tenderness, referred to as diabetic myalgia (Gill et al., 1986). In some, a raised sedimentation rate may suggest a diagnosis of polymyalgia but the symptoms do not respond to steroids. The authors did not comment on the presence or absence of polyneuropathy and it is possible that the muscle pain was of neurogenic origin.

Muscle infarctions can also be found on biopsy in patients with vasculitis, and myalgia may be prominent in polyarteritis and rheumatoid disease for example, but such infarcts are usually small and neurogenic pain usually predominates.

Muscle infarction and fibre necrosis can also occur during sickle cell crises. The resulting secondary fibrosis can produce multifocal atrophy and induration with contractures. Valeriano-Marcet and Kerr (1991) reported four typical patients who suffered recurrent episodes of proximal myalgia and muscle swelling as major features of crises. Muscle biopsies from affected muscles revealed acute myonecrosis with little inflammation, together with marked collagen deposition between fibres.

Diffuse muscle pain

The differential diagnosis of diffuse myalgia is determined by the presence or absence of accompanying weakness. The presence of weakness, particularly if associated with other laboratory evidence of disease such as a raised serum CK level, increases the likelihood that a disease process, such as an inflammatory myopathy, infection or metabolic/endocrine disorder, will be found to be the cause (Mills and Edwards, 1983). Again, drugs and toxins can produce diffuse myalgia, and hypokalaemia caused by drugs or unusual dietary proclivities is of particular importance (Nielsen and Mazzone, 1999).

The development of proximal myalgia in elderly patients is especially challenging because of the wide differential diagnosis. Polymyalgia rheumatica may have atypical features, such as peripheral synovitis, distal extremity pain and mild weakness, and the sedimentation rate may not be increased. If no clear alternative diagnosis is made after careful investigation, which should include muscle biopsy to exclude polymyositis, a therapeutic trial with low-dose steroids is justified (Brooks and McGee, 1997).

Unfortunately, it is much more often the case that a patient presents with diffuse myalgia, not exclusively related to exercise although often worsened by exertion, in the absence of demonstrable weakness. The probability of reaching a specific diagnosis through investigation in such patients is low. Pourmand (1997) reviewed previous studies and reported a retrospective personal series of 100 consecutive patients who underwent muscle biopsy for investigation of myalgia, with normal findings on clinical examination: 25% had elevated serum CK levels and 16.5% had 'myopathic' electromyographs (EMG). A diagnosis was reached in only five: two patients had polymyositis, with raised serum CK and increased erythrocyte sedimentation rate (ESR); two had McArdle's disease, with raised serum CK levels and myopathic EMGs, and one patient had light microscopic and ultrastructural features of a mitochondrial myopathy. About 25% of the other patients had nonspecific changes on biopsy, including increased fibre diameter variability, scattered angulated fibres, moth-eaten fibres and type II fibre atrophy (see also exertional muscle pain syndrome (EMPS), below).

Myofasciitis

Several diseases characterized by inflammatory infiltration of the skin, subcutaneous tissues and often the muscle connective tissues have been described. Diffuse or multifocal myalgia is typical in such patients and is often the presenting feature.

Shulman's syndrome (eosinophilic fasciitis)

Shulman's syndrome usually presents with a short prodromal illness characterized by myalgia, fatigue and arthralgia with low-grade fever, followed by progressive thickening of the subcutaneous tissues and tightening of the skin, resulting in a *peau d'orange* effect (Shulman, 1975). In some patients, muscle may be involved, resulting in polymyositis with weakness and raised serum CK levels (Bjelle et al., 1980). The ESR is increased and an intermittent eosinophilia may be found. Full thickness skin and muscle biopsy shows fascial thickening and infiltration by mononuclear cells, notably eosinophils and macrophages. The condition may remit spontaneously and usually responds to steroids. The cause is unknown but there are similarities between this condition and the eosinophilia-myalgia syndrome induced by contaminated L-tryptophan, chiefly in the USA in 1974 and 1989 (Martin et al., 1990). However, in that disorder, muscle fibre involvement was much less prominent; ESR and serum CK levels were not increased and there was evidence of a peripheral nerve disorder rather than myopathy (Martin et al., 1990; Verity et al., 1991).

Macrophagic myofasciitis

A number of cases of myofasciitis characterized by macrophage infiltration of muscle connective tissues have been reported from France. Gherardi et al. (1998) described 14 patients ascertained through five myopathology centres. Mild to moderate chronic diffuse myalgia was the commonest feature, present in 86% of patients. Arthralgia, particularly affecting large joints, occurred in 64%, and 43% had mild to moderate weakness. Four of the patients had fever. No visible skin changes were noted. About half of the patients had raised serum CK levels and increased ESRs and a third had myopathic EMGs. Muscle biopsy showed infiltration of the subcutaneous tissues, epimysium, perimysium and perifascicular endomysium by sheets of large macrophages with a finely granular periodic acid–Schiff base-positive content. On ultrastructure, the macrophages showed aggregates of dense spicules, some membrane-bound. Subsequent investigation showed that these macrophagic inclusions resulted from deposition of phosphate crystals, from the use of aluminium as an adjuvant in hepatitis vaccines injected intramuscularly. Similar inclusions were induced in rats injected with these vaccines (Coquet et al., 1999). However, this group have since described dermatomyositis characterized by marked macrophagic infiltration of fascia and endothelial tuloreticular inclusions, in which macrophagic aluminium inclusions were not seen except in two patients who showed histological and ultrastructural features of both macrophagic myofasciitis and dermatomyositis (Coquet et al., 2000).

Myalgia with prominent fatigue: fibromyalgia and chronic fatigue syndrome

When fatigue is predominant in patients with myalgia without significant weakness, patients may be found to fulfil operative criteria for a diagnosis of fibromyalgia or chronic fatigue syndrome. While many patients with these conditions also fulfil accepted criteria for recognized psychiatric disorders, there is increasing evidence that the symptoms experienced have 'organic' determinants, and these clinical syndromes are likely to be heterogeneous with regard to aetiology and pathogenesis.

Fibromyalgia

Fibromyalgia is characterized by numerous tender 'trigger points' in muscle. Soernson et al. (1998) recently found that patients with fibromyalgia had significantly lower muscle pressure pain thresholds than normal individuals, even in muscles that were not affected by spontaneous pain or tenderness. By contrast, thresholds for cutaneous pain evoked by electrical stimulation did not differ. Hypertonic saline consistently evoked muscle pain of longer duration and wider distribution in fibromyalgic patients than in controls, and it was concluded that there is a state of central hyperexcitability in the muscle nociceptive system in these patients. This observation is in keeping with an earlier study of isokinetic dynamometry in patients with fibromyalgia, in which muscle relaxation characteristics were observed in patients after performing 100 consecutive shoulder flexions (Elert et al., 1992). The patients demonstrated inability to relax all active muscles between contractions. Patients with work-related trapezius myalgia showed a similar inability to relax that was confined to the affected trapezius muscle. An inability to relax muscle during repetitive movements may, therefore, play an important role in initiating and sustaining muscle pain.

However, it should not be assumed that a diagnosis of fibromyalgia is appropriate, even if recognized criteria for the condition are met. Gotze et al. (1998) recently reported the case of a middle-aged woman who presented to a rheumatology clinic with joint pains and muscle stiffness and was found to have multiple tender points in muscles typical of fibromyalgia. However, she was also noted to have weakness and her son and several close relatives were found to have similar symptoms. Investigation showed that this family had hyperkalaemic periodic paralysis.

Chronic fatigue syndrome

Muscle pain is often a feature in patients with chronic fatigue syndrome, although fatigue is the predominant symptom. A full discussion of this complex illness is outside the scope of this chapter, but there is increasing evidence that it is a heterogeneous condition, and some patients have evidence of defective muscle energy metabolism (Lane et al., 1998a). This does not seem to cause static muscle weakness but presumably affects dynamic function and endurance, and this might be a factor in the delayed recovery after exercise observed in some patients (Paul et al., 1999). The origin of myalgia in chronic fatigue syndrome has not been studied to the same extent as fatigue, and its origins are unclear at present. In one study, increased fibre density on single-fibre EMG and nonspecific biopsy abnormalities of extensor digitorum communis were significantly more common in patients with chronic fatigue in whom myalgia was particularly prominent (Connolly et al., 1993).

Paroxysmal muscle pain: cramp, contracture and myotonia

Cramp

Cramp is a spasmodic, painful, visible or palpable involuntary focal muscle contraction, often accompanied by secondary abnormal posturing of related joints. It can be relieved by stretching the muscle. On EMG, the contracted area exhibits high-frequency motor unit discharges, generally of normal morphology. There is good evidence that cramps are of neurogenic origin. They are commonly encountered in anterior horn cell diseases and sometimes in radiculopathies and polyneuropathies; they are often associated with or preceded by fasciculations or myokymia, which are also considered to be neurogenic. True cramp is not a feature of myopathies however, although patients may describe pain in myopathy as being caused by 'cramp'.

Cramp is caused by central processes involving the motor nerve cell body, and by peripheral mechanisms involving ephaptic transmission in distal axon branches. Consequently, cramp can be induced by repetitive nerve stimulation distal to a peripheral nerve block and relieved by stretching the muscle, without invoking any central processes (Bertolasi et al., 1993). However, studies on patients with refractory cramps and myokymia suggest that the somatodendritic membrane of the anterior horn cells in such patients might exhibit bistable polarization characteristics, in which inputs from low-threshold afferents such as those from muscle spindles would shift membrane potential to a second stable state that would allow repetitive discharges, resulting in cramp or myokymia depending on the size of the motor neuron pool involved (Baldissera et al., 1994). Such a mechanism predicts that strong afferent inputs to the motor pool, sufficient to excite high-threshold pain and tactile fibres, might reverse the process. Mills et al. (1982) reported that stimulation of the skin by ice, mechanical vibration and transcutaneous nerve stimulation was effective in a patient with severe refractory cramps.

Joekes (1982) produced a simple classification of cramps based on precipitating factors (Table 34.2). They can occur in normal subjects as a result of exercise (effort cramps), at rest (particularly in the elderly and in pregnancy) and as a result of fluid and electrolyte disturbances (as with excessive sweating and in intestinal and renal disorders causing electrolyte losses). Rest cramps are generally felt to result from alterations in the ionic milieu of nerve endings, and cramps related to hypo-osmolality can be relieved by infusions of hypertonic saline or glucose (Neal et al., 1981). However, electrolyte imbalance is rarely the cause of cramps in other circumstances, and in most the origin is unclear (Miles and Clarkson, 1994). Cramp and myalgia, caused by magnesium deficiency may be particularly severe and difficult to treat (Bilbey and Prabhakaran, 1996). Cramps occurring in neurogenic diseases, and diseases such as uraemia, dysthyroidism, hypoadrenalism and cirrhosis, are qualitatively similar to cramps occurring in normal subjects. Tetany induced by hypocalcaemia and by hyperventilation results in cramp that, when severe, can manifest as carpopedal spasm.

Finally, familial forms of muscle pain and cramp have been described (Jusic et al., 1972; Lazaro et al., 1981) that are similar to isolated cases of idiopathic muscle pain fasciculation syndrome (Denny-Brown and Foley syndrome) (Hudson et al., 1978).

Cramps have to be distinguished clinically from focal dystonias (e.g. writer's cramp), reflex muscle spasm (owing to neck pain for example) and from disorders characterized by motor unit hyperactivity, such as tetanus, stiffman syndrome and neuromyotonia (Auger, 1994). Neuromyotonia (Isaac's syndrome) is a generic term for a syndrome of diverse aetiology resulting in muscle stiffness, cramps, myokymia and delayed muscle relaxation (Hart and Newsom-Davis, 1996). This, in turn, has to be distinguished from conditions such as benign cramp–fasciculation syndrome and the rare Brody's disease (sarcoplasmic calcium ATPase deficiency, see below).

Insulin resistance, acanthosis nigricans and acral hypertrophy (Flier's disease)

Flier's disease is a rare endocrine disorder in which cramps and eventually chronic diffuse or multifocal myalgia are the dominant and often the presenting symptoms (Flier et al., 1980; Kingston, 1983). It occurs sporadically but can be familial and is presumably autosomal recessive. It is mainly encountered in obese black females with features of masculinization (hirsuitism, clitoromegaly and masculine habitus). The acanthosis is usually generalized and accompanied by numerous skin tags in areas of altered pigmentation, and the hands are typically enlarged. The cause of the cramps is unclear but they can be severe, lasting up to 30 minutes or more, and can lead to muscle fibre damage and chronic myalgia. The cramps evolve in frequency and severity over weeks to months and typically affect large proximal muscles and are worse after exercise. Weakness is not a feature but muscle hypertrophy may be observed in the hands, legs and feet.

Serum CK levels are often increased but EMG between episodes of cramps is usually normal, and muscle biopsy shows only nonspecific changes. Plasma insulin levels are inappropriately high while glucose tolerance is normal or only mildly impaired. This may be the result of inherited insulin receptor abnormalities (type 1 insulin resistance) or caused by antibodies to the insulin receptor in patients with associated autoimmune diseases (type 2 insulin resistance). Hyperinsulinaemia results in ovarian overstimulation, causing polycystic ovary disease and hyperandrogenism, with high levels of plasma testosterone.

Satoyoshi syndrome

Satoyoshi syndrome is an extremely rare disorder (particularly in Caucasians) characterized by progressively more frequent and severe painful muscle spasms, skeletal abnormalities including dysplasia and multiple fractures (which may result in part from the spasms), malabsorption, alopecia and amenorrhoea, with uterine and gonadal aplasia but normal breast development (Ehlayel and Lacassie, 1995; Haymon et al., 1997). It is not yet clear whether the muscle spasms are true cramps, since they may be associated with myoclonus. Muscle hypertrophy may occur. Most cases reported to date have been female and the disorder may be autoimmune in origin. Steroids and intravenous immunoglobulin have been found to be beneficial while acetazolamide and botulinum toxin may help to control spasms (Arita et al., 1996; Haymon et al., 1997).

Contracture

Contracture is a physiological rigor. Clinically and symptomatically, it is similar to cramp but always results from repeated muscle contraction, and it never occurs at rest. The most fundamental distinction however, is that contracture is electrically silent, in contrast to the high-frequency EMG discharges seen during cramp. Such 'dynamic' contractures must obviously be distinguished from the fixed contractures of muscle resulting from muscle fibre degeneration and fibrosis, which can develop in some forms of myopathy and dystrophy.

Contracture has most often been described and studied in diseases of the glycolytic pathway, particularly McArdle's disease and PFK deficiency. Indeed, contracture is unique to this group of energy metabolism disorders and is not seen in disorders of lipid metabolism or mitochondrial myopathies. Perhaps the lack of intracellular acidosis typical of glycolytic disorders is important in this regard. For example, contracture produced in experimental systems in which CK activity or glycolysis was inhibited was not related to decreases in ATP or phosphocreatine levels but to high free ADP levels, which would enhance actin and myosin interaction (Ruff and Weissman, 1989).

Contracture is also a feature of certain rare conditions characterized by failure of the muscle relaxation mechanism. This may be seen in paramyotonia congenita, in which the duration of muscle contracture may outlast the period of myotonic discharge (Haass et al., 1981), in Brody's disease and in 'rippling muscle disease' (see below).

Brody's disease

Brody's disease is a rare metabolic myopathy that results from a deficiency in activity of calcium ATPase in the sarcoplasmic reticulum, principally of fast twitch type II muscle fibres (Hiel et al., 1996). This deficiency results in a failure in re-uptake of calcium ions from the sarcoplasm following muscle contraction, causing a state of protracted actomyosin interaction. The enzyme is encoded by a gene on chromosome 16 and both autosomal recessive and dominant forms of the disease have been reported.

Patients usually develop symptoms of exertional myalgia, stiffness and difficulty with muscle relaxation affecting the limbs in childhood. Typically, they have difficulty loosening handgrip, and activities such as typing and playing the piano lead to stiffening up and freezing of the fingers. After a few seconds, further exercise is possible but the time required for muscle relaxation increases progressively. In the later stages, muscles of the trunk and face may be involved, with difficulty opening the eyelids after forced closure. The symptoms are usually worse in the cold; in extremely cold conditions, exercise can result in rhabdomyolysis.

Serum CK levels are typically normal. Although the symptoms are reminiscent of myotonia, there is no percussion myotonia and EMG is either normal or mildly myopathic, and silent during contractures.

Rippling muscle disease

Rippling muscle disease is a very rare autosomal dominant disease first described by Torbergsen in 1975. Many cases appear to result from a mutation at 1q41 but no linkage to this locus was found in other families so the condition seems to be genetically heterogenous (Stephan et al., 1994).

Symptoms typically begin in childhood. A blow to a muscle belly, such as biceps, results in unusual focal pain, with myoedema (the mounding phenomenon) lasting several seconds, followed by a persistent indentation in the same area that lasts for minutes. Patients also experience myalgia when they carry out a sudden movement, such as a deep squat, after a period of rest. Such pains disperse with repeated contraction and can be avoided by 'warming up'. In adolescence and later life, muscle stiffness becomes an increasing problem, again often precipitated by sudden activity after a period of rest. Such pain is associated with a peculiar 'rippling' effect across the muscle. This rippling effect can be demonstrated clinically, for example by having the patient exert maximal quadriceps extension followed by abrupt knee flexion. Spontaneous rippling waves of muscle contraction will be seen to traverse the muscle at right angles to the long axis of the quadriceps. The muscles are also sensitive to other simple mechanical stimuli such as squeezing or tapping with a tendon hammer, which produces percussion contraction and mounding, followed by indentation. As the years pass, however, the symptoms and signs typically become less prominent and may resolve completely. Serious cardiac disease has been reported in conjunction with this syndrome and drugs such as verapamil and membrane stabilizers, which might be useful to treat the myalgia, should be used with caution (Ricker et al., 1989).

Serum CK levels are usually mildly increased but may be 6–17 times normal (Ricker et al., 1989). On EMG, increased insertional activity may be noted, but during a rippling contraction, there is electrical silence. The rippling wave travels at approximately 0.6 m/s, about ten times slower than muscle fibre action potential. Cooling and potassium challenge have no effect (Ricker et al., 1989).

The rippling muscle sign is not confined to this inherited disorder, however, and was reported in a patient with myasthenia gravis and associated thymoma (Ansevin and Agamanolis, 1996).

Myotonia

Myotonia is a condition of prolonged muscle contraction, with subsequent slowed relaxation, following activation either voluntarily or through electrical or mechanical stimulation. It results from inherited or acquired abnormalities of the cable properties of the sarcolemma, causing electrical instability, which is manifest as myotonic runs on EMG. Myotonia is a feature of a number of diseases and is most commonly described as a muscle 'stiffness' rather than a pain, but muscle pain owing to myotonia can be prominent in some myotonic disorders, such as certain sodium channelopathies, potassium-aggravated myotonic syndromes, including acetazolamide-responsive myotonia, myotonia fluctuans and myotonia permanens (Orrell et al., 1998), and proximal myotonic myopathy (PROMM). These conditions are discussed fully in Chapter 30.

Exertional myalgia

Finally, there are a large number of patients who present with muscle pain that is precipitated by or made worse by exercise. In rare instances, such exertional myalgia may be associated with rhabdomyolysis and frank myoglobinuria, with a marked increase in serum CK levels. If so, the probability of finding an underlying metabolic myopathy is high.

Disorders of muscle energy metabolism

Glycogenolytic (e.g. McArdle's disease) and glycolytic (e.g. PFK deficiency) diseases typically present with exertional myalgia, which when severe may be associated with contracture, usually described by patients as cramp or prolonged and severe stiffness in working muscles, and sometimes rhabdomyolysis. McArdle's disease is by far the most common of these conditions, but this syndrome has been described with deficiency of each of the enzymes in the glycolytic pathway. Myalgia typically develops with rapid, high-intensity exertion that stresses the glycolytic pathway; it can be reduced or avoided to some extent in McArdle's disease by gentle warm-up or pretreatment with fructose, ribose or glucagon to stimulate alternative energy pathways in some patients. Such strategies cannot be used for diseases involving more distal enzymes in the pathway. Patients with lipid storage myopathies who present with exertional myalgia (as opposed to myopathic weakness or other systemic metabolic problems) experience symptoms after prolonged, steady-state exercise, which utilizes free fatty acids preferentially. Rhabdomyolysis and myoglobinuria may be the presenting features in such patients, particularly with carnitine palmityltransferase deficiency. Curiously, mitochondrial myopathies only rarely present with exertional myalgia. Inherited myoadenylate deaminase deficiency presents with exertional myalgia that is similar to that seen in glycolytic disorders. The clinical features, pathophysiology,

investigation and management of these conditions are discussed in Chapters 28 and 29.

Dystrophinopathies

The broad phenotypic spectrum of the dystrophinopathies is increasingly recognized, and many examples of exertional myalgia as the predominant or even the sole expression of in-frame mutations of the dystrophin gene have been reported. Indeed, exertional 'cramp' and myalgia is often a prominent symptom in patients with classical Becker dystrophy. Samaha and Quinlan (1996) emphasized the importance of rigorously excluding dystrophin deficiency in any male patient presenting with exertional myalgia. They reported 12 patients with exertional myalgia, each of whom was shown to have dystrophin deficiency typical of Becker dystrophy. All had normal muscle strength and five had normal EMGs and normal routine muscle histology. Furthermore, four had normal serum CK levels and four had levels only twice the upper normal limit. Prognosis and symptomatology has been found to be related to the size and position of in-frame deletions (Angelini et al., 1996; Ishigaki et al., 1996). For example, deletion or duplication of the 5′ end of the gene is associated with a poor prognosis, while the course of the disease is more benign in patients with large deletions or duplications in the proximal rod region. Such patients typically suffer 'cramps' and myalgia and may develop rhabdomyolysis.

Exertional muscle pain syndrome

Unfortunately, detailed investigation frequently fails to identify a cause for exertional myalgia. While psychogenic causes may be invoked in some cases, patients with EMPS often have nonspecific abnormalities on laboratory tests, such as mildly raised serum CK levels, 'myopathic' EMGs and nonspecific abnormalities on muscle biopsy (Lane et al., 1986). Certain biopsy features are found in EMPS more commonly than expected, including internalized capillaries (Gutman et al., 1989) and tubular aggregates and cylindrical spirals (Danon et al., 1989). A deficiency of type I muscle fibres with a reduced type I/type II fibre ratio has been noted both in EMPS (Lane et al., 1986) and in some patients with chronic fatigue syndrome (Lane et al., 1998b). The significance of such observations is not yet clear.

Principles of management

Physical treatments and diet

The management of myalgia occurring in the course of defined neuromuscular diseases is largely determined by the treatment of the primary condition, for example the use of antibiotics in pyomyositis and steroids in inflammatory myopathy. Certain dietary manipulations or supplements may be helpful in disorders of intermediary metabolism and mitochondrial myopathies, as discussed in the relevant chapters dealing with these conditions. Comorbid endocrine disorders, such as hypothyroidism, acromegaly and insulin resistance, and electrolytic disorders, such as hypokalaemia and hypomagnesaemia, may worsen myalgia and cramp and should be detected and treated. Fasting and increases in plasma potassium will exacerbate symptoms in sodium channelopathies.

In myalgia of uncertain origin, a diary can help to determine factors associated with symptoms and the effects of therapeutic interventions (Lane et al., 1986). It may be possible to identify and reduce activities that stress muscle, particularly eccentric contractions. Regular stretching and warm-up exercises may be helpful (Bertolasi et al., 1993), as may simple physical measures such as warm or cold packs, ultrasound or transcutaneous nerve stimulation (TENS). The successful use of TENS in refractory cramp has already been mentioned (Mills et al., 1982).

Drug treatment

Myalgia that is thought to be caused by chemical mediators may respond to simple and nonsteroidal anti-inflammatory analgesics, perhaps in combination with a tricyclic antidepressant. There are no clinical trials of such interventions however. As mentioned, myalgia resulting from eccentric contraction damage does not seem to respond to such strategies. Exertional myalgia and cramp will sometimes respond to calcium antagonists such as verapamil and nifedipine. Nifedipine was reported to alleviate cramp induced by exercise (Sufit and Peters, 1984) and haemodialysis (Peer et al., 1983), and verapamil improved symptoms in a controlled trial in patients with EMPS (Lane et al., 1986).

Verapamil is also the treatment of choice in Brody's disease (Taylor et al., 1988). Symptoms failed to respond to a large number of other drugs, including membrane stabilizers such as phenytoin and carbamazepine, nonsteroidal analgesics and vasodilators (Walton, 1981). Verapamil inhibits the normal release of calcium ions from the sarcoplasmic reticulum by blocking the dihydropyridine–ryanodine receptor complex, preventing cytosolic calcium overload. It would be expected that dantrolene would be similarly effective.

Quinine remains the treatment of choice for cramp, and its effectiveness has been confirmed in a meta-analysis of published trials (Man-Son-Hing and Wells, 1995). Many other drugs are also helpful, including diazepam, dantro-lene, phenytoin and procainamide (Anon., 1983). A study of cramp in cirrhosis concluded that the symptom was related to a reduction in plasma volume, and a placebo-controlled trial showed that a weekly infusion of albumin significantly reduced the frequency of cramps (Angeli et al., 1996). The treatment of myotonia is considered in Chapter 30.

References

Angeli, P., Albino, G., Carraro, P. et al. (1996). Cirrhosis and muscle cramps: evidence of a causal relationship. *Hepatology* **23**, 264–273.

Angelini, C., Fanin, M., Freda, M. P. et al. (1996). Prognostic factors in mild dystrophinopathies. *J. Neurol. Sci.* **142**, 70–78.

Anon. (1983). More on muscle cramps. *Drugs Therapeut. Bull.* **21**, 83–84.

Ansevin, C. F. and Agamanolis, D. P. (1996). Rippling muscles and myasthenia gravis and rippling muscles. *Arch. Neurol.* **53**, 197–199.

Arendt-Nielsen, L., Graven-Nielsen, T., Svensson, P. and Jensen, T. S. (1997). Temporal summation in muscles and referred pain areas: an experimental study. *Muscle Nerve* **20**, 1311–1313.

Arita, J., Hamano, S., Nara, T. and Maekawa, K. (1996). Intravenous gammaglobulin therapy of Satoyoshi syndrome. *Brain Dev.* **18**, 409–411.

Auger, R. G. (1994). Diseases associated with excess motor unit activity. *Muscle Nerve* **17**, 1250–1263.

Baldissera, F., Cavallari, P. and Dworzak, F. (1994). Motor neurone 'bistability'. A pathogenetic mechanism for cramps and myokymia. *Brain* **117**, 929–939.

Banker, B. Q. and Chester, C. S. (1973). Infarction of thigh muscle in the diabetic patient. *Neurology* **23**, 667–677.

Bertolasi, L., DeGrandis, D., Bongiovanni, L. G., Zanette, G. P. and Gasperini, M. (1993). The influence of muscular lengthening on cramps. *Ann. Neurol.* **33**, 176–180.

Bilbey, D. L. and Prabhakaran, V. M. (1996). Muscle cramps and magnesium deficiency: case reports. *Can. Fam. Physician* **42**, 1348–1351.

Bjelle A., Henriksson, K-G. and Hofer, P-A. (1980). Polymyositis in eosinophilic fasciitis: review and case report. *Eur. Neurol.* **19**, 493–517.

Bjornskov, E. K., Carry, M. R., Katz, F. H., Lefokowitz, J. and Ringel, S. P. (1995). Diabetic muscle infarction: a new perspective on pathogenesis and management. *Neuromus. Dis.* **5**, 39–45.

Brooks, R. C. and McGee, S. R. (1997). Diagnostic dilemmas in polymyalgia rheumatica. *Arch. Intern. Med.* **157**, 162–168.

Bushby, K. M. D., Pollitt, C., Johnson, M. A., Rogers, M. T. and Chinnery, P. F. (1999). Muscle pain as a prominent feature of facioscapulohumeral muscular dystrophy (FSHD): four illustrative case reports. *Neuromusc. Dis.* **8**, 574–579.

Coquet, M., Authier, F. J., Moretto, P. et al. (1999). Adjuvant of vaccination aluminium in macrophagic myofasciitis. *Neuromusc. Disord.* **9**: 476–477.

Coquet, M., Lechapt, E., Authier, F. J. et al. (2000). Dermatomyositis with acute diffuse macrographic infiltration: a differential diagnosis of macrographic myofasciitis. *Neuromusc. Disord.* 10: 358.

Connolly, S., Smith, D., Doyle, D. and Fowler, C. J. (1993). Chronic fatigue: electromyographic and neuropathological evaluation. *J. Neurol.* 240, 435–438.

Cook, D. B., O'Connor, P. J., Eubanks, S. A., Smith, J. C. and Lee, M. (1997). Naturally occurring muscle pain during exercise: assessment and experimental evidence. *Med. Sci. Sports Exercise* 29, 999–1012.

Croisier, J. L., Camus, G., Deby-Dupont, G. et al. (1996). Myocellular enzyme leakage, polymorphonuclear neutrophil activation and delayed muscle soreness induced by isokinetic eccentric exercise. *Arch. Physiol. Biochem.* 104, 322–329.

Danon, M. J., Carpenter, S. and Harati, Y. (1989). Muscle pain associated with tubular aggregates and structures resembling cylindrical spirals. *Muscle Nerve* 12, 265–272.

Ehlayel, M. S. and Lacassie, Y. (1995). Satoyoshi syndrome: an unusual postnatal multisystemic disorder. *Am. J. Med. Genet.* 57, 620–625.

Elert, J. E., Rantapaa-Dahlqvist, S. B., Henriksson-Larsen, K., Lorentzon R. and Gerdle, B. U. (1992). Muscle performance, electromyography and fibre type composition in fibromyalgia and work-related myalgia. *Scand. J. Rheumatol.* 21, 28–34.

Farinon, A. M., Marbini, A., Gemignani, F. et al. (1984). Skeletal muscle and peripheral nerve changes caused by chronic arterial insufficiency. *Clin. Neuropathol.* 3, 240–252.

Flier, J. S., Young, J. B., Landsberg, L. (1980). Familial insulin resistance with acanthosis nigricans, acral hypertrophy and muscle cramps. *N. Eng. J. Med.* 303, 970–973.

Friden, J. (1984). Muscle soreness after exercise: implications of morphological changes. *Int. J. Sports Med.* 5, 57–66.

Gherardi, R. K., Coquet, M., Cherin, P. et al. (1998). Macrophagic myofasciitis: an emerging entity. *Lancet* 352, 347–351.

Giamberardino, M. A., Dragani, L., Valente, R., Di-Lisa, F., Saggini, R. and Vecchiet, L. (1996). Effects of prolonged L-carnitine administration on delayed muscle pain and CK release after eccentric effort. *Inter. J. Sports Med.* 17, 320–324.

Gill, G. V., White, M. and Anderson, J. (1986). Diabetic myalgia? *Diabet. Med.* 3, 90–91.

Gleeson, M., Almey, J., Brooks, S., Cave R., Lewis, A. and Griffiths, H. (1995). Haematological and acute-phase responses associated with delayed-onset muscle soreness in humans. *Eur. J. Appl. Physiol.* 71, 137–142.

Golding, D. N. (1968). Brachial neuralgia and the carpal tunnel syndrome. *Br. Med. J.* 3, 803.

Gotze, F. R., Thid, S. and Kyllerman, M. (1998). Fibromyalgia in hyperkalemic periodic paralysis. *Scand. J. Rheumatol.* 27, 383–384.

Graven-Nielsen, T., Arendt-Nielsen, L., Svensson, P. and Jensen, T. S. (1997a). Quantification of local and referred muscle pain in humans after sequential i.m. injections of hypertonic saline. *Pain* 69, 111–117.

Graven-Nielsen, T., McArdle A., Phoenix, J. et al. (1997b). In vivo model of muscle pain: quantification of intramuscular chemical, electrical, and pressure changes associated with saline-induced muscle pain in humans. *Pain* 69, 137–143.

Gutman, L., Wolf, R., Nix, W., Goebel, H. H., Schochet, S. S., Hopf, H. C. and Kramer, G. (1989). Internalised myofibre capillaries: observations on their origin and clinical features. *Muscle Nerve* 12, 191–196.

Haass, A., Ricker, K., Rudel, R. et al. (1981). Clinical study of paramyotonia congenita with and without myotonia in a warm environment. *Muscle Nerve* 4, 388–395.

Hamilton, A. L., Killian, K. J., Summers, E. and Jones, N. L. (1996). Quantification of intensity of sensations during muscular work by normal subjects. *J. Appl. Physiol.* 81, 1156–1161.

Harriman, D. G. F. (1977). Ischaemia of peripheral nerve and muscle. *J. Clin. Pathol.* 11(Suppl.), 94–104.

Hart, I. K. and Newsom-Davis, J. (1996). Neuromyotonia (Isaac's syndrome). In: *Handbook of Muscle Disease*, ed. R. J. M. Lane, pp. 355–363. New York: Marcel Dekker.

Haymon M., Willis R. B., Ehlayel, M. S. and Lacassie, Y. (1997). Radiological and orthopedic abnormalities in Satoyoshi syndrome. *Ped. Radiol.* 27, 415–418.

Hiel, J. A. P., Jongen, P. J. H., Peols, P. J. E. et al. (1996). Sarcoplasmic reticulum Ca^{2+}-adenosine triphosphatase deficiency (Brody's disease). In: *Handbook of Muscle Disease*, ed. R. J. M. Lane, pp. 473–478. New York: Marcel Dekker.

Hockaday, J. M. and Whitty, C. W. M. (1967). Patterns of referred pain in the normal subject. *Brain* 40, 481–496.

Hudson A. J., Brown, W. F. and Gilbert, J. J. (1978). The muscular pain fasciculation syndrome. *Neurology* 28, 1105–1109.

Ishigaki, C., Patria, S. Y., Nishio, H., Yabe, M. and Matsuo, M. A (1996). Japanese boy with myalgia and cramps has a novel in-frame deletion of the dystrophin gene. *Neurology* 46, 1347–1350.

Issberner, U., Reeh, P. W. and Steen, K. H. (1996). Pain due to tissue acidosis: a mechanism for inflammatory and ischaemic myalgia? *Neurosc. Lett.* 208, 191–194.

Joekes, A. M. (1982). Cramp. *J. Roy. Soc. Med.* 75, 546–549.

Jusic A., Dogan, S. and Stojanovitch, V. (1972). Hereditary persistent distal cramps. *J. Neurol. Neurosurg. Psychiatry* 35, 379–384.

Kellgren, J. H. (1937/38). Observations of referred pain arising from muscle. *Clin. Sci.* 3, 175–190.

Kellgren, J. H. (1939). On the distribution of pain arising from deep structures with charts of segmental pain areas. *Clin. Sci.* 4, 35–46.

Kingston, W. J. (1983). Endocrine myopathies. *Semin. Neurol.* 3, 258–264.

Kummel, B. M. and Zazanis, G. A. (1973). Shoulder pain as the presenting complaint in carpal tunnel syndrome. *Clin. Orthoped,* 92, 227–230.

Lane, R. J. M., Turnbull, D. M., Welch, J. L. and Walton, J. N. (1986). A double-blind, placebo-controlled, crossover study of verapamil in exertional muscle pain syndrome. *Muscle Nerve* 9, 635–641.

Lane, R. J. M., Barrett, M. C., Taylor, D. J., Kemp, G. J. and Lodi, R. (1998a). Heterogeneity in chronic fatigue syndrome: evidence from magnetic resonance spectroscopy of muscle. *Neuromusc. Dis.* 8, 204–209.

Lane, R. J. M., Barrett, M. C., Woodrow, D., Moss, J., Fletcher, R. and Archard, L. C. (1998b). Muscle fibre characteristics and lactate responses to exercise in chronic fatigue syndrome. *J. Neurol., Neurosurg. Psychiatry* **64**, 362–367.

Lazaro, R. P., Rollinson, R. D. and Fernichel, G. M. (1981). Familial cramps and muscle pain. *Arch. Neurol.* **38**, 22–24.

Lewis, T. (1932). Pain in muscular ischaemia. *Arch. Intern. Med.* **49**. 713–727.

Lindahl, O. and Hamberg, J. (1981). Angina pectoris symptoms caused by thoracic spine disorders. Neuro-anatomical considerations. *Acta Med. Scand.* **664**, 81–83.

Man-Son-Hing, M. and Wells, G. (1995). Meta-analysis of efficacy of quinine for treatment of nocturnal leg cramps in elderly people. *Br. Med. J.* **310**, 13–17.

Marchettini, P. (1993). Muscle pain: animal and human experimental and clinical studies. *Muscle Nerve* **16**, 1033–1039.

Martin, R. W., Duffy, J., Engel, A. G. et al. (1990). The clinical spectrum of the eosinophilia-myalgia syndrome associated with L-tryptophan ingestion: clinical features in 20 patients and aspects of pathophysiology. *Ann. Intern. Med.* **113**, 124–134.

Matre, D. A., Sinkjaer, T., Svensson, P. and Arendt-Nielsen, L. (1998). Experimental muscle pain increases the human stretch reflex. *Pain* **75**, 331–339.

Mense, S. (1991). Considerations concerning the neurological basis of muscle pain. *Can. J. Physiol. Pharmacol.* **69**, 610–666.

Miles, M. P. and Clarkson, P. M. (1994). Exercise-induced muscle pain, soreness and cramps. *J. Sports Med. Physical Fitness* **34**, 203–216.

Mills, K. R. and Edwards, R. H. T. (1983). Investigative strategies for muscle pain. *J. Neurol. Sci.* **58**, 73–88.

Mills, K. R., Newham, D. J. and Edwards, R. H. T. (1982). Severe muscle cramps relieved by transcutaneous nerve stimulation; a case report. *J. Neurol., Neurosurg. Psychiatry* **45**, 539–542.

Mills, K. R., Newham, D. J. and Edwards, R. H. T. (1985). Muscle pain. In: *Textbook of Pain*, ed. P. D. Wall and R. Melzak, pp. 319–330. New York: Churchill Livingstone.

Myers, D. E., Shaikh, Z. and Zullo, T. G. (1997). Hypoalgesic effect of caffeine in experimental ischemic muscle contraction pain. *Headache* **37**, 654–658.

Neal, C. R., Renikoff, E. and Unger, A. M. (1981). Treatment of dialysis-related muscle cramps with hypertonic dextrose. *Arch. Intern. Med.* **141**, 171–173.

Newham, J. J., Jones, D. A. and Edwards, R. H. T. (1983a). Large delayed plasma creatine kinase changes after stepping exercise. *Muscle Nerve* **6**, 380–385.

Newham, J. J., McPhail, G., Mills, K. R. and Edwards, R. H. T. (1983b). Ultrastructural changes after concentric and eccentric contractions of human muscle. *J. Neurolog. Sci.* **61**, 109–122.

Nielsen, C. and Mazzone, P. (1999). Muscle pain after exercise. *Lancet* **353**, 1062.

Orrell, R. W., Jurkat-Rott, K., Lehmann-Horn, F., Lane, R. J. M. (1998). Familial cramp due to potassium-aggravated myotonia. *J. Neurol., Neurosurg. Psychiatry* **65**, 569–572.

Patel, S. R., Olenginski, T. P., Perruquet, J. L. and Harrington, T. M. (1997). Pyomyositis: clinical features and predisposing conditions. *J. Rheumatol.* **24**, 1734–1738.

Paul, L., Wood, L., Behan, W. M. H., and Maclaren, W. M. (1999). Demonstration of delayed recovery from fatiguing exercise in chronic fatigue syndrome. *Eur. J. Neurol.* **6**, 63–69.

Peer, G., Blum, M. and Avirum, A. (1983). Relief of haemodialysis-induced muscular cramps by nifedipine. *Dialysis Transplant.* **12**, 180–181.

Pourmand, R. (1997). The value of muscle biopsy in myalgia. *Neurologist* **3**, 173–177.

Ricker, K., Moxley, R. T. and Rohkamm, R. (1989). Rippling muscle disease. *Arch. Neurol.* **46**, 405–408.

Ruff, R. L. and Weissman, J. (1989). Possible role of ADP in contracture of muscle with impaired myoglycolysis. *Neurology* **39** (Suppl.), 360.

Samaha F. J. and Quinlan, J. G. (1996). Myalgia and cramps; dystrophinopathy with wide-ranging laboratory findings. *J. Child Neurol.* **11**, 21–24.

Shulman L. E. (1975). Diffuse fasciitis with eosinophilia: a new syndrome? *Trans. Assoc. Am. Phys.* **88**: 70–86.

Soernson, J., Graven-Nielsen, T., Henriksson, K. G., Bengtsson, M., and Arendt-Nielsen, L. (1998). Hyperexcitability in fibromyalgia. *J. Rheumatol.* **25**, 152–155.

Spillane, J. D., Nathan, P. W., Kelly, R. E. and Marsden, C. D. (1971). Painful legs and moving toes. *Brain* **94**, 541–556.

Stephan, D. A., Buist, N. R. M., Chittenden, A. B., Ricker, K., Zhou, J. and Hoffman, E. P. (1994). A rippling muscle disease gene is located to 1q41: evidence for multiple genes. *Neurology* **44**, 1915–1920.

Sufit, R. L. and Peters, H. A. (1984). Nifedipine relieves exercise-exacerbated myalgias. *Muscle Nerve* **7**, 647–649.

Svensson, P., Beydoun A., Morow, T. J. and Casey, K. L. (1997). Human intramuscular and cutaneous pain: psychological comparisons. *Exp. Brain Res.*, **114**, 390–392.

Sylven, C., Jonzon, B., Fedholm, B. B. and Kaijser, L. (1988). Adenosine injection into the brachial artery produces ischaemia-like pain or discomfort in the forearm. *Cardiovasc. Res.* **22**, 674–678.

Taylor, D. J., Brosnan, M. J., Arnold, D. L. et al. (1988). Ca^{2+}-ATPase deficiency in a patient with exertional muscle pain syndrome. *J. Neurol., Neurosurg. Psychiatry* **51**, 1425–1433.

Torbergsen, T. A. (1975). Family with dominant hereditary myotonia, muscular hypertrophy, and increased muscular irritability, distinct from myotonia congenita thomsen. *Acta Neurol. Scand.* **51**, 225–232.

Torebjork, H. E., Ochaoa, J. L. and Schady, W. (1984). Referred pain from intraneural stimulation of muscle nerve fascicles in the median nerve. *Pain* **18**, 145–156.

Valeriano-Marcet, J. and Kerr L. D. (1991). Myonecrosis and myofibrosis as complications of sickle cell anemia. *Ann. Intern. Med.* **115**, 99–101.

Verity, M. A., Bulpitt, K. J. and Paulus, H. E. (1991). Neuromuscular manifestations of L-tryptophan-associated eosinophilia-myalgia syndrome: a histomorphological analysis of 14 patients. *Hum. Pathol.* **22**, 3–11.

Walton, J. N. (1981). Diffuse exercise-induced muscle pain of undetermined cause relieved by verapamil. *Lancet* **i**, 993.

Part IV

The principles of management of muscle disease

35

Genetic counselling in muscle disease

Kate Bushby

Introduction

This chapter aims to focus on the applications of genetic analysis and counselling to some of the many inherited forms of muscle disease. Since the last edition of this book was published, the majority of the genes involved in inherited muscle disease have been identified, with a corresponding range of mutational mechanisms recognized. The ability to establish the underlying molecular pathology of these disorders has led to huge advances in our understanding of their pathogenesis, and as such is described in detail in many other chapters of this book. A continuously updated summary of the current state of knowledge of the genes involved in inherited muscle disease can be found in each edition of the journal *Neuromuscular Disorders*. Other sources of up-to-date information include the websites at OMIM (http://www3.nabi.nlm.nih.gov/omim/) and Leiden (http://www.dmd.nl) (the Leiden muscular dystrophy database).

So instead of providing an overview of the factual information that can be found elsewhere, this chapter aims to provide a practical guide to addressing the various questions of genetic counselling that may be raised in some of these conditions, and especially those conditions where particularly difficult problems may be involved either in the counselling itself or in the application of the genetic technology. Using the available molecular data to allow families to make informed choices about their lives and reproductive decisions is only a part of the process of genetic counselling. The diagnosis of an inherited disorder carries major implications beyond the index case, and the family consequences of such diagnoses, therefore, can be wide-ranging. Issues of recurrence, presymptomatic or prenatal diagnosis, and the establishment of carrier status may apply to a large number of family members, and the

multidisciplinary approach to the management of muscle disease cannot ignore these wider issues. Precision of genetic information has added enormously to answering many of these questions (Table 35.1) and thereby also allows the patient and his family the opportunity to make informed and autonomous decisions in many areas. Added to this is the much more widespread availability of DNA analysis of chorion villous biopsy samples taken in the first trimester of pregnancy for a variety of disorders, allowing earlier prenatal diagnosis. Preimplantation diagnosis is theoretically available for some muscle diseases, though as yet on a very small scale. Not all family members will accept the offer of addressing issues of genetics, nor the offer of any genetic testing, but it is a responsibility of the physician to ensure that the option of discussing such issues is at least offered.

Critical to the provision of genetic counselling is correct diagnosis, and this is an area where the ability to look directly at the gene or protein involved in a particular condition has brought clear gains. In fact, the ability to determine the genetic faults underlying particular conditions has in many disorders superseded previously available diagnostic tools completely, and in some instances provided a challenge to the traditional understanding of the conditions, leading to the establishment of new classifications based on molecular pathology rather than symptomatology. This has been notably so for some of the muscular dystrophies and the ion channel disorders. This approach has its proponents and detractors, but in any case has revealed an intriguing and unexpected level of heterogeneity at every level. It must also be borne in mind that while the major benefits of precise diagnosis at present are to provide prognostic and genetic information, in the future any move towards gene-based therapies will have to have as a prerequisite a diagnosis based on the specific genetic fault itself.

Table 35.1. Current state of applicability of molecular testing in skeletal muscle disease

Disorder	Heterogeneity	Mode of inheritance	Feasibility of genetic analysis	Feasibility of protein analysis	Comments
Dystrophinopathy (DMD/BMD)	Clinical variability within group	XR	+++	+++	Basic tests (deletion analysis) widely available; more specialized analysis may be needed in some situations (see text)
Limb girdle muscular dystrophy	>14 different forms	AR/AD	+ (some types)	++ (some types)	Specialized analysis necessary to confirm different forms; testing limited in some types (see text)
Facioscapulohumeral muscular dystrophy	One predominant locus on 4q; others inferred but not known	AD	++	−	Common deletion allows DNA diagnosis in absence of knowledge of gene defect; however, test is not always simple
Emery–Dreifuss muscular dystrophy	Two genes identified	AD/XR, AR (uncommon)	+ (AD/XR)	++ (XR only)	Specialized analysis may be necessary to complete diagnosis; AR and AD disease are caused by mutations in the same gene
Congenital muscular dystrophy	>6 different forms	AR	+ (some types)	++ (some types)	Analysis feasible only in defined subgroups (see text)
Congenital myopathy	>6 different types	AR/AD/XR	+	−	Analysis limited to a few types (see text)
Distal myopathy	Many different forms	AR/AD	+ (MM only)	+ (MM only)	Linkage only tool in majority of subtypes
Spinal muscular atrophy	One predominant form; rest very heterogeneous	AR	+++	−	Single mutation type in vast majority of chromosome 5-linked disease
Myotonic dystrophy	One predominant form; other loci defined by linkage only	AD	+++	−	Single mutation type (triplet repeat) in most common form
Ion channel disorders	Several genes involved	AD/AR	++	−	DNA analysis superseding other more traditional diagnostic tools

Notes:

AR, autosomal recessive; AD, autosomal dominant; XR, X-linked recessive MM, Miyoshi myopathy; DMD, Duchenne muscular dystrophy; BMD, Becker muscular dystrophy.

+, testing problematic, for example because genes harbour very few recurrent mutations, because of the need to look at a number of different genes, because linkage analysis is the only option or because tests may relate only to a few forms of the condition (see text). In this situation, analysis is likely to be available only through laboratories with a research interest in the topic.

++, testing technically feasible but may be restricted to specialized laboratories. This may be because of the relative rarity of the conditions, the need to look for a range of mutations or use a range of antibodies or because the test itself is more technically challenging.

+++, testing likely to be widely available and relatively easy to perform.

Having said that these molecular discoveries have changed the approach to diagnosis and extended the range of tests available to patients and their families, a note of caution must be added. The widespread application to the clinical setting of these molecular findings may be rapid or maybe more problematic, depending on a number of disease- and test-related findings. The major disease-related factors that affect how quickly a novel molecular finding is brought into service include the frequency of a particular disorder and the burden of the disease. The demand for a service may be especially great if a disorder is relatively common and inevitably fatal. At the other extreme, some molecular findings may apply to a single family only and, despite coverage in the scientific literature, will therefore never be more widely applicable. From the technological perspective, a test will be much more widely applied if it is simple and relatively cheap to perform: ideally, if a single type of mutation, detectable by the polymerase chain reaction (PCR), accounts for all cases of a disease. Testing becomes much more problematic if many genes, each with a range of potential mutations, may be involved. All of these considerations are inevitably played out against a background of the requirements to fund an ever-increasing range of gene-based tests, which will vary from country to country and even area to area within a single country, potentially challenging the equity of access to a full range of genetic analyses.

Modes of inheritance

Dominantly inherited muscle diseases

There are many examples of muscle diseases that are inherited in an autosomal dominant manner. For many of these disorders, genetic issues may on the face of it be relatively simple: an affected individual will have a 50% chance of transmitting the disorder to his or her offspring in any pregnancy, irrespective of their sex. Simple though this information is, its impact should never be underestimated. For some affected individuals, the burden of guilt that can be felt about the possibility of transmitting the disease to their offspring may be greater than the burden of the disease itself.

In some autosomal dominant disorders, the mutation is essentially always inherited (for example in myotonic dystrophy). However, in other conditions, the ability to perform direct molecular investigations has led to the increasing recognition of new dominant mutations (that is, the diagnosis of a dominant disorder in an individual where neither parent can be shown to have the same con-

dition). Notable examples include facioscapulohumeral muscular dystrophy (FSHD) and autosomal dominant Emery–Dreifuss muscular dystrophy (EDMD). Despite the fact that they are not somatic carriers of the mutation, the risk of recurrence to the parents of an affected individual is not always negligible as there is frequently a population of gametes in the germline bearing the mutation. This 'germline mosaicism' can be difficult to quantify and currently available figures vary from gene to gene based on observed data. Germline mosaicism risks apply in a single generation only: the risk to the offspring of the affected person will be 50/50.

Increasing precision of diagnosis means that presymptomatic testing may be available to people at risk of an autosomal dominant disorder (for example the offspring of an affected individual). Most models of predictive testing for late-onset and incurable diseases are based on the experience in predictive testing for Huntington's disease. People have various reasons for seeking predictive testing, which may include the relief of uncertainty, the ability to make plans for the future and, often overwhelmingly, to obtain information relating to risk to their own offspring and allow childbearing decisions to be made in an informed manner. Embarking on predictive testing requires the appreciation of the specific circumstances of this type of test and should include pre- and post-test counselling including full discussion of all of the implications (including to potential insurers) and limitations of a test. Current guidelines acknowledge that predictive testing in childhood poses particular problems, except where a disorder may have clinical implications in childhood. It is, therefore, generally recommended that testing asymptomatic children for a late-onset autosomal dominant disorder is not desirable, and that testing should be restricted to individuals who can be counselled as to the full implications of the disorder and a positive test result. This point should be made to parents who bring their young children for such testing, often (understandably) through a desire to relieve their own anxiety. In practice, this translates in many countries into a policy of offering testing in young adulthood, when the issues of insurance implications, risks to their offspring in turn and the various pros and cons of certainty versus uncertainty can be discussed in an informed way, a process that may take several sessions to ensure that all of the implications are understood. Most families accept this approach after careful counselling.

The availability of specific genetic tests, which can be easily applied in pregnancy, adds to the choices available to individuals who are concerned about risks to their offspring, but it may also add to the dilemmas faced by families and their doctors, especially where prenatal diagnosis is sought for late-onset disorders where severity cannot be predicted with certainty. Here an individual's experience of a disease will inevitably colour their approach to the risk of recurrence, and issues of choice must be seen within this context and respected as such.

Autosomal recessive muscle disease

In autosomal recessive diseases, an affected individual has, by definition, inherited a faulty copy of the disease gene in question from each parent. Such parents will have a 1 in 4 risk of having a similarly affected child in each pregnancy thereafter. The healthy sibling of an affected person has a 2/3 chance of being a carrier of the same gene. The risk to an affected individual, or to any other carrier in the family, of having an affected child depends on the frequency of the disease gene in their community. In most Caucasian populations, the most frequent autosomal recessive disease of muscle is spinal muscular atrophy (SMA) with a carrier frequency of around 1 in 50. An affected individual with SMA, therefore, has a 1 in 100 risk of having an affected baby with an unrelated partner, while the risk to their siblings will be 1 in 120. Unfortunately, as described later, although there is a common mutation type in SMA, testing for carriers is not necessarily easy. For individual autosomal recessive disorders in isolated populations, the frequency of a particular mutation may be much higher; for example, there is a particularly common dysferlin mutation in the Libyan Jewish population, with its frequency as high as 1 in 10 of the population. Here, testing for the common mutation is relatively straightforward; carrier testing in noninbred populations is less so, especially in genes with large numbers of reported mutations. In these situations, molecular analysis may realistically have little to add to the general reassurance that with uncommon recessive diseases the risk of having an affected child is likely to be small.

X-linked muscle diseases

There are various features of X-linked recessive diseases that raise particular issues for genetic counselling. Because of the mode of inheritance, most affected patients are male, while females in the family related through the maternal line may be carriers of the disease and at risk of having affected sons. In most X-linked recessive disease, there is a significant rate of new mutations and the phenomenon of germline mosaicism, as discussed above, may also be observed in families with apparently 'new mutation' cases of X-linked recessive disease. The inactivation of the X chromosome in females, which leads to a single X chromosome being active in any particular cell, can deviate from random, leading to some female carriers having symptoms or signs of the disease. Most such carriers will have minor manifestations of the condition; however, the severity of the disease in such 'manifesting carriers' can be very variable. This phenomenon also led in the past to the development of a variety of indirect tests for carrier status; for example, in Duchenne muscle dystrophy (DMD) and Becker muscular dystrophy (BMD) various techniques for detecting minor subclinical manifestations of the carrier state were tried and mostly abandoned, though measurement of serum creatine kinase incorporated with other information is useful in some families. The availability of precise molecular information in X-linked diseases has led to increasing certainty in carrier detection in many situations; although this is not yet applicable to all families, for many the result is much better information on which to base reproductive decisions than was previously available.

Mitochondrial inheritance

Mitochondrial DNA (mtDNA) mutations or rearrangements have been reported in a number of patients presenting with muscle-related symptoms, especially myopathy or exercise intolerance, though the proportion of patients with mtDNA abnormalities who present with a 'pure' myopathic phenotype is very small. A larger proportion will have a myopathy associated with external ophthalmoplegia or multisystem disease. It is also important to recognize that biochemical evidence of mitochondrial abnormalities may be the result of nuclear DNA mutations. A record of the mutations described to date in mtDNA can be found in the journal *Neuromuscular Disorders*, as well as on the web at http://www.gen.emory.edu/mitomap.html. There is considerable heterogeneity associated with most mtDNA mutations: similar mutations may produce widely different phenotypes and similar phenotypes may result from different mutations. Part of the variability in expression relates to the varying load of mtDNA mutations in different individuals and in different cells in the same individual (heteroplasmy). The level of mutant mtDNA found in a muscle biopsy (which is generally much more reliable for this type of analysis than a blood sample) has been shown generally to correlate with disease severity, though sampling problems and the variability of mutant DNA load with time in the same person make it hard to use this kind of analysis to offer definitive prognostic advice (Chinnery et al., 1999).

The particular behaviour of mtDNA presents specific

problems for genetic counselling. Mitochondria are essentially exclusively maternally inherited. Maternal inheritance may not, however, be immediately obvious from examination of the pedigree as it may mimic X-linked or dominant inheritance (though never with male–male transmission). Additional problems may arise in pedigree assessment from differences in penetrance and through assessment of the significance of the presence of nonspecific features in some family members (for example, short stature, deafness and diabetes may be associated with mitochondrial disease but equally may be entirely nonspecific incidental findings in a family). The different types of pathogenic mtDNA mutation also carry variable risks for children. Thus mtDNA deletions are not transmitted to offspring though duplications may be, and such duplications can predispose to the formation of deletions in the offspring. Point mutations in mtDNA may be transmitted from mother to child. With transmissible mutations, there are two factors that are particular imponderables at the present time. One relates to the amount of mutant mtDNA in the oocyte, and the second is the way that the mtDNA segregates in development. During oocyte maturation, there is an initial restriction in the numbers of mtDNA followed by an amplification. This results in a high level of variability in the level of mutated DNA transmitted to the subsequent generation. This has been referred to as a 'genetic bottleneck' (Poulton et al., 1998). Models have been proposed that begin to allow prediction of the mutant load transmitted based on the study of animal models and human oocytes, with one study demonstrating skewing of the proportion of mutant mtDNA in oocytes (Blok et al., 1997) though this interpretation of events remains controversial (Chinnery et al., 1998a). Unfortunately, this variability is further compounded by the differential rates of replication and segregation of mutated mtDNA during maturation of the fetus. Current advice, therefore, to families with a mtDNA disorder is necessarily uncertain. Data are beginning to accumulate on the relationship between mutant load in the mother and clinical problems in her offspring, though with few exceptions such correlations are as yet not well enough established to be clinically useful (Chinnery et al., 1998a,b, 1999; White et al., 1999). The collection of complete and prospective data offers the prospect of more definitive information in the future.

Not surprisingly, while correlations in adults between mutant load and phenotype remain so poorly understood, the situation with prenatal testing is even more hazardous. Problems of interpretation of the results of chorion villus biopsies or preimplantation tissue renders such analyses of little practical use at the present time, and highly specialized advice needs to be sought relating to the circumstances of specific families who may be seeking such testing. While more definitive data are awaited on which to base more precise risks, the challenge of genetic counselling in mitochondrial disorders is that it still has more to do with helping families come to terms with uncertain risks than dealing with definitive investigations.

Commonly encountered conditions and genetic issues

Dystrophinopathy

With the ability to demonstrate dystrophin abnormalities in muscle and to detect mutations in the dystrophin gene, the spectrum of clinical phenotypes associated with this locus has expanded beyond the classically recognized DMD and BMD, with some conclusions possible about genotype–phenotype correlations.

In DMD, affected boys are typically confined to a wheelchair by the age of 12 years. The genotype and phenotype both at the protein and clinical level in DMD is relatively homogeneous. Over 90% of mutations in DMD (of which about 60% will be deletions) disrupt the open reading frame of the gene, resulting in the inability to produce a functional protein (Bakker and van Ommen, 1999). In at least 50% of DMD cases, no dystrophin at all is detected on immunocytochemical analysis of muscle biopsies (Nicholson et al., 1993a–c). The rest produce either some dystrophin in isolated fibres or a low level on most fibres. The latter is associated statistically with a slightly better prognosis (Nicholson et al., 1993d). In BMD, a higher proportion of mutations are deletions (about 80%) of which nearly all are in-frame, most occurring in the mid-rod domain. Here a slightly smaller protein of reduced abundance can be detected in muscle (Bushby et al., 1993) and the abundance of protein produced is much greater than seen in DMD. Occasionally very mildly affected (presenting only with muscle cramps for example (Gospe et al., 1989)) or even asymptomatic 'BMD' patients' are discovered with the same kind of genotype and protein pattern. There is no clear explanation for why they have a different presentation of disease. However, in the few patients where dystrophinopathy presents as a predominant or isolated cardiomyopathy (Muntoni et al., 1994, 1997; Milasin et al., 1996; Ferlini et al., 1998), the mutations reported have been unusual (Muntoni et al., 1994, 1997; Milasin et al., 1996; Ferlini et al., 1998), most sited in or around the muscle promoter, sparing the brain and Purkinje cell promoter, and allowing upregulation of their products to a degree in muscle that is sufficient to prevent any symptomatic muscle weakness. Those patients with dystrophinopathy and cardiac disease alone do, however, represent a very specific group: it is important to realise that in all affected male patients with dystrophin abnormalities, there is a risk of cardiac involvement to some extent, irrespective of the site of the mutation (Nigro et al., 1994; Ishikawa et al., 1995; Melacini et al., 1996). The situation in respect to cardiac involvement in dystrophinopathy carriers is less clear-cut, though some studies show a very high proportion of carriers having cardiomyopathy (Politano et al., 1996). Intellectual impairment is another part of the phenotype of dystrophinopathy that appears to show no clear correlation with mutation site or type (Appleton et al., 1991; Hodgson et al., 1992; Bresolin et al., 1994; North et al., 1996). It may also be variable within families.

The following discussion will focus on DMD, as this is the condition for which genetic counselling and testing is overwhelmingly sought. The principles, however, apply equally to the investigation of the dystrophin gene and protein in families with milder disease.

The approach to a family with DMD
Establish the diagnosis, generate prognostic information and define the mutation
The diagnosis of DMD should be straightforward and in establishing the diagnosis and prognosis gene and protein analysis are complementary. A muscle biopsy from a patient with DMD will always show a severe reduction in the level of dystrophin. Residual levels may correlate with a slightly better than average prognosis and as such be useful information for the family and their physician. There are some features of genetic analysis in dystrophinopathy that are extremely straightforward, while others are very complex. At least part of this complexity reflects the fact that the dystrophin gene is exceptionally large (with 79 exons) (Roberts et al., 1992). However, in 60% of cases, a deletion will be present in the dystrophin gene. Deletions tend to cluster in two particular regions of the gene, with up to 35% of deletions in a proximal 'hotspot' and 65% in the central rod domain, a fact that is exploited in the sets of multiplex PCR primers which have been developed to study the dystrophin gene (Chamberlain et al., 1988; Beggs et al., 1990). Using a combination of these sets of primers, and relying on the presence of these hot spots, means that approximately 98% of all deletions will be detected using this cheap and simple test. Where a deletion is identified by PCR, this is a very useful piece of information. However, the use of this test alone has its limitations: for example, missing rarer deletions, outside the most typical hotspots. It will also not define the extent of all deletions, again a point of some importance in helping to determine progno-

sis. From a practical viewpoint, it is important to realise that even patients with milder forms of dystrophinopathy may present early (Bushby and Gardner-Medwin, 1993); consequently, it is vital to obtain as much prognostic information as possible for counselling the family. No single result will determine prognosis alone, but assessment of a child's physical prowess compared with other affected children of the same age, combined with knowledge of the extent and type of deletion (frameshifting or not) and also the abundance of protein produced, will give the best possible guide to outcome.

If PCR analysis fails to predict the effect of the deletion found on the open reading frame, or if no deletion is detected by PCR at all, then further analysis (typically by Southern blotting in the first instance) is required. A number of cDNA probes are used to cover all the exons of the gene, allowing analysis of exons not included in the PCR sets. These techniques may also be successful at clarifying the presence of duplications in the dystrophin gene (present in around 5% of all cases) though more specialized analysis such as pulsed field gel electrophoresis (PFGE) may be better for the identification of duplications.

If none of these methods is successful in determining the mutation, the techniques needed to search for point mutations, which account for the remaining pathogenic mutations in the gene, are much more complex and specialized, and are generally available through a few laboratories only. Techniques that have been applied to searching for dystrophin point mutations include SSCP (single-strand conformation polymorphism), DGGE (denaturing gradient gel electrophoresis) and PTT (the protein truncation test) (Bakker and van Ommen, 1999). As with most scenarios where several techniques have been applied to solve a problem, none is perfect and all are very time-consuming, partly because there is no clustering of point mutations in the deletion hotspots or elsewhere in this huge gene. A record of the point mutations detected in the dystrophin gene and the methods used to identify them is available through the Leiden muscular dystrophy database (http://www.dmd.nl). Despite the difficulties in this analysis, there is no doubt that finding a mutation by one of these means may dramatically simplify things for the counselling of family members (see Figure 35.3, below). In some scenarios then, it is worthwhile pursuing this expensive search to its limits. It may also become the case that direct detection of the mutation is a prerequisite for treatment if gene-based therapy becomes a reality.

Carrier status of at-risk female relatives
The new mutation rate in DMD is high. Now that carrier testing has been available to affected families for many

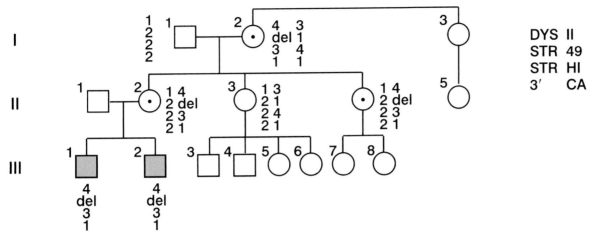

Fig. 35.1. The diagnosis of Duchenne muscular dystrophy (DMD) in child 1 of the third generation (III₁) was established by absent dystrophin and a deletion of exon 46–52 in muscle biopsy at the age of 4½ years. His parents had been concerned about his mobility for 2 years before the diagnosis was made but he was not referred for diagnosis until he started school, at which stage his teachers noticed that he could not get up from the floor without difficulty. At the time of his diagnosis, his parents expressed concerns about their younger son III₂ then aged 1½ years. Subsequent analysis of serum creatine kinase in this child revealed a level of 20 000 Iu/l, confirming that he too was affected. The delay in the diagnosis in III₁ denied the parents the opportunity for the family to seek prenatal diagnosis in their second pregnancy (Bushby, 1999). Molecular analysis in II₂ subsequently confirmed that not only she but also her mother (I₂) and one of her two sisters (II₄) were carriers of the same deletion, despite there having been no prior family history of DMD. Testing can now be offered to I₃ and her daughter, and to III₇ and III₈ when they are old enough, while the risk to III₅ and III₆ can be excluded.

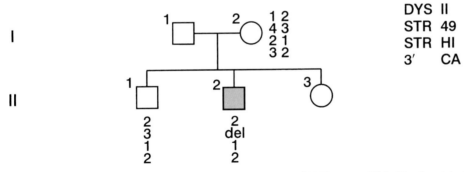

Fig. 35.2. Child II₂ has Duchenne dystrophy (DMD); the diagnosis of DMD was established by absent dystrophin in his biopsy and by the demonstration of a dystrophin deletion of exons 47–53. Subsequent examination of his mother demonstrated that she was heterozygous for STR 49 which is within her son's deletion. Therefore, she is not a somatic carrier of the mutation in her son. Her sisters and other female relatives in the family are not at risk of being carriers. The risk to her daughter depends on which X chromosome has been transmitted to her, as the possibility of germline mosaicism for the mutation exists. If she has inherited the same maternal X chromosome as her brother, her risk of being a carrier will be up to 20%, though the theoretically lower risk of germline mosaicism with distal dystrophin deletions means that this figures is probably an overestimate. This can be tested directly using these markers including STR 49 when she is old enough. For I₂ the risk in a subsequent male pregnancy of having an affected boy also relates to the risk of germline mosaicism, which can be tested directly by looking for the deletion in a chorion villus biopsy sample.

years, the vast majority of affected boys are born to mothers with no previous family history of the disorder. Having said that, these women may still be carriers of DMD. They may have inherited the DMD mutation from their mother, who even in the absence of a family history may still be a carrier (Figure 35.1). Alternatively, the affected child's mother may have a new mutation of the dystrophin gene, which may be on either the grandmaternal or grandpaternal chromosome. Finally, it is possible that the mutation arose in the maternal germline, with the mother not being a somatic carrier at all (Figure 35.2). Each scenario carries significantly different risks for the rest of

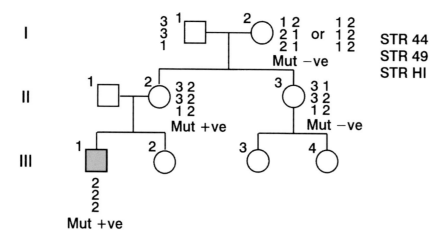

Fig. 35.3. Individual III₁ was diagnosed as having Duchenne muscular dystrophy (DMD) at the age of 3½ years with absent dystrophin on his muscle biopsy. Deletion analysis first by polymerase chain reaction and subsequently by Southern blotting showed no deletion. Haplotypes across the dystrophin gene were constructed for his mother, grandmother and aunt as shown. A crossover between STR 44 and STR 49 complicated the identification of the X chromosome at risk in this family, with II₃ sharing the X chromosome with her sister II₂ and nephew III₁ 3′ to STR 49. As serum creatine kinase levels were moderately elevated in both his mother (II₂) and aunt (II₃), no definitive reassurance about their carrier status could be offered to either. Point mutation analysis in III₁ revealed a G–A transversion in exon 50 present in his mother but not his grandmother or aunt. Here, resolving the issue of carrier status relied completely on the direct illustration of the point mutation, with its absence in I₂ and II₃ proving that the mutation was de novo in II₂.

the family, and the key issue to resolve first is the carrier status of the mother.

In the presence of a known dystrophin gene deletion in the affected child, this may be relatively straightforward (Peters et al., 1997). Various techniques exist to establish carrier status where a deletion is known, including analysis of common polymorphisms (short tandem repeats or STRs) across the dystrophin gene. If a polymorphism exists that is within the deletion, then it is often very straightforward to establish if a woman is heterozygous (implying she is not a carrier) or hemizygous (implying that she is) at that locus (Figs. 35.1 and 35.2). Dosage analysis may also be practical, particularly if automated analysis is available (Abbs and Bobrow, 1992). FISH (fluorescence in site hybridization) analysis using cosmid clones within a deletion is also an excellent method for establishing carrier status, providing the facilities exist, and PFGE (pulsed field gel electrophoresis) is an alternative technique (Cockburn and Miciak, 1992). Once a point mutation has been found in an affected male patient, the same mutation can be sought in females at risk of being carriers (Fig. 35.3) (Lenk et al., 1994). In short, the relative ease of being able to determine carrier status in women at risk of being carriers of DMD where the mutation in the family is known means that establishing the mutation in an affected individual in the family is of paramount importance.

If the mutation cannot be established in an affected indi-

vidual either because of methodological restrictions or because no samples are available from affected relatives, the absolute determination of carrier status may be much more difficult. A number of specialized tests have been proposed to detect unknown mutations in females at risk, but none is universally available (Roberts et al., 1990; Roest et al., 1993). Indirect tests such as haplotype analysis using the many polymorphisms that are present across the dystrophin gene allows the X chromosome at risk to be identified, but the high rate of recombination across the gene may lead to pitfalls in this analysis (Fig. 35.3) (Peters et al., 1997; Bakker and van Ommen, 1999). Inevitably, families still come to light where affected individuals died without samples being stored for DNA analysis. Occasionally stored Guthrie cards or frozen muscle biopsy material may be found, providing the template for direct mutation detection, and such material may be invaluable. Without such samples, direct mutation analysis in individuals at risk of being carriers may be successful (Fig. 35.4), though the limitations of the tests available at this stage means that even a negative result (no mutation found) does not rule out carrier status absolutely.

Germline mosaicism is of much more than theoretical importance in dystrophinopathy. Even where the mother of an affected boy has been shown not to be a somatic carrier of the dystrophin deletion, there is a risk of around 14–20% of having another affected child associated with

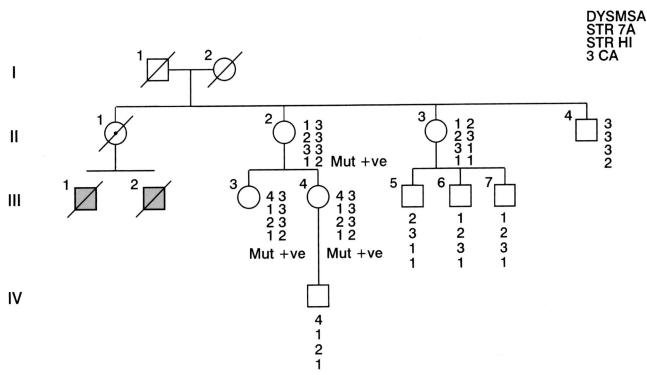

Fig. 35.4. In this family, individual III$_4$ presented when her son was a few weeks old, having just found out about the family history of DMD in her cousins who had died many years before. Her son's creatine kinase levels were normal, excluding DMD in him, but with her anxiety levels raised, she was keen to pursue further genetic testing, as was her sister. Haplotypes were constructed for the extended family, including all available living males. Individual II$_3$ could be reassured that she was not a carrier, as she had transmitted both of her X chromosomes to healthy sons. Individual II$_2$ shared an X chromosome in common with her unaffected brother; however, consistently high serum creatine levels in II$_2$, III$_3$ and III$_4$ led to problems in excluding carrier risk in these women. Samples were, therefore, analysed for the presence of their unknown mutation by pulsed field gel electrophoresis and a duplication in the 3′ end of the gene was found in II$_2$, III$_3$ and III$_4$, confirming that they were all carriers. It is likely that I$_2$ was a germline mosaic for this mutation on the chromosome identified by the haplotype 3-3-3-2.

the transmission of the X chromosome in their affected son (Bakker et al., 1989; van Essen et al., 1992). It would appear that this reflects a tendency for dystrophin deletions to occur at an early stage of mitotic germline proliferation. It has been calculated that the risk of germline mosaicism is different depending on the site of the deletion, with a 30% recurrence risk associated with proximal deletions and a 4% risk for distal deletions (Passos-Bueno et al., 1992), suggesting possibly that proximal deletions may be more prone to occur earlier in germline proliferation.

In any case, this relatively high frequency of germline (and in fact also somatic) mosaicism for dystrophin mutations does translate into a very important practical message for genetic counselling. The mother of an affected boy can never be reassured completely that she has no risk of having another affected child, though usually very specific prenatal diagnosis will be available. Any daughters

will also be at risk of being carriers (see Fig. 35.2). Equally, in a sibship where a woman has been found to be the first somatic carrier of a mutation, her sisters will be at risk of being carriers as well if they have inherited the at-risk haplotype. This appears to be irrespective of whether the mutation is on the maternal or paternal chromosome.

It is very important to realise that with changing molecular techniques the message given to a family may have altered over time. This may not always be unmitigated good news for the family. Women may in the past have been given a high risk of being a carrier based on the best possible information at the time, for example pedigree analysis in association with creatine kinase estimations. Based on this advice, women may have chosen not to have children or may have opted for prenatal diagnosis by fetal sexing resulting in male terminations. With the benefit of new molecular information, some of these women will be shown not to be carriers. While this may be good news for the future, the emotional stress of finding out this kind of information at a stage when irretrievable life decisions have been made needs to be taken into account in the counselling situation.

Prenatal diagnosis

Prenatal diagnosis, typically by DNA analysis of material obtained at chorionic villous biopsy, is usually readily available to carriers or suspected carriers of dystrophinopathy; it may be up to 100% accurate based on the mutation known in the family. Where haplotyping is used, the accuracy depends on the number of informative markers used across the gene to minimize the chance of a recombination in the gene going undetected. Preimplantation diagnosis is technically feasible but as yet of limited availability (Holding et al., 1993). If carrier testing issues cannot be resolved prior to a pregnancy, or if the mutation cannot be defined, then two methods may be useful during pregnancy itself. Fetal muscle biopsy at around 18 weeks of gestation has been shown to be useful in determining the affected status of a fetus at high risk (for example, as determined by fetal sexing and haplotype analysis by chorionic villous biopsy earlier in the pregnancy) (Bieber et al., 1989). However, the relatively late stage at which this has to be performed, coupled with a predicted high risk for the procedure, has led to few centres generally adopting the technique.

Alternatively, if a pregnancy is terminated after a 'high risk' prediction on haplotype analysis of chorion villous biopsy material, the examination of dystrophin in the fetal muscle can give a definitive answer about carrier status, as well as providing material for direct demonstration of the mutation for future pregnancies (Fig. 35.5) (Ginjaar et al., 1991).

Dystrophinopathy: differential diagnosis

Dystrophinopathy remains the most likely diagnosis in a child or adult presenting with progressive proximal muscle weakness and elevated serum creatine kinase especially in males. However, there may occasionally be problems in confirming the diagnosis.

- Where DNA analysis is used alone and no mutation is found. As most laboratories have access only to deletion analysis by PCR (with or without Southern blotting) for DNA diagnosis of dystrophinopathy, the diagnosis cannot be confirmed in the 40% of patients who do not have a deletion. Here the combined use of protein analysis (on muscle biopsy) and DNA analysis is essential.
- Where the sarcoglycanopathy occurs. The sarcoglycanopathies (see below) may clinically resemble dystrophinopathy and may cause particular confusion as

dystrophin may occasionally be mildly abnormal. Appropriate diagnostic techniques, as described below, should discriminate the various types of limb girdle muscular dystrophy (LGMD); again it is likely that a combination of DNA and protein analysis will be necessary to provide a full diagnosis.

- Where the patient is an isolated manifesting carrier of a dystrophinopathy. The proportion of carriers of DMD who may manifest symptoms of the disease is traditionally quoted as at least 10%, though most will have only minor symptoms and only a very small proportion will have disease of severity comparable to that in male patients. Diagnosis is particularly difficult in isolated manifesting carriers of dystrophinopathy, leading to problems in genetic counselling. The discovery of a mosaic pattern of dystrophin labelling on immunological analysis of muscle biopsy sections in a female patient with muscular dystrophy is suggestive of a diagnosis of manifesting carrier of dystrophinopathy (Hoffman et al., 1992) though particular care needs to be taken in distinguishing this diagnosis from sarcoglycanopathy (see Fig. 35.9 below). In an isolated female patient with a diagnosis of manifesting carrier, this may be supported by the finding of skewed X-inactivation. The finding of the dystrophin mutation in an isolated female is essential to confirm the diagnosis; however, as already discussed, this may be problematic. In the absence of a known mutation, providing genetic counselling to a manifesting carrier and her female relations can be extremely difficult.

Myotonic dystrophy

Myotonic dystrophy is a relatively common autosomal dominant disease (incidence approximately 1 in 8500) (Brewster et al., 1998), and one that carries a number of important implications for genetic counselling. A single mutation type can be identified as responsible for all cases of myotonic dystrophy worldwide and may in fact be able to be traced to only a few ancestral chromosomes. Very few new mutations are known. A CTG expansion in the 3′ region of a gene designated *DMPK* (myotonic dystrophin protein kinase) is pathognemonic for the disorder, though as this expansion may influence the expression of a number of surrounding genes the molecular pathogenesis of the disease remains unclear (Boucher et al., 1995; Klesert et al., 1997; Sabourin et al., 1997). Myotonic dystrophy, therefore, represents an example of a disease where a very precise molecular diagnosis is possible and often technically straightforward (Fig. 35.6) without there being as yet a totally clear idea of how this mutation causes disease. There are a number of unusual observed features of the

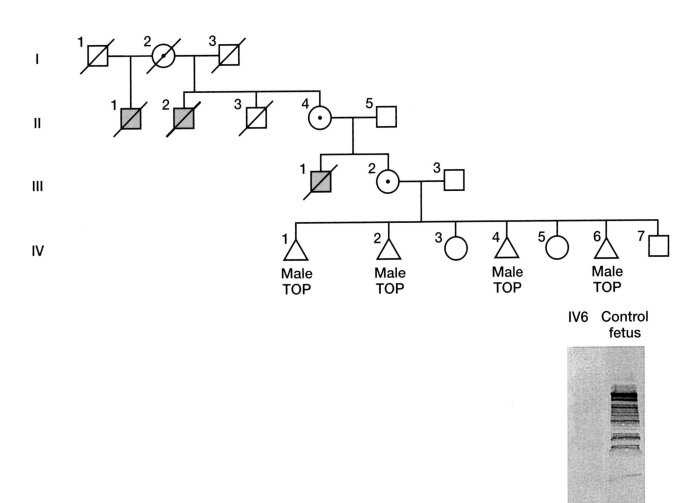

Fig. 35.5. This large family had had many affected members with Duchenne dystrophy (DMD) in the past and individual II_4 is an obligate carrier. Her daughter III_2 was found to have very high serum creatine kinase levels ($>700\,IU/l$) and was counselled that she was at high risk of being a carrier of DMD. Unfortunately, no samples were stored from III_1 who died before molecular analysis was possible. As DNA probes became available, a high-risk haplotype could be identified in II_4 and III_2, and III_2 was advised that prenatal diagnosis would be available with an accuracy of 90% allowing for the possibilities of intragenic recombination with the DNA probes available at that stage. Given the trauma that III_2 associated with growing up with a brother with DMD, she perceived a 10% risk of error as too high to contemplate. She therefore chose to terminate male pregnancies even where prenatal diagnosis on chorionic villous biopsy showed a male fetus to have inherited the low-risk haplotype, which occurred on two occasions (IV_2 and IV_4). Pregnancy IV_6 was a male predicted to have inherited the high-risk haplotype, and following the termination of this pregnancy, muscle from the fetus was examined for dystrophin. This confirmed that the fetus was affected and DNA was extracted and a deletion of exons 19–23 was identified. Based on the 'perfect' DNA test possible in subsequent pregnancies, III_2 was happy to proceed with her seventh pregnancy, which resulted in the birth of a healthy male baby. TOP, termination of pregnancy.

genetics of myotonic dystrophy, some of which can be explained by its being a triplet repeat disorder.

Genotype–phenotype correlation

Myotonic dystrophy is clinically a highly heterogeneous disease. The mildest disease manifestation may be minimal features such as early cataracts or frontal balding.

In the adult-onset form, myotonia may be symptomatic, together with symptoms such as tiredness and muscle weakness. There is around an 80% chance of becoming wheelchair bound in the classical adult myotonic dystrophy, with survival typically to a mean age of around 60 years (de Die-Smulders et al., 1998). The most severe form of myotonic dystrophy is a devastating congenital disease

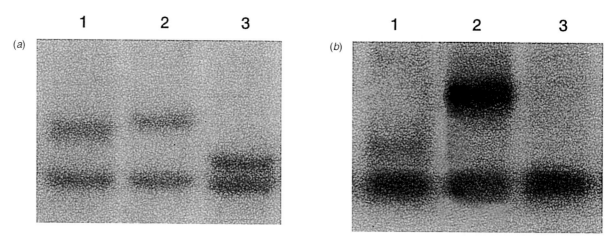

Fig. 35.6. DNA analysis for myotonic dystrophy may be very straightforward. The smallest expansions may be detectable by the polymerase chain reaction (not shown); for larger deletions Southern blotting using a variety of restriction enzyme digests are used. (*a*) DNA digested with *Eco*RI. Lane 1 shows a small expansion in an adult patient with myotonic dystrophy (upper band) and lane 2 an increased expansion in a child with childhood-onset myotonic dystrophy. The lower band in both lanes represents the normal 9 kb allele. Lane 3 shows two normal bands of 9 and 10 kb. (*b*) DNA digested with *Pst*I. Again a moderate expansion in an affected adult is seen in lane 1 and an increased expansion in a child with myotonic dystrophy in lane 2. Lane 3 has only a band of normal size.

with intellectual handicap as well as profound muscle weakness; survival is usually restricted to less than 30 years (Reardon et al., 1993). Affected patients are at risk from cardiac arrhythmias and anaesthetic complications. The clinical variability in myotonic dystrophy is frequently seen in members of the same family, with a tendency for the condition to worsen with successive generations (anticipation). This, and other features of the disease that perplexed those dealing with it for many years, can now be at least partly explained by the behaviour of the CTG expansion. In more than 80% of parent–child pairs, the age of disease onset is younger and CTG size is greater in the children than the parents (Harley et al., 1993; Ashizawa et al., 1996). When CTG repeat length is studied in large populations of affected and unaffected people, a number of conclusions can be drawn about the behaviour of the repeat and broad genotype–phenotype correlations can be determined. In the normal population, a range of 5 to 38 triplet repeats are seen. Typically 42 to around 180 repeats are seen in very-late-onset disease with minor manifestations. In classical or adult-onset disease, the range of repeats observed is very wide, from a few hundred to several hundred repeats, while in congenital myotonic dystrophy typically over 1000 triplets are seen (Cheng et al., 1996; Hamshere et al., 1999). These correlations are not absolute and relate more to populations than to individual patients, especially as somatic instability of the CTG expansion is a feature of the disease (Joseph et al., 1997). This leads to continued uncertainty in the interpretation of individual test results especially where prenatal diagnosis

has been requested, where the critically important question is whether a child will be congenitally affected or not. Presymptomatic testing is less problematic in these respects as individuals who are truly asymptomatic in adult life are unlikely to experience very severe disease; however, the size of any expansion detected will not absolutely predict severity. It can be argued that there may be some benefits to at-risk individuals in knowing affected status in terms of avoidance of anaesthetics and monitoring for cardiac complications, as well as for the implications for their offspring.

Risks to offspring

Risks to individuals with myotonic dystrophy planning to have a family can be given based partly on the results of molecular analysis and partly on the observations made over many years of families with this condition. Various considerations need to be taken into account when counselling affected women in particular. There is a significantly higher incidence of neonatal deaths to these mothers, with 16% of all liveborn of affected mothers dying within a few days compared with 1.9% in the normal population; obstetric complications are common (Brewster et al., 1998; Rudnik-Schoneborn et al., 1998). The risk of having a congenitally affected child for any female gene carrier is 3–9%. This risk rises in a classically affected mother or a mother with a previously congenitally affected child to as high as 20–37%. Counselling of affected women is a key part of the management of families with myotonic dystrophy. This process can be complicated by the intellectual difficulties that can be seen in myotonic dystrophy, as well as the altered affect, which may be a part of the condition (Bungener et al., 1998; Delaporte, 1998). Very few cases of congenitally affected children born to affected fathers have been reported (Nakagawa et al., 1994; de Die-Smulders et al., 1997); a factor in this may be the reduced fertility in affected males with large expansions. Specific issues also relate to the difference in the transmission of the triplet repeat in males compared with females, with the CTG repeat behaving differently in the male and female germline. Overall, there is at least a 90–95% chance of enlargement in repeat size with any transmission of alleles greater than 80 CTGs in size (Harley et al., 1993; Ashizawa et al., 1994a,b; Monketon et al., 1995). Expansions of over 20 times the parental repeat length can be seen, but only where the parental allele is greater than 100 CTGs in length. Expansion lengths of over 1000 triplets continue to expand only in the female germline, with an apparent barrier to this huge expansion in the male germline. This contrasts to the situation with small repeats, where expansions can be greater on male transmission. Just as the triplet repeat length can increase with germline transmission, so it can contract as well, with the greatest tendency to contraction being in males with large repeat size (contraction of repeat size is seen in only around 3% of female transmission compared with about 10% of male transmissions) (Ashizawa et al., 1994a,b; Magee and Hughes, 1998).

At present, therefore, the presence of an easily detectable mutation in myotonic dystrophy has become the main diagnostic tool and allows the identification of gene carriers in known families, with the benefits of health surveillance and genetic counselling that can accrue from this information. Prenatal diagnosis is also widely offered, especially to affected women. However, while the issues of intergenerational instability in this disorder remain incompletely understood, there are continued elements of uncertainty in risk assessment. Future developments will include the improved precision of this process.

Myotonic dystrophy: differential diagnosis

In the vast majority of patients with typical features of myotonic dystrophy, the characteristic DNA abnormality will be found. Where the CTG repeat expansion is not present, however, there are a number of differential diagnoses to be considered.

- In congenitally affected children, myotubular myopathy may show phenotypic overlap (see below).
- A second myotonic dystrophy locus on chromosome 3 (DM2) has been reported (Ranum et al., 1998). The family in which linkage was demonstrated have a number of clinical features in common with those of myotonic dystrophy, including cataracts, baldness and predominantly distal muscle weakness and wasting; however, there was only electrophysiological evidence of myotonia.
- An autosomal dominant disorder known as proximal myotonic myopathy (PROMM) has been recognized and is likely itself to be heterogeneous. The key clinical features of this condition include proximal weakness mainly affecting the thighs, variable myotonia or stiffness, cataracts identical to those seen in myotonic dystrophy and frequent muscle pain (Moxley, 1996; Abbruzzese et al., 1996). These patients are at risk of cardiac conduction defects and anaesthetic complications similar to those with myotonic dystrophy, and may show additional features such as endocrine disturbance, white matter changes on magnetic resonance imaging and cognitive disturbance (Moxley et al., 1998a,b). At least some PROMM families show linkage to the DM2 locus on chromosome 3, suggesting that there may be allelic heterogeneity at this locus or that there may be overlapping phenotypes within a spectrum of disease (Ricker et al., 1999)
- While they may present with myotonia as a prominent sign, the nondystrophic myotonias (ion channel disorders, see below) frequently show major clinical differences from myotonic dystrophy, especially in their lack of multisystem involvement; they should not cause major diagnostic confusion.

Facioscapulohumeral muscular dystrophy

FSHD is another autosomal dominant muscle disease for which molecular genetic testing has become the diagnostic 'gold standard', even in the absence of an absolute understanding of its molecular pathology. The vast majority of families with FSHD are associated with linkage to chromosome 4q35, though there remain a few families in whom linkage to chromosome 4 has probably been excluded. No alternative locus has been identified in these families (Padberg, 1999).

Molecular analysis

Although the FSHD gene has not yet been cloned, the demonstration of a disease-associated deletion of an integral number of copies of a tandemly repeated 3.3 kb sequence on chromosome 4q35 can be used in diagnosis of FSHD with 95% specificity and sensitivity (Bakker et al., 1996). Affected individuals typically show a DNA fragment size of <30 kb and unaffected individuals a DNA fragment of >40 kb detected using a double digest system and a DNA probe known as p13E-11. This test is robust provided appropriate safeguards are taken: there is an important 'grey area' in allele size as between 33 and 40kb it can be hard to designate absolutely affected status (Ott, 1985; Lunt, 1998). In addition, the region deleted on chromosome 4q35 is highly homologous to a region on chromosome 10q26, with the degree of homology between the two regions such that up to 20% of the population will have exchanged material between the two chromosomes, leading to potential difficulties in interpretation of the test results (van Deutekom et al., 1996). This underlines the fact that, while this is a highly specific and sensitive test for FSHD, the test is still not directly assessing the FSHD gene itself, and as such it counts as an indirect rather than a truly 'direct' test for the gene. The complexity of the region means that some results will be difficult to interpret definitively. Providing these caveats are taken into account, this analysis has taken a rightful place in the diagnostic setting, with an important role in clinical diagnosis, presymptomatic testing and prenatal diagnosis, where this is sought.

The ability to diagnose FSHD in this way has led to the recognition of a high rate of new mutations. Before a specific test for FSHD was available, it could be hard to decide whether a minor degree of facial or shoulder girdle weakness in a parent of an affected child was significant or not, and the occurrence of two or more affected children in families without a clearly affected parent led to the suggestion that there might be an autosomal recessive form of the disease. When apparently de novo cases are reappraised in the light of molecular genetic testing, the deletion is found in a nonpenetrant parent in around 12% of cases (Ricci et al., 1999). It can now be demonstrated directly that the proportion of new mutations ranges between 9.6% (probably an underestimate) and 33% (perhaps a somewhat biased group) (Wijmenga et al., 1992; Zatz et al., 1995; Bakker et al., 1996). Germline and somatic mosaicism for the deletion have now frequently been reported; consequently even in the absence of an affected parent siblings of an isolated case probably have a risk in the region of 10% of being affected as well (Bakker et al., 1996). In the vast majority of parents mosaic for the mutation, the mother was the mosaic parent (Ricci et al., 1999).

Genotype–phenotype correlation
FSHD is a highly variable disease. It can occasionally present in an early-onset, or infantile, form where facial weakness is usually extreme, progression of muscle weakness may in some cases be very rapid, and there is a frequent association with hearing loss and retinal telangiectasia, associated signs that can also be found but

which are rarely symptomatic in less severely affected individuals (Brouwer et al., 1991, 1994, 1995). These children may present major problem in rehabilitation because of the combination of profound hip extensor weakness, hip flexion contractures and extreme lumbar lordosis (Shapiro et al., 1991). Overall, however, presentation in the first 5 years of life is seen in only around 5% of all gene carriers, with penetrance rising to 21% for ages 5–9, 58% for 10–14, 86% for 15–19 and 95% for ages 20 years and over, though these figures have not been revisited in the light of molecular diagnosis, which may reveal a higher than previously suspected rate of nonpenetrance (Lunt and Harper, 1991). There is a sex difference in severity of the disease, with mean age of onset slightly lower in males and a higher proportion of females than males amongst asymptomatic cases (Padberg, 1982; Zatz et al., 1998). A statistical correlation appears to exist between fragment size and severity especially in sporadic cases (Lunt et al., 1995a,b), with the smallest fragments (and therefore the largest deletions) detected in the youngest onset and most severely affected, who often tend to be de novo cases (Fig. 35.7). This correlation has been extended to predict a severe course in patients with the largest deletions (Ricci et al., 1999). This does not, however, account for all of the variability seen in the disease; certainly within families, where all affected individuals have the same fragment size, a huge range of severity may be seen, with some reports suggestive of a degree of anticipation even in the absence of any evidence for a dynamic mutation (Zatz et al., 1995). Consequently the counselling of a family must include the lack of certainty about likely progression of the disease: while a gene carrier can be identified through the use of DNA testing, this carries with it no prediction as to the likely course of the disease. This is a critical point for discussion in families planning presymptomatic or prenatal diagnosis. It remains to be seen whether the identification of the FSHD gene itself and its pathological mechanism will add further information to the testing available.

Facioscapulohumeral dystrophy: differential diagnosis
The clinical phenotype associated with FSHD, though variable, is usually very characteristic, and in most cases the diagnosis is readily confirmed by DNA analysis. In the cases where a chromosome 4q35 deletion cannot be demonstrated, further molecular analysis will not necessarily be easily available or practical, though it must be stressed that until the absolute mechanism for disease production in FSHD is elucidated, these patients may still have 4q35-

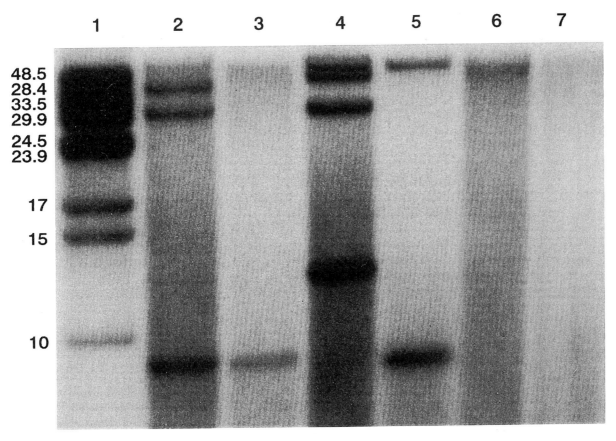

Fig. 35.7. Double-digest Southern blot probed with p13E11, which detects a short band in chromosome 4q35-linked facioscapulohumeral dystrophy. Lane 1 shows size markers; lanes 2 and 3 contain DNA from the father of the affected girl, whose DNA is in lanes 4 and 5. Her mother's DNA is in lanes 6 and 7. The bands at around 9 kb in the father's samples are constant bands of cross-reacting DNA from the Y chromosome. In the daughter's sample, a short band of approximately 12 kb, which reduced further on double digest, can be clearly seen. This band is not present in either of her parents, thereby proving that her disease is the result of a new dominant mutation.

linked disease. Potential problems in diagnosis occur in the occasional sporadic case or family with atypical clinical features – especially where facial weakness is very minor or absent. These patients are likely to have been misdiagnosed as 'scapulohumeral' muscular dystrophy, or a form of LGMD.

Spinal muscular atrophy

SMA is by far the most common autosomal recessive neuromuscular disorder, with a carrier frequency in most populations as high as 1/50 (Pearn, 1973). Variability in the severity of the disease led to the classification of SMA into three broad groups, with type I the most severe, presenting within the first six months of life. These children never achieve independent sitting and typically die by the age of 2 years. In type II SMA, children present before the age of 18 months and are unable to stand or walk. Type III SMA is most variable of all, characterized by onset after the age of 18 months with chronic proximal muscle weakness and variable disease course (Munsat, 1991; Dubowitz, 1991). Consistent reports of intrafamilial variation, as well as the continuum of severity which is seen in SMA, have always suggested that the varying degrees of severity in fact involve different expression of the same or similar genetic fault, and linkage to chromosome 5q in all three child-hood types of SMA was confirmed in 1990 (Gilliam et al., 1990; Davies et al., 1991; Brahe et al., 1995). By contrast,

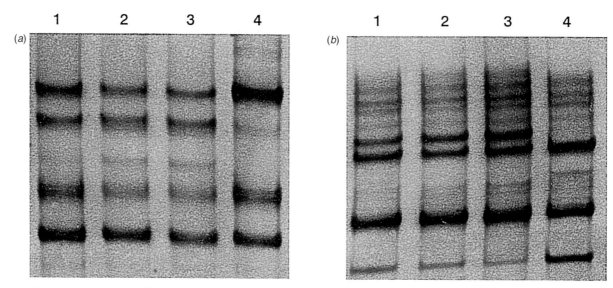

Fig. 35.8. Analysis of the gene *SMN*, which is associated with spinal muscular atrophy. (*a*) Analysis of exon 7 and (*b*) analysis of exon 8. The different band patterns in lane 4 of each part of the figure illustrate a homozygous deletion.

adult-onset and complicated forms are much more heterogeneous and there is no clear understanding of the molecular basis of the non-5q-linked SMAs at this stage (Brahe et al., 1995; Vuopala et al., 1995; Zerres et al., 1995; Zerres and Davies, 1999). In milder SMA, the later the age at onset, the less likely it is that a chromosome 5q deletion will be found. Types of early-onset SMA that are now felt to be other than chromosome 5q-linked diseases include diaphragmatic SMA and SMA and olivopontocerebellar atrophy. However, a few cases of SMA associated with large chromosome 5q deletions may present with a severe neo-natal onset, often with congenital contractures. These unusual presentations are relatively rare, and most of the issues relating to genetic counselling in SMA are centred around childhood-onset disease, and in particular type I and type II families.

Molecular genetics

The identification of two SMA-associated genes (the survival motor neuron gene *SMN* and the neuronal apoptosis inhibitory protein gene *NAIP* (Lefebvre et al., 1995; Roy et al., 1995; Melki, 1998)) has revealed a striking degree of complexity of the SMA region on chromosome 5. A third gene p44 (Burglen et al., 1997; Carter et al., 1997) in the same region has also been identified. All three genes are present in at least two copies, referred to as telomeric or centromeric depending on their relative position on chromosome 5q within the SMA critical region. Telomeric *SMN* is generally regarded as most closely linked with the production of an SMA phenotype. The telomeric copy of

SMN produces mainly full-length transcripts, while the transcripts produced from the centromeric copy are much more variable, with a range of isoforms seen. Subtle nucleotide differences between the telomeric and centromeric copies of *SMN* allow the two to be distinguished, thereby permitting the detection of homozygous deletions of exons 7 and 8 of the telomeric copies of *SMN* (Fig. 35.8). This is the type of mutation found in 93% of patients with SMA, with a further 5.6% having a homozygous deletion of exon 7 only. In rare patients without homozygous deletions, a range of missense mutations or microdeletions have been described (Talbot et al., 1997; reviewed in Biros and Forrest, 1999). The pattern of deletions or mutations of telomeric *SMN* do not distinguish between the various types of SMA, though in the vast majority of cases the detection of a homozygous *SMN* deletion is confirmatory of the diagnosis. There is a broad correlation of the number of copies of the centromeric gene in the absence of the telomeric copy with severity of the disease (Zerres and Davies, 1999). This is not, however, currently of use in clinical practice.

Functional telomeric *NAIP* has a centromeric pseudo-copy that can be distinguished by the absence in the centromeric copy of two exons. Homozygous telomeric *NAIP* deletions are seen in about 45% of patients with type I SMA and in only 12–18% of those with type II and type III. No mutations other than homozygous deletions have been described in *NAIP*. *SMN* is also homozygously deleted in 98% of patients with *NAIP* deletions; data are lacking, however, on whether the remaining 2% had another type of

SMN mutation. In a clinically typical patient it may, therefore, be worthwhile to look for an *NAIP* deletion even if an *SMN* deletion has not been detected.

The role of p44 in SMA is not clear. It is probably deleted in large-scale deletions that also include *SMN* and *NAIP*.

Applications to genetic counselling

Linkage of SMA to chromosome 5q was quickly taken into clinical practice for prenatal diagnosis, with a high uptake of this test once it was made available (Daniels et al., 1992). Following the discovery of the SMA-associated genes, the homozygous absence or mutation in the telomeric copy of *SMN* in the presence of clinical symptoms has become the major diagnostic tool. If both copies of the telomeric *SMN* are present, the diagnosis is highly unlikely. The only confounding factor is the small number of asymptomatic parents or siblings of patients with SMA who have been shown to be homozygously deleted for the telomeric copy of *SMN* as well, suggesting that in a few cases other factors may compensate for homozygous loss of telomeric *SMN* (Hahnen et al., 1995; Wang et al., 1996; Somerville et al., 1997). In around 2% of patients with SMA, a de novo mutation not present in either parent will be found in the child (Wirth et al., 1997). Despite the molecular complexity of the SMA region on chromosome 5, the subtle differences between the centromeric and telomeric copies of *SMN* and *NAIP* allow relatively simple DNA tests based on SSCP analysis or PCR followed by restriction enzyme digestion to confirm diagnosis in an individual with a clinical phenotype suggestive of SMA or to allow specific prenatal diagnosis in a family with a proven history of SMA (Fig. 35.8). Given the possibility of parental homozygosity for the telomeric deletion, linkage is often performed alongside deletion analysis.

These applications represent a tremendous advance in options available to families affected with SMA who are seeking prenatal diagnosis, but carrier testing unfortunately remains problematic (Wang et al., 1996; McAndrew et al., 1997; Zerres and Davies, 1999). The determination of dosage of the telomeric copy of *SMN* should theoretically be a relatively straightforward analysis. However, given the complexity of the region, stringent safeguards need to be followed to confirm heterozygosity, including the incorporation of internal controls (typically amplification of the cystic fibrosis gene). A further potential cause of confusion will be the proportion of individuals who have more than one telomeric copy of *SMN* on a single chromosome. This has been estimated to be 3–4%. These limitations need to be taken into account in offering carrier testing, which at present is available only through specialized laboratories.

Heterogeneity: different genes for apparently similar diseases and different diseases caused by mutations in the same gene

Heterogeneity is a major area where pitfalls can be encountered in genetic counselling; this applies to a greater or lesser extent to most groups of muscle diseases. In some diseases, the heterogeneity can be resolved fairly readily, while in others it may take a complex series of investigations to determine the exact nature of a particular problem. In other situations this cannot yet be done, leaving the situation inevitably uncertain.

Relatively minor heterogeneity may be encountered where a predominant gene or gene defect is responsible for the vast majority of cases of a clinically recognizable disorder. So as already discussed, there are rare reports of patients with FSHD who are clinically indistinguishable from those with a chromosome 4 deletion (see above) where molecular genetic analysis has not been informative; in these cases at present no further testing can be offered. Most patients with myotonic dystrophy have a CTG expansion on chromosome 19 (as discussed in more detail above), but rare families have a clinically similar disorder that maps elsewhere. Again, beyond excluding the most common form of myotonic dystrophy, no further testing will be available to these families except if they are large enough for linkage analysis, and even there analysis would only be able to be carried out in research laboratories with a special interest in these disorders. Almost all patients with childhood-onset SMA will be found to have an *SMN* deletion on chromosome 5 (see above), though adult-onset disease may present more problems in achieving a precise diagnosis. Clinical heterogeneity in common muscle diseases is a further consideration. For example in dystrophinopathy, clinical presentation may range from the typical Duchenne presentation, with marked and rapidly progressive muscle weakness and wasting, through the Becker phenotype with much less progressive muscle disease, to a cardiomyopathy phenotype only, or even to asymptomatic disease detected only on investigation. The variation in severity of myotonic dystrophy and its relationship to triplet repeat length is another example of clinical heterogeneity.

Major heterogeneity is encountered in many groups of muscle diseases, and here fairly complex investigations may be necessary to provide a precise diagnosis before any genetic counselling can be provided. Examples of these groups of disorders include the LGMDs, EDMD, congenital muscular dystrophies (CMDs), congenital myopathies and ion channel disorders of muscle. In these conditions, an unqualified diagnosis carries in itself no implications for genetic counselling, and further investigation is imperative before the correct advice can be given. Having said that, investigations may be variably successful at resolving these issues. Moving towards an understanding of the underlying defect in these heterogeneous groups of conditions has elucidated both common and diverse mechanisms of disease: for example the involvement of the various components of the sarcoglycan complex in a relatively clinically similar group of diseases (the LGMDs), and the nuclear envelope proteins emerin and lamin A in the X-linked and autosomal dominant forms of EDMD, respectively. These conclusions have allowed new classifications of these genetic disorders of skeletal muscle.

The limb girdle muscular dystrophies

Under the 'umbrella' category of LGMD, currently 14 different genetic entities can be defined at least by their chromosomal localization, and at least seven are defined directly by the involvement of a particular gene (Table 35.2) (Bushby, 1999). These conditions may be either dominant or recessive and as such carry hugely different implications for recurrence. It is impossible, therefore, to offer any kind of advice to a patient presenting with a simple diagnosis of LGMD in the absence of further information. By contrast, with additional information from the history and examination, as well as most importantly from specialized investigations, a precise diagnosis can probably be reached in the majority of patients with LGMD, provided DNA and even more critically a muscle biopsy sample are available for study. LGMD illustrates an extreme example of heterogeneity at every level: many genes potentially involved, each of which is multiexonic and may contain a large number of different mutations, with very few predominant mutations reported except in some rare founder populations. The prospect of searching for a potentially novel mutation that might reside in any one of a number of different genes is simply not practical, so mutation analysis must be directed by other techniques, chiefly the study of a muscle biopsy with antibodies to the various proteins involved in LGMD. In families of a suitable structure, haplotype analysis may also be helpful in directing the search towards the appropriate gene. Last, but not least, some simple clinical guidelines are also emerging that are beginning to allow the predominant phenotype of the various types of LGMD to be recognized. These conclusions can be integrated into a practical guide to achieving the correct diagnosis.

Diagnostic steps

Step 1 Are alternative diagnoses excluded?
Most forms of LGMD are individually relatively rare in most populations. Therefore, exclusion of more common types of muscular dystrophy remains an important (though no longer the only) part of the diagnostic pathway (Tachi et al., 1990). Dystrophinopathy remains an important differential diagnosis, especially with the sarcoglycanopathies (Jones et al., 1998; Passos-Bueno et al., 1999). In families with dominant disease, the most frequent confusion arises with FSMD (van der Kooi et al., 1994; Bushby, 1999).

Step 2 Is it likely to be recessive or dominant disease?
The autosomal recessive types of LGMD are much more common than the autosomal dominant disorders. However, dominant disease cannot automatically be discounted even in the absence of a positive family history because of the possibility of new dominant mutations. Potential pointers to the presence of dominant disease include a relatively low serum creatine kinase (typically elevated to a far greater degree in recessive disease, but often within the normal range or just above in the genetically defined types of dominant LGMD) or the presence of marked contractures with relatively slowly progressive muscle weakness. Cardiac disease in other family members, even in the absence of a clear history of neuromuscular problems, may indicate the presence of an autosomal dominant type of LGMD and should be investigated further (van der Kooi et al., 1997).

Step 3 How likely is a particular diagnosis?
Because of the rarity of some of the types of LGMD, which to date have been described only in single or a few families, there are practically a smaller number of diagnoses to consider in the individual patient. For example, LGMD1A, which is associated with dysarthria and tight Achilles tendons as well as a proximal myopathy, has been described in a single large North American family only. LGMD1C, where mutations in the gene for caveolin 3 have been described (McNally et al., 1998; Minetti et al., 1998), also appears to be very rare, and LGMD1D, 1E, 2G, 2H and 2I (all, apart from LGMD2G (resulting from mutations in the gene for telethonin), defined so far only by genetic loci) are apparently not common (Moreira et al., 1997; Weiler et al., 1998; Speer et al., 1999). All of the other types of LGMD have been reported worldwide, though with some regional differences in their frequency. Founder mutations have been described for most types of autosomal recessive LGMD, though overall nonrecurrent and highly variable mutations are more common (Bushby, 1999). Epidemiological data based on the ability to diagnose these different groups at the molecular level are still awaited.

Step 4 Precise diagnosis: clinical correlates and diagnostic tools

Some broad conclusions can be drawn about the phenotypes usually associated with the more common genetically defined subgroups of LGMD and these can be used to direct confirmation of the diagnosis.

Autosomal dominant limb girdle dystrophy: type 1B and Emery–Dreifuss dystrophy

LGMD1B results from mutations in the gene for lamin A/C (van der Kooi et al., 1997; Bonne et al., 1999). There is phenotypic heterogeneity for mutations in this gene. Some patients have an Emery–Dreifuss phenotype (see below) with humeroperoneal weakness, contractures at the elbows, Achilles tendons and spine and a prominent cardiac conduction defect, which will require pacing and which may progress to a dilated cardiomyopathy. Other affected individuals may have only cardiac disease or a much more 'pure' LGMD presentation with proximal muscle weakness without contractures (van der Kooi et al., 1996). New dominant mutations in this disease appear to be common, as does germline mosaicism. This is a graphic illustration of the dangers of assuming that siblings with unaffected parents always have recessive disease.

Differential diagnosis

Differential diagnosis of LGMD1B/autosomal dominant EDMD includes several disorders.

- Other forms of autosomal dominant LGMD. At present, apart from caveolin 3 deficiency, which can be demonstrated by mutations in the caveolin 3 gene but seems to be rare, the other autosomal dominant subtypes are so far defined by loci only (Table 35.2).
- X-linked EDMD can be excluded by examination of skin or muscle with antibodies to emerin or by mutation analysis in the emerin gene (Bione et al., 1994; Manilal et al., 1996). Lamin A and emerin are both proteins of the nuclear envelope, suggesting a common pathway for these related diseases.
- Bethlem myopathy involves contractures (typically of the ankles, elbows and fingers) as the predominant presentation (Jobsis et al., 1999). There is an associated degree of muscle weakness that may be progressive. This disorder may present with contractures or torticollis at birth. This is itself a genetically heterogeneous group, with mutations described in each of three genes for collagen VI in different families (*COL6A1, COL6A2, COL6A3*) (Jobsis et al., 1996; Lamande et al., 1998; Pepe et al., 1999).
- Laminin β1-chain deficiency is a secondary manifestation found in adult biopsies in association with a number of different primary muscle diseases. Most frequently, contractures are an important part of the phenotypes in these patients (Taylor et al., 1997). Laminin-β1 deficiency has now been reported as a secondary phenomenon in patients subsequently proven to have either Bethlem myopathy or mutations affecting lamin A (Bonne et al., 1999; Merlini et al., 1999). Whether all patients with this phenotype and secondary laminin-β1 deficiency will turn out to have these primary diseases remains to be seen. Meantime, if laminin-β1 deficiency is seen on a biopsy, there should be a high index of suspicion that this is a dominant disease, especially if the phenotype includes contractures.

Diagnostic tools

Diagnosis of LGMD1B or autosomal dominant EDMD rests on the demonstration of a lamin A mutation. Lamin A staining on a muscle biopsy does not distinguish these cases. As indicated above, reduction of laminin-β1 on a muscle biopsy may in some cases be a clue to the diagnosis.

Autosomal recessive limb girdle dystrophy: type 2A/calpainopathy

A fairly characteristic phenotype has been described in association with calpainopathy (Fardeau et al., 1996; Urtasun et al., 1998). Typically, onset in this disease is between the ages of 8 and 15 years, though presentation in early childhood and much later adult life have both been described. Early involvement of the posterior thigh muscles, early scapular winging and striking preservation of the hip abductors are typical. Calf hypertrophy is rare, and the disease tends to be predominantly atrophic. A subgroup of patients present with Achilles tendon and elbow contractures and rigidity of the spine (Pollitt et al., unpublished data). Progression is never as severe as in DMD, but those with the earliest onset disease may be confined to a wheelchair in early adulthood. Scoliosis is not a common complication and cardiac involvement is not so far described, though respiratory impairment can be seen late in the course of the disease.

Differential diagnosis

- Other types of LGMD may be hard to distinguish from calpainopathy, especially in the late stages of the disease when the clear specificity of the pattern of muscle involvement has been lost.
- Where presentation is with prominent contractures and spinal rigidity, calpainopathy may be difficult to distinguish from the phenotypes associated with contractures described above. On the whole, however, serum creatine kinase tends to be higher in calpainopathy.

Table 35.2. The limb-girdle muscular dystrophies and associated conditions

Locus name (gene symbol)	Distribution	Genetics	Protein	Key clinical features
Dominant disease				
LGMD1A	Single large US family	Linkage to chr. 5q; candidate gene under investigation	Myotilin	Proximal weakness, slow progression, possible anticipation
VPDMD	Single large US family	Overlapping candidate region with LGMD1A; haplotypes not shared	Not yet	Aspiration, nasal voice, distal muscle involvement
LGMD1B (*LMNA*)	First described in Dutch families	Mutations identified in lamin A/C	Lamin A/C	Proximal weakness, cardiac conduction defects
ADEDMD (*LMNA*)	Worldwide	Mutations identified in lamin A/C gene – may be new dominant mutations	Lamin A/C involved but expression not reduced in patients with mutations	Humeroperoneal weakness, dominant contractures, cardiac conduction defects
LGMD1C (*CAV3*)	Few reports	Mutations reported in gene for caveolin 3 on chr. 3p25; mutations predominantly located in scaffolding domain of protein;	Caveolin 3 implicated: expression in affected patients probably abnormal	Proximal muscle weakness, calf hypertrophy
LGMD1D (*FDC–CDM*)	One large family (>25 affected)	Locus on chr. 6q22	Not yet	Cardiac complications important.; skeletal and cardiac problems worse in males
LGMD1E	Two families	Linkage to chr. 7q	Not yet	Atrioventricular conduction disturbance: presentation as young adults
Recessive disease				
Sarcoglycanopathy, LGMD2C–2F (*SGCA*, *SGCG*, *SGCB*, *SGCD*)	Worldwide, regional differences in different types	1. α-R77C seen in 42% chr. 2. γ-SG two predominant mutations, in N. African and gypsy populations otherwise mutations very heterogeneous 3. Missense mutations in all SGs mainly in extracellular domain.	Overall variable patterns of primary and secondary reduction 1. Dystrophin may be mildly abnormal (most often with γ-SG) 2. May see selective reduction of the SGs if γ- and α-SG mutated 3. With mutated β and δ-SG mostly see depletion of all sarcoglycans	Calf (and other muscle) hypertrophy common; scapular winging common at onset; highly variable onset and progression but mostly onset in childhood. Intrafamilial variability often marked

Calpainopathy (LGMD2A) CAPN3	Worldwide, some isolates (e.g. Reunion, Amish, Basque)	Mutations widely distributed, few recurrent; all types of mutation seen, large deletions rare; changes may be nonpathogenic; except in homozygotes, it is difficult to correlate mutation type with rate of progression	Calpain 3 detectable by monoclonal antibody on blots: absent or reduced in calpainopathy	Onset typically 8–15 years; posterior thigh, scapular weakness early; often hip abductor sparing and calf hypertrophy is rare
Dysferlinopathy (LGMD2B/MM) DYSF	Worldwide; founder effect in Libyan Jewish population; ? others	Mutations widely distributed, few so far recurrent; no clear genotype–phenotype correlations so far	Dysferlin detectable on sections and blots: absent or reduced in dysferlinopathy	Onset usually late teens; onset may involve proximal or distal muscle or a mixture of the two; little shoulder girdle involvement, calf hypertrophy rare
LGMD2G	Brazil	Linkage to chr. 17q	Telethonin	Distal involvement seen as prominent feature
LGMD2H	Manitoba Hutterites	Linkage to chr. 9q31–33	Not yet	Proximal symptoms often in mid 20s, slow progression
LGMD2I	Tunisian families	Linkage to chr. 19q13.3	Not yet	Variable at onset and clinical course

Notes:

SG, sarcoglycan; chr, chromosome; LGMD, limb girdle muscular dystrophy; EDMD, Emery–Dreifuss muscular dystrophy; AD, autosomal dominant.

Table 35.3. Distal muscular dystrophies or myopathies with known gene locations

Muscular dystrophy	Inheritance	Gene locus	Gene product
Tibial muscular dystrophy	AD	2q31	
Distal myopathy of 'Laing'	AD	14q11	
Welander distal myopathy	AD	2p13	
Miyoshi myopathy	AR	2p13	Dysferlin
Miyoshi myopathy 2	AR	10q	
Dermatomyositis with rimmed vacuoles	AR	9p1-q1	
Hereditary inclusion body myopathy	AR	9p1-q1	

Notes:
AD, autosomal dominant; AR, autosomal recessive.

- Usually the pattern of muscle involvement will distinguish BMD from calpainopathy, especially the weakness of the hamstrings relative to the quadriceps muscles in calpain deficiency, which is the opposite to the pattern seen in dystrophinopathy. In the occasional patients with calf hypertrophy, distinction may be more difficult.

Diagnostic tools
Monoclonal antibodies to calpain 3 are commercially available but work only on immunoblotting, not on muscle biopsy sections (Anderson et al., 1998). The confirmation of the diagnosis rests on the demonstration of mutations in the gene for calpain 3. As these mutations are highly variable, with very few recurrent mutations reported in this large gene, mutation detection without clinical and/or protein information to guide it is a difficult task (Richard et al., 1997, 1999).

Autosomal recessive limb girdle dystrophy: type 2B/dysferlinopathy
The typical phenotype seen in association with dysferlinopathy is variable to some degree, in particular the mode of presentation, which may be either in the distal (typically gastrocnemius in the Miyoshi myopathy type presentation) or proximal muscles (Bashir et al., 1998; Liu et al., 1998). The type of mutation does not distinguish the different modes of presentation and in fact patients homozygous for the same mutation may present with either distal or proximal muscle involvement (Illarioshkin et al., 1996; Weiler et al., 1999). Having allowed for this degree of variability, there are some common factors in dysferlinopathy. These include usual onset in the late teens or early twenties often with good motor prowess beforehand, and predominant lower limb involvement at onset with a lack of scapular winging, but sometimes asymptomatic selective loss of biceps (Mahjneh et al., 1996). Contractures are not a feature of the disease, and to date cardiac or respiratory complications have not been reported. Progression is usually fairly slow, though with some exceptions.

Differential diagnosis
- Serum creatine kinase in these patients may be massively elevated at presentation, and inflammatory features are relatively commonly seen on biopsy. Amongst our patients, the commonest previous diagnosis was polymyositis. There appears to be, however, no response to steroids.
- Other forms of distal myopathy may be confused with patients presenting with a distal onset. However, such a marked elevation of serum creatine kinase is not typical in other distal myopathies and the exact pattern of muscle involvement may be informative. The distal myopathies in themselves comprise a group of genetically distinct disorders. As yet, however, none of these distal myopathy genes has been cloned (Table 35.3). In patients with a proximal onset, the differential diagnosis will include the other forms of LGMD, which in most cases can be shown to have a subtly different pattern of muscle involvement on examination.

Diagnostic tools
Examination of dysferlin staining on a muscle biopsy section is now possible (Anderson et al., 1999) and can be used to identify patients in whom mutation analysis is likely to be successful. Again, the dysferlin gene is very large (55 exons) and mutations are widely dispersed (Aoki et al., unpublished data). Neither mutation type nor position correlates with proximal or distal onset. The pattern of staining of dysferlin in muscle does not distinguish the different presentations.

Autosomal recessive limb girdle dystrophy: types 2C–2F/sarcoglycanopathies
While there may be subtle differences between the different sarcoglycanopathies at the clinical level, at present there is

insufficient experience of the different entities to be clear about this. There, however, are some broad conclusions that can be drawn about the group. Sarcoglycanopathy is more common amongst childhood-onset muscular dystrophy than adult onset, though presentation may be at any age (Eymard et al., 1997; Ozawa et al., 1998; Angelini et al., 1999; Passos-Bueno et al., 1999). Hypertrophy of the calves or other muscles is usually seen, as are scapular winging and lumbar lordosis at onset, both of which may be more marked than in a patient with dystrophinopathy at a similar stage. Scoliosis and respiratory impairment may be important complications, and cardiomyopathy, possibly reflecting smooth muscle disease and probably less common than in dystrophinopathy, can be seen (Angelini et al., 1999; van der Kooi et al., 1998).

Diagnostic tools
Diagnostic antibodies to each of the four sarcoglycans implicated in LGMD are available. However, because of the close association of the various members of the complex, use of a single antibody may be misleading. Some patients with sarcoglycanopathy also have a secondary reduction in dystrophin labelling (Fig. 35.9, colour plate) (Bushby et al., 1997; Jones et al., 1998; Ozawa et al., 1998; Passos-Bueno et al., 1999). In general, with primary involvement of either β- or δ-sarcoglycan, there is often a complete loss of the other complex members (Duggan et al., 1997b; Duclos et al., 1998). The pattern of secondary deficiencies seen with primary involvement of α- or γ- sarcoglycan is much more variable. Use of a full range of sarcoglycan antibodies will, therefore, give the best chance of defining which gene harbours the primary genetic defect, and multiplex Western blotting offers an alternative method of evaluating the pattern of deficiencies simultaneously (Anderson and Davison, 1999). Definition of the gene defect itself is of course necessary if prenatal diagnosis or carrier testing is sought. As with all of the LGMD genes, a range of different mutations have been reported in each of the sarcoglycan genes, with a common recurrent mutation present only in α-sarcoglycan (Carrie et al., 1997; Duggan et al., 1997a,b; Fanin et al., 1997).

Differential diagnosis
As suggested above, the major differential diagnosis is with dystrophinopathy. The distinction probably cannot be made with absolute certainty at the clinical level, though there may be subtle differences as above. In addition, the intellectual retardation that is so commonly seen in dystrophinopathy is not a part of the sarcoglycanopathy phenotype.

Limb girdle dystrophy: conclusions
For people seeking a precise diagnosis in LGMD for prognostic or genetic counselling purposes, a combined approach integrating clinical examination, analysis of the muscle biopsy and DNA analysis may be very fruitful (Bushby, 1999). In the autosomal recessive types of LGMD, pivotal to making the diagnosis is the examination of a muscle biopsy using a range of antibodies to the various LGMD proteins. This is the only logical route to targeting the appropriate gene for mutation detection in these recessive diseases. Outside rare founder populations, mutations in all of the LGMD genes are highly variable and cannot be predicted; with the single exception of α-sarcoglycan (Carrie et al., 1997) there are no hotspots to focus down the analysis. This diversity of mutations (and, in fact, also of neutral polymorphisms) in these genes means that testing unrelated partners of patients or potential carriers in known families is extremely difficult and essentially cannot be done at the present time. As the frequency of these disorders in most populations is probably fairly low, the risk of recurrence in offspring will be low providing affected individuals do not marry a relative. Serum creatine kinase estimations are not helpful in determining carrier status; occasional but rare reports of elevated creatine kinase in carriers of all of the recessive types of LGMD make it a pointless exercise.

Emery–Dreifuss muscular dystrophy

The core phenotype
The phenotype of EDMD is highly characteristic, and clinical distinction between the various reported modes of inheritance (X-linked, autosomal dominant and autosomal recessive) may be impossible in the absence of a family history. The key features of the phenotype are humeroperoneal muscle weakness, which may be relatively mild but which is accompanied by joint contractures). These contractures typically involve the Achilles tendons, elbows and spine. In some patients they may be extremely progressive and debilitating; in others, they may be much less severe. All patients with EDMD are at risk of cardiac disease, which is almost invariably seen in the late teens, most often presenting with rhythm disturbances that require pacing. Especially in autosomal dominant EDMD, the arrhythmias may be hard to control and require an implantable defibrillator. It has also been reported that the cardiac disease in autosomal dominant EDMD may progress to a dilated cardiomyopathy, and indeed cardiac disease may be seen in some family members in the absence of any muscle symptoms or signs (see discussion above of LGMD1B, which is allelic to autosomal dominant EDMD). X-linked EDMD results from mutations in *STA*, which encodes emerin (Bione et al., 1994). Autosomal dominant and recessive EDMD are caused by mutations in the gene for lamin A/C (Bonne et al., 1999). Both emerin

and lamin A/C are components of the nuclear envelope, illustrating a common molecular pathological mechanism in these clinically overlapping disorders.

Distinguishing the mode of inheritance

As the clinical phenotypes involved with the different modes of inheritance do not distinguish them, investigations are necessary to allow the provision of correct genetic counselling, though some clues may be gained from careful attention to the family history as, particularly in autosomal dominant EDMD, there may be a history of sudden cardiac death in family members. In all forms of EDMD, serum creatine kinase is typically fairly mildly elevated, though in some cases a more marked elevation may be seen. The histological analysis of the muscle biopsy does not distinguish the different types; however, in the X-linked form of EDMD, immunochemical analysis of emerin in the skin or muscle (with lack or reduction of the normal nuclear labelling pattern) provides evidence of the diagnosis in all but very rare cases where mutations do not disrupt localization of the protein (Manilal et al., 1996). Emerin analysis of a skin or muscle biopsy sample may also demonstrate carrier status in some patients with a mosaic pattern of labelling, but the absence of a mosaic staining pattern does not definitively exclude the carrier state. Some carriers of EDMD do develop symptoms and in particular may be at risk of cardiac disease, so determining the carrier state through direct demonstration of the emerin mutation in the family is necessary to provide the relevant surveillance as well as to offer appropriate genetic advice. Mutations in the gene for emerin tend to be family specific and have been identified in all regions of the gene (Bione et al., 1994). In autosomal dominant EDMD, emerin analysis is normal, though a direct interaction between these two components of the nuclear envelope has recently been described (Fairley et al., 1999) and the lamin A knock-out mouse has mislocalization of emerin (Sullivan et al., 1999). Immunostaining for lamin A/C in muscle or other tissues is normal in autosomal dominant EDMD, though a secondary reduction in laminin-$\beta 2$ staining in muscle is seen in some adult biopsies. This is not specific to this disorder; consequently confirmation of the diagnosis relies on the direct demonstration of the causative mutation. Autosomal recessive EDMD is felt to be very rare, with only a single case confirmed so far. By contrast, mutations in lamin A/C present heterozygously and have been described in an increasing number of patients with no previous family history; germline mosaicism for new dominant mutations has also relatively frequently been described in the cases so far characterized. It follows, therefore, that where X-linked inheritance has been excluded dominant inheritance is the most likely and the risk to the offspring of a new patient is likely to be 50%. In view of the risk of germline mosaicism, the recurrence risk to the parent of a new sporadic case cannot be dismissed, though a figure based on anything other than empirical data is hard to calculate.

Genotype–phenotype correlations

The clinical features in an individual case of EDMD will not distinguish emerin or lamin A/C involvement; however, on the whole, X-linked on the whole EDMD is more uniform and more classically conforms to the 'typical' pattern of humeroperoneal weakness and contractures. Different emerin mutations produce clinically similar disease, and there is no clear correlation between the type or distribution of the mutation affecting the emerin molecule and the predicted course of the disease.

By contrast, mutations affecting lamin A/C are responsible for a number of different phenotypes. Families with a typical EDMD phenotype are described (Bonne et al., 2000), as are families with a much more limb girdle type pattern of muscle weakness in the absence of prominent contractures (Muchir et al., 2000). Other families have had pure cardiac disease (Fatkin et al., 1999). With all of these presentations, families may have relatively homogeneous disease or present variably; this variability especially relates to the presence and distribution of muscle weakness and contractures, while cardiac disease appears in essentially all gene carriers in these families and may be the only manifestation of disease. Mutations throughout the gene for lamin A/C have been described in families with any of these presentations and intrafamilial variability may be very marked.

Familial partial lipodystrophy does not involve either skeletal or cardiac muscle and is the other disorder described in association with mutations of lamin A/C. It does appear to show some selectivity of mutations, with all mutations so far described located in exon 8 or exon 11 (Cao and Hegele, 2000; Speckman et al., 2000). These patients develop a patchy loss of adipose tissue as well as a variety of endocrine disturbances. Lamin A/C (like emerin) is expressed in all tissues, and the reason why such diverse yet very highly tissue-specific diseases are associated with mutations in this single gene is not yet understood. It is of note that the lamin A/C knock-out mouse has a phenotype in the homozygous state that includes absence of white fat with dystrophic muscle and cardiac disease (Sullivan et al., 1999).

The congenital muscular dystrophies

The CMDs are by definition autosomal recessive diseases, characterized by very early onset, with hypotonia usually manifesting in the first year of life. A number of genetically defined entities within this group have been recognized, with significant molecular genetic progress within the last few years. There appears to be a major geographical variation in the incidence of some of these groups. The first major distinction in determining precise diagnosis in this group is the predominance of muscle or brain involvement.

'Classical' congenital muscular dystrophy

Patients with classical CMD have no significant symptomatic central nervous system (CNS) problems. They can be further subdivided on the basis of absence or deficiency of the laminin α2-chain (merosin).

Primary laminin-α2 deficiency

Primary laminin-α2 deficiency occurs in approximately half of all cases of classical CMD and can be defined on three parameters. First, they have total or partial deficiency of laminin-α2 (which can be demonstrated in muscle or skin) (Sewry et al., 1996). Second, white matter changes on brain magnetic resonance imaging (MRI) manifest as abnormally high T_2 signals (typically seen in patients older than six months of age) (Philpot et al., 1995; van der Knaap et al., 1997); these are asymptomatic. Third, mutations in *LAMA2* on chromosome 6q24 can be demonstrated (Helbling-Leclerc et al., 1995). In practice, the large size of the gene and the widespread distribution of mutations makes the third criterion in isolation impractical for routine diagnosis. In patients fulfilling these criteria, prenatal diagnosis is available based on examination of laminin-α2 in chorion villous samples combined with linkage or mutation analysis where possible (Voit et al., 1994; Anderson et al., 1999).

Secondary laminin-α2 deficiency

Various groups of patients with CMD have been described where a reduction in laminin-α2 is not caused by mutations in *LAMA2*. They do not have the typical white matter MRI changes seen in primary laminin-α2 deficiency, though some subgroups with secondary laminin-α2 deficiency may show other structural brain abnormalities. Secondary deficiency of laminin-α2 is likely to be a heterogeneous group, the definition of which is only just beginning (Dubowitz, 1991, Tomé et al., 1999). At present the important distinction is that prenatal diagnosis is not likely to be reliable in this group (see above). Further practical help awaits the molecular delineation of these syndromes.

Classical CMD with normal laminin-α2

Patients with classical CMD but normal laminin-α2 also form a highly heterogeneous group at the clinical level and likely to comprise a number of genetic entities. The majority of these patients are clinically essentially indistinguishable from those with laminin-α2 deficiency though on average their disease tends to be milder (Philpot et al., 1995; Mahjneh et al., 1998). Others have associated features, the most consistent of which is spinal rigidity. A locus for CMD and rigid spine syndrome has been identified on chromosome 1p35 (Moghadaszadeh et al., 1998); however, this does not account for all families with this rigid spine phenotype.

Differential diagnosis

- Problems may arise in determining whether a partial deficiency of laminin-α2 is primary or secondary. This may be resolved by using a number of antibodies to different domains of laminin-α2 and to different laminins (Cohn et al., 1998), and also by the examination of the brain MRI. In all cases of true primary laminin-α2 deficiency, the brain MRI shows typical abnormalities (van der Knaap et al., 1997). This is a key distinction to make, as prenatal diagnosis based on partial laminin-α2 deficiency is not reliable in the absence of likely linkage to chromosome 6q.
- Without laminin-α2 examination in muscle or skin, it is not possible to distinguish the different subgroups of CMD on clinical grounds.
- Patients with partial laminin-α2 deficiency may be very mildly affected and clinically resemble a childhood-onset LGMD (Tan et al., 1997).

Congenital muscular dystrophy with prominent central nervous system involvement

Patients with CMD with prominent CNS involvement have a constellation of CMD, structural abnormalities of the brain (typically within the spectrum of the neuronal migration defects) and ocular abnormalities (Fig. 35.10). The abnormalities may dominate the phenotype to such an extent (with severe mental retardation) in these patients that in some cases the muscle phenotype may be missed if not specifically sought by estimation of serum creatine kinase and muscle biopsy. There are three relatively clearly defined groups within this category. However, many children with combined cerebral, ocular and muscle problems may be seen that do not fit absolutely into any of these categories. The relatedness or not of these various groups awaits a clear understanding of their molecular pathology.

Fukuyama congenital muscular dystrophy

Fukuyama CMD (FCMD) is seen at high frequency in Japan and much more rarely elsewhere. Severity is variable, but all have profound muscle weakness though a proportion attain independent ambulation for a while. CNS

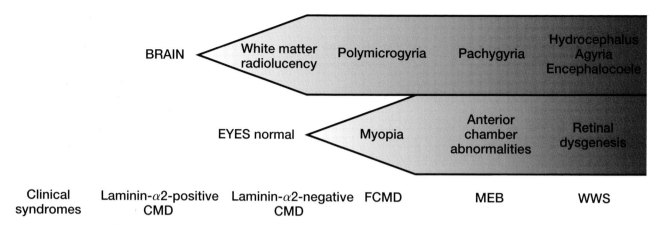

Fig. 35.10. The spectrum of congenital muscular dystrophy as determined by the variable involvement of the central nervous system and eyes. CMD, congenital muscular dystrophy; FCMD, Fukuyama congenital muscular dystrophy; MEB, muscle–eye–brain disease; WWS, Walker Warburg syndrome.

changes typically include polymicrogyria, and affected children have major intellectual impairment. Eye abnormalities may be minor. The gene for FCMD is known (*fukutin*) and a common retrotransposon insertion is responsible for almost all Japanese cases of the disease (Kobayashi et al., 1998). A few point mutations have been described, but to date there are no reported cases with two noninsertion mutations. In the Japanese population, these findings translate into a straightforward test for diagnosis, carrier status and prenatal diagnosis.

Muscle–eye–brain disease
Muscle–eye–brain disease (MEBD) is a form of CMD described mainly in Finnish patients; it is associated with more marked cerebral abnormalities than FCMD, including cobblestone cortex, cerebral atrophy and a small cerebellar vernis and brainstem. Ocular abnormalities are variable and tend to start with myopia progressing to retinal degeneration and cataracts. Serum creatine kinase levels are high. Chromosome 1p linkage has been described in MEBD but the gene is not yet known. Most patients are from Finland.

Walker Warburg syndrome
Walker Warburg syndrome (WWS) represents the most severely affected children within this group. The spectrum of abnormalities is dominated by very marked brain malformations, including typically type II lissencephaly but also sometimes ventricular dilatation and encephalocoele. A range of ocular abnormalities can be seen including anterior chamber abnormalities, corneal opacities and microphthalmia. Serum creatine kinase levels are elevated. Affected children typically die before the age of 2 years. No molecular basis for this group is yet defined.

The congenital myopathies

The congenital myopathies are classified according to the presence of specific histopathological characteristics detected on examination of the muscle biopsy. As yet, molecular methodologies have not superseded these traditional techniques. Within the groups of myopathies characterized by these various findings, however, there exists further heterogeneity. Constant reappraisal of the current levels of knowledge about these disorders is necessary to provide the correct genetic counselling.

Nemaline myopathy

From the clinical perspective, cases of nemaline myopathy may be encountered with congenital onset (often causing neonatal death), classical onset in the first months of life with hypotonia, respiratory and feeding difficulties but more prolonged survival, and childhood or adult onset (Wallgren-Pettersson et al., 1995a, 1998; North et al., 1997). Childhood onset outside the neonatal period appears to be rare, and adult-onset disease with muscle weakness associated with nemaline rods in the biopsy is probably a very heterogeneous group indeed, not all of which may be genetic. Autosomal dominant and recessive groups are recognized, and examination of the parents or parental muscle biopsies is notoriously unreliable in trying to distinguish the two modes of inheritance. Mutations in the gene for α-tropomyosin (*TPM3*) on chromosome 1 have been found in a single Australian family with dominant childhood-onset disease and also in one person of recessive disease (Laing et al., 1995; Tan et al., 1999). Also in autosomal recessive nemaline myopathy, the gene for nebulin on chromosome 2q has recently been shown to be involved in a number of families, though the extremely large size of this gene makes mutation detection extremely difficult (Hilpela et al., 1999).

Table 35.4. Ion channel disorders of skeletal muscle

Ion channel	Disorder	Inheritance	Gene (standard nomenclature)	Chromosome
Skeletal muscle sodium channel	HyperKPP	Dominant	SCN4A	17q23–2
	PMC	Dominant		
	PAM	Dominant		
	?NormoKPP	Dominant		
Skeletal muscle dihydropyridine-sensitive calcium channel	HypoKPP	Dominant	CACLN1A3	1q31–32
	MH	Dominant		
Skeletal muscle ryanodine calcium channel	MH	Dominant	RYR1	19q13.1
	Central core disease	Dominant		
Skeletal muscle chloride channel	Myotonia congenita			
	Thomsen's disease	Dominant	CLCNA1	7q35
	Becker's myotonia	Recessive		

Notes:

HyperKPP, hyperkalaemic periodic paralysis; PMC, paramyotonia congenita; PAM, potassium-aggravated myotonia; Normo KPP, normokalaemic periodic paralysis; HypoKPP, hypokalaemic periodic paralysis; MH, malignant hyperthermia.

A third genetically defined group with nemaline myopathy have mutations in the gene for actin (Nowak et al., 1999), but not all cases are yet accounted for. All of these findings are very recent and, in these rare disorders, have yet to become fully available as diagnostic investigations. As the heterogeneity in this disease becomes better understood, however, this is likely to become more feasible.

Myotubular myopathy

In the X-linked form of myotubular myopathy, genetic analysis has revealed consistent involvement of the same gene (Wallgren-Pettersson and Clarke, 1998). Many mutations, most found in only a single family, have now been described in the gene for myotubularin, a member of a tyrosine phosphatase family with genes on chromosome Xq28 (Laporte et al., 1996). Fairly frequent germline mosaicism has now been established for mutations in this gene, and these may account for apparently previously discrepant families (Wallgren-Pettersson et al., 1995b; Helliwell et al., 1998; Vincent et al., 1998; Wallgren-Pettersson, 1998). The major differential diagnosis for the X-linked form of myotubular myopathy is congenital myotonic dystrophy, easily excluded by testing for the presence of the chromosome 19 CTG repeat characteristic of this disorder. No genetic cause has yet been identified for the proposed autosomal dominant or recessive forms of this condition, which are relatively poorly characterized.

Central core disease

Central core disease is an autosomal dominant myopathy. Most cases are associated with mutations in the gene for the ryanodine receptor (RYR1) (Quane et al., 1993; Lynch et al., 1999) though routine mutation analysis is hampered by the heterogeneity of the mutations in this gene. The finding of these mutations confirms the observed association between central core disease and malignant hyperthermia (Frank et al., 1980). This association is not absolute, however: only around 28% of patients with central core disease are at risk of malignant hyperthermia, and most patients with malignant hyperthermia have histologically normal muscle. Where families have been described with both conditions, the presentation may be complex, with either manifestation being present alone or both present together (Busby and Squier, 1998). Not all malignant hyperthermia families have ryanodine receptor gene mutations. An alternative association with other mutations affecting calcium channels has been described in some of these patients (Table 35.4) (Monnier et al., 1997)

Multicore myopathy

No clear guidance can yet be given on the genetics of multicore myopathy. Autosomal recessive inheritance is most likely, but no information is available on the molecular pathology in this group. Collection of potentially informative families with this condition is currently underway.

Congenital myopathy without a specific histopathological diagnosis

More commonly than any of the specific histopathological subtypes of congenital myopathy are encountered, a diagnosis of congenital myopathy without diagnostic features will be made. Other potential entities defined histopathologically have been reported so rarely that their identity as separate conditions cannot be confirmed (Goebel and Anderson, 1999). At a practical level, these patients need to be kept under review as numerous examples exist of patients in whom biopsy changes became clearer with time; for example, a biopsy taken in early childhood may show only nonspecific features while a later biopsy may be diagnostic. In the meantime, these patients are at potential risk of the complications of these disorders including possibly respiratory failure, scoliosis, joint contractures and cardiomyopathy. Genetic advice is always difficult in the absence of a definitive diagnosis, but many congenital myopathies may be autosomal dominant in inheritance and new dominant mutations are increasingly recognized. Therefore, while the risk cannot easily be quantified, it is not appropriate to give a negligible risk.

The ion channel disorders of muscle

Molecular genetic testing in those with disorders of muscle ion channels has led to a complete reclassification of the nondystrophic myotonias and paroxysmal muscle diseases such as hyper- and hypokalaemic periodic paralysis (hyperKPP and hypoKPP, respectively; Table 35.4). Heterogeneity is an important feature of this group, with disorders previously considered to be separate entities now known to be caused by mutations in the same gene. For patients suspected of having one of these diseases, DNA analysis is proving a reliable first-line test (Hanna et al., 1998) and certainly safer (and more comfortable) than neurophysiology and provocation testing.

The periodic paralyses, paramyotonia congenita and the potassium-aggravated myotonias

The gene involved in hyperKPP was identified as encoding the skeletal muscle subunit of the voltage-gated sodium channel (*SCN4A*) by a candidate approach, following electrophysiological evidence of the involvement of this channel. Different mutations, leading to different effects on the expression of the gene and function of the channel, cause paramyotonia congenita and the potassium-aggravated myotonias. By contrast, the gene for hypoKPP encodes a muscle-voltage gated calcium channel (*CACNL1A3*), in which three major mutations predominate. Molecular genetic analysis is of growing importance in this group as evidence is beginning to accumulate that some drugs may be potentially helpful in genetically determined subgroups of patients. Diagnosis is also important to counsel the avoidance of potential participating factors (Hanna et al., 1998).

Myotonia congenita

Myotonia congenita exists in a more common recessive form (Becker's generalized myotonia) or in the milder and less frequent dominant form (Thomsen's disease). Both forms of myotonia congenita, which are characterized clinically by myotonia from childhood (but unaccompanied by involvement of other systems, as seen in myotonic dystrophy), result from different mutations in the gene for the human skeletal muscle chloride channel (*CLCN1*). The recessive mutations typically cause loss of function of the protein, while the effect of the dominant mutations may be either via haploid insufficiency or via a dominant negative effect. Mutation detection in *CLCN1* is difficult because of the wide range of different point mutations described.

Summary

Molecular genetic investigation of the disorders discussed in this chapter now underpins a whole new classification of genetically determined muscle disease. The knowledge on which genetic counselling is based in any disease does not stand still, and this is overwhelmingly true for the inherited disorders of skeletal muscle. Many previously research-based findings are now in regular use to aid in genetic counselling for these families all over the world, and as more technological and basic advances continue, it is likely that an even wider range of analyses will become available with time. A continued challenge to genetic counselling is to use these tests wisely, with sensitivity and in partnership with the families involved at all times.

References

Abbruzzese, C., Krahe, R., Liguori, M. et al. (1996). Myotonic dystrophy phenotype without expansion of (CTG)*ₙ* repeat: an entity distinct from proximal myotonic myopathy (PROMM). *J. Neurol.* **243**, 715–721.

Abbs, S. and Bobrow, M. (1992). Analysis of quantitative PCR for the diagnosis of deletion and duplication carriers in the dystrophin gene. *J. Med. Genet.* **29**, 191–196.

Anderson, L. V. B. and Davison, K. (1999). Multiplex Western blotting for the analysis of muscular dystrophy proteins. *Am. J. Pathol.* **154**, 1017–1022.

Anderson, L. V. B., Davison, K., Moss, J. A. et al. (1998). Characterisation of monoclonal antibodies to calpain 3 and protein expression in muscle from patients with limb-girdle muscular dystrophy type 2A. *Am. J. Pathol.* **153**, 1169–1179.

Anderson, L. V. B., Davison, K., Moss, J. A. et al. (1999). Dysferlin is a plasma membrane protein and is expressed early in human development. *Hum. Mol. Genet.* **8**, 855–861.

Angelini, C., Fanin, M., Freda, M. P., Duggan, D. J., Siciliano, G. and Hoffman, E. P. (1999). The clinical spectrum of sarcoglycanopathies. *Neurology* **52**, 176–179.

Appleton, R. E., Bushby, K., Gardner-Medwin, D., Welch, J. and Kelly, P. J. (1991). Head circumference and intellectual performance in patients with Duchenne muscular dystrophy. *Dev. Med Child Neurol.* **33**, 884–890.

Ashizawa, T., Anvret, M., Baiget, M. et al. (1994a). Characteristics of intergenerational contractions of the CTG repeat in myotonic dystrophy. *Am. J. of Hum. Genet.* **54**, 414–423.

Ashizawa, T., Dunne, P. W., Ward, P. A., Seltzer, W. K. and Richards, C. S. (1994b). Effects of the sex of myotonic dystrophy patients on the unstable triplet repeat in their affected offspring. *Neurology* **44**, 120–122.

Ashizawa, T., Monketon, D. G., Vaishnav, S., Patel, B. J., Voskova, A. and Caskey, C. T. (1996). Instability of the expanded $(CTG)_n$ repeats in the myotonin protein kinase gene in cultured lymphoblastoid cell lines from patients with myotonic dystrophy. *Genomics* **36**, 47–53.

Bakker, E. and van Ommen, G. J. B. (1999). Duchenne and Becker muscular dystrophy (DMD and BMD). In: *Neuromuscular Disorders: Clinical and Molecular Genetics*, ed. A. E. H. Emery, pp. 59–86. Chichester: Wiley.

Bakker, E., Veenema, H., den Dunnen, J. T. et al. (1989). Germinal mosaicism increases the recurrence risk for 'new' Duchenne muscular dystrophy mutations. *J. Med. Genet.* **26**, 553–559.

Bakker, E., van der Wielen, M. J. R., Voorhoeve, E. et al. (1996). Diagnostic, predictive and prenatal testing for facioscapulohumeral muscular dystrophy: diagnostic approach for sporadic and familial cases. *J. Med. Genet.* **33**, 29–35.

Bashir, R., Britton, S., Strachan, T. et al. (1998). A gene related to *Caenorhabditis elegans* spermatogenesis factor *fer-1* is mutated in limb-girdle muscular dystrophy type 2B. *Nat. Genet.* **20**, 37–42.

Beggs A. M., Koenig M., Boyce F. M. and Kunkel L. M. (1990). Detection of 98% of DMD/BMD gene deletions by polymerase chain reaction. *Hum. Genet.* **86**, 45–48.

Bieber, F. R., Hoffman, E. P. and Amos, J. A. (1989). Dystrophin analysis in Duchenne muscular dystrophy: use in fetal diagnosis and in genetic counseling. *Am. J. Hum. Genet.* **45**, 362–367.

Bione, S., Maestrini, E., Rivella, S. et al. (1994). Identification of a novel X-linked gene responsible for Emery–Dreifuss muscular dystrophy. *Nat. Genet.* **8**, 323–327.

Biros, I. and Forrest, S. (1999). Spinal muscular atrophy: untangling the knot? *J. Med. Genet.* **36**, 1–8.

Blok, R. B., Gook, D. A., Thorburn, D. R. and Dahl, H. M. (1997). Skewed segregation of the mtDNA nt 8993 (T-G) mutation in human oocytes. *Am. J. Hum. Genet.* **60**, 1495–1501.

Bonne, G., di Barletta, M. R., Varnous, S. et al. (1999). Mutations in the gene encoding lamin A/C cause autosomal dominant Emery–Dreifuss muscular dystrophy. *Nat. Genet.* **21**, 285–288.

Bonne, G., Mercuri, E., Muchire, A. et al. (2000). Clinical and molecular genetic spetrum of autosomal dominant Emery–Dreifuss muscular dystrophy due to mutations of the lamin A/C gene. *Ann. Neurol.* (in press).

Boucher, C. A., King, S. K., Carey, N. et al. (1995). A novel homeodomain-encoding gene is associated with a large CpG island interrupted by the myotonic dystrophy unstable $(CTG)_n$ repeat. *Hum. Mol. Genet.* **4**, 1919–1925.

Brahe, C., Servidei, S., Zappata, S., Ricci, E., Tonali, P. and Neri, C. (1995a). Genetic homogeneity between childhood-onset and adult-onset autosomal recessive spinal muscular atrophy. *Lancet* **346**, 741–742.

Bresolin, N., Castelli, E., Comi, G. P. et al. (1994). Cognitive impairment in Duchenne muscular dystrophy. *Neuromusc. Disord.* **4**, 359–369.

Brewster, B., Groenen, P. J. T. A. and Wieringa, B. (1998). Myotonic dystrophy: clinical and molecular aspects. In: *Neuromuscular Disorders: Clinical and Molecular Genetics*, ed. A. E. H. Emery, pp. 323–364. Chichester: Wiley.

Brouwer, O. F., Padberg, G. W., Ruys, C. J. M., Brand, R., de Laat, J. A. P. M. and Grote, J. J. (1991). Hearing loss in facioscapulohumeral muscular dystrophy. *Neurology* **41**, 1878–1881.

Brouwer, O. F., Padberg, G., Wijmenga, C. and Frants, R. (1994). Facioscapulohumeral muscular dystrophy in early childhood. *Arch. Neurol.* **51**, 387–394.

Brouwer, O. F., Padberg, G. W., Bakker, E., Wijmenga, C. and Frants, R. R. (1995). Early onset facioscapulohumeral muscular dystrophy. *Muscle Nerve* **2**, S67–72.

Bungener, C., Jouvent, R. and Delaporte, C. (1998). Psychological and emotional deficits in myotonic dystrophy. *J. Neurol. Neurosurg. Psychiatry.* **65**, 353–356.

Burglen, L., Seroz, T., Miniou, P. et al. (1997). The gene encoding p44, a subunit of the transcription factor TFIIH, is involved in large scale deletions associated with Werdnig–Hoffman disease. *Am. J. Hum. Genet.* **60**, 72–79.

Busby, M. and Squier, M. (1998). Central core disease. In: *Neuromuscular Disorders: Clinical and Molecular Genetics*, ed. A. E. H. Emery, pp. 277–288. Chichester: Wiley.

Bushby, K. (1999). Making sense of the limb-girdle muscular dystrophies. *Brain* **122**, 1403–1420.

Bushby, K. and Gardner-Medwin, D. (1993). The clinical, genetic and dystrophin characteristics of Becker muscular dystrophy. 1. Natural History. *J. Neurol.* **240**, 98–104.

Bushby, K., Gardner-Medwin, D., Nicholson, L. et al. (1993). The clinical, genetic and dystrophin characteristics of Becker muscular dystrophy. 2: Correlation of phenotype with genetic and protein abnormalities. *J. Neurol.* **240**, 105–112.

Bushby, K., Anderson, L. V. B., Sewry, C. et al. (1997). Dystrophinopathy or sarcoglycanopathy – the importance of a full diagnostic assessment in suspected manifesting carriers of Duchenne and Becker muscular dystrophy. *J. Med. Genet.* **34**, S54.

Cao, H. and Hegele, R. A. (2000). Nuclear lamin A/C R482Q mutation in Canadian kindreds with Dunnigan-type familial partial lipodystrophy. *Hum. Mol. Genet.* **9**, 109–112.

Carrie, A., Piccolo, F., Leturcq, F. et al. (1997). Mutational diversity and hot spots in the α-sarcoglycan gene in autosomal recessive muscular dystrophy (LGMD2D). *J. Med. Genet.* **34**, 470–475.

Carter, T. A., Bonnemann, C. G., Wang, C. H. et al. (1997). A multi-copy transcription-repair gene, BTF2p44, maps to the SMA region and demonstrates SMA associated deletions. *Hum. Mol. Genet.* **6**, 229–236.

Chamberlain, J. S., Gibbs, R. A., Ranvier, J. E., Nguyen, P. N. and Caskey, C. T. (1988). Deletion screening of the Duchenne muscular dystrophy locus via multiplex DNA amplification. *Nucl. Acids Res.* **16**, 11141–11156.

Cheng, S., Barcelo, J. M. and Korneluk, R. G. (1996). Characterization of large CTG repeat expansions in myotonic dystrophy alleles using PCR. *Hum. Mutat.* **7**, 304–310.

Chinnery, P., Howell, N., Lightowlers, R. N. and Turnbull, D. M. (1998a). Genetic counselling and prenatal diagnosis for mtDNA disease. *Am. J. Hum. Genet.* **63**, 1908–1910.

Chinnery, P. F., Howell, N., Lightowlers, R. N. and Turnbull, D. M. (1998b). MELAS and MERRF: the relationship between maternal mutation load and the frequency of clinically affected offspring. *Brain* **121**, 1889–1894.

Chinnery, P., Howell, N., Andrews, R. M. and Turnbull, D. M. (1999). Clinical mitochondrial genetics. *J. Med. Genet.* **36**, 425–436.

Cockburn, D. J. and Miciak, A. (1992). Accurate carrier detection for Duchenne muscular dystrophy (DMD) by pulsed field gel electrophoresis. *Clin. Cytogenet. Bull.* **2**, 16.

Cohn, R. D., Herrmann, R., Sorokin, L., Wewer, U. M. and Voit, T. (1998). Laminin α2 chain-deficient congenital muscular dystrophy. *Neurology* **51**, 94–101.

Daniels, R., Suthers, G., Morrison, K. et al. (1992). Prenatal prediction of spinal muscular atrophy. *J. Med. Genet.* **29**, 165–170.

Davies, K., Thomas, N., Daniels, R. and Dubowitz, V. (1991). Molecular studies of spinal muscular atrophy. *Neuromusc. Disord.* **1**, 83–85.

de Die-Smulders, C. E. M., Smeets, H. J. M., Loots, W. et al. (1997). Paternal transmission of congenital myotonic dystrophy. *J. Med. Genet.* **34**, 930–933.

de Die-Smulders, C. E. M., Howeler, C. J., Thijs, C. et al. (1998). Age and causes of death in adult-onset myotonic dystrophy. *Brain* **121**, 1557–1563.

Delaporte, C. (1998). Personality patterns in patients with myotonic dystrophy. *Arch. Neurol.* **55**, 635–640.

di Barletta, M. R., Ricci, E., Galluzzi, G. et al. (2000). Different mutations in the LMNA gene caused autosomal dominant and autosomal recessive Emery–Dreifuss muscular dystrophy. *Am. J. Hum. Genet.* **66**, 1407–1412.

Dubowitz, V. (1991). Chaos in classification of the spinal muscular atrophies of childhood. *Neuromusc. Disord.* **1**, 77–80.

Duclos, F., Broux, O., Bourg, N. et al. (1998). β-Sarcoglycan: genomic analysis and identification of a novel missense mutation in the LGMD2E Amish isolate. *Neuromusc. Disord.* **8**, 30–38.

Duggan, D. J., Gorospe, J. R., Fanin, M., Hoffman, E. P. and Angelini, C. (1997a). Mutations in the sarcoglycan genes in patients with myopathy. *N. Engl. J. Med.* **336**, 618–624.

Duggan, D. J., Manchester, D., Stears, K. P., Mathews, D. J., Hart, C. and Hoffman, E. P. (1997b). Mutations in the δ-sarcoglycan gene are a rare cause of autosomal recessive limb-girdle muscular dystrophy (LGMD2). *Neurogenetics* **1**, 49–58.

Eymard, B., Romero, N. B., Leturcq, F. et al. (1997). Primary adhali-nopathy (α-sarcoglycanopathy): clinical, pathologic and genetic correlation in 20 patients with autosomal recessive muscular dystrophy. *Neurology* **48**, 1227–1234.

Fairley, E. A. L., Kendrick-Jones, J. and Ellis, J. A. (1999). The Emery–Dreifuss muscular dystrophy phenotype arises from aberrant targeting and binding of emerin at the inner nuclear membrane. *J. Cell Sci.* **112**, 2571–2582.

Fanin, M., Duggan, D. J., Mostacciuolo, M. L. et al. (1997). Genetic epidemiology of muscular dystrophies resulting from sarcolgy-can gene mutations. *J. Med. Genet.* **34**, 973–977.

Fardeau, M., Hillaire, D., Mignard, C. et al. (1996). Juvenile limb-girdle muscular dystrophy. Clinical, histopathological and genetic data on a small community living in the Reunion Island. *Brain* **119**, 295–308.

Fatkin, D., MacRae, C., Sasaki, T. et al. (1999). Missense mutation in the rod domain of the lain A/C gene as causes of dilated cardiomyopathy and conduction-system disease. *N. Engl. J. Med.* **341**, 1715–1724.

Ferlini, A., Galie, N., Merlini, L., Sewry, C., Branzi, A. and Muntoni, F. (1998). A novel alu-like element rearranged in the dystrophin gene causes a splicing mutation in a family with X-linked dilated cardiomyopathy. *Am. J. Hum. Genet.* **63**, 436–446.

Frank, J. P., Harati, Y., Butler, I. J., Nelson, T. E. and Scott, C. I. (1980). Central core disease and malignant hyperthermia syndrome. *Ann. Neurol.* **7**, 11–17.

Gilliam, T., Brzustowicz, L., Castilla, L. et al. (1990). Genetic homogeneity between acute and chronic forms of spinal muscular atrophy. *Nature* **345**, 823–825.

Ginjaar, I., Soffers, S., Moorman, A. et al. (1991). Fetal dystrophin to diagnose carrier status. *Lancet* **338**, 257–258.

Goebel, H. H. and Anderson, J. R. (1999). Workshop report: the 56th ENMC sponsored international workshop on structural congenital myopathies (excluding nemaline myopathy, myotubular myopathy and desminopathies). *Neuromusc. Disord.* **9**, 50–57.

Gospe, S. M., Lazaro, R. P., Lava, N. S., Grootscholten, P. M., Scott, A. B. and Fischbeck, K. H. (1989). Familial X-linked myalgia and cramps: a non-progressive myopathy associated with a deletion in the dystrophin gene. *Neurology* **39**, 1277–1280.

Hahnen, E., Forkert, R., Marke, C. et al. (1995). Molecular analysis of candidate genes on chromosome 5q13 in autosomal recessive spinal muscular atrophy: evidence of homozygous deletions of the SMN gene in unaffected individuals. *Hum. Mol. Genet.* **4**, 1927–1933.

Hamshere, M. G., Harley, H., Harper, P., Brook, J. D. and Brookfield, J. F. Y. (1999). Myotonic dystrophy: the correlation of (CTG) repeat length in leucocytes with age at onset is significant only for patients with small expansions. *J. Med. Genet.* **36**, 59–61.

Hanna, M. G., Wood, N. W. and Kullmann, D. M. (1998). Ion channels and neurological disease: DNA based diagnosis is now possible and ion channels may be important in common paroxysmal disorders. *J. Neurol. Neurosurg. Psychiatry.* **65**, 427–431.

Harley, H. G., Rundle, S. A., MacMillan, J. C. et al. (1993). Size of the unstable CTG repeat sequence in relation to phenotype and parental transmission in myotonic dystrophy. *Hum. Mol. Genet.* **4**, 1–8.

Helbling-Leclerc, A., Zhang, X., Topaloglu, H. et al. (1995). Mutations in the laminin α_2-chain gene (*LAMA2*) cause merosin-deficient congenital muscular dystrophy. *Nat. Genet.* **11**, 216–218.

Helliwell, T. R., Ellis, I. H. and Appleton, R. E. (1998). Myotubular myopathy: morphological, immunohistochemical and clinical variation. *Neuromusc. Disord.* **8**, 152–161.

Hilpela, P., Pelin, K., Donner, K. et al. (1999). Mutations in the nebulin gene associated with autosomal recessive nemaline myopathy. *Proc. Natl. Acad. Sci. USA* **96**, 2305–2310.

Hodgson, S. V., Abbs, S., Clark, S. et al. (1992). Correlation of clinical and deletion data in Duchenne and Becker muscular dystrophy, with special reference to mental ability. *Neuromusc. Disord.* **2**, 269–276.

Hoffman, E. P., Arahata, K., Minetti, C. et al. (1992). Dystrophinopathy in isolated cases of myopathy in females. *Neurology* **42**, 967–975.

Holding, C., Bentley, D., Roberts, R., Bobrow, M. and Mathew, C. (1993). Development and validation of laboratory procedures for preimplantation diagnosis of Duchenne muscular dystrophy. *J. Med. Genet.* **30**, 903–909.

Illarioshkin, S. N., Ivanova-Smolenskaya, I. A. et al. (1996). Clinical and molecular analysis of a large family with three distinct phenotypes of progressive muscular dystrophy. *Brain* **119**, 1895–1909.

Ishikawa, Y., Bach, J. R., Sarma, R. J. et al. (1995). Cardiovascular considerations in the management of neuromuscular disease. *Semin. Neurol.* **15**, 93–108.

Jobsis, G. J., Keizers, H., Vreijling, J. P. et al. (1996). Collagen VI mutations in Bethlem myopathy, an autosomal dominant myopathy with contractures. *Nat. Genet.* **14**, 113–115

Jobsis, G. J., Boers, J. M., Barth, P. G. and de Visser, M. (1999). Bethlem myopathy: a slowly progressive congenital muscular dystrophy with contractures. *Brain* **122**, 649–655.

Jones, K. J., Kim, S. S. and North, K. N. (1998). Abnormalities of dystrophin, the sarcoglycans and laminin α_2 in the muscular dystrophies. *J. Med. Genet.* **35**, 379–386.

Joseph, J. T., Richards, C. S., Anthony, D. C., Upton, M., Perez-Atayde, A. R. and Greenstein, P. (1997). Congenital myotonic dystrophy pathology and somatic mosaicism. *Neurology* **49**, 1457–1460.

Klesert, T. R., Otten, A. D., Bird, T. D. and Tapscott, S. J. (1997). Trinucleotide repeat expansion at the myotonic dystrophy locus reduces expression of DMAHP. *Nat. Genet.* **16**, 402–406.

Kobayashi, K., Nakahori, Y., Miyake, M. et al. (1998). An ancient retrotransposal insertion causes Fukuyama-type congenital muscular dystrophy. *Nature* **394**, 388–392.

Laing, N. G., Wilton, S. D., Akkari, P. A. et al. (1995). A mutation in the α tropomyosin gene *TPM3* associated with autosomal dominant nemaline myopathy. *Nat. Genet.* **9**, 75–79.

Lamande, S. R., Bateman, J. F., Hutchison, W. et al. (1998). Reduced collagen VI causes Bethlem myopathy: a heterozygous COL6A1 nonsense mutation results in mRNA decay and functional haploinsufficiency. *Hum. Mol. Genet.* **7**, 981–989.

Laporte, J., Hu, L., Kretz, C., Mandel, J. et al. (1996). A gene mutated in X-linked myotubular myopathy defines a new putative tyrosine phosphatase family conserved in yeast. *Nat. Genet.* **13**, 175–182.

Lefebvre, S., Burglen, L., Reboullet, S. et al. (1995). Identification and characterization of a spinal muscular atrophy-determining gene. *Cell* **80**, 155–165.

Lenk, U., Hanke, R. and Speer, A. (1994). Carrier detection in DMD families with point mutations, using PCR-SSCP and direct sequencing. *Neuromusc. Disord.* **4**, 411–418.

Liu, J., Aoki, M., Illa, I. et al. (1998). Dysferlin, a novel skeletal muscle gene, is mutated in Miyoshi myopathy and limb girdle muscular dystrophy. *Nat. Genet.* **21**, 31–36.

Lunt, P. W. (1998). Workshop report: the 44th ENMC international workshop on facioscapulohumeral muscular dystrophy: molecular studies. *Neuromusc. Disord.* **8**, 126–130.

Lunt, P. W. and Harper, P. S. (1991). Genetic counselling in facioscapulohumeral muscular dystrophy. *J. Med. Genet.* **28**, 655–664.

Lunt, P. W., Jardine, P. E., Koch, M. et al. (1995a). Phenotypic-genotypic correlation will assist genetic counselling in 4q35-facioscapulohumeral muscular dystrophy. *Muscle Nerve* **2**, S103–S109.

Lunt, P. W., Jardine, P. E., Koch, M. C. et al. (1995b). Correlation between fragment size at D4F104S1 and age at onset or at wheelchair use, with a possible generational effect, accounts for much phenotypic variation in 4q35-facioscapulohumeral muscular dystrophy (FSHD). *Hum. Mol. Genet.* **4**, 951–958.

Lynch, P. J., Tong, J., Lehane, M. et al. (1999). A mutation in the transmembrane/luminal domain of the ryanodine receptor is associated with abnormal Ca^{2+} release channel function and severe central core disease. *Proc. Natl. Acad. Sci. USA* **96**, 4164–4169.

Magee, A. C. and Hughes, A. E. (1998). Segregation distortion in myotonic dystrophy. *J. Med. Genet.* **35**, 1045–1046.

Mahjneh, I., Passos-Bueno, M. R., Zatz, M. et al. (1996). The phenotype of chromosome 2p-linked limb-girdle muscular dystrophy. *Neuromusc. Disord.* **6**, 483–490.

Mahjneh, I., Bushby, K., Anderson, L. V. B. et al. (1998). Merosin-positive congenital muscular dystrophy: a large inbred family. *Neuropaediatrics* **30**, 22–28.

Manilal, S., Nguyen thi Man, Sewry, C. A. and Morris, G. E. (1996). The Emery–Dreifuss muscular dystrophy protein, emerin, is a nuclear membrane protein. *Hum. Mol. Genet.* **5**, 801–808.

McAndrew, P. E., Parsons, D. W., Simard, L. R. et al. (1997). Identification of proximal spinal muscular atrophy carriers and patients by analysis of *SMN*T and *SMN*C gene copy number. *Am. J. Hum. Genet.* **60**, 1411–1422.

McNally, E. M., de Sa Moreira, E., Duggan, D. J. et al. (1998). Caveolin-3 in muscular dystrophy. *Hum. Mol. Genet.* **7**, 871–877.

Melacini, P., Fanin, M., Danieli, G. A. et al. (1996). Myocardial involvement is very frequent among patients affected with subclinical Becker's muscular dystrophy. *Circulation* **94**, 3168–3175.

Melki, J. (1998). Spinal muscular atrophy. In: *Neuromuscular disorders: Clinical and Molecular Genetics*, ed. A. E. H. Emery, pp. 421–432. Chichester: Wiley.

Merlini, L., Villanova, M., Sabatelli, P., Malandrini, A. and Maraldi, N. M. (1999). Decreased expression of laminin β1 in chromosome 21-linked Bethlem myopathy. *Neuromusc. Disord.* **9**, 326–329.

Milasin, J., Muntoni, F., Severini, G. M. et al. (1996). A point mutation in the 5′ splice site of the dystrophin gene first intron responsible for X-linked dilated cardiomyopathy. *Hum. Mol. Genet.* **5**, 73–79.

Minetti, C., Sotgia, F., Bruno, C. et al. (1998). Mutations in the caveolin-3 gene cause autosomal dominant limb-girdle muscular dystrophy. *Nat. Genet.* **18**, 365–368.

Moghadaszadeh, B., Desguerre, I., Topaloglu, H. et al. (1998). Identification of a new locus for a peculiar form of congenital muscular dystrophy with early rigidity of the spine, on chromosome 1p35–36. *Am. J. Hum. Genet.* **62**, 1439–1445.

Monketon, D. G., Wong, L. C., Ashizawa, T. and Caskey, C. T. (1995). Somatic mosaicism, germline expansions, germline reversions and intergenerational reductions in myotonic dystrophy males: small pool PCR analyses. *Hum. Mol. Genet.* **4**, 1–8.

Monnier, N., Procaccio, V., Stieglitz, P. and Lunardi, J. (1997). Malignant hyperthermia susceptibility is associated with a mutation of the α_1-subunit of the human dihydropyridine-sensitive L-type voltage-dependent calcium-channel receptor in skeletal muscle. *Am. J. Hum. Genet.* **60**, 1316–1325.

Moreira, E. S., Vainzof, M., Marie, S. K., Sertie, A. L., Zatz, M. and Passos-Bueno, M. R. (1997). The seventh form of autosomal recessive limb-girdle muscular dystrophy is mapped to 17q11–12. *Am. J. Hum. Genet.* **61**, 151–159.

Moxley, R. T. (1996). Proximal myotonic myopathy: mini-review of a recently delineated clinical disorder. *Neuromusc. Disord.* **6**, 87–93.

Moxley, R. T., Udd, B. and Ricker, K. (1998a). Workshop report: the 54th ENMC international workshop on PROMM (proximal myotonic myopathies) and other proximal myotonic syndromes. *Neuromusc. Disord.* **8**, 508–518.

Moxley, R. T., Udd, B. and Ricker, K. (1998b). Proximal myotonic myopathy (PROMM) and other proximal myotonic syndromes. *Neuromusc. Disord.* **8**, 519–520.

Muchir, A., Bonne, G., van der Kooi, A. J. et al. (2000). Identification of mutations in the gene encoding lamins A/C in autosomal dominant limb girdle muscular dystropy with atrioventricular conduction disturbances (LGMD1B). *Hum. Mol. Gen.* **9**, 1453–1459.

Munsat, T. (1991). Workshop report: international SMA collaboration. *Neuromusc. Disord.* **1**, 81.

Muntoni, F., Melis, M. A., Ganau, A. and Dubowitz, V. (1994). Transcription of the dystrophin gene in normal tissues and in skeletal muscle of a family with X-linked dilated cardiomyopathy. *Am. J. Hum. Genet.* **56**, 151–157.

Muntoni, F., di Lenarda, A., Porcu, M. et al. (1997). Dystrophin gene abnormalities in two patients with idiopathic dilated cardiomyopathy. *Heart* **78**, 608–612.

Nakagawa, M., Yamada, H., Higuchi, I., et al. (1994). A case of paternally inherited congenital myotonic dystrophy. *J. Med. Genet.* **31**, 397–400.

Nicholson, L. V. B., Johnson, M. A., Bushby, K. M. D. et al. (1993a). Integrated study of 100 patients with Xp21-linked muscular dystrophy using clinical, genetic, immunochemical and histopathological data. Part 1. Trends across the clinical spectrum. *J. Med. Genet.* **30**, 728–736.

Nicholson, L. V. B., Johnson, M. A., Bushby, K. M. D. et al. (1993b). Integrated study of 100 patients with Xp21-linked muscular dystrophy using clinical, genetic, immunochemical and histopathological data. Part 2. Correlations within indiviual patients. *J. Med. Genet.* **30**, 737–744.

Nicholson, L. V. B., Johnson, M. A., Bushby, K. M. D. et al. (1993c). Integrated study of 100 patients with Xp21-linked muscular dystrophy using clinical, genetic, immunochemical and histopathological data. Part 3. Differential diagnosis and prognosis. *J. Med. Genet.* **30**, 745–751.

Nicholson, L., Johnson, M., Bushby, K. and Gardner-Medwin, D. (1993d). The functional significance of dystrophin-positive fibres in Duchenne muscular dystrophy. *Arch. Dis. Child.* **68**, 632–636.

Nigro, G., Politano, L., Nigro, V., Petretta, V. R. and Comi, L. I. (1994). Mutation of dystrophin gene and cardiomyopathy. *Neuromusc. Disord.* **4**, 371–379.

North, K. N., Miller, G., Iannaccone, S. T. et al. (1996). Cognitive dysfunction as the major presenting feature of Becker's muscular dystrophy. *Neurology* **46**, 461–465.

North, K. N., Laing, N. G. and Wallgren-Pettersson, C. (1997). Nemaline myopathy: current concepts. *J. Med. Genet.* **34**, 705–713.

Nowak, K. J., Wattanasirichaitoon, D., Goebbel, H. H. et al. (1999). Mutations in the skeletal muscle actin gene in patients with acta myopathy and nemaline myopathy. *Nat. Genet.* **23**, 208–212.

Ott, J. (1985). *Analysis of Human Genetic Linkage.* Baltimore, MD: Johns Hopkins University Press.

Ozawa, E., Noguchi, S., Mizuno, Y., Hagiwara, Y. and Yoshida, M. (1998). From dystrophinopathy to sarcoglycanopathy: evolution of a concept of muscular dystrophy. *Muscle Nerve* **21**, 421–438.

Padberg, G. (1982). Facioscapulohumeral disease. (Thesis) Leiden: University of Leiden.

Padberg, G. W. (1999). Facioscapulohumeral muscular dystrophy. In: *Neuromuscular Disorders: Clinical and Molecular Genetics*, ed. A. E. H. Emery, pp. 105–122. Chichester: Wiley.

Passos-Bueno, M. R., Bakker, E., Kneppers, A. et al. (1992). Different mosaicism frequencies for proximal and distal Duchenne muscular dystrophy (DMD) mutations indicate difference in etiology and recurrence risk. *Am. J. Hum. Genet.* **51**, 1150–1155.

Passos-Bueno, M. R., Vainzof, M., Moreira, E. S. and Zatz, M. (1999). Seven autosomal recessive limb-girdle muscular dystrophies in the Brazilian population: form LGMD2A to LGMD2G. *Am. J. Med. Genet.* **82**, 392–398.

Pearn, J. (1973). The gene frequency of acute Werdnig–Hoffman disease (SMA type I): a total population survey in north-east England. *J. Med. Genet.* **10**, 260–265.

Pepe, G., Giusti, B., Bertini, E. et al. (1999). A heterozygous splice site mutation in *COL6A1* leading to an in-frame deletion of the

α1(VI) collagen chain in an Italian family affected by Bethlem myopathy. *Biochem. Biophys. Res. Comm.* **258**, 802–807.

Peters, M. F., O'Brien, K. F., Sadoulet-Puccio, H. M., Kunkel, L. M., Adams, M. E. and Froehner, S. C. (1997). β-Dystrobrevin, a new member of the dystrophin family. *J. Biolog. Chem.* **272**, 31561–31569.

Philpot, J., Sewry, C., Pennock, J. and Dubowitz, V. (1995). Clinical phenotype in congenital muscular dystrophy: correlation with expression of merosin in skeletal muscle. *Neuromusc. Disord.* **5**, 301–305.

Piccolo, F., Jeanpierre, M., Leturcq, F. et al. (1996). A founder mutation in the γ-sarcoglycan gene of gypsies possibly predating their migration out of India. *Hum. Mol. Genet.* **5**, 2019–2022.

Politano, L., Nigro, V., Nigro, G. et al. (1996). Development of cardiomyopathy in female carriers of Duchenne and Becker muscular dystrophies. *JAMA* **275**, 1335–1338.

Poulton, J., Macaulay, V. and Marchington, D. R. (1998). Mitochondrial genetics 1998. Is the bottleneck cracked? *Am. J. Hum. Genet.* **62**, 752–757.

Quane, K. A., Healy, J. M. S., Keating, K. E. et al. (1993). Mutations in the ryanodine receptor gene in central core disease and malignant hyperthermia. *Nat. Genet.* **5**, 51–55.

Ranum, L. P. W., Rasmussen, P. F., Benzow, K. A., Koob, M. D. and Day, J. W. (1998). Genetic mapping of a second myotonic dystrophy locus. *Nat. Genet.* **19**, 196–198.

Reardon, W., Newcombe, R., Fenton, I., Sibert, J. and Harper, P. S. (1993). The natural history of congenital myotonic dystrophy: mortality and long term clinical aspects. *Arch. Dis. Child.* **68**, 177–181.

Ricci, E., Galluzi, G., Deidda, G. et al. (1999). Progress in the molecular diagnosis of facioscapulohumeral muscular dystrophy and correlation between the number of Kpn1 repeats at the 4q35 locus and clinical phenotype. *Ann. Neurol.* **45**, 751–757.

Richard, I., Brenguier, L., Dincer, P. et al. (1997). Mutliple independent molecular etiology for limb-girdle muscular dystrophy type 2A patients from various geographical origins. *Am. J. Hum. Genet.* **60**, 1128–1138.

Richard, I., Roudaut, C., Saenz, A. et al. (1999). Calpainopathy – a survey of mutations and polymorphisms. *Am. J. Hum. Genet.* **64**, 1524–1540.

Ricker, K., Grimm, T., Koch, M. C. et al. (1999). Linkage of proximal myotonic myopathy to chromosome 3q. *Neurology* **52**, 170–171.

Roberts, R. G., Bentley, D. R., Barby, T. F. M., Manners, E. and Bobrow, M. (1990). Direct diagnosis of carriers of Duchenne and Becker muscular dystrophy by amplification of lymphocyte RNA. *Lancet* **336**, 1523–1526.

Roberts, R., Coffey, A., Bobrow, M. and Bentley, D. (1992). Determination of the exon structure of the distal portion of the dystrophin gene by vectorette PCR. *Genomics* **13**, 942–950.

Roest, P. A. M., Roberts, R. G., Sugino, S., van Ommen, G. J. B. and den Dunnen, J. T. (1993). Protein truncation test (PTT) for rapid detection of translation-terminating mutations. *Hum. Mol. Genet.* **2**, 1719–1721.

Roy, N., Mahadevan, M. S., McLean, M. et al. (1995). The gene for neuronal apoptosis inhibitory protein is partially deleted in individuals with spinal muscular atrophy. *Cell* **80**, 167–178.

Rudnik-Schoneborn, S., Nicholson, G. A., Morgan, G., Rohrig, D. and Zerres, K. (1998). Different patterns of obstetric complications in myotonic dystrophy in relation to the disease status of the fetus. *Am. J. Med. Genet.* **80**, 314–321.

Sabourin, L. A., Tamai, K., Narang, M. A. and Korneluk, R. G. (1997). Overexpression of 3′-untranslated region of the myotonic dystrophy kinase cDNA inhibits myoblast differentiation in vitro. *J. Biol. Chem.* **272**, 29626–29635.

Sewry, C. A., Philpot, J., Sorokin, L. M. et al. (1996). Diagnosis of merosin (laminin-2) deficient congenital muscular dystrophy by skin biopsy. *Lancet* **347**, 582–584.

Shapiro, F., Specht, L. and Korf, B. R. (1991). Locomotor problems in infantile facioscapulohumeral muscular dystrophy. *Acta Orthopod. Scand.* **62**, 367–371.

Somerville, M. J., Hunter, A. G., Aubry, H. L., Korneluk, R. G., MacKenzie, A. E. and Surh, L. C. (1997). Clinical application of the molecular diagnosis of spinal muscular atrophy: deletions of neuronal apoptosis inhibitor protein and survival motor neuron genes. *Am. J. Med. Genet.* **69**, 159–165.

Speckman, R. A., Garg, A., Du, F. et al. (2000). Mutational and haplotype analyses of families with familial lipodystrophy (Dunnigan variety) reveal recurrent missense mutations in the globular c-terminal domain of lamin A/C. *Am. J. Hum. Genet.* **66**, 1192–1198.

Speer, M. C., Vance, J. M., Grubber, J. M. et al. (1999). Identification of a new autosomal dominant limb-girdle muscular dystrophy locus on chromosome 7. *Am. J. Hum. Genet.* **64**, 556–562.

Sullivan, T., Escalante-Alcalde, D., Bhatt, H. et al. (1999). Loss of A type lamin expression comprises nuclear envelope integrity leading to muscular dystrophy. *Cell Biol.* **147**, 913–919.

Tachi, N., Tachi, M., Sasaki, K., Nagata, N. and Chiba, S. (1990). Dystrophin analysis in the differential diagnosis of autosomal recessive muscular dystrophy of childhood and Duchenne muscular dystrophy. *Pediatr. Neurol.* **6**, 265–268.

Talbot, K., Ponting, C. P., Theodosiou, A. M., Ridrigues, N. R., Surtees, R., Mountford, R. and Davies, K. E. (1997). Missense mutation clustering in the survival motor neuron gene: a role for a conserved tyrosine and glycine rich region of the protein in RNA metabolism? *Hum. Mol. Genet.* **6**, 497–500.

Tan, E., Topaloglu, H., Sewry, C., et al. (1997). Late onset muscular dystrophy with cerebral white matter changes due to partial merosin deficiency. *Neuromusc. Disord.* **7**, 85–89.

Tan, P., Briner, J., Bolthsauser, E., Davis, M. R. et al. (1999). Homozygosity for a nonsense mutation in the alphatropomyosin slow gene *TMP3* in a patient with severe infantile nemaline myopathy. *Neuromusc. Disord.* **9**, 573–579

Taylor, J., Muntoni, F., Robb, S., Dubowitz, V. and Sewry, C. (1997). Early onset autosomal dominant myopathy with rigidity of the spine: a possible role for laminin beta-1. *Neuromusc. Disord.* **7**, 211–216.

Tomé, F. M. S., Guicheney, P. and Fardeau, M. (1999). Congenital muscular dystrophies. In: *Neuromuscular Disorders: Clinical and Molecular Genetics*, ed. A. E. H. Emery, pp. 21–57. Chichester: Wiley.

Urtasun, M., Saenz, A., Roudaut, C. et al. (1998). Limb-girdle muscular dystrophy in Guipuzcoa (Basque Country, Spain). *Brain* **121**, 1735–1747.

van der Knaap, M. S., Smit, L. M. E. and Barth, P. G. (1997). Magnetic resonance imaging in classification of congenital muscular dystrophies with brain abnormalities. *Ann. Neurol.* **42**, 50–59.

van der Kooi, A. J., de Visser, M. and Barth, P. G. (1994). Limb-girdle muscular dystrophy: reappraisal of a rejected entity. *Clin. Neurol. Neurosurg.* **96**, 209–218.

van der Kooi, A. J., Ledderhof, T. M., de Voogt, W. G. et al. (1996). A newly recognised autosomal dominant limb girdle muscular dystrophy with cardiac involvement. *Ann. Neurol.* **39**, 636–642.

van der Kooi, A. J., van Meegen, M., Ledderhof, T. M., McNally, E. M., de Visser, M. and Bolhuis, P. A. (1997). Genetic localisation of a newly recognised autosomal dominant limb-girdle muscular dystrophy with cardiac involvement (LGMD1B) to chromosome 1q11–21. *Am. J. Hum. Genet.* **60**, 891–895.

van der Kooi, A. J., de Voogt, W. G., Barth, P. G. et al. (1998). The heart in limb girdle muscular dystrophy. *Heart* **79**, 73–77.

van Deutekom, J. C., Bakker, E., Lemmers, R. J. L. F. et al. (1996). Evidence for subtelomeric exchange of 3.3 kb tandemly repeated units between chromosomes 4q35 and 10q26: implications for genetic counselling and etiology of FSHD1. *Hum. Mol. Genet.* **5**, 1997–2003.

van Essen, A. J., Abbs, S., Bauget, M. et al. (1992). Parental origin and germline mosaicism of deletions and duplications of the dystrophin gene: a European study. *Hum. Genet.* **88**, 249–257.

Vincent, M. C., Giuraud-Chaumeil, C., Laporte, J., Manouvrier-Hanu, S. and Mandel, J. L. (1998). Extensive germinal mosaicism in X-linked myotubular myopathy stimulates genetic heterogeneity. *J. Med. Genet.* **35**, 241–243.

Voit, T., Fardeau, M. and Tomé, F. M. S. (1994). Prenatal detection of merosin expression in human placenta. *Neuropaediatrics* **25**, 332–333.

Vuopala, K., Makela-Bengs, P., Suomalainen, A., Herva, R., Leisti, J. and Peltonen, L. (1995). Lethal congenital contracture syndrome (LCCS), a fetal anterior horn cell disease, is not linked to the SMA 5q locus. *J. Med. Genet.* **32**, 36–38.

Wallgren-Pettersson, C. (1998). Workshop report: the 58th ENMC Workshop on myotubular myopathy. *Neuromusc. Disord.* **8**, 521–525.

Wallgren-Pettersson, C. and Clarke, A. (1998). Myotubular myopathy. In: *Neuromuscular Disorders: Clinical and Molecular Genetics*, ed. A. E. H. Emery, pp. 263–276. Chichester: Wiley.

Wallgren-Pettersson, C., Hiilesmaa, V. and Paatero, H. (1995a). Pregnancy and delivery in congenital nemaline myopathy. *Acta Obstet. Gynaecol. Scand.* **74**, 659–661.

Wallgren-Pettersson, C., Clarke, A., Samson, F. et al. (1995b). The myotubular myopathies: differential diagnosis of the X-linked recessive, autosomal dominant and autosomal recessive forms and present state of DNA studies. *J. Med. Genet.* **32**, 673–679.

Wallgren-Pettersson, C., Beggs, A. H. and Laing, N. G. (1998). Workshop report: the 51st ENMC international workshop on nemaline myopathy. *Neuromusc. Disord.* **8**, 53–56.

Wang, C. H., Xu, J., Carter, T. A. et al. (1996). Characterisation of survival motor neuron (*SMN*) gene deletions in asymptomatic carriers of spinal muscular atrophy. *Hum. Mol. Genet.* **5**, 359–365.

Weiler, T., Greenberg, C. R., Zelinski, T. et al. (1998). A gene for autosomal recessive limb-girdle muscular dystrophy in Manitoba Hutterites maps to chromosome region 9q31–33: evidence for another limb-girdle muscular dystrophy locus. *Am. J. Hum. Genet.* **63**, 140–147.

Weiler, T., Bashir, R., Anderson, L. V. B. et al. (1999). Identical mutation in patients with limb girdle muscular dystrophy type 2B or Miyoshi myopathy suggests a role for modifier gene(s). *Hum. Mol. Genet.* **8**, 871–877.

White, S. L., Collins, V. R., Wolfe, R. et al. (1999). Genetic counselling and prenatal diagnosis for the mitochondrial DNA mutations at nucleotide 8993. *Am. J. Hum. Genet.* **65**, 000–000.

Wijmenga, C., Hewitt, J., Sandkuijl, L. et al. (1992). Chromosome 4q DNA rearrangements associated with facioscapulohumeral muscular dystrophy. *Nat. Genet.* **2**, 26–30.

Wirth, B., Schmidt, T., Hahnen, E. et al. (1997). De novo rearrangements found in 2% of index patients with spinal muscular atrophy: mutational mechanisms, parental origin, mutation rate and implications for genetic counselling. *Am. J. Hum. Genet.* **61**, 1102–1111.

Zatz, M., Marie, S. K., Passos-Bueno, M. R. et al. (1995). High proportion of new mutations and possible anticipation in Brazilian facioscapulohumeral muscular dystrophy families. *Am. J. Hum. Genet.* **56**, 99–105.

Zatz, M., Marie, S. K., Cerqueira, A., Vainzof, M., Pavanello, R. C. M. and Passos-Bueno, M. (1998). The facioscapulohumeral muscular dystrophy (FSHD1) gene affects males more severely and more frequently than females. *Am. J. Med. Genet.* **77**, 155–161.

Zerres, K. and Davies, M. E. (1999). Workshop report: the 59th ENMC international workshop on spinal muscular atrophies: recent progress and revised diagnostic criteria. *Neuromusc. Disord.* **9**, 272–278.

Zerres, K., Rudnik-Schoneborn, S., Forkert, R. and Wirth, B. (1995). Genetic basis of adult-onset spinal muscular atrophy. *Lancet* **346**, 1162.

36

The principles of treatment, prevention and rehabilitation and perspectives on future therapies

Giovanni Meola, George Karpati and Robert C. Griggs

Introduction

This chapter deals with both the medical treatment of patients with muscle disease and strategies for prevention of disease. It also briefly summarizes practical aspects of physical therapy and surgical treatment of neuromuscular disease. The chapter concludes with perspectives on future treatment of muscle disease. Specific treatment is now available for many muscle diseases and is considered in appropriate detail in the chapters dealing with each disease. An overview of specific treatments for muscle disease are summarized below.

Treatments for muscle diseases

In most hereditary neuromuscular diseases in which the causal gene, or genes, has been located and characterized and in which the missing or abnormal gene product has been identified, there are new opportunities for studying the efficacy of treatment strategies made possible by the ability to define diseases accurately. Even now, clinical trials have begun to define successful treatment. Table 36.1 lists treatments considered effective in the myopathies and indicates those for which there are data from well-controlled clinical trials.

Use of corticosteroids in patients with neuromuscular disease

Corticosteroids have been shown in randomized controlled trials to increase strength and muscle mass in patients with Duchenne dystrophy (Mendell et al., 1989; Griggs et al., 1991; Fenichel et al., 1991) and are anecdotally effective in Becker dystrophy. They are widely used in the inflammatory myopathies dermatomyositis and polymyositis despite the lack of evidence from placebo-controlled studies supporting their use. Patients with neuromuscular disease are especially vulnerable to the side effects of corticosteroids. Most severe complications and many side effects can be prevented with appropriate considerations of (i) choice of agent; (ii) method of administration and dosage; (iii) concomitant medications and illness; and (iv) preventive strategies with medications, diet and exercise.

Intermittent corticosteroid administration schedules are less toxic than daily or multiple daily doses. However, there are no adequate therapeutic trials comparing the effectiveness of specific schedules for most disorders. Moreover, where disease response is readily measured objectively, daily schedules have usually been found to be more effective: examples include giant cell arteritis, rheumatoid arthritis and Duchenne dystrophy. For giant cell arteritis, the superiority of daily over alternate-day corticosteroids in controlling disease activity has been objectively demonstrated by clinical symptoms and by measurements of sedimentation rate. High-dose (1 g) intravenous methylprednisolone is sometimes used with acute exacerbations of myositis and other disorders. It has been suggested that such 'bolus' methylprednisolone (1 g/day for three days) will induce rapid improvement in the patient with an acute exacerbation without subjecting patients to the long-term consequences of high-dose corticosteroids. Certain side effects (e.g. osteopenia) may, however, appear rapidly in bolus-treated patients (Rodillo et al., 1991).

The concomitant administration of agents inducing the cytochrome P450 system (e.g. phenobarbitone (phenobarbital) and phenytoin) will lower blood corticosteroid levels (Chalk et al., 1984) and diminish corticosteroid therapeutic and toxic effects. Cyclosporin (cyclosporine) decreases the clearance of corticosteroids and increases their effect. Hypoalbuminaemia increases the free corticosteroid level

Table 36.1. Specific treatments for skeletal muscle diseases

Disease	Treatment
Duchenne dystrophy	Corticosteroids[a] (slight–moderate benefit)
Dermatomyositis	Corticosteroids, azathioprine, methotrexate
Polymyositis	Corticosteroids, azathioprine, methotrexate
Acute metabolic myopathies	Resolve with correction of derangement, (e.g. hypokalaemia)
Toxic myopathy	Most resolve with drug/toxin elimination
Endocrine deficiency/excess	Hormone replacement/reduction
Hypokalaemic periodic paralysis	Acetazolamide, dichlorphenamide[a]
Hyperkalaemic periodic paralysis	Acetazolamide, thiazides, dichlorphenamide[a]
Myotonia	
Autosomal dominant	Phenytoin,[a] quinine, procainamide
Autosomal recessive	Mexiletine
Carnitine deficiency	Corticosteroids, riboflavine carnitine, propanolol
Malignant hyperthermia	Dantrolene

Note:
[a] Established by controlled clinical trials.

and increases steroid effect. Azathioprine and other cytotoxic agents may have a 'steroid-sparing' effect and permit reduction in corticosteroid dosage.

Preventing side effects of corticosteroids
Osteopenia
Older women and growing children are especially prone to develop bony complications of corticosteroid use. The two major factors predisposing to osteoporosis in the older woman are low bone mass at menopause and an accelerated rate of bone loss after menopause. If menopause is early, if bone mass is reduced and if the rate of bone loss is accelerated, aggressive preventive strategies are indicated (Bente, 1991). Bone mass can be assessed by single (forearm) or dual (spine) photon absorptiometry. Bone loss can be assessed by deoxypyridinoline excretion (Reid and Ibbertson, 1986). The administration of calcium supplements with or without vitamin D has been shown to improve calcium balance and to prevent osteopenia. Calcium carbonate sufficient to give 1 g elemental calcium, and vitamin D 50 000 units per week are often used. It is essential to monitor both serum and urinary calcium during such therapy. Exercise increases bone mass in normal individuals and may be beneficial in preventing corticosteroid osteopenia. Weight bearing may be equally important. Other measures that increase bone mass such as fluoride, androgens and oestrogens are of uncertain benefit in steroid-induced osteopenia. The androgen- or oestrogen-deficient individual should receive appropriate replacement therapy.

Bisphosphonates are synthetic analogues of pyrophosphate. They are poorly absorbed and they bind avidly to bone mineral, are retained in mineralized tissue (or excreted in the urine) and tend to inhibit bone resorption. They have been shown to decrease bone loss in postmenopausal women, immobilized patients with spine fractures and corticosteroid-treated patients.

Muscle wasting
The majority of patients receiving pharmacological doses of corticosteroids will eventually develop muscle atrophy. Many develop atrophy within only 12 weeks of therapy. Muscle atrophy can be improved and prevented, at least to some extent, by exercise (Garrel et al., 1988). There is both computed tomographic and ergometric documentation of a prevention or reversal of muscle atrophy and weakness with exercise. Hypokalaemia, occasionally profound, may complicate corticosteroid therapy and cause weakness. Whether moderate depletion of total body potassium is a cause of muscle weakness in corticosteroid-treated patients is unknown.

A variety of other strategies can prevent or improve corticosteroid atrophy, including aggressive treatment of pain (e.g. from joints), which limits activity. Testosterone levels are low in corticosteroid-treated men. Testosterone replacement may be justifiable if levels are low. Fluorinated corticosteroids should be avoided if long-term use is needed since they are more likely to cause myopathy (Dropcho and Soong, 1991).

Ocular complications
Cataracts may develop rapidly and in young individuals are to some extent potentially reversible. Careful surveillance for cataracts is essential, particularly if their presence would influence duration or dosage of corticosteroid therapy. Glaucoma occurs in approximately 10% of

corticosteroid-treated individuals and is probably an idiosyncratic response based on either a hereditary susceptibility to corticosteroid effect or a hereditary predisposition to glaucoma. Proptosis is common with corticosteroid use.

Ulcer prevention

Corticosteroids do not, by themselves, cause peptic ulcer disease (Conn and Blitzer, 1976; Carson et al., 1991). Neurological diseases being treated with corticosteroids (head injury, stroke, myositis) are often associated with ulcer. The use of histamine H_2 receptor blockade has become routine in patients symptomatic with peptic disease. Patients receiving corticosteroids should be prophylactically treated with histamine H_2 blockers only if another factor associated with peptic disease is present. Use of H_2 blockers causes positive occult blood tests.

Lipomatosis

Corticosteroid-induced enlargement of adipose tissue can result in a variety of complications that must be anticipated. Fat deposits affected include epidural fat, producing myelopathy or a cauda equina syndrome; retro-orbital fat, producing exophthalmos; pericardial fat, producing an 'enlarging mediastinum'; peripheral fat in the wrist, producing carpal tunnel syndrome; intra-abdominal fat, producing pseudoascites; and popliteal fossa fat, simulating Baker cysts. Most patients that develop lipomatosis have received excessive corticosteroid dosage. The recognition of spinal cord involvement in the patient with neuromuscular disease requiring high-dose corticosteroids is often delayed; while uncommon, it must be considered in any patient who has a progression of weakness despite corticosteroids.

Developing new treatment

There are excellent prospects for the development of new treatments for chronic, progressive neuromuscular disease. The steps necessary for such discovery have been carefully reviewed in the past (Brooke et al., 1981, 1983; Edwards et al., 1984; Griggs, 1994). In general, the first step in developing therapy is to characterize the course of the untreated disease by charting the natural history. Such natural history studies must:

- be longitudinal (i.e. following patients for many months or even years depending on the rate of disease progression)
- be cross-sectional (i.e. determining the findings of a large group of patients at each age and stage of disease)

- be conducted in a homogeneous defined population of patients with the disease
- employ quantitative measures that can be used to derive statistically analysable data.

Reproducible measurements for weakness include forced vital capacity (Griggs, 1990), manual muscle testing (Brooke et al., 1983; Florence et al., 1992), quantitative myometry (Edwards et al., 1987; Brussock et al., 1992; Personius et al., 1994; Tawil et al., 1994) and timed functional testing (Brooke et al., 1983).

Once natural history data have been obtained, it is then possible to (i) determine the variability of a quantitative measurement between different tests in the same patient, between tests by different examiners and between patients; (ii) determine the rate of change of the measurement over time; and (iii) determine the number of patients and extent of treatment response necessary to produce a significant change in the natural history over any specified interval of time (Brooke et al., 1983; Tawil et al., 1994).

The introduction of a putative therapeutic modality is usually conducted in a small group of patients to establish safety. Even a single patient, carefully studied, can provide important information. If the natural history has been charted, it is possible to perform a relatively small controlled therapeutic trial using historical controls (Mendell et al., 1987). The randomized, double-masked controlled trial remains the 'gold standard' for therapeutic trials but can seldom be performed until there is preliminary evidence for safety and efficacy of the proposed treatment. Fortunately, many clinicians have begun to address the quantification of the natural history of many of the muscle diseases, including Duchenne dystrophy, myotonic dystrophy, the limb girdle dystrophies, facioscapulohumeral dystrophy, oculopharyngeal dystrophy, periodic paralysis and inclusion body myositis.

Supportive treatment: physical therapy

The patient with progressive, disabling weakness for whom there is no specific, pharmacological treatment presents a major challenge to the physician. Patients who require a wheelchair may even be unable to reach the physician's surgery. Much can be done to maintain function in such patients despite inexorably progressive weakness. The consequences of immobility reduce dramatically the life quality in patients and add to the burden imposed upon caregivers: obesity, constipation and gastrointestinal problems, bone loss and pressure sores are all preventable and most are treatable.

Physical therapy of neuromuscular diseases

The physical management of muscle disease depends upon the age of onset of the specific disease and whether the disease is progressive or nonprogressive. The role of physical therapy is supportive and usually focuses on preventing the consequences of weakness such as contractures and deformity, while maintaining function through the use of compensatory mechanisms, appropriate orthoses and aids to mobility. The goals of rehabilitation programmes for muscle disease are to maintain or improve muscle strength; to promote or prolong ambulation and other functions; to prevent tendon contractures, deformity and other consequences of weakness; and to facilitate psychosocial development and interaction.

The methods of treatment used in managing the patient with a muscle disease are exercise, passive stretching, the provision of night splints and the provision of orthoses or, where applicable, aids to mobility (Brooke et al. 1989). As a general rule, patients with neuromuscular disease benefit from a daily exercise programme that includes both stretching to maintain a full range of motion about each joint and a judicious general endurance component. All muscles, whether diseased or normal, respond in a graded fashion to exercise stress; strengthening occurs if 35% of maximal tension is exceeded, while atrophy develops if muscle contractions fall below 20% of maximal tension. Excessive work performed near maximal tension may lead to muscle damage. In myopathy, the therapeutic window is reduced; since there are fewer available muscle fibres, only a submaximal exercise response is possible. However, in patients with relatively stable weakness or only slow decline, up to 50% increase in work capacity and endurance has been recorded with exercise such as stationary bicycling and swimming. *Eccentric* contraction during exercise (contraction of a muscle while it is lengthening) is particularly likely to injure weak muscles in patients with neuromuscular disease. An example of eccentric contraction is the exercise of descending stairs: muscles lengthen as the patient steps downward. Electrical stimulation of weakened muscles is often suggested by physiotherapists. In general, such strategies are likely to cause excessive tension on injured fibres, further injuring the muscle. The most sensible programme is the regular performance of tasks that are a part of normal activities of daily living. One clear exception is the value of therapeutic standing in patients who are no longer able to walk. The provision of assistance and protective support against falling will allow patients to maintain bone mass and cardiovascular autoregulation. Walking (with supervision) in a swimming pool serves the same value.

Respiratory management

Two important points pertaining to the respiratory system in all patients with chronic progressive neuromuscular disease are recognition of a second and treatable coincidental illness and recognition of the presence of atypical manifestations of the underlying neuromuscular disease that might suggest a second diagnosis to the unwary or naive clinician. In the second instance, inappropriate diagnostic and therapeutic measures may be applied. Both considerations require familiarity with the spectrum of medical illness complicating neuromuscular disease. As an example of coincidental illness that might be overlooked, a patient with severe, wheelchair-bound facioscapulohumeral muscular dystrophy who presents with acute respiratory symptoms, hypoxia and carbon dioxide retention might be considered to have end-stage neuromuscular disease. However, since facioscapulohumeral muscular dystrophy seldom results in ventilatory failure (Griggs and Donohoe, 1982), it is overwhelmingly likely that a treatable intercurrent illness is present. In this instance, aggressive respiratory support would be indicated and a search for an additional diagnosis is warranted. As an example of a typical or often-unexpected manifestation of the underlying neuromuscular disease, a child with myotonic dystrophy who presents with colicky abdominal pain and is found to have elevated liver function test results including γ-glutamyltransferase might be suspected of having liver disease. Although a coincidental illness *could* be present, unexplained abdominal pain is a frequent manifestation of childhood myotonic dystrophy (Harper, 1989) and the γ-glutamyltransferase and other liver function studies are often elevated in myotonic dystrophy. In practice, one would simply follow the patient with myotonic dystrophy to see if the symptoms and laboratory abnormalities were progressive.

Table 36.2 lists the chronic neuromuscular disorders that characteristically cause respiratory insufficiency. The availability of techniques for home management of what was once considered 'terminal respiratory failure', and the increasing awareness that ventilator dependency can be prevented for many years by appropriate treatment, has prompted careful study of the mechanisms leading to ventilatory failure in patients with muscular dystrophy (Smith et al., 1991).

Patients with neuromuscular disease characteristically develop a restrictive defect with a reduction in total lung capacity (Newsom-Davis et al., 1976; Roussos and Macklem, 1982). This fall in lung capacity is the result of a combination of factors. Impaired ventilatory musculature leads to chest wall stiffness through a combination of

Table 36.2. Restrictive lung disease in the neuromuscular diseases

Type of disorder	Diseases
Anterior horn cell disease	Amyotrophic lateral sclerosis,[a] spinal muscular atrophy (especially Werdnig–Hoffman disease), late progression of poliomyelitis
Peripheral neuropathy	Charcot–Marie–Tooth disease, inflammatory demyelinating peripheral neuropathy
Neuromuscular junction disorders	Myasthenia gravis,[a] Lambert-Eaton syndrome[a]
Myopathies	
Muscular dystrophies	Duchenne dystrophy and other dystrophinopathies, myotonic dystrophy,[a] limb girdle dystrophy (several types), facioscapulohumeral dystrophy[b] (very rare), scapuloperoneal dystrophy
Metabolic disorders	Acid maltase deficiency,[a] carnitine deficiency
Congenital myopathies	Centronuclear myopathy, nemaline myopathy, congenital fibre type disproportion, polymyositis/dermatomyositis[b]

Notes:

[a] May present with respiratory failure prior to other signs of weakness.

[b] Respiratory muscle insufficiency uncommon.

kyphoscoliosis, fibrosis of dystrophic chest muscles, pulmonary microatelectasis, aspiration and impaired clearing of secretions because of reduced ability to cough (McCool et al., 1986; Smith et al., 1991). The inability to expand the lungs by a sigh as well as inability to shift posture may contribute to restrictive lung disease. The earliest detectable abnormality easily recognized by clinical tests is a reduction in static pressures: maximum expiratory pressure is reduced to a greater extent than maximum inspiratory pressure (Black and Hyatt, 1971; Saunders et al., 1978; Griggs et al., 1981). Other factors contributing to respiratory difficulties include ineffective cough because of impaired glottic function as well as respiratory muscle weakness, impaired central nervous system ventilatory drive and upper airway obstruction during sleep. Sleep-related respiratory abnormalities often play a role in ventilatory failure; nocturnal hypoxaemia develops and contributes to cardiac failure (cor pulmonale), and hypercapnia. Nocturnal hypoxaemia first occurs during REM sleep and may be present when other signs of hypoxaemia such as daytime hypoxaemia, carbon dioxide retention and associated symptoms are lacking (Coakley et al., 1990). Duchenne dystrophy (Carroll et al., 1991; Smith et al., 1988, 1989), myotonic dystrophy (Gilmartin et al., 1991) as well as other myopathies (Ellis et al., 1987) have sleep-related hypoxaemia well in advance of other signs of ventilatory failure. Since treatment of this process with nocturnal respiratory support is now practical (Garay et al., 1981; Ellis et al., 1987; Heckmatt et al., 1990) and since studies to detect hypoxaemia can be obtained with no morbidity and can

even be done as an outpatient (Carroll et al., 1991), patients with neuromuscular disease must be followed prospectively for the possibility of impending ventilatory difficulties.

Acute respiratory failure

Acute respiratory failure is usually precipitated by a readily apparent event such as pneumonitis, bronchitis, atelectasis, aspiration, pneumothorax, congestive heart failure or other intercurrent process (Griggs and Donohoe, 1985). In following patients with neuromuscular disease, when the forced vital capacity falls below 30% of normal, the patient and family should be warned of the risk of both acute and chronic ventilatory failure, and management options should be discussed. A decision about providing ventilatory assistance is complex and depends upon the availability of caregivers, the patient's economic situation, the tempo of the disease, the lifestyle and the wishes of the patient and caregivers (Goldblatt, 1984; Madorsky et al., 1984; Mendell and Vaughn, 1984; Silverstein et al., 1991).

Prevention of respiratory complications

In neuromuscular diseases where respiratory muscle involvement is expected (Table 36.2) the forced vital capacity should be assessed at least annually. If respiratory symptoms develop, both forced vital capacity and static pressure (particularly maximum expiratory pressure) should be obtained. A reduction of forced vital capacity with the preservation of maximum expiratory pressure indicates that the respiratory symptoms are not caused by the restrictive disease of neuromuscular weakness (Griggs et al., 1981; Griggs and Donohoe, 1985). A coincidental process is likely to be present. Chronic obstructive lung disease, for example, is present in at least 25% of patients over the age of 50 years and is frequently confused with 'end-stage' restrictive lung disease. In this case, the obstructive disease may be the cause or may contribute to apparent terminal neuromuscular disease with respiratory insufficiency.

If the forced vital capacity is reduced to less than 50% of normal, respiratory exercises should be instituted, and a chest roentgenogram and electrocardiogram should be obtained. All patients should receive one-time immunization for pneumococcal infections (Schwartz, 1982) and in patients with a vital capacity of less than 30%, annual immunization for influenza viral infection should be administered (Belshe, 1999). The major exception for use of respiratory exercises is in disorders characterized by fatiguability, such as myasthenia gravis, where exercise may pose hazards. Although intermittent positive pressure breathing (IPPB) has been recommended in the past as a means of improving lung compliance, it is ineffective in long-term treatment of patients with neuromuscular disease (McCool et al., 1986). It may have role in the acute illness for delivery of inhaled bronchodilators.

Detecting incipient respiratory failure

Patients with neuromuscular disease often tolerate developing hypoxaemia and carbon dioxide retention without air hunger. Symptoms that should suggest respiratory insufficiency include morning headache, insomnia, increasing ankle oedema, weight loss or fatigue. Signs on examination include those of chronic carbon dioxide retention: retinal vein engorgement, and occasionally papilloedema, somnolence and tremors, myoclonus or asterixis. Patients with Duchenne dystrophy may exhibit glossopharyngeal breathing: the use of the tongue and glottic muscles to force air into the lungs. This remarkable strategy enables a patient to cough or shout and can increase a dwindling vital capacity from 300–400 ml to an apparent value of 1500–1800 ml. An unwary technician or physician finding such a forced vital capacity may totally overlook severe restrictive lung disease as a consequence.

Routine laboratory tests are extremely sensitive to impending respiratory failure. A depression of serum chloride implies a compensation for carbon dioxide retention

and is an ominous sign in amyotrophic lateral sclerosis (Stambler et al., 1998) and other neuromuscular diseases. In the nonsmoker, a rising haematocrit indicates hypoxaemia. The carboxyhaemoglobin of the chronic smoker provides a stimulus for erythropoietin.

Blood gases may be measured by either invasive or non-invasive methods. Oxygen saturation can be measured by using a transcutaneous electrode; it is useful for evaluating a patient for acute decompensation (indicating acute infection or mucus plug) and for comparison of response after therapy. In order to get an accurate value for the partial pressure of oxygen, one must take an arterial blood sample (for estimation of arterial blood gases), an uncomfortable procedure often accompanied by hyperventilation, which artificially lowers the partial pressure of carbon dioxide. One can measure end-tidal carbon dioxide pressure at the nose or mouth to get an estimate of the blood level. Measurement of capillary blood gases offers a compromise and if done with appropriate techniques (warming the hand, avoiding clotting of blood) may be quite accurate.

Expectant management of respiratory failure

Patients with amyotrophic lateral sclerosis, Duchenne dystrophy and the late stages of other neuromuscular diseases need to be told the risk of both acute and chronic ventilatory failure and management options should be discussed. It is important that a plan of action (or inaction) be charted and discussed carefully. Patients, including boys with Duchenne dystrophy, are generally well aware of the likelihood that respiratory failure will develop eventually and are reassured rather than frightened by such discussions. Moreover, patients with progressive neuromuscular disease may often mistakenly anticipate that death is imminent at a time when their respiratory function is adequate or even normal.

Management of acute respiratory failure

Patients who are obtunded or dyspnoeic associated with hypoxia and hypercapnia usually require emergency endotracheal intubation. If hypoxia alone (without carbon dioxide retention) is present and the patient is alert, low flow oxygen (less than 1 l/min) may correct hypoxia without causing hypercapnia. Special equipment is often necessary to provide reliable low flow rates. If oxygen is administered in the acute setting, it is essential to obtain blood gases frequently to exclude the development of hypercapnia. Oxygenation can be monitored by digital oximetry. Patients with respiratory muscle weakness are often intermittently hypercapnic, and the administration of oxygen may further depress already decreased ventilatory drive and worsen hypoventilation (Weinberger et al., 1989). Specific treatment of ventilatory failure depends on the cause. The commonest event to precipitate ventilatory failure is atelectasis, which can be improved by ventilatory support, appropriate suctioning of secretions, hydration and postural drainage. Pathogens are seldom cultured from bronchial secretions at the time of acute presentation. Antibiotics are indicated if the sputum is purulent or there are other clinical findings to support the presence of infection.

Long-term ventilatory support

Negative pressure ventilation such as the cuirass (Holtackers et al., 1982) and plastic 'raincoat' (Griggs and Donohoe, 1982) devices are occasionally helpful but are not well tolerated by alert patients with normal sensation. Positive pressure nasal mechanical ventilation during sleep has been applied with success to patients with neuromuscular disease. Duchenne dystrophy (Rideau et al., 1981; Heckmatt et al., 1990), amyotrophic lateral sclerosis and many other disorders (Ellis et al., 1987) are amenable to such treatment. If glottic function impairs cough, the retention of secretions ultimately poses an insurmountable problem for the use of negative pressure ventilators or positive pressure nasal ventilation, and in this situation tracheostomy is necessary. Many end-stage patients with Duchenne dystrophy, myotonic dystrophy and Becker dystrophy will ultimately require tracheostomy and positive pressure ventilation. Tracheostomy permits normal speech and provides an easy means of clearing tracheal secretions. If tracheostomy is performed, it must be done in hospital and usually requires one to three days of treatment in an intensive care unit and subsequently one to two weeks of training for patients and caregivers to develop the necessary skills for outpatient management. Atelectasis often develops in the postoperative period and may necessitate longer respiratory care in the hospital. The goal of ventilatory support is to return the patient to an active lifestyle and permit both patient and family to maintain activities outside the home. With lightweight, portable, rechargeable ventilators, portable suction equipment, and a wheelchair that accommodates the equipment, patients who require ventilatory support can often continue attending school and even maintain employment. The possibility of providing long-term ventilatory support for patients with neuromuscular disease poses both ethical and economic issues that have been considered in reviews (Goldblatt, 1984; Goldblatt and Greenlaw, 1989; Silverstein et al., 1991). The account of the

decision taken by one patient with Duchenne dystrophy to pursue ventilatory support makes compelling reading (Eberhardt, 1988).

Cardiac complications

Symptomatic cardiac disease is relatively uncommon in neuromuscular disease (Table 36.3). Histopathological, electrocardiographic and ultrasonographic studies, however, indicate that myocardial involvement is extremely frequent in myopathies (Reeves et al., 1980; Nippoldt et al., 1982). Primary myocardial involvement with a congestive cardiomyopathy occurs in a subset of patients with Duchenne and Becker muscular dystrophy (Brooke et al., 1989). Prospective studies indicate that patients with relatively preserved ambulation are more likely to develop clinical cardiac disease (Brooke at al., 1989). Cardiomyopathy is occasionally the presenting manifestation of a neuromuscular disorder (Table 36.3) (Norris et al., 1966). In such patients, as in all instances of apparent primary myocardial disease in association with neuromuscular disease, the possibility that cardiac failure may be the direct result of respiratory insufficiency and consequent cor pulmonale must be carefully pursued. Oximetry should be performed in all instances. Even patients with normoxaemia during the day may have severe sleep apnoea or hypoventilation with nocturnal hypoxia (see above). Night-time respiratory support that eliminates this hypoxia will correct heart failure.

If cardiac failure is indeed present as a result of myocardial involvement, medical treatment options are limited. Fluid restriction, diuretics such as frusemide (furosemide) and afterload reduction with agents such as the angiotensin-converting enzyme inhibitors may be of benefit. Patients with ejection fractions of less than 25% should receive anticoagulation therapy to prevent emboli.

Cardiac transplantation

In the dystrophinopathies, cardiac muscle disease is invariably present, but in Duchenne dystrophy it is symptomatic only very late in the course of the disease. A substantial subset of patients with Duchenne appear particularly vulnerable (Brooke at al., 1989). The severity of the weakness of these patients and the imminent threat of respiratory failure precludes consideration for cardiac transplantation. There are a number of milder phenotypes of dystrophinopathy in which cardiomyopathy dominates the phenotype. If skeletal muscle weakness is moderate and there is severe cardiac failure, transplantation has

Table 36.3. Chronic neuromuscular diseases with cardiac disease

Cardiac disease	Neuromuscular diseases
Congestive cardiomyopathy	Muscular dystrophies: limb girdle, myotonic, Duchenne, Becker, Emery–Dreifuss[a] Congenital myopathies: nemaline Metabolic myopathies: acid maltase deficiency (infantile disease), carnitine deficiency, lysosome-associated membrane protein 2 defect Inflammatory myopathy: polymyositis
Cor pulmonale	Muscular dystrophies: Duchenne, Becker, myotonic, limb-girdle Congenital myopathy: nemaline Metabolic myopathy: acid maltase deficiency
Arrhythmias	Muscular dystrophies: myotonic,[a] limb girdle, Emery Dreifuss[a] Metabolic myopathies: Kearn–Sayre syndrome, Andersen's syndrome,[a] hyperkalaemic periodic paralysis Inflammatory myopathy: polymyositis
Mitral valve prolapse	Muscular dystrophies: myotonic, Duchenne, limb girdle (various)

Note:

[a] May present with cardiac disease

been performed with excellent restoration of function. Patients with dystrophinopathy and cardiomyopathy without any appreciable skeletal muscle weakness have received successful transplants (Donofrio et al., 1989).

Most other neuromuscular diseases with life-threatening cardiomyopathy are sufficiently disabling that cardiac transplantation is not a consideration. The two exceptions are the unusual X-linked glycogen storage disease lysosome-associated membrane protein 2 deficiency, where transplantation has been performed (Nishino et al., 2000). Similarly, there are patients with acid lysosomal glycogen storage who have undergone successful transplantation (Dworzak et al., 1994).

Cardiac arrhythmias commonly complicate several neuromuscular diseases. Complete heart block requiring pacemaker implantation is frequent in myotonic dystrophy (Griggs et al., 1975; Moorman et al., 1985), Emery–Dreifuss muscular dystrophy and mitochondrial myopathies. Life-threatening tachyarrhythmias are infrequent in most myopathies but are characteristic of Andersen's syndrome (periodic paralysis with bidirectional tachycardia) (Sansone et al., 1997a). Patients with myotonic dystrophy, Duchenne dystrophy, Becker dystrophy, and occasional patients with humeroperoneal or scapulo-peroneal dystrophy can have atrial or ventricular arrhythmias that mandate therapy.

Prevention of oedema

Oedema of the feet, ankles or, in the bed-bound patient, the presacral region is frequent in the severely immobilized patient with neuromuscular disease. The new appearance of oedema should prompt clinical evaluation for respiratory failure and cor pulmonale; cardiomyopathy; or a coincidental illness such as renal disease, hypoalbuminaemia or drug-related fluid retention. In most patients with neuromuscular disease over 25–30 years of age, however, ankle oedema is the combined result of a loss of muscle pumping action and the dependency of the legs. Oedema is a particular nuisance in patients with neuromuscular disease because it increases the weight of the extremities, further compromising mobility. It also eventuates in tissue damage leading to skin infection and ulceration.

Prevention and treatment of ankle oedema

Medications that cause or worsen ankle oedema should be avoided: amitriptyline and other tricyclic antidepressants, nonsteroidal anti-inflammatory agents, β-adrenergic blocking agents and calcium channel blocking agents are particularly likely to precipitate or exacerbate ankle oedema. Wheelchair-bound patients should have elevating leg rests to avoid the complete dependency of lower

Table 36.4. Gastrointestinal manifestations of neuromuscular disease

Manifestations	Disorders
Abnormalities of deglutition	
Nasal regurgitation	Myasthenia gravis, amyotrophic lateral sclerosis, Kennedy syndrome
Dysphagia: pain	Dermatomyositis, polymyositis
Dysphagia: Inability to swallow	Dermatomyositis, polymyositis, myotonic dystrophy
Cricopharyngeal achalasia	Oculopharyngeal muscular dystrophy, inclusion body myositis, dermatomyositis, polymyositis, myotonic dystrophy
Oesophageal hypomotility	Dermatomyositis, polymyositis, myotonic dystrophy
Abnormalities of gastrointestinal function	
Gastroparesis or gastric dilatation	Duchenne dystrophy, mitochondrial myopathies
Intestinal hypomotility	Pseudo-obstruction; Duchenne dystrophy; Becker dystrophy; mitochondrial myopathies
Megacolon	Myotonic dystrophy; mitochondrial myopathies
Constipation	Duchenne dystrophy; Becker dystrophy; myotonic dystrophy; most neuromuscular diseases resulting in loss of ambulation
Biliary tract disease	Myotonic dystrophy

extremities. Elevation of the foot of the bed at night by placing a cushion between a mattress and innerspring (not under the legs themselves) is often well tolerated and will lessen oedema in patients who can spend a period of the day in bed. Elastic support stockings may decrease oedema but are often uncomfortable and require frequent reapplication; consequently, both patient and caregivers are reluctant to use them. Sodium restriction has theoretical benefits but is often unacceptable to patients. Patients often request diuretics; anecdotally, furosemide is effective in eliminating ankle oedema. Diuretic treatment poses the risk of electrolyte imbalance and should be avoided where possible.

Gastrointestinal complications

All portions of the alimentary system are subject to involvement by one or more neuromuscular disease (Table 36.4). Although most myopathies have their major impact on skeletal muscle, emerging data on diseases such as Duchenne muscular dystrophy, where it is clear that dystrophin is deficient in smooth muscle, indicate that major, symptomatic involvement of the gastrointestinal tract is a direct consequence of the disease (Barohn et al., 1988). In other instances, gastrointestinal complications may be the result of immobility.

Abnormalities of deglutition

Patients with bulbar weakness may develop nasal regurgitation of liquids when they swallow. Myasthenia gravis,

Kennedy syndrome (bulbar spinal muscular atrophy) and congenital myasthenic disorders are notable examples. Impaired function of pharyngeal muscles results in pooling of secretions in the hypopharynx and usually leads to aspiration. Atelectasis and pulmonary infection may result. However, they are not frequent unless there is coincidental weakness of respiratory and glottic muscles that impairs cough. Patients with abnormalities of swallowing usually recognize their problem and localize the difficulty. Patients with oculopharyngeal muscular dystrophy, inclusion body myositis and dermatomyositis are susceptible to cricopharyngeal achalasia and indicate the site of obstruction by pointing to the submental and glottic regions. These disorders affect the striated muscle of the upper one-third of the oesophagus. If the obstruction or motility disturbance is located in the lower portion of the oesophagus (as occurs in scleroderma, the mixed connective tissue syndrome and, uncommonly, in dermatomyositis), the patient will point to the substernal region as the site of obstruction or pain.

Occasionally patients with severe swallowing dysfunction have no spontaneous complaints referable to deglutition. Such unrecognized difficulty with swallowing is frequently seen in oculopharyngeal muscular dystrophy and myotonic dystrophy. Patients may present with unexplained cough, unexplained dyspnoea at mealtime, recurrent pulmonary infection because of aspiration and, remarkably, may even lose weight to the point of inanition while not directly complaining of swallowing difficulties.

Cricopharyngeal achalasia

Cricopharyngeal achalasia is important to recognize because it can be surgically corrected. If the cricopharyngeus muscle does not contract normally, food remains in the hypopharynx. Cricopharyngeal achalasia is frequent in oculopharyngeal muscular dystrophy (Brais et al., 1999) and occurs in other syndromes with progressive external ophthalmoplegia. It is also prominent in a subset of patients with polymyositis and inclusion body myositis (Palmer, 1976; Kagen et al., 1985; Verma et al., 1991). Patients with these diseases should be followed expectantly for the development of swallowing difficulties. Patients with oculopharyngeal muscular dystrophy, in particular, should have studies of swallowing function once their disease has reached the point of marked ptosis and ophthalmoparesis (Brais et al., 1999).

Patients with neuromuscular disease and abnormal swallowing function who develop severe weight loss or recurrent aspiration need studies of swallowing function and often require an invasive procedure to provide adequate nutrition. Percutaneous gastrostomy is now the procedure of choice for virtually all patients with the inability to maintain alimentation. The sole exceptions are patients with previous gastric surgery, and the ambulatory patient with selective involvement of muscles of deglutition such as occasionally seen in dermatomyositis, polymyositis and inclusion body myositis. Here, a formal gastrostomy is necessary in order to position the feeding tube high in the abdomen (avoiding problems of acid reflux).

Gastric and intestinal abnormalities

Patients with Duchenne dystrophy have impaired gastric motility and may present with severe gastric dilatation and intestinal pseudo-obstruction (Barohn et al., 1988). Treatment consists of decompression of the dilated stomach with a nasal gastric tube and parenteral fluids. Low-dose metaclopramide 10–20 mg/day has been helpful in preventing this complication in our anecdotal experience. In the MNGIE syndrome (mitochondrial myopathy, peripheral neuropathy, gastrointestinal disease and encephalopathy), involvement of intestinal muscles results in episodes of pseudo-obstruction caused by visceral neuropathy (Cevera et al., 1988). The syndrome occurs with cytochrome oxidase deficiency and may well reflect a mitochondrial disorder of visceral nerves. Dermatomyositis, particularly in childhood, is associated with a vasculitis that can culminate in intestinal perforation (Banker and Victor, 1966). This complication is rarely encountered in adequately treated patients. Patients with polymyositis and inclusion body myositis are not suscep-tible to this complication. Other disorders of gastric and oesophageal function also occur in various myopathies (Swick 1981; Yoshida et al., 1988).

Constipation

Management of constipation represents a major treatment problem in most bed-bound patients with neuromuscular disease. The inconvenience of toileting results in most patients electing to restrict their own fluids severely (often to less than 500 ml a day) and choosing a low-residue, low-fibre diet. Patients can be encouraged to reduce constipation by taking larger fluid amounts and eating high-residue foods only if there is sufficient attention to making it easy for them to void and defecate. Medications are usually necessary. Stool softeners and natural or synthetic cellulose moistening agent are preferable to bowel-irritating laxatives. Magnesium-containing preparations such as magnesium sulphate are often necessary on an intermittent basis. Magnesium-containing agents are potentially hazardous in patients with neuromuscular junction diseases or any neuromuscular disorder associated with coincidental renal insufficiency.

Both children and adults always have questions concerning bowel function that they will raise in a private, supportive office setting. It is our impression that adequate attention to these questions will prevent the severe constipation which is unfortunately common in end-stage neuromuscular disease. Rectal suppositories, various forms of enema and manual disimpaction often become necessary if preventive measures are delayed. Lactulose (30 ml one to three times a day) and pyridostigmine bromide (15–60 mg) have the potential hazards of electrolyte imbalance and parasympathetic toxicity but are occasionally helpful. In following patients with neuromuscular disease, it is important to prevent hypokalaemia since it will lead to intestinal ileus. Patients with gastric dilatation, intestinal pseudo-obstruction or those that require frequent enemas are particularly vulnerable to this problem.

Dietary treatment and prevention of obesity

There is no evidence that any dietary modification improves muscle strength or function in patients with neuromuscular disease. Prevention of obesity in both young and old patients with neuromuscular disease is extremely important and requires careful prospective dietary management and follow-up of weight. Excessive weight is both cosmetically disabling as well as limiting to mobility. It is difficult, but no less important, to determine the weight of wheelchair-bound and bed-bound adult patients. Patients must be followed by facilities that have wheelchair-weighing and bed-weighing capability. If patients are not losing weight as their disease progresses, they are gaining adipose tissue. As with children, prospective dietary counselling is essential. Once obesity is established, severe dietary restriction is necessary, depriving the patient of one of their few physical pleasures. Severe dietary restriction can, however, reduce obesity without compromising muscle strength (Edwards et al., 1984). The normal growth and development charts used by clinical nutritionists and dieticians make no allowance for the progressive loss of muscle that occurs in childhood muscular dystrophy or spinal muscular atrophy. Unless the child appears somewhat cachectic, excess body fat is almost certainly present.

Only a limited number of studies of metabolic rate have been performed but these confirm that metabolic rate declines in the wasted patient with diseases such as myotonic dystrophy. Muscle mass as assessed by creatinine excretion correlates well with the reduction in metabolic rate (Jozefowicz et al., 1987). In practice it is more important to follow weight than to assess muscle mass in following patients.

Pressure-related (decubitus) ulcers

Patients with progressive neuromuscular disease cannot 'fidget' and reposition themselves normally. They are also unable to turn themselves at night, in contrast to normal subjects where unconscious repositioning occurs 10–20 times per night. Normal subjects awaken only one to three times per night and such movements are largely unconscious. Patients with neuromuscular disease, in contrast, awaken because they are uncomfortable and as a result have severe interruption of sleep. Patients are, however, surprisingly free of decubitus ulcers unless sensory involvement decreases the awareness of pressure. Duchenne dystrophy and amyotrophic lateral sclerosis, the most common neuromuscular diseases resulting in quadriplegia, do not usually result in the development of pressure-related ulcers. The patient with Duchenne dystrophy, in particular, becomes increasingly difficult to manage because of his need to be repositioned frequently at night – often at 20 to 30 minute intervals, a trial for the patient and parents.

However, in diseases where sensation is disturbed, pressure necrosis is common and must be prevented by appropriate precautions. Older patients with diseases sparing sensory systems, including amyotrophic lateral sclerosis and myasthenia gravis, commonly have coincidental peripheral nerve, spinal cord or central nervous system disease that decreases the perception of pain or increases pain tolerance.

Alert young patients demand frequent repositioning, and caregivers will be equally insistent on finding aids to decrease the need for repositioning. Older, immobile patients should be provided with the same equipment to prevent pressure necrosis. Electrical alternating pressure mattresses for night-time use are helpful. Waterbeds or equally weight-distributing (but expensive) bead-filled mattresses are helpful in improving sleep quality and decrease the number of repositionings necessary. Wheelchair-bound patients benefit from gel cushions in the chair. Body jackets used to treat scoliosis and calipers (braces) must be carefully padded and skin must be inspected regularly.

Patients with peripheral neuropathy (or their caregiver) must be taught to inspect areas of pressure. The feet are vulnerable in hereditary neuropathies with decreased distal sensation. Perforating ulcers, osteomyelitis and Charcot joints are frequent. Not uncommonly, the first and presenting symptom of a foot ulcer that penetrates deeply to the bone is that the feet are malodorous. Patients should inspect the soles of their feet with a mirror daily. The inside of shoes must also be inspected and palpated (by someone other than the patient if hand sensation is reduced) for small nails and pebbles.

Surgical treatment

Many of the consequences of muscle weakness can be improved by surgical strategies: scoliosis, joint contractures, scapular winging, ptosis, exposure of the cornea and dysphagia (Table 36.5). In general, surgery on weak muscles can be expected to further weaken a transplanted muscle. Consequently, transplanting tendons from strong, redundant muscles to replace weakened muscles is unwise in rapidly progressive muscle disease.

Surgical correction of progressive scoliosis can be of great benefit in patients with Duchenne dystrophy (Giranata et al., 1996). Patient appearance and comfort are often improved and ventilatory function may be stabilized. Not all patients require surgery since scoliosis is not severe in many. Surgery should not be performed in certain patients despite severe scoliolis: those with incipient respiratory failure, those with massive obesity and in some with severe intellectual and emotional disability. The correct timing of surgery requires careful sequential monitoring of the degree of scoliosis and the forced vital capacity. Patients who are ambulatory do not need scoliosis surgery. Once patients are confined to a wheelchair,

Table 36.5. Corrective surgical treatments for skeletal muscle diseases

Complications	Modality	Diseases considered
Scoliosis	Lucke instrumentation	Duchenne and congenital dystrophies, nemaline myopathy
Scapular winging	Costal ligatures	Facioscapulohumeral, scapuloperoneal dystrophies
Joint contractures	Tenotomy	Duchenne dystrophy, Becker dystrophy, severe limb girdle dystrophy
Lagophthalmus and corneal exposure	Gold weights, tarsorrhaphy	Facioscapulohumeral dystrophy
Ptosis	Sling procedures	Facioscapulohumeral dystrophy, mitochondriopathies, other causes of progressive external ophthalmoplegia
Dysphagia	See p. 747	

they should be followed with physical examination for scoliosis; if it develops, serial X-ray examination for scoliosis and measurement of forced vital capacity should be initiated.

Joint contractures are usually seen only in patients with severe, progressive weakness. In patients with inflammatory myopathies such as dermatomyositis, physical therapy must be initiated immediately and accompany corticosteroid and other treatment. Surgery is necessary in only rare instances. In Duchenne dystrophy, and less frequently in Becker dystrophy, heel cord or ileotibial band contractures commonly develops despite physical therapy. Release of tendons is often necessary for patients to be able to stand (supported) with long leg braces. Night splints of ankles often delays the development of heel-cord contractures.

Eyelid surgery can correct lagophthalmus and prevent corneal drying and exposure keratitis (Sansone et al., 1997b). Ptosis in patients with progressive external ophthalmoplegia can be corrected temporarily by resection of redundant lid tissue. Ptosis almost invariably returns in 6–24 months following lid resection. Various 'sling' procedures are used to lift the lids. Cosmesis is usually excellent and often permanent. Sling procedures have the added advantage should facial weakness supervene, with resulting lagophthalmus, in that the sling can be removed. Lid resection is potentially hazardous in patients with progressive facial weakness.

Psychosocial treatment

The Muscular Dystrophy Group of Great Britain, the Muscular Dystrophy Association (in the USA and Canada) and similar organizations in other countries provide an important and practical source of education and support as well as an opportunity to work towards the goal of rational treatment of the disease and, where possible, its prevention.

Support groups where patients and families can share the experience of dealing with practical problems in everyday life are helpful to some patients and families. Neuromuscular disease clinics play a valuable role in giving specialist diagnostic services and treatment, and genetic counselling.

The later years

For the patient with Duchenne muscular dystrophy, it is distressing to see his contemporaries deteriorating and eventually dying while he becomes aware of his own progressive weakness and further disability. So far little has been done formally to explore the attitudes of the patient to his impending demise. Our own discussions with individuals who have approached their end with more or less equanimity indicate a progressive weariness with the struggles of life.

Future perspectives

Several new therapeutic approaches are likely to develop in the foreseeable future for muscle diseases (Karpati et al., 1999).

Cell and gene therapy

For genetic muscle diseases, cell therapy in the form of myoblast transfer has been tested in patients with Duchenne muscular dystrophy (Karpati et al., 1993a; Mendell et al., 1995). Large numbers of pure, fusion-competent myoblasts derived from a healthy male donor (usually the father) have been injected into a single muscle of immunosuppressed patients with Duchenne dystrophy and various end-points were monitored for therapeutic success (dystrophin, force generation, etc.). Thus far, no convincing therapeutic success has been reported, presumably because of rapid elimination of most of the injected myoblasts before they had a chance to fuse with each other, or into the host fibres (Huard et al., 1994). Future efforts are focused on using stem cells with myogenic potential for transplantation (Gussoni et al., 1999).

Various modalities of direct gene therapy are being tested in experimental models for recessive muscle diseases, such as Duchenne dystrophy (Acsadi et al., 1996), sarcoglycanopathies (Holt et al., 1998) and McArdle's disease (Karpati et al., 1999). The most common form of gene therapy is somatic cell gene replacement. In this modality, a normal variant of cDNA (corresponding to the mutated gene) is introduced into muscle either by direct injection or by a vascular route. The most promising gene vectors for skeletal muscle are genetically modified adenovirus (AV) (Gao et al., 1996) or adeno-associated virus (AAV) (Xiao and Samulski, 1996). In the *mdx* mouse and dystrophin-deficient dystrophic dogs, mediated dystrophin gene transfer was found to be very efficient in creating abundant dystrophin-positive muscle fibres and improving force generation (Lochmüller et al., 1996). The use of a new generation adenovirus vector ('gutted' AV vector) has eliminated the immunological handicap that compromised gene transfer by earlier AV vectors (Clemens et al., 1996). AAV, which is a better gene vector than AV for skeletal muscle fibres, is only capable of transferring smaller cDNAs than AV vectors (Fisher et al., 1997) and is suitable for the introduction of sarcoglycan cDNAs into sarcoglycan-deficient muscles (Holt et al., 1998). Such an approach has been successful in correcting δ-sarcoglycan deficiency in dystrophic hamsters (Holt et al., 1998). Preliminary human trials are underway (Dr J. Mendell, personal communication 1999).

Another possible approach to genetic therapy would be a substantial upregulation of utrophin in muscles of patients with Duchenne dystrophy (Tinsley and Davies, 1993). Utrophin is a molecular and functional homologue of dystrophin, and its gene is intact in these patients (Tinsley, 1998). However, utrophin is only expressed in normal muscle at the neuromuscular and myotendinous junctions (Karpati et al., 1993b). If utrophin is overexpressed, it appears throughout the sarcolemma, as is the case in transgenic *mdx* mice or after AV-mediated utrophin gene transfer (Tinsley, 1996, Gilbert et al., 1999). In such models, the dystrophic pathology was corrected and force generation was improved (Deconinck et al., 1997). Intensive efforts are underway to identify small nontoxic molecules the administration of which could sufficiently upregulate utrophin in muscle to have therapeutic benefits.

Recently, gentamicin administration was shown to result in dystrophin production in *mdx* mouse muscles (Barton-Davis et al., 1999), presumably by negating the effect of the mutant stop codon at the translational level. Whether this will ever be applicable for the treatment of some patients with Duchenne dystrophy involving a stop codon resulting from a single base change is doubtful because of the prohibitive toxicity of large doses of gentamicin in humans.

Immunotherapy

Another area where marked advances are expected in the future is immunotherapy. This would be important because several major muscle diseases have an autoimmune pathomechanism (inflammatory myopathies, myasthenia gravis, Lambert–Eaton syndrome, etc.). Presently, most immunotherapies (i.e. pharmacological agents, plasma exchange, high-dose intravenous immunoglobulin administration, thymectomy, etc.) are nonspecific and, therefore, suboptimal. Future immunotherapies will be specific with regard to a defined antigen, a subset of primed immune cells or a specific antibody, cytokine or chemokine. Gene transfer can also be used to introduce a stable gene reservoir for the production of 'good' cytokines to mitigate or frustrate the pathogenic immune responses.

Customized drugs

The understanding of the cellular and molecular pathology of muscle diseases will open up possibilities for designing drugs with the specific mission of negating or counteracting effects of an abnormal or missing protein. The most illustrative examples are ion channel disorders, where an abnormal ion channel protein alters the channel function with deleterious consequences (Fukudome et al., 1998). Designing and producing drugs to alleviate or correct the identified dynamic disturbance has become possible by advanced chemical and molecular techniques.

Prenatal diagnosis

A useful approach to the prevention of genetic muscle disease is prenatal diagnosis, which offers an option of terminating the pregnancy (Lissens and Sermon, 1998). However, in the future, fetal gene therapy may be contemplated. Prenatal diagnosis is possible by demonstrating a deficient protein or a particular gene mutation in a sample of the chorionic villus. A more refined form of prenatal diagnosis is preimplantation diagnosis where the identification of a gene mutation is made in a single blastomere of an eight-cell stage embryo. If no mutation is found in a particular gene of interest in a single blastomere, the seven-cell implanted embryo is capable of developing into a normal fetus.

References

Acsadi, G., Lochmüller, H., Jani, A. et al. (1996). Dystrophin expression in muscles of *mdx* mice after adenovirus-mediated in vivo gene transfer. *Hum. Gene. Ther.* **7**, 129–140.

Banker, B. Q. and Victor, M. (1966). Dermatomyositis (systemic angiopathy) of childhood. *Medicine* **45**, 261–269.

Barohn, R. J., Levin, E. J., Olson, J. O. and Mendell, J. R. (1988). Gastric motility in Duchenne's muscular dystrophy. *N. Engl. J. Med.* **319**, 15–18.

Barton-Davis, E. R., Cordier, L. and Shoturmo, D. L. et al. (1999) Aminoglycoside antibodies restore dystrophin functions to skeletal muscle of *mdx* mice. *J. Clin. Invest.* **104**, 375–381.

Belshe, R. B. (1999). Influenza prevention and treatment: current practices and new horizons. *Ann. Intern. Med.* **131**, 621–623.

Bente, J. R. (1991). Biochemical markers of bone turnover in diagnosis and assessment of therapy. *Am. J. Med.* **91**(Suppl. 5B), 645–685.

Black, L. F. and Hyatt, R. E. (1971). Maximal static respiratory pressures in generalized neuromuscular disease. *Am. Rev. Resp. Dis.* **103**, 641–650.

Brais, B., Rouleau, G. A., Bouchard, J-P., Fardeau, M. and Tomé, F. M. S. (1999). Oculopharyngeal muscular dystrophy. *Semin. Neurol.* **19**, 59–66.

Brooke, M. H., Griggs, R. C., Mendell, J. R., Fenichel, G. M., Shumate, J. B. and Pellegrino, R. J. (1981). Clinical trials in Duchenne muscular dystrophy. 1. The design of the protocol. *Muscle and Nerve* **4**, 186–197.

Brooke, M. H., Fenichel, G. M., Griggs, R. C., et al. (1983). Clinical investigation in Duchenne muscular dystrophy: 2 Determination of the 'power' of therapeutic trials based on the natural history. *Muscle and Nerve* **6**, 91–103.

Brooke, M. H., Fenichel, G. M., Griggs, R. C. and the CIDD Group (1989). Duchenne muscular dystrophy: patterns of clinical progression and effects of supportive therapy. *Neurology,* **39**, 475–481.

Brussock, C. M., Haley, S. M., Munsat, T. L. and Bernardt, D. B. (1992). Measurement of isometric force in children with and without Duchenne's muscular dystrophy. *Phys. Ther.* **72**, 105.

Carroll, N., Bain, R. J. I., Smith, P. E. M., Saltissi, S., Edwards, R. H. T. and Calverley, P. M. A. (1991). Domiciliary investigation of sleep-related hypoxaemia in Duchenne muscular dystrophy. *Eur. Resp. J.* **4**, 434–440.

Carson, J. L., Strom, B. L., Schinnar, R., et al. (1991). The low risk of upper gastrointestinal bleeding in patients dispensed corticosteroids. *Am. J. Med.* **91**, 223–228.

Cevera, R., Bruix, J., Bayes, A. et al. (1988). Chronic intestinal pseudoobstruction and ophthalmoplegia in a patient with mitochondrial myopathy. *Gut* **29**, 544–547.

Chalk, J. B., Ridgeway, K., Brophy, T., Yelland, J. D. and Eadie, M. J. (1984). Phenytoin impairs the bioavailability of dexamethasone in neurological and neurosurgical patients. *J. Neurol. Neurosurg. Psychiatry* **47**, 1087–1090.

Clemens, P. R., Kochanek, S., Sunada, Y. et al. (1996). In vivo muscle gene transfer of full-length dystrophin with adenoviral vector that lacks all viral antigenes. *Gene. Ther.* **3**, 965–972.

Coakley, J. H., Edwards, R. H. T. and Calverley, P. M. A. (1990). Sleep and breathing pattern in myotonic dystrophy: effect of mazindol. *Thorax* **45**, 336.

Conn, H. O. and Blitzer, B. L. (1976). Non-association of adrenocorticosteroid therapy and peptic ulcer. *N. Engl. J. Med.* **294**, 473–479.

Deconinck, N., Tinsley, J. M., de Backer, F. et al. (1997). Expression of truncated utrophin leads to major functional improvements in dystrophin-deficient muscles of mice. *Nat. Med.* **3**, 1216–1221.

Donofrio, P. D., Challa, V. R., Hackshaw, B. T., Mills, S. A. and Cordell, A. R. (1989). Cardiac transplantation in a patient with muscular dystrophy and cardiomyopathy. *Arch. of Neurol.* **46**, 705–707.

Dropcho, E. J. and Soong, S. J. (1991). Steroid-induced weakness in patients with primary brain tumors. *Neurology* **41**, 1235–1239.

Dworzak, F., Casazza, F., Mora, M. et al. (1994). Lysosomal glycogen storage with normal acid maltase: a familial study with successful heart transplant. *Neuromusc. Disord.* **4**, 243.

Eberhardt, M. (1988). *Mark's Test.* New York: Vantage.

Edwards, R. H. T., Round, J. M., Jackson, M. J., Griffiths, R. D. and Liburn, M. F. (1984). Weight reduction in boys with muscular dystrophy. *Dev. Med. and Child Neurol.* **26**, 384–390.

Edwards, R. H. T., Chapman, S. J., Newham, D. J. and Jones, D. A. (1987). Practical analysis of variability of muscle function measurements in Duchenne muscular dystrophy. *Muscle Nerve* **10**, 6.

Ellis, E. R., Bye, P. T. P., Bruderer, J. W. and Sullivan, C. E. (1987). Treatment of respiratory failure during sleep in patients with neuromuscular disease. *Am. Rev. of Resp. Dis.* **135**, 148–152.

Fenichel, G. M., Mendell, J. R., Moxley, R. T. et al., (1991). A comparison of daily and alternate-day prednisone therapy in the treatment of Duchenne muscular dystrophy. *Arch. Neurol.* **48**, 575–579.

Fisher, K. J., Jooss, K., Alson, et al. (1997). Recombinant adenoassociated virus vector. *J. Virol.* **3**, 306–312.

Florence, J. M., Pandya, S., King, W. M. et al. (1992). Intrarater reliability of manual muscle test (Medical Research Council Scale) grades in Duchenne's muscular dystrophy. *Phys. Ther.* **72**, 115–122.

Fukudome, T., Ohno, K., Brengman, J. M. and Engel, A. G. (1998). AchR channel blockade by quinidine sulfate reduces channel open duration in the slow-channel congenital myasthenic syndrome. *Ann. N.Y. Acad. Sci.* **841**, 199–202.

Gao, G-P., Yang, Y. and Wilson, J. M. (1996). Biology of adenovirus vectors with E1 and E4 deletions for liver-directed gene therapy. *J. Virol.* **70**, 8934–8943.

Garay, S. M., Turino, G. M. and Goldring, R. M. (1981). Sustained reversal of chronic hypercapnia in patients with alveolar hypoventilation syndromes: long-term maintenance with noninvasive nocturnal mechanical ventilation. *Am. J. Med.* **70**, 269.

Garrel, D. R., Delmas, P. D., Welsh, C., et al., (1988). Effects of moderate physical training on prednisone-induced protein wasting: a study of whole-body and bone protein metabolism. *Metabolism* **37**, 257–262.

Gilbert, R., Nalbantoglu, J., Petrof, B. et al. (1999). Adenovirus-mediated utrophin gene transfer mitigates the dystrophic phenotype of *mdx* muscles. *Hum. Genet. Ther.* **10**, 1299–1310.

Gilmartin, J. J., Cooper, B. G., Griffith. C. J. et al. (1991). Breathing during sleep in patients with myotonic dystrophy and non-myotonic respiratory muscle weakness. *Q. J. Med.* **78**, 21–31.

Goldblatt, D. (1984). Decisions about life support in amyotrophic lateral sclerosis. *Semin. Neurol.* **4**, 104.

Goldblatt, D. and Greenlaw, J. (1989). Starting and stopping the ventilator for patients with amyotrophic lateral sclerosis. *Neurol. Clin.* **7**, 789–806.

Granata, C., Merlini, L., Cervellati, S., Ballestrazzi, A. et al. (1996). Long-term results of spine surgery in Duchenne muscular dystrophy. *Neuromusc. Disord.* **6**, 61–68.

Griffiths, R. D. and Edwards, R. H. T. (1988). A new chart for weight control in Duchenne muscular dystrophy. *Arch. Dis. Child.*, **63**, 1256–1258.

Griggs, R. C. (1990). The use of pulmonary function testing as a quantitative measurement for therapeutic trial. *Muscle and Nerve* **13**, 530–534.

Griggs, R. C. (ed.) (1994). Developing new treatments for muscle disease: prospects and promise. *Curr. Opin. Neurol.* **7**, 422–426.

Griggs, R. C. and Donohoe, K. M. (1982). The recognition and management of respiratory insufficiency in neuromuscular disease. *J. Chron. Dis.* **35**, 497–500.

Griggs, R. C. and Donohoe, K. M. (1985). Emergency management of neuromuscular disease. In: *Handbook of Critical Care Neurology and Neurosurgery*, eds. R. J. Henning and D. L. Jackson, p. 201. New York: Praeger.

Griggs, R. C., Davis, R. J., Anderson, D. C. and Dove, J. T. (1975). Cardiac conduction in myotonic dystrophy. *Am. J. Med.* **59**, 37–42.

Griggs, R. C., Donohoe, K. M., Utell, M. J., Goldblatt, D. and Moxley, R. T., III. (1981). Evaluation of pulmonary function in neuromuscular disease. *Arch. Neurol.* **38**, 9–12.

Griggs, R. C., Moxley, R. T., Mendell, J. R., et al. (1991). Prednisone in Duchenne dystrophy: a randomized, controlled trial defining the time course and dose response. *Arch. Neurol.* **48**, 383–388.

Gussoni, E., Soneoka, Y. Strickland, C. D. et al. (1999). Dystrophin expression in the *mdx* mouse restored by stem cell transplantations. *Nature*, **401**: 390–394.

Harper, P. S. (1989). *Myotonic dystrophy*, 2nd edn. Philadelphia, PA: Saunders.

Heckmatt, J. Z., Loh, L. and Dubowitz, V. (1990). Clinical Practice. Night-time nasal ventilation in neuromuscular disease. *Lancet*, **335**, 579–582.

Holt, K. H., Lim, H. E., Straub, V. et al. (1998). Functional rescue of the sarcoglycan complex in the BIO 14.6 hamster using δ-sarcoglycan gene transfer. *Mol. Cell.* **1**, 841–848.

Holtackers, T. R., Loosbrock, L. M. and Gracey, D. R. (1982). The use of the chest cuirass in respiratory failure of neurologic origin. *Resp. Care* **27**, 271.

Huard, J., Acsadi, G., Jani, A., Massie, B. and Karpati, G. (1994). Gene therapy into skeletal muscles by isogenic myoblasts. *Hum. Gene. Ther.* **5**, 949–958.

Jozefowicz, R. F., Welle, S. L., Nair, K. S., Kingston, W. J., Griggs, R. C. (1987). Basal metabolic rate in myotonic dystrophy: evidence against hypometabolism. *Neurology* **37**, 1021–1025.

Kagen, L. J., Hochman, R. B. and Strong, E. W. (1985). Cricopharyngeal obstruction in inflammatory myopathy (polymyositis/dermatomyositis): report of three cases and review of literature. *Arthritis Rheum.* **28**, 630–636.

Karpati, G., Ajdukovic, D., Arnold, D. et al. (1993a). Myoblast transfer in Duchenne muscular dystrophy. *Ann. Neurol.* **34**, 8–17.

Karpati, G., Carpenter, S., Morris, G. E., Davies, K. E., Guerin, C. and Holland, P. (1993b). Localization quantification of chromosome 6-encoded dystrophin-related protein in normal and pathological muscle. *J. Neuropath. Exp. Neurol.* **52**, 112–119.

Karpati, G., Pari, G. and Molar, M. J. (1999). Molecular therapy for genetic muscle diseases – status 1999. *Clin. Genet.* **55**, 1–8.

Lissens, W. and Sermon, K. (1998). Preimplantation genetic diagnosis: current status and new developments. *Hum. Reprod.* **12**, 1756–1761.

Lochmüller, H., Petrof, B., Pari, G. (1996). Transient immunosuppression by FK506 permits a sustained high-level dystrophin expression after adenovirus-mediated dystrophin minigene transfer to skeletal muscles of adult dystrophic (*mdx*) mice. *Gene Ther.* **3**, 706–716.

Madorsky, J. G. B., Radford, L. M. and Newman, E. M. (1984). Psychosocial aspects of death and dying in Duchenne muscular dystrophy. *Arch. Phys. Med. Rehab.* **65**, 79–82.

McCool, F. D., Mayewski, R. J., Shayne, D. S., Gibson, C. J., Griggs, R. C., and Hyde, R. W. (1986). Intermittent positive pressure breathing in patients with respiratory muscle weakness. Alterations in total respiratory system compliance. *Chest* **90**, 546–552.

Mendell, J. R. and Vaughn, J. (1984). Duchenne muscular dystrophy: ethical and emotional considerations in long-term management. *Semin. Neurol.* **4**, 98.

Mendell, J. R., Province, M., Moxley, R. T. et al. (1987). Clinical investigation of Duchenne dystrophy. A methodology for therapeutic trials based on natural history controls. *Arch. Neurol.* **44**, 808–811.

Mendell, J. R., Moxley, R. T., Griggs, R. C. et al. (1989). Randomized double-blind six-month trial of prednisone in Duchenne muscular dystrophy. *N. Engl. J. Med.* **320**, 1592–1597.

Mendell, J. R., Kissel, J. T., Amato, A. A. et al. (1995). Myoblast transfer in the treatment of Duchenne's muscular dystrophy. *N. Engl. J. Med.* **333**, 832–838.

Moorman, J. R., Coleman, R. E., Packer, D. L. et al. (1985). Cardiac involvement in myotonic muscular dystrophy. *Medicine* **64**, 371–387.

Newsom-Davis, J., Goldman, M., Loh, L. and Casson, M. (1976). Diaphragm function and alveolar hypoventilation. *Q. J. Med.* **45**, 87–100.

Nippoldt, T. B., Edwards, W. D., Holmes, D. R. Jr, et al. (1982). Right ventricular endomyocardial biopsy: clinicopathologic correlates in 100 consecutive patients. *Mayo Clin. Proc.* **57**, 407–418.

Nishino, I., Fu, J., Tanji, K. et al. (2000). Primary LAMP-2 deficiency causes X-linked vacuolar cardiomyopathy and myopathy (Danon disease). *Nature* **406**, 906–910.

Norris, F. H. Jr, Moss, A. J. and Yu, P. N. (1966). On the possibility that a type of human muscular dystrophy commences in myocardium. *Ann. N. Y. Acad. Sci.* **138**, 342–355.

Palmer, E. D. (1976). Disorders of the cricopharyngeus muscle: a review. *Gastroenterology,* **71**, 510–519.

Personius, K., Pandya. S., Tawil, R., King, W. M,, McDermott, M. P. and the FSH-DY Group (1994). Facioscapulohumeral dystrophy natural history study: standardization and reliability of testing procedures. *Phys. Ther.* **74**, 253–263.

Reid, I. R. and Ibbertson, H. K. (1986). Calcium supplements in the prevention of steroid-induced osteoporosis. *Am. J. Clin. Nutrit.* **44**, 287–290.

Reeves, W., Griggs, R. C., Nanda, N. C., Thomson, K. and Gramiak, R. (1980). Echocardiographic evaluation of cardiac abnormalities in Duchenne dystrophy and myotonic muscular dystrophy. *Arch. Neurol.* **37**, 273–277.

Rideau, Y., Jankowski, L. W. and Grellet, J. (1981). Respiratory function in the muscular dystrophies. *Muscle Nerve* **4**, 155–164.

Rodillo, E., El-Meleigy, D. and Heckmatt, J. Z. (1991). Multifocal avascular necrosis following high dosage steroid treatment of juvenile dermatomyositis. A case report. *Neuromusc. Disord.* **1**, 55–57.

Roussos, C. and Macklem, P. T. (1982). The respiratory muscles. *N. Engl. J. Med.* **307**, 786–797.

Sansone, V., Griggs, R. C. and Meola, G. et al. (1997a). Andersen's syndrome: a distinct periodic paralysis. *Ann. Neurol.* **42**, 305–312.

Sansone, V., Boynton, J. and Palenski, C. (1997b). Use of gold weights to correct lagophthalmos in neuromuscular disease. *Neurology.* **48**, 1500–1503.

Saunders, N. A., Rigg, J. R. A., Pengelly, L. D. and Campbell, E. J. M. (1978). Effect of curare on maximum static PV relationships of the respiratory system. *J. Appl. Physiol.* **44**, 589–595.

Schwartz, J. S. (1982). Pneumococcal vaccine: clinical efficacy and effectiveness. *Ann. Intern. Med.* **96**, 208–220.

Silverstein, M. D., Stocking, C. B. and Antel, J. P. (1991). Amyotrophic lateral sclerosis and life-sustaining therapy: patients' desires for information, participation in decision making, and life-sustaining therapy. *Mayo Clin. Proc.* **66**, 906–913.

Smith, P. E. M., Calverley, P. M. A. and Edwards, R. H. T. (1988). Hypoxemia during sleep in Duchenne muscular dystrophy. *Am. Rev. Resp. Dis.* **137**, 884.

Smith, P. E. M., Calverley, P. M. A. and Edwards, R. H. T. (1989). Ventilation and breathing pattern during sleep in Duchenne muscular dystrophy. *Chest* **96**, 1346.

Smith, P. E. M., Edwards, R. H. T., Calverley, P. M. A. (1991). Mechanisms of sleep-disordered breathing in chronic neuromuscular disease: implications for management. *Q. J. Med.* **296**, 961.

Stambler, N., Charatan, M. and Cedarbaum, J. M. (1998). Prognostic indicators of survival in ALS. ALS CNTF Treatment Study Group. *Neurology* **50**, 66–72.

Swick, H. M., Werlin, S. L., Dodds, W. J. and Hogan, W. J. (1981). Pharyngoesophageal motor function in patients with myotonic dystrophy. *Ann. Neurol.* **10**, 454–457.

Tawil, R., McDermott, M. P., Mendell, J. R., and the FSH-DY Group (1994). Facioscapulohumeral muscular dystrophy (FSHD): design of natural history study and results of baseline testing. *Neurology* **44**, 442–446.

Tinsley, J. (1996). Amelioration of the dystrophic phenotype of *mdx* mice using a truncated utrophin transgene. *Nature* **384**, 349–353.

Tinsley, J. (1998). Utrophin or dystrophin: which is the better potential gene therapeutics agent for Duchenne muscular dystrophy? *Curr. Res. Mol. Ther.* **1**, 695–700.

Tinsley, J. M., and Davies, K. E. (1993). Utrophin: a potential replacement for dystrophy? *Neuromusc. Disord.* **3**, 537–539.

Verma, A., Bradley, W. G., Adesina, A. M., Sofferman, R. and Pendlebury, W. W. (1991). Inclusion body myositis with cricopharyngeus muscle involvement and severe dysphagia. *Muscle Nerve* **14**, 470–473.

Weinberger, S. E., Schwartzstein, R. M. and Weiss, J. W. (1989). Hypercapnia. *N. Engl. J. Med.* **321**, 1223–1231.

Xiao, X., Li, J. and Samulski, R. J. (1996). Efficient long-term gene transfer into muscle tissue of immunocompetent mice by adeno-associated virus vector. *J. Virol.* **70**, 8089–8108.

Yoshida, M. M., Krishnamurthy, S., Wattchow, D. A., Furness, J. B. and Schuffler, M. D. (1988). Megacolon in myotonic dystrophy caused by a degenerative neuropathy of the myenteric plexus. *Gastroenterology* **95**, 820–827.

Index